NORMAL CLINICAL PATHOLOGY DATA

Normal values of laboratory data vary widely, depending on the patient's sex, breed and age, and on the laboratory. The values in these tables are approximations for use as guidelines only.

These tables are normal data from clinical laboratory sheets used at the N.Y.S. Veterinary College, Cornell University.

Routine Chemistry

GENERAL	DOG	CAT
Bilirubin, total (mg./dl.)	0.07–0.61	0.15–0.20
direct (mg./dl.)	0.0–0.14	–
indirect (mg./dl.)	0.07–0.61	–
BSP (% ret.) at 30 min.	5.0	–
Cholesterol (mg./dl.)	125–250	75–151
Creatinine (mg./dl.)	1–2	1–2
Glucose (mg./dl.)	60–100	64–118
Iron (μg./dl.)	94–122	68–215
TIBC (μg./dl.)	280–340	170–400
PSP (μg./dl.) plasma clearance at 60 min.	60–100	–
Urea N. (mg./dl.)	10–20	20–30
Uric acid (mg./dl.)	0–1.0	1.0–1.9
GOT (SF U.)	<50	<50
GPT (SF U.)	<50	<50
CPK (IU)	0–70	10–60
LDH (BB U.)	<600	
Alk. Phos. (S U.)	<5	<5
Lipase (ST U.)	<1	<1
Amylase (Som. U.)	<800	<800
Proteins total, serum (gm./dl.)	5.4–7.1	5.4–7.8
Fibrinogen (mg./dl.)	300–600	300–600
A:G	0.8–1.7	0.4–1.7
Albumin (gm./dl.)	2.3–3.2	2.1–3.3
Globulin (gm./dl.)	2.7–4.4	2.6–5.1
ACID–BASE		
pH (units)	7.31–7.42	7.24–7.40
pCO$_2$ (mm. Hg)	29–42	29–42
Base excess (mEq./l.)	±2.5	±2.5
Bicarbonate (mEq./l.)	17–24	17–24
ELECTROLYTES		
Sodium (mEq./l.)	140–155	147–156
Potassium (mEq./l.)	3.7–5.8	4.0–4.5
Chloride (mEq./l.)	105–115	117–123
Osmolality (mOsm./l.)	280–305	280–305
Calcium (mg./dl.)	8.4–11.2	7.0–10.0
Phosphorus (mg./dl.)	2.5–5.0	4–7
Magnesium (mg./dl.)	1.8–2.4	2–3
SPECIAL CHEMISTRY		
δ-ALA (μg./dl.)	<500	–
Blood lead (μg./dl.)	0–20	–
T-4 (μg./dl.)	2.0–6.0	1.5–4.0
Cortisol (μg./dl.)	5–10	–

Hematology

	DOG	CAT
PCV (%)	37–55	24–45
WBC ($\times 10^3/\mu$l.)	6–17	5.5–19.5
Neutrophil, segmented ($\times 10^3/\mu$l.)	3–11.5	2.5–12.5
Neutrophil, band ($\times 10^3/\mu$l.)	0–0.3	0–0.3
Eosinophils ($\times 10^3/\mu$l.)	0.1–1.2	0–1.5
Basophils ($\times 10^3/\mu$l.)	Rare	Rare
Monocytes ($\times 10^3/\mu$l.)	0.1–1.4	0–0.8
Lymphocytes ($\times 10^3/\mu$l.)	1.0–4.8	1.5–7.0
Hemoglobin (gm./dl.)	12–18	8–15
RBC ($\times 10^6/\mu$l.)	5.5–8.5	5–10
MCV ($\mu.^3$)	60–77	39–55
MCH ($\mu\mu$g.)	19.5–24.5	13–17
MCHC (%)	32–36	30–36
Platelets ($\times 10^5/\mu$l.)	2–9	3–7
Reticulocytes (%)	0–1.5	0–1.0
Plasma Protein (gm./dl.)	6.0–7.8	6–7.5

Normal Values, Urinalysis

	DOG	CAT
Color	Light yellow	Light yellow
Turbidity	Clear	Clear
Specific gravity	1.015–1.045	1.015–1.060
Volume	24–40 ml./kg./day	22–30 ml./kg./day
Protein, ketones, glucose, hemoglobin, urobilinogen	Negative	Negative
Bilirubin	Negative –Trace	Negative
pH	5.0–7.0	5.0–7.0

Abbreviations

dl. = deciliter
mg. = milligram
SF u. = Sigma-Frankel unit
IU = International unit
BB u. = Berger-Broida unit
S u. = Sigma unit
Som. u. = Somogyi unit
gm. = gram
mm. = millimeter
Hg. = hemoglobin
mEq. = milliequivalent
mOsm. = milliosmol
μg. = microgram
$\mu.^3$ = cubic micron
$\mu\mu$g. = micromicrogram
ST u. = Sigma-Tietz unit
TIBC = total iron binding capacity
l. = liter
μl. = microliter

With contributions by

Dennis T. Crowe, Jr., D.V.M.

Diplomate, American College Veterinary Surgeons
Assistant Professor of Surgery
University of Georgia
School of Veterinary Medicine;
Staff Surgeon and Director, Shock and Trauma Team
University of Georgia Small Animal Clinic.

N. Joel Edwards, D.V.M.

Diplomate, American College of Veterinary Internal
   Medicine, Specialty of Cardiology
Adjunct Professor of Internal Medicine and Cardiology
New York State College of Veterinary Medicine
Cornell University
Ithaca, New York

Alexander deLahunta, D.V.M., Ph.D.

Diplomate, American College of Veterinary Internal
   Medicine, Specialty of Neurology
Professor of Veterinary Anatomy
Director of Department Clinical Studies
New York State College of Veterinary Medicine
Cornell University
Ithaca, New York

Marc Raffe, D.V.M.

Diplomate, American College of Veterinary
   Anesthesiologists
Assistant Professor, Department of Clinical Studies
University of Minnesota School of Veterinary Medicine;
Director, Anesthesia Services, University of Minnesota
School of Veterinary Medicine
St. Paul, Minnesota

William Hornbuckle, D.V.M.

Diplomate, American College of Veterinary Internal
   Medicine
Associate Professor, Department of Small Animal Medicine
and Surgery
New York State College of Veterinary Medicine
Cornell University
Ithaca, New York

HANDBOOK OF
VETERINARY PROCEDURES & EMERGENCY TREATMENT

FOURTH EDITION

ROBERT W. KIRK, B.S., D.V.M.

Diplomate, American College of
  Veterinary Internal Medicine
Diplomate, American College of
  Veterinary Dermatology
Professor of Medicine
Director, Veterinary Medical
  Teaching Hospital
New York State College of
  Veterinary Medicine
Cornell University
Ithaca, New York

STEPHEN I. BISTNER, B.S., D.V.M.

Diplomate, American College of
  Veterinary Ophthalmologist
Professor
Department of Clinical Medicine
School of Veterinary Medicine
University of Minnesota
St. Paul, Minnesota

W. B. Saunders Company   1985

Philadelphia/London/Toronto/Mexico City/Rio de Janeiro/Sydney/Tokyo/Hong Kong

W. B. Saunders Company: West Washington Sqaure
Philadelphia, PA 19105

Library of Congress Cataloging in Publication Data

Kirk, Robert Warren, 1922–

Handbook of veterinary procedures & emergency treatment.

Includes index.

1. Veterinary medicine—Handbooks, manuals, etc.   2. First aid for animals—
   Handbooks, manuals, etc.   I. Bistner, Stephen I.   II. Title.   III. Title:
   Handbook of veterinary procedures and emergency treatment.

SF748.K57 1985   636.089   85–1945

ISBN 0–7216–1264–4

Listed here is the latest translated edition of this book together
with the language of the translation and the publisher.

French (2nd Edition)—Editions Vigot Frères, Paris, France

Italian (2nd Edition)—Edizioni Ermes, Milan, Italy

Japanese (1st Edition)—Ishiyaku Publishers, Inc., Tokyo, Japan

Spanish (2nd Edition)—Salvat, Editores, S.A., Barcelona, Spain

Handbook of Veterinary Procedures
and Emergency Treatment   ISBN   0-7216-1264-4

Last digit is the print number: 9   8   7   6   5   4   3   2   1

PREFACE

This handbook is dedicated to the many colleagues who have influenced our professional lives over the years. Their influence continues, and new information continues apace—hence, another expanded edition. The book is jammed to the capacity of a single volume of the pocket-sized format. To conserve space, the section on poisoning has been condensed and organized into tables and charts for ready reference, but directions are given for better use of the poison control centers for detailed information. This released space has allowed us to expand and emphasize sections on shock, cardiac, and anesthetic emergencies as well as the chapters on interpretation of laboratory tests. The entire text has been updated.

Knowledge expands at a bewildering rate, but we have been blessed with a host of talented colleagues who have added expertise to the handbook, which is becoming a multi-authored project.

In this edition, we are particularly indebted to Drs. D. Crowe, A. deLahunta, J. Edwards, W. Hornbuckle, and M. Raffe; but also to Drs. S. Center, T. Crimmi, A. Dietze, R. Gleed, W. Horn, R. Johnson, F. Kallfelz, D. Lein, M. Morris Jr., S. Shinn, E. Trotter, D. Walton, and J. Zimmer. All have been generous with their time and talents.

Helen and Diana, our wives, helped plan and coordinate our efforts in the production of this edition.

As always, the W. B. Saunders Company staff has provided cheerful expertise in interpreting and polishing our message into its final form.

We hope you find the fruits of our labors useful in your everyday practice.

ROBERT W. KIRK
STEPHEN I. BISTNER

CONTENTS

SECTION **2** **Interpreting Signs of Disease**	225

SECTION **6** **Charts and Tables**	835

NOTICE

Extraordinary efforts have been made by the authors, the editors, and the publisher of this book to insure that dosage recommendations are precise and in agreement with standards officially accepted at the time of publication.

It does happen, however, that dosage schedules are changed from time to time in the light of accumulating clinical experience and continuing laboratory studies. This is most likely to occur in the case of recently introduced products.

It is urged, therefore, that you check the manufacturer's recommendations for dosage, especially if the drug to be administered or prescribed is one that you use only infrequently or have not used for some time.

THE AUTHORS

Emergency Care

PRIORITY OF EVALUATION AND TREATMENT

The practicing veterinarian is often faced with emergency situations that are extremely difficult to evaluate and treat. Because of the nature of these emergencies, it is important that: (1) a portion of the hospital be set up to contain drugs and equipment needed in handling these cases, (2) a triage of treatment be formulated, and (3) a plan for initial evaluation of the severely injured animal be established and followed.

Seventy-five per cent of all emergency cases have been attributed to motor vehicle accidents, with 25 per cent of these cases involving injuries in more than one region of the body. Numerous other forms of injury, however, can take place.

The following conditions are considered serious and require immediate attention.

PRIORITY OF EVALUATION FOR THE SEVERELY INJURED ANIMAL

1. **Very severe** (act within seconds to a few minutes)
   Cardiopulmonary arrest
   Airway obstruction
   Respiratory arrest
   Rapid arterial or venous hemorrhage
2. **Severe** (must act within a few minutes to 1 hour at most)
   Multiple deep lacerations with hypovolemia
   Profound shock from any cause
   Penetrating wounds of thorax or abdomen
   Head injuries with progressive loss of consciousness
   Blunt trauma with profound shock
   Respiratory distress or embarrassment
   Spinal trauma with neurologic damage
3. **Serious** (must act within the first few hours)
   Multiple deep lacerations
   Thoracic or abdominal injury with moderate degree shock
   Spinal cord injury with paralysis
   Massive musculoskeletal injuries
   Open fractures of major bones
   Open wounds to joints involving major nerves, tendons, and vessels
   Acute to overwhelming infections
4. **Major** (must act within 24 hours)
   Fractures of long bones, pelvis without shock
   Luxation and ligament injuries
   Deep laceration puncture wounds

LIFE—THREATENING AND SERIOUS MEDICAL EMERGENCIES

Anaphylaxis
Coma and loss of consciousness
Rapid-acting poisons (Table 1)
Acute overwhelming bacteremia or toxemia

Table 1. EQUIPMENT USEFUL IN THE TREATMENT OF CHEMICAL POISONING

Mechanical respirator. The Bird Respirator is recommended.
Tube sizes for toxicologic procedures.*

Weight of Animal	Endotracheal Tubes†	Stomach Tubes‡	Colon Tubes§
2 kg	3.0– 4.5 mm	⅛–¼ in. OD	⅛ in. OD
2– 5 kg	3.5– 6.0 mm	¼ in. OD	¼ in. OD
5–10 kg	5.0– 7.5 mm	⅜ in. OD	⅜ in. OD
10–20 kg	7.5–11.0 mm	½ in. OD	⅜ in. OD
20–30 kg	8.5–15.0 mm	⅝ in. OD	½ in. OD

Aspirator bulbs. Assorted sizes commensurate with the stomach capacity of various animals should be on hand. Large syringes can also be used for gastric lavage.
Venostomy (scalp vein infusion) sets. A wide variety of kits containing instruments suitable for dissecting veins that may be difficult to locate are available.
Intravenous (IV) catheters and stylets. A plastic catheter is left in the vein. This procedure is useful for prolonged IV administration of fluids or repetitive injections.
Miscellaneous equipment: syringes, needles, clinical thermometers, stethoscope, urinary catheters, and adhesive tape.
Collection of tissues for toxicologic analysis: an assortment of unused wide-mouth plastic bottles and plastic bags with capacities of 4 oz (100 ml) to 1 qt (1 L).

*The largest tube diameter possible should always be used. The tube diameters given for dogs and cats of various weights are presented only as a guide.
†Cuffed endotracheal tubes are recommended. The size is based on internal diameter.
‡Clear polyethylene tubing or rubber is satisfactory.
§Soft rubber tubes are recommended.
From Aronson, A. L.: Emergency and general treatment of poisonings. *In* Kirk, R. W. (ed.): Current Veterinary Therapy V, Philadelphia, W. B. Saunders Company, 1974.

EMERGENCY INFORMATION, EQUIPMENT, AND DRUGS

The supplies needed will vary with the type of practice, but the following items should be in the office and readily available.

ESSENTIAL EQUIPMENT

Aspirator bulbs or 50-ml syringes for gastric lavage
Bandages—1, 2, and 3 inch widths
Blankets and towels
Blood specimen tubes—clean
Catheters, urinary—canine male and female
Catheters, urinary—feline male and female
Colon tubes—1/4, 3/8, and 1/2 inch OD, 5-ft rubber
Culture tubes—sterile
Endotracheal tubes (cuffed) and, for cats, cole tubes; sizes from 3.0 to 15.0 mm internal diameter

Enema can and tubing
Finger cots
Forceps—for removal of foreign objects; large and small Forrester sponge
 forceps or alligator forceps
Forceps—obstetrical, clam shell
Forceps—sponge, rongeur
Hypodermic needles
Intravenous (IV) catheters and stylets (see also p. 610)
Lubricating jelly
Mechanical respirator (e.g., Bird respirator; see also pp. 82–86)
Minor surgical pack, sterile—
 Bachus towel clamps, 4
 Catgut—plain and chromic
 Eye spud, 1
 Forceps—splinter, small, 1
 Forceps—Adson
 Forceps—Debakey cardiovascular forceps
 Hemostat—Carmalt, 2, curved
 Hemostat—Kelly, 4, curved
 Needle holder, 1
Oxygen tank, reducing valves, flowmeters, Ambu bag
Pliers—side-cutting, for removal of foreign objects
Rubber gloves—nonsterile
 Rubber gloves—sterile
 Scalpel blades—assorted sizes
 Scalpel handle, 1
 Scissors—Mayo, monofilament nylon 0 to 6-0 sizes
 Scissors—Metzenbaum, curved
Specimen collecting bottles—plastic, wide-mouth, 4 ounce to 1 pint
Stethoscope
Stomach tubes—1/4, 3/8, and 1/2 OD, clear polyethylene
 Suture material—silk on cutting needle 0 to 4-0
Syringes—assorted sizes
Tape—adhesive, 1 inch width
Thermometers—clinical
Venostomy set—regular IV
Venostomy set—scalp vein infusion

Miscellaneous

Tracheostomy sets—small, medium, and large; metal and plastic
Aero-flo tip suction catheters—5, 8, 12, 14, and 18 F sizes
Face masks—small, medium, and large
Laryngoscope with small, medium, and large blades
Endotracheal tube stylet—made from SS welding rod
Mouth speculums

Esophageal stethoscope and earpiece
Flashlight
Argyle trochar catheters—8, 10, 16, and 28 F sizes
Heimlich chest drain valve
Pleur-evac water trap aspiration and collection sets
Argyle double seal chest drainage unit
Thermometers—clinical and electronic
Nonsterile fecal cups and caps
Plastic garbage bags—small, medium, and large
Tie-down ropes
"K-pad" hot water heating blankets and controls
Fleece pads—small, medium, and large; long and square
Newspaper
Kimwipe disposable wipers
Buckets—SS
Waste containers—plastic
Hair clippers
Open-ended stomach tubes—small, medium, and large
Closed-ended stomach tubes—small, medium, and large
Large animal stomach pump
Dose syringes—30, 50, and 100 ml
Funnels
Adhesive tape—1, 2, and 3 inch widths
Cling-curity stretch wrapping—2, 3, and 4 inch widths
Cotton padding—2 and 3 inch wide rolls
Rolled gauze—1, 2, 3, and 4 inch widths
Gauze sponges—2 × 2 inch and 4 × 4 inch sizes
Vetrap—self-clinging wrap; 3 and 4 inch widths
Cast padding
Plaster of paris or fiberglass rolls—2, 3, and 4 inch widths for splints and
    casts
Suction unit—portable, Yankauer suction tip
Peritoneal dialysis catheter (see p. 619)
Foley catheters—5, 8, 12, 16, 24, and 30 F sizes
Chest tubes—12, 16, 20, 26, 30, and 36 F sizes
Nasogastric tubes—12, 16, and 18 F sizes (see also p. 578)

DRUGS AND SOLUTIONS (See also Cardiovascular Emergency Tray, pp. 38–39)

Acetic acid, 0.5 per cent
Activated charcoal
Aminophylline, 25 mg per ml
Ammonia water, 0.2 per cent
Apomorphine
Atropine sulfate—parenteral, 0.4 mg per ml

Bretylium (Bretolol)
Bemegride, 3 per cent
Calcium gluconate—parenteral, 10 per cent
Charcoal—activated
Chlorpromazine hydrochloride, 25 mg per ml
Cimetidine
Desoxycorticosterone
Dexamethasone—dexamethasone sodium phosphate, 2 and 4 mg per ml
Dextran (regular and low molecular weight)
Dextrose in water, 5 and 50 per cent solution
Diazepam (Valium), 5 mg per ml
Digoxin
Dimercaprol (BAL)
Diphenhydramine hydrochloride (Benadryl)—parenteral 10 mg per ml
Diphenylthiocarbazone
Doxapram hydrochloride, 20 mg per ml
Edetic acid (EDTA)
Epinephrine hydrochloride, 1:10,000, 0.1 mg per ml, 1:10,000, 1.0 mg
   per ml
Ethanol, 50 per cent
Furosemide (Lasix)
Heparin—parenteral
Hydrocortisone sodium succinate—ampules
Hydrogen peroxide, 3 per cent
Isoproterenol
IV forms of antibiotics—gentamicin, ampicillin Na, cephalosporins, Na
K-Y Jelly—individual sterile packages penicillin (see p. 928)
Ketamine hydrochloride
Levallorphan
Lidocaine HCl, 2 per cent (20 mg/ml) without epinephrine; also spray
Mannitol ampules, 30 per cent
Meperidine hydrochloride (Demerol)
Metaraminol bitartrate (Aramine)—parenteral
Methylprednisolone
Milk of magnesia
Mineral oil
Morphine hydrochloride
Nalorphine hydrochloride
Naloxone (Narcan), 0.4 mg per ml
Norepinephrine
Novin-dipyrone, 500 mg per ml
Olive oil emollient
Ouabain
Oxymorphone
Oxytocin (Pitocin)

D-Penicillamine
Pentothal sodium, 2.5 per cent solution
Pentobarbital sodium—parenteral
Phenobarbital sodium—parenteral (Luminal), 130 mg per ml
Phenylephrine hydrochloride—parenteral
Potassium chloride (2 mEq/ml)
Potassium permanganate, 1:5,000
Prednisolone—prednisolone sodium succinate, 100 mg per 10-ml vial
Procainamide hydrochloride (Pronestyl)
Propranolol (Inderal)
Pyridine-2-aldoxime (2-PAM)
Quinidine gluconate, 80 mg per ml
Ringer's lactate and 1/2 strength Ringer's lactate with 2.5 per cent dextrose
    solution
Sodium bicarbonate
Sodium chloride, 0.9 per cent
Sodium-nitroprusside dihydrate, 10 mg per ml
Sodium sulfate, 20 per cent solution and salt
Tannic acid, 1:400
Thiamylal sodium
Vitamin K₁ (AquaMephyton injection)

INITIAL EMERGENCY EXAMINATION AND MANAGEMENT

The examination of the acutely injured animal, that is, unconscious, in shock, or suffering from acute hemorrhage or respiratory distress, must proceed simultaneously with life-saving treatment. There is no time for a detailed history taking. Diagnosis is based on physical examination and simple diagnostic aids and must be carried out quickly. The process of examination and rapid classification of emergency cases by the urgency with which treatment is required is known as *triage*. For the following conditions, immediate recognition and prompt treatment are lifesaving:

Emergency Measures

1. Relieve asphyxiation.
    a. Clear air passage by rolling the tongue forward, and remove any mucous debris obstructing the passageway; suction may be necessary.
    b. Perform a tracheotomy or tracheal intubation, if indicated.
    c. Cover any open wounds of the throat or chest, and perform thoracocentesis or tube thoracostomy, if needed. Use a cover dressing with antibiotic or povidone-iodine ointment.
    d. Institute artificial respiration, if necessary.
    e. Administer oxygen, if necessary.
2. Stop hemorrhage by pressure or direct clamping.
3. Establish a large-bore IV line (see pp. 610–617).

4. Administer whole blood, plasma, plasma expanders, or fluids in conjunction with other forms of treatment for shock (see p. 622).
5. Temporarily immobilize fractures. Attempt to keep animal in lateral recumbency. Place animals suspected of having spinal cord injuries on boards to be moved. Cover open wounds using pressure to control bleeding where necessary.
6. Relieve pain by the judicious use of analgesics.
7. Perform an initial physical examination in order to assess the degree of injury. Use the following pneumonic to evaluate all areas of animal (from D.T. Crowe):

A CRASH PLAN

A—Airway	C—cardiovascular	P—pelvic (rectal)
	R—respiratory	L—limbs
	A—abdomen	A—arteries and veins
	S—spine	N—peripheral nerves
	H—head	

THE INITIAL RAPID SURVEY EXAMINATION IN THE EMERGENCY CASE

General Examination

Examine the animal to detect any obvious abnormalities in body conformation, evidence of external bleeding, skin color, rate and quality of pulse and respiration, temperature, state of consciousness, and unusual odors.

Head and Neck

Examine the animal for injuries of the face and skull, neck rigidity and pain, the appearance of the pupils and their response to light, fluid, or blood coming from the nose or ears, color of the mucous membranes of the mouth, position of the tongue, and displacement of the teeth. Gently palpate the neck to detect local pain, muscle spasm, crepitus, swelling, hematoma, subcutaneous emphysema, and unusual arterial pulsation.

Throat and Thorax

Examine the animal for external evidence of injury, sucking wounds, and rib fractures. Palpate the rib cage for asymmetry, pain, fractures, and subcutaneous emphysema. With a pressure dressing, immediately seal any sucking wounds of the chest. Perform percussion and auscultation for the presence of fluid or air in the thoracic cavity, breathing pattern, cardiac arrhythmias or murmurs, and areas of thoracic dullness. Palpate brachial or femoral artery while auscultating the heart.

Abdomen

Examine the animal for external evidence of injury, presence of tenseness and pain, generalized expansion, absence of bowel sounds, and palpation of bladder and kidney areas.

Extremities and Spine

Examine the animal to assess the color and position of the extremities. Palpate the extremities to reveal possible fractures or dislocations. Compress the wings of the ilium and prominences of the tuber ischii to check for pelvic fractures; palpate the cervical, thoracic, lumbar, and sacral spine; and perform a rectal examination to evaluate pelvic fracture if there is no evidence of spinal pain.

Neurologic Examination

Restlessness and agitation exhibited by the injured animal are often associated with hypoxia, hypovolemia, and pain. Prudent use of sedatives and pain relievers is indicated, although overdosage may lead to more profound respiratory or central nervous system (CNS) depression. Examine the animal to assess the deep and superficial reflexes, the presence of flaccidity or rigidity of the limbs, and the presence of paralysis, coma, or paresis (see pp. 422–447). Evaluate deep pain sensation with toe pinch and toe web pinch in each of the extremities. Perform a more complete neurologic examination (see p. 422). After completing the initial physical examination, evaluate the following questions: (1) Is immediate surgical intervention indicated? (2) Is additional supportive care indicated prior to surgery? (3) Are additional diagnostic procedures indicated, and, if so, what procedures? (4) What anesthetic risks are evident? (5) Should an additional period of observation be instituted before further definitive treatment plans are undertaken?

References and Additional Readings

Parker, H. R.: Equipping and operating small animal intensive care unit. Proc. 49th American Animal Hosp. Assoc. Mtg., 481, 1982.

Sattler, F. P., Knowles, R. P., and Whittick, W. G.: Veterinary Critical Care. Philadelphia, Lea & Febiger, 1981.

Schwartz, G. R., Safar, P., Stone, J. H., et al.: Principles and Practice of Emergency Medicine. Philadelphia, W. B. Saunders Company, 1978.

Zaslow, I. M.: Veterinary Trauma and Critical Care. Philadelphia, Lea & Febiger, 1984.

Emergency Treatment of Specific Conditions

ACUTE ABDOMEN

The syndrome of acute abdomen may have many different causes but is commonly characterized by the sudden onset of acute abdominal pain, vomiting, diarrhea, negative or marked peristaltic activity, fever, dyspnea, anorexia, depression, shock, coma, and death. Occasionally, onset of acute abdominal pain may be insidious, as with rupture of the bile duct or slow necrosis of a strangulated loop of bowel. It may be difficult to distinguish between the acute surgical abdomen and other less fulminating conditions requiring medical treatment.

Rapid differential diagnosis with radiography and diagnostic peritoneal lavage are most useful in arriving at a diagnosis. Exploratory celiotomy may be indicated.

GENERAL DIAGNOSTIC PROCEDURES

History

Carefully question owners of young animals about the signs of acute infection, the ingestion of foreign bodies or poisons, or the possibility of a traumatic incident. For older animals, a careful history may reveal the possibility of a chronic infection, a slowly progressive neoplasm, or a vascular disorder. Question the owner with regard to his pet and:

Any previous infectious disease or trauma.

Any previous abdominal surgery.

Any exposure to foreign bodies or toxins.

Any excessive weight change.

The activity status of the animal and the time of its latest feeding.

How quickly the present signs have developed.

General Physical Examination (See pp. 310–319)

1. Inspect the abdomen for size and symmetry. Hair may have to be clipped to visualize puncture wounds or abdominal bruising. Look for grease or tire marks on the hair.
2. Auscultate the abdomen for normal or abnormal peristaltic sounds. For example, in advanced peritonitis, peristalsis is absent, and in acute gastritis, peristalsis is hyperactive.
3. Percuss the abdomen for tympany (the sound associated with accumulation of gas in a hollow organ, e.g., gastric distention).

4. Carefully palpate the abdomen. Splinting and rigidity of the abdominal musculature may indicate severe abdominal pain; however, spinal or pelvic trauma, spinal disc protrusions, and acute soft-tissue injuries of muscle and skin may produce signs of referred abdominal pain. Palpation may reveal an enlarged liver, spleen, kidneys, foreign body, intussusception, cystic calculi, enlarged uterus, abdominal masses, or abdominal fluid. During palpation, try to locate one specific area of pain, because it may be a clue to the organ that is primarily affected.
5. Perform a rectal examination, and note the color and consistency of the stool. In male animals, palpate the prostate and the testicles. Torsion of a retained testis often causes sudden severe abdominal pain.

Differential Diagnosis

Gastrointestinal System
Acute gastroenteritis—M*
Hemorrhagic gastroenteritis—M
Acute pancreatitis—MS†
Pancreatic abscess—S‡
Canine parvovirus enteritis—M
Gastric distention—MS
Gastric torsion—volvulus complex—SM
Gastrointestinal foreign body—S
Intestinal volvulus—S
Peritonitis—S
Acute trauma with ruptured hollow viscus – S
Ruptured spleen—splenic volvulus—S, splenic abscess—S
Diaphragmatic hernia—S
Internal or external herniation and strangulation—S

Liver
Cholangiohepatitis—biliary obstruction—S
Ruptured liver—S
Hepatic abscess—S
Ruptured gall bladder—S
Acute hepatitis—M

Renal
Acute pyelonephritis—MS
Acute nephritis—M
Renal calculus—S
Ruptured kidney, avulsed ureter—S
Obstructed ureters via calculus—S

---

*M—medical emergency
†MS—either medical or surgical emergency, with the first listed being the most common
‡S—surgical emergency

Urethral obstruction—S
Urethral rupture—S
Ruptured urinary bladder—S
Reproductive System
Acute prostatitis—M
Prostatic abscess—S
Acute metritis—pyometra – SM
Uterine torsion—S
Retained testicle with torsion—S
Ruptured gravid uterus—S

CLINICAL LABORATORY PROCEDURES (See pp. 671, 737, and 812)

The following tests are not meant to be run on every patient. Rather, a careful history taking and physical examination will enable the clinician to select those tests that will provide the most valuable information.

Laboratory Screening Tests

1. Blood tests including blood chemistries:
   Hematocrit; total white blood count and differential count; erythrocyte sedimentation rate (see p. 671), bilirubin test; serum glutamic–oxaloacetic (aspartate) transaminase (SGOT); serum glutamic–pyruvic (alanine) transaminase (SGPT); serum urea nitrogen (SUN) (see p. 737); serum amylase, serum lipase levels; blood clotting time (see p. 709); prothrombin time; and alkaline phosphatase. Serum electrolytes and blood glucose should be performed.
2. Urinalysis (see p. 812).
3. Stool analysis (see p. 798).
4. Abdominal paracentesis (see p. 522).
5. Diagnostic peritoneal lavage (see pp. 19–20).
   Both abdominal paracentesis and diagnostic peritoneal lavage should be done following radiographic evaluation of the abdomen.

RADIOGRAPHIC EXAMINATION (See pp. 567–578)

Survey radiographs of the abdomen may permit confirmation of a tentative diagnosis without extensive manipulation of the patient. However, more specific radiologic procedures may be required to confirm a diagnosis. If indicated, evacuate the alimentary tract by mild warm saline enema. Enemas are contraindicated in acute intestinal obstructions, intussusceptions, or other conditions in which normal bowel vitality has been impaired. Take lateral and ventrodorsal radiographic views of the abdomen. Standing lateral radiographs are suggested for demonstrating air-fluid interfaces as seen, for example, in obstruction or free air in the abdomen. The entire abdomen should be visible on the radiograph. Systematically examine all the organ systems for any abnormalities. Also examine the diaphragm, caudal lung fields, spine, inguinal area, external genitalia, and pelvis because lesions involving these organs may produce referred pain.

In the initial screening radiographs of the abdomen, pay careful attention to the overall relationship of abdominal structures to each other, the overall abdominal density patterns, the distribution of the intestinal loops within the abdomen, the appearance of gas patterns within the bowel, the intraluminal contents, the appearance and contour of the bowel wall, and the diameter of the bowel. Search for evidence of free gas within the peritoneal cavity. Free gas will accumulate in the subdiaphragmatic area between the liver and diaphragm. Also look for small areas of entrapped air in the mesentery.

Determine whether the appearance of the intestinal lumen correlates with the history and findings on physical examination. Determine whether any ileus is evident (see p. 14).

If the first films fail to clearly reveal the normal pattern of intestinal loops and if the patient's condition permits it, a contrast study can be performed (see pp. 567–569). Examine the outlines, densities, and size of all solid abdominal organs.

1. Examine the normal outline of the kidneys (see p. 408). Look for densities within the kidneys indicating calculi formation. An increase in the size of a kidney may be associated with hydronephrosis, tumor formation, or subcapsular accumulation of blood, transudates or urine. An irregular outline of the kidney with free gas or increased soft-tissue density in the sublumbar area may indicate renal trauma. Intravenous (IV) excretory urography (see p. 570) will be needed to visualize the ureters.

2. Examine the posterior abdomen for presence of a bladder shadow. The absence of bladder shadow may indicate a rupture of the bladder (see pp. 27–28). Examine the prostatic shadow in male animals. Increased densities or blurring of the prostatic shadow may indicate presence of an enlarged prostate (benign prostatic hypertrophy) or a prostatic cyst or abscess. In female animals, masses in the caudal abdomen may be indicative of pyometra, mucometra, torsion of a gravid uterus, or pregnancy.

3. If the patient's condition permits, a contrast study (see p. 569), a pneumocystogram (see p. 373), a pneumoperitoneum, or an excretory pyelogram may be of value (see p. 570).

The differential diagnosis of animals with gas in the small bowel is difficult. Include the clinical signs and history when establishing a differential diagnosis. When there is excessive gas with distention of bowel loops and when the diameter of the bowel has increased to 50 per cent over normal, a condition of dynamic or adynamic ileus exists. The most common cause of segmental gas accumulation with distention is foreign body obstruction (see pp. 110–111). A standing lateral radiograph is an important aid in diagnosis.

An obstructive condition of the intestine is called *ileus*. This results in abnormal accumulation of gas and intestinal fluids. Ileus is either mechanical or functional. Mechanical ileus is also called *dynamic* or *obstructive ileus*. Ileus that is functional (not due to strangulation or mechanical obstruction) is called *paralytic* or *adynamic ileus*.

Differential Diagnosis of Intestinal Gas Pattern*

Ileus confined to one or several small segments of intestinal loops.

Mechanical ileus—obstruction by a foreign body, neoplasm, intussusception, or pressure from the outside exerted by incarceration, adhesion, or neoplasms.

Spastic ileus—persistent contraction or spastic contractions of the intestines. Stringlike foreign bodies, bowel ruptures forming adhesions, and inflammatory changes within and outside a segment of the intestines.

Irritation of intestinal wall causing persistent abnormal patterns without signs of gaseous distention. "Beading" in cats; stiffened, unpliable, or asymmetrical intestinal wall in tumors (lymphosarcomas); or inflammation within or adjacent to the intestinal wall (pancreatitis, abscesses).

Ileus generalized, involving all or large sections of the intestinal tract; few, but long, gas levels can be seen.

Adynamic or paralytic ileus (reflex inhibition) superimposed on a prolonged obstruction of the mechanical or spastic type, or following impairment of blood supply. Volvulus, torsion of stomach, peritonitis, abdominal hemorrhage, intestinal inflammation, acute renal diseases, bladder rupture, abdominal and spinal trauma, rupture of the pyometra, abdominal surgery, diabetic crisis, cholecystitis, hepatitis, neoplasia, constipation, toxemias, intoxications, and thrombosis may also cause generalized ileus.

Transient ileus and generalized abdominal distention may follow simple procedures such as enemas, rectal examinations, and IV urograms. Excitation, swallowing of gas, or dyspnea result in a "pseudo-ileus."

DIFFERENTIAL DIAGNOSIS

There are three general groups of acute abdominal disorders:

1. Those requiring immediate surgical intervention with acute medical management initially. Specific disorders of this type include acute intestinal (see pp. 110–111), urinary (see pp. 122–138), and biliary (see p. 755) obstructions; foreign bodies with or without perforations (see pp. 108–109); rupture of a hollow viscus (see pp. 27–28); torsion of the intestine, spleen, testis, or stomach (see pp. 108–122); vascular occlusion (see p. 210), incarcerated hernia (see p. 116); acute abscess (see p. 220); and aortic and portal thrombosis. In all these instances, it is important to *stabilize* the patient with adequate fluid support, to normalize electrolyte and acid-base balance as best as possible, and in general improve the operative risk for the patient. Thus, *immediate medical care* must precede surgery.

2. Those requiring immediate medical treatment. Disorders of this type include pancreatitis, cystitis, hepatitis, nephritis, prostatitis, lymphadenitis, and trauma.

---

*Adapted from Suter, P. F.: Acute abdominal diseases: possibilities and limitations of radiographic examination in small animals. Proc. 39th Am. Anim. Hosp. Assoc. Mtg., 262, 1972.

3. Those that may require medical or surgical treatment. Included in this group are passive congestion of the liver or spleen, diaphragmatic hernia, abdominal tumors, peritonitis, metritis, abdominal adhesions, lead poisoning, and neoplasms of visceral or mesenteric nodes.

Acute Peritonitis

Peritonitis, localized or general, is the most important complication of a wide variety of acute abdominal disorders. Peritonitis can be caused by the following: infection or chemical irritants, direct contamination of the abdomen from septic abdominal surgery, bowel puncture from trauma, damage to the renal or biliary system with escape of free bile or urine into the abdominal cavity, extension of inflammation from other areas (such as drainage of a septic process in the prostate or liver), and chemical or foreign bodies within the peritoneal cavity producing an intense inflammatory response. Regardless of etiology, certain signs and symptoms are usually present. Systemic reactions include nausea, vomiting, leukocytosis, electrolyte imbalances, toxemia, shock, and increased temperature, pulse, and respiration rates. These signs are not always present in peritonitis, especially in very young animals, old animals, and severely debilitated animals.

Abdominal signs include
1. Pain and tenderness, which may be variable in degree.
2. Muscle rigidity (splinting), which may be absent in subsequent stages when toxemia develops.
3. Paralytic ileus, resulting in a decrease or absence of peristalsis and progressive abdominal distortion.
4. Fluid accumulation, the amount depending on the degree of inflammation and its duration. When the peritonitis is associated with bile or urine accumulation in the abdomen, aspiration of this material is indicated (see pp. 19–20).

In diffuse peritonitis, three components appear to be necessary to produce the highly fatal form: (1) a diffuse inflammatory response; (2) live bacteria; and (3) presence of materials that enhance bacterial virulence—namely, bile salts, hemoglobin, foreign material, and white blood cells. Mixed bacterial floras of aerobic and anaerobic organisms usually found in diffuse peritonitis enhance their virulence by a synergistic effect. Protein substances and hemoglobin found within the peritoneal cavity also enhance virulence. A severe toxemia can develop in peritonitis.

RADIOGRAPHIC FINDINGS

Peritonitis may be seen as a localized or diffuse soft-tissue density that permits only poor visual delineation of the loops of the bowel and organs. The increased density may be regional or generalized, depending on the origin of the lesion. Localized, poorly defined increased densities in the cranial abdomen may be consistent with pancreatitis, neoplasia, perforated stomach or proximal duodenum, extension of hepatic abscess, lacerated liver or spleen, and rupture of gallbladder or common bile duct. Densities in the central abdomen may indicate neoplasia, perforated jejunum or ileum, and lacerated spleen. Caudal abdominal densities may indicate prostatic infection, rupture of large bowel or urinary bladder, torn urethra, and ruptured uterus. Suter reports, "if peritonitis is suspected from the radiographs, the foremost problem is to decide whether it resulted from a perforated inflammatory disease or rupture of a hollow viscus, or whether it is due to a nonperforating inflammatory disease such as pancreatitis. It is still all too often assumed that free gas should be present in the abdomen following intestinal ruptures. Unfortunately, this is not so. Significant amounts of free gas can sometimes be found after gastric, colonic and rectal ruptures. The small amount of gas normally found in the small intestine, the rapid absorption of gas by the peritoneal surfaces and the sealing of a perforated area by adhesions to the mesentery or omentum make the presence of free gas a very unreliable sign of bowel rupture."* The wall of the bowel may appear thicker than normal owing to edema and inflammation, and loops of bowel may be fixed in place because of adhesions.

PARACENTESIS AND DIAGNOSTIC PERITONEAL LAVAGE
(See Table 2)

Abdominal paracentesis and diagnostic lavage combined with cytologic examination of abdominal fluid are extremely helpful. Examine peritoneal fluid for bile with an ictotest reaction and creatinine or urea nitrogen indicating possible ruptured bladder. Also inspect the fluid for any evidence of spillage from the gastrointestinal tract, including bacteria, vegetable fibers, intracellular bacteria, and polymorphonuclear leukocytes (see pp. 19–20).

TREATMENT OF ACUTE PERITONITIS

The measures used in the treatment of acute peritonitis are, in general, applicable to most acute abdominal disorders. The basic aims of treatment are to control infection by the use of antibiotics, to manage metabolic changes, and to use surgical intervention if necessary. Diagnostic peritoneal lavage is the most important test, coupled with radiographic evaluation in determining whether an exploratory celiotomy is indicated (see pp. 29–30). Indications for celiotomy are abdominal hemorrhaging, soiling of the abdomen from bowel contamination, bile in the abdomen, urine in the abdomen, and free air with evidence ruptured hollow viscus.
1. Provide effective body system support.
   a. Ensure that adequate ventilation is available and supply additional oxygen tension if possible.

---

*From Suter, P. F.: Acute abdominal diseases: possibilities and limitations of radiographic examination in small animals. Proc. 39th Am. Anim. Hosp. Assoc. Mtg., 262, 1972.

Table 2. COMMON CAUSES OF ABDOMINAL EFFUSION

Transudate	**Serosanguineous Exudate**
Hypoproteinemia	Feline infectious peritonitis
Intestinal malabsorption	Urine peritonitis
Intestinal protein loss	Bile peritonitis
Glomerular disease	Pancreatic peritonitis
Lymphangiectasia	Gastric perforation
Neoplasia	Steatitis
Obstructing lymph drainage	
Hepatopathies	**Hemorrhagic Effusion**
Chronic active hepatitis	Traumatic injury to major vessel,
Diaphragmatic hernia	spleen, liver
Abdominal neoplasia	Neoplasm
	Hemangiosarcoma
Modified Transudate	Vascular tumor
Congestive heart failure	Tumor eroding a vessel
Postsinusoidal (thoracic	Pheochromocytoma
vena cava) obstruction	Bleeding disorders
Portal venous obstruction	Warfarin toxicity
Abdominal neoplasia	Thrombocytopenia
Purulent Exudate	Thrombosis
Intestinal perforation	Torsion
Penetrating wounds	Stomach
Ruptured pyometra	Spleen
Ruptured (intraabdominal or	
retroperitioneal) abscess	
Bacterial (septic) peritonitis	

Modified from Scott, R. C., et al.: Abdominal paracentesis and cystocentesis. Vet. Clin. North Am., 4:413, 1974.

    b. Correct fluid and electrolyte imbalances (see pp. 591–617).

    c. Severe acidosis and accumulation of tissue debris can result in the protein binding of calcium. Before administering doses of bicarbonate, monitor the serum calcium level and potassium; correct any fluid and acid-base disturbance (see p. 593).

    d. Control infection. Surgically drain acute abscesses; this usually involves exploratory celiotomy. Antibiotics should be started prior to exploratory celiotomy and should be administered by the IV route: For gram-positive anaerobes—ampicillin or clindamycin; gram-negative aerobes—tobramycin or gentamycin. After celiotomy has been performed, abdominal cultures should be obtained (see p. 499).

    e. Control any shock state that may exist (see pp. 60–61).

2. Treat the specific cause (remove foreign bodies, correct torsions, and repair ruptured hollow viscera).

3. The use of intermittent peritoneal lavage has proved valuable in the treatment of diffuse peritonitis if exploratory celitomy is not performed and

if the abdomen is left closed. Place a multiple-fenestrated Silastic drain in the abdomen through a subcutaneous tunnel and two paramidline abdominal incisions approximately 2 to 3 inches from the midline. Two tubes are placed into the gutteral furrows. With the animal in lateral recumbency, infusion fluid is placed in the top tube and aspirated through the lower tube. When the animal is rolled over, the same procedure is followed. Secure the tube to the skin with a purse-string suture of nonabsorbable material, bandage, and place a collar on the affected animal. To make the initial lavage solution, add 10 ml of 1 per cent titratable Betadine solution to 1 L of warmed lactated Ringer's solution. Allow this lavage fluid to run into the abdomen for 30 minutes, and then drain. Repeat the procedure three times a day. Electrolyte balance must be watched during lavage, because hypokalemia may develop. Effective supportive therapy—replacement of protein loss and energy demands must be met by IV administration (plasma, 4.5 per cent amino acids, 20 per cent dextrose); (see also p. 617).

4. Correct fluid, electrolyte, and nutritional disorders. Avoid giving solid food and medication by mouth; substitute fluids and electrolytes as needed (see pp. 591–617). If septic shock develops, treat as indicated (see p. 59).

5. Provide adequate ancillary care. Hospitalize and keep the animal as comfortable as possible. Use pain relievers and sedatives judiciously. Relieve excessive build-up of gas in the intestines and the stomach by nasogastric intubation (see p. 582).

See Exploratory Celiotomy (pp. 29–30)

ABDOMINAL INJURIES

NONPENETRATING ABDOMINAL INJURIES

Nonpenetrating injuries are very common, especially following automobile accidents, and may be accompanied by various degrees of shock, hemorrhage, and peritonitis. They present a diagnostic challenge because (1) they are often consequences of other serious trauma (such as fractures and coma), (2) relatively minor abdominal trauma may produce rupture of a hollow viscus, and (3) the absence of any external wounds on the abdomen may be deceptive. When an animal has suffered from nonpenetrating abdominal injury, the presenting signs often reflect multiple organ damage. The signs of blunt abdominal trauma are associated with blood loss, bruising and tearing of solid organs, and leaking of irritating juices from hollow abdominal organs. A rapid pulse and rising temperature with acute abdominal pain could indicate peritonitis or bowel obstruction with infarction.

Careful and gentle palpation of the injured abdomen is helpful. Abdominal masses following blunt trauma occur late in the course of the clinical signs, and such a mass may represent a hematoma of the liver, spleen, mesentery, or kidney. Auscultation may be of value; despite extensive intra-abdominal injury and bleeding, peristaltic sounds may be heard. Peristaltic sounds heard in the chest may aid in the diagnosis of traumatic diaphragmatic hernia.

The following are diagnostic techniques that help determine the extent of injury in blunt abdominal trauma:

1. Inspect the abdomen and caudal chest wall for evidence of penetrating injuries, muscle contusions, and hematomas or for evidence of being hit by a car or other vehicle. A red or bluish circle at the umbilicus indicates the presence of free intra-abdominal blood and the same discoloration in the inguinal region indicates retroperitoneal hemorrhage most commonly associated with pelvic fractures.

2. Palpate the abdomen, both superficially and deeply, in an organized manner, starting with the right and left caudal abdominal quadrants, the midabdominal area, and cranial right and left quadrants. Generalized abdominal discomfort that is consistent on palpation can be a sign of serious visceral injury. Referred pain from a more superficial injury can also cause pain on palpation. Following abdominal palpation, carefully perform rectal palpation to evaluate the pelvis and pelvic urethra.

3. Percussion combined with palpation can be used to detect free fluid within the abdominal cavity. Percussion can also be used to detect abnormal abdominal sounds such as hyperresonant or tympanic, as occurs with distention of a hollow viscus, or increased dullness, as occurs over an organ that is misplaced or a partially fluid-filled abdomen.

4. Auscultation can prove helpful in diagnosing intra-abdominal injury. Bowel sounds are produced from the movement of fluid and air in the intestinal tract. Three types of intestinal movement have been described in the dog: (1) segmenting contractions, (2) pendular movement, and (3) peristaltic waves. Normal peristaltic sounds in the dog are 3 to 4 per minute; in the cat, there are 5 to 6 per minute following eating. Changes in bowel sounds following abdominal trauma can be highly variable and serial. Repetitive examinations can be more significant than a single examination. In the early stages of peritonitis and obstruction, an increase in peristaltic sounds may be heard. As peritonitis proceeds, shock ensues, increasing pain develops, and decreased bowel activity becomes evident. Findings on auscultation should be coupled with other diagnostic signs such as abdominal pain, vomiting, lassitude, and fever in order to make a diagnosis of severe abdominal injury and to determine whether to proceed with exploratory celiotomy.

5. Abdominal paracentesis can be a helpful technique in collecting fluid from the peritoneal space and analyzing cellular appearance. Place the animal in dorsal recumbency, and clip the ventral abdomen from the xiphoid to the pubis. Manually express the bladder and prepare the abdomen aseptically. Use an 18-gauge, 1½-inch spinal needle to make either a two-quadrant or four-quadrant tap. In a two-quadrant tap, 2 ml of xylocaine are infiltrated into the skin on each side of the abdominal musculature, 1 to 2 inches below the umbilicus and lateral to the boundary of the rectus muscle. In the four-quadrant tap, the area of the abdomen from the umbilicus to pubis

is divided into four quadrants, and four separate taps are made in the middle of each quadrant. Allow the needle to penetrate the peritoneum. A popping sensation will be felt and further penetration will become suddenly easier. Collect fluid through the hub of the needle by pressing the abdomen. Analyze the fluid collected by making a smear and staining with Wright's and Gram's stain and performing creatinine and amylase determinations and an Ictotest. False negative results, characterized by the inability to obtain fluid from the abdomen, are frequently seen with a needle tap. More accurate results have been obtained using the technique of diagnostic peritoneal lavage. To effectively perform this technique, a peritoneal dialysis catheter* should be used. Prepare the abdomen for surgery as previously described, with the animal in left lateral recumbency. Inject 2 per cent xylocaine into the abdomen 1/2 to 2 inches below the umbilicus on the midline of the abdomen. Make a small incision through the skin and ventral abdominal musculature. Control bleeding with gauze sponges and pressure. Insert the dialysis catheter into the abdominal cavity, and note the presence of fluid entering the catheter. Attach a syringe to the catheter to remove fluid. If no abdominal fluid is obtained, institute abdominal lavage by instilling 22 ml per kg of warm lactated Ringer's solution. Roll the animal over on its back to distribute and mix the fluid within the abdomen, then collect via the catheter using gravity and/or suction. Evaluate the returning fluid grossly as well as through samples taken for microhematocrit, cytology, creatinine amylase, and Ictotest. Remove the catheter and close the abdominal incision. If frank blood is obtained in the catheter following its passage into the abdomen and 2 ml of blood can be collected for every 5 kg of body weight, a diagnosis of intra-abdominal injury can be made.

Other evidence of intra-abdominal injury can be: (1) microhematocrit of the lavage fluid over 5 per cent; (2) red blood cell (RBC) count of fluid over 100,000 per cu mm, white blood cell (WBC) count over 500 to 1000 per cu mm; and (3) creatinine level of the lavage fluid, if higher than that of the serum, indicates uroabdomen. The spleen, liver, stomach, intestines, and pancreas are vulnerable to blunt injury. Cytologic examination and the finding of many polymorphonuclear neutrophils (PMNs) and free and intracellular bacteria indicate septic peritonitis. Injury may result when the viscus is crushed against the vertebral column or is suddenly displaced from its normal mesenteric attachment.

Abdominal Hemorrhage

When abdominal paracentesis or lavage indicates continued abdominal bleeding, septic contamination, or bile, an exploratory celiotomy is indicated. Abdominal pain may or may not be present, and distention of the abdomen may not be evident. Severe intra-abdominal hemorrhage is often associated

---

*Trocath, adult size; McGaw Laboratories.

with splenic or hepatic injury. Prior to bringing the animal to surgery, hemorrhage may be reduced by:

1. Applying abdominal counterpressure. An additional 22 ml per kg of warmed lactated Ringer's solution is placed in the abdomen, and an abdominal bandage is placed on the animal. Ventilation must be carefully observed, because abdominal pressure may result in decreased thoracic tidal volume. The animal should be taken to surgery as rapidly as possible if continuous severe bleeding is suspected.
2. Autotransfusion can be helpful in severe abdominal bleeding. Blood may be collected aseptically from the abdomen in CPD bags or blood bottles. If possible, a filter* should be used when returning the blood via jugular catheter to the animal. The blood can be removed via a peritoneal dialysis catheter or it can be autotransfused during surgery, using a "trap" bottle with ACD, CPD, or 2 per cent citrate added. The blood is aspirated into the bottle via suction.

Urinary Tract Trauma

Pelvic trauma, including fractures and luxations, are frequently seen in both cats and dogs. In one large study of pelvic trauma, 39 per cent of dogs had concurrent urinary tract trauma that included ureteral avulsions, ruptured bladders, urethral ruptures, mucosal irregularities of the bladder wall and blood clot formation, urinary bladder herniations and hydroureter/hydronephrosis. Signs of concurrent urinary tract injury may include dysuria, hematuria, abdominal pain, and evidence of abdominal trauma. The extent of urinary tract injury is not well correlated with the extent of pelvic injury. An important fact found during this study was that one third of all urinary tract trauma cases associated with pelvic injury were clinically unsuspected. Although survey radiographs are an important screening procedure in pelvic and abdominal injury, 60 per cent of these tests may be negative for clinical abnormalities, whereas contrast radiography, that is, excretory urograms (see p. 570) or positive contrast retrograde urethrography will reveal lesions not seen on flat films. The most consistent radiographic findings on flat films in cases of urinary trauma are increased retroperitoneal density changes that could indicate ureteral avulsions, bladder ruptures, or urethral ruptures. Although hematuria is a clinical sign that is often seen following pelvic trauma, it is most often associated with mucosal wall hemorrhage of the bladder and hemorrhage into the bladder. The *most important* factor in urinary tract trauma associated with pelvic injury is to detect early those cases requiring surgical intervention, such as bladder rupture, ureteral rupture, and urethral rupture.

If urinary tract injury is 12 to 24 hours old and if the abdomen has been contaminated with urine for this time, initial medical supportive treatment is recommended prior to surgery. Place a peritoneal dialysis catheter in the

---

*Micropore Filter, Swank-Sorensen Research, Inc., Salt Lake City, Utah.

abdomen, and dialyse for 12 hours while maintaining fluid and electrolyte balance.

Rupture of the Kidney

Renal injuries may range from mild ecchymosis, bruises, or contusions to lacerations or rupture. Rupture of large renal arteries and veins or avulsion of the renal artery and vein from the renal hilus may result in hemorrhage and sudden death from shock. A rent in the renal parenchyma may extend into the collecting system, with blood clots obstructing urine flow. Connection of the collecting system with the abdominal cavity or retroperitoneal tissue may be associated with inflammation caused by the extravasation of urine. The most frequent type of renal injury in dogs and cats appears to be contusions, with the formation of subcapsular hematomas. Abdominal counterpressure with bandage wrap may be initially helpful in controlling hemorrhage until the animal can be stabilized.

Signs. Clinical signs are variable and depend partly on the extent of damage. The animal may feel pain in the kidney, but it may be obscured by pain from other lesions. Hematuria is usually present and may be accompanied by shock, oliguria, or anuria. A mass palpated in the sublumbar area may represent either a hematoma or an infiltration of urine into surrounding soft tissues.

Laboratory Findings. Abnormalities associated with primary renal failure will not develop if only one kidney is affected. Urinalysis will reveal gross or microscopic hematuria and proteinuria. There is not good correlation between the degree of hematuria and kidney damage. Abdominal paracentesis or diagnostic lavage may reveal blood or extravasated urine. A negative tap does not eliminate the possibility of severe renal damage. Negative diagnostic lavage is rarely associated with isolated retroperitoneal urine leakage or bleeding.

Radiographic Findings. Striated sublumbar density obliterating the kidney shadow and depressing the colon is typical of sublumbar hematoma and renal or ureteral rupture. Other radiographic signs that may indicate renal damage are fractured ribs at lumbar vertebrae adjacent to the kidneys and displacement or abnormalities in the symmetry of the kidneys. As soon as shock has been treated, an intravenous pyelogram (IVP) should be taken. Because frequently there is associated nephron damage and poor renal perfusion in injury, the standard method of performing an IVP may not provide sufficient dye in the collecting system. High dosage excretory urograms (give 250–900 mg of iodine/kg body weight using an aqueous organic iodide medium) may be helpful in these situations (see pp. 570–572). If the urogram shows evidence of injury to one kidney, it is important to note whether the other kidney is normal, because an emergency nephrectomy may have to be performed.

Differential Diagnosis. Trauma to the lumbar region and rib and spinal fractures may cause local signs that suggest renal injury; however, hematuria is usually absent and urograms are normal.

Treatment
1. Treat for shock and hemorrhage.
2. Follow the progress of the patient carefully for 48 hours. Measure urine volume for the first 24 hours. If renal trauma is associated with gross hematuria, institute appropriate fluid therapy to induce a marked diuresis to minimize blood clot formation in excretory pathways. Subcapsular and perirenal hematomas usually undergo spontaneous resorption in 7 to 10 days. Surgical intervention is indicated during the first 24 hours if IVPs reveal a ruptured kidney, kidney laceration, or ruptured ureter or if the patient continues to decline despite intensive treatment, as evidenced by a falling hematocrit, rising temperature, and signs of deepening shock.
3. Consider nephrectomy only if the contralateral kidney appears normal. Some kidney lacerations can be sutured; however, swelling and loss of normal kidney parenchyma may make this very difficult. Excessively tight sutures through the kidney parenchyma may result in further kidney laceration and necrosis. If severe injury is confined to one pole of the kidney, consider performing a partial nephrectomy using the transverse technique of amputation.
4. Nephritic infections and abscesses may follow initial kidney damage. Peritonitis resulting from extravasation of urine into the peritoneum may also follow kidney trauma. These complications usually develop 2 to 4 days after the initial trauma.

Rupture of the Ureter

This is not a common condition, but some of the signs may resemble those of kidney trauma. Unless both ureters are involved, signs of uremia will not develop. Leakage of urine results in inflammation. Obstruction of the ureter may result in the development of hydronephrosis. Common results are abdominal pain, oliguria, anuria, hematuria, shock, progressive signs of uremia, and toxemia.

Laboratory Findings. Evaluation of lavage fluid from the abdomen may reveal elevated creatinine above serum creatinine.

Radiographic Findings. A plane film of the abdomen may reveal loss of soft-tissue detail if urinary extravasation and peritonitis have occurred. Sublumbar densities may indicate concurrent kidney trauma. Conclusive diagnosis can be reached only by the use of IVP (see p. 570).

Treatment
1. Treat for hemorrhage and shock. Control secondary infections.
2. If the contralateral kidney is normal, nephrectomy may be considered.
3. Reanastomosis of the ureter over a splinting catheter may be attempted. Ruptures of the distal end of the ureter may permit reimplantation of the proximal end into the bladder.

Complications. Ureteral stenosis, hydronephrosis, renal infection, peritonitis, and ureteral abscess are frequent complications.

Rupture of the Spleen

A rupture of the spleen may follow any sudden, severe blow to the abdomen or may be associated with splenic tumors such as hemangioma or hemangiosarcoma. Small tears in the spleen may cause continuous or recurrent bleeding. Some tears only involve the splenic capsule, producing subcapsular hematomas. These can produce severe bleeding if they rupture spontaneously.

Additionally, the gastric dilatation volvulous complex may result in twisting of the splenic pedicle, causing acute venous obstruction and thrombosis with massive splenic infarction.

Signs. Pain may center over the anterior quadrant of the abdomen, or it may be restricted to the left anterior quadrant. There may be signs of blood loss and shock, palpable swelling in the left anterior quadrant of abdomen, fluid-free blood (possibly within the abdomen), mild peritoneal irritation, and ileus.

It is important to remember that subcapsular splenic hemorrhage may occur without extravasating into the free peritoneal cavity. Also, delayed or intermittent splenic hemorrhage may occur 10 to 30 days following the initial insult. Multiple abdominal paracentesis and lavage (see pp. 19–20) should be performed and can be helpful in making a diagnosis.

In the case of ruptured hemangiomas or hemangiosarcomas, there is usually no history of trauma; however, signs of debilitation, chronic anemia, abdominal distention, and dyspnea may have been developing over a protracted period of time.

Radiographic Findings. Loss of normal outline of perisplenic region, separation of intestinal loops associated with fluid accumulation, caudal displacement of the splenic flexure of the colon, gastric dilatation, possible fractured ribs, and abnormal motion of the diaphragm are common findings.

Laboratory Findings. Hematocrit (Hct) and hemoglobin (Hb) levels fall. Because of blood loss, a mild leukocytosis or anemia may develop. If blood loss is prolonged, there may be evidence of bone marrow hyperplasia. Diagnostic abdominal paracentesis may be helpful when free, unclotted blood is present within the peritoneal cavity (see pp. 522–523); however, a negative tap does not rule out the possibility of a ruptured spleen. The diagnosis of intra-abdominal bleeding is almost 100 per cent accurate when diagnostic peritoneal lavage is used.

Treatment

1. Treat for shock and control secondary infections. Begin treatment for septic shock using intravenous (IV) antibiotics, that is, gentamicin 1 mg per lb of body weight IV every 8 hours and ampicillin or clindamycin for anaerobes. Stabilize the patient. Always take chest radiographs in all trauma cases.
2. In cases of tumor, radiographically evaluate the thorax, and if surgery is performed, carefully evaluate the entire abdomen for any indication of metastasis.
3. Perform a splenectomy.

Splenic Torsion

Splenic torsion that is not accompanied by gastric torsion is rarely seen in dogs. When present, it may present as an acute emergency with signs of shock, collapse, and an acutely painful abdomen, with pale mucous membranes and splenomegaly. In the more chronic form, there is anorexia, depression, splenomegaly, vomiting, and abdominal pain. The problem is usually seen in large, deep-chested breeds of dogs, especially Great Danes. Clinical pathology may reveal anemia, with extensive fragmentation of red blood cells, hemoglobinemia, hemoglobinuria, elevated serum alkaline phosphatase, development of disseminated intravascular coagulation (see p. 63), and ventricular arrhythmias. Urinalysis may show hemoglobinuria, proteinuria, and bilirubinuria. Survey abdominal radiographs are rarely diagnostic of splenic torsion, and only splenomegaly may be observed; diagnosis is usually confirmed on the basis of exploratory celiotomy.

The differential diagnosis of enlarged spleen should include neoplasia such as hemangiosarcoma, lymphosarcoma, splenic hematoma, extramedullary hematopoiesis, passive congestion, amyloidosis, reticuloendothelial stimulation, autoimmune hemolytic anemia (AIHA), granulomatous splenitis associated with infection, and, rarely, splenic abscessation. In cats, mast cell sarcomas have also been observed.

Rupture of the Liver

Rupture of the liver is characterized by a history of trauma followed either immediately or after several hours by anterior abdominal pain and tenderness, signs of hemorrhage, shock, coma, and death. Various types of traumatic injuries to the liver may occur: (1) single or multiple lacerations in the capsule and parenchyma, (2) deep disruption of the parenchyma, and (3) disruption and fragmentation of one or more liver lobes. Intra-abdominal bleeding is characteristic of hepatic rupture and liver fractures. Bile peritonitis may develop 24 to 72 hours following the initial injury. In some cases, free blood may be aspirated from the abdomen by abdominal paracentesis. Rupture of the liver involving the biliary ducts produces a characteristic "motor oil" type of exudate. Rupture of the liver should be suspected in all cases of abdominal trauma. The best method of diagnosing biliary-free damage with abdominal leakage bile is by diagnostic peritoneal lavage and an Ictotest.

Laboratory Findings. Hct and Hb levels drop as hemodilution occurs. The WBC is elevated. Transient relief of shock and hypotension may occur following the IV administration of fluids and electrolytes; however, with continued hepatic bleeding, hypovolemia and shock again develop.

Treatment. Treatment of hepatic rupture varies with the degree of injury. In cases in which intra-abdominal bleeding has been diagnosed, some degree of control of bleeding may prove very helpful while the animal is being stabilized and prepared for possible abdominal exploration. Abdominal counter pressure bandage or a torso wrap may be helpful. The use of intra-abdominal infusions of norepinephrine may be helpful in this regard. Dilute 4 ml of norepinephrine solution with 100 to 200 ml 5 per cent dextrose in water. Table 3 shows dosages recommended for use in dogs and cats. Hepatic lacerations that continue to bleed require exploratory surgery, suturing, and abdominal drainage. Rupture of or extensive damage to a large portion of the liver may require excision of a portion or the entire lobe of the liver.

Injuries to the Gallbladder

Traumatic rupture of the gallbladder and bile ducts is usually associated with other abdominal trauma. Damage to the gallbladder may be indicated on paracentesis by the finding of a heavy, greenish-brown fluid in the abdomen or may be found only at the time of exploratory laparotomy. In peritoneal lavage or paracentesis, perform an Ictotest on the fluid to detect the presence of bile. The gallbladder may rupture following obstruction caused by calculi or abscesses. The degree of severity and rapidity of onset of bile-induced peritonitis is dependent on the presence of anaerobic bacteria from the intestinal tract and on the rate at which bile is leaking out of the biliary system.

Treatment depends on the location and the extent of the damage to the biliary system. If one of the divisional bile ducts is damaged, repair may be attempted. If the common duct is ruptured primary suturing and anastomosis should be attempted. These repairs may involve the use of reimplantation of the bile duct; cholecystoduodenostomy, indwelling polyethylene catheter, and cholecystectomy. Cholecystoduodenostomy or cholecystojejunostomy can be used if the bile duct cannot be repaired. The duct is ligated above and below the tear.

Peritonitis will develop in all cases in which bile escapes into the abdominal cavity. Thorough irrigation of the abdomen with warm Ringer's solution, adequate abdominal drainage, and intensive treatment for peritonitis are very important.

Table 3. DOSAGE OF NOREPINEPHRINE FOR INTRA-ABDOMINAL INFUSION*

Animal Weight (kg)	Solution Volume (ml)	Norepinephrine Dose (mg)
All cats	50	2
Dogs up to 10 kg	50	2
Dogs 10 to 40 kg	100	3
Dogs 40 to 80 kg	100–150	4
Dogs greater than 80 kg	200–300	6–8

*Note: Only effective for capillary or venule arteriolar bleeding, not for major venous or arterial bleeding where abdominal pressure bandage and/or exploratory celiotomy is indicated.

From Ewing, G. O.: Abdominal trauma. Canine Practice, 2:22, 1975.

Pancreatic Injuries

Traumatic damage to the pancreas may be associated with blunt abdominal trauma. Damage to the pancreas may result in intra-abdominal hemorrhage and, frequently, in the delayed development of focal peritonitis associated with the escape of digestive enzymes. Clinical signs of increasing abdominal pain, vomiting, anorexia, depression, and shocklike syndrome can develop. Radiographically, a dense, mottled area appears between the stomach and distended, gas-filled loops of the small intestine. There is dorsal or dorsomedial displacement of the duodenum and corrugation and spasticity of the duodenal wall. Laboratory tests utilizing serum lipase and amylase values can be very helpful (see pp. 742 and 753). The diagnosis of traumatic or hemorrhagic pancreatitis is confirmed on exploratory laparotomy.

Diaphragmatic Hernias (See pp. 217–218)

RUPTURED HOLLOW VISCERA

If signs of peritonitis develop within 24 to 48 hours following blunt abdominal trauma, perforation of a hollow viscus of the gastrointestinal tract should be suspected. The signs usually consist of increasing abdominal pain, muscle spasm, ileus, elevated temperature, increased pulse and respiration rates, pallor, vomiting, shock, toxemia, and collapse. This condition may result in death. Diagnosis of ruptured hollow viscus can be made early by diagnostic peritoneal lavage (see pp. 19–20).

Laboratory Findings. If concurrent hemorrhage is present, there may be a decrease in the Hct and Hb levels. Peritonitis causes leukocytosis. A diagnostic abdominal tap may reveal an exudate and the presence of intestinal contents within the peritoneal cavity. Peritoneal lavage may indicate plant material, free bacteria, and degenerating neutrophils.

Radiographic Findings. Free fluid or air may also be seen in the peritoneal cavity; however, this is not seen in many early cases of peritonitis. Horizontal radiographs are helpful in locating free air in the abdomen.

Rupture of the Bladder

Rupture of the bladder is most frequently associated with blunt trauma to the pelvis and can be seen in both male and female dogs. The extent of pelvic trauma is not related to the presence or absence of urinary tract trauma. Rupture of the bladder can develop with only mild pelvic or abdominal injury. Rupture of the bladder is also more frequently seen in obstructed male cats. Because of the anatomic location of the bladder in dogs and cats, rupture of the bladder wall usually communicates with the peritoneal cavity. Traumatic rupture of the bladder does not always cause acute abdominal pain. Pain is more severe when there is associated cystitis and peritonitis because of bladder rupture.

Signs. Signs of bladder rupture are abdominal pain and tenseness. In severe cases, vomiting, progressive uremia and toxemia, and increased temperature, pulse, and respiration occur. There may be anuria or oliguria, possibly incipient hematuria followed by collapse, coma, and death. Large amounts of hypertonic urine collecting in the peritoneal cavity lead to the development of severe hemoconcentration and electrolyte abnormalities. Additionally, hypertonic urine in the peritoneal cavity produces peritonitis. Some animals with a ruptured bladder may be completely anuric; others may continue to pass small quantities of blood-tinged urine. Still others pass what appears to be a normal amount of urine that appears normal; however, this is not as common as the other situations.

Laboratory Findings. There may be leukocytosis and, if uremia is present, an elevated blood urea nitrogen (BUN) level. The packed cell volume (PCV) may be markedly elevated because of the hemoconcentration present when urine accumulates in the peritoneal cavity. A scanty amount of urine may be obtained. Urinalysis reveals the presence of RBCs. Abdominal paracentesis should reveal the presence of fluid with a high content of urea.

Radiographic Findings. Survey radiographs usually fail to reveal the outline of a normal bladder. Loss of normal abdominal detail around the bladder occurs, with a ground-glass appearance to the abdomen caused by urine and developing peritonitis. There is a high incidence of pelvic fractures that can be recognized along the bladder rupture. There may be an associated increase in soft-tissue density around the pelvic area secondary to trauma. Positive contrast retrograde cystography is the technique of choice for demonstrating bladder rupture. Only sterile triiodinated organic iodine products should be used where bladder rupture is suspected. Ventrodorsal, lateral, and two oblique views of the posterior abdomen should be taken. (See Radiographic Techniques on pp. 567–578.)

GENERAL TREATMENT OF NONPENETRATING ABDOMINAL WOUNDS

A period of close observation may be necessary before the diagnosis of an intra-abdominal lesion can be made. During this observation period, the following procedures may be carried out:

1. Hospitalize the animal, watch all vital signs carefully, and observe for increasing abdominal findings or development of deepening shock. Do not dose too heavily with pain relievers, because this will cause abdominal signs to be masked.
2. Do not administer food orally, and maintain patient on parenteral fluids intravenously (see p. 519).
3. Treat shock, if indicated (see pp. 60–61).
4. Perform serial hematocrit, WBC, and differential tests (see p. 671).
5. Failure to respond to treatment for shock and blood loss or relapse into shock after an initial treatment period usually indicates continuing major blood loss, the development of a fulminating infection, or pelvic fractures

with extensive retroperitoneal bleeding. Diagnostic peritoneal lavage will confirm intra-abdominal hemorrhage. Radiographs of the chest and abdomen are indicated.

6. Indications for an exploratory celiotomy in any nonpenetrating abdominal injury are as follows: (a) the presence of pneumoperitoneum, as evidenced by radiographs; (b) abdominal paracentesis or diagnostic peritoneal lavage yielding blood (not by puncture of the spleen) or evidence of contamination from contents of a hollow viscus (stomach contents, bile, feces, or urine); (c) secondary collapse, following recovery from post-traumatic shock, if associated with suggestive abdominal signs confirmed by radiography or diagnostic peritoneal lavage; (d) the presence of an enlarging mass within the abdomen; (e) when abdominal signs are obscure, and there is a continuation or recurrence of signs with an increase in severity or frequency. An unnecessary exploratory celiotomy is often far less dangerous than the failure to intervene surgically in the case of a ruptured hollow or solid viscus.

PENETRATING ABDOMINAL WOUNDS

Any sharp, pointed object or projectile that could have penetrated the free peritoneal cavity must be assumed to have lacerated a hollow viscus. Thus, exploratory celiotomy is indicated in all penetrating abdominal wounds. The probing of a penetrating wound is not a reliable means of assessing the extent of the injury. Diagnostic peritoneal lavage can be used if there is any question about abdominal cavity penetration. All patients with rupture of a hollow viscus should be treated for peritonitis.

Exploratory Celiotomy

The abdomen, once opened from xyphoid to near the pubis on the ventral midline should be explored in a systematic manner. If gross contamination and peritonitis exist, irrigation of the abdominal cavity with warm, sterile lactated Ringer's solution and water-soluble antibiotics such as crystalline penicillin or kanamycin is indicated. In cases of peritonitis, the abdominal wound should not be closed but should be packed open using sterile laparotomy sponges or wound pads followed by sterile dressings and cling wrap around the abdomen. The bandage will have to be changed, because drainage soaks through; however, as the peritonitis is brought under control, drainage will be reduced and the abdomen can be closed using nonabsorbable suture materials.

Systematic Exploration of the Abdominal Cavity

If the abdomen is full of blood and continued bleeding is suspected, systematic exploration of the abdominal cavity should be carried out. As soon as the abdomen is entered, the blood is aspirated quickly (into a sterile fluid trap containing an anticoagulant of sodium citrate, 2 per cent, 15 ml/500 ml of blood). A hand is introduced into the abdomen, and the left adrenal gland is palpated. Then the celiac artery is palpated (2–3 cm cranial to the adrenal). The aorta-celiac artery is compressed in a downward movement; this maneuver effectively stops all arterial flow into the abdominal cavity. The abdomen is then opened the rest of the way (xyphoid to pubis) and packs (towels, lap pads, or sponges) are inserted into the abdomen and packed into the area of continued bleeding. The packs are slowly removed after blood pressure has been stabilized as suction is continued and the point of hemorrhaging is determined and controlled as needed.

1. **Cranial Left Quadrant**
   a. Begin with the examination of the left lateral and medial lobes of the liver, esophageal hiatus, and the rest of the central and left diaphragm.
   b. Examine the fundus of the stomach and its greater curvature, the spleen, and the left limb of the pancreas.
   c. Examine the left adrenal gland, and palpate the celiac and cranial mesenteric artery.

2. **Caudal Left Quadrant**
   a. Begin by picking up the descending colon and inspecting it and its mesentery. With this as a natural barrier and holding the small intestine to the right, inspect the left vertebral gutter, caudal mesenteric artery, left kidney, ureter, and left uterine horn and ovary in females. Palpate the aorta.
   b. Inspect the urinary bladder.

3. **Cranial Right Quadrant**
   a. Begin by examining the right diaphragm, the dome of the right lateral and middle lobes, and the rest of the liver, including its underside, and the gallbladder and the biliary tree.
   b. Inspect and palpate the pylorus, the lesser curvature of the stomach, and antrum.
   c. Inspect the proximal duodenum by elevating it.
   d. Inspect the adjacent pancreas and associated mesentery.
   e. With this maneuver, the mesoduodenum acts as a barrier for the intestines and the right adrenal gland, caudal vena cava, and the cranial pole of the right kidney can be inspected.
   f. Expose the epiploic foramen, and inspect the hepatic artery and portal vein.

4. **Caudal Right Quadrant**
   a. With the duodenum still elevated, elevate the colon. These structures and the duodenocolic ligament will act as an intestinal barrier, allowing inspection of the rest of the right kidney, right ureter, and caudal vena cava.
   b. Inspect the right uterine horn and ovary, if the animal is a female.
   c. Examine the remaining small and large intestine, cecum, and root of the mesentery. Inspect the intestine by palpation and visualization, beginning at the pelvic flexure of the duodenum and working distally until reaching the descending colon.

References and Additional Readings

Berzon, J. L.: Surgical repair of traumatic injuries to the biliary system: case report and discussion. J. Am. Anim. Hosp. Assoc., *17*(3):421, 1981.

Bjorling, D. E., Crowe, D. T., Kolata, R. J., and Rawlings, C. A.: Penetrating abdominal wounds in dogs and cats. J. Am. Anim. Hosp. Assoc., *18*(5):742, 1982.

Bjorling, D. E., Latimer, K. S., Rawlings, C. A., et al.: Diagnostic peritoneal lavage before and after abdominal surgery in dogs. J. Am. Vet. Res., *44*(5):816, 1983.

Blass, C. E.: Surgery of extra hepatic biliary tree; Compendium on Continuing Education, 5(10):801, 1983.

Bojrab, M. J. (ed.): Current Techniques in Small Animal Surgery, 2nd ed. Philadelphia, Lea & Febiger, 1983.

Crane, S. W.: Exploratory celiotomy in diagnosis of gastrointestinal diseases: Vet. Clin. North Am., *13*(3):477, 1983.

Crowe, D. T.: Autotransfusion in the critically injured patient. J. Vet. Crit. Care, *4*:14, 1981.

Crowe, D. T.: Peritoneum and peritoneal cavity. *In* Slatter, D. H. (ed.): Textbook of Small Animal Surgery. Philadelphia, W. B. Saunders Company, 1985.

Crowe, D. T.: Diagnostic abdominal paracentesis techniques: clinical evaluation; 129 dogs and cats. J. Am. Anim. Hosp. Assoc., *20*(2):228, 1984.

Dillon, A. R., and Apano, J. S.: The acute abdomen. Vet. Clin. North Am., *13*(3):461, 1983.

Selcer, B. A.: Urinary tract trauma associated with pelvic trauma. J. Amer. Anim. Hosp. Assoc., *18*(5):785, 1982.

Stevenson, S., Chew, D., and Kociba, G.: Torsion of the splenic pedicle in a dog: a review. J. Am. Anim. Hosp. Assoc., *17*(2):239, 1981.

ALLERGIC REACTIONS

Allergic reactions that require emergency care may be divided into two main categories: anaphylactic shock and angioneurotic edema (urticaria).

ANAPHYLACTIC OR ANAPHYLACTOID SHOCK

This is an immediate type of hypersensitivity reaction in which death may occur rapidly owing to respiratory and circulatory collapse. In animals, anaphylactic shock rarely develops without the interference of man. An exception is the condition that results from the stings of bees or wasps.

The main signs are attributable to the effect of the activation of the complement system (especially C5a) with intensive vascular dilatation of smooth muscle. The release of additional chemical mediators, that is, histamine, slow-reacting substance (SRS), serotonin, heparin, acetylcholine, and bradykinin increases the severity of the problem. In dogs, the most common signs are restlessness, diarrhea, vomiting, circulatory collapse, epileptiform seizures, coma, and death.

Agents that may cause anaphylaxis are penicillin, streptomycin, tetracyclines, chloramphenicol, erythromycin, vancomycin, foreign serums (antitoxins), adrenocorticotropic hormone (ACTH), insulin, Pitocin, vaccines, penicillinase, procaine, benzocaine, tetracaine, lidocaine, salicylates, antihistamines, tranquilizers, iodinated contrast media, vitamins, heparin, stinging insects, food, and allergens (hypersensitization and skin testing).

Treatment

In severe cases, immediately administer an intravenous (IV) injection of 1:10,000 epinephrine hydrochloride (Adrenalin), 0.5 to 1.0 ml. If indicated, repeat in 20 to 30 minutes. Infiltrate subcutaneously (SQ) the entrance site of the allergen (insect bites) with 1:10,000 epinephrine, 0.3 ml.

1. Ensure a clear air passage, and administer oxygen by endotracheal tube or face mask if necessary.
2. Establish an IV line, and begin lactated Ringer's saline or D5W.
3. If the reaction is mild to moderate, give 0.2 to 0.5 ml of epinephrine SQ and another 0.2 to 0.5 ml by deep SQ injection elsewhere. One 0.5 ml dose may be repeated in 20 minutes if manifestations of anaphylaxis have not subsided.
4. Administer an IV injection of a rapidly acting steroid, such as hydrocortisone sodium succinate (Cortef sterile solution), 100 to 500 mg, or prednisolone sodium hemisuccinate, 50 to 200 mg. Repeat the injection in 3 to 4 hours, if necessary.
5. Give an IV injection of an antihistamine such as diphenhydramine hydrochloride (Benadryl), 1.0 to 2.0 mg per kg, slowly.
6. Hospitalize and observe the patient closely following the aforementioned procedures. If recovery occurs within 5 to 10 minutes following this intensive treatment, the prognosis is good.
7. In dogs with atopy, avoid the use of potential sensitizing drugs.

ANGIONEUROTIC EDEMA OR URTICARIA

Angioneurotic edema or urticaria is characterized by swelling of the soft tissues of the head, especially around the eyes, mouth, and ears. An ocular discharge may develop, and the animal frequently rubs its mouth and eyes on the ground or with its paws. This type of allergic reaction may develop within 20 minutes after contact with the inciting allergen and is very alarming to the owner, although it seldom causes serious damage to the animal.

Etiology

Food allergies, ingestion of spoiled protein material, blood transfusions, plasma transfusions, insect bites, and contact with certain chemicals are the primary causes.

Treatment

1. Try to ascertain the cause and remove the irritating substance if possible (laxatives and high colonic enemas are indicated in food allergies). Stop

blood or plasma transfusions. Wash the animal free of any known chemical residues. Pretreatment with antihistamines is a good idea prior to the administration of blood or plasma transfusions.

2. Administer high doses of rapidly acting steroids and antihistamines. Administer Adrenalin only if angioneurotic edema is very severe, that is, if swelling interferes with normal respirations.

3. Less serious allergic conditions may be manifested as gastroenteritis or skin problems. Acute hemorrhagic gastroenteritis may be associated with the ingestion of proteins such as horse meat, milk, or garbage. It is characterized by the sudden onset of acute vomiting, diarrhea, which may be bloody, anorexia, and depression. This condition usually responds well to symptomatic treatment. Skin allergies may present an emergency situation because of self-mutilation; however, they usually require a protracted course of diagnostic work-up and therapy once the emergency treatment has been instituted.

TREATMENT OF SKIN ALLERGIES

1. If possible, separate the animal from its allergen.
2. Sedate the animal with tranquilizers.
3. Clip and clean the area of the skin that has been traumatized.
4. Compresses using aluminum acetate (Burow's solution, Domboro tablets), in a 1:20 dilution or potassium permanganate, diluted 1:5,000, may be helpful in reducing inflammation.
5. Apply topical antibiotic–steroid preparations.
6. Administer steroids and antihistamines systemically with prednisolone, 2 mg per kg intramuscularly (IM) or IV, or diphenhydramine hydrochloride, 1.0 to 2.0 mg per kg IM or IV.
7. Control secondary infections by systemic administration of antibiotics.

BURNS

Causes

Most burns result from the patient's contact with hot water, grease, hot tar, or other liquids (scalds); from chewing wires (electrical burns, see p. 168); or from entrapment in burning buildings (smoke inhalation) or chemical exposure.

Severity

The most severe burns are those involving very young and very old subjects and those that involve the airway, head, perineum, oral cavity, eyes, and joints and result in the formation of scar tissue.

Prognosis

Burns causing extensive damage to less than 15 per cent of the body have a reasonable prognosis. Those in which 15 to 50 per cent of the body is involved cause severe complications and the prognosis is only fair to poor. Burns that involve more than 50 per cent of the body have a very poor prognosis; almost all patients in this group die within 2 weeks, and attendant suffering is great. Serious consideration should be given to prompt euthanasia without treatment unless there are compelling circumstances to the contrary.

Classification

Depth of Burn

Group I: Superficial. Group I burns involve the entire epidermis with variable damage to the dermis and accessory structures. The lesion is painful, and erythematous and vesicles *may* be present. The hair may be singed but still firmly attached. Healing is rapid after epithelial desquamation has occurred.

Group II: Partial Thickness. Loss of skin substance is greater than in Group I burns but less than in Group III burns. The lesion is painful, but the hair may be intact. Severe subcutaneous edema subsequently develops, followed by the appearance of a dry, tan crest. Healing occurs slowly after sloughing but without grafting.

Group III: Full Thickness. The entire skin is destroyed. The lesion is painless, hair falls out, and the eschar may be black or pearly white. Healing is slow unless grafting is performed. A full thickness burn is four times as serious as Group II lesions of similar size.

Group IV: Deep Full Thickness. The burn involves deep musculature and bone. The eshar is black, and charcoal-like tissues are evident. Loss of involved limbs is common, and amputation is a most realistic course. Débridement and rotational pedicle flaps are used for treatment of localized areas involving the trunk.

Extent of Burned Area

Use a metric ruler to measure the area of burned tissue.

$$\frac{\text{Area burned (sq cm)}}{\text{Total body area (sq cm)}} \times 100 = \text{Percentage of body burned}$$

Principles of Treatment

1. Make a rapid evaluation of the other body systems.
2. Elicit vital signs: note especially respiratory involvement (type of respirations, history of steam or smoke inhalations), degree of shock, and the length of time between the burn and treatment. Determine urine output and hematocrit, and examine for hemoglobinuria.
3. Decide the prognosis early; perform euthanasia if the case is hopeless.
4. For Group I burns:
   a. Use pain relievers such as morphine or oxymorphone p.r.n.

   b. Clip and cleanse the area gently (using saline and Betadine solution, 5 per cent).

   c. If the burn is recent, apply cold water or ice compresses for 20 minutes (ice compresses should be used on no more than 5 per cent of the burn area).

   d. Débride any obviously necrotic skin that may be present.

   e. Apply topical antimicrobial ointment such as silver sulfadiazine (sylvadine cream), Betadine ointment, or sulfamylon cream (if the burn area is small).

   f. Apply a topical burn dressing, and tape in place.

5. For Group II burns and less than 50 per cent involvement:

   a. Establish an adequate airway and ventilation. Give oxymorphone, 0.1 mg per kg IV via catheter, and intubate if necessary (see also p. 629).

   b. Treat for shock (see pp. 60–61).

   c. Administer pain relievers (morphine or oxymorphone) IV.

   d. Use the following formula to determine the volume of solution required:

$$\text{body weight (kg)} \times \text{percentage of body burned} = \text{volume (ml) of lactated Ringer's solution required in 24 hours.}$$

     Give 50 per cent of the solution during the first 8 hours, and 25 per cent during both the second and third 8-hour periods. Adequate rehydration should be based on maintenance of good blood pressure, color capillary refill time, and urine output (see p. 812). All oral fluids should be withheld for 48 hours. In severe burn cases, the use of plasma expanders or whole blood transfusions can be helpful in restoring plasma oncotic pressure, especially 2 to 3 days following initial treatment. Whole blood transfusions should be delayed for the first 24 hours following injury unless the patient shows signs of carbon monoxide poisoning.

   e. Cleanse the wound with cool saline compresses with 3 to 5 per cent Betadine solution, débride loose flesh, and remove any foreign material. Repeat daily.

   f. Apply antibiotic dressing such as silver sulfadiazine, 1 per cent cream, or gentamicin cream. Mafenide (Sulfamylon cream) is also an excellent product, although it may be irritating. Apply a topical burn dressing over the wound, and tape it in place. Keep the patient in an ambient temperature of 24° C (75° F) and on a soft clean blanket bedding. Provide adequate nutritional support during the convalescent period.

   g. Further management of extensive burn wounds involves the use of skin grafts to decrease healing time. Porcine heterografts have been used with success in dogs as a temporary dressing.

   h. The prevention of burn-wound sepsis is an important part of treating this type of wound. The use of systemic antibiotics is apparently not of much help in this regard; however, good nursing care and the use of sterile dressings, sterile instruments, masks, and gloves when changing dressings is essential.

6. For Group III burns treat as Group II burns except:
   a. If the burned area is extensive, explain to the owner that the prognosis is very poor and prolonged treatment and grafting are necessary.
   b. If a small area is involved, excision and suture or early surgical and enzymatic débridement may be helpful. Surgical excision of those portions of the eschar that are no longer adherent is performed without sharp dissection. Sulfamylon cream, 10 per cent, should be applied twice daily.
   c. If sepsis develops, begin IV antibiotics. The eschar should be removed daily (very painful), and wet dressing changes should be completed every 8 hours.
   d. Hydrotherapy daily in warm water containing Betadine solution is helpful. It stimulates healing, is gently cleansing, and accomplishes débridement. It also facilitates initial mobilization of the patient.

References and Additional Readings

McKeever, P. J.: Thermal injuries. *In* Kirk, R. W. (ed.): Current Veterinary Therapy 8: Small Animal Practice. Philadelphia, W. B. Saunders Company, 1983.

Schwartz, G. R., Safar, P., Stone, J. H., et al.: Principles and Practice of Emergency Medicine. Philadelphia, W. B. Saunders Company, 1978.

CARDIAC EMERGENCIES
by N. Joel Edwards*

Cardiac emergencies seldom allow the luxury of a well-pondered response. Irreversible brain damage usually occurs within 3 1/2 to 4 minutes following cardiac arrest. Consequently, being adequately prepared is the most important step in managing a cardiac emergency.

Preparation

1. Maintain an adequately stocked emergency cart or kit (see Tables 4 and 5 for contents).
2. Know how to intubate and begin respirations.
3. Know how to record an electrocardiogram (ECG) and be able to identify arrythmias.
4. Be familiar with drugs used, location of equipment.
5. Know how to administer external cardiac massage.
6. Develop a system of signaling hospital staff that an emergency exists.
7. Practice the team approach until each member of the team is confident.
8. Hold regular emergency "drills" to maintain competence.

---

*This section was contributed by N. Joel Edwards, D.V.M., Diplomate A.C.V.I.M., Adjunct Associate Professor of Small Animal Medicine, New York State College of Veterinary Medicine, Cornell University, Ithaca, New York, and Gary R. Bolton, D.V.M., deceased.

Table 4. DRUGS TO TREAT CARDIAC ARRHYTHMIAS IN THE CAT

Drug	Dosage and Route of Administration	Indications
Atropine sulfate, 0.4 mg/ml injectable	SC, IM, IV: 0.04 mg/kg BW every 4 to 6 hours	Sinus bradycardia, AV block
Calcium chloride*	IC, IV: 0.05 to 0.10 ml of 10% solution/kg BW	Ventricular asystole (to increase cardiac irritability), electrical-mechanical dissociation
Digoxin (Lanoxin), 0.125 mg tablets; 0.05 mg/ml elixer	Oral: 0.0055 mg/kg BW, BID; (e.g., ¼ of a 0.125 mg tablet twice daily for a 6-kg cat)	Congestive heart failure, APCs, atrial tachycardia, atrial fibrillation, atrial flutter
Epinephrine hydrochloride* (Adrenalin), 1:1000 solution; 1 mg/ml injectable	IC: 6 to 10 μg/kg BW IV: 0.05 to 0.1 mg of 1:10,000 dilution	Ventricular asystole, changing fine ventricular fibrillation to coarse fibrillation
Isoproterenol (Isuprel), 0.2 mg/ml injectable	IV: 0.5 mg/250 ml of D5W and titrate to effect	Sinus bradycardia, complete AV block
Potassium chloride*	IC: 0.25 to 0.75 mEq followed by calcium chloride	Depolarization of the heart, chemical defibrillator
Propranolol (Inderal), 10 mg tablets; 1 mg/ml injectable	Oral: 2.5 mg every 8 to 12 hours for average 5-kg cat; higher doses to effect IV: 0.25 mg diluted in 1 ml of saline, given as 0.2 ml boluses to effect	Sinus tachycardia, supraventricular tachycardia, and ventricular arrhythmias, preexcitation arrhythmias, and with digoxin for atrial fibrillation.

*Drugs for cardiac arrest.
Code: IV—intravenous; IM—intramuscular; SC—subcutaneous; IC—intracardiac.
Modified from Tilley, L. P.: Essentials of Canine and Feline Electrocardiography. St. Louis, The C. V. Mosby Co., 1979, p. 214.

Table 5. CARDIOVASCULAR EMERGENCY TRAY

1. *Levarterenol bitartrate (norepinephrine)* (Levophed)
   Winthrop Laboratories (Division of Sterling Drugs Inc.)—2 mg/ml in ampules.
   Give in an IV drip to effect. Dilute 1 to 2 ml in 250 ml of drip. Used as a potent
   vasopressor to increase blood pressure. Does have some chronotropic and inotropic
   effects on the heart.

2. *Epinephrine HCl*—1:10,000
   Give 1 to 5 ml intracardially (IC). Used primarily in an attempt to convert cardiac
   standstill to either ventricular fibrillation or a normal heart beat. Epinephrine
   causes coarse ventricular fibrillation, which can be more successfully converted to
   sinus rhythm by direct current electric shock. Fine fibrillations may be converted
   to coarse fibrillations by the IC administration of epinephrine.

3. *Isoproterenol* (Isuprel)
   Winthrop Laboratories (Division of Sterling Drugs Inc.)—1 and 5-ml ampules, 0.2
   mg/ml. Give IV in a drip. Dilute 1 mg in 250 ml of solution, and give as needed to
   maintain heart rate between 80 and 140 beats per minute. Isoproterenol is used for
   its positive inotropic and chronotropic effects. It also causes peripheral vasodilatation.

4. *Phenylephrine HCl* (Neo-Synephrine)
   Winthrop Laboratories (Division of Sterling Drugs Inc.)—1-ml ampules, 2 mg/ml.
   Give 0.15 mg/kg IV. Phenylephrine is used to raise blood pressure because of its
   potent vasopressure action. It has no direct effect on the heart.

5. *Doxapram HCl* (Dopram)
   A. H. Robins Company, Inc.—20 mg/ml. Give 1.0 mg/kg IV as a potent analeptic
   to reverse respiratory depression. May need to be repeated frequently. (Can use
   up to 5 to 10 mg/kg IV in barbiturate intoxication.)

6. *Atropine sulfate*—60.5 mg/ml
   Give 0.05 mg/kg of body weight IV to block vagal reflexes and prevent severe
   bradycardias.

7. a. *Calcium gluconate*—10% solution
      Give 5 to 10 ml IV or IC.
   b. *Calcium chloride*—10% solution
      Give 1 to 2 ml IV or IC.
   Calcium solutions strengthen myocardial contraction. They also increase myocardial
   excitability, which may be helpful during cardiac arrest.

Table continued on opposite page

Table 5. CARDIOVASCULAR EMERGENCY TRAY *(Continued)*

8. *Lidocaine HCl* (Xylocaine)—WITHOUT EPINEPHRINE!
   Astra Pharmaceutical—20 mg/ml. Give 1 mg/kg IV bolus and follow with a 30 to 50 μg/kg/minute IV drip if needed. Xylocaine is used as an antiarrhythmic drug to control ventricular arrhythmias. It may be used if ventricular fibrillation tends to recur.

9. *Procainamide HCl* (Pronestyl)
   Squibb—100 or 500 mg/ml. Give 100 mg IV bolus, followed by 10 to 40 μg/kg/minute IV drip. Useful for rapid conversion of ventricular tachycardia.

10. *Ouabain*—0.25 mg/ml
    Eli Lilly—Initial dose is 25% of calculated total dose, given IV. Total dose is 0.04 mg/kg. Repeat in 30 minutes if necessary. Digitalis strengthens myocardial contraction, increases cardiac output, and thus controls congestive heart failure. It controls supraventricular tachycardias by delaying conduction through atrioventricular node and by vagal effects on the sinoatrial node.

11. *Sodium bicarbonate*
    Abbott Laboratories—44.6 mEq/50 ml. Given in an IV drip. Dilute 7.5 mEq in 250 ml of drip. May give 10 to 20 mEq IC. The administration of sodium bicarbonate helps alleviate acidosis during cardiac arrest.

12. *Aminophylline*
    Searle—250 mg/ml, ampules of 2 ml. Give 4 to 8 mg/kg IV—must be diluted in 20 ml of D5W and given slowly. Aminophylline causes bronchodilation for effective exchange of gases, and it has a myocardial stimulatory effect.

13. *Dopamine HCl* (Intropin)
    Arnar-Stone—200 mg/5 ml; give 2 to 8 μg/kg/min IV drip. Dilute 40 mg in 500 ml lactated Ringer's solution; give 1 drop/kg/min or to effect. Has positive inotropic effects, minimal effect on heart rate or peripheral vascular resistance. Preserves renal blood flow.

14. *Dobutamine HCl* (Dobutrex)
    Eli Lilly—250 mg/vial. Add 250 mg (1 vial) to 1,000 ml of D5W—Inferior rate 1 drop/kg/min (2.5 μg/kg/min).

Modified from Bolton, G.: Cardiovascular emergencies. Vet. Clin. North Am., 2:414, 1972.

The Response
1. Recognize that an emergency exists.
2. Identify the type of emergency.
3. Begin your response.
4. Signal for help.

Reliable Signs of Cardiopulmonary Emergencies
1. Absence of heart sounds or pulse
2. Absence of respirations
3. Cyanosis of mucous membranes
4. Dilated or fixed pupils

Premonitory Signs of an Impending Cardiopulmonary Emergency
1. Darkening of venous blood
2. Increased rate and shallowness of respirations
3. Pulse irregularities and/or marked changes in blood pressure
4. Coldness of the extremities and skin
5. ECG abnormalities such as S-T segment and/or T-wave changes, marked increase or decrease in heart rate, and the appearance of ventricular arrhythmias

Response Protocol — "A B C D E"
This should be an automatic response by the emergency team.

1. "A" — Establish an airway
2. "B" — Breathe: positive pressure respiration
            Begin ECG evaluation
3. "C" — Cardiac massage: external, internal
4. "D" — Drug therapy, fluids, bicarbonate, defibrillation
5. "E" — Evaluate status, monitor, ECG, CVP, maintenance therapy

Remember two very important points:
1. Don't panic.
2. In an emergency, the first pulse to take is your own.

Management

Time is of the essence! Classification of the type of emergency is critical.

CARDIAC ARREST (Fig. 1)

1. Verify the arrest.
   a. Check carotid or femoral pulse.
   b. Listen for heart sounds.
2. Establish an airway and breath.
   a. 20 to 40 breaths per minute.
   b. 1:1 inspiratory/expiratory time
   c. 20 to 25 cm H_2O inspiration pressures
3. External cardiac massage.

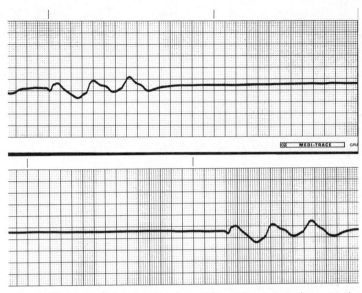

Figure 1. Cardiac arrest may be seen as a straight even line or (as in this case) with some evidence of bizarre electrical activity that does not generate mechanical contraction.

    a. 60 per minute, compress for a count of 2, release for a count of 1. "Compress one thousand, two one thousand, release one thousand."
    b. Check for adequate femoral pulse.
    c. Round-chested dogs in dorsal recumbency, narrow-chested dogs in lateral recumbency
4. Check rhythm with ECG.
    a. Asystole
       1. Inject 0.1 to 2.0 ml 1:10,000 epinephrine intracardially (IC).
       2. Continue massage.
       3. Start rapid IV drip of lactated Ringers' solution with 15 mEq $NaHCO_3$ per 500 ml fluid.
       4. If still no heartbeat, inject 1 ml per 10 kg of 10 per cent calcium chloride or gluconate IC.
       5. If still cardiac arrest, continue massage plus 10 mEq $NaHCO_3$ IC and repeat epinephrine and calcium.
       6. If unable to establish a pulse or ventricular fibrillation within 2 minutes, open the chest at the left sixth intercostal space and begin cardiac massage. Do not incise phrenic nerve.
          a. Cup heart in hand and compress and release 70 to 90 times per minute allowing for ventricular filling each time. Digital occlusion of the descending aorta will improve cerebral perfusion.

7. If mechanical systole returns but the heart rate is below normal, begin IV isoproterenol 1 mg (5 ml) in 500 ml of D5W at a rate of 0.01 μg per kg per minute, approximately 1 drop per kg per minute using a standard microdrip infusion system. Adjust the drip to maintain heart rate between 80 and 140 beats per minute.
8. If mechanical systole returns and the heart rate is normal, administer dobutamine HCL at a rate of 2.5 μg per kg per minute IV by adding 250 mg (1 vial) to 1,000 ml of D5W at an infusion rate of approximately 1 drop per kg per minute using a standard microdrip infusion system.

VENTRICULAR FIBRILLATION (Either initially or following asystole; Fig. 2)

1. Initiate or continue cardiac massage.
2. Defibrillate.
   a. DC defibrillator; if unsuccessful double the energy dose; if still unsuccessful repeat epinephrine and NaHCO₃ and repeat defibrillation. Be sure to use adequate amounts of electrode paste on the skin. **DO NOT USE ALCOHOL,** because it is flammable. If using internal defibrillation, moisten heart with saline.

DC Defibrillation	<7 kg	7–40 kg	>40 kg
External	2 watt–sec/kg	5 watt–sec/kg	5–10 watt–sec/kg
Internal	0.2 watt–sec/kg	0.3 watt–sec/kg	0.4 watt–sec/kg

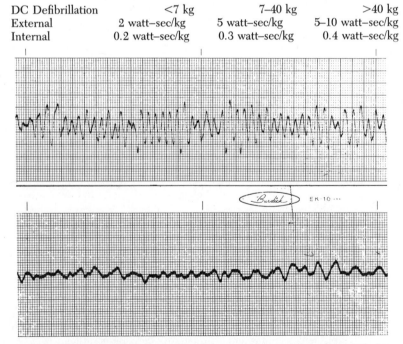

Figure 2. Ventricular fibrillation may be coarse as in the upper tracing or fine as in the lower tracing. Patients with coarse ventricular fibrillation are easier to defibrillate.

b. Chemical defibrillation—mix potassium chloride at 1 mEq per kg with acetycholine at 6 mg per kg, and inject IC, or give potassium chloride at 1 mEq per kg followed by 2 ml of calcium chloride or 8 ml calcium gulconate IC.

HEARTBEAT FOLLOWING RESUSCITATIVE EFFORTS

1. Verify rhythm.
2. Continue respirations.
3. Continue IV fluids with 10 to 20 mEq $NaHCO_3$.
4. Administer dobutamine HCL 2.5 μg per kg per minute IV.
   Continue administration of dobutamine HCL, isoproterenol, or dopamine HCL (inactivated by $NaHCO_3$) until the patient is stable, then gradually withdraw inotropic support.
5. Administer heparin, 100 U per kg IV every 2 to 4 hours.

Frequently, hearts that have undergone cardiac massage will show ectopic activity, but this is usually self-limiting and therapy is generally not needed.

Other Cardiac Arrhythmias Requiring Emergency Treatment

VENTRICULAR ECTOPIC ARRHYTHMIAS

Ventricular arrhythmias (ventricular premature beats, ventricular tachycardia) occur and cause clinical signs relatively frequently in dogs. They signify that the animal has myocarditis or myocardial degeneration. Myocarditis is usually a sequela of some other disease process. It has been associated with most bacterial, viral, mycotic, and protozoan infections. In addition, myocarditis may occur with toxemias caused by such disease conditions as pyometra, uremia, pancreatitis, intestinal foreign bodies, and poisoning, or it may be secondary to advanced congestive heart failure. Tumors at the base of the heart, hemangiosarcomas, lymphosarcomas, and other tumors that invade the myocardium can cause myocarditis. It may be secondary to severe chest trauma with myocardial bruising, or it may be caused by digitalis overdose. Myocarditis has been associated with chronic mitral valvular fibrosis, congenital aortic stenosis, and idiopathic cardiomyopathy. Autoimmune diseases, hypothyroidism, hyperthyroidism, and excessive catecholamine release may also cause myocardial disease. Electrolyte disorders such as hyper- or hypokalemia may lead to ectopic ventricular arrhythmias.

Occasionally, an animal may present with severe myocarditis of no known origin. This animal is then referred to as having primary or idiopathic myocarditis. A thorough evaluation of the entire patient should be made. Similarly, auscultation of the heart for arrhythmias should be performed on any animal that has a severe disease or that presents with unexplained weakness, fatigue, or collapse.

Clinical signs can range from weakness and fatigue to collapse and sudden death, depending on the severity of the arrhythmias. The diagnosis is made by auscultating an arrhythmia and/or detecting a femoral pulse deficit. The ECG is used in diagnosing the type of arrhythmia present (Fig. 3). Because treatment is critical, it is essential to do an ECG to determine the type of arrhythmia.

Treatment

The urgency of the treatment depends on the status of the patient.
1. Emergency: The patient is weak, collapsed, or comatose with ventricular tachycardia or frequent ventricular premature beats. Treatment should consist of:
    a. Lidocaine (without epinephrine) given IV 1 mg per kg bolus, followed by a steady IV drip of 30 to 50 μg per kg per minute—1 mg per kg bolus may be repeated every 20 minutes, up to a total of 8 mg per kg (not to cats).
    b. Procainamide given slowly IV, 100 mg bolus, followed by a steady IV drip of 10 to 40 μg per kg per minute.
    c. Begin oral maintenance therapy when possible:
        1. Quinidine sulfate tablets, 200-mg tablets, 8 to 20 mg per kg orally every 6 to 8 hours.
        2. Quinidine polygalacturonate (Cardioquin, Purdue-Frederick), 8 to 20 mg per kg orally every 8 to 12 hours.

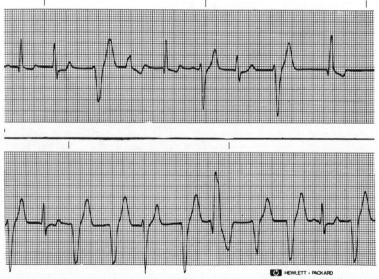

Figure 3. Four or more ventricular premature complexes (VPCs) in succession constitute ventricular tachycardia. Multifocal VPCs are more serious than those that are unifocal.

3. Quinidine gluconate (Quinaglute, Cooper), 8 to 20 mg per kg orally every 8 to 12 hours.
   d. Propranolol is the drug of choice in cats with arrhythmias (see Table 4, p. 37 for dosage).
2. Urgent, but oral therapy is adequate: Patient is showing moderate weakness or fatigue with ventricular premature complexes.
   a. Begin quinidine, procainamide, or disopyramide orally. Monitor ECG at hourly intervals.
   b. A summary of these drugs follows:

Quinidine
1. Preparations
   Quinidine sulfate—200-mg tablets
   Cardioquin (Purdue-Frederick)—275-mg tablets
   Quinaglute (Cooper)—324-mg tablets
   Quinidine gluconate (Lilly)—80 mg per ml injection
2. Dose
   All forms—8 to 20 mg per kg
   Oral
      Quinidine sulfate—TID or QID
      Cardioquin, Quinaglute—BID or TID
   Injectable
      Quinidine gluconate—IM, given TID
3. Toxicity
   Vomiting, diarrhea
   Depression
   Seizures (rare)
   Prolonged QRS duration greater than 25 per cent of normal

Procainamide
1. Preparations
   Pronestyl (Squibb)—250-, 375-, and 500-mg tablets or capsules, 100, 500 mg per ml injection
   Procan SR (Parke-Davis)—250- and 500-mg tablets
2. Dose
   Oral—10 to 12 mg per kg
      Pronestyl—QID
      Procan SR—TID
   IM—10 to 12 mg per kg
      IV bolus—1 to 5 mg/kg every 5 minutes until effect or until toxicity
      Steady-state IV drip—10 to 40 μg per kg per minute
3. Toxicity same as quinidine

Propranolol
1. Preparations
   Inderal (Ayerst)—10-, 40-, and 80-mg tablets, 1 mg per ml injection
2. Dose
   Oral—dog, 0.2 to 1.0 mg/kg TID; cat, 2.5 to 5 mg TID
   IV— (use caution) give slowly 0.04 to 0.06 mg/kg until effect or toxicity
3. Toxicity: bradycardia, hypotension, bronchoconstriction, congestive heart failure

Diphenylhydantoin
1. Preparations
   Dilantin (Parke-Davis)—30-, and 100-mg capsules, 125 mg per ml suspension
2. Dose
   Oral—8 to 15 mg per kg TID
   IV (use caution)—50 to 100 mg over a 5-minute period (maximum total dose 24 mg per kg)
3. Toxicity
   Oral—none
   IV—sinus bradycardia, ventricular arrest, and fibrillation

Disopyramide
1. Preparations
   Norpace (Searle)—100- and 150-mg capsules
2. Dose
   6 to 15 mg per kg TID
3. Toxicity (Same as quinidine, but better tolerated)

Lidocaine (without epinephrine)
1. Preparations
   Xylocaine (Astra)—2 per cent (20 mg/ml)
   Xylocaine IM (Astra)— 10 per cent (100 mg/ml)
2. Dose
   IM—2.5 mg per kg every 2 hours as needed
   IV bolus—1 mg per kg every 10 to 15 minutes up to a total of 8 mg per kg
   Rapid IV infusion—use 500 ml of D5W, add 50 ml of 2 per cent lidocaine. Give rapidly by IV drip until conversion or toxicity. Use drip as needed to control the arrhythmia.
   Steady-state IV infusion—30 to 50 μg per kg per minute
3. Restlessness, trembling, excitement
   Seizures (controlled with Valium)

3. Patient is asymptomatic, has few or many ventricular premature beats, and may have ventricular tachycardia.
   a. Any ventricular arrhythmia must be regarded as potentially dangerous if it occurs frequently (pairs, runs, paroxysms) or is multifocal.
   b. Oral therapy with long-acting quinidine, procainamide, or disopyramide is adequate.

A paradoxical situation sometimes occurs and may cause a therapeutic dilemma. On the one hand, severe congestive heart failure may cause hypoxic myocarditis; on the other hand, a dog with severe myocarditis may first have ventricular tachycardia, and then may develop congestive heart failure secondary to the tachycardia. Thus, in a dog that has both congestive heart failure and a severe ventricular arrhythmia, it may be difficult to determine which of the two problems came first. If congestive heart failure is primary, therapy with one of the digitalis glycosides will generally improve the arrhythmia. However, if the myocarditis is primary, digitalis glycosides are apt to increase myocardial irritability and increase the frequency and severity of ventricular arrhythmias. *Correct treatment is essential.*

There are several signs that are helpful in making the correct diagnosis. First, most dogs with severe myocarditis collapse or die suddenly without developing congestive heart failure. Therefore, if heart failure is present, the probability is that the heart failure came first. Secondly, treatment can be used as a diagnosis. Give furosemide (Lasix), 2 mg per kg IV, IM, or SC. Give aminophylline, 4 to 8 mg per kg. Dilute aminophylline in 20 ml of D5W, and give slowly IV. Administer 1 mg per kg of morphine SC (dogs only). Place the animal in an oxygen cage.

As the treatment alleviates the heart failure and oxygenation improves, the arrhythmia should be resolved. If there is no improvement in 30 minutes, antiarrhythmic therapy using lidocaine, quinidine, procainamide, or disopyramide may be needed.

Supraventricular Tachycardia (Fig. 4)

This type of arrhythmia is usually associated with primary atrial myocarditis or toxicities or toxemias. Occasionally, invasive processes may cause tachycardia of supraventricular origin.

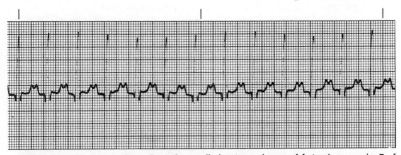

Figure 4. Supraventricular tachycardia usually has some degree of fusing between the T of the previous complex and the P of each succeeding complex, often forming an M-shaped configuration between R waves. The heart rate here is approximately 240 beats per minute. Note the very regular R-R interval.

Therapy consists of:
1. Eliminate toxicity or toxemia.
2. Reduce the rapid ventricular response.
    a. Occular or carotid massage
    b. Digoxin, 0.011 mg per kg BID
    c. Propranalol, 0.04 to 0.06 mg/kg slowly IV or .20 to 1.0 mg/kg orally TID.
    d. Verapamil, 0.1 to 0.3 mg per kg IV slowly, not to exceed 5 mg total dose. Maintain with oral dose of 1 to 3 per kg TID or QID
    e. Edrophonium, 0.11 to 0.22 mg per kg IV (dogs only)

ATRIOVENTRICULAR HEART BLOCK

Complete third-degree heart block occurs uncommonly and causes excessively slow heart rates. At rates below 60 beats per minute, an animal may show clinical signs ranging from weakness and fatigue to collapse and sudden death. Generally, the animal does well at rest but may experience symptoms while attempting to move about. This is because the animal cannot increase its heart rate, usually above 60 beats per minute, to meet the increased demands on cardiac output. Heart rates may go as low as 15 to 20 per minute.

Complete heart block may be caused by digitalis toxicity, hyperkalemia, myocarditis, AV nodal fibrosis, neoplastic invasion of the AV node, and, occasionally, by excessive vagal tone. Often the precise cause cannot be identified. The diagnosis is made by auscultating the bradycardia and recording an ECG (Fig. 5).

Treatment

1. Hospitalize the animal and keep at cage rest.
2. Try atropine first to rule out vagal causes. Give 0.5 mg per kg IV. This is usually unsuccessful.
3. Isoproterenol (Isuprel, Winthrop; Proternol tablets, Key).
    a. Isuprel injection (0.2 mg/ml), 0.1 to 0.2 mg SC every 6 hours. Monitor for ventricular tachycardia.

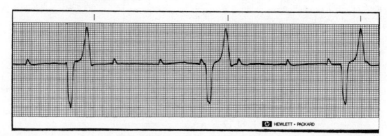

Figure 5. Third-degree atrioventricular heart block. Seven P waves and 3 ventricular depolarizations are seen. There is no correlation between them. The heart rate here is approximately 40 beats per minute.

b. Proternol tablets (10 or 30 mg), 15 to 30 mg orally every 4 to 6 hours.

Usually, medical therapy is not effective, because oral absorption is poor. The isoproterenol may at least increase the heart rate to over 70 beats per minute so that the dog can have moderate exercise without symptoms.

The treatment of choice for complete heart block is the installation of a cardiac pacemaker. One of the most readily available pacemakers is the ventricular–inhibited pulse generator VVI model No. 5995 Medtronic with sutureless epicardial lead.* Temporary transvenous pacing via the jugular to the right ventricle is advised both to ascertain the beneficial effects of pacing and to regulate heart rate during the anesthesia and surgical implantation procedure for permanent pacemaker therapy.

If digitalis is the cause of arrhythmia, withdraw the digitalis completely until the arrhythmia ceases. If the heart rate is excessively slow or if the symptoms are severe, the treatment just outlined may be needed while digitalis levels recede. When the arrhythmia abates, resume the digitalis at a lower dosage.

ATRIAL STANDSTILL

This arrhythmia occurs with hyperkalemia or SA nodal dysfunction, as in the persistent silent atrial syndrome. Hyperkalemia in the dog is usually due to adrenal insufficiency or severe uremia. In the cat, urethral obstruction is the most common cause of hyperkalemia. The excessive serum potassium causes very slow heart rates and thus accounts for symptoms of weakness' fatigue, collapse, or death. The arrhythmia may be overlooked if the heart is not auscultated. The diagnosis is made by auscultating a bradycardia and recording an ECG (Figs. 6 and 7). Other arrhythmias, such as complete heart block or ventricular tachycardia, may occur with hyperkalemia.

Treatment. Treatment may be instituted even before a final diagnosis of the primary disease is made.

1. Correct the underlying disease when possible. Relieve urethral obstruction in the cat.

---

*Medtronic, Inc., Minneapolis, Minnesota 55455

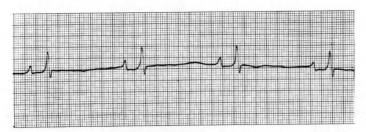

Figure 6. Atrial standstill. A slow heart rate (60 to 70 beats per minute) and a steady, quiet baseline with no P waves. The ECG is from a six-year-old standard poodle suffering from adrenal insufficiency. The serum potassium was 8.5 mg per 100 ml.

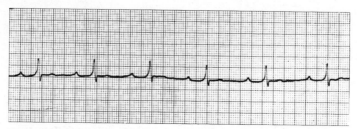

Figure 7. ECG friom poodle in Figure 6 following therapy for acute adrenocortical insufficiency. Treatment consisted of hydrocortisone, 100 mg intravenously; DOCA acetate, 2 mg intramuscularly; sodium chloride with 5 per cent dextrose fluids intravenously; and 10 units of regular insulin subcutaneously.

2. Begin rapid IV drip of 5 per cent dextrose in saline.
3. Give 1 mEq per kg $NaHCO_3$ IV immediately; add 3 mEq per kg to the drip. If blood gas capabilities are available, the following formula can be used to estimate bicarbonate replacement:

$$HCO_3 \text{ replacement (mEq)} = \text{body weight (kg)} \times (25\text{-plasma bicarbonate [mEq/L])} \times 0.3.$$

Bring serum bicarbonate levels less than 15 mEq per L back to 15 mEq per L immediately, and correct the remainder of the calculated deficit over 6 to 12 hours. Without blood gas measurements, use as a rule of thumb: mild, moderate, and severe acidotic states with base deficits of 5, 10, and 15, require replacement with 3, 6, or 9 mEq of bicarbonate per kg of body weight.
4. Give 100 mg hydrocortisone IV and another 100 mg in the IV drip.
5. Give DOCA IM, 1 mg per 12 kg of body weight.
6. If the animal is in serious condition and the arrhythmias are severe, give 1 to 10 ml of 20 per cent calcium gluconate slowly by IV to effect (4 mg/kg). Monitor with ECG. The effect of calcium gluconate is transient. The drug should be administered over a 10-minute period. If bradycardia occurs, the drug should be discontinued.
7. Regular insulin has been used when the animal's condition is severe. Give 0.25 units of regular insulin per lb of body weight with 2 gm dextrose per unit of insulin. The glucose (50 per cent glucose—each ml, contains 0.5 gm of glucose) can be added to 0.9 per cent saline. Mix insulin in the drip or give it SC. More prolonged control of potassium is provided by cation exchange resin. Kayexelate, 0.2 gm per kg orally in three divided doses, in combination with 5 to 10 ml of 70 per cent sorbitol. One gm of resin exchanges 1 mEq of Na for 1 mEq of K. Kayexelate can be given by enema 32–50 gm per 100 ml water repeated every 6 hours.

Regardless of the cause of the hyperkalemia, the treatment just described will improve the situation, usually within 15 to 30 minutes. The hydrocortisone is repeated every 2 to 4 hours; the DOCA is given once a day. The fluids establish renal function or elimination of potassium from the body. The treatment of the primary disease must, of course, be continued beyond these emergency procedures.

VENTRICULAR FIBRILLATION IN THE CAT

Cardiac arrest due to ventricular fibrillation is less complicated to treat in the cat than in the dog. The patient will usually respond to cardiac massage for 5 to 10 minutes and to being well ventilated. Propranolol is the drug of choice if needed (see p. 37).

Acute Congestive Heart Failure

Acute congestive heart failure occurs when the patient no longer has cardiac reserves and the heart, failing to maintain adequate blood flow, cannot meet the requirements of the body for oxygen. The clinical manifestations are influenced by the nature of the etiologic defect and by its effects upon circulatory dynamics and may show great variation from animal to animal. Signs that usually remain constant are dyspnea, tachycardia, cardiomegaly, circulatory collapse, pulmonary edema, cyanosis, ascites, hepatomegaly, decrease in systolic blood pressure, and collapse, leading ultimately to death.

Fortunately, chronic congestive heart failure is much more common than acute failure in small animals. The following are instances when acute congestive failure develops:

1. Dogs that develop congestive heart failure because of mitral insufficiency may do well for long periods of time on treatment and then have flare-ups of acute congestive heart failure. These flare-ups almost always occur at night during sleeping hours and require emergency therapy.
2. Rupture of chordae tendineae can result in an acute onset of congestive heart failure either in a previously symptomatic or asymptomatic patient.
3. Canine idiopathic cardiomyopathy (congestive-dilated) frequently presents as an apparent acute onset of congestive heart failure, presumably associated with the onset of atrial fibrillation.
4. Puppies that chew electric cords and receive a shock may have acute congestive heart failure.
5. Cats with cardiomyopathy tend to develop acute congestive heart failure during times of stress. Often the stress is due to arterial embolization, another feature of the cardiomyopathy complex.

The animal with acute congestive heart failure has severe dyspnea. It may sit on its haunches and support its weight on its forelegs. Its head is extended as it breathes, and pulmonary edema fluid may bubble out of its mouth and nose. Hemoptysis is often present. Its eyes are glazed, and it does not notice the activity around it. Its breathing sounds are rattling and bubbling, and moist rales can be auscultated. The heart rate is usually very rapid, and murmurs or gallop rhythms may or may not be auscultated. The animal with acute congestive heart failure cannot move, nor can it tolerate being moved or restrained. It cannot eat or drink; all its energies are being consumed in breathing enough air to stay alive.

Treatment

Any unnecessary stress (such as attempts at oral medication, restraint for radiography, electrocardiography, or blood sample collection) may lead to irreversible respiratory and cardiac arrest. Upon admission to the hospital, the dog or cat in acute congestive heart failure should be placed in an oxygen unit. No additional stress should be placed on the animal. Medical therapy should include:

1. Aminophylline, 4 to 8 mg per kg, which must be diluted with 20 ml of D5W and given slowly IV, or if available in oil, given as an IM injection.
2. Furosemide (Lasix), 2 to 4 mg per kg IM.
3. Morphine, 1.0 mg per kg SC (dogs only).

Place the animal in an oxygen cage. If the animal is going to survive, it will show improvement within 30 minutes to an hour. The aminophylline and furosemide may be repeated in 2 hours. If the dog continues to fail despite therapy, institution of IV dobutamine HCL therapy at a rate of 2.5 μg per kg per minute to effect may be helpful in improving cardiac output by increasing contractility and, to a lesser extent, heart rate. *Dobutamine must be diluted prior to use.* An initial infusion of 250 mg (1 vial in 1,000 ml of D5W delivered at a rate of 1 drop per kg per minute using a standard microdrip infusion system is usually effective. Newer inotropic agents may be available in the near future for use in these patients.

$$\mu g/kg/min \times kg = \mu g/min$$
$$\mu g/min - \mu g/ml = ml/min$$

Digitalization for the dog may be accomplished IM or IV (see Table 6). In the IM approach, inject digoxin (0.01 mg/kg) every 6 to 12 hours until effect or toxicity (vomiting; diarrhea, arrhythmias). The maximum total dose is 0.04 to 0.06 mg per kg. The maintenance dose is one fourth of the total amount that produced effect or toxicity, given s.i.d.

IV administration of Ouabain (Lilly) should not be used without an ECG. Inject 0.01 mg per kg IV every 30 minutes to effect or toxicity (arrhythmias). The maximum total dose is 0.02 to 0.04 mg per kg. The maintenance dose is one fourth of the total amount that produced effect or toxicity. Give every 3 hours, or switch to digoxin IM. *Note:* Ouabain is not recommended for use in cats.

To administer digoxin intravenously, give 0.01 mg per kg IV every hour until effect or toxicity. The maximum dose is 0.04 to .06 mg per kg. The maintenance dose is one fourth of the amount that produced effect or toxicity. (These dosages of digoxin do not apply to cats.) See Table 4, p. 37.

When possible, switch the dog to oral maintenance therapy with digoxin.

Table 6. RAPID DIGITALIZATION FOR THE DOG—PARENTERAL FORMS

Therapeutic Indices	Ouabain Injection U.S.P.	Digoxin Injection U.S.P.
Size of vial	0.5 mg/2 ml	0.5 mg/2 ml
Method of administration	IV only	IV or IM (IM causes local pain; if used, preferred site is lumbar muscles)
Total dose	0.02–0.04 mg/kg*	0.04–0.06 mg/kg*
Division of dosage	25 to 50% initially, then 25% every 30 min until intoxication or desired effect is reached	25 to 50% initially, then 25% every hour (IV) or 6 to 12 hr. (IM) until intoxication or desired effect is reached
Time for administration to onset of effect	3 to 10 min†‡	5 to 30 min† 10 to 30 min‡
Time from administration to maximum effect	30 min to 2 hr† 30 min‡	1½ to 5 hr† 1 to 2 hr‡
Maximum duration of intoxication	2 to 6 hr‡	12 to 36 hr‡
Maintenance therapy required	Longer-acting glycosides required immediately after treatment to maintain the effect	25% of total dose required for digitalization is given once daily to maintain the effect.

*Detweiler, 1965.
†Moe and Farah, 1965.
‡Rubin, Gross, and Arbeit, 1968.
Adapted from Ettinger, S. J., and Suter, P. F.: Canine Cardiology. Philadelphia, W. B. Saunders Company, 1970, p. 236.

Oral maintenance is 0.011 mg per kg per q12h. The oral maintenance dose for cats is 0.0055 mg per kg q12h.

Adjunctive Therapy

Venoclysis. Bleeding the animal may help by reducing blood volume and venous return. One may safely remove about 5 to 8 ml of blood per kg of body weight. It is best to monitor central venous pressure during this procedure, provided that the procedure is not too stressful to the patient (see p. 564).

Rotating Tourniquets. Placing a tourniquet on two of the legs effectively reduces blood volume by the amount that is in the legs. These tourniquets should be rotated every 20 minutes.

Paracentesis (either thorax or abdomen). Remove as much fluid as possible provided the patient can tolerate the manipulation necessary for this procedure.

Vasodilators. Vasodilators improve overall pump function by (a) decreasing afterload—resistance to forward flow of blood through the arterial system; (b) decreasing preload—the amount of blood returned to the heart and hence the amount needed to be pumped; and (c) decreasing both afterload and preload. With mitral insufficiency, these drugs reduce the volume of blood being pumped from the left ventricle to the left atrium during systole (regurgitant fraction).

Currently Reliable Vasodilators for Use in Acute Congestive Heart Failure
Hydralazine (Apresoline, Ciba Pharmaceutical Co.)
1. Oral dose
    Dog—0.5 to 3 mg per kg q12h
    Cat—2.5 mg per cat q12h
    IV dose
    Dog—0.15 to 0.2 mg per kg q6h. Blood pressure and heart rate must be monitored, and drug must be given over 30-minute IV infusion time.
2. Titration protocol*
    a. Obtain baseline chest radiograph, venous oxygen tension or capillary refill time, and systemic arterial blood pressure, if available.
    b. If the venous oxygen tension is less than 30 mm Hg or the capillary refill time is greater than 2 seconds and the mean blood pressure is greater than 80 mm Hg, administer 1 mg per kg of hydralazine orally.
    c. Repeat blood pressure measurement in 1 hour, venous oxygen tension measurement in 2 to 3 hours, or capillary refill time in 3 to 5 hours.
    d. If the mean blood pressure is 70 to 80 mm Hg and/or the venous oxygen tension is less than 30 mm Hg or the capillary refill time is less than 1 second, do not administer any more drug. Repeat this dosage every 12 hours.
    e. If an adequate response is not seen, administer another 1 mg per kg dose and repeat c. If the criteria in d. are still not met, give another 1 mg per kg dose.

---

*From Kittleson, M: Concepts and therapeutic strategies in the management of heart failure. *In* Kirk, R. W. (ed.): Current Veterinary Therapy 8: Small Animal Practice. Philadelphia, W. B. Saunders Company, 1983.

f. Do not exceed 3 mg per kg.

3. Complications

Tachycardia, hypotension, anorexia, vomiting exacerbation of arrhythmias

4. Action

Predominately an arterial vasodilator

Prazosin (Minipress; Pfizer Laboratories)

1. Oral dose

1 to 5 mg per dog q8h

Not recommended for cats

2. Titration

Initial dose of 1 mg per dog q8h, with subsequent increase if needed

3. Complications

Tachycardia, hypotension, tachyphylaxis, gastrointestinal disturbances

4. Action

Both arterial and venous dilator

Captopril (Capoten; E. R. Squibb and Sons, Inc.)

1. Oral dose

Dog—0.5 to 2.0 mg per kg q8h

Cat—0.5 to 1.0 mg per kg q8h

2. Titration

Begin at low end of dose range and increase as needed

3. Complications

Proteinuria, neutropenia/agranulocytosis, systemic lupus erythematosus (SLE), hypotension, dysgeusia (loss of taste), gastrointestinal disturbances (do not use in patients with concurrent renal disease)

4. Action

Angiotensin-converting enzyme inhibitor consequently has both afterload and preload effects

Nitroglycerin paste 2 per cent (Nitrol Ointment; Kremers-Urban)

1. Dose

Dog—1/8 to 1 inch applied topically q6h

Cat—1/8 to 1/2 inch applied topically q6h. Either inside the ear pinna or inguinal or axillary regions are best because there is not much hair in these regions.

2. Titration

Begin at low to mid range and adjust upward per dose if needed.

3. Complications

Skin irritation, hypotension, headache

4. Action

Predominately a venous vasodilator

The following vasodilators may also prove to be of value for veterinary patients; however, at the present time they are not recommended for use because of inadequate study and clinical experience:

Sodium nitroprusside—Roche Laboratories

Isosorbide dinitrate—Ives Laboratories

Pindolol—Sandoz
Cyclandilate—Ives Laboratories
Dibenzyline—Smith Kline and Beckman
Papavarine HCL—Marion Laboratories
Isoxsuprine HCL—Mead Johnson Pharmaceuticals

Thromboembolism (see p. 210)

Thromboembolism may occur (1) secondary to cardiomyopathy in the cat, (2) as a pulmonary emboli of unknown etiology, (3) iatrogenically, associated with IV catheter use, (4) secondary to neoplasia, (5) subsequent to vascular injury, or (6) secondary to vegetative valvular disease.

Therapy is designed to reduce inadequate perfusion of downstream tissues and to relieve pulmonary edema or pleural effusion, if present.
1. Furosemide, 2 to 4 mg per kg IV or IM
2. Aspirin, 5 mg per kg per day; every other day for the cat
3. Thrombolynic enzymes (streptokinase, urokinase). Initial human dose is 4,400 U per kg IV over a 10-minute period, followed by 4,400 U per kg per hour for 12 hours by continuous IV infusion. The author has used this protocol successfully in dogs. However, the drug is not cleared for animal use, and an appropriate veterinary dosage regimen has not been determined.
4. Heparin, 200 U per kg q8h SC
5. Corticosteroids (Dexamethasone), 0.125 to 0.5 mg IM q12h

Thrombolytic enzymes and heparin should not be used simultaneously. Clotting parameters, especially activated coagulation time (ACT) and activated partial thrombplastin time (APTT) should be monitored.

	Dog	Cat
APTT should not be prolonged beyond	30 sec	25 sec
ACT should not be prolonged beyond	140 sec	90 sec

In all cases, a primary etiology should be pursued diagnostically as well as a thorough evaluation of those structures or body organs being affected by the alteration in blood supply.

Pericardial Effusion (Table 7)

Pericardial effusion can be recognized by the following signs:
1. Muffled heart sounds
2. Jugular pulse
3. Peripheral venous distention
4. Decreased R wave amplitudes with electrical alternans on the ECG
5. Enlarged globoid round heart shadow radiographically
6. Ascites and/or pleural effusion may be present.
7. Weakness, dyspnea

Table 7. DIFFERENTIAL DIAGNOSIS OF PERICARDIAL EFFUSION

Type of Pericardial Effusion	Etiology	Characteristic Features
Blood	Heart base tumors	Usually brachycephalic breeds over 8 years old, blood usually nonclotting
	Other neoplasia (metastatic)	
	Left atrial rupture	Usually occurs in male dogs of smaller breeds, over 8 years old
	Physical trauma	
	Iatrogenic trauma	Due to cardiac puncture or cardiac catheterization
Transudate	Congestive heart failure	Effusion not commonly recognized by physical or radiographic examination
	Hypoproteinemia	
	Secondary to peritoneopericardial diaphragmatic hernia	
Exudate (pericarditis)	Benign idiopathic pericardial effusion	Fluid serosanguineous: port wine color, nonclotting, and sterile (Luginbühl and Detweiler, 1965)
	Infectious pericarditis	Serous exudate in distemper and leptospirosis; sanguineous exudate in tuberculosis (Labie, 1962); or in conjunction with pleuritis and coccidioidomycosis.

From Ettinger, S. J., and Suter, P. F.: Canine Cardiology, Philadelphia, W. B. Saunders Co., 1970, p. 404.

8. Weak, thready femoral pulse

Response to pericardial effusion should include

1. Sedation, if necessary
2. Surgical prep and local anesthesia using 2 per cent Xylocaine at the left 4th intercostal space just above the costochondral junction
3. Record ECG and leave ECG unit attached to patient. An occasional VPC will be observed upon entry into the pericardial sac or contact by the needle or catheter with the epicardium. VPCs usually do no require therapy.
4. Use Venocath 16 gauge or IV Intrafusor.* Advance the needle through the

---

*Sorenson Research Company, Salt Lake City, Utah

intercostal muscle into the pericardial sac. Thread the catheter through the needle into the pericardial sac. Withdraw the needle. Drain the pericardial sac using a three-way stopcock and a closed collection system. Save a sample of the pericardial fluid for chemical and cytologic examination (see p. 807).

5. CO_2 can be injected through the catheter following pericardiocentesis, and a pneumopericardiograph can be taken to aid in determining the etiologic diagnosis. Do not use room air.

6. If the pericardium refills with fluid within 30 days, exploratory pericardectomy is advisable.

Postcaval Syndrome of Heartworm Disease

Postcaval syndrome of heartworm disease is recognized by the following signs:

1. Acute renal and hepatic failure
2. Enlarged right atrium and posterior vena cava
3. Ascites
4. Hemoglobinuria
5. Anemia
6. Acute collapse, dyspnea
7. Disseminated intravascular coagulation
8. Jugular pulse
9. Circulating microfilaria

Response to this syndrome should include:

1. Surgical removal of adult worms from the right atrium and caudal vena cava with long alligator forceps through the right jugular vein under local anesthesia.
2. Digitalization—digoxin, 0.011 mg per kg q12h
3. Peritoneal dialysis, if needed, following normalization of circulating fluid volume
4. Corticosteroids—dexamethasone, 5 mg per kg IV
5. Furosemide, 2 to 4 mg per kg q12h, if needed
6. Routine heartworm therapy following stabilization of the effects of post-caval obstruction

References and Additional Readings

Bolton, G.: Cardiovascular emergencies. Vet. Clin. North Am., 2:411, 1972.

Bonagura, J. D.: Feline cardiovascular emergencies. Vet. Clin. North Am., 7:385, 1977.

Ettinger, S. J., and Suter, P. F.: Canine Cardiology. Philadelphia, W. B. Saunders Company, 1970.

Gibbs, C., Gaskell, C. J., Darke, G. G., and Wotton, P. R.: Idiopathic pericardial hemorrhage in dogs. J. Small Anim. Pract. 23:483, 1982.

Haskins, S. C.: Cardiopulmonary resuscitation. Compendium on Continuing Education 4(2):170, 1982.

Hill, B.: Canine idiopathic congestive cardiomyopathy. Compendium on Continuing Education 3(7):615, 1981.

Jackson, R. F., et al.: Surgical treatment of the caval syndrome of canine heartworm disease. J.A.V.M.A. *171*:1065, 1977.

Schaer, M.: Hyperkalemia in cats with urethral obstruction: electrocardiographic abnormalities and treatment. Vet. Clin. North Am., 7:407, 1977.

Tilley, L. P.: Essentials of Canine and Feline Electrocardiography. 2nd ed. Philadelphia, Lea & Febiger, 1984.

Tilley, L. P., et al.: *In* Ettinger, S. J. (ed.): Textbook of Veterinary Internal Medicine, 2nd ed. Philadelphia, W. B. Saunders Company, 1983, pp. 1029–1051.

SHOCK

Shock is a clinical syndrome characterized by ineffective perfusion of tissues with blood and resultant cellular hypoxia. There can be numerous causes of shock, including hypovolemia; and inadequate peripheral resistance, causing distributive shock (neurogenic shock, septic shock, anaphylactic shock); cardiogenic causes and tension pneumothorax, causing obstructive shock (blood flow is impeded).

PATHOPHYSIOLOGY

The body responses in shock involve both neurogenic and hormonal mechanisms, and these changes account for the clinical signs seen in the shock patient.

Hypotension associated with hemorrhage results in constriction of the arterial wall at the carotid sinus, with diminished inhibitory afferent impulses from the carotid sinus, and subsequent stimulation of sympathetic regulators, causing arterioles and veins to constrict and the heart to beat faster and more forcefully, causing transient hypotension.

Neuroendocrine stimulation causes release of increased amounts of catecholamines, antidiuretic, adrenocorticotropic growth hormones. Activation of the renin-angiotensin system releases aldosterone. In addition, glycogen breakdown increases; inhibition of the cellular use of glucose and suppression of insulin occur, resulting in hyperglycemia.

Redistribution of cardiac output decreases blood flow to the skin, muscles, and kidneys; however, blood supply to the brain and heart is maintained. Inadequate tissue perfusion results in poor oxygenation and the development of anaerobic glycolysis with excess lactic acid production, intracellular acidosis, and extracellular acidemia, which results in an increase in thromboxane, which acts as a stimulus to the synthesis of an unidentified negative inotrope. Inadequate perfusion of the pancreas causes the release of a myocardial depressant factor.

Redistribution of the blood supply to the brain, with mean pressures between 45 and 50 mm, can result in changes in levels of consciousness; for example, initial excitement followed by a comatose state. Prolonged hypotension, with pressures in the 30 to 35 mm range for more than 2 hours, can result in ischemic brain damage. Altered blood flow to the splanchnic circulation, particularly the mesenteric circulation, results in intestinal ischemia. A common finding in dogs, following volume replacement in shock, is intestinal necrosis and hemorrhage, with bloody diarrhea and toxemia.

Renal function can be severely compromised during the hypotension of shock. Decrease in renal blood flow decreases the glomerular filtration rate and results in decreased cortical tubular function. Renal function is also affected when severe tissue damage has occurred, resulting in circulating myoglobin and/or hemoglobin. There is increased danger of renal damage from these products if the patient is acidotic. Renal hypotension results in the release of vasoactive hormones such as renin-angiotensin and catecholamines, with resultant renal vasoconstriction and renal tubular damage. Changes in renal function are clinically characterized by oliguria, polyuria, isosthenuria, glycosuria, renal tubular necrosis, and developing azotemia.

CLINICAL SIGNS

The classic signs of shock are related to the physiologic changes associated with hypotension and hypoxia: tachypnea, tachycardia, reduced pulse pressure, poor capillary refill and pallor, decreased mean arterial pressure, muscle weakness, depressed sensorium, hyperventilation, and decreased urinary output.

TREATMENT

The classic approach to initial shock management is ventilation, infusion, and perfusion. After the initial assessment of the patient in shock has been made, the following priorities of management should be established: (1) ensure adequate ventilation and oxygenation, (2) arrest hemorrhage if present, (3) begin volume replacement, and (4) regulate acid-base disturbances.

Estimate alveolar ventilation by observing rate, depth, sound, and force of ventilation. If difficulty in breathing is encountered and there is an altered state of consciousness, establish an airway with endotracheal intubation. Evaluate the general status of the pulmonary system following trauma (see p. 447). Institute intermittent positive pressure ventilation with a volume-cycled respirator or by hand, using an Ambu bag and 100 per cent oxygen. Tidal volumes of greater than 10 to 12 ml per kg and rates of 8 to 12 breaths per minute at 20 cm of water inspiratory pressure are required. Severe traumatic parenchymal lung disease may require minute volumes one and one half to twice the tidal volume last mentioned, with an initial inspiratory pressure of 35 cm of water. Hyperventilation in the shock patient is often very important (see p. 202).

Provide temporary oxygen therapy for the noncomatose (although depressed) animal via a nasal catheter. Place 2 to 3 drops of 2 per cent Pontocaine solution in the nasal canal. Coat a soft, flexible rubber catheter with Xylocaine jelly, and pass the catheter through the nasal canal to a level of the nasopharynx. Tape the tube to the bridge of the nose. Oxygen, 100 per cent, at a flow rate of 2 to 6 L is bubbled through a nebulizer, and humidified oxygen is delivered to the catheter. More prolonged administration of oxygen requires an oxygen cage (see p. 633). More severe pulmonary problems may exist in shock cases, especially those associated with trauma and pulmonary edema or traumatic lung syndrome may be present (see p. 209).

Fluid Replacement. The aim of fluid replacement is to restore and maintain tissue perfusion. The fluids to be administered may be crystalloids, blood, or plasma. Ringer's solution with lactate, gluconate, or acetate is the crystalloid of choice in most shock cases. In the following situations, alternate methods of fluid replacement must be considered (see also p. 591).

When the hematocrit falls to below 20 per cent or when clinical estimates indicate blood loss of 30 ml per kg (especially in hypovolemia associated with trauma), packed cells are needed. Four units of fluids to 1 unit of fresh whole blood may be given at a rate of 12 to 20 ml per kg (see p. 622). If the total amount of solids fall below 4 gm per 100 ml, plasma is needed.

In cases of azotemia, a potassium-free solution is needed until diuresis occurs (see p. 607).

The administration of fluids in shock cases must be rapid and requires a large-bore (14- to 18-gauge) intravenous (IV) catheter. In large dogs, two such catheters may be required. A jugular catheter is helpful, because central venous pressure can also be monitored (see p. 610). A cutdown procedure is helpful to place a large-bore No. 5–8 French red rubber feeding tube in the jugular vein. Administer fluids while monitoring the physiologic parameters previously discussed until a degree of homeostasis is achieved. Then continue fluids at a slower rate. Evaluate the acid-base status (see p. 593). Circulatory support from balanced electrolyte solutions lasts approximately 60 to 120 minutes. The initial severity and phase of shock will determine how much fluid is initially needed. In the dog, initial doses of 60 to 90 ml per kg of buffered Ringer's solution per kg of body weight is often needed during the first 5 to 30 minutes. Monitoring of central venous pressure (CVP) is helpful during initial rapid fluid administration (see p. 564). If the packed cell volume (PCV) is 20 per cent or below, whole blood should be used. The rate of infusion of fluids and the amount infused is regulated by establishing a return to cardiovascular stability. The rate of infusion should be as rapid as possible and monitored by CVP, palpation of pulse rate and pressure, and evaluation of tissue perfusion.

If the CVP rises (to a level of 13 to 15 cm) while the circulatory state declines, as judged by mucous membrane function, pulse rate, and urinary output, cardiogenic factors may be present. Dobutamine HC1 can be used in a drip (see p. 39).

When poor perfusion remains despite an elevated CVP, increased peripheral vasoconstriction may be present. An alpha blocking agent such as chlorpromazine, 0.01 to 0.1 mg per kg, as needed, given slowly IV, may produce vasodilation and improve peripheral circulation.

A rapid rise in CVP levels to between 10 and 15 cm may lead to pulmonary edema. This is especially true if urine output is less than 1 ml per kg per hour in the dog and 0.5 ml per kg per hour in the cat. In these cases, furosemide, 1 to 2 mg per kg should be given. (See also flow chart on pulmonary edema, p. 209.)

In shock, the fall in systolic blood pressure to levels of 50 to 60 mm Hg can precipitate renal shutdown, oliguria, or anuria. Following fluid replacement and elevation of blood pressure, it may be necessary to help stimulate urine output. IV mannitol has the following effects: (1) it increases circulating blood volume via an osmotic effect; (2) it increases renal blood flow; and (3) it reduces cellular edema (see Urinary Emergencies, p. 123).

Use of Glucocorticosteroids. Massive doses of aqueous soluble salts of selected glucocorticosteroids must be given very early in shock cases. Methylprednisolone sodium succinate (Solu-Medrol), 20 mg per kg IV or prednisolone sodium succinate (Solu-delta-cortef), 10 to 30 mg per kg IV may be used. The water-soluble steroids prednisolone sodium succinate are much more effective in shock cases than dexamethasone in a polyethylene glycol carrier (Azium).

Broad-spectrum antibiotic therapy in shock cases is recommended for prophylactic reasons. If an offending organism has been the cause of septic shock, specific antibiotic therapy may be indicated. Give chloramphenicol succinate, 25 mg per lb of body weight, gentamicin, 1 mg per lb, or high levels of crystalline penicillin (sodium salt, 1 to 4 million units) IV.

Use of naloxone as an opiate antagonist blocks the action of endorphine release and its associated cardiac depressant effects. The drug, 2 mg per kg per hour, is used to increase cardiac output, aortic pressure, and left ventricular function and has proved to be effective in hemorrhagic shock model systems. The expense of the drug greatly limits its use, however.

Septicemia or Bacteremia. Shock resulting from either hypovolemia or inadequate peripheral resistance may develop into septic or endotoxic shock. The patient is weak and comatose, with a rapid, weak pulse and slightly blanched or muddy membranes. The rectal temperature is usually subnormal, and the desquamating rectal mucosa appears as "raspberry jam" on the thermometer. The packed cell volume is often 65 to 75 per cent, and the erythrocyte sedimentation rate is very rapid.

This form of shock is often a late stage of other types. Particularly serious problems are severe acidosis, low pO_2, high PCV, and disseminated intravascular coagulation (DIC).

Attempt to remove or drain any specific known causes of sepsis. Débride necrotic or infected tissue.

Generally follow the treatment outlined for hypovolemic shock. Use steroids in high concentrations as previously described.

Lower blood viscosity (PCV). Blood is contraindicated. Low molecular weight dextran (Rheomacrodex, 20 ml/kg IV) may be used *with* buffered lactated Ringer's solution to reduce viscosity.

Correct the bacteremia and reduce endotoxin production. Gentamicin sulfate, 4.5 mg per kg in a lactated Ringer's IV drip, should be administered as a loading dose over a 75-minute period. Repeat gentamicin IV, 1.0 mg per kg IV, at 3 and 5 hours and 4.0 mg per kg IV at 7 1/4 hours following initial IV loading dose and at 8-hour intervals after this, provided that renal function is normal. IV treatment with ampicillin or clindamycin (Cleocin) should be simultaneously begun to control anaerobic infections.

Compensate for the severe acidosis. Use assisted ventilation with 40 per cent oxygen. Give 0.4 per cent solution of $NaHCO_3$ in an IV drip.

Consider the use of heparin, 3 to 5 U per kg IV every 4 hours, to prevent microemboli formation.

Begin therapy with cyclo-oxygenase inhibitor to reduce the production of prostaglandins. Flunixin meglumine (Banamine) can be used IV, 1 mg per kg, repeated no more than once at 12 to 18-hour interval.

Intracellular hypoglycemia may develop during the course of endotoxic shock. The IV administration of glucose, regular insulin, and potassium may help correct this condition. The glucose dosage is 1 gm per kg per hour IV, using 50 per cent glucose in lactated Ringer's solution, 0.3 U of regular insulin per 1 gm of glucose and 0.15 mg of potassium per gm of glucose (Rawlings and Crowe, 1983).

Sludging and capillary stasis predispose to DIC. Improved perfusion will help prevent this (see p. 65).

Cardiogenic Causes. To evaluate the role of cardiac disease in shock production, monitor ECG and heart rate, measure blood pressure, if possible, or CVP, measure urinary output, and monitor fluid input. If cardiac arrhythmias or myocardial disease presents, attempt to correct them (see pp. 123–125).

DISSEMINATED (DIFFUSE) INTRAVASCULAR COAGULATION

Disseminated intravascular coagulation (DIC) is a disorder associated with generalized activation of the clotting mechanism resulting from the release of coagulation-initiating factors from damaged tissues, cells, or vasculature. The release of tissue thromboplastin (from a wide variety of causes) can induce activation of extrinsic clotting mechanisms. Platelet aggregation and metamorphosis, which also are involved with various types of tissue damage, can induce the activation of intrinsic clotting mechanisms. In the DIC process, prothrombin, fibrinogen, or platelets, and several other coagulation factors (including factors V and VIII) are consumed in the formation of intravascular thrombi. When the clotting system is activated in the circulation, plasminogen is activated as a secondary but almost simultaneous event. Plasmin digests fibrinogen and attacks factors V and VIII. The digestion of fibrinogen produces fibrin split products that impair clot formation and platelet function. When these clotting abnormalities become generalized and severe, the available store of labile coagulation factors and platelets can be severely depleted, leading to widespread bleeding and diathesis.

The triggering mechanism for DIC can be extremely varied and may involve any of the following factors:

1. Injury to endothelial cells activates the Hageman factor (factor XII) and the intrinsic clotting system.
2. Tissue injury releases thromboplastin, and the presence of factor VII activates the extrinsic clotting system.
3. Erythrocyte, leukocyte, and platelet injury results in release of phospholipids, triggering both intrinsic and extrinsic clotting systems.
4. Hypercoagulable states may also be seen in the nephrotic syndrome where

antithrombin III is reduced and increased fibrinogen and factor VIII concentrations are present. There may be evidence of thrombosis in these nephrotic syndromes, especially thoracic thromboembolism (see pp. 210–211). Loss of proteinuria in the nephrotic syndrome may result in the loss of proteins of low molecular weight and the retention of high molecular weight hemostatic factors. Increased factor VIII may also be produced by systemic inflammation. The ratio of fibrinogen (per cent normal) to antithrombin III (per cent normal) can be used to help determine whether a hypercoagulable state with antithrombin III loss may be present. In one study, the normal ratio was reported at 0.5 to 1.5.

5. Transfusion of stored blood may activate intrinsic clotting mechanisms.
6. Bacterial cell walls and endotoxin activate complement and platelet aggregation.

DIC can be associated with trauma, poisonings, hemolytic syndromes, bacterial endotoxemia and septicemia, hemorrhagic shock, and a variety of diseases (see Table 8).

The symptoms of DIC are a combination of simultaneous thrombotic and hemorrhagic events. The presenting signs depend on which of the pathological processes is predominating. The initiating process is thrombosis, with thrombotic infarctions occurring in numerous areas in the body.

Tests demonstrating the presence of fibrin split products in the circulation are confirmative for fibrinolysis. Measurement of coagulation time, using activated coagulation time (see p. 712), reveals prolonged clotting time, and dissolution of the clot is evidence of active fibrinolysis. The most consistent laboratory test changes are the following: prolonged one-stage prothrombin time, prolonged partial thromboplastin time, thrombin time prolonged in

Table 8. DISEASES ASSOCIATED WITH DIC IN DOGS OR CATS

Infections	Miscellaneous
Septicemia	Shock
Infectious canine hepatitis	Endotoxemia
Leptospirosis	Heat stroke
Panleukopenia	Hemorrhagic pancreatitis
Trypanosomiasis	Hemolytic disease
Rocky Mountain spotted fever	Nephrotic syndrome
	Gastric torsion
Neoplasia	Heartworm disease
Carcinoma	Hemorrhagic enteritis
Lymphosarcoma	Hepatic necrosis
Hemangiosarcoma	Extracorporeal circulation
Granulocytic leukemia	Autotransfusions
	Surgical trauma
	Diaphragmatic hernia

Adapted from Kociba, G. J.: Disseminated intravascular coagulation. *In* Kirk, R. W. (ed.): Current Veterinary Therapy VI. Philadelphia, W. B. Saunders Company, 1977, p. 449.

severe cases associated with circulating FDPs, low blood fibrinogen level, thrombocytopenia, increased level of fibrin split products, abnormal bleeding tendencies, and decreased levels of factors (i.e., I, II, V, VIII, and X; Table 9). Fragmented red blood cells (shistocytes) may appear on smears. (See p. 894 for normal values.)

In treating DIC, first consider: (1) controlling the primary disease entity; (2) supporting blood volume and preventing further deterioration associated with shock by providing adequate fluid support (see p. 591) to correct hypovolemia and prevent vascular stasis and to dilute the thrombin and fibrin degradation products and activators of fibrinolysis; (3) maintaining adequate respirations; (4) preventing severe acidosis from developing; and (5) if direct evidence of thrombosis or bleeding begins to develop, drugs to inhibit intravascular thrombosis (heparin) and replace used up coagulation products (platelets, plasma, or cryoprecipitate) are indicated. Heparin potentiates the action of plasma antithrombin III.

Heparin has a very short active pharmacologic effect when given IV to the dog (2 hours). The initial loading dose can be given IV. Dosage recommendations for heparin (1 mg of heparin equals 100 IU) in DIC are the following: Mini doses of heparin used repeatedly IV are indicated. Give an initial loading dose of 10 to 20 U per kg, then 5 U per kg every 3 hours IV. As the primary disease condition is brought under control, the heparin dosage can be given over a more extended period of time, and the subcutaneous (SC) route can be used. If heparin activity needs to be antagonized, protamine sulfate can be given, 1 mg for every 100 U of heparin administered. SC therapy with heparin in the dog at 500 U per kg every 8 hours maintains the activated partial thromboplastin time at 1.5 to 2.5 over the normal values and the activated coagulation time (ACT) values at 1.2 to 2.5 times the normal values.

Replacement of platelets and plasma or plasma cryoprecipitate is indicated in patients with DIC (see p. 622). Blood replacement should be fresh. The blood being transfused should be pre-treated in the bag with heparin (2 U per ml of blood transfused).

MONITORING TECHNIQUES IN EVALUATING SHOCK

Temperature

The temperature of the shock patient can vary widely. Monitor the temperatures with a continuous reading rectal thermometer, if possible. If the patient becomes hypothermic, rewarm with hot water bottles or with a water blanket. Rewarm replacement fluids to 37°C (98.6°F). Rectal temperature should be above 38°C (100°F), if possible.

Pulse

Check the pulse by monitoring the femoral, lingual, and jugular arteries. Return of pulse rate rhythm to normal with shock therapy is a good prognostic sign.

Table 9. LABORATORY FINDINGS IN STAGES OF DIC

Stage of DIC	Platelet Cells/mm³ × 10³	Activated Coagulation Time (sec)*	Other Coagulation Test Findings	Clinical Signs
Normal values	*150 to 500*†	*< 120 (dog)* *< 75 (cat)*	*FDP < 30 μ/ml (dog)* *< 8 μg/ml (cat)*	
Early, low-grade, or chronic	Decreased ≦ 100	Normal < 120 (dog) < 75 (cat)	FDP, PT, PTT, TT: normal Plasminogen, antithrombin III: normal to decreased Coagulation factors‡: normal to increased	Petechial hemorrhages, hemolysis
Acute	Decreased < 100	Slightly to moderate prolongation 120–200 (dog) 75–120 (cat)	FDP: moderate increase PT, PTT, TT: moderate prolongation Plasminogen, antithrombin III, coagulation factors: marked decrease	Variable, organ dysfunction, hemorrhagic diathesis, hematomas, petechiae, hemolysis
End-stage	Decreased < 75	Marked prolongation > 200 (dog) > 120 (cat)	FDP: marked increased PT, PTT, TT: marked prolongation Plasminogen, antithrombin III, coagulation factors: marked decrease	Severe hemorrhagic diathesis, petechiae, hematomas, body cavity effusions, frank hemorrhage

*ACT values are a rough guideline and should not be taken as absolutes.
†Values apply to dogs and cats unless specified.
‡Factors XIII, XII, XI, VIII, V, II, and I.
From Kirk, R. W. (ed.): Current Veterinary Therapy VIII: Small Animal Practice. Philadelphia, W. B. Saunders Company, 1983.

Respiration

Evaluate the respiratory rate and rhythm, and note any increase in the rate that may indicate hypoxia, pulmonary edema, or atelectasis. Auscultate the lungs and listen for any adventitious sounds (see p. 449).

Capillary Circulation

Determine capillary refill by pressing oral mucosa until blanching occurs. A rapid return to pink color indicates good capillary circulation; a slow return indicates poor circulation. A capillary refill time of more than 2 seconds is abnormal and may signify hypovolemia, hypotension, or peripheral vasoconstriction. Note also the color of the mucous membranes. Cyanosis (see pp. 275–277) may be present in the late stages of hypoxemia.

Vital Organ Circulation

The rate of urine production is proportional to the glomerular filtration rate (GFR) and is a measure of renal perfusion. When arterial pressure falls below 60 mm Hg, GFR ceases.

Place an indwelling catheter in the urinary bladder. The rate of urine flow (normally, 1.0 to 2.0 ml/kg/hr in dogs and 0.5 ml/kg/hr in cats) parallels the rate of perfusion of the kidneys, which normally receive 25 per cent of cardiac output, and parallels the GFR.

Circulating Blood Volume

Determine the circulating blood volume clinically. Firm, full, femoral pulse, rapid capillary refill, and filled veins are good signs.

The CVP is used as a measure of circulating blood volume and cardiac output. CVP is measured via a catheter placed in the external jugular vein (see pp. 564–566).

Packed Cell Volume—Total Solids

Serial measurements of PCV and total solids are helpful in monitoring shock patients. Changes in the normal PCV (35 to 48 per cent) and total solids (5.5 to 8.0 gm/100 ml) are helpful in evaluating red cell plasma ratios, and total solids are an indication of plasma protein levels.

Acid-Base Balance

Shock usually causes severe tissue acidosis. Although this can be managed by assisted ventilation and IV administration of sodium bicarbonate, it requires careful and complex monitoring. The degree of acidosis has an important bearing on shock.

The measurement of lactate concentrations in the peripheral blood can be used as an indication of the general state of tissue oxygenation. Blood lactate levels can be measured in blood samples collected in sodium fluoride–potassium oxalate anticoagulant. Lactate concentrations in normal dogs at rest is 5 to 20 mg per dl of venous blood and 12.6 to 36 mg per dl of plasma.

Blood Pressure

Blood pressure can be monitored by either direct or indirect means. Hypotension is one of the last signs of shock to appear.

Toe Web Temperature

Measurement of toe web temperature is a good measurement of peripheral perfusion. Place a temperature probe between the toes of the rear foot, and keep it in place with a light dressing. Record the rectal temperature simultaneously. The toe web temperature is compared with the rectal temperature. A normal change in temperature (RT-TT) is less than 7°F; if there is greater than 10°F change in temperature, the animal will be in shock; and if there is greater than 20°F change, the animal will be in deep shock. A poor prognosis exists when there are persistent large temperature differences. Major changes in peripheral temperature are proportional to changes in cardiac output.

The mental status of the patient should be continually evaluated.

References and Additional Readings

Feldman, B.: Disseminated intravascular coagulation. Compendium of Continuing Education, 3(1):46, 1981.

Haskins, S.C.: Shock. In Kirk, R. W. (ed.) Current Veterinary Therapy VIII: Small Animal Practice. Philadelphia, W. B. Saunders Company, 1983.

McAnulty, J. F.: Septic shock in the dog: a review. J. Am. Anim. Hosp. Assoc. 19(6):824, 1983.

Rawlings, C. A., and Crowe, D. T.: Shock and anesthesia management of the emergency patient. Proc. Am. Anim. Hosp. Assoc. 107, 1983.

Shoemaker, W. C.: Pathophysiology and therapy of shock syndromes. In Shoemaker, W.C., Thompson, W.L., and Holbrook, P.R. (eds.): The Society of Critical Care Medicine: Philadelphia, W. B. Saunders Company, 1984.

White, G. L., White, G. S., Kosanke, S. D., et al.: Therapeutic effects of prednisolone sodium succinate vs. dexamethosone in dogs subjected to E. coli septic shock. J. Am. Anim. Hosp. Assoc. 18(4):639, 1982.

ANESTHETIC COMPLICATIONS AND EMERGENCIES
by Marc Raffe, D.V.M., M.S.*

Most anesthetic complications or emergencies are associated with one of the following problems: (1) equipment failures, (2) respiratory problems, (3) cardiovascular problems, or (4) human error.

In evaluating the patient under anesthesia, adequate monitoring can be very important (see pp. 72–76). If the anesthetic level of the patient becomes too deep, the following signs may be noted: dilated pupils, lack of muscle tone, absence of reflexes, bradycardia, diminished tidal volume, hypotension, and slow capillary refill. If the anesthetic level becomes too light, the following signs may be noted: response to painful stimuli, muscular movement, marked reflex activity, rapid respiration, tachycardia, and hypertension.

EQUIPMENT FAILURES

Endotracheal Tube Problems

Signs Observed
1. Inability to keep patient anesthetized
2. Difficulty in breathing—increased ventilatory effort
3. Erratic breathing cycles
4. Cyanosis

Problems
1. Tube placed in the esophagus
2. Leak in the cuff or cuff improperly inflated
3. Primary bronchial intubation—length too long
4. Endotracheal tube too small
5. Obstructed endotracheal tube
6. Kinked endotracheal tube
7. Endotracheal tube disconnected from gas machine

Vaporizer Problems

Signs Observed
1. Inability to keep patient anesthetized
2. Animal may be excessively deep

Problems
1. No anesthetic in vaporizer
2. Incorrect vaporizer dial setting
3. Wrong anesthetic put into vaporizer
4. Calibration of vaporizer not accurate

---

*Associate Professor of Veterinary Anesthesiology, College of Veterinary Medicine, University of Minnesota.

Anesthetic Machine Problems

Signs Observed
1. Inadequate gas flow through flow meter
2. Hypoxemia or cyanosis in patient
3. Increased ventilatory effort or rate
4. Undesirable light plane of anesthesia

Problems
1. No gas in reservoir cylinders
2. Inappropriate flow meter settings or mechanical failure of flow meter
3. Machine leaks at vaporizer—machine connection
4. Breathing system leaks
   a. Perforation of corrugated tubing or reservoir bag
   b. Worn out gaskets or seals
   c. Incomplete seal of "pop-off" valve
   d. Poor connection to endotracheal tube
5. Exhaustion of CO_2 absorbant
6. Breathing system obstruction
   a. Unidirectional valve sticking or misassembled
   b. Misassembly of breathing circuit components

RESPIRATORY SYSTEM

In evaluating respiration during anesthesia in the patient with assisted but not controlled ventilation, the respiratory rate alone is not a reliable determinant of adequate ventilation. The tidal volume or minute volume (tidal volume × respiratory rate) is more important than the respiratory rate alone. Most anesthetic agents cause a progressive decrease in tidal volume and minute volume as the level of anesthesia deepens. The tidal volume can be estimated by observing either the excursions of the reservoir bag on the anesthetic machine or chest wall excursions. Clinical signs of inadequate ventilation may be: tachypnea and bradypnea; tachycardia and hypertension, followed by bradycardia and hypotension (late stages); cardiac arrhythmias; cyanosis (not usually visible if inhalation agents and oxygen are used); bradycardia; and cardiac arrest.

Problems in Respiratory–Induced Anesthetic Complications

1. Inadequate ventilation for or by the patient.
   a. Neuromuscular—CNS depression from general anesthesia; CNS edema from hypoxia, trauma, fluids, and muscle relaxants; thoracic wall problems; anesthesia-related muscle weakness
   b. Upper airway obstruction—laryngeal edema, collapsing trachea or larynx, improper use of endotracheal tube, problems in brachycephalic breeds, aspiration of gastric contents
   c. Intrathoracic obstruction—hydrothorax, hemothorax; pneumothorax; diaphragmatic hernia

    d. Parenchymal disease—atelectasis; edema, pneumonia, neoplasia; trauma hemorrhage in the lung

    e. Anesthetic equipment—increased resistance to ventilation, increased dead space from machine to patient interface, improper oxygen concentration or flow rates.

2. Pulmonary atelectasis

Causes

  1. General anesthesia

  2. Pleural space disease

  3. Disruption of alveolar stability (i.e., pneumonia, edema, emphysema, ventilating too vigorously)

Problems

  1. Improper gas exchange with pulmonary capillaries resulting in hypercapnia, hypoxemia, and increased ventilatory effort in awake animals

3. Abnormal breathing pattern during anesthesia

Causes

  1. Anesthetic drugs—may be species related

  2. Surgical positioning or maneuvers that compromise ventilation

  3. Inadequate or excessive anesthetic depth

  4. Inadequate gas exchange—hypercapnia, hypoxemia

  5. Equipment malfunction or exhaustion of CO_2 absorbant

  6. Thoracic wall or diaphragmatic injury, penetration

  7. CNS injury to respiratory centers

  8. Agonal breathing—death imminent

Problems

  1. Poor gas exchange

  2. Poor uptake and distribution of inhalation anesthetic drugs

  3. Atelectasis

4. Postoperative depression of ventilation

Causes

  1. Anesthetic drugs

  2. Overventilation during intraoperative support

  3. Surgical techniques that may compromise ventilation

  4. Postoperative dressing on abdomen or chest too tight

  5. Increased ventilatory "effort" when the animal is fatigued

  6. Hypothermia

  7. CNS injury

Problems

  1. Poor gas exchange—hypoxemia or hypercapnia

  2. Pulmonary tissue atelectasis

  3. Retarded elimination of volatile anesthetic agents

5. Postoperative dyspnea

Causes

  1. Pulmonary tissue disease or injury

  2. Pleural space injury or accumulation of air or fluid therapy

  3. Upper airway obstruction or compromise—may be anatomic defect, a

result of intubation injury, or related to neurogenic or myoneurogenic cause of lack of muscular "tone" to pharynx and tongue
Problems
1. Increased "work" of breathing
2. Poor gas exchange—hypoxemia, hypercapnia
3. Cyanosis

CARDIOVASCULAR SYSTEM PROBLEMS
(See pp. 36–59)

Bradycardia

In this condition, the pulse rate is below normal (normal levels in large dogs, 70 to 120 beats/min; medium dogs, 90 to 140 beats/min; small dogs, 100 to 150 beats/min; and domestic cats, 140 to 250 beats/min).
Problems
1. Anesthetic drug related—use of narcotics or xylazine
2. Animal too deeply anesthetized—check other parameters
3. Increased vagal tone—atropine effect dissipated
4. Hypothermia—patient may need warming
5. Hypoxia—in later stages, bradycardia

Tachycardia

In this condition, the pulse rate is markedly above normal.
Problems
1. Anesthetic level too light for patient or for the degree of surgical stimulation
2. Hypercapnia or hypoxemia (hypercarbia or increased CO_2 retention, hypoxia)
3. Hypotension and/or shock
4. Drug induced—usually associated with the use of vagolytic drugs such as atropine, glycopyrrolate, and ketamine or sympathomimetic drugs such as Isuprel, epinephrine, and dopamine
5. Hyperthermia (increased temperature)

Hypotension

Hypotension is the development of low blood pressure and poor tissue perfusion associated with hypovolemia, diminished cardiac output, and/or peripheral vasodilatation.
Problems
1. Decreased cardiac output associated with any of the following: decreased venous return to the heart resulting from hypovolemia, excessive surgical manipulation of viscera; decreased myocardial contractility associated with anesthetic agents, hypoxemia or toxemia; bradycardia; cardiac arrhythmias.
2. Hypovolemia or decreased circulating blood volume associated with fluid deficits during surgery, excessive bleeding at surgical site, vasodilation of venules.
3. Peripheral vasodilation, which may be associated with administration of preanesthetic agents (promazine derivatives or gaseous anesthetics, namely, halothane or enflurane), hypoxia, and toxemia.

Recognition
1. Evaluation of peripheral pulse by palpation, mucous membrane color, and capillary refill time
2. Oliguria or anuria
3. Measurement of blood pressure by direct or indirect methods
   Normal: systolic, 100–160 mm Hg
   diastolic, 60–90 mm Hg
   mean (1/3S + 2/3D), 80–120 mm Hg

Cardiac Arrhythmias

Adequate monitoring of the patient under general anesthesia is very important. ECG monitoring can detect the early development of cardiac arrhythmias and lead to their early treatment. Signs of cardiac arrhythmias may include irregular pulse rate and/or pressure; abnormal or irregular heart sounds; pallor, cyanosis, and hypotension; and abnormal ECG tracing. Continuous monitoring of the surgical patient with an ECG monitor can be very helpful. The following parameters should be observed:
1. Rhythm and rate of the heart
2. Identification of P waves: Is atrial activity regular and uniform?
3. Recognition of QRS complex—morphology, rate, and uniformity. Is there evidence of ectopic beats?
4. Relationship between P waves and QRS complexes. Is the atrioventricular conduction time normal?

Some of the commonly recognized causes of cardiac arrhythmias include the following:
1. Sensitization of the myocardium by anesthetics to catecholamines released from fear, excitement, stress, on intubation, or pain.
2. Acidosis and hypercarbia
3. Myocardial hypoxia
4. Electrolyte imbalances—hyperkalemia, hypokalemia
5. Vagal reflexes or sympathetic reflexes
6. Oculocardiac reflexes
7. Surgical stimulation
8. Prolonged anesthesia (see also pp. 36–59).

Arrhythmias may be categorized by several different methodologies. The site of origin and the rate are two types of classification. Because monitoring will usually be provided with a provision for evaluation of rate, the present discussion will use this criteria for classification. Using this scheme, arrhythmias with rates of less than 65 beats per minute are called *bradyarrhythmias,* arrhythmias with rates greater than 170 beats per minute (200 beats per minute in cats) are called *tachyarrhythmias,* and arrhythmias between 65 and 170 beats per minute are *arrhythmias with near normal rates.*

The following factors can be observed in arrhythmias during anesthesia:
1. Poor preoperative preparation, including attention to fluid balance, electrolytes, and acid-base status will predispose to arrhythmias.
2. A high percentage of arrhythmias are associated with anesthetic induction

and occur during the first 5 minutes of anesthesia, many of which are initiated with endotracheal tube placement.

3. Controlled respiration and preoxygenation decrease the tendency to develop acidosis and resultant arrhythmias.

4. Stimulation of the sympathetic and parasympathetic nervous system may lead to arrhythmias and can be induced by painful stimuli (perceived because the patient is too light) such as traction on abdominal structures, manipulation of extraocular muscles, tube thoracostomy, and tracheal intubation.

5. A higher level of arrhythmias can be seen in dogs during the initial preanesthetic stage with atropine.

6. Certain anesthetic agents have been associated with anesthesia-related arrhythmias. Xylazine (Rompun) is associated with sinoatrial and atrioventricular blockade and potentiates cardiac sensitization to epinephrine and halothane. The thiobarbiturates (thiamylal sodium) are arrhythmogenic and may be associated with ventricular premature complexes. Lower percentage concentrations of thiamylal sodium (2.5 per cent) or slower rates of administration are less likely to produce arrhythmia. Halothane can produce arrhythmias, and this effect is greatly potentiated if epinephrine is used unless acepromazine is given as a preanesthetic.

To prevent anesthetic-related arrhythmias, the following guidelines should be observed:

1. Evaluate preoperative patient to detect and stabilize preexisting arrhythmias, electrolyte or acid-base disturbance, and hydration status prior to anesthesia.

2. Select appropriate preanesthetic agent to allay apprehension to anesthesia.

3. Be aware of pharmacologic effects of anesthetic drugs upon the myocardium and autonomic nervous system.

4. Ensure adequate anesthetic depth and good oxygenation prior to endotracheal intubation

5. Ensure adequate ventilatory support during anesthesia

6. Ensure adequate anesthetic depth prior to surgical stimulation

7. Avoid surgical manipulation to heart or great vessels for a prolonged period of time

8. Avoid vascillations in anesthetic depth

9. Avoid hypothermia

In treating anesthesia-related arrhythmias (see also pp. 43–51), some general considerations should be kept in mind. Treat the underlying cause, if known, rather than indiscriminately using antiarrhythmic drugs. Correction of oxygenation, carbon dioxide levels, and acidemia of metabolic origin, as well as electrolyte correction, will aid in the treatment. Use of anticholinergic, cholinergics, or adrenergic agents when indicated may, in addition, prove beneficial.

One must try to avoid errors in judgement of anesthetic depth. Reconfirm the appropriate plane of surgical anesthesia. Ensure that adequate ventilation and IV support are present.

Administration of drugs that alter automaticity (epinephrine, atropine, thiobarbiturates, xylazine, potassium) concurrently with agents that sensitize myocardium (halothane) may induce arrhythmias. Avoid these combinations or treat arrythmias with specific counteractive pharmacologic agents.

The following types of arrhythmias dictate therapy:

1. *Atrial origin.* In general, those that interfere with efficient ventricular function should be treated. Examples include atrial tachycardia, fibrillation, paroxysmal atrial tachycardia, sinus bradycardia, and atrioventricular blocks.
2. *Ventricular origin.* Arrhythmias that present an "R-on-T" potential (ventricular fibrillation) should be treated. Those that impede efficient hemodynamics should also be resolved.
3. *Multiform ectopic ventricular beats.* These arrhythmias require therapy because of the possibility of uncoordinated Purkinje system depolarization, resulting in ventricular fibrillation.
4. *Ventricular ectopic beats that occur in "salvo" greater than three beats in succession.* Predisposition in ventricular fibrillation is present.
5. *Ventricular ectopic beats greater than 12 per minute.* A parasystolic focus with repetitive depolarization occurs. Interference with hemodynamics as well as predisposition to more significant arrhythmias.

Antiarrhythmic drugs include the following:

1. *Atropine,* 0.04 to 0.08 mg per kg, 1/3 to 1/2 given IV initially and the remainder given subcutaneously (SC) or intramuscularly (IM) for bradycardias and second-and third-degree heart blocks. Atropine can also be given via the airway, diluting the amount needed with an equal volume of sterile saline and given down the endotracheal tube. This technique is of value if an IV is not in place.
2. *Lidocaine* is still the drug of choice for therapy of ventricular origin arrhythmias. The dose is 1 to 2 mg per kg IV until the effect is achieved. In cats, epinephrine should not be used if at all possible, or if it must be used, use with extreme care at 1 mg per kg or less. An infusion rate of 40 to 60 μg per kg per minute may be used to maintain an antiarrythmic effect. Lidocaine can also be given transtracheally (2–4 mg/kg, with an equal volume of saline injected into the tracheal tube).
3. *Procainamide* is an effective agent for ventricular arrhythmias. It is parenterally administered IM; IV administration may be accompanied by hypotension. It may be used in conjunction with lidocaine for arrhythmia suppression. Dose range is wide, 6 to 20 mg per kg q6h has proved effective.
4. *Quinidine* is effective for both supraventricular and ventricular arrhythmias. Quinidine depresses both the depolarization rate and the conduction velocity, decreasing the automaticity of secondary pacemakers. Mild decreases in blood pressure may be noted. Side effects include bradyarrhythmias and gastrointestinal signs (nausea, vomiting). Dose schedule is 6 to 10 mg per kg TID or QID. Both oral and parenteral forms are commercially available.
5. *Propanolol* is an effective beta-adrenergic blocking drug. Propanolol is indicated in supraventricular tachyarrhythmias, with a secondary role in ventricular arrhythmias. A lidocaine-like effect on the cell membrane produces a delayed atrioventricular conduction, lengthened diastolic depolarization and depresses automaticity of ventricular tissue. Decreased cardiac output and hypotension may be noted with its use. Propanolol may be

administered orally or IV. IV administration should occur under ECG monitoring. An initial dose of 0.04 mg per kg is administered and may be repeated until desirable effects are noted.

6. *Potassium* administration in conjunction with lidocaine may accentuate antiarrhythmic activity. Rapid shifts in transcellular potassium concentration may alter automaticity, thus suppressing ectopic activity. Potassium may be safely administered at 20 to 40 mEq K^+ per 500 ml in conjunction with lidocaine. Do not give more than 1 mEq per kg per hour.

Increased oxygen ventilation may be very beneficial in severe arrhythmias.

Management of acute renal dysfunction during general anesthesia is similar to management of the acute renal failure patient. Measurement of urine output by closed collection of urine may be considered in preanesthetic, anesthetic, or postanesthetic cases or in animals with preexisting renal disease. The approach to management is described on pages 122–138.

Administration of anesthesia (Tables 10 and 11) is only as safe as the weakest "link." In many cases, the weak link is the anesthetist. Several surveys reporting preventable mishaps cite the person monitoring the anesthesia as the most frequent failure. Factors associated with preventable mishaps include unfamiliarity with equipment or the discipline of anesthesia, poor communication, haste, carelessness, fatigue, failure to perform a proper check or history, visual field restriction, "first time" incident. All these factors could be attributable to incidents occurring in veterinary practice.

In order to avoid mistakes (1) be familiar with the equipment and check it out prior to *each* anesthetic administration, (2) ensure that the proper equipment is maintained and available, (3) recognize and neutralize precursors of errors, and (4) organize materials.

Based on case studies accumulated at the University of Minnesota, accidents of human error occur at the following times and percentages:

Preinduction	6%
Induction	22%
Beginning of surgery	22%
Middle of surgery	38%
End of surgery	10%
After surgery	3%

OXYGEN FLOW RATES

Semi-Open Systems	Oxygen Flow Rate
Ayre's T-piece	2.0–2.5 × minute volume
Norman elbow	
Stephens-Slater	2.0–2.5 × minute volume
	1 × minute volume

Note: Minute volume is a product of tidal volume and resting respiratory rate. Tidal volume is approximately 22 ml per kg multiplied by body weight in kg.

Semi–Closed Systems	
Circle system	greater than 10 ml per kg per minute

Closed Systems	
Circle system	10 ml per kg per minute

Table 10. RECOMMENDED DOSAGES OF ANESTHETIC DRUGS

Agent	Dosage (mg/kg)	
	Dog	*Cat*
PREMEDICATION (all IM route unless noted)		
Anticholinergics		
Atropine sulphate	0.02–0.04	same
Glycopyrrolate	0.01–0.02	same
Ataractics		
Major		
Acepromazine	0.1–0.2	same
Promazine	0.6–1.0	1.0–3.0
Chlorpromazine	0.2–0.4	same
Droperidol	0.2–1.0	0.2–1.0
Minor		
Diazepam	0.25–0.5 IV	0.25–0.5 IV
Sedative		
Xylazine	0.4–1.0	0.4–1.0
Pentobarbitol	1–3	—
Narcotic agonists		
Morphine	0.4–1.5	0.1
Oxymorphone	0.11–0.22	0.04–0.22
Meperidine	2–6	2–4
Pentazocine	1–2	same
Fentanyl	0.02–0.04	—
Butorphanol	0.4	—
Nalbuphine	2	—
Dissociative		
Ketamine	6–10 (use with ataractic)	4–10
NEUROLEPTANALGESICS		
Fentamyl and droperidol (Innovar-Vet)	1 ml/10–30 kg IM	—
Acepromazine	0.1	0.05–0.1
Oxymorphone	0.1–0.2	0.02–0.2
Acepromazine	0.1	0.1
Meperidine	2–6	2–6
Diazepam	0.1 IV	0.1 IV
Oxymorphone	0.1–0.2	0.02–0.2
Acepromazine	0.05–0.1	—
Fentanyl	0.04–0.06	—
COMBINATION		
Ketamine	5–10	same
Acepromazine	0.1–0.2	same

Table continued on following page

Table 10. RECOMMENDED DOSAGES OF ANESTHETIC DRUGS
(Continued)

Agent	Dosage (mg/kg)	
	Dog	*Cat*
Ketamine	5–10	same
Diazepam	0.5–1.0 IV	same
Ketamine*	5–10	same
Xylazine*	0.4–1.0	same
Phenobarbital	2 IV	—
Diazepam	0.5 IV	—
Innovar	1 ml/20 kg	—
Pentobarbital	2–6	—
Narcotic/neuromuscular blocking agent	see individual dose schedules	
MAINTENANCE		
Inhalation Agents	MAC† *value (Vol %)*	
Methoxyflurane	0.23	same
Halothane	0.87	1.19
Enflurane	2.2	2.37
Isoflurane	1.5	1.61
Nitrous oxide	188	150
INDUCTION		
Sedative-hypnotics		
Thiamylal	12–18	same
Thiopental	12–18	same
Methohexital	10–12	—
Pentobarbital	20–25	same
Neuroleptanalgesics		
Fentanyl/droperidol (Innovar)	1 ml/10–30 kg	—
Oxymorphone	0.2	0.2
Acepromazine	0.1	0.1
Oxymorphone	0.2	0.1–0.2
Diazepam	0.2–0.5	0.1–0.2
Meperidine	4–6	4–6
Acepromazine	0.1	0.1
Dissociative		
Ketamine‡	—	10–20 IM
		10 IV

*This combination may cause a high incidence of serious heart block.

†MAC—The minimum alveolar concentration of anesthetic at 1 atmosphere that produces immobility in 50 per cent of the animals exposed to a noxious stimulus.

Note: Induction "dose" of 2.5–3.0 × MAC is used for all agents except N_2O. The maintenance level of 1.5–2.0 × MAC is usually satisfactory. Nitrous oxide is mixed with oxygen in a 1:1 to 2:1 ratio and may decrease levels required of other inhalation agents.

‡The preanesthetic usage of Valium, 0.1 mg/kg prior to Ketamine is suggested.

Table 11. ANESTHETIC REVERSAL

Agent	Dosage (mg/kg)
NARCOTIC ANTAGONISTS	
Naloxone	0.04–0.06 IV or IM
Levallorphan	0.1–0.2 IV
Nalorphine	0.2–1.0 IV
AROUSAL AGENTS	
Doxapram	0.5–1.0 IV

INJECTABLE AGENTS

All induction techniques may be supplemented by continued incremental dose administration to maintain anesthesia. In general, redosing at one half the original amount as necessary is prudent.

A combination of injectable agents at low doses plus inhalant agents will produce satisfactory patient anesthesia. Examples include:
1. Narcotic + muscle relaxant + $N_2O:O_2$.
2. Narcotic + muscle relaxant + IMAC inhalant agent.
3. Neuroleptanalgesic + muscle relaxant + $N_2O:O_2$.
4. Dissociative agent + ataractic + inhalant.
Consult individual dose schedules for guidelines of usage.

Table 12. FACTORS THAT ALTER ANESTHETIC REQUIREMENT—MAC

Factor	Effect	
	Increase	*Decrease*
Body temperature		
-hypothermia	—	×
-hyperthermia	×	—
Age		
-newborn (24 hr)	—	×
-6 months	×	—
-adult	—	—
-geriatric	—	×
Thyroid function		
-hyperthyroidism	×	—
-hypothyroidism	—	×
Anesthetic adjuvants and other drugs		
-Atropine	—	×
-Scopolamine	—	×
-Narcotics	—	×
-Diazepam	—	slight ×
-Nitrous oxide	—	×
-CNS stimulants	×	—
-CNS depressants	—	×

Table 13. IMPORTANT CHARACTERISTICS OF COMMON
NEUROMUSCULAR BLOCKING AGENTS

Generic Name	Succinylcholine chloride	Gallamine triethiodide	Pancuronium bromide
Trade Name	Sucostrin or Anectine	Flaxedil	Pavulon
Manufacturer	E. R. Squibb & Sons, Inc., New York, NY 10022	Davis & Geck American Cyanamid Co., Pearl River, NY 10965	Organon, Inc., West Orange, NJ 07052
Mode of Action	Depolarizing	Nondepolarizing	Nondepolarizing
Dose, initial (mg/ kg); repeat	0.1–0.4; 100 mg in 500 D5W*	1.0–2.0 0.1	0.06–0.10 0.01
Metabolism and Excretion			
Major	Plasma	Renal	Renal
Minor	—	—	Liver
Cardiovascular Effects	Some blood pressure ↑ due to ganglionic stimulation	Marked increase in heart rate; mild increase in blood pressure	Slight ↑ heart rate due to vagal block
Time of onset	0.75 min	1.5–2.0 min	0.75–1.0 min
Duration of Effect	20–30 min—dog 3–5 min—cat	30 min	45–60 min

*Start with minidrip set where 60 drops = 1 ml, and begin rate at 0.003–0.01 mg/ kg/min = 1–3 drops/kg/min.

Table 13. IMPORTANT CHARACTERISTICS OF COMMON NEUROMUSCULAR BLOCKING AGENTS *(Continued)*

Tubocurarine chloride	Dimethyltubocurarine	Atracurium besylate	Vercuronium (ORGNC45)
Tubocurarine	Metubine Iodide	Tracrium	Norcuron
Abbott Labs, North Chicago, IL 60064	Eli Lilly, Indianapolis, IN	Burroughs, Wellcome Co., Research Triangle Pk., NC 27709	Organon, Inc., West Orange, NJ 07052
Nondepolarizing	Nondepolarizing	Nondepolarizing	Nondepolarizing
0.2–0.4	0.2–0.4 mg	0.2–0.4 mg	0.05 mg
0.05	0.1–0.1 mg	0.2 mg	
Renal	Renal	Plasma cholinesterase Metabolism	Liver
Liver	Liver		Kidney
Slight heart rate ↑; hypotension from histamine release	Some blood pressure changes due to ganglionic blocking ↓; slight increase in heart rate	Slight decrease in blood pressure	—
2.0–4.0 min	1.5–2.0 min	1.5–3.0 min	1.5–4.0 min
60–90 min	30–45 min	30–45 min	30–45 min

CONTROLLED VENTILATION
by A. J. Crimmi*

Controlled ventilation is used for (1) drug-induced respiratory depression; (2) thoracic trauma (chest wall or lung) or neuromuscular disease; (3) chest-filling defects (tumors, pneumothorax, hemothorax, pleural effusion); (4) diaphragmatic compromise due to abdominal pressure caused by a gas-filled gastrointestinal tract, tumors, pyometra, diaphragmatic hernias, or fetuses presented for cesarean section; and (5) cardiac resuscitation.

Assisted vs Controlled Ventilation

Assisted ventilation refers to situations in which the patient directly controls either the respiratory rate or the tidal volume. Controlled ventilation refers to situations in which the respiratory rate and the tidal volume are controlled by the ventilator. For practical purposes, controlled ventilation is usually used. The depressant effects of anesthetic drugs coupled with stretch receptor reflexes will result in patients in an assisted mode of ventilation, being hypoventilated. Mechanical ventilation of any sort requires CNS depression, to nearly a medium anesthetic plane, or paralysis.

Physiologic Parameters

The following physiologic parameters must be considered:
1. Normal tidal volumes are 15 to 20 ml per kg of ideal body weight.
2. Normal respiratory rates are 8 to 12 breaths per minute.
3. Normal peak airway pressures are 12 to 20 cm H_2O.
4. Normal inspiratory time is 1.5 to 2 seconds.
5. Normal time of active expiration is 2 to 3 seconds.

Objective of Controlled Ventilation

The objective of controlled ventilation is to "mimic" normal ventilation, that is, determine rate, tidal volume, and inspiratory/expiratory time.

Rate is determined by a timing mechanism. Tidal volume is determined by directly limiting bag or bellows displacement or indirectly by limiting inspiratory pressure or inspiratory flow rate.

Inspiratory time is controlled indirectly by varying the flow rate of gas driving the bellows or directly by rate of displacement when hand bagging. Expiratory flow rate can be passively controlled (dependent on chest wall compliance) or actively controlled (dependent on a weighted bellows or negative expiratory pressure).

Hand Bagging vs Mechanical Ventilation

Hand bagging is preferred during (1) brief periods of ventilatory support; (2) external cardiac massage, due to the interference of the massage on

*Assistant Scientist, Department of Anesthesiology, College of Veterinary Medicine, University of Minnesota, St. Paul, Minnesota.

mechanical ventilator function; and (3) situations in which the demands of the patient are beyond the capability of available mechanical ventilators, such as variable airway leaks and conscious resistance to ventilation.

Mechanical ventilation is preferred during (1) extended periods of support (Machines are very repeatable in their functions whereas humans fatigue both physically and mentally.); (2) situations in which patient management is more than the available personnel can handle. (Under these circumstances, ventilators function as helping hands.); and (3) situations that demand support functions that hand bagging cannot supply, such as negative expiratory pressures.

Basic Ventilator Design

All ventilators *must* have controls to vary the rate, tidal volume, and inspiratory time. Additionally, ventilators *may* have controls to start and stop, alter expiratory flow rate, allow for patient override of ventilatory rate, and allow for operator override of tidal volume. This feature allows for occasional sighing or inspiratory hold. Some ventilators allow the interchanging of hand bagging and mechanical ventilation.

Pitfalls of Mechanical Ventilation

It must be remembered that mechanical ventilators are simply machines that are designed to mindlessly perform a few tasks, within a limited range of flexibility. They are capable of failure and dependably reproduce any human error in their setup. Ventilators are not tools that diminish the need for patient monitoring; the adequacy of patient ventilation must still be continuously monitored. In fact, if one chooses to use a ventilator, one's monitoring chores will be more difficult because, in addition to the patient, one now also has a machine to monitor. Some common problems encountered in the use of mechanical ventilators include:

1. Leaks caused by patient disconnect, airway/endotracheal tube leaks, open pop-off valves on anesthetic machines, deterioration of rubber goods
2. Erratic performance due to dirty driving gas
3. Disruptions of driving gas supply

Adverse Effects of Mechanical Ventilation

1. Positive intrathoracic pressure decreases venous return and cardiac filling.
2. Excessive positive pressure can rupture pulmonary tissues.
3. Positive pressure ventilation can cause gas trapping. Pneumothorax can be severely aggravated in the closed chest and ventilated patients with airway obstruction can have gas trapping within the lungs themselves.

Ventilators Available for Veterinary Use

Bird MK7 Ventilator
Description
The bird MK7 ventilator exists as an integral part of a complete anesthesia machine or alone for respiratory therapy, but it is not interfaced with a separate

anesthetic machine. It has six controls, some of which are interrelated. Disregard all numbers on the controls, because they are used for machine calibration only. Three controls are located on the front of the ventilator, two are located on the left side, and the remaining control is located on the right side.

Setup and Check-out Prior to Patient Attachment

Check for integrity of gas supply by turning the *flow rate knob* counterclockwise 180 degrees. This control is located on the top front of the ventilator. Depress the *hand timer rod* on the left hand side of the machine; the ventilator should cycle. During this check, the *sensitivity arm*, located on the left side of the machine, should be in a vertical position.

If using the ventilator as an anesthesia machine, check O_2 flow meter, sodasorb, and inhalant level; and check for leaks by cycling the ventilator as just described, with the O_2 flow meter off. When the ventilator stops the inspiratory part of the cycle, occlude the end of the patient Y-piece and observe the bellows; it should not fall. During this check and during subsequent use, the *air-mix knob* should be pulled out. This knob is located in the center of the front panel.

Allow the ventilator to cycle, on its own, for 60 seconds, and determine the number of cycles per minute. Adjust the cycling rate to the desired respiratory rate by increasing or decreasing the *expiratory time* (time between breaths). The longer the expiratory time, the fewer breaths per minute. Clockwise rotation of this knob increases the time between breaths. The control is located toward the bottom of the front panel.

Occlude the patient Y-piece at the end of expiration, and keep it occluded through one entire cycle. Watch the pressure manometer on the front of the ventilator. Adjust the pressure that the ventilator achieves by turning the *pressure limit arm*, located on the right side of the ventilator, either clockwise (increases pressure) or counterclockwise (decreases pressure).

Setup After Patient Attachment

Adjust the inspiratory time to the desired interval by turning the flow rate knob either clockwise (increases inspiratory time) or counterclockwise (decreases inspiratory time). Check the patient's tidal volume by observing for adequate chest excursion. The tidal volume may be either increased or decreased by increasing or decreasing the inspiratory pressure. Recheck the respiratory rate; it may be greater than initially set as a result of patient override. If the rate is greater than that set, either the patient is too light or he is being ventilated improperly.

Pitman-Moore Metomatic Ventilator

Description

This unit must be interfaced with a separate anesthetic machine. Connecting this unit directly to a patient's endotracheal tube will result in certain death. This ventilator has eight controls; seven are located on the front of the control box, the eighth is located near the top of the bellows assembly.

Setup and Check-out Prior to Patient Attachment

Check for integrity of gas supply by turning the *on-off knob* to the on position. This control is located on the lower left front of the control box. If the ventilator does not immediately cycle, depress and release the *manual trigger button*. This button is located on the top of the hex-nut located on the right center front of the control box. During this check, the indicator on the *inspiratory trigger effort knob* should be in a vertical position. This control is located on the lower right front of the control box.

Allow the ventilator to cycle, on its own, for 60 seconds, and determine the number of cycles per minute. Adjust the cycling rate to the desired respiratory rate by increasing or decreasing the *expiratory time* (time between breaths). The longer the expiratory time, the fewer breaths per minute. This control is located on the upper right front of the control box.

Set the desired tidal volume by raising or lowering the bottom of the bellows. This is accomplished by turning the *tidal volume knob*, located near the top of the bellows. The amount of bellows displacement is determined by using the volume scale located on the front of the bellows canister. The bellows should be set to displace approximately 200 ml more than the intended tidal volume, because some is "lost" in the expansion of the patient circuit hoses during inspiration. Allow the ventilator to cycle several times after adjusting the bellows. Due to the design of this control, it has a tendency to self-adjust during the first few cycles, During this check, the indicator on the *inspiratory pressure knob* should be in a vertical position. This control is located on the lower right front of the control box.

Adjust the inspiratory time to the desired interval by turning the *inspiratory flow rate knob* either clockwise (decreases inspiratory time) or counterclockwise (increases inspiratory time). This control is located on the upper right front of the control box.

Adjust the expiratory time to the desired interval by turning the *expiratory flow rate knob* either clockwise (decreases expiratory time) or counter clockwise (increases expiratory time). This control is located on the upper left front of the control box.

Attach the patient circuit hose on the ventilator to the bag fitting on the anesthesia machine. Close the pop-off valve on the anesthesia machine, and connect your waste gas scavenging hose to the port located near the top of the bellows assembly.

Setup After Patient Attachment

Check the patient's tidal volume by observing for adequate chest excursion. At this time, the inspiratory pressure knob should be adjusted, so that the yellow line on the bellows travels all the way to the zero mark. The bellows should not hang up at the top, however, at the end of inspiration. The tidal volume may be either increased or decreased by increasing or decreasing the volume that the bellows displaces.

Recheck the respiratory rate; it may be greater than initially set due to patient override. If the rate is greater than that set, either the patient is too light or he is being ventilated improperly.

Drager AV Anesthesia Ventilator

Description

This unit must be interfaced with a separate anesthesia machine. Connecting this unit directly to a patient endotracheal tube will result in certain death. This ventilator has four controls; three are located on the front of the control box, the fourth is located near the bottom of the bellows assembly.

Setup and Check-out Prior to Patient Attachment

Check for integrity of gas supply by turning the *on-off knob* to the on position. This control is located on the left front of the control box. The ventilator should cycle.

Allow the ventilator to cycle for 60 seconds, on its own, and determine the number of cycles per minute. Adjust the cycling rate to the desired respiratory rate by adjusting the *frequency knob* located in the center front of the control box. Clockwise rotation of the knob increases the frequency of breaths per minute.

Set the desired tidal volume by raising or lowering the bottom of the bellows. This is accomplished by turning the *tidal volume knob* located near the bottom of the bellows assembly. The amount of bellows displacement is determined by using the volume scale located on the front of the bellows canister. The bellows should be set to displace approximately 200 ml more than the intended tidal volume, because some is "lost" in the expansion of the patient circuit hoses during inspiration.

Attach the patient circuit hose on the ventilator to the bag fitting on the anesthesia machine. Close the pop-off valve on the anesthesia machine, and connect your waste gas scavenging hose to the port located near the top of the bellows assembly.

Setup After Patient Attachment

Adjust the inspiratory time to the desired interval by turning the *flow control knob* either clockwise (decreases inspiratory time) or counterclockwise (increases inspiratory time). This control is located on the right front of the control box. This control should always be set such that the bellows reaches the upper stop.

Check the patient's tidal volume by observing for adequate chest excursion. The tidal volume may be either increased or decreased by increasing or decreasing the volume that the bellows displaces.

EAR EMERGENCIES

Foreign bodies within the ear canal, foxtails for example, may result in acute inflammation and pressure necrosis of the tissue of the external auditory meatus, causing severe pain and discomfort. Acute inflammation of the external auditory meatus or middle ear may result in sudden pain and discomfort for the animal.

Adequate examination and treatment of the ear in an animal in pain requires the use of a short-acting anesthetic, such as thiamylal sodium, or a neuroleptanalgesic agent. Examine the ear canal as described on page 394. Carefully remove visible foreign bodies with alligator forceps. Obtain samples of pus or exudates in the ear canal and perform bacterial and/or fungal cultures (see p. 499), then gently irrigate the external ear canal with warm, sterile saline, removing debris and exudates. When irrigating, do not allow excessive pressure (over 50 mm Hg) to build up, because it may rupture an inflamed tympanic membrane. After all detritus and exudate has been removed and the ear canal has been dried, inspect the tympanic membrane. Inflammation of the external ear canal requires instillation of antibiotic-steroid ointment such as Panalog and the use of narcotics if pain is severe.

Characteristics of otitis media involving the inner ear are head rotation with the affected ear down, circling to the affected side, falling or rolling to the affected side, nystagmus, fever, depression, and severe pain. Most cases of otitis media are accompanied by a severe otitis externa, which must be treated simultaneously. The most common cause of otitis media is bacterial infection with staphylococcus sp, streptococcus sp, pseudomonas, *Escherichia coli* or proteus sp. Otitis media can develop by infection spreading across the tympanic membrane from the external ear canal, through the eustachian tubes (rare), or through the blood to the middle ear. In most cases of otitis media, the tympanic membrane is ruptured. If the tympanic membrane is not ruptured but is swollen and hyperemic, a myringotomy should be performed. A culture of debris and exudate from the tympanic cavity should be obtained, and a sensitivity test should be performed. The tympanic cavity is then cleaned and a liquid antibiotic such as chloramphenicol solution is instilled. If otitis media persists despite initial treatment, radiographic examination of the bullae is of value in better defining the pathology involved. Surgical drainage of the tympanic bulla may be required.

References and Additional Reading

Neer, M. T., and Howard, P. E.: Otitis media. Compendium of Continuing Education, 4(5):410, 1982.

Spreull, J. S. A.: Otitis media of the dog. *In* Kirk, R. W. (ed.): Current Veterinary Therapy V. Philadelphia, W. B. Saunders Company, 1974.

Venker-van Hagen, A. J.: Managing diseases of the ear. *In* Kirk, R. W. (ed.): Current Veterinary Therapy 8: Small Animal Practice. Philadelphia, W. B. Saunders Company, 1983.

OCULAR EMERGENCIES*

An ocular emergency is any serious situation that threatens or has already caused loss of vision or severe pain and deformity. The following ocular emergencies should be treated within one to several hours following injury:

Penetrating injuries of the globe
Proptosis of the globe
Acute corneal abrasion or ulcer
Ocular foreign bodies
Acute iritis

*This section is adapted from Bistner, S. I., and Aguirre, G. D.: Management of ocular emergencies. Vet. Clin. North Am., 2:359, 1972.

Hyphema
Descemetocele
Lid laceration
Pupillary block glaucoma (acute glaucoma)
Orbital cellulitis
Corneal laceration
Chemical burns

ASSESSMENT OF OCULAR INJURIES

A carefully performed ocular examination is necessary to assess the degree of ocular injury. Frequently, adequate sedation or a short-acting general anesthetic will be required to permit a complete examination. The following equipment is needed:

Loupe
Direct ophthalmoscope with rechargeable handle and Finoff transilluminator
Fine-tooth forceps
Lid retractors
Lacrimal probes
Sterile eye wash solution in irrigating bottle
Fluorescein-impregnated sterile strips
"Weck-cel" sponges
Topical anesthetic (proparacaine, 0.5 per cent)
Culture swabs and culture media
Schiötz tonometer
Short-acting mydriatic (tropicamide, 1 per cent)

Procedure

1. Obtain an adequate history. This may reveal the existence of previous eye disease, the instillation of some chemical irritant, or the occurrence of trauma. Try to determine when the injury occurred and if any medication or eye wash has been used.
2. Examine the eye for any discharge, blepharospasm, or photophobia. If discharge is present, note the type. If the animal is in extreme discomfort with the eye completely closed, *do not* try to force the lids open.
3. Note the position of the globe within the orbit. If the eye is exophthalmic, there is frequently strabismus and protrusion of the third eyelid, exposure keratitis, and, in cases of retrobulbar or zygomatic salivary gland inflammation, pain on opening the mouth. Note any displacement of the globe medially or temporally.
4. Note any swelling, contusions, or lacerations of the lids. Note whether the lids are able to cover the cornea. In cases of lid lacerations, try to determine the depth of the laceration. Penetrating lid lacerations may be associated with secondary injury to the globe,
5. Palpate the orbital margins, feeling for fractures, crepitus, air, and cellulitis.

6. Examine the cornea and sclera for evidence of partially penetrating or completely penetrating injuries. The use of lid retractors in these cases can be very helpful. If the wound is completely penetrating, look for loss of uveal tissue, lens, or vitreous. Do not put pressure on the globe, because intraocular herniation will result.

7. Examine the conjunctiva for hemorrhage, chemosis, lacerations, or foreign bodies. Examine the superior and inferior conjunctival cul-de-sacs for foreign bodies. Occasionally, topical anesthesia and a sterile cotton swab can be used to "sweep" the conjunctival fornix in order to pick up foreign bodies. Use a small, fine-toothed forceps to pick up the third eyelid, and examine its bulbar aspect for foreign bodies.

8. Examine the cornea for opacities, ulcers, foreign bodies, abrasions, or lacerations. A loupe and a good focal source of illumination are important in conducting this examination.

9. Record pupil size, shape, and response to light, both direct and consensual.

10. Examine the anterior chamber, and note its depth and the presence of hyphema, iridodonesis, or iridodialysis.

11. If indicated and if the cornea is undamaged, measure intraocular pressure.

12. Examine the posterior ocular segment using a short-acting dilating agent and a direct or indirect ophthalmoscope to look for intraocular hemorrhage, retinal hemorrhage or edema formation, and retinal detachment.

When examining an animal with an ocular emergency, the history may indicate sudden loss of vision occurring unilaterally or bilaterally. The following conditions can produce sudden loss of vision (see also p. 233):

Hyphema or vitreous hemorrhage

Traumatic lid swelling

Extensive corneal edema or exposure keratitis

Acute congestive glaucoma

Retinal hemorrhage or extensive retinal edema

Retinal detachment

Extensive trauma to or avulsion of the optic nerve

Intracranial damage secondary to hemorrhage, ischemia, or anoxia, resulting in the interruption of visual pathways

Proptosis of the globe

The following basic surgical instruments should be at hand to treat ocular lacerations and other types of emergencies:

Castroviejo or Barraquer lid speculum

Bishop-Harmon tissue forceps

Stevens tenotomy scissors—standard

Castroviejo corneal scissors

Castroviejo needle holder—standard jaws with lock

Beaver knife handle and No. 64 blades

Lacrimal cannula—straight 22 gauge

Barraquer iris repositor

Foreign body spud

Enucleation scissors—medium curve

Suture material—6-0 silk, 4-0 nylon, 7-0 collagen, or 6-0 ophthalmic gut, 7-0 nylon

Injuries of the Lids

Lid contusions and lacerations are most commonly associated with bite wounds or automobile trauma. Basic principles of surgical treatment of lid lacerations are similar to other areas of the body; however, very careful primary repair must be undertaken to ensure adequate physiologic and cosmetic results.

The puncta lacrimalia are located in the mucocutaneous junction, 2 to 4 mm from the medial canthus of both the upper and lower lids. The puncta are slitlike openings frequently surrounded by a small amount of pigment. In correcting eyelid lacerations, the surgeon must keep in mind the location of the puncta and maintain their normal function.

The lids can be considered a two layered structure, with the anterior layer composed of skin and orbicularis muscle and the posterior layer composed of tarsus and conjunctiva. The openings of the meibomian glands in the lid margin form the approximate line separating the lids into anterior and posterior segments. Splitting the lid into these two components facilitates the use of sliding skin flaps to close wound defects. Large defects in the conjunctiva and tarsus can be corrected by transposing the lid tissue with the same tissue from the opposing lid.

The conjunctiva is a mucous membrane that covers the posterior surface of the lids (palpebral conjunctiva) and reflects onto the globe (bulbar conjunctiva) at the fornix. The natural looseness of the conjunctiva permits extensive mobilization for surgical repairs.

Gentle cleansing and careful and thorough irrigation are necessary preoperative routines before correcting lid lacerations. Use sterile intravenous (IV) saline to irrigate the wound. The conjunctival sac is also irrigated and foreign bodies are removed. A solution of Betadine can be used on the skin. Draping the wound with eyedrapes is necessary to prevent further contamination.

In lid lacerations, ragged wound margins should be trimmed and very conservative tissue débridement should be performed. However, *as much tissue as possible should be saved* to minimize wound contracture and lid deformity. When correcting a ragged lid margin, trim the tarsus in a slightly curved fashion to permit slight overcorrection and "pouting" of the suture incision when the lid is sutured vertically. This helps to ensure tight lid closure and prevents excessive scarring.

Close small wounds of the lid margin with a figure-of-eight or a two-layered simple interrupted suture of 4-0 or 5-0 silk, polypropylene, or nylon. The lid margins must be absolutely apposed to prevent postoperative lid notching.

In more extensive lacerations, splitting the lid along the margin just anterior to the meibomian gland openings permits mobilization of the skin, orbicularis muscle layer, and a two-layered closure. Suture the conjunctiva with 6-0 or 7-0 gut or collagen. Use an interrupted pattern, with the knots tied so as not to touch the cornea. Suture the skin in a different plane, using 6-0 ophthalmic silk, polypropylene, or nylon.

Ecchymosis of the Lids

Because of the excellent vascular supply to the eyelids, direct blows may cause ecchymosis. Associated ocular injury such as orbital hemorrhage, proptosis, or corneal laceration may occur. Trauma, allergic reactions, and internal or external hordeolum may also result in lid ecchymosis.

Treat lid ecchymosis initially with cold compresses, followed later by warm compresses. Resorption of blood may occur in from 3 to 10 days. Ocular allergies respond to topical and systemic administration of corticosteroids, such as 0.1 dexamethasone ointment TID or QID, plus the application of cold compresses.

Conjunctival Lacerations

Conjunctival lacerations and contusions are common following trauma. It is important to carefully examine conjunctival lacerations for evidence of underlying pathologic conditions. The conjunctiva may have to be carefully dissected away from the underlying sclera to provide a better view of any abnormalities. Undue pressure should not be placed on the globe when performing this dissection in order to prevent herniation of intraocular contents through a scleral wound.

Repair of large conjunctival lacerations can be accomplished by the use of 6-0 gut or collagen using an interrupted or continuous suture pattern. The margins of the conjunctiva should be carefully approximated to prevent inclusion cysts from forming. When large areas of conjunctiva have been damaged, conjunctival advancement flaps may be used to close the defect.

Subconjunctival Hemorrhage

Subconjunctival hemorrhage is a common sequela to head trauma. In itself, it is not a serious problem. However, it may indicate the presence of more severe intraocular damage; therefore, a complete eye examination is indicated. Subconjunctival hemorrhage also may be associated with various types of blood dyscrasias and systemic diseases, including thrombocytopenia, autoimmune hemolytic anemia, hemophilia, leptospirosis, severe systemic infections, and difficult or prolonged labor (dystocia).

Uncomplicated subconjunctival hemorrhage usually clears within 14 days. If the conjunctiva is exposed because of the hemorrhage, use a protective ophthalmic antibiotic ointment. Methylcellulose drops or hydroxymethylcellulose drops also can be used until the chemosis is reduced.

Chemical Injuries

Chemical injuries of the eye are arbitrarily classified into toxic, acid, or alkali. The severity of ocular burns from chemical injury is dependent on the concentration of the chemical, the duration of exposure, and the pH of the solution.

Weak acids do not penetrate biologic tissues very well. The hydrogen ion precipitates protein on contact, providing some protection to the corneal stroma and intraocular contents. Precipitation of the epithelial proteins produces a ground glass appearance of the cornea.

Alkalis (and very strong acids) penetrate tissues rapidly, saponify plasma membranes, denature collagen, and cause vascular thromboses in the conjunctiva, episclera, and anterior uvea.

The severe pain, blepharospasm, and photophobia accompanying chemical ocular injury results from direct stimulation to free nerve endings located in the epithelium of the cornea and the conjunctival lining. Severe burns with alkalis produce a rise in intraocular pressure; intraocular prostaglandin release; increase in aqueous humor pH; alteration in blood-aqueous barrier and secondary uveitis; and intraocular uveitis with secondary synechia formation, eventual chronic glaucoma or phthisis, secondary cataract, and corneal perforation.

Early repair of epithelial defects is accomplished by sliding and increased mitosis of epithelial cells. Healing of the epithelial surface is usually accompanied by vascularization. Severe corneal stromal burns heal by degradation and removal of necrotic debris and replacement of collagenous matrix and cells. Polymorphonuclear response can result in degranulation of these cells with release of agents such as collagenase, endopeptidases, and cathepsins, that serve to further break down the corneal stroma. In very severe corneal burns, only PMNs may be present in the corneal stroma and fibroblasts may never invade the stroma.

Initial Treatment

All chemical burns should receive copious lavage with any clean aqueous solution available. Remove any sticky paste or powder (e.g. lime) from the conjunctival sac by cotton-tipped applicators that can be soaked in EDTA, 0.01 molar solution.

In very severe burns with alkali, paracentesis of the anterior chamber and replacing fluid with balanced salt solution may help bring the pH back toward normal.

Begin mydriasis and cycloplegia with topical atropine, 1 per cent drops or ointment. Begin antibiotic therapy with gentamicin ointment 4 or 5 times a day. Secondary glaucomas can be treated with carbonic anhydrase inhibitors. Analgesics are needed for pain. Keep the conjunctival cul-de-sacs free of proteinaceous exudate to avoid fibrinous adhesions and symblepharon formation.

Persistent epithelial erosions can be treated with a conjunctival flap left in place for 3 to 4 weeks. Topical antibiotics, mydriatics, and lubricants such as Adapt drops or Lacrilube ointment should be used.

Corneal stromal loss is most likely to develop in eyes burned with strong alkali or strong acids. Although the type of treatment is controversial, the use of acetylcysteine, 10 per cent (Mucomyst), or EDTA, 0.2 molar solution dropped onto the cornea 5 times a day is used to inhibit mammalian collagenase activity.

The use of topical steroids after the ocular chemical burn is very controversial. The advantage of steroid use such as prednisolone acetate, 1 per cent drops topically, is to reduce intraocular inflammation. The disadvantage is the retardation of wound healing by inhibiting fibroblast formation. It is best to avoid topical steroids if possible, especially 7 to 10 days after an alkali burn.

Corneal Abrasions

Corneal epithelial abrasions are exceedingly painful and are characterized by intense blepharospasm, lacrimation, and photophobia. Movement of the eyelids or third eyelid seems to cause more discomfort. Animals in such discomfort are difficult to examine until effective relief from pain is achieved. Topical use of 0.5 per cent proparacaine hydrochloride will permit relaxation of the lids so that the eye can be examined. Using a focal source of illumination and an eye loupe, examine the inferior and superior conjunctival fornices and medial aspect of the membrana nictitans for foreign bodies. Place a drop of sterile saline on a sterile paper strip impregnated with fluorescein and touch the superior conjunctiva. The fluorescein spreads rapidly in the tear film to cover the cornea. Irrigate the excess fluorescein from the eye with sterile saline. Areas of corneal epithelial damage will remain green.

Barring complications, minor corneal epithelial abrasions rapidly heal. A cycloplegic (1 per cent atropine) is used to make the eye more comfortable and to reduce the effects of the secondary iridocyclitis that usually develops. A broad-spectrum antibiotic ointment is used 6 times a day to prevent secondary infections. The animal is kept out of bright light, and an analgesic is administered if pain is severe. The eye is re-examined in 48 hours. Topical anesthetics or antibiotic-steroid-anesthetic combinations are not dispensed. These products tend to retard healing and may lead to superinfection.

Penetrating Corneal Lacerations

Penetrating corneal lacerations may result in prolapse of intraocular contents. Frequently, pieces of uveal tissue or fibrin effectively but temporarily seal the wound and permit the anterior chamber to reform. Manipulation of these wounds should be avoided until the animal has been anesthetized. Care should be used in anesthetizing an animal with a corneal laceration, because struggling and/or excitement during administration of anesthesia may result in loss of the temporary seal in the corneal laceration and extrusion of intraocular contents.

Preparation for repair of a corneal laceration should be as meticulous as for any intraocular surgery. Superficial corneal lacerations need not be sutured. However, if the laceration extends through 50 per cent or more of the cornea or if it is more than 3 to 4 mm in length, sutures are required to close the wound.

Careful, accurate suturing is essential to maintain a watertight corneal wound and to minimize scar formation. Use of magnification by the surgeon is advantageous in properly placing sutures in the cornea. Silk sutures, 7-0 or 8-

0, collagen sutures, 7-0 or 8-0, or fine sutures, 8-0 to 9-0 nylon, all with micropoint spatula type needles, are effective in closing corneal wounds. Sutures are tied individually and are left in place for a minimum of 3 weeks. Many corneal wounds are jagged in appearance or the cornea is edematous and tight closure is not possible. In these cases, a thin conjunctival flap is pulled down (or up) over the corneal wound to help seal it and prevent aqueous loss. Sutures must never be placed through the entire full thickness of the cornea but should cross into the middle third of the stroma.

Following closure of the corneal wound, the anterior chamber must be reformed to prevent synechia formation and the resulting secondary glaucoma. Taking care to avoid injury to the iris, insert a 25- or 26-gauge needle into the anterior chamber at the limbus. Gently instill sterile saline solution to reform the anterior chamber. Defects in the suture line will be recognized by leakage of fluid, and they should be repaired. The anterior chamber should not be overfilled for fear of inducing secondary glaucoma, nor should the eye be left hypotonic.

Incarceration of uveal tissue in corneal wounds presents a difficult surgical problem. Persistence of incarcerated uveal tissue predisposes to a chronic filtering wick in the cornea, shallow anterior chamber, chronic irritation, edema and vascularization of the cornea, and intraocular infection, leading to panophthalmitis.

Occasionally, the use of a mydriatic agent (e.g., 1 per cent atropine and/or 10 per cent phenylephrine) permits removal of a small tag of uveal tissue from a corneal wound. This is only possible soon after the injury, before synechiae have formed (usually within 24 to 48 hours).

Incarcerated uveal tissue (usually iris) can be surgically removed from a corneal wound in several ways. The uveal tissue can be trimmed from the corneal wound using an electroscalpel and/or scissors and the wound swept with a blunt cyclodialysis spatula to free further adhesions. Repair the corneal wound as previously described.

Conjunctival flaps can be used in the correction of large corneal lacerations and in deep stromal ulceration or perforation.

Ocular Foreign Bodies

The most common foreign bodies associated with ocular injuries in small animals are birdshot, B-B pellets, and glass. The site of intraocular penetration of these foreign bodies may be obscured by the eyelids.

A foreign body entering the eye may penetrate the cornea and fall into the anterior chamber or become lodged in the iris. Foreign bodies may penetrate the anterior capsule of the lens, producing cataracts. Some metallic, high-speed foreign bodies may pass through the cornea, iris, and lens to lodge in the posterior wall of the eye or in the vitreous cavity. Occasionally, a foreign body may pass entirely through the eye and remain within the orbit.

There are numerous techniques available to determine the presence and location of ocular foreign bodies. Direct visualization of a foreign body is the best means of localization. Examination of the eye with the biomicroscope or indirect ophthalmoscope may prove invaluable in locating foreign bodies. The anterior chamber and anterior drainage angle can be directly viewed with the aid of a gonioprism. A careful ocular examination should be performed as early as possible before secondary ocular inflammation or cataract formation opacifies the ocular media.

Indirect demonstration of an intraocular foreign body may be achieved by radiographic techniques. At least three radiographic views should be taken.

In addition to radiography, the more refined technique of ultrasonography may be used to locate foreign bodies.

Intraocular penetration by a foreign body always results in a guarded prognosis, and the outcome largely depends on the foreign body's chemical nature and its position within the eye. Foreign bodies composed of iron or copper can produce extensive ocular inflammation.

When considering removing any foreign body from an eye, weigh the dangers of leaving the foreign body in the eye against those of surgically removing it. Foreign objects in the anterior chamber are much easier to remove than objects at the posterior pole. Magnetic foreign bodies are easier to remove than nonmagnetic ones. Attempted removal of foreign bodies from the vitreous cavity of animals has consistently produced poor results. In many cases, the eye has been enucleated.

Ocular Traumatic Injuries

Blunt trauma to the eye can result in luxation or subluxation of the lens. The subluxated lens may move anteriorly, thus shallowing the anterior chamber. Trembling of the iris (iridodonesis) may be noticed when the lens is subluxated. In complete luxation, the lens may come to lie in the anterior chamber, thus causing obstruction to aqueous outflow, or may be lost in the vitreous cavity. Luxation of the lens is almost always associated with rupture of the hyaloid membrane and herniation of the vitreous through the pupillary space.

Emergency surgery for lens dislocation is required if the lens is entirely within the anterior chamber or incarcerated within the pupil, thus causing a secondary pupillary-block glaucoma. This elevation of intraocular pressure can result in severe visual loss within 48 hours; thus lens removal should be accomplished as quickly as possible. Incarceration of the vitreous in the pupil can also produce pupillary block glaucoma. Recognition of vitreous herniation into the anterior chamber prior to surgery is important. Complications of vitreous loss may then be minimized by administering systemic hyperosmotic agents or by aspiration of liquid vitreous at the pars plana. Intravitreal dislocation of the lens is a serious problem; however, do not routinely operate on these cases, because postoperative results are uniformly poor.

Surgical management of dislocated lenses is a difficult problem with many complications, chief of which is loss of vitreous. Preoperative management is extremely important. If the lens is in the anterior chamber, take measures to prevent the lens from falling into the posterior chamber during surgery.

Constriction of the pupil prior to surgery by the use of 2 per cent pilocarpine drops may help to "trap" the lens in the anterior chamber. Intraocular tension should be reduced by the use of IV mannitol just prior to surgery. This also helps to shrink the vitreous body, aiding in the prevention of vitreous loss.

Severe Trauma to the Globe

Severe trauma to the globe or a direct blow to the head can result in retinal and/or vitreous hemorrhage. There may be large areas of subretinal or intraretinal hemorrhage. Subretinal hemorrhage usually assumes a discrete, globular form, and the blood appears reddish-blue in color. The retina is detached at the site of hemorrhage. Superficial retinal hemorrhage may assume a flame-shape appearance, and preretinal or vitreal hemorrhage assumes a bright red amorphous appearance, obliterating the underlying retinal architecture. Retinal and vitreous hemorrhage associated with trauma usually resorbs spontaneously over a 2- to 3-week period. Unfortunately, vitreous hemorrhage, as it organizes, can produce vitreous traction bands that may eventually produce retinal detachment.

Expulsive choroidal hemorrhage can occur at the time of injury and usually leads to retinal detachment, severe visual impairment, and total visual loss.

Treatment of retinal and vitreous hemorrhage involves rest and the correction of factors that may predispose to intraocular hemorrhage. Local measures are of little value in aiding in the resorption of blood.

Hyphema refers to blood in the anterior chamber of the eye. Its most common cause is trauma resulting from automobile injuries. Hyphema may also be present secondary to penetrating intraocular wounds.

Blood within the eye may come from the anterior and/or posterior uveal tract. Trauma to the eye may result in iridodialysis or a tearing of the iris at its root, permitting excessive bleeding from the iris and ciliary body.

Usually, simple hyphema resolves spontaneously in 7 to 10 days and does not cause visual loss. Loss of vision following bleeding into the anterior chamber is associated with secondary ocular injuries including glaucoma, traumatic iritis, cataract, retinal detachment, endophthalmitis, or corneal scarring.

Treatment of hyphema must be individualized; however, there are several general principles of treatment.

1. Arrest continuing bleeding and control recurrent bleeding.
2. Aid in the elimination of blood from the anterior chamber.
3. Control secondary glaucoma.
4. Treat associated injuries, including traumatic iritis.
5. Detect and treat late complications of hyphema.

Unfortunately, little can be done to arrest and prevent rebleeding in the eye. The iris stroma has marked fibrinolytic activity, and this may be associated with the failure of fibrin clots to effectively occlude damaged ocular vessels. The role of movement by the iris and ciliary body in producing recurrent ocular bleeding is a controversial one.

In cases of early hyphema, it is advisable to keep the affected animal confined and to prohibit active exertion. If the hyphema is so extensive that it may produce a secondary glaucoma, observe the animal while it is hospitalized.

Daily examination of the animal with hyphema should be conducted. Rebleeding may occur within the first 5 days following injury. The intraocular pressure should be closely observed.

After 5 to 7 days, the blood in the anterior chamber changes from a bright red color to a bluish-black color (eight-ball hemorrhage). If the total hyphema persists and an elevation in ocular pressure is evident despite medical therapy, surgical intervention is indicated. Continued presence of blood in the anterior chamber under increased pressure may lead to blood staining of the cornea.

Primary escape of red blood cells from the anterior chamber is via the anterior drainage angle, with iris absorption and phagocytosis accounting for minor removal of blood elements. Because of the associated traumatic iritis in hyphema, topical corticosteroids such as 1 per cent prednisolone acetate should be used to control anterior segment inflammation. In addition, a cycloplegic agent such as 1 per cent atropine should be used.

The hyphemas secondary to retinal detachment (e.g., Collie ectasia syndrome) and end-stage glaucoma are extremely difficult to treat medically and have a poor prognosis.

One of the most serious complications of hyphema is secondary glaucoma. Glaucoma of this type is due to angle obstruction by blood clots. Large hyphemas producing eight-ball hemorrhage may effectively block the anterior drainage angle.

Control of glaucoma secondary to hyphema may prove extremely difficult. Carbonic anhydrase inhibitors such as acetazolamide or dichlorphenamide decrease aqueous secretion and may effectively reduce intraocular pressure if the trabecular outflow system is still functioning to 40 per cent of capacity. An eye with glaucoma and a completely blocked trabecular outflow system will respond poorly to a carbonic anhydrase inhibitor. Osmotic agents, such as oral glycerol, or IV mannitol may be helpful in controlling glaucoma secondary to hyphema. Reduction in vitreous volume deepens the anterior chamber and may increase aqueous fluid outflow.

Evacuation of blood or blood clots from the anterior chamber is not advisable unless there is secondary glaucoma that cannot be controlled medically or if there is no indication over a prolonged period that blood resorption is occurring. Experimentally, it has been shown that irrigation of the anterior chamber that contains fresh blood clots (1 to 2 days old) with 1250 IU per ml of fibrinolysin will help to lyse the blood clots. This treatment is ineffective in treating older, organized blood clots.

It is important to emphasize that surgical intervention and blind probing of the anterior chamber in an attempt to remove blood or blood clots may cause serious surgical complications such as rebleeding, luxated lens, extensive iris damage, and damage to the corneal endothelium.

Proptosis of the Globe

Proptosis of the globe secondary to trauma is not uncommon, especially in brachycephalic breeds. Proptosis of the globe in the dolicocephalic breeds requires a greater degree of initiating contusion than in the brachycephalic breeds. Therefore, secondary damage to the eye and central nervous system (CNS) associated with proptosis of the globe may be far greater in the Collie than in the Pekingese.

When presented with a case of proptosis of the globe, careful evaluation of the cardiovascular system for evidence of shock and examination of the respiratory and nervous systems should be carried out. Establish an adequate airway, treat shock, control overt bleeding, and so on, before replacing the eye in the orbit. While the initial examination and treatment are being carried out, protect the proptosed globe against further exposure and drying. This can be accomplished by using sponges soaked in cold, hypertonic solution (hypertonic 10 per cent dextrose) to reduce ocular edema and prevent corneal drying.

Proptosis of the globe can be associated with severe intraocular problems such as iritis, chorioretinitis, retinal detachment, luxation of the lens, and avulsion of the optic nerve.

It is advisable to attempt to replace most of the proptosed globes encountered despite the severity of the condition. Exceptions to this are eyes in which the intraocular contents have been extruded, when massive destruction of the intraocular contents has taken place, or if the owner wishes to have the eye removed because of cosmetic or economic considerations.

Surgical replacement of the proptosed globe should be carried out under general anesthesia. Carefully evaluate the patient to determine whether general anesthesia can be tolerated. Make a lateral canthotomy incision to widen the palpebral fissure. The canthotomy incision can extend from the canthus to the orbital ligament. It is not a good policy to cut the canthal ligament; however, if the globe cannot be replaced by enlarging the palpebral fissure with a canthotomy, the canthal ligament can be partially severed.

Using gentle pressure applied to the globe with a moistened, sterile sponge, replace the globe into the orbit. Do not probe the retro-orbital space with a needle or attempt to reduce intraocular pressure by paracentesis. When the eye is replaced in the orbit, place a nictitating membrane flap in position. Three nonpenetrating mattress sutures are placed in the lid margins but not drawn taut. Gently replace the eye in the orbit and tighten the nictitating membrane and lid sutures. Use small pieces of rubber tubing under the sutures to prevent pressure necrosis of the skin overlying the lids. The nictitating membrane sutures are also tied over a piece of rubber tubing.

After replacing the eye in the orbit, inject 2 to 4 mg of methylprednisolone acetate into the retrobulbar space to aid in reducing inflammation.

Postoperative treatment is aimed at controlling traumatic iritis and the extensive corneal damage that is associated with proptosis and exposure keratitis. Systemic broad-spectrum antibiotics are indicated. One per cent atropine is used TID; 1 per cent prednisolone acetate drops and gentamicin ophthalmic ointment are used 6 times a day. If it is believed that trauma to an eye has been extensive, the topical steroids will be supplemented with systemic steroids for a 1-week period.

Leave the sutures in place until intraorbital swelling is markedly reduced—usually 10 days to 2 weeks. After this time, remove the sutures and inspect the globe. If proptosis recurs, replace the sutures and remove after an additional 2 weeks.

Extraocular muscle injury and resultant strabismus are very commonly seen following proptosis. The most frequent deviation observed is upward and outward, indicating possible paralysis or rupture of the medial rectus, superior oblique and inferior rectus muscles, or an over-action of the lateral superior rectus muscles. The strabismus is most noticeable immediately following removal of the lid sutures. Surprisingly, in most cases, return to a relatively normal visual axis occurs in 3 to 4 months following the initial injury.

Acute Glaucoma

Acute glaucoma (a rise in intraocular pressure not compatible with normal ocular function) is commonly recognized by veterinarians. Unfortunately, owners many times fail to recognize the cardinal signs of glaucoma: sudden onset of pain, photophobia, lacrimation, deep episcleral vascular engorgement, an edematous ("steamy") and insensitive cornea, shallowing of the anterior chamber depth, a dilated and unresponsive pupil, and loss of visual acuity.

Most glaucomas in small animals are secondary and are associated with other ocular problems, such as luxated lenses, uveitis, hemorrhage, and so on. However, it is beyond the scope of this book to discuss, in depth, the differential diagnosis of secondary glaucoma or the concepts involved in primary glaucoma.

Intraocular pressure may be reduced by three medical methods: (1) improve the facility of aqueous outflow, (2) reduce ocular volume by the use of osmotic agents, (3) reduce aqueous formation.

1. A miotic agent such as 2 or 4 per cent pilocarpine drops is used in an attempt to increase outflow through the anterior drainage angle. It must be stressed that most cases of acute congestive glaucoma in the dog are associated with a narrowed drainage angle and in many cases, beginning anterior synechia. The topical use of pilocarpine on an emergency basis in most of these cases will be of little benefit and, in the case of uveitis, may make the condition worse. Excessive treatment with pilocarpine may lead to the development of toxic systemic side effects due to cholinergic stimulation. The dilated pupil in acute galucoma associated with very high intraocular pressure (above 60 mm Hg) may be unresponsive to pilocarpine therapy because of paralysis of the sphincter muscle.

   If angle-closure glaucoma is secondary to forward displacement of the lens, as occurs in lens subluxation, miotic therapy is contraindicated, because it may worsen the glaucoma by increasing pupillary block and further narrowing the angle.

2. Osmotic agents can be used to reduce the size of the vitreous body and to reduce the amount of aqueous present. These agents create an osmotic gradient between intraocular fluids and the vascular bed, thus acting independently of the aqueous outflow and inflow system. Oral glycerol (50 per cent) can be used, 0.6 ml per kg every 8 hours, to effectively reduce intraocular pressure. IV mannitol therapy (20 per cent) 2 gm per kg will

rapidly (within 1 hour) reduce intraocular pressure. If the filtration mechanism is open and working, pressure may be controlled medically. If increased intraocular pressure rapidly recurs following osmotic therapy, there is extensive obstruction to the aqueous drainage mechanism and filtering procedures or other types of glaucoma surgery such as cyclocryosurgery are indicated.

3. The third method of glaucoma control uses carbonic anhydrase inhibitors to reduce aqueous secretion. This method of controlling greatly increased elevated levels of intraocular pressure in narrow angle glaucoma is not very effective, because secretory inhibition by carbonic anhydrase inhibitors is incomplete, decreasing aqueous production by only 50 to 60 per cent. If the aqueous drainage apparatus is so severely damaged that it cannot handle 40 per cent of its normal drainage function, the carbonic anhydrase inhibitors will not be able to control intraocular pressure effectively. Thus, the use of carbonic anhydrase inhibitors alone in acute, narrow angle glaucoma will not effectively control and stabilize intraocular pressure.

Glycerol, 50 per cent, may be helpful in the evaluation of acute glaucoma when it is applied topically to the eye. Application of hypertonic glycerol does not have any effect on intraocular pressure; however, it may rapidly clear corneal edema, thus permitting greater visualization of the anterior chamber. Prior to the use of glycerol, several drops of topical anesthesia should be placed in the eye. Reduction in corneal edema will help in examining the anterior ocular segment and in performing gonioscopy so that an etiologic diagnosis can be made and effective medical or surgical therapy can be instituted.

References and Additional Readings

Bistner, S. I., and Aguire, G.: Management of ocular emergencies. Vet. Clin. North Am., 2; 359, 1972.

Freeman, H. M.: Ocular Trauma. Norwalk, Connecticut, Appleton-Century-Crofts, 1979.

Paton, D., and Goldberg, M. F.: Injuries of the Eye, the Lids and the Orbit. Philadelphia, W. B. Saunders Company, 1968.

Pfister, R. R.: Chemical injuries of the eye. Ophthalmology, 90(10):1246, 1983.

ENVIRONMENTAL EXPOSURE

Cold Injuries

FROSTBITE

Local freezing is most commonly experienced in peripheral tissue (ears, tail) that may be sparsely covered with hair, poorly vascularized, or previously traumatized by cold.

Immediate treatment includes rapid rewarming by moist heat applications at 29.5° C (85° F) or by immersion in warm baths. Analgesics may be needed to alleviate pain and administration of prophylactic antibiotics must be considered. The injured areas should be gently dried and protected from trauma.

Do not rub or apply pressure dressing or ointments. Do not use corticosteroids, and do not be in a hurry to amputate or débride the frozen area. Many tissues recover which do not appear to be viable on first examination. Because intravascular coagulation is a common problem, dextran 40 (10% low molecular weight dextran) (100 to 200 ml) given IV and repeated every 12 hours for 2 days may reduce the extent of tissue necrosis.

HYPOTHERMIA

Chilling of the entire body from exposure results in a decrease in physiologic processes that becomes irreversible at a body temperature of about 24° C (75° F). The duration of exposure and the animal's physical condition influence its ability to survive.

If the body temperature is low, rapid, careful rewarming by warm water baths or careful heating by electric heaters may be necessary. An effective mechanism to warm a very cold patient is via peritoneal dialysis, 20 ml per kg of lactated Ringer's solution, warmed to 103° F and repeating dialysis at 30-minute intervals until the body temperature is 98° to 100° F. The body temperature always increases slowly. The body's response to drugs is unpredictable, so medications should be avoided if possible until the body temperature approaches normal.

A urinary catheter should be inserted and fluids given intravenously (IV) only after renal function is re-established.

The heart should be monitored for arrhythmias, and appropriate therapy should be administered.

Heat Injuries

HEAT STROKE

Heat stroke occurs in dogs exposed to a high environmental temperature and placed under stress (such as confinement in an enclosed space or overexertion). Brachycephalic breeds, obese dogs, and older dogs with cardiovascular disease are particularly affected. Hyperthermia is indicated by a rectal temperature of 41° to 43° C (105° to 110° F). Dogs presenting with hyperthermia have congested mucous membranes and tachycardia and are panting rapidly. Heat stroke can be associated with alterations of all organs and systems of the body. There is generalized cellular necrosis associated with heat denaturization of cellular proteins. Severe hypotension may develop, and renal failure and hypotensive shock may be seen. The most frequently seen signs are panting, vomiting, diarrhea, dehydration, oliguria, and proteinuria. More profound changes such as shock, disseminated intravascular coagulation (DIC) and coma develop rapidly.

Dogs with heat stroke will pant excessively, leading to respiratory alkalosis. As the respiratory exertion continues, metabolic acidosis develops. These abnormalities of blood and tissue pH can lead to cerebral edema and death. A marked increase in packed cell volume also occurs with heat stroke.

Immediate treatment is aimed at lowering the patient's temperature. This can be accomplished by immersion of the animal in cold water. Monitor the rectal temperature, because hypothermia can develop rapidly. Prevent the development of cerebral edema by administering dexamethasone, 1.0 to 2.0 mg per kg of body weight IV. IV mannitol is indicated if stupor or coma is present and is caused by cerebral edema (see Neurologic Emergency, pp. 149–168). Start an IV drip of lactated Ringer's solution. Determine the acid-base status by a study of blood gases; however, if this is not feasible, IV administration of fluids coupled with supportive care often proves beneficial in controlling pH abnormalities (see pp. 591–617). Caution must be used in administering fluids if oliguria is present. Furosemide can be used to induce diuresis. Evidence of progressive primary renal disease may develop following correction of the acute temperature rise. Look for evidence of DIC, such as hemorrhagic diathesis and melena, and begin treatment (see pp. 63–65).

Following initial emergency treatment, keep affected animals in a well-ventilated cool room and confine them so they do not become overactive. If available, a cool 22° C (70° F) oxygen chamber can be used for small dogs, provided that excessive CO_2 build-up does not develop (see Oxygen Section, pp. 633–636).

References and Additional Readings

Dieterich, R. A.: Cold injury. In Kirk, R. W. (ed.): Current Veterinary Therapy VIII. Philadelphia. W. B. Saunders Company, 1983.

Elder, P. T.: Accidental hypothermia. In Shoemaker, W. C., Thompson, W. L, and Holbrook, P.R. (eds.): The Society of Critical Care Medicine: Textbook of Critical Care. Philadelphia, W. B. Saunders Company, 1984.

Schall, W. D.: Heatstroke. In Kirk, R. W. (ed.): Current Veterinary Therapy VIII: Small Animal Practice. Philadelphia, W. B. Saunders Company, 1983.

Zenoble, R. D.: Accidental hypothermia. In Kirk, R. W. (ed.): Current Veterinary Therapy VIII: Small Animal Practice. Philadelphia, W. B. Saunders Company, 1983.

FRACTURES AND MUSCULOSKELETAL TRAUMA

The conditions at the site of fracture are very important in formulating general principles of fracture management. A simple greenstick fracture is handled differently from a compound, comminuted fracture. Treatment will also depend on whether the animal is examined and treated immediately after injury, a few days after injury, during the peak of an inflammatory reaction, or a few weeks after the injury occurred.

IMMEDIATE CARE

1. Maintain an adequate open airway for respiration and assist respiration, if necessary.
2. Control hemorrhage by applying pressure dressings over the bleeding area or apply direct pressure over the brachial artery or femoral artery. Temporary splinting of the fracture should be done if fracture is lower to mid radius and below stifle. A temporary splint of rolled newspaper can be used and wrapped around the leg. The ability to place a temporary splint on the animal depends on the degree of pain that the animal is in and the temperament of the animal.
3. Treat shock (see pp. 60–61).
4. Ascertain whether there are other life-threatening injuries present that may need immediate attention such as diaphragmatic hernia, pneumothorax, severe skull or spinal cord fractures, and associated neurologic signs.

INITIAL TREATMENT OF MUSCULOSKELETAL INJURIES

1. The possibility of either multiple fractures or injury to the spinal column, head, thorax, and abdomen must constantly be kept in mind when dealing with musculoskeletal injuries.
2. Use care and gentleness when handling a broken limb, and avoid unnecessary handling.
3. Splint the fractured limb before moving the patient, especially fractures below the elbow and below stifle and any closed fracture in danger of becoming an open fracture.

INITIAL EXAMINATION

In addition to examining for a fracture, determine:
1. Whether the circulation at or distal to the site of injury has been seriously injured by noting color, extremity temperature, and pulse.
2. Whether there has been any associated nerve injury by testing pain sensation.
3. Whether there has been a dislocation at an associated joint. It is often difficult to differentiate between fractures in or near joints and luxations.
4. The presence and extent of any injuries to adjacent tendons, muscles, and ligaments.
5. Whether there is evidence of trauma to adjacent soft-tissue structures. Pelvic fractures may produce ruptured bladders and urethra; pelvic, hindlimb trauma may also result in intra-abdominal trauma; and forelimb fractures can produce intrathoracic trauma. Animals with multiple orthopedic fractures should have the adjacent soft-tissue cavities, abdominal and thoracic, radiographed for evidence of possible injury.

It is good general practice to radiograph the chest in all cases of serious long bone or pelvic fractures or where there is a history of blunt trauma to more than just an isolated body area.

The basic differences between a "strain" and a "sprain" are as follows. A strain is damage to some part of a muscle-tendon unit usually associated with activity that places unusual stress on the tissues. Sudden hyperextension or hyperflexion of muscle-tendon units can produce acute strain, causing damage to tendon or muscle and possibly avulsing the muscle attachments. Strain results in pain, lameness, and discomfort that develops its most acute form usually 2 to 3 days following the injury. A sprain is an injury to a ligament associated with stressing of the ligamentous attachments to the point that the ligaments and/or their attachments are damaged.

The presence or absence of a fracture can be diagnosed by an examination carried out in the following sequence:

Inspection

Inspection of the injury may reveal swelling, ecchymosis, deformity, and inability to use the injured part. In some fractures, however, there is no deformity and the animal may continue to have limited use of the affected part.

Palpation

Palpation may reveal a local point of tenderness, bony crepitus, false point of motion of a bone, and irregularity of bone contour. Crepitus and motion within a bone should not be deliberately tested for; it is exceedingly painful and may cause more injury.

Comparative Measurements

Comparative measurements of the length of the extremities may be a valuable diagnostic aid.

Physical Changes

Swelling, an increase or loss of normal skin temperature, change in color of the skin, and changes in sensation of the skin may help to localize a point of fracture.

Radiographs

Radiographs are a necessary part of all complete examinations for fractures. In making the films, the injured part should not be moved excessively. A bone with a suspected fracture should be examined along its entire length, including the associated proximal and distal joints. It may be of value to take radiographs of the opposite limb for comparison.

TREATMENT OF MUSCULOSKELETAL INJURIES

Fractures fall into three classifications, according to the need for repair.

1. *Critical fractures* require immediate repair to maintain life or normal physiologic function of the structure involved. This category includes skull fractures, spinal fractures, open fractures, and certain types of luxations.

2. *Semicritical fractures* may give rise to severe problems and abnormal function if not treated quickly. These fractures include those of joint surfaces or of epiphyseal growth plates; luxations of the femoral head, shoulder, and elbow; fractures of the mid and distal thirds of the humerus; pelvic fractures, and fractures os penis.

3. *Noncritical fractures* do not require early reduction. Examples are scapular and pelvic fractures, greenstick fractures, and closed fractures of the shafts of long bones.

Until definitive treatment is determined, a temporary dressing on the injury and immobilization of the part will: (1) prevent further comminution of fragments, (2) prevent additional trauma to nerves, blood vessels, and soft tissues, (3) decrease pain, (4) prevent further bacterial contamination, (5) decrease edema and circulatory impairment, and (6) prevent extension of a closed fracture into an open (compound) fracture.

The modified Robert Jones dressing is readily made of sterile material. It is a heavily padded splint with multiple layers of a wound dressing held on by cast padding, 1 or 2 pounds of rolled cotton uniformly wound around the entire extremity, leaving the last two phalanges of the two middle toes exposed, so that circulation checks can be made and compressed with several rolls of conforming gauze, and a final layer of Elasticon, adhesive tape, or elastic bandage. With small dogs and cats, rolls of cast padding may be substituted for the cotton. Although this splint appears bulky, it gives support without interfering with the circulation. This form of temporary fixation is not for fractures above the stifle or elbow. The toes should be left open so that the temperature of the tissues can be felt, ensuring that circulation is adequate.

Temporary immobilization may also be achieved with metasplints, folded newspapers, or towels. Air splints (pneumatic splints) are very applicable for large dogs with fractures of the radius, ulna, or metacarpals.

Reduce fractures with displacement as soon after the injury as possible and before excessive swelling and muscle traction develop. Fractures that can be managed by closed reduction include greenstick fractures of the radius, ulna, and tibia and simple fractures of these bones and of metacarpals and metatarsals. Most often, fractures will require open reduction and fixation. Carry out closed reductions as gently as possible with the animal under general anesthesia. If manipulation of the fractured bone is necessary, radiographs should be available while the bone fragments are manipulated. It is important to remember that a splint does not reduce a fracture but only maintains the reduction that has previously been attained. Use open reduction when the expected results will be superior to those of closed reduction. (The methods of reduction are beyond the scope of this discussion.)

Open Fractures

The extent of the severity of injury in compound fractures can be categorized as follows:

Grade 1—Skin and muscle penetration occurs by a bone fragment from within going outward.

Grade 2—An external force causes skin and muscle penetration and crushing tissue injury.

Grade 3—Severe soft-tissue damage to skin, muscle, and nerves from abrasions and bone fracture, as occurs when an animal is dragged by a car.

The following procedures should be carried out during the initial management of compound wounds:

1. Establish a patent intravenous (IV) catheter, and begin fluid administration with lactated Ringer's solution. Immediately start IV administration of appropriate antibiotics. The most effective period for antibiotic administration is within 6 hours of the initial injury. At the initial time of examination of the wound, cultures for aerobic as well as anaerobic microorganisms should be taken. *Staphylococcus aureus* is a frequent isolate from infected orthopedic wounds in dogs. Other organisms more frequently isolated are coliforms, anaerobes, including Bacteriodes and Fusobacterium, clostridium and pasteurella sp. Organisms of *S. aureus* resistant to penicillin are not infrequently found, and the initial antibiotics of choice are clindamycin, methicillin, cephalothin, and chloramphenicol. A good choice would be clindamycin and gentamycin, both initially given IV as a loading dose.
2. Cover the wound with sterile gauze. Control any associated shock and fluid abnormalities. Treat minor lacerations, and evaluate the general systemic condition.
3. Administer anesthetic or neuroleptanalgesic of choice. Take the patient to the operating room.
4. Clip (remove hair from) the entire limb, using sterile technique, with the animal under anesthesia. Use K-Y jelly over the wound, then cover the wound with sterile gauze before clipping. Surgically prepare the skin with Betadine scrub. Enlarge the wound so that the extent of the injury can be seen.
5. Excise any damaged muscle and/or tendon, and remove tissue debris.
6. Irrigate the wound by lavaging it with sterile saline or lactated Ringer's solution, either of which has 2 to 3 million units of crystalline penicillin G added to it. Sterile saline with povodine-iodine, 1 part to 9 parts saline, can be used to irrigate the wound. Use copious irrigation to remove as much foreign matter as possible. Avoid detergents and soaps in the wound, because they are often cytotoxic.
7. Cover the wound with a sterile dressing.
8. Complete radiographic evaluation.

The decision whether to perform primary closure of the wound and repair the fracture or to leave the wound open and attempt later repair depends on the degree of contamination of the wound. Wherever possible, primary repair should be attempted, because it will result in better healing of the fractures and the vascular supply of soft tissues can be maintained.

The most important adverse influences over good fracture healing are: (1) adequate lack of reduction, (2) failure to adequately immobilize the fracture, (3) presence of foreign bodies, (4) infection, and (5) poor blood supply.

Treatment of Specific Musculoskeletal Injuries

Coxofemoral (Hip) Luxations

Do not attempt reduction of a coxofemoral luxation until the relationship of the bones of the hip has been established and the extent of the injury has been assessed. Radiographs are absolutely necessary to rule out fractures of the pelvis or femoral head. The most common form of displacement of the hip is in the cranial dorsal position. The affected limb is held in the adducted position, with the paw externally rotated. The toes may touch the ground, but weight is not borne on the leg. Palpate the greater trochanter, which in anterior dorsal hip luxation will be higher in position than a line drawn from the iliac crest to the tibial tuberosity. In the dorsal recumbency position, the luxated limb will be shorter. Closed reduction of the luxated joint may not be possible when soft tissue is interposed in the joint cavity and should not be performed when coexisting fractures are present. Luxations should be reduced as soon as possible. A general anesthetic will be required to overcome pain and muscle spasm.

Place the animal in lateral recumbency, with the luxation uppermost. The pelvis must be restrained either manually by using an oversized Schroeder Thomas splint or by passing a padded rope or heavy piece of gauze over the medial side of the thigh and anchoring it to the table. If the luxation is anterior or dorsal, grasp the leg just below the stifle and flex the joint. The other hand is used to palpate the trochanter major and acetabulum. Abduct the leg and rotate it outward so that the femoral head will be dorsal to the acetabulum and the femoral neck and the shaft will be anterior. By applying slow, steady traction at the stifle and guiding the femoral head with the opposite hand, the luxation should reduce. With a posterior luxation, the same procedure can be followed except that the leg is rotated inward. Confirm reductions by palpation and roentgenography. Temporary splintage such as an Ehmer sling should be used to maintain the reduction.

Another method used to reduce posterior coxofemoral luxations is to manipulate the luxation to the anterior dorsal position, grasp the leg below the stifle joint, and rotate the limb outward to dislodge the femoral head. Pull downward and backward at a 45-degree angle with the spine with adduction. When the femoral head has reached the rim of the acetabulum, inward rotation of the leg and abduction should permit the femoral head to enter the acetabulum again.

Luxations of the Elbow

Supination of the elbow joint to any degree in the dog indicates a fracture or luxation in the elbow region. Luxation of the elbow joint frequently involves injury to the radius and ulna. A roentgenogram should be taken in the anteroposterior (AP) and lateral positions.

If there are no fractures involving the joint and the luxation is amenable to closed reduction, place the animal under surgical anesthesia and flex the affected limb. With the angle of the elbow less than 45 degrees, rotate the foot so that the semilunar notch faces medially. Apply traction at the olecranon to force it beyond the epicondyle of the humerus. At the same time, the ulna and radius are forced medially. A full pin may have to be drilled through the olecranon to permit the application of sufficient traction to the radius and ulna.

References and Additional Readings

Alexander, J.: Coxofemoral luxation in the dog. Comp., Cont. Ed., 4:575, 1982.

Arnoczky, S. P.: Surgery of the hip. Proc. Am. Anim. Hosp. Assoc., 401, 1983.

Brinker, W. O., Piermattei, D. L., and Flo, G. L.: Handbook of Small Animal Orthopedics and Fracture Treatment. Philadelphia, W. B. Saunders Company, 1983.

Dueland, R.: Emergency treatment of limb fractures. Vet. Clin. North Am., 5:305, 1975.

Hirsh, D. C., and Smith, T. M.: Osteomyelitis in the dog: microorganisms isolated and susceptibility to antimicrobial agents. J. Small Anim. Pract. 19:679, 1978.

Nunamaker, D. M.: Treatment of open fractures in small animals. Compendium of Continuing Education, 1:66, 1979.

Slatter, D. H. (ed.): Textbook of Small Animal Surgery. Philadelphia, W. B. Saunders Company, 1984.

GASTROINTESTINAL EMERGENCIES

This section includes treatments for emergencies involving foreign bodies, obstructions, perforations of the intestinal tract, gastric dilatation–volvulus complex, fractured teeth, hemorrhage from the mouth and rectum, hernias, prolapse of the rectum, acute gastritis, and acute pancreatitis.

Foreign Bodies

Foreign bodies are the most common cause of intestinal obstructions in dogs and cats and are most prevalent in young animals. History of the animal can be very helpful in making a diagnosis. Not all foreign bodies are visible radiographically, especially the plastics that are commonly ingested.

The clinical signs that follow the ingestion of a foreign object depend on the degree of gastrointestinal blockage and the location in the intestinal tract. Foreign objects that produce only partial obstruction may result in intermittent episodes of vomiting and anorexia.

In general, foreign bodies in the intestine produce dilation of the bowel that can be recognized radiographically. The accumulation of gastric, duodenal, pancreatic, and biliary fluid plus venous stasis and transudation increases intraluminal pressure proximal to the obstruction. Foreign bodies causing blockage of pylorus or duodenum generally lead to profuse vomiting with no air in the duodenum. Contrast media may be necessary to identify high bowel obstruction and occasional lower bowel partial obstructions or esophageal foreign bodies (see p. 567). Standing lateral radiographs can be an important diagnostic aid in detecting foreign body obstructions.

Foreign bodies in the mouth, esophagus, and stomach can often be removed without great difficulty. Foreign bodies in the mouth should be removed, anesthetizing the patient, if necessary. The mouth should then be thoroughly inspected, and any local trauma should be treated. Although the oral mucosa is susceptible to infection, it heals rapidly, and local débridement or suturing, together with antibacterial treatment, is advisable.

Foreign bodies in the esophagus and stomach should be accurately located by radiographs. In any animal with signs of difficulty in swallowing, regurgitation, or history of possibly swallowing a foreign object, radiographs of the cervical, thoracic, and abdominal regions should be taken and the mouth should be examined. Small objects (stones, buttons, needles, and pins) may pass through the alimentary tract, although feeding the animal an indigestible substance (such as cotton wads) to surround the objects may facilitate their passage. An object will usually pass within three days. If the object stops or if the patient shows signs of tenseness, vomiting, or fever, an exploratory operation should be done immediately. With the patient anesthetized, some rounded, dull objects can be removed from the esophagus with gastric forceps or by using endoscopy and biopsy forceps.

A common nonobstructive foreign body often found in the cat is string. The string, with perhaps a needle attached, becomes lodged in the mouth, especially around the base of the tongue. The end of the string is usually swallowed, and if it passes through the pylorus, it may become lodged in the intestinal tract. Contractions of the intestine around the string may cause the intestines to become plicated, and eventually the string may produce intestinal necrosis. Radiographic findings associated with lineal foreign bodies are accordion-like pleating of the small bowel, a shortened small bowel in the midventral region of the abdominal cavity, and peritonitis secondary to laceration of the bowel wall. If the string is found lodged in the mouth, it should be cut, but it should *not* be pulled out; this may produce further gastric or intestinal damage. The animal should then be carefully observed for the development of any signs associated with gastrointestinal obstruction, the stool should be carefully examined to see if the string has been passed. If the string appears at the rectum, it should *not* be pulled out. If a string cannot be passed, it must be removed by a series of enterotomy incisions.

Foreign objects in the rectum or colon may have become embedded during passage but are more likely the work of sadists. The object must be carefully removed with the patient anesthetized. Local infection by perianal fistulas is a common sequela; therefore, systemic antibiotics together with neomycin and Sulfathalidine should be administered orally for 7 days.

Obstructions

An obstruction of the intestinal tract is any condition that produces interference with or depresses the movement of the gastrointestinal contents in an orderly physiologic manner. Bowel obstructions may be simple where there is luminal blockage or strangulated where there is an obstruction to mesenteric blood supply. Strangulations of the bowel can produce severe necrosis, and septic shock can develop suddenly (see p. 59). Causes of obstructions include foreign bodies, tumors, torsion, intussusception, strangulated hernias, pyloric stenosis, and fecal impactions. In general, high intestinal obstructions (pylorus, duodenum, and proximal jejunum) cause more acute problems than low intestinal problems (distal jejunum, ileum, colon, and rectum). High intestinal obstructions are usually associated with persistent vomiting and severe fluid and electrolyte disturbances (see p. 593). Persistent vomiting due to pyloric obstruction can cause hypochloremic alkalosis, which can be quite severe. Persistent vomiting from intestinal obstruction in the duodenum and jejunum produces metabolic acidemia, hypovolemia, prerenal azotemia, and lactic acidosis.

If a foreign body is able to pass through the pylorus, it will usually pass through the duodenum and the first one third of the jejunum, where it will become lodged at the point at which the intestinal lumen narrows. Occlusion of normal intestinal blood supply and local edema formation may lead to intestinal necrosis. Signs and symptoms associated with intestinal obstruction vary greatly, depending on the type and degree of obstruction. Those frequently seen include vomiting, depression, dehydration, abdominal pain, abdominal distention, fever, restlessness, and reduced production of feces. In many cases, careful and thorough abdominal palpation (see p. 330) will reveal evidence of a foreign body. Both scout films and contrast studies of the abdomen should be used when necessary (Table 14). No enemas should be given prior to radiographs, because additional gas will be produced in the intestine. Flat abdominal and standing lateral radiographs should be used. The differential diagnosis between paralytic ileus and mechanical obstruction must be made.

Table 14. RADIOGRAPHIC SIGNS OF MECHANICAL OBSTRUCTION

Varying degrees of distention or ballooning of the small bowel with bowel lumen being double or more in size

Retention of ingesta above obstruction and evacuation of bowel below obstruction

Hairpin turning of the distended loop, with "layering" or loops lying parallel to one another

Squaring off of distended loops of bowel

Gas-capped fluid levels seen on standing lateral projection. Unequal levels of fluid in the inverted U-shaped loops are suggestive of a mechanical ileus

Hyperperistalsis (early stages) of loops proximal to obstruction

Increased volume of peritoneal fluid

Modified from O'Brien, T. R.: Radiographic Diagnosis of Abdominal Disorders in the Dog and Cat. Philadelphia, W. B. Saunders Company, 1978, p. 304.

In paralytic ileus the entire small intestinal tract is usually gas filled, whereas in mechanical obstruction, only that portion proximal to the obstruction is dilated with fluid and gas. In strangulated obstructions, that portion of the bowel that is strangulated becomes distended. Barium by mouth should *not* be used to demonstrate small bowel obstruction, because it flocculates, is difficult to see, and may get into the abdomen if a break in the intestinal tract exists. Water-soluble contrast agents should be used by mouth, and barium should be reserved for barium enemas (see p. 569).

Intraluminal bowel distention develops proximal to the mechanical obstruction. Intraluminal gas pressure increases and may be 10 to as high as 50 or 60 mm Hg, which severely compromises intestinal circulation and viability. The distended, obstructed bowel loses its ability to absorb fluids, and varying amounts of fluids are secreted into the bowel lumen. The loss of bicarbonate, dehydration, and not eating lead to metabolic acidosis.

Intestinal obstruction and loss of normal vascular supply alter the type, concentration, and distribution of bacteria within the intestinal tract. The major exotoxin production comes from overgrowth of *Escherichia* and *Clostridia sp.* The pathogenicity of *E. coli* is increased by the presence of hemoglobin, which develops with mucosal necrosis and hemorrhage. Because of the devitalized intestinal wall, bacterial exotoxins diffuse transmurally into the peritoneal cavity and enter the circulation, resulting in endotoxic shock and hypovolemia. The fluid in the intestinal tract becomes very dark and foul smelling.

The following clinical signs may be evidence of intestinal strangulation: abdominal pain, development of endotoxic shock, bloody diarrhea, hypovolemia, increased respiratory rate, subnormal temperature, increased heart rate, acute collapse, and bloody septic peritoneal fluid. Palpation reveals distended bowel loops.

Treatment of gastric or intestinal obstruction involves surgical celiotomy; however, emergency preoperative support is critical and includes (1) treating fluid and electrolyte losses (see p. 591), (2) treating endotoxic shock (see pp. 60–61), and (3) administering antibiotics systemically to control the growth of aerobic and anaerobic intestinal bacteria (see p. 119).

In general, if the diagnosis of a foreign body is uncertain and the animal's condition is becoming progressively worse, it is better to perform exploratory surgery on the abdomen immediately, because delay may cause the animal's condition to deteriorate rapidly, with a greatly added surgical risk.

INTUSSUSCEPTION

Intussusception is an invagination of the proximal portion of the intestine into the area immediately distal. As the intussusception enlarges, the proximal portion is pushed further into the dilated distal portion. Intussusceptions can occur within the small intestine (enteroenteric), large intestine (colocolic), and small and large intestine (ileocolic), or as an invagination of the cecum into the colon or ileum. Intussusception develops frequently in the area of the ileocecal valve. Additionally, the intussuscepted bowel may protrude through the anus;

the condition must be differentiated from a rectal prolapse (see p. 116). The signs associated with intussusception are variable and depend on whether or not a complete intestinal obstruction exists and how long the intussusception has been present. Signs frequently seen are abdominal pain, emesis, bloody diarrhea, and the presence of a palpable, sausage-shaped mass in the cranial dorsal portion of the abdomen. The severity of clinical signs is related to the degree of vascular interruption and the level of bowel where the intussusception has occurred.

Abdominal radiographs may reveal gas accumulation anterior to a cylindrical soft-tissue mass. Radiographs reveal distention of bowel loops, with gas and fluid proximal to the intussusception and an empty bowel distal to the intussusception. Contrast radiography is usually needed to outline the level of bowel obstruction. Direct intussusception can best be identified by a barium enema. Obstruction of the intestinal tract produces dynamic or mechanical ileus. Very severe obstructions of the intestinal tract that results in occlusion of blood vessels results in severe shock and death within 6 hours. Dilation of the bowel secondary to obstruction occurs because of the presence of swallowed air and saliva and the accumulation of mucosal secretions in the intestinal tract. Pressure on the bowel wall by gas accumulation results in atony and pressure necrosis.

Treatment for intussusception is exploratory laparotomy and surgical correction. Fluid therapy and correction of electrolyte abnormalities are very important preoperatively.

OBSTIPATION

Fecal impactions often must be broken up by forceps and removed by colonic irrigations, a procedure that requires light anesthesia. Usually such cases should not be worked on for longer than 30 minutes at a time because of trauma. Daily administration of dioctyl sodium sulfosuccinate orally and by enema helps water to penetrate and soften the fecal mass. Severe obstipation may produce toxemia and septic shock. Appropriate antibiotics and fluids should be given in such cases.

Perforations of the Gastrointestinal Tract

Perforations may result from internal causes, such as foreign bodies, ulcers, and trauma, or from external causes, such as penetrating wounds and other severe (blunt) trauma.

External wounds that penetrate the abdomen must always be explored to determine the extent of damage and to repair any perforated organs. Antibiotic therapy should be instituted presurgically.

Internal perforations may present bizarre signs, but common signs are peritonitis, shock, and free air in the abdomen (radiographic evidence). Patients who manifest such signs require emergency surgical exploration and shock therapy (see pp. 29–30 and 60–61).

Gastric Dilatation–Volvulus Complex in the Dog

Acute gastric dilatation with or without volvulus occurs primarily in large, deep-chested dogs such as Great Danes, Irish Setters, Doberman Pinchers, German Shepards, Irish Wolfhounds, and Boxers. The age of most cases is between 4 and 7 years, with a mean of 5.2 years; mortality may approach 47 to 50 per cent. Two conditions are necessary for gastric dilatation to occur: (1) a source for the distending gas and/or fluid, and (2) an obstruction that prevents relief of the distention by eructation, emesis, absorption, or passage of the gastric contents into the small bowel.

The source and composition of the air that accumulates in gastric dilatation–volvulus complex remain controversial and may include (1) aerophagia; (2) bacterial fermentation of substrate materials, such as various foods; and (3) reaction of gastric acid and basic pancreatic secretions. Gastric dilatation can develop very rapidly and precipitate a chain of events leading to anatomic and physiologic alterations that produce severe hypovolemic shock.

ANATOMIC CHANGES

With the dog in dorsal recumbency and the surgeon looking at the stomach from a caudal to cranial direction, in gastric dilatation there is a 90- to 180-degree clockwise turning of the stomach about the distal esophagus. The pylorus comes to lie dorsally and to the left. The distal esophagus may be twisted 90 degrees and is not completely occluded. As the stomach fills with gas, it moves to fill the long axis of the abdominal cavity as it distends. In simple dilation of the stomach, the spleen remains on the left side and the duodenum is not compressed.

As dilatation progresses and volvulus develops, the stomach turns clockwise about the distal esophagus, varying from 90 to 360 degrees. The duodenum becomes incarcerated between the distal esophagus and the dilated stomach. The position of the spleen can vary from left posterodorsal to right anterodorsal, depending on the degree of volvulus. In severe torsions of 180 degrees or more, the distal esophagus become occluded and the gastric wall becomes edematous and infarcted. The area most susceptible to infarction with necrosis is left greater curvature.

PHYSIOLOGIC CHANGES

The following physiologic changes occur in gastric dilatation–volvulus complex:
1. Complete blockage of the portal vein can occur.
2. Injury to the gastric wall, with congestion and venous stasis.
3. Marked splenic congestion and congestion of the small intestines leads to ileus, endotoxic shock, and septicemia, with production of coagulation factors that can lead to disseminated intravascular coagulation (DIC).
4. Pressure of the dilated stomach on the diaphragm leads to diminished ventilatory capacity, decreased tidal volume, increased respiratory rate, and

cyanosis. In the early stages of the disease, 60 per cent of the cases develop respiratory alkalosis, and hyokalemia is present. Most cases have normal blood gases unless they present late in the course of the disease.

5. Decreased cardiac output with resulting shock. Central venous pressure, cardiac output, and mean arterial pressure fall rapidly. Hypovolemia and shock develop.

6. Development of pancreatic ischemia and hypoxia leads to the formation of myocardial depressant factor leading to a form of cardiogenic shock.

7. Development of metabolic acidosis in the *late* stages of the disease.

8. Cardiac arrhythmias, consisting of premature atrial depolarizations and fibrillation, premature ventricular depolarizations, paroxysmal ventricular tachycardia, and ventricular tachycardia. Arrhythmias frequently develop 12 to 36 hours after the onset of dilatation–volvulus, which is a serious and a common complication.

Clinicopathologic findings are hyperphosphatemia and increased SGPT, SGOT, CPK, BUN, creatinine, and packed cell volume. Most cases first exhibit hypokalemia because K^+ ions pool in the stomach. Following correction, hyperkalemia may develop as K^+ ions are released; this is thought to contribute to cardiac abnormalities.

MANAGEMENT OF ACUTE DILATATION–VOLVULUS COMPLEX

Methods of treating gastric dilatation and volvulus are controversial; however, the following regimen of emergency care is advocated:

1. Confirm the diagnosis. Percuss the abdominal wall behind the last rib on both sides. If the abdominal wall is tense and tympanic sound is heard, there is gas under pressure in the stomach.

2. Attempt to pass a stomach tube of the largest diameter possible (in large dogs 3/4 inch diameter colt [large animal] stomach tube; see p. 3). If the animal is comatose, pass an endotracheal tube first before passing a stomach tube. If the tube cannot be passed into the stomach, perform a gastrocentesis with an 18-gauge 2- to 3-inch needle. The use of an 18-gauge 5- or 10-inch angiocath with the catheter on the outside of needle is also very effective in allowing trapped gas to escape from the stomach.

3. If the tube can be placed into the stomach, aspirate air and any gastric contents. Remove the tube, and place a nasogastric tube with an extension (see p. 582). Aspirate air and fluid from the stomach through the nasogastric tube every hour. The tube should be left in place for 24 to 48 hours.

4. Administer Maalox down the nasogastric tube q4h and Tagamet, 10 mg per kg QID, if the pH of the aspirated fluid is lower than 4.

5. To assist in passing a stomach tube in an animal in whom a tube cannot be initially passed (a) Establish an intravenous (IV) connection via a large-bore IV catheter (see p. 610). (b) Begin supportive treatment (fluids, etc.) for shock (see p. 59). Begin infusion of lactated Ringer's solution, 80 ml per kg; inject glucocorticosteroids–dexamethasome phosphate, 4 mg per kg or prednisolone sodium succinate, 10 to 20 mg per kg. These are

minimum doses, which some surgeons increase greatly. Administer high doses of systemic antibiotics. (c) It is especially important that adequate pulmonary ventilation be maintained throughout the time of acute treatment procedures (see p. 82). (d) Sedate the animal with oxymorphone, 0.1 mg per kg, plus Valium, (see p. 77).

6. Hold the animal up by front feet and attempt to pass stomach tube again. The weighted stomach falls away from the diaphragm and may allow the tube to pass. If the tube still *cannot* be passed, emergency gastrotomy should be performed.

7. Begin cardiac antidysrhythmic therapy if indicated by giving an initial IV bolus of lidocaine hydrochloride, 4 mg per kg, or a lidocaine drip, 1 gm in 500 ml dextrose in water (D/W), or procainamide hydrochloride, 2 mg per kg, or procainamide drip, 500 mg in 500 ml D/W at 3 to 25 ml per minutes. The lidocaine drip should be maintained at 60 µgm per kg per minute. To the same 500 ml of D/W of lactated Ringer's or saline that contains lidocaine, add 20 to 40 mEq K^+. Dogs in the early stage of torsion or volvulus are often alkalotic (respiratory alkalosis) and hypokalemic.

8. To perform a gastrostomy through a right paracostal incision, use local anesthesia in the abdominal wall. Suture the wall of the stomach to the skin with continuous suture, isolating the stomach from the peritoneal cavity. Place two purse-string sutures in the stomach wall, one inside the other. Enter the stomach cavity with a small incision, and place a No. 35 French Foley catheter or a No. 20–25 French chest tube into the stomach. Suture it in place by pulling the purse-string sutures tight. Tie the ends of the sutures around the tube. Gently lavage the stomach, and force out all the food possible.

9. After gastrostomy has been performed, exploratory surgery will have to be carried out (should be done within 2 to 3 hours after gastrostomy when the animal has been stabilized).

10. If the stomach tube *can* be passed and if gastrostomy is *not* required, following decompression stomach, radiographs of the abdomen are indicated for position of the stomach (use barium to evaluate stomach position if necessary), possibility of free air in the abdomen or free fluid, any evidence of bowel torsion or abnormal gas patterns in the bowel, and position and size of the spleen.

11. If the animal does not respond well to shock therapy, lavage the abdomen for further clinical diagnosis (see pp. 19–20). If blood +3, vegetable fibers, bacteria, and so on are found on lavage, fluid exploratory celiotomy must be performed.

12. Watch for any evidence of cardiac arrhythmias over the next 72 hours.

Fractured Teeth

Fractures of the teeth can be classified into 3 categories:
Class I—Fractured but no exposure of pulp; fracture above the crown.

Class II—Fractured but dental pulp exposed; fracture above the crown.

Class III—Fracture into dental pulp at the level of the crown or below.

Transverse fractures leave razor-sharp tooth edges. Under anesthesia, these edges can be filed down easily with a fine-tooth carpenter's file if the fracture is Class I. In Class II and III fractures, if the owner wishes to save the tooth, endodontic surgery with tooth capping is possible by a veterinarian or a dentist (in conjunction with a veterinarian) trained in and knowledgeable about this procedure (see pp. 320–327). If there is no desire to save the tooth in Class II or III fractures, extracting the tooth is probably the most practical alternative.

Hemorrhage from the Mouth and Rectum

Fresh, frank blood from the mouth is usually the result of trauma. If there are no skin or mucosa petechiae or bleeding from other body openings, which might indicate systemic disease, local trauma should be suspected. Inspection of the mouth under general anesthesia is usually necessary. Good suction apparatus should be available, with a Yankauer oral suction tip, and there must be good illumination to localize the source of bleeding. Always intubate and inflate the endotracheal cuff to prevent blood from entering the lungs. When extubating, aspirate all blood from the posterior pharynx. Esophagoscopy or bronchoscopy may be necessary to find the source of the bleeding. Cold packs, ice water lavage, sutures, transfusions, or shock therapy may be needed, depending on the cause and location of the bleeding.

Hemorrhage from the anus usually results from granulomatous colitis, neoplasia, poisonings, traumatic injury or shock, and pooling of blood in the splanchnic vessels, with resulting necrosis of the intestinal mucous membrane. Emergency treatment is usually conservative and confined to spasmolytics, antibiotics, or blood transfusions if blood loss is severe. Proctoscopy is subsequently indicated if the cause of hemorrhage is not evident.

Hernias

Hernias are emergencies only when structures such as the intestines or uterus are incarcerated within the hernial ring. Immediate herniorrhaphy is indicated in such cases. Traumatic hernias require that an exploratory celiotomy be performed so that other internal injuries can be found, if present.

Prolapse of the Rectum

Prolapse of the rectum may occur in puppies. This condition may be associated with rectal foreign bodies, neoplasms, rectal diverticula, colitis, dystocia, or sadism. The young, debilitated animal with persistent diarrhea seems most prone to develop this condition. It may be either a true prolapse, partial, or complete, or the extra-anal protrusion of an intussusception of the bowel. To differentiate a true rectal prolapse from a protrusion of an intussuscepted piece of bowel, insert a blunt object such as glass or a metal rod between the prolapsed mass and the anus. If the rod *cannot* be inserted, a true rectal prolapse exists. If the glass rod or thermometer *can* be inserted, an intussusception is present (see p. 111). If the rectum is prolapsed, lubrication and immediate replacement may be effective. However, purse-string sutures should be placed in the anus for 3 to 7 days. Pull the purse-string sutures down over a pencil inserted into the rectum. This will allow a small hole for escape of gas and fluids. Colopexy is indicated if prolapse recurs. If intussusception is diagnosed, a laparotomy should be performed to inspect and completely correct the problem. Colopexy may also be indicated here to prevent recurrence, or an enteroplication can be done from the proximal jejunum to the proximal colon.

Acute Gastritis

Acute gastritis in small animals is usually associated with overeating or with ingesting garbage and spoiled foods. In puppies, overeating—especially with highly fermentable, low digestible foods—can precipitate acute gastritis. Eating of foreign materials such as bone and other garbage is frequently seen in puppies. Diarrhea often develops following gastritis and may be hemorrhagic. Severe hemorrhagic gastroenteritis may precipitate a shocklike syndrome, with a rapidly rising hematocrit. Various toxins, such as heavy metals, arsenic, thallium, or ethylene glycol, may also produce severe gastric irritation. Gastritis is characterized by pain in the anterior abdomen, vomiting, excessive water drinking, depression, and dehydration.

A careful history and examination of the vomitus may be helpful in arriving at a differential diagnosis (see Vomiting, p. 259). Persistent severe vomiting can be very debilitating and may lead to severe dehydration and electrolyte imbalances. The following supportive steps are helpful until a more conclusive diagnosis can be reached:

1. Withhold oral fluids and solids for the first 24 hours.
2. Correct fluid and electrolyte imbalances (see p. 591).
3. Control vomiting with antiemetics such as prochlorperazine (Compazine), chlorpromazine (Thorazine), perphenazine (Trilafon), and trimethobenzamide (Tigan).
4. With severe vomiting, especially when disruption of the mucosal wall of the stomach is suspected, high doses of systemic antibiotics are indicated to treat both aerobic and anaerobic bacteria.
5. Antacids (i.e., Mylanta liquid) TID or QID can reduce gastric activity and irritation. Anticholinergics are not effective in either inhibiting the vomiting reflex or in reducing gastric acidity.
6. In gastritis associated with azotemia (see p. 124), increased secretion of gastrin, and H_2 receptor stimulation, the use of cimetidine is indicated (see p. 125).

7. Locally acting medication containing bismuth subsalicylate (Pepto Bismol) may be helpful in reducing gastric irritation associated with prostaglandin release (1 ml/lb QID Pepto Bismol).
8. When oral fluids and food can be tolerated, a very bland diet such as ID (see p. 863) should be fed in small quantities.

SALMON POISONING

This acute gastrointestinal disease is seen primarily in dogs that have ingested raw salmon, trout, lampreys, sculpins, and redside shiners carrying rickettsial-infected metacercariae of the fluke *Nanophyetus salmincola*. The rickettsial organism *Neorickettsia helminthoeca* is the infecting organism. A second rickettsia-like organism, "Elokomin fluke fever" agent *Neorickettsia elokominica*, can also be involved in salmon poisoning.

The intestinal fluke *N. salmincola* is both the vector and the reservoir in this disease. Eggs passed in the feces of dogs, foxes, coyotes, bears, and raccoons hatch into miracidia, which infect snails. Cercariae released from snails infect salmon and encyst to form metacercariae.

Clinical signs of the disease develop after an incubation period of 5 to 7 days following the ingestion of fish. The clinical signs are characterized by (1) high fever of 39.7 to 41.7° C (103.5 to 107.0° F); (2) acute vomiting and diarrhea; (3) marked dehydration; (4) lymph node enlargement; and (5) prostration, coma, and death.

Diagnosis is based on finding fluke eggs in the feces and rickettsia-like bodies in the aspirates of lymph nodes.

Treatment in this disease includes using systemic oxytetracycline IV and supporting fluid therapy (see p. 591). Affected animals should be hospitalized and kept warm and dry.

HEMORRHAGIC GASTROENTERITIS

This is an acute gastrointestinal upset usually seen in small breed dogs (e.g., Poodles, Dachshunds, Miniature Schnauzers) 2 to 4 years of age. The history usually reveals that the dogs have been in good health and are well cared for. Signs develop rapidly and include vomiting, fetid diarrhea with hemorrhage, and "jam"-like consistency of stool. Dehydration may be severe, and hematocrit may be from 55 to 70 ml per 100 ml. The patient is depressed and hypovolemic; it strains when defecating but shows no marked abdominal pain. Fluid and electrolyte abnormalities develop if the diarrhea is prolonged. Bleeding may be associated with the development of DIC.

The definitive etiology of this condition is unknown. There is evidence that it is most likely an immune-mediated problem and is not associated with acute overt bacterial infection. Acute, fulminating diarrhea associated with coronavirus or parvovirus may mimic these signs and is highly contagious.

Treatment is aimed at restoring fluid and electrolyte balance and eliminating invasion by bacterial organisms that can produce septicemia or more severe enteritis. Treatment is usually given for at least 48 hours and includes the following steps:

1. Correct fluid deficits with IV fluids administered via catheter.
2. Allow no oral food for 48 hours. If vomiting is controlled, small amounts of electrolyte solutions can be given orally in small, divided amounts.
3. Increases in gastric motility can be controlled with paregoric or *Lomotil* (diphenoxylate hydrochloride). Lomotil is a schedule V drug. Administer 2.5 mg of diphenoxylate HCl per 7 to 15 kg every 4 to 6 hours as needed. A disadvantage of the motility-controlling agents is that they may inhibit clearance of intestinal toxicants and prolong a bacterial-induced enteritis. These agents should be used in the more severe diarrheas, especially when cramping and severe pain appear evident.
4. Antimicrobial therapy—antibiotics effective against gastrointestinal anaerobes, such as systemic injections of penicillin—should be used. Administer antibiotics effective against aerobes that can elaborate endo- and exotoxins. Give kanamycin intramuscularly (IM).
5. Corticosteroids are used systemically to treat the shocklike syndrome (see pp. 60–61).
6. The animal should be carefully observed for DIC and treated with systemic heparin if indicated (see pp. 63–65).
7. When systemic signs are controlled, the return to oral food should be very gradual; cooked white rice and cottage cheese, plus very small amounts cooked lamb are acceptable. Commercially prepared prescription diets such as ID are helpful.

Acute Pancreatitis

Pancreatitis occurs most frequently in middle-aged, obese female dogs and is often associated with the feeding of a meal high in fat content. Pancreatitis can also be drug induced. Glucocorticoids are the drugs most incriminated. Glucocorticoids can increase the viscosity of pancreatic secretions and induce ductal proliferation, thus narrowing the pancreatic duct lumen, resulting in obstruction. Pancreatitis can also occur following penetrating or blunt trauma.

Acute pancreatitis usually produces sudden and severe vomiting, abdominal pain, marked depression, hypotension, and a shocklike syndrome. Vascular damage to the pancreas resulting in ischemia can also produce acute inflammation. Hypovolemic shock and DIC can contribute to vascular alteration. The blood supply to the pancreas is critical in determining whether edematous pancreatitis progresses to hemorrhagic necrotic pancreatitis. Embolization of blood vessels supplying the pancreas leads to necrosis. Diarrhea can follow vomiting and is associated with duodenal irritation. Pain may be very acute, especially on palpation of the right upper abdominal quadrant. Some dogs will show only minimal pain on abdominal palpation. The major differential diagnosis is the same as that for acute abdomen (see pp. 10–15). The pathophysiology of inflammation in acute pancreatitis involves destruction of pancreatic cellular barriers and release of activated pancreatic enzymes. The initial inflammatory reaction is complement mediated. Destruction of cellular membranes allows the release of proenzymes and activated trypsin that induces the conversion of chymotrypsinogen to chymotrypsin, prophospholipase A to phospholipase A, prekallikrein to kallikrein, and the subsequent release of bradykinin.

The most common complications of pancreatitis are fluid and electrolyte abnormalities, profound hypotension, and peritonitis. Hypotension results from the actions of bradykinin, phospholipase A and elastate release, vomiting and diarrhea, endotoxic shock, DIC, and release of vasoactive polypeptide myocardial depressant factor and activation of the complement, which activates the clotting cascade, activating platelets and causing release of serotonin and histamine, producing vasodilation and distributive shock. A toxic peptide called *myocardial depressant factor* can further lead to shock, hyperemia, cardiomyopathy, and cardiac arrhythmia. Toxins produced by intestinal bacteria, especially if there is ileus, can lead to shock and toxemia. Electrolyte imbalances can develop because of persistent vomiting; potassium loss by this mechanism can be severe. Localized chemical peritonitis can develop, producing intestinal ileus and diarrhea. Hepatic lesions, characterized by hepatic necrosis, fatty infiltration, congestion, and less-than-normal hepatic architecture, may develop.

Laboratory examination is essential for an accurate diagnosis. Serum amylase performed by the amyloclastic method and lipase are the tests of choice (see pp.742 and 753). Both serum amylase and lipase are excreted in the urine, and renal insufficiency can result in elevations of both. Hyperamylasemia must always be interpreted after renal function has been evaluated. Amylase values are *not* as specific for acute pancreatitis as are lipase values, and some clinicians do not use amylase in their minimum data base for acute pancreatitis. Serum amylase levels rise to abnormal levels (two to six times greater than normal) early in the course of the disease. Serum lipase levels also become elevated, and the amylase and lipase tests can be run concurrently. Hypotension and prerenal azotemia result in an elevated BUN. There is frequently serum hyperlipemia, and there may be hyperglycemia. Hemorrhagic pancreatitis has been associated with elevated levels of methemalbumin, which is formed as the released pancreatic enzyme acts on hemoglobin at the site where pancreatic hemorrhage is present. Hypocalcemia and hypoproteinemia may be observed in acute pancreatitis.

Urinalysis and specific gravity are indicated to determine whether azotemia is renal or prerenal in origin. A hemogram usually reveals a mild to moderate leukocytosis, with stress response. Hemoconcentration is usually present, despite extensive fluid therapy.

Ventrodorsal and lateral radiographic views should be taken. Diagnostic peritoneal lavage can be a distinct aid in acute pancreatitis. Increasing amylase levels in lavage fluid has a very high correlation with acute pancreatitis. Additionally, elevated white blood cell (WBC) counts 1,000 cells per mm, and the presence of bacteria or toxic neutrophils indicate septic pancreatic necrosis, requiring exploratory celiotomy and usually indicating pancreatic abscessation.

The following radiographic changes may be seen: (1) increased density, diminished contrast, and granularity in the right cranial abdomen; (2) stomach displaced toward the left or pyloric antral border; (3) mass medial to the proximal descending duodenum or duodenal displacement toward the right flank; (4) gastric gas pattern in or thickened walls of the descending duodenum; and (5) static gas pattern in or caudal displacement of the transverse colon.

Diabetes mellitus is a common complication of pancreatic disease, and transitory changes in blood glucose levels can be present during acute stages of pancreatitis.

Therapy in acute pancreatitis is designed to provide symptomatic relief and reduce inflammation. The most critical period in the course of the disease is 24 to 48 hours after the onset of pancreatitis. Treatment should include the following measures:

1. Correct shock, fluid, electrolyte, and acid-base abnormalities (see p. 59). Use low-dose heparin with fluid therapy (see p. 63).
2. Systemic penicillin, a cephalosporin, and gentamicin should be administered IV to control growth of aerobic and anaerobic bacteria. Renal functions should be normal before using aminoglycosides; otherwise, aminoglycoside levels should be adjusted (see p. 129).
3. Suppression of pancreatic secretion can be accomplished by complete restriction of all oral materials, including food, water, and medications. As the clinical condition improves, confine oral intake to nutrients that will stimulate pancreatic secretion the least (e.g., boiled rice as a carbohydrate source and cottage cheese or cooked eggs as a source of high biologic value proteins).

Anticholinergic drugs to control pancreatic secretion (atropine) are of questionable value. Anticholinergics may reduce intestinal motility in an already atonic intestinal tract with ileus. Vomiting can be controlled with antiemetics such as prochlorperazine or chlorpromazine. Caution is advised if severe hypovolemia is already present. Inhibition of pancreatic trypsin by Trasylol in dogs may be helpful, but unfortunately, it is expensive.

Peritoneal lavage has been discussed for use as a diagnostic aid, but it can also be used as treatment in animals who are not septic and not responding to therapy for pancreatitis. Lavage the peritoneal cavity every 6 hours with 20 ml per kg of warm lactated Ringer's solution for 1 day and once each additional day if needed.

4. Give an analgesic to reduce pain. Nalbuphine (Nubain-Endo Laboratories), 1 to 2 mg per kg IM every 4 to 6 hours as needed, is a good non-narcotic analgesic.
5. The use of glucocorticosteroids is controversial. Steroids cause hyperplasia of the pancreatic ductular epithelium and changes in pancreatic secretions, which have produced pancreatitis in experimental animals. Glucocorticosteroids should be reserved for cases with toxic shock. In experimentally induced pancreatitis, there is no evidence that the systemic administration of corticosteroids reduces the inflammation or shortens the course of the disease.

6. Sequelae include pancreatic exocrine enzyme deficiency and diabetes mellitus.

References and Additional Readings

DeHoff, W. D., Greene, R. W., and Greiner, T. P.: Surgical management of abdominal emergencies. Vet. Clin. North Am. 2:301, 1972.

Feldman, B. F., Attix, E. A., Strombeck, D. R., and O'Neill, S.: Biochemical and coagulation changes in a canine model of acute necrotizing pancreatitis. Am. J. Vet. Res., 42(5): 805, 1981.

Fets, J. F., Fox, P. R., and Burk, R. L.: Thread and sewing needles as gastrointestinal foreign bodies in the cat: A review of 64 cases. J. Am. Vet. Med. Assoc., 184:56, 1984.

Horne, W. A., Gilmore, D. R., Dietze, A. E., et al.: Effects of gastric dilatation–volvulus on coronary blood flow and myocardial oxygen consumption in the dog. Am. J. Vet. Res., 1984.

Johnson, R. G., Barrus, J., and Greene, R. W.: Gastric dilatation volvulus: recurrence rate following tube gastrotomy. J.A.A.H.A., 20(1): 33, 1984.

Kleine, L. J., and Hornbuckle, W. E.: Acute pancreatitis: radiographic findings in 182 dogs. J. Am. Vet. Radiol. Soc., 19:02, 1978.

Lantz, G. C.: The pathophysiology of acute mechanical small bowel obstruction. Compendium of Veterinary Clinical Education, 3(10):910, 1981.

Matthiesen, D. T.: The gastric dilation—volvulus complex: medical and surgical complications. J.A.A.H.A., 19(6):925, 1983.

Morgan, R.: Acute gastric dilatation—volvulus syndrome. Compendium of Continuing Education, 4(8):677, 1982.

Muir, W. W., and Weisbrode, S. E.: Myocardial ischemia in dogs with gastric dilatation–volvulus. J.A.V.M.A., 181(4): 363, 1982.

Polzin, D. J., Osborne, C. A., Stevens, J. B., and Hayden, D. W.: Serum amylase and lipase activities in dogs with chronic primary renal failure. Am. J. Vet. Res., 44(3): 404, 1983.

GENITOURINARY EMERGENCIES

Emergency treatments for uremic crisis, retention of urine, paraphimosis, acute mastitis, acute metritis, prolapsed uterus, vaginal hyperplasia, mismating, and dystocia are discussed in this section.

Uremic Crises

Azotemia is the presence of abnormally high concentrations of urea, creatinine, and other nonprotein nitrogenous substances in the blood. Azotemia may be caused by factors not directly related to the urinary system (increased liver synthesis urea or increased intake creatinine or muscle breakdown creatinine). Azotemia is not a synonym for renal failure or uremia. *Uremia* refers to abnormal amounts of urine products caused by primary generalized renal disease and its associated systemic complications.

Death from uremia is due to the retention of toxic levels of electrolytes and other metabolites and to pH and fluid abnormalities. The objectives of emergency treatment are as follows:

1. Determine whether the uremia is prerenal, renal, or postrenal. If renal, determine the degree of renal dysfunction. Determine the state of hydration (see p. 599). Determine the ability of the kidneys to concentrate or dilute urine by determining urine specific gravity. Urine with specific gravity values between 1.006 and 1.029 in dogs and between 1.006 and 1.034 in cats when associated with clinical dehydration and azotemia suggest primary renal failure. The most critical differential diagnosis here is adrenocortical insufficiency (see p. 147). Azotemia associated with hypersthenuria usually indicates prerenal azotemia.

2. Correlate the urine production (anuria, oliguria, or polyuria) with the disease process. Oliguria is defined as urine volume of less than 0.5 ml per lb (1.0 ml/kg) per hour in the dog and 0.25 ml per lb in the cat. Defective tubular function results in failure to conserve sodium or to concentrate urinary solutes such as urea and creatinine.

3. Initially manage the azotemia by correcting the renal abnormality, improving renal function to its maximum capacity, and applying supportive and symptomatic treatment to modify the lethal metabolic abnormalities.

PRERENAL UREMIA

The cause of prerenal uremia is decreased renal perfusion of normal kidneys. Causes may be shock, hypovolemia, adrenocortical insufficiency, hypotension owing to anesthetic agents, severe cardiac failure, cardiac arrhythmias, and cardiac tamponade. Frequently, prerenal disease is a complicating factor in an animal with compensated chronic renal disease. Treatment should include the following procedures:

1. Correct the extrarenal cause (shock, hypotension) rapidly, before renal damage develops: (a) correct fluid and electrolyte imbalances (see p. 591); (b) monitor input of fluids and establish an intravenous (IV) catheter (see p. 610); (c) record urine output (see p. 812); and (d) monitor urine specific gravity (see p.814).

2. Place IV catheters and rehydrate.

3. Treat shock vigorously (see p. 59). Evaluate urine production following correction of prerenal uremia.

ACUTE RENAL FAILURE

The prognosis and type of treatment for acute renal failure depend on whether the renal lesion is reversible and whether three fourths of the nephrons have been completely destroyed. Emergency treatment should correct dehydration, reduce acidosis, correct hyperkalemia, and provide caloric support.

There are a wide variety of possible causes of acute renal failure (Table 15). In veterinary medicine, the most common etiologies seen are heavy metal poisonings, ethylene glycol poisoning, hypercalcemia nephropathy, and drug toxicity to aminoglycosides. Serum chemistry profiles, urine volume measure-

Table 15. CAUSES OF ACUTE INTRINSIC RENAL FAILURE

Infections	**Nephrotoxins**
Leptospirosis	Organic compounds
Diffuse bacterial pyelonephritis	Ethylene glycol
Ischemia–Hypoxemia	Carbon tetrachloride
Hypovolemia resulting from surgery, burns,	Trichloroethylene
or trauma with hemorrhage	Heavy metals
Hypotension	Bismuth
Vascular abnormalities	Uranium
Embolism	Arsenic
Thrombosis	Lead
Hypersensitivity Reactions	Silicone
Anaphylaxis	Mercury
Vasculitis	Pigments
Nephrotoxins	Myoglobin
Drugs	Hemoglobin
Aminoglycosides	Others
Sulfonamides	Iodides
Amphotericin	Hypercalcemia (> 12 mg/100 ml)
Methoxyflurane	

ment, and urinalysis are essential to confirm the diagnosis. Patients with oliguria, high urinary sodium concentration (>40 mEq/L), fixed urine specific gravity (1.007 to 1.017), elevated SUN and serum creatinine, and low urine-to-plasma creatinine ratio ($<5:1$) have acute renal failure.

Treatment for acute renal failure involves the following measures:

1. Weigh the animal and estimate the state of dehydration (see p. 599). Attempt to determine whether the animal is urinating, how often, and approximately how much by inserting a urinary catheter.
2. Place an IV catheter (see p. 610).
3. Begin fluid replacement to correct dehydration. Carefully observe changes in body weight, and monitor for any signs of pulmonary edema (see p. 209). Most oliguric renal failure patients are volume contracted from gastrointestinal losses. The volume deficit should be replaced in the first 2 to 3 hours.
4. Evaluate acid-base status, and obtain an ECG for possible evidence of electrolyte abnormalities. Administer sodium bicarbonate, if needed (see p. 608).
5. If possible, blood pressure should be measured. Estimates are that 60 per cent of dogs with nonglomerular renal failure and 80 per cent of dogs with glomerular failure have elevated blood pressures.
6. In the oliguric or anuric patient, begin efforts to increase urine flow. Start 20 per cent dextrose drip IV, 25 to 65 ml per kg, at a rate of 2 ml per minute for 10 to 15 minutes. Monitor urine production with an indwelling catheter. If adequate urine flow is obtained, continue osmotic diuretic at a rate of 1 ml per minute. Alternate the administration of fluid replacement

therapy with osmotic diuresis. IV mannitol is another hypertonic agent that could be used at a dosage of 1 gm per kg IV. Failure to stimulate a urine flow of greater than 3 ml per kg per hour after 2 to 4 hours of fluid replacement in oliguric patients indicates significant renal parenchymal damage. *Do not* administer additional mannitol or other osmotic diuretic if diuresis cannot be established; otherwise, serious vascular overload may develop.

An attempt to begin diuresis can be made by the administration of furosemide (2 mg/kg) given IV. The drug dosage may be doubled in 2 hours if no diuresis occurs. If diuresis cannot be established, peritoneal dialysis may be needed to maintain the patient (see p. 619). If diuresis is established, renal blood flow and glomerular filtration must be maintained by supporting extracellular fluid volume with maintenance fluids. Monitor electrolytes, particularly potassium with ECG and serum levels. In severe renal failure, hyperkalemia may develop. (For correction of hyperkalemia, see Cardiac emergencies, p. 35.)

7. Treat any underlying specific etiologies that can be found (e.g., ethylene glycol poisoning; see p. 194).
8. A renal biopsy may be required to establish a prognosis (see p. 530).
9. Reduce dietary intake of phosphorus and sodium, and use a high biologic value low-protein diet (see p. 872). Care must be taken not to suddenly place animals on restricted diets but to gradually place them on lower protein and sodium restriction. Provide free access to water. Control hypertension if measurements indicated blood pressure of 180/95 or greater. Gradually reduce oral intake of sodium in the diet.
10. Use aluminum hydroxide gel (Amphogel) orally as a phosphorus binding agent; Dogs should receive 5 to 15 ml with their food TID; cats should receive 1 to 5 ml with their food TID.
11. Use cimetidine (Tagamet) to decrease uremic gastritis and offset the effects of increased gastrin secretion, which occurs in renal failure. Cimetidine is available as tablets, as an oral liquid, and as an injectible. In severe gastropathy, the initial dosage can be given IV, 10 mg per kg TID, followed by 5 mg per kg BID. Home usage can be oral, 5 mg per kg BID to once a day as needed. If acute renal failure is possibly reversible, the use of ambulatory peritoneal dialysis (see p. 619) is a possibility.

POSTRENAL UREMIA

Obstructions and ruptures of the urinary system may prevent excretion of urine from the body. This condition, if acute and complete, may cause death in 3 to 5 days due to the accumulation of metabolic wastes. Causes are trauma, calculi, neoplasia, stricture, and congenital anomalies. In most cases, definitive treatment is surgery. Immediate treatment should re-establish urine flow, support, and correct metabolic imbalances.

After the release of complete urinary obstruction, a dramatic diuresis develops and persists for several days. During this diuresis, large sodium and potassium losses occur. Extracellular fluid volume must be maintained during this diuretic phase. The fluids should contain sodium, and sodium bicarbonate should be used to correct acidosis (see p. 610).

Retention of Urine

CAUSES

Ruptured Bladder (See p. 27)

The initial treatment of bladder rupture depends on the status of the animal when it is initially presented for examination. Animals with elevated potassium levels, elevated BUN and creatinine, and those in severe uremia must initially be supported with fluids and peritoneal dialysis for at least 24 hours to make them a better anesthetic risk. Exploratory celiotomy is then indicated. An indwelling urinary catheter should be positioned during critical care therapy.

The utmost care in administering anesthesia and treatment of shock is crucial to a successful repair. Epidural or local block anesthesia may be best for toxic patients. Steroid, antibiotic, and adequate fluid or transfusion support is essential.

The peritoneum should be thoroughly lavaged to remove all traces of residual urine.

Following repair, fluid intake should be promoted to encourage renal function and to correct the uremia.

Urethral Occlusion

Obstruction of the urethra is most frequently associated with urolithiasis but also may be associated with tumors, infection, strictures, and inflammation. The condition is most frequently recognized in male dogs and occurs when calculi become trapped behind the os penis bone. Strictures of the urethra may be associated with previous urethostomy. Clinical signs of urethral obstruction are dysuria, hematuria, anuria, progressive depression and azotemia, and enlarged bladder on abdominal palpation.

Initial treatment centers around catheterization and bladder expression. Often, the site of obstruction can be distinguished as the catheter is passed. If urethral calculi block passage of the catheter, try the technique of urohydropropulsion. Place the dog under sedation. Compress the proximal urethra on the pelvic floor with a finger in the dog's rectum while saline is injected under pressure into the distal urethra. Use a catheter and compress the distal urethra around it. Withdraw the catheter suddenly to release the pressure (be sure to maintain the occlusion of the urethra in the pelvic canal), and the saline and calculi commonly are ejected distally. This procedure, which may be repeated several times, often removes the obstructing stones.

If the urethral calculi are too large to pass the os penis, the procedure can be modified and pressure on the distal urethra can be maintained while pressure on the pelvic urethra is rapidly released. This enables larger calculi to be flushed back into the bladder where they can be removed by cystotomy.

If this method fails, perform aseptic cystocentesis with a 22-gauge 2-inch needle for temporary relief. Corrective surgery can often be delayed to prepare the patient as a better surgical risk. If all these steps fail, definitive surgical removal should be performed immediately.

FELINE UROLOGIC SYNDROME
(Lower Urinary Tract Disease of Cats)

Feline urologic syndrome (FUS) is comprised of cystitis, urethritis, cystic calculi, and urethral obstruction. The disease can occur in both male and female cats, although males between the ages of 1 and 5 years predominate. The etiology of FUS is complex, and all the factors involved are not yet understood.

Ninety to 99 per cent of all uroliths in cats are primarily magnesium-ammonium-phosphate (struvite). From 0.5 to 3 per cent of uroliths in cats are urate and oxalate, and 3 to 5 per cent are amorphous gelatinous plugs (if they contain mineral, it is usually struvite).

Secondary causes of FUS are involved in the production of struvite uroliths in the bladder and urethra. Urinary pH greater than 6.8, reduced water intake and urine volume with increased urinary concentration of minerals, and diets high in dry foods or ash content predispose to struvite accumulations. Increased intake of urolith-forming constituents in the diet can increase chances of urolithiasis, that is, dietary magnesium levels of 0.37 to 0.4 per cent (dry matter), as can diets with greater than 5 per cent ash content (dry matter) when combined with a high magnesium content. Magnesium and ash content are more likely to be higher in commercial dry and soft, moist cat foods. Feeding cats dry to semimoist cat foods free choice throughout the day increases urinary pH in cats predisposing to struvite calculi.

Clinical signs may include dysuria, urinating with increased frequency or in unusual places, and hematuria. The most severe problem is urethral obstruction.

The penile urethra in the male cat is the site of urethral blockage. However, urethral strictures or urethral or cystic calculi may occur and require retrograde contrast urethrography to demonstrate the lesion (see p. 572). The most frequent signs are: straining to urinate and bloody urine. Additional clinical signs include licking of the penis and perineal area; swollen, bluish, discolored penis with mucous-struvite plug; enlarged painful bladder on palpation; and concentrated bloody urine containing struvite crystals.

Urinary obstruction that persists in the cat for longer than 24 hours results in severe postrenal uremia. The following changes are life threatening: severe dehydration, especially associated with vomiting; hyperkalemia; metabolic acidosis; elevated BUN and serum creatinine; and cardiac arrhythmias.

Treatment is as follows:

Rapid relief of urethral obstruction. Obstructed cats are frequently azotemic, hyperkalemic, and dehydrated. Great care must be used in sedating them to attempt to relieve the urethral blockage and/or perform cystocentesis and pass a catheter.

1. Do not use IV barbiturates; avoid ketamine in severe acidotic, azotemic cats.
2. Use inhalation anesthesia if possible (nitrous oxide, oxygen, halothane-balance; see pp.69–81); be ready to intubate the cat (see p. 629).
3. If severe uremia and acidosis are present, begin fluid therapy (see p. 610) before dislodging the blockage and passing the urethral catheter.
4. Support the animal's body temperature with a thermal water blanket, towels, or blankets.

To remove the blockage, (a) gently massage the penis to dislodge plugs in the penile urethra and (b) perform reverse flushing of the urethral lumen with sterile saline, lactated Ringer's solution, or dilute solutions of acetic acid (Walpole's solution). Prepare Walpole's solution by mixing 57 ml of 0.2 molar acetic acid with 43 ml of 0.2 molar sodium acetate. Because it may support bacterial growth, pass the solution through a millipore filter to remove debris and to sterilize the solution prior to use.

The type of catheter used in back flushing is important, because metal catheters can produce severe urethral trauma. Use only sterile catheters.

A variety of different types of tomcat catheters that can be used as indwelling urinary catheters are available. A catheter having an open end and enough length to reach the preprostatic urethra, but not the bladder lumen, should be used. Long catheters protruding into the bladder can produce excessive irritation and hemorrhage. A catheter of 11 cm in length, 3.5 French, is usually sufficient to reach the preprostatic urethra. A 3.5 French rubber urethral catheter lubricated with Xylocaine jelly or sterile petrolatum will result in less trauma than some plastic catheters. The end of the indwelling catheter is wrapped with adhesive tape and then sutured to the prepuce. An Elizabethan collar should be used on the cat to prevent it from removing the catheter. Kitty litter should be removed from the toilet box and replaced with paper towels. If the catheter is left in the urethra, a closed drainage system should be established and the cat should be started on systemic antibiotics that will achieve urine levels.

If urethral catheterization and back flushing of the urethral plug are not successful, cystocentesis is indicated to drain the bladder (see p. 549). Prolonged obstruction requires measures to prevent the development of severe metabolic defects.

Principles for correcting fluid-metabolic defects caused by urethral obstruction include:

1. Estimate the degree of dehydration and correct with appropriate fluid therapy (see p. 610).
2. Correct metabolic acidosis (see p. 593).
3. Correct underlying severe hyperkalemia as evidenced by electrocardiographic (ECG) changes (see p. 49). Correct the urinary blockage, and give fluids to correct hyperkalemia.

In selected severe cases, insulin and dextrose can be used to decrease extracellular levels of potassium. Give insulin IV at a dosage rate of 0.5 units per kg, followed by 2 gm of dextrose per unit of insulin IV. Twenty-five per cent of this dosage of dextrose is administered over a 5-minute period, with the remainder placed in fluids to make a solution of 2.5 per cent dextrose.

It must be stressed that not all urethral blockages nor the inability of some cats to urinate should be treated in the same manner. It is important to (1) evaluate for the presence of cystic or urethral calculi; (2) determine whether any urethral defects or damage exists (retrograde urethrography; see p. 572); and (3) look for predisposing causes, that is, bacterial cystitis, persistent urachal diverticulum of the bladder, and changes in pH of the urine.

Following relief of obstruction, the glomerular filtration rate may be 20 to 50 per cent of normal and may remain decreased for up to 7 days.

As renal function resumes, a period of diuresis will occur. During this period, dehydration, hyponatremia, and hypokalemia may develop. Encourage water consumption by adding fluids to the regular diet, by salting the food (¼ tsp per day), or by giving the animal a 1-gm salt tablet per day in divided doses. Daily fluid supplementation via subcutaneous fluid administration is often needed.

Although most cases of FUS do not involve bacterial cystitis, the use of an indwelling catheter can cause a bacterial infection, and prophylactic antibiotics should be used. The type of antibiotic selected should be assessed in regard to the degree of renal function present, because some antibiotics are nephrotoxic. Calculi present in the urinary tract may be relieved by surgery or by the feeding of a calculolytic diet, which reduces urinary magnesium and maintains an acidic urine. This can be a home-made diet (see p. 872) or feline s/d diet (Hill's), which has less than 20 mg of magnesium per 100 kcal, maintains urine pH near 6.0 3 to 5 hours after eating, and promotes water consumption. The diet should not be used for longer than 6 months (see p. 872). A diet that contains not more than 20 mg of magnesium per 100 kcal or 0.10 per cent magnesium in its dry matter or greater than 5 per cent ash in the dry matter should then be used. The addition of 1 gm of ammonium chloride or 1.5 gm per dl of methionine can be added daily to further acidify the urine.

DRUG ADMINISTRATION IN ANIMALS WITH RENAL DISEASE
(See also p. 812)

Unmetabolized drugs may accumulate in the body when drugs that are normally eliminated or excreted by the kidneys are not metabolized properly by abnormal renal function. The half-life of drugs eliminated mainly by the kidneys is relatively normal until the glomerular filtration rate (GFR) is 30 to 40 per cent of normal.

To avoid accumulation, doses of drugs eliminated by the kidney must be reduced when renal insufficiency is present. If the GFR, as measured by creatinine clearance (cl_{cr}) is known, the dosage of medication to be administered can be given at increased intervals or reduced levels.

Interval extension method—^{T}*renal failure $= ^{T}$normal $\times \dfrac{\text{normal cl}_{cr}}{\text{patient cl}_{cr}}$

Dose reduction method—^{D}†renal failure $= ^{D}$normal $\times \dfrac{\text{patient cl}_{cr}}{\text{normal cl}_{cr}}$

If the creatinine clearance is not known, the use of serum creatinine can provide a rough estimate of how to decrease the dosage of a drug. Normal serum creatinine in dogs and cats is usually considered to be 1.0.

PARALYSIS OF BLADDER MUSCULATURE
(See Urinary Incontinence, p. 281)

Paralysis of bladder musculature causes retention of urine with overflow and commonly occurs when a housebroken dog is confined for long periods of time. Urine may dribble, giving the appearance of incontinence. It is imperative to catheterize or express urine from the greatly dilated bladder and to keep the bladder nearly empty for roughly 2 weeks by frequent compression or catheterization. Healing usually occurs. Smooth muscle stimulation with bethanechol chloride (5 to 25 mg every 8 hours orally) may also be helpful. Bladder musculature dysfunction is also frequently seen with neurologic abnormalities, especially those of traumatic origin.

Renal Trauma (See also Abdominal Injuries)

Because the kidneys are well protected and somewhat pendulous, they are not commonly injured. However, sudden compressive forces against the abdominal wall can force the kidneys against the paralumbar musculature. Trauma can be extreme and may rupture large renal vessels, with death occurring in minutes. Less severe trauma may produce intracapsular damage or hematomas, which usually heal spontaneously. In such cases, hematuria may result and thrombosis of vessels may cause infarction and permanent loss of some renal tissue. Hemorrhage through the renal parenchyma and capsule with bleeding into the retroperitoneal space or peritoneal cavity can cause shock, severe hypovolemia, and anemia. The use of a body or torso wrap may be helpful in controlling internal bleeding while initial shock is being managed and prior to exploratory celiotomy.

If the renal capsule is torn, blood and urine may escape into the peritoneal cavity. Paracentesis and peritoneal lavage may be useful in checking for urea and red blood cells. If in doubt, exploratory surgery may be necessary to detect the type of injury. Partial or complete nephrectomy or renal capsule repair with Gelfoam or cellulose strips may be indicated.

---

*T = dose interval
†D = amount of drug

Paraphimosis

Paraphimosis is invariably the result of coitus. Gentle cleaning with Betadine and water, thorough lubricating with K-Y jelly or Lubritine, and replacing the prepuce over the penis usually correct paraphimosis in the early stages. No further treatment is needed.

Severe edema, hemorrhage, and lacerations of the penis may require cold packs or hypertonic solutions to reduce tumescence. A small incision in the dorsal commissure of the sheath may be needed to replace the sheath. In rare cases, the penis may have to be amputated.

Genital Trauma

Genital trauma usually involves male dogs, because the female genitalia are well protected. Contusions and lacerations of the sheath, penis, and scrotum are common. Small injuries to the scrotum prompt the dog to lick them, resulting in acute infection. In all cases, sedation and/or restraint to prevent this are important. Most areas are highly vascular, and careful ligature of vessels, tunicae, and fasciae may be necessary to control hemorrhage. Urethral trauma may also be involved, so drains or catheters should be used to prevent tissue infiltration of extravasated blood and urine leakage. A Foley catheter works well in larger breeds. A more proximally located urethrotomy may bypass urine and allow the traumatized area to heal. Heavy sedation and avoidance of sexual stimulation are necessary to avoid penile erection. Most wounds are infected, so the use of topical and systemic antibacterial medications is desirable.

Other genital emergencies that may be seen in the male dog are:

1. *Severe orchitis,* an extremely painful condition, is characterized by acute scrotal swelling. An initial clinical sign may be lameness. Acute septic orchitis can lead to rapid development of septic shock and should be managed accordingly (see p. 59). Initial treatment with corticosteroids will reduce the swelling, and broad-spectrum antibiotics (such as tetracyclines) should be administered for 14 to 21 days. Evaluate all dogs with orchitis and scrotal dermatitis for *Brucella canis* infection.

2. *Testicular torsion* usually involves a retained abdominal testicle that may be enlarged because of tumor development. The rotation of the testicle on its cord precipitates severe venous occlusion, marked swelling, pain, and tenesmus. Most cases of torsion of an intra-abdominal testicle present with clinical signs resembling acute intestinal obstruction: anorexia, vomiting, acute abdominal pain, and possible palpable abdominal mass. Careful physical examination can reveal the problem, and exploratory laparotomy is indicated. Supportive treatment and control of shock are indicated. The involved testicle must be surgically removed in most cases.

3. *Acute prostatic disease,* associated with either severe prostatic hypertrophy or prostatic infection, can lead to marked pain, difficulty in defecation,

and urine retention with partial urethral obstruction. In these cases, catheterization of the bladder is indicated. Additionally, enemas and stool softeners (such as dioctyl sodium sulfosuccinate) should be used. Treat to reduce the prostatic hypertrophy and to control infection.

Acute Mastitis

In dogs and cats, the common condition of acute mastitis is an acute inflammation with localization (abscess formation) in one breast. In the cat, acute mastitis is usually related to parturition and lactation. The glands affected are most often posterior in location. Streptococcus and Staphylococcus microorganisms are usually involved. The first signs of mastitis are a swollen breast and weak pups or kittens because of abnormal milk. The patient is febrile and septic. Start antibiotic therapy with cephalosporins plus cold compresses. Obtain a bacterial culture and a gram stain of milk sediment. Obtain both aerobic and anaerobic cultures (see p. 499). Incise and drain abscesses as soon as localization develops. Remove suckling animals and feed them as orphans; tape the affected breast, so that it cannot be nursed. Recovery is usually uncomplicated.

Acute Metritis

Acute metritis is often associated with dystocia, obstetric manipulations, abortions, or retained placenta or fetus. The normal postpartum vaginal discharge is a blood-tinged mucoid discharge. Normal placentas should be expelled by 12 to 24 hours postpartum. Evidence of a foul-smelling vaginal discharge, fever, depression, and inability to nurse is evidence of developing metritis.

Acute metritis is seen several days after whelping and is a febrile, highly fatal septicemia. Start antibiotic therapy with cephalosporins (1st generation) or penicillin-gentamicin or ampicillin-gentamicin, all administered IV. Institute fluid therapy, and treat septic shock if it exists. Obtain culture and sensitivity of the uterine discharge.

Drain the uterus of all fluids by inserting a catheter through the cervix, by using postural drainage, or by irrigating. Furacin solution (15 to 30 ml) should be left in utero. Remove suckling animals, and raise them as orphans.

In both metritis and pyometra, the administration of prostaglandin F_2alpha-THAM at a level of 250 μg per kg and given subcutaneously, coupled with medical treatment, may avoid the necessity of ovariohysterectomy.

Pyometritis

Pyometritis in the bitch and queen can be secondary to any infectious process. It may follow postpartum metritis, postcopulation, or postinsemination infections; a mismating injection of estrogens, especially estradiol; or the indiscriminate use of exogenous progesterone therapy. It most frequently is a final sequela of cystic endometrial hyperplasia-endometritis-pyometritis complex. This complex occurs following several nonpregnant cycles in the bitch and queen and increases in frequency with age.

Pyometra is often associated with bacterial toxins, producing glomerular damage and renal complications of considerable severity. The early phase of cystic endometrial hyperplasia, accompanied or followed by endometritis, may show a clinical vaginal discharge that varies from blood-tinged to mucopurulent. There are two types of pyometra, open and closed cervix. The latter type has no vaginal discharge and is usually more toxic. In the open form, a mucopurulent and possibly blood-tinged or serosanguinous vaginal discharge is present. In closed pyometras, severe septicemia and elevated WBC develops. History in both forms indicates polydysia, polyuria, a recent heat cycle, parturition, or sex steroid–hormonal injections. Radiographs of the abdomen are indicated to visualize the uterus.

If a bitch or queen with pyometritis is not a valuable breeder, ovariohysterectomy is the preferred treatment. Antibiotic therapy and uterine drainage plus supportive therapy for shock, dehydration, and acidosis may be necessary. Surgical patients must be carefully evaluated for the aforementioned conditions and to determine the safest anesthesia for the individual case.

In breeding animals, when it is important to produce more offspring, prostaglandin therapy combined with antibiotics can be attempted. Antibiotic therapy (based on sensitivity tests performed on cultures of deep vaginal exudate when possible) should begin 24 hours prior to prostaglandin therapy. Prior to sensitivity results, antibiotics such as chloramphenicol that combat *Escherichia coli* infections are the best choice. Therapy should continue for 10 to 21 days.

The most widely used prostaglandin (PG) in the bitch and queen has been $PGF_{2\alpha}$ (dinoprost, Lutalyse*) The dose regimen is variable. Successful treatment has been reported with twice daily intramuscular (IM) injections of 25 to 50 mcg per kg of body weight of $PGF_{2\alpha}$. These animals are hospitalized and usually started on the low dose to observe side reactions and to start cervical opening and uterine contractions. Most animals are treated for 3 to 5 days, depending on reduction in the size of the uterus, the tone of the uterus, disappearance of discharge, and general improvement of the patient. Daily douching of the deep vagina with 250 ml of a warm 1 per cent tamed iodine solution (Betadine) is helpful during $PGF_{2\alpha}$ therapy.

A higher dosage in the bitch, 250 mcg per kg, IM of $PGF_{2\alpha}$ in one to four treatments daily or every 48 hours, has been reported. This has been used in nonhospitalized, less critical cases with good results. The higher the dose, the more severe the side effects. Major side effects are seen within minutes to within 90 or 120 minutes in the more severe reactions. These reactions include salivation, loose stool, vomiting, anxiety, dyspnea, tachycardia, ataxia, and

---

*Upjohn Company, Kalamazoo, Michigan.

collapse. The median lethal dose (LD 50) in the dog is 5.13 mg per kg of body weight.

All bitches and queens diagnosed as having cystic endometrial hyperplasia-endometritis-pyometritis complex who are treated, should be rechecked clinically and cultured prior to the next estrus and bred if normal or retreated if still showing clinical signs of uterine infection. Bitches and queens not to be used for breeding can be ovariohysterectomized before the next estrus.

Prolapsed Uterus

Prolapsed uterus occurs after whelping and is an emergency of the utmost concern. Treatment requires anesthesia and replacement of the organ. In some cases, this can be done easily; however, it is essential that the entire organ be unfolded properly in the abdomen. If there is doubt that it has been unfolded properly, a laparotomy must be performed to complete proper restoration of the uterus. Pitocin can then be given to cause contraction of the uterus. The lips of the vulva can be sutured; however, if the uterus has contracted, there is usually no recurrence. Antibiotics should be administered, and shock should be treated, if necessary.

If severe edema is present in the prolapsed uterus, applying hypertonic glucose or saline solution, kneading, and massaging will help remove the fluid. If the uterus cannot be effectively replaced or if it is cyanotic or appears necrotic and/or gangrenous, an ovariohysterectomy should be performed. In this case, the uterus is not returned to the abdomen but is removed per vaginal incision using an episiotomy to allow better exposure.

Vaginal Hyperplasia

Vaginal hyperplasia occurs during estrus in large breeds of dogs. This is not a real emergency, because commonly, only a small amount of tissue protrudes from the vulva. Frequent application of ointments to keep the exposed tissue soft, protected, and viable is recommended until surgical correction is carried out or hormonal (progesterone) effects are evident. The condition often recurs at subsequent estral cycles, so ovariohysterectomy is often performed for permanent cure.

Mismating

Some bitches can be receptive in proestrus and bred as early as 3 days before their pituitary release of luteinizing hormone (LH) or 5 days before ovulation and 10 days before oocytes are destined to be released from the oviduct. A bitch may also not be receptive and bred until as late as 6 days after the LH peak or 4 days after ovulation and, thus, only 1 to 2 days before oocytes are destined to be released into the uterus. Dog spermatozoa are capable of fertilization for 6 to 7 days and possibly 11 days after ejaculation into the female reproductive tract. Canine ova are ovulated from follicles as primary oocytes about 36 to 48 hours after the LH peak but undergo maturation in the oviduct for as long as 2 to 3 days later. Fertilization probably occurs no earlier than 3 days after the LH peak. Thus, gestation periods based on the first breeding may range from 57 to 72 days. Transportation of ova through the oviduct takes 8 to 10 days from the LH peak.

In the queen, ovulation is induced by coitus, which causes release of sufficient pituitary LH in 25 to 30 hours. Following ovulation, oocytes remain viable for up to 48 hours. Oviductal transport of fertilized oocytes to the uterus takes 4 to 5 days.

The object of treating mismating with estrogens is to delay passage of oocytes in the oviduct and to create a hostile environment for them in the oviduct and uterus.

In the queen, the best time to administer estrogen is within 2 to 5 days after observed coitus, while the oocytes are in the oviducts. In the bitch, the optimal time is 3 to 6 days after ovulation or the LH peak. Because some bitches can be bred in proestrus, this is not a good period to administer estrogens; they may delay her release of LH and ovulation, thus permitting subsequent fertility. Recent research indicates that estrogens administered to bitches at proestrus breeding are less likely to prevent pregnancy. The use of vaginal smears and/or vaginoscopic examination for estrous cycle determination and timing of a mismating injection are highly useful.

Using vaginal cytology, the administration of estrogens for mismating in the bitch is best late in estrus when the cytology is changing from fully cornified cells to containing some noncornified cells. If the smear is one of proestrus or early estrus, a delay of 3 to 6 days before administering estrogens may be considered; if the smear is very late estrus or early metestrus (containing a mixture of cornified and noncornified cells, parabasal, and small intermediate cells with large nuclei and a small to large number of leukocytes), an immediate administration of estrogen should be given.

No drugs are legally labeled for mismating in dogs or cats. Injectible estradiol cyponiate is usually used at a single IM injection level of 0.125 to 1.0 mg depending on the size of the dog and 0.125 to 0.25 mg in the cat. Oral diethylstilbestrol tablets are available in 0.1 to 5.0 mg tablets. In the bitch, oral administration of 5 mg the first day, followed by daily oral dose of 1 to 3 mg for 5 days has been suggested.

Symptoms of estrus may be prolonged following administration of estrogens, and owners should be cautioned to confine their animal during this period to avoid further mating. Estrogens are toxic in both the dog and cat and can cause bone marrow depression, thrombocytopenia, followed by a hemorrhagic syndrome and death. Uterine infection and pyometritis may also develop secondarily to estrogen administration, and owners should be warned of abnormal vaginal discharges or the development of septic pyometritis 2 to 6 weeks posttreatment.

Both the bitch and queen can be aborted in late pregnancy. $PGF_{2\alpha}$ is luteolytic in the bitch if administered repeatedly from midpregnancy period until term. After a diagnosis of pregnancy has been made by palpation at 25 to 30 days, doses of 25 to 50 mcg per kg are given IM twice daily, with most bitches aborting in 3 to 7 days. Cessation of treatment before abortion or before all pups are aborted can result in no or incomplete abortion, with the remainder of the litter going to term and being delivered as normal pups.

Termination of pregnancy in cats with $PGF_{2\alpha}$ has been reported from 40 days of gestation to term, with 0.50 to 1.00 mg of $PGF_{2\alpha}$ per kg of body weight, given once or twice in 24-hour intervals. In both bitches and queens, various side effects of $PGF_{2\alpha}$, including anxiety, salivation, vomiting, diarrhea, tachycardia, and dyspnea, can be seen shortly after administration.

Dystocia*

The normal onset of labor is marked by the following events:
1. Milk may appear in the breasts from 4 to 5 days to just before parturition.
2. 24 hours before—bitch goes off to hide and make a nest.
3. 12 hours before—bitch refuses food. A white vaginal discharge may appear (cervical seal). It may appear several days before whelping.
4. 12 to 8 hours before—bitch's rectal temperature drops at least 1° C often to 37° C (98° F).
5. 4 hours before—cervix begins rapid dilatation.
6. 1 hour before—cervix dilates and labor pains begin.

The presence of a greenish-black discharge indicates placental separation and may appear before or after the first fetus is delivered.

If no puppy is delivered within 4 hours after the onset of labor, a pelvic examination is indicated. Two puppies are usually presented in close succession, followed by a pause of 1 to 2 hours. Delivery of the entire litter may take 24 to 30 hours. Fetal membranes may be eaten by the bitch, but they often produce a gastroenteritis lasting 8 to 12 hours.

Dystocia can exist (1) when no delivery of a fetus occurs within 4 to 6 hours after the onset of stage 2 labor; (2) if more than 4 to 5 hours have elapsed following the last delivery of a fetus and no attempt is made to deliver more, despite the presence of more fetuses in the uterus; (3) if weak and infrequent labor contractions are present; (4) if depression, weakness, and signs of toxemia are developing; (5) if no puppies are born by about the 72nd day of gestation; (6) if no puppies are born 2 to 3 hours after the amniotic-allantoic membranes have ruptured; and (7) if no puppies are born after 2 to 3 hours of active labor.

Dystocias may be either maternal or fetal. Maternal dystocias can include primary and secondary uterine inertia, pelvic abnormalities, psychologic dis-

---

*These comments pertain to the canine species. Many are also appropriate to the feline species. Dystocia in the queen usually is due to uterine inertia and is rare. Parturition is usually an easy process in the queen.

turbances, inguinal herniation, and uterine torsion. Fetal dystocias can include oversized fetuses (often owing to small number of fetuses), and abnormal presentation (remember that both anterior and posterior presentations are normal in dogs and cats). The most common problems are transverse presentations and breech presentations. The latter is posterior, with both legs directed anteriorly.

If dystocia is diagnosed, further digital exploration of the pelvic canal is indicated. The perineum should be clipped and cleaned, and digital palpation should be done with a sterilized gloved hand. Sterile lubricant such as K-Y jelly can be used. Determine the position of the fetus if in the pelvic inlet, the size of the pelvic inlet, and the degree of dilatation of the cervix. In large breeds, the latter may be determined only by endoscopic examinations.

Primary uterine inertia is common in pampered toy bitches, especially the Dachshund, Scottish terrier, Chihuahua, Yorkshire terrier, and Toy poodles. Begin initial treatment of primary inertia with 10 per cent calcium gluconate 1 ml per 5 kg IV, followed by Pitocin, 2 to 20 units IM. Pitocin can be repeated, if necessary. In nervous bitches, IM injections of meperidine HCL, 2 to 4 mg per kg, may promote labor by its analgesic and relaxing effect. Feathering (scratching the dorsal vaginal wall with a gloved index finger) may also stimulate labor. If no results are obtained following these procedures, a cesarean section should be considered.

When only one or two puppies are to be delivered, medical attempts at stimulating uterine contractions or forceps manipulations are worth exploiting. However, if a large number of pups are involved, a cesarean section usually offers the best chance for successful delivery of viable offspring. This procedure tends to conserve the strength of the bitch (and her attendants).

Secondary uterine inertia results from fatigue due to obstruction of the pelvic canal. Fetal malposition and pelvic measurement of less than 1.5 inches lateral are the usual causes. It is usually best managed by cesarean section unless only one fetus is retained and can be removed manually.

References and Additional Readings

Barsanti, J. A., and Finco, D.: Feline urologic syndrome. *In* Kirk, R. W. (ed.): Current Veterinary Therapy VIII: Small Animal Practice, Philadelphia, W. B. Saunders Company, 1983.

Bennett, D.: Normal and abnormal parturition. *In* Morrow, D. (ed.): Current Therapy in Theriogenology. Philadelphia, W. B. Saunders Company, 1980, pp. 595–606.

Burke, T. J.: Prostaglandin $F_{2\alpha}$ in the treatment of pyometra-metritis. Vet. Clin. North Am., *12*(1): 107, 1982.

Colby, E., and Soijka, N. J.: Feline reproductive diseases. *In* Morrow, D. (ed.): Current Therapy in Theriogenology. Philadelphia, W. B. Saunders Company, 1980.

Concannon, P. W.: Fertility regulation in the bitch: contraception, sterilization, and pregnancy termination. *In* Kirk, R. W. (ed.): Current Veterinary Therapy VIII: Small Animal Practice. Philadelphia, W. B. Saunders Company, 1983, pp. 901–909.

Cowgill, L. D.: Diseases of the kidney. *In* Ettinger, S. J.: Textbook of Veterinary Internal Medicine: Diseases of the Dog and Cat, 2nd ed. Philadelphia, W. B. Saunders Company, 1983, pp. 1793–1879.

Lein, D. H.: Pyometritis in the Bitch and Queen. *In* Kirk, R. W. (ed.): Current Veterinary Therapy VIII: Small Animal Practice. Philadelphia, W. B. Saunders Company, 1983, pp. 942–944.

Lewis, L., and Morris, M., Jr.: Small Animal Clinical Nutrition, Topeka, Kansas, Mark Morris Associates, 1983.

Nachreiner, R. F., and Marple, D. N.: Termination of pregnancy in cats with prostaglandin $F_{2\alpha}$. Prostaglandin, 7:303, 1974.

Nelson, R. W., Feldman, E. C., and Stabenfeldt, G. H.: Treatment of canine pyometra and endometritis with prostaglandin $F_{2\alpha}$. J.A.V.M.A., *181*(9): 899, 1982.

Osborne, C. A., Johnston, G. A., et al.: Feline urologic syndrome. J.A.A.H.A., *20*(1): 17, 1984.

Shille, V. M.: Canine reproductive diseases. *In* Morrow, D. (ed.): Current Therapy in Theriogenology, Philadelphia, W. B. Saunders Company, 1980.

Soderberg, S. F., and Olson, P. N.: Abortifacents. *In* Kirk, R. W. (ed.): Current Veterinary Therapy VIII: Small Animal Practice. Philadelphia, W. B. Saunders Company, 1983, pp. 945–946.

Sokolowski, J. H.: Prostaglandin $F_{2\alpha}$-THAM for medical treatment of endometritis, metritis, and pyometritis in the bitch. J.A.A.H.A., *16*: 119, 1980.

METABOLIC EMERGENCIES

Emergency treatments for hyperglycemia (diabetic ketoacidosis), hypoglycemia, puerperal tetany (canine eclampsia), adrenocortical insufficiency, and acidosis are discussed in this section.

Diabetic Ketoacidosis

Diabetic ketoacidosis is the terminal result of insulin insufficiency and possible glucagon excess. Early in the disease, patients exhibit the typical signs of diabetes mellitus. Diabetic ketoacidosis is characterized by vomiting, dehydration, hypotension, oliguria, severe depression, Kussmaul's breathing, diarrhea, weight loss, and coma.

Initial physical examination reveals:

1. Dehydration (not always).
2. Prerenal azotemia.
3. Severe depression, possibly progressing to coma.
4. Fever (not always).
5. Shock, hypovolemia.
6. Rapid, Kussmaul's-type breathing.
7. Blood glucose usually greater than 300 mg per kg, urine glucose 4 +, urine ketones 4 +, elevated BUN (prerenal), urine specific gravity 1.030 or greater (see p. 664).
8. Hyperosmolarity of the serum (sometimes; see p. 601).
9. Plasma may be lipemic (can produce false hyponatremia).
10. Plasma sodium is usually increased.
11. Deficit in total—body potassium is present. There may be a normal serum

potassium, because acidosis results in translocation of intracellular potassium to extracellular space (see p. 602).

12. Acute pancreatitis may be present (see p. 119).
13. Liver enzymes may be elevated, associated with altered glucose metabolism and fatty liver.
14. Metabolic acidosis is present—elevated levels of β-hydroxybutyric acid, H^+—respiratory compensation for the metabolic acidosis is being attempted, thus the Kussmaul's-type respiratory pattern.
15. A large anion gap is present, along with the metabolic acidosis (see   ).
16. Diabetics are more sensitive to infections, thus cystitis, pyelonephritis, and metritis may be present.

Treatment

Draw blood for hemogram, glucose, BUN, and ketones. Monitor blood pH, bicarbonate, sodium, potassium, and chloride, if possible. Collect urine for glucose, pH, and ketone determinations. Maintain an adequate airway passage and, if necessary, insert an endotracheal tube. Place an indwelling catheter in either the jugular or cephalic vein. Start an intravenous (IV) infusion of 0.9 per cent NaCl or 2.5 per cent fructose in 0.45 per cent NaCl. If serum sodium is over 155 mEq per L, use 0.45 per cent saline. Replace 50 per cent of the calculated fluid loss over the first 12 hours; however, fluids should not be administered faster than 70 ml per kg per hour, so that the vascular compartment can adjust and until renal perfusion and renal output are adequate. Add 10 to 20 mEq of sodium bicarbonate per L of fluid if bicarbonate levels cannot be measured. The potassium deficit can be estimated at 3 mEq per kg, and plans should be made to replace the deficit over a 24-hour period. Do not exceed more than 40 mEq per L (see also p. 604).

Attempt to measure the acid-base balance. Ideally, pCO_2 and pH should be measured; however, if not available, total CO_2 can be measured using a kit (see p. 593).

Insulin administration can be begun by either low-dose IV or low-dose IM method. In the low-dose IV method, begin insulin administration by continuous low-dose infusion. Add 5 units of regular insulin to 250 ml of lactated Ringer's solution; administer insulin, using a pediatric infusion drip, at a rate of 0.5 to 1.0 unit of regular insulin per kg per hour for dogs and 0.1 to 0.2 units of insulin per kg per hour for cats. More rapid administration of noninsulin solutions is performed by using a second vein to maintain hydration. When the blood glucose begins to fall, do not administer more insulin until the full effect of the last dose is known (Table 16).

In the low-dose IM method, the following chart can be used. Blood glucose levels should be estimated hourly using Ames dextrometer and Dextrostix.

Body Weight (kg)	Initial Dose	Hourly Dose
<10	2 units (total)	1 unit
>10	0.25 units/kg	0.1 unit/kg

Table 16. INSULIN PREPARATIONS

Type of Insulin	Appearance	Type of Action	Peak Activity*†	Duration (hours)†	Available Concentration	Species Available	Modifying Agent	Mixed with Regular Insulin	Route of Administration
Crystalline zinc insulin (regular)	Clear	Rapid	2–4	5–8	U-40 U-100	Beef and pork	None	—	SQ, IM, IV
NPH	Cloudy	Intermediate	8–12	18–26	U-40 U-100	Beef and pork	Protamine	Yes	SQ
Semilente	Cloudy	Rapid	4–8	12–16	U-40 U-100	Beef and pork	None	Yes	SQ
Lente	Cloudy	Intermediate	8–16	18–28	U-40 U-100	Beef and pork	None	Yes	SQ
Ultralente	Cloudy	Prolonged	16–24	24–36	U-40 U-100	Beef and pork	None	Yes	SQ
PZI	Cloudy	Prolonged	14–24	24–36	U-40 U-100	Beef and pork	Protamine	No	SQ

*Hours postadministration.
†These data are from human studies.
Note: Canine insulin has the identical amino acid content as pork insulin, and both are different from beef insulin by two amino acids. Purified pork insulin may act as a homologous insulin in dogs and is not antigenic as is beef or pork-beef insulin.

From Schaer, M: Insulin treatment for the diabetic dog and cat. Compendium of Continuing Education, 5(4):580, 1983. Used by permission.

Administer these doses of insulin until blood glucose level falls from 250 or higher mg per dl to 150 mg per dl. Then change fluids to 5 per cent dextrose, with 4 to 8 mEq per L of potassium chloride. If the blood sugar is 150 to 250 mg per dl, give fluids and potassium chloride as previously, but add 0.5 units of regular insulin per kg subcutaneously until the animal is stabilized. Then begin therapy with Lente insulin.

Measure blood glucose, urine volume, urine pH, glucose, and ketones every hour. Perform an ECG or take blood samples to assess potassium needs. As urine volume increases, begin lactated Ringer's solution IV.

As the animal begins to respond to insulin, carefully monitor for hypoglycemia and hypokalemia. Insulin facilitates movement of potassium from the extracellular fluid compartment into the cell, and hypokalemia may result. Potassium supplementation will be needed, and in most cases, the oral route, being safe, is preferred. Potassium gluconate can be given orally every 6 hours if urine output is adequate. In severe cases of hypokalemia, 30 mEq of potassium can be added to each L of IV fluids administered only if renal function is re-established. IV potassium should not be given at a rate exceeding 1 mEq per kg per hour.

Major problems that kill ketoacidic dogs are:
1. Cerebral edema caused by rapid decline blood glucose or by hypotonic fluids.
2. Hypokalemia caused by insulin and bicarbonate administration.
3. Iatrogenic hypoglycemia or insulin shock.

When the blood glucose has decreased to below 200 mg per cent and urine ketones have decreased, neutral protein Hagedorn (NPH) insulin can be administered. After the patient has been stabilized, maintenance therapy for chronic diabetes mellitus can be initiated (see Table 16).

If insulin syringes are not available and one has only 1-ml tuberculin syringes, how can one calculate the amount of insulin to administer?

$$\frac{\text{desired amount of drug}}{\text{strength on hand}} = \frac{\text{unknown quantity (x)}}{\text{known quantity drug}}$$

If 25U of U40 regular are ordered, how many ml will be adminstred with a 1-ml tuberculin syringe.

$$\frac{25U}{40U} = \frac{xml}{1\text{-ml}} x = \frac{5}{8} \text{ or } 0.625 \text{ ml}$$

Cats are very sensitive to insulin, especially when in diabetic ketoacidosis. In the severely dehydrated cat that is hypotensive, initial insulin treatment should be crystalline zinc insulin administered via slow infusion in fluids, using a pediatric drip set to give ¼ to 1 unit per hour. Blood glucose should be monitored using Dextrostix and glucometer until blood glucose levels are in the range of 200 to 300 mg per dl, then regular insulin can be used subcutaneously (SC) to further stabilize the animal, finally going to NPH–Lente split dosage every 12 hours.

UNCOMPLICATED DIABETES MELLITUS

Uncomplicated diabetic cases are those animals whose serum–fasting blood glucose is greater than 200 mg per dl and who are not ketonuric, although they are glycosuric. They are not severely ill with their diabetes, that is, not ketoacidotic. The following points are important in regulating these diabetic cases with insulin:

1. Insulin, usually NPH, is administered early in the morning, so that peak insulin activity occurs in the late afternoon and a mild hyperglycemia is present in the morning.
2. The dose of insulin administered to dogs and cats is variable, depending on size, activity, food intake, and environmental stress.
3. Dosage of NPH is usually started at ½ to ⅔ unit per kg SC. Cats are very sensitive to insulin and should be started at ½ unit per kg SC. NPH Iletin insulin in cats has a peak concentration and activity between 2 and 6 hours postinjection, with a duration of action of less than 12 hours. Protamine zinc has a peak action of 6 to 12 hours, with a duration of action longer than NPH Iletin. Diabetic cats treated with NPH Iletin require insulin twice daily. Protamine, zinc, and Iletin could be used once daily. At peak insulin activity, the plasma glucose content should be between 125 and 175 mg per dl.
4. Insulin is administered in the early morning. During the regulation period, blood samples for glucose may be checked at peak insulin time (late afternoon) and in the early morning. Diet and exercise should be kept constant, if possible.
5. Evaluate urine glucose in the morning (see p. 818) and attain a 1 + glucose. If urine spillage of glucose is elevated in the morning, the insulin dosage may be adjusted upwards.

PROBLEMS ENCOUNTERED IN REGULATING THE DIABETIC

1. *Giving too much insulin*, so that hypoglycemia develops during the peak action of insulin, is a significant problem. Additional glucose can be supplied by using Karo syrup or, in a hospitalized animal, beginning an IV drip of 10 per cent dextrose and water. In acute collapse from insulin reaction, 50 per cent dextrose, 1 ml per kg IV can be bolused, and then, an IV dextrose drip of 5 to 10 per cent can be maintained.
2. *Widely fluctuating blood glucose levels* may develop in some dogs being given insulin. When the blood glucose levels are taken infrequently and found to be abnormally elevated, increased levels of insulin are administered. These increased insulin levels cause an outpouring of glucogen, cortisol, and epinephrine during the hypoglycemic phase, resulting in a paradoxical hyperglycemic response. This syndrome (Somogyi effect) results in insulin overdosing.

When there appear to be widely fluctuating blood glucose levels or insulin-induced posthypoglycemic hyperglycemia is suspected, serial measurements of

blood glucose should be done every 2 hours from the time of insulin administration until it has peaked. This can be done using a blood glucose analyzer
(Miles Laboratories; see p. 749). Demonstration of hypoglycemia (<60 mg/dl)
followed by hyperglycemia confirms the diagnosis of a Somogyi effect. Treatment for this problem is reduction in insulin administration to achieve a blood
glucose in the 70 to 110 mg per dl range, with spillage of 1+ glucose in the
morning.

3. *Insulin resistance* may develop in unspayed bitches during estrus, pregnancy, or anestrus, associated with growth hormone increases (see p. 664).
   These female diabetics can be better managed following ovariohysterectomy.
4. *Underlying hyperadrenocorticoidism and hypothyroidism* can make diabetic
   animals more difficult to control (see p. 648).
5. *Other management problems* may include the improper use of the wrong
   type of insulin or the wrong dosage, fluctuations in caloric intake, fluctuations
   in exercise and stress, and production of antibodies against beef insulin
   derivatives.
6. Some dogs and especially cats metabolize insulin more rapidly, thus insulin
   peaks early and its effects decline more rapidly. In these cases, several
   regimens of treatment can be tried: (a) Split the insulin dose of NPH so that
   one dose is given in the early morning and a second dose is given 8 to 10
   hours later. The morning blood glucose is used to determine the evening
   insulin dosage, and the evening blood glucose determines the morning insulin
   dosage. (b) Use Lente insulin because it has a longer duration of action (see
   p. 140). (c) Use protamine zinc insulin (PZI) because of its longer duration of
   action (see p. 140).

Hyperosmolar, Nonketotic Diabetic Coma

Coma can develop in association with increased serum osmolality. In
diabetes, the hyperosmolality can be associated with severe hyperglycemia and
hypernatremia. Normal canine osmolality is approximately 300 mOsm per kg
of serum, and hyperosmolality can be suspected when serum osmolality is
above 340 mOsm. If equipment for determining serum osmolality is not
available, serum osmolality can be estimated from the formula:

$$\text{serum osmolality (mOsm/kg)} = 2(Na + K) + \frac{\text{blood glucose}}{18} + \frac{BUN}{2.8}$$

With severe dehydration, hyperglycemia, dehydration, and hyperosmolality
without ketosis, cerebral edema results. The treatment should be aimed at
bringing the glucose levels down slowly and rehydrating the animal.

Hypotonic fluids, such as half-strength saline or 2.5 per cent dextrose in
water, should be used in the therapy of hyperosmolar diabetic ketoacidosis.
Start potassium supplementation using conservative dosage after the initial
rehydration period.

Hypoglycemia

Hypoglycemia is not a specific diagnosis but a manifestation of various systemic abnormalities that can involve the intestinal absorption of nutrients, hepatic production of glucose, normal function of liver enzymes, and adequate peripheral glucose utilization. Blood glucose is maintained at normal levels by hormones secreted by the adrenal glands, pituitary gland, pancreas, intestine, and thyroid glands. Hepatic glycogenolytic and gluconeogenic enzymes are important in the control of blood glucose. Deficiencies of enzymes such as phosphorylase, amylo-1,6-glucosidase, or glucose-6-phosphatase can result in glycogen storage disease, with accumulations of hepatic glycogen.

In the fasting dog, the primary source of energy is ketones from fatty acids and glucose that are synthesized from pyruvate and alanine. Low levels of pyruvate and alanine can lead to inability of the liver to synthesize adequate levels of glucose.

The clinical manifestations center around the dependency of the brain on glucose oxidation for energy and its inability to store quantities of glucose. Clinical signs can be extremely variable and may include weakness, ataxia, muscular twitching, incoordination, visual disturbances, generalized seizures, and other neurologic abnormalities. Blood glucose levels of 45 mg per dl or lower may precipitate clinical signs of hypoglycemia. The coupling of clinical signs just described, a low blood glucose, and response to the administration of glucose is known as Whipple's triad.

Several factors are important to consider when evaluating hypoglycemia: (1) age of onset; (2) the nature of the hypoglycemia episode (transient, persistent, or recurrent); and (3) the pattern, as indicated by the patient's history (for example, is it induced by stress, fasting, or physical exertion?).

Hypoinsulinemia produces increased lipolysis of adipose tissue, altered ketogenic capacity of the liver, and decreased utilization of organic acids by muscle tissue. The major blood ketone acid is β-hydroxybutyrate, which is present in a ratio of 3:1 compared with acetoacetate. Acetone results from the decarboxylation of acetoacetate and is not a ketone acetate.

Laboratory Evaluation

1. Rapid blood glucose with Ames dextrometer.
2. Urinary ketones—nitroprusside reaction is not always an accurate assessment of ketoacidosis, which can be present with little change in blood pH if the ketones are being adequately buffered and excreted. Nitroprusside reaction reacts best with acetoacetic acid and not with acetone or β-hydroxybutyric acid. If high quantities of β-hydroxybutyric acid are contributing to ketoacidosis, the nitroprusside test may not be strongly positive.
3. Calculate the anion gap (see p. 603). Increased anion gap in diabetic patients with little or no detectable ketones is usually associated with β-hydroxybutyric acid, increased lactic acid, or retained organic acids of uremia.
4. Estimate serum osmolality (see p. 601).

Causes

Hypoglycemia is caused by either accelerated glucose removal or failure of glucose secretion. Both causes are broken down into specific factors as follows:

Accelerated Glucose Removal
1. Insulin overdose
2. Functional islet cell tumor
3. Toxicity of oral hypoglycemic drugs
4. Renal glycosuria
5. Hepatoma
6. Endotoxemia, septic shock

Failure of Glucose Secretion
1. Functional hypoglycemia
2. Glycogen storage diseases
3. Adrenal insufficiency
4. Hepatic insufficiency
5. Malabsorption and starvation
6. Large mesodermal tumors that use larger quantities of glucose than can be maintained by glyconeogenesis
7. Sepsis
8. Increased extrahepatic utilization of glucose substrates
9. Hematomas
10. Hepatic abscesses

Treatment

Treatment of hypoglycemia includes the following measures:
1. Fluids—half-strength lactated Ringer's solution, 0.45 per cent NaCl, 5 per cent dextrose.
2. Give 2 to 4 ml per kg of 50 per cent glucose IV or 20 ml per kg of 10 per cent glucose.
3. Potassium supplementation for moderate or severe hypokalemia, using potassium chloride (KCl) added to fluids. *Do not rush* into potassium supplementation aggressively. Stabilize the animal first. Give potassium very slowly. Monitor hypokalemia with ECG. Prolongation of the Q-T interval to >0.22 seconds in the dog and greater than 0.16 seconds in the cat is suggestive of hypokalemia.
   a. *Mild hypokalemia* (serum K+ = 3.0 to 3.5 mEq/L): give 1 to 3 mEq KCl per kg of body weight over 24 hours.
   b. *Moderate hypokalemia* (serum K+ = 2.5 to 3.0 mEq/l): give 3 to 5 mEq KCl per kg of body weight over 24 hours.
   c. *Severe hypokalemia* (serum K+ <2.5 mEq/L): give 5 to 10 mEq KCl per kg of body weight over 24 hours.
4. When the patient recovers, begin frequent administration of food.
5. Watch closely for relapse.
6. Schedule the patient for tests to determine the cause of hypoglycemia.

Puerperal Tetany
(Canine Eclampsia)

The history and clinical signs of puerperal tetany are usually diagnostic and result from the reduction of serum calcium to levels below 7 mg per 100 ml. Because the disease is seen primarily in small, excitable dogs, a stress factor may be involved in the etiology.

Calcium supplementation is available as calcium chloride (CaCl) or calcium gluconate solutions, 10 per cent solutions. One ml of 10 per cent CaCl is equal to 27.2 mg (1.36 mEq), whereas 1 ml of calcium gluconate is equal to 9.3 mg (0.46 mEq) of calcium.

Treatment

Treatment of puerperal tetany involves the following steps:

1. Administer calcium gluconate IV at a dosage rate of 10 to 15 mg per kg per hour. Administer calcium slowly, and monitor the heart rate during administration.

2. If tetany persists, sedate the patient with barbiturates given IV or Valium may be given IV.

3. If hyperthermia is present, cool the patient (see p. 101).

4. Administer oral calcium therapy (see p. 659) and vitamin D (see p. 928) to elevate calcium levels.

Hypercalcemia (See p. 659 for etiology)

The renal, gastrointestinal, and nervous systems are most severely affected by hypercalcemia. Hypercalcemic values of greater than 16.0 mg per dl coupled with hypokalemia and hyperphosphatemia cause the most severe systemic disease. Soft-tissue mineralization develops when the serum calcium level multiplied by the serum phosphate level exceeds 60.

Hypercalcemia produces muscle weakness, vomiting, seizures, coma, and muscle twitching. Cardiac conduction abnormalities include prolongation of the P-R interval, shortening of the Q-T interval, and ventricular fibrillation. Renal complications can be very serious and include defects in renal concentrating ability, polyuria-polydypsia, elevation BUN and creatinine, decreased glomerular filtration rate (GFR) and renal blood flow. GFR and renal blood flow are most compromised at calcium levels of 20 mg per dl or greater. The extent of the renal lesions, namely the degree of renal mineralization, the presence of adequate numbers of functional nephrons, and the presence of intact tubular basement membrane, determine whether the renal lesions are reversible.

Treatment

Emergency treatment is indicated with severe renal decompensation, cardiac disease, and systemic disease associated with hypercalcemia in the 15 to 20 mg per dl range and if calcium × phosphorus is greater than 60.

1. Give fluids to increase extracellular fluid (ECF) volume and to increase GFR fluids of choice; 0.9 per cent NaCl may require potassium supplementation (see p. 604).
2. Search for the underlying etiology of hypercalcemia and decide whether to treat it. The most common cause is lymphosarcoma, but it may be difficult to determine the primary tumor focus (anterior mediastinal, intestinal, bone marrow; see p. 494 for further discussion of calcium metabolism).
3. Begin diuretic therapy with furosemide. Give initial IV bolus at 5 mg per kg, with IV fluid maintenance levels 5 ml per kg per hour. Observe the urine volume and ensure that the patient is well rehydrated.
4. Glucocorticoids reduce calcium levels by decreasing bone resorption calcium, decreasing intestinal absorption calcium, and increasing renal excretion calcium. Do *not* use high doses of steroids (unless absolutely necessary) before performing a biopsy and looking for the source of lymphosarcoma.
5. In very high serum calcium levels (20 mg/dl or greater) with accompanying cardiovascular abnormalities, the IV use of sodium EDTA as a calcium chelating agent can be used, 25 to 75 mg per kg per hour. The dosage is regulated by observing the serum calcium level and monitoring with an ECG.

Acute Adrenocortical Insufficiency (See also p. 648)

Hypoadrenocorticism is a disease seen most frequently in young and middle-aged female dogs. The major clinical signs are associated with deficiencies of both aldosterone and cortisol. The signs seen with adrenal insufficiency may develop slowly; adrenal gland reserve function is not lost until the point at which 90 per cent or more of the adrenal glands are nonfunctional and complete adrenal collapse (Addisonian crisis) can develop. Lack of aldosterone results in impaired ability to conserve sodium and excrete potassium (see pp.   for further discussion).

The most significant clinical signs associated with hypoadrenocorticism are (1) depression and lethargy, (2) weakness, (3) anorexia, (4) shaking and shivering, (5) vomiting, (6) diarrhea, (7) weight loss, (8) abdominal pain, (9) polydypsia-polyuria, (10) reluctance to walk, (11) weak pulse and bradycardia, and (12) dehydration.

Diagnosis

1. Hyperkalemia: The serum potassium levels may be greatly elevated (6.0 to 9.5 mEq) and produce typical cardiovascular changes (see p. 49).
2. Hyponatremia: The serum sodium levels are greatly reduced (115 to 130 mEq). A decrease in the sodium-potassium ratio from 33:1 normal to 25:1 or below is present and usually diagnostic.
3. Cardiovascular changes: (a) bradycardia (less than 60 beats/min), (b) weak pulse, (c) an elevated, spiked T wave, (d) decreased amplitude of p waves and atrial arrest, and (e) a widening of the QRS complex.

Treatment of Addisonian Crisis

Treatment involves the following steps:
1. Establish a patent IV catheter.
2. Obtain blood samples for baseline cortisol and electrolyte levels. Record an ECG; perform an ACTH response test (see p. 648).
3. Begin a rapid IV infusion of 0.9 per cent sodium chloride or 2.5 per cent glucose in 0.45 per cent sodium chloride (see p. 610). Inject 2 to 10 mg per kg of hydrocortisone hemisuccinate IV. Add 1 to 2 mg per kg of dexamethasone to the IV fluids being administered. A wide variety of glucocorticoids are available in the crisis situation, although the hydrocortisone sodium hemi-succinate and prednisolone sodium succinate work most rapidly.
Hydrocortisone sodium hemisuccinate—10–20 mg/kg IV
Prednisolone sodium succinate—11–25 mg/kg IV
Dexamethasone (Azium alcohol based)—2–4 mg/kg IV
Prednisolone acetate—0.1–0.2 mg/kg IM of 8–12h
Hydrocortisone acetate—0.1–0.2 mg/kg IM of 8–12h
Dexamethasone phosphate—1–3 mg/kg IV
4. Continue therapy until blood pressure rises and urine output has returned to normal.
5. Administer the mineralocorticoid, desoxycorticosterone acetate in oil, 1 to 5 mg IM q24h, or fludrocortisone acetate, 0.1 to 0.6 mg per os q24 h.
Fludrocortisone acetate:
small dog: 0.1–0.2 mg/day/po
medium dog: 0.2–0.3 mg/day/po
large dog: 0.4–0.6 mg/day/po
giant breed: 0.6–1.2 mg/day/po
6. Continue DOCA injections daily, and monitor serum sodium and potassium levels. Give hydrocortisone acetate IM every 12 hours. Salt the food heavily.
7. Obtain ECG tracing (see pp. 49–51). If serum electrolyte levels and ECG tracings indicate severe hyperkalemia (greater than 8.0 mEq per L), rapid lowering of the potassium levels by the use of IV glucose and insulin should be considered (see p. 50).
8. Evaluate the acid base status of the patient (see p. 593). Sodium bicarbonate therapy is often needed because of the acidosis.
9. When the crisis has been controlled and the serum electrolytes are normal, begin therapy for chronic adrenal insufficiency.

Iatrogenic secondary adrenocortical insufficiency is a common sequela to glucocorticosteroid therapy in the dog. The primary problem is the development of ACTH insufficiency secondary to either the sudden withdrawal of long-term exogenous glucocorticosteroids or the presence of acute stress reaction in an animal that has been on low-dose daily maintenance glucocorticosteroids. The normal mineralocorticoid function of the zona glomerulosa of the adrenal gland is not affected, so that the classic signs of Addison's disease are not seen. Failure to compensate for stress, marked hypotension, weakness, and collapse can characterize the clinical signs. These animals require IV glucocorticoids.

For more chronic forms of treatment, oral replacement of hydrocortisone, 0.2 to 0.5 mg per kg once a day between 7:00 and 10:00 A.M., is the treatment of choice.

References and Additional Readings

Allen, T. A.: Canine Hypoglycemia. *In* Kirk, R. W. (ed.): Current Veterinary Therapy VIII: Small Animal Practice. Philadelphia, W. B. Saunders Company, 1983.

Breitschwerdt, E. B., et al.: Hypoglycemia in four dogs with sepsis. J.A.V.M.A., *178*(10): 1072, 1981.

Chew, D. J., and Meuten, D. J.: Disorders of calcium and phosphorus metabolism. Vet. Clin. North Am., *12*(3):411, 1982.

Church, D. B.: Diabetes mellitus. *In* Kirk, R. W. (ed.): Current Veterinary Therapy VIII: Small Animal Practice. Philadelphia, W. B. Saunders Company, 1983.

Feldman, E. C., and Tyrrell, B.: Hypoadrenocorticism. Vet. Clin. North Am., 7:555, 1977.

Moise, S. N., and Reimers, T. J.: Insulin therapy in cats with diabetes mellitus. J.A.V.M.A., *182*(2):158, 1983.

Nelson, R. W., Feldman, E. C., and Karam, J. H.: Comparison of immunogenicity of pork insulin versus beef-pork insulin in dogs with spontaneous insulin–dependent diabetes mellitus. Proc. Am. Coll. Vet. Intern. Med. 1983, p. 38.

Rosenthal, R. D., and Wilcke, J. R.: Glucocorticoid therapy. *In* Kirk, R. W. (ed.): Current Veterinary Therapy VIII: Small Animal Practice. Philadelphia, W. B. Saunders Company, 1983.

Turnwald, G. H., and Troy, G. C.: Hypoglycemia; Parts I and II. Compendium of Continuing Education, 5(11): 932–934, 1983, and 6(2):115–123, 1984.

NEUROLOGIC EMERGENCIES
Alexander deLahunta

Although infrequently seen, neurologic emergencies can seriously jeopardize an animal's life. In this section, four conditions that constitute neurologic emergencies are discussed: (1) head injuries, (2) injuries of the spinal cord and spinal column, (3) coma, and (4) seizures.

Head Injuries

Head injuries may include skin and superficial lacerations, concussions, fractures (including extracranial, linear, and depressed intracranial) and extra- and intracranial hemorrhage (including extradural, subdural, subarachnoid, and intracerebral).

Immediate Care

The animal must be handled carefully so that it does no harm to the handler or further injury to itself. Tranquilizers (in minimal dosages) and pain

---

*This section contributed by Alexander deLahunta, D.V.M., Ph. D., Professor of Veterinary Anatomy and Chairman of Department of Clinical Sciences, New York State College of Veterinary Medicine, Cornell University, Ithaca, New York.

relievers may have to be administered if the animal cannot be evaluated without chemical restraint. Morphine should be used in minimal amounts, because it depresses respiration and vital signs in an animal that is already severely depressed owing to injury to the central nervous system (CNS).

Hypoxia is one of the most common causes of death following severe head trauma. An adequate airway and exchange of air must therefore be maintained. In the comatose animal, an endotracheal tube should be inserted and oxygen administered. Hyperventilation is very helpful in maintaining cerebral blood flow and helping to prevent CNS edema. If severe head trauma has resulted in laryngeal edema or marked dyspnea associated with blockage of the upper airway, a tracheostomy will have to be performed. An intermittent positive pressure apparatus like the Bird respirator may be necessary to assist respiration. Oxygen may also be administered by the use of a face mask, oxygen tent, nasopharyngeal tube, or transtracheal catheter (see pp. 60–61). The level of oxygenation of the brain may be reflected in the state of consciousness of the animal.

Control any bleeding and treat shock (see pp. 60–61).

Frequently examine and elicit vital signs such as pulse, respirations per minute, depth of respiration, and temperature, and evaluate the neurologic status, including the state of consciousness, size and response of pupils, pain perception, and voluntary motor activity. Progressively dilating pupils usually indicate brain stem edema. Any deterioration of the aforementioned neurologic data usually indicates progressive brain stem edema and anoxia. With an initial rapid rise in intracranial pressure, the pulse and respirations become slowed and the temperature is elevated. If intracranial pressure continues to rise and reduced cerebral circulation leads to progressive hypoxia, vital signs may become reversed, producing a rapid pulse, rapid respirations, and an elevated temperature. Cheyne-Stokes respirations occur with diencephalic lesions. Central neurogenic hyperventilation follows mesencephalic lesions. Irregular or ataxic respirations occur with medullary lesions and precede arrest.

Initial Examination

In order to follow the patient's course, a baseline neurologic assessment must be made as soon as possible, and the neurologic status must be continually re-evaluated.

Initial neurologic examination should include evaluation of the following parameters:

1. *State of consciousness.* Examine the animal's state of consciousness and elicit the response to commands, to painful stimuli such as a pinch on the toe, and to movement of people in the room. The various levels of consciousness may be described as: *coma* (unconscious with no response to painful stimuli); *semicoma* (unconscious but responsive to painful stimuli); *delirium; confusion; depression;* and *alertness.* Initial consciousness followed by unconsciousness generally indicates severe brain stem injury. In dogs, hemorrhages into the midbrain and pons are relatively frequent, producing

coma and decerebrate rigidity. Brain stem compression can also be associated with compressed skull fractures, extradural or subdural hematomas, or cerebral edema.

2. *Pupil size and response.* Bilateral mydriatic pupils in an unconscious animal are a very grave sign and indicate severe midbrain contusion and usually an irreversible condition. Bilateral miotic pupils occur with diffuse cerebral or diencephalic lesions. Miotic pupils that become mydriatic indicate a progressive midbrain lesion and a poor prognosis. Asymmetric pupils occur with rostral brain stem lesions and can change rapidly. A change from dilated to constricted to normal indicates a favorable prognosis. Unresponsive pupils that are fixed in midposition occur with lesions extending into the medulla and are a grave sign. Examine the eyes, because the pupillary dilation may be due to ocular lesions and not the brain stem.

3. *Vision.* Visual defects are common in intracranial injury. Less severe lesions limited to the cerebrum will produce contralateral menace deficits with normal pupil response to light. Bilateral cerebral edema will cause blindness with normal pupillary response to light if the midbrain is not disturbed. A severely depressed recumbent animal may not respond to menacing gestures, even though visual pathways are intact. Ocular, optic nerve, chiasm, or optic tract lesions will interfere with vision as well as pupillary responses to light. Brain stem contusion and cerebral edema may produce blindness and dilated unresponsive pupils from oculomotor neuronal disturbance.

4. *Other cranial nerves.* Initial evidence of cranial nerve abnormality indicates direct contusion-laceration of the neurons within the brain stem or where they pass through the skull. Cranial nerves that initially are normal and subsequently lose their function indicate a progressive expanding lesion. Prognosis must be guarded when specific cranial nerve deficits are present.

Petrosal bone and/or cerebellomedullary lesions commonly produce signs of vestibular neuron disturbance with rolling to one side or torsion and head tilt to one side and abnormal nystagmus. Petrosal bone fractures often cause bleeding from the external ear canal. If the lesion is limited to the membranous labyrinth, the loss of balance will be toward the injured side and the quick phase of the nystagmus will be toward the opposite side.

Normal or abnormal nystagmus requires a pathway to be intact from the medullary vestibular nuclei to the nuclei of the cranial nerves that innervate the extraocular muscles (III, IV, VI). Severe brain stem lesions will disrupt this pathway. This is indicated by the inability to produce a normal nystagmus on moving the head from side to side. Occasionally, this cannot be elicited in severely depressed animals.

5. *Posture and motor function.* Opisthotonos and extensor rigidity of all four limbs indicate a severe caudal midbrain or pontine lesion or rostral cerebellar lesion. Opisthotonos, with extended forelimbs and hind limbs extended forward with hips flexed, occurs with rostral cerebellar lesions. Tetraplegia indicates a pontomedullary or cervical spinal cord lesion. Be aware that the intracranial injury may be accompanied by a cervical vertebral fracture and spinal cord injury. These animals must be handled with care. If uncertain,

radiograph the cervical vertebrae before manipulating the patient. Hemiplegia usually indicates an ipsilateral pontomedullary or cervical spinal cord lesion. Hemiparesis can be caused by similarly located lesions in the opposite rostral brain stem or cerebrum. With the latter lesions, the hemiparesis usually resolves in 1 to 3 days. Severe neck torsion or turning of the head and neck to one side may accompany contralateral midbrain–pontine tegmental lesions.

Evaluation of cranial nerve function repeated at frequent intervals may reveal an initial nerve injury or the presence of a progressive, expanding lesion of the brain (see p. 424). Signs of severe vestibular disorientation, marked head tilt, and nystagmus occur with contusion of the membranous labyrinth, which is usually associated with a fracture of the petrosal bone. Hemorrhage may occur from the external ear canal. Alterations in respirations may be present with head injuries. Cheyne-Stokes respirations are seen in diencephalic lesions, hyperventilation in mesencephalic lesions, and irregular respirations with medullary lesions. Rolling movements usually indicate a cerebellar-medullary vestibular system lesion.

Paralysis or weakness of one side of the body following head injury can result from laceration or contusion of the ipsilateral pons or medulla.

Convulsions following head injury may be associated with intracranial hemorrhage and an expanding intracranial mass. Medical treatment to control the convulsive state should be instituted. If necessary, give intravenous (IV) injections of diazepam, 5 to 10 mg, or phenobarbital, 2 to 4 mg per kg. If convulsions persist despite this treatment, IV pentobarbital should be administered to produce light general anesthesia (see p. 78). See Tables 17 and 18.

Special Studies

Special studies useful in the management of animals with head injuries include roentgenographic examination of the head and chest and diagnostic peritoneal lavage to rule out occult injuries. Roentgenographic studies of the skull should be taken only after all other emergency procedures have been initiated. If the animal is not cooperative and sedation and the use of a short-acting anesthetic are contraindicated, radiographs should be delayed until diagnostic films can be safely obtained. Roentgenograms of both skull and cervical vertebrae are indicated in traumatic injuries of the head.

Treatment of Specific Head Injuries

The hysterical, delirious animal may be sedated with diazepam or phenobarbital. Seizures may occur, associated with intracranial lesions, and should be treated with IV diazepam (5–10 mg) or phenobarbital (2–4 mg/kg). If these agents are ineffective, IV pentobarbital should be administered to produce a light, general anesthesia (see p. 78).

Brain edema commonly occurs with intracranial injury. The disruption of vascular endothelium produces vasogenic edema, which is extracellular and

Table 17. LOCALIZING SIGNS OF CNS TRAUMA

Level	Consciousness	Pupils	Eye Movements	Motor	Anatomic
Early diencephalic	Apathy	Small but reactive	Normal	Hemiparesis	Normal to irregular respiration
Late diencephalic	Stupor	Same	Same	Hemiparesis to tetraparesis	Cheyne-Stokes
Midbrain	Coma	Dilated bilaterally	Poor physiologic nystagmus	Decerebrate rigidity	Hyperventilation
Pons	Coma	Midposition unresponsive	Physiologic nystagmus absent	Flaccid paralysis	Rapid, shallow respiration
Medulla	Coma	Midposition, dilated terminally	Absent	Flaccid paralysis	Irregular to apnea; pulse slowing

Modified from Oliver, J. E.: Neurologic emergencies in small animals. Vet. Clin. North Am., 2:348, 1972.

Table 18. DIFFERENTIAL FEATURES OF TENTORIAL HERNIATION
AND BRAIN STEM HEMORRHAGE

	Brain Stem Hemorrhage	Tentorial Herniation
Onset	Early	Delayed
Course	Static to progressive	Progressive
Pupils	Constricted early, dilated late	Unilateral dilation, progression to bilateral dilation
Consciousness	Stuporous to comatose	Alert or apathetic, progressing to coma
Muscle tone	Decerebrate rigidity or flaccid paralysis	Normal or weak, progressing to decerebrate rigidity or flaccid paralysis
Reflexes	Usually symmetric	Often unilateral asymmetry

From Oliver, J. E.: Neurologic emergencies in small animals. Vet. Clin. North Am., 2:344, 1972.

predominantly in the white matter. The glucocorticosteroid dexamethasone should be administered to treat this edema at an IV dose of 2 to 4 mg per kg at 6-hour intervals for the first 1 to 3 days, followed by a decreased oral dosage. (Some clinicians advocate a lower initial dose of 0.2 mg/kg).

Dimethylsulfoxide (DMSO) has experimentally been effective in reducing or preventing vasogenic edema without some of the side effects of glucocorticoids. The dose is 1 to 2 gm per kg IV, diluted 50 per cent with dextrose in saline and administered slowly over 30 minutes. This can be repeated 2 to 3 times in the first 24 hours. This drug is not approved for veterinary use, and client permission should be obtained. The hypoxia that occurs secondary to the vascular compromise and vasogenic edema causes cytotoxic edema with neuronal and glial swelling. This is best treated with mannitol at 2 gm per kg IV, using a 20 per cent solution over 15 minutes. This can be repeated once at 3 to 4 hours. If there has been extensive blood loss or intracranial hemorrhage is apparent from epistaxis, if there is bleeding from the ear canal, or if there are palpable skull fractures, mannitol should be avoided.

If possible, keep the animal in an oxygen-rich environment. If there are skull fractures, broad-spectrum antibiotics should be administered. If the animal is hyperthermic, cold water baths and cool enemas should be used to lower the temperature to normal or slightly subnormal. Insert an indwelling catheter into the bladder to avoid bladder distention, which may occur during unconsciousness.

The vital and neurologic signs should be monitored closely every few hours. If the signs worsen, more vigorous medical therapy is indicated or decompressive surgery can be considered.

Surgery is usually limited to depressed fractures of the calvaria that compress the brain. These can be diagnosed by careful palpation and radiography. When the patient is stabilized on medical therapy, the surgery to remove this compression can be performed. Surgery to decompress the brain where fractures are not apparent and clinical signs are severe or progressing is rarely performed because of the poor prognosis and results. The surgery involves making several 1- to 2-cm diameter openings into the cranial cavity over the cerebrum (burr holes). Blood clots can be removed through these openings. For most effective decompression, a large portion of the calvaria (bone flap) is removed.

The most common lesion present in animals that present initially with severe brain stem signs is contusion, with laceration and hemorrhage in the midbrain and pons. This is irreversible, and the prognosis is hopeless. Subdural or extradural hemorrhages with space-occupying blood clots are uncommon. If the hemorrhage slowly accumulates in these sites, repeated neurologic examinations will reveal a deteriorating patient. If the signs can be lateralized to one cerebrum, burr holes or bone flap surgery can be performed to relieve the hemorrhage.

Prognosis of Head Injuries

1. Prognosis is always initially guarded.
2. Initial care (first 30 minutes) is most critical in preventing severe cerebral edema.
3. Head trauma cases may require extensive nursing care over a prolonged period of time (months) before recovery is seen. Often, people do not give animals enough time to recover before deciding in favor of euthanasia.
4. Early cerebral decompression is important if progressive loss of consciousness is developing.

Spinal Cord Injuries

Spinal cord injuries are usually associated with disc ruptures, fractures, or dislocations of the vertebral column.

Initial Handling and Management

Move animals suspected of having spinal injuries with extreme care and caution. All animals rendered unconscious following an injury are regarded as having cervical or thoracolumbar injury until ruled out by radiographs. They should be moved on a wide board or a rolling cart, and flexion, extension, or torsion of the spinal cord should be avoided. The vertebral column should be kept as immobile as possible from the time of injury to the time of repair.

Sedation with tranquilizers and pain relievers may be required before the animal can be moved safely. Narcotics should be used in amounts necessary only to relieve pain, because if more than minimal amounts are used, respiration and other vital signs may also be depressed.

Treat shock, respiratory embarrassment, and open wounds immediately, as required.

Initial Examination

In the initial examination, try to identify the location and evaluate the extent of the spinal lesion and establish an initial prognosis for the case.

The presence of pain, edema, hemorrhage, or a visible deformity may localize an area of spinal injury.

Identifying the location of spinal cord injuries will require a neurologic examination (see p. 436). This examination should be carried out without excessive manipulation of the animal.

Good roentgenographic visualization of the area of spinal cord injury is essential to achieve an early diagnosis and to institute treatment. In almost all cases, the animal must receive a short-acting anesthetic (thiamylal sodium) so that good radiographs can be taken without causing further injury. Myelography may be needed to more clearly delineate the area of spinal injury (see p. 574).

Prognosis in spinal cord injury depends on the extent of the injury and the reversibility of the damage. Perception of pain on the part of the animal when stimulus is applied caudal to the level of the lesion is a good sign. To give pain, firm pressure to a toe may be applied with hemostatic forceps. Flexion of the limb is a spinal reflex and is not a significant response unless the animal exhibits evidence of pain perception. Absence of pain response following recovery from spinal shock (1 to 2 hours) is a very poor prognosis.

Focal lesions in one or more of the spinal cord segments from the third thoracic to the fourth lumbar may cause complete dysfunction of the injured tissue from concussion, contusion, or laceration. The degree of structural damage cannot be determined from the neurologic signs. Focal lesions result in paraplegia, with intact pelvic limb spinal reflexes and analgesia of the body and limbs caudal to the lesion.

These lesions are usually associated with vertebral fractures and displacements of the vertebral canal. The most common site is the caudal thoracic and cranial lumbar region. Lesions here often result in the Schiff-Sherrington syndrome, which is characterized by rigidly extended hypertonic thoracic limbs and flaccid hypotonic paralyzed analgesic pelvic limbs with intact spinal reflexes. The thoracic limbs have normal voluntary motor function, despite their marked hypertonia. They can perform all the postural reactions and spinal reflexes and have intact sensation.

Severe injury to the spinal cord from the fourth lumbar through the caudal segments causes a flaccid paraplegia with atonia, areflexia, and analgesia of the pelvic limbs, anus, and tail. Injuries to the spinal cord from the sixth cervical to the second thoracic segments will cause tetraparesis or tetraplegia, with depressed spinal reflexes from the thoracic limbs and hyperactive spinal reflexes from the pelvic limbs. Horner's syndrome (miosis, protruded third eyelid, smaller palpebral fissure, and enophthalmos) occurs with lesions in the first three thoracic segments. Injuries cranial to the sixth cervical segment will cause spastic tetraparesis or tetraplegia, with hyperactive reflexes in all four limbs. If the injury is severe, death will occur from respiratory failure. Assess the patient for respiratory function and supplement, if necessary. Care should be taken in handling animals with cervical fractures, because displacement of fractures may cause deterioration of neurologic signs.

Initial Therapy

The treatment for spinal cord injury is the same as for brain injury (see pp. 152–154). If there is palpable and/or radiographic evidence of a vertebral lesion compressing the spinal cord, surgery is indicated unless the vertebral displacement has compromised most or all of the vertebral canal. Displacements through 50 to 100 per cent of the vertebral canal have a poor prognosis. In the absence of a radiographic lesion and the persistence of severe neurologic deficit, exploratory surgery is indicated to determine the extent of spinal cord injury, to remove blood clots, and to lavage the segments, and to consider the possibility of a myelotomy.

Prior to surgical stabilization of the injured vertebrae, it is important to restrict any movement of the vertebral column by using a padded back brace or splint taped around the body and over the vertebral column. All activity of the animal must be severely restricted.

An animal with severe spinal cord injury must receive special care with respect to bowel and bladder function. Retention of urine develops quickly after many spinal cord injuries and may not cause any distress to the animal because of associated loss of sensory innervation to the bladder. Urinary retention leads to bladder infections and loss of the normal tonicity of the bladder wall. Frequent manual expression of the urine and washing the hindquarters with warm water may be enough to keep the bladder empty. Repeated catheterizations (two to three times daily), especially in males, may be necessary to prevent urinary retention. This often predisposes to infection; thus, these animals should receive appropriate antibiotic and urinary antiseptic therapy. Indwelling catheters of soft rubber should be used. Betadine ointment should be placed in the prepuce and on the penis at the entry site of the catheter. The catheter should be stabilized in the urethra by suturing the end to the prepucial orifice, and a collar should be placed on the dog so that the catheter cannot be pulled out. A collecting vessel or plastic bag should be attached to the catheter and urine should be prevented from flowing back into the catheter.

Paralytic ileus and fecal retention are also frequent complications of spinal cord injury. The correction of fluid and electrolyte imbalances, together with the ingestion of small amounts of highly digestible foods, will help to relieve the ileus. Mild enemas (Fleet enema) will help to control the fecal retention. A nasogastric tube may be needed to prevent gas retention in the stomach.

Dexamethasone should be used only for a short period of time, probably the initial 24 to 72 hours of treatment. This is especially true in nonambulatory paretics or in dogs with sensory and motor paralysis associated with ruptured intervertebral discs or other trauma. Treatment of these dogs with dexamethasone for 3 or more days may precipitate bloody diarrhea, vomiting, gastrointestinal ulceration, colonic ulceration, peritonitis, and death. This form of gastrointestinal complication has been estimated to occur in 15 to 20 per cent of all intervertebral disc cases treated with dexamethasone.

Special care of the skin is also required in spinal cord injuries. Areas of decubital ulceration may develop rapidly and lead to ischemic necrosis of dermal and muscle tissue. Place the injured animal on an air mattress or foam rubber pad, and change the body position frequently. Preventing excessive moisture such as urine from accumulating on the skin over pressure points will also help to prevent decubital sores. Following bowel movement, enemas, expression of urine, or catheterization of the bladder, clean and dry the perineum or preputial area. The use of a warm whirlpool bath may be exceedingly valuable by providing hydromassage in paralytic animals and by keeping the skin clean.

The initial handling of fractures of the vertebral column or ruptures of the intervertebral discs is discussed earlier in this section. (See also Table 19). Acute compression of the spinal cord is a surgical emergency. In this situation, permanent damage to the spinal cord can only be prevented if decompression is performed soon after the initial insult. If pain response persists after injury, the prognosis is improved.

If the vertebral canal is displaced at the site of the injury, realignment and/or laminectomy should be performed. If there is a complete discontinuity of the vertebral canal, nothing can be done for the patient to recover the lost neurologic function. Displacements of 50 to 100 per cent of the vertebral canal have a very poor prognosis.

INJURIES TO THE PERIPHERAL NERVOUS SYSTEM
(See Examination of the Neurologic System, pp. 420–421)

Radial Nerve

The radial nerve innervates all the extensors of the elbow, carpus, and digits. The radial nerve supplies the only sensory innervation to the distal cranial and lateral surface of the forearm and dorsal surface of the forepaw. Injuries to the radial nerve at the level of the elbow result in the inability of the animal to extend its carpus and digits; the animal walks supporting its

Table 19. PROTOCOL FOR TREATMENT OF THORACOLUMBAR DISK PROTRUSION

Categories, as Determined by History and Neurologic Examination	Therapy
Pain only, first attack	Medical
Pain only, recurrent attacks	Fenestration
Mild paresis and ataxia (grade 4), first attack	Medical
Mild paresis and ataxia (grade 4), recurrent attacks	Fenestration
Moderate paresis and ataxia (grade 3)	Fenestration *or* decompression
Severe paresis (grades 2 and 1) and paraplegia (grade 0)	Decompression

From Trotter, E. J.: Canine intervertebral disk disease. *In* Kirk, R. W. (ed.): Current Veterinary Therapy VI. Philadelphia, W. B. Saunders Company, 1976, p. 844.

weight on the dorsal surface of the paw. Additionally, there is loss of cutaneous sensation. Injuries of the radial nerve in the shoulder area result in the inability of the animal to extend the elbow and bear weight on the affected leg.

Brachial Plexus

Injuries to the brachial plexus (Roots C6–T2) are involved predominantly with signs of radial nerve paralysis. Other nerves may also be injured, resulting in the following signs: musculocutaneous—inability to flex the elbow; axillary and/or thoracodorsal—dropped elbow; and median and ulnar nerves—loss of flexor ability of carpal and digital muscles and loss of sensation of caudal surface of forearm and palmar and lateral surfaces of forepaw.

Contusion or avulsion of the brachial plexus may involve nerve roots C8–T1 (radial, median, and ulnar nerves) or C6 and C7 (musculocutaneous, suprascapular, and axillary). Horner's syndrome can be seen associated with damage to the area of C7–T1.

Sciatic Nerve (L6–S1)

The sciatic nerve innervates the caudal thigh muscles, which primarily flex the stifle and extend the hip. Its tibial nerve branch innervates the caudal leg muscles that extend the tarsus and flex the digits. The tibial nerve provides the sole cutaneous sensory nerves to the plantar surface of the paw. The peroneal branch of the sciatic nerve innervates the cranial leg muscles, flexors of the tarsus and extensors of the digits. The sciatic nerve is the sole cutaneous innervation to the dorsal surface of the paw. With sciatic nerve injury, there is decreased stifle flexion, the hock is overflexed (tibial), and the animal walks on the dorsal surface of the paw (peroneal). Sciatic nerve injury occurs with pelvic fractures, especially those that involve the body of the ilium at the greater ischiatic notch, or with sacroiliac luxations that contuse the L6 and L7 spinal nerves, which pass ventral to the sacrum to contribute to the sciatic nerve.

The signs of tibial and/or peroneal nerve deficit follow femoral fractures, with displacement of fragments caudally or the inadvertent injection of drugs in or around the nerve in the caudal thigh muscles.

Femoral Nerve (L4–L6)

The femoral nerve innervates the extensors of the stifle, and its saphenous nerve branch supplies the sole cutaneous innervation to an area on the medial side of the distal thigh, the leg, and the paw. The nerve is protected by muscles and rarely is injured by pelvic fractures. Clinical signs of injury are the inability to support weight on the pelvic limb, absence of the patellar reflex, and analgesia in the area of sole cutaneous innervation.

References and Additional Readings

Averill, D. R., Jr.: Intracranial injuries. *In* Kirk, R. W. (ed.): Current Veterinary Therapy V. Philadelphia, W. B. Saunders Company, 1974.

Ballinger, W. F., Rutherford, R. B., and Zuidema, G. D.: Management of Trauma, 2nd ed. Philadelphia, W. B. Saunders Company, 1973.

Bunch, S.: Anticonvulsant therapy in companion animals. *In* Kirk, R. W. (ed.): Current Veterinary Therapy VIII: Small Animal Practice. Philadelphia, W. B. Saunders Company, 1983.

Christman, C. L.: Problems in Small Animal Neurology. Philadelphia, Lea & Febiger, 1982.

deLahunta, A.: Veterinary Neuroanatomy and Clinical Neurology, 2nd ed. Philadelphia, W. B. Saunders Company, 1983.

Hoerlein, B. F.: Canine Neurology, 3rd ed. Philadelphia, W. B. Saunders Company, 1978.

Hoerlein, B. F., et al.: Evaluation of dexamethasone, DMSO, mannitol and solocoseryl in acute spinal trauma. J.A.A.H.A., *19*:216, 1983.

Moore, R. W., and Withrow, S. J.: Gastrointestinal hemorrhage and pancreatitis associated with intervertebral disk disease in the dog. J.A.V.M.A., *180*(12):1443, 1982.

Oliver, J. E.: Neurologic emergencies in small animals. Vet. Clin. North Am., 2:341, 1972.

Oliver, J. E., and Lorenz, M. D.: Handbook of Veterinary Neurologic Diagnosis. Philadelphia, W. B. Saunders Company, 1983.

Prata, R. G.: Cervical and thoracolumbar disc disease in the dog. *In* Kirk, R. W. (ed.): Current Veterinary Therapy VIII: Small Animal Practice. Philadelphia, W. B. Saunders Company, 1983.

Rucker, N. C.: Spinal cord trauma. Am. J. Vet. Res., *42*(7):1138, 1981.

Coma

Coma is the complete loss of consciousness, with no response to painful stimuli, and is a symptomatic expression of disease (see p. 293). In some animals presented in a stuporous or comatose state, the cause will be apparent. However, in most instances, a careful diagnostic work-up must be performed.

Initial Treatment

Initial treatment of coma involves the following procedures:

1. Maintain a clear airway and provide respiratory assistance if needed; treat shock and control existing hemorrhage.

2. Take as complete a history as possible from the owner, especially noting the presence of trauma or previous convulsive or comatose episodes.

3. Begin the physical examination by taking the animal's temperature, pulse, and respiration. An elevated temperature suggests a systemic infection such as pneumonia or hepatitis, or a brain lesion with loss of normal temperature control. Very high temperatures associated with signs of shock are indicative of heat stroke. A lowered body temperature is seen in barbiturate intoxication and circulatory collapse. Slow breathing can be seen in barbiturate intoxication or with elevated intracranial pressure. A rapid respiratory rate may indicate pneumonia and diabetic or uremic acidosis.

Examine the skin and note any bruises, ecchymoses, swellings, or lacerations that may signify a traumatic incident. Examine the mucous membranes, noting the presence of pallor, indicative of possible internal hemorrhage, or the presence of icterus, indicative of possible liver disease. Smell the breath for the odor of spoiled fruit, indicative of diabetic acidosis, for uremic odor, or for the musty odor associated with hepatic coma.

4. Following the initial examination, a more complete physical examination, including neurologic evaluation, should be conducted. Any indication of asymmetric neurologic signs suggests an intracranial structural lesion such as an injury, acute hemorrhage, or neoplasm. Toxicities and metabolic disease will not produce asymmetric signs, and cerebral signs predominate. Pupils are usually normally responsive in metabolic encephalopathy and in most toxicities.

5. The following laboratory tests may be of value:
   a. A urinalysis, which should include tests for specific gravity, sugar, acetone, and albumin. Urine of high specific gravity, glycosuria, and acetonuria are indicative of diabetic coma. Urine of low specific gravity with an elevated protein content is found in uremia together with high fevers. Urine may be saved for specific tests such as determining barbiturate intoxication. Urine sediment should be examined for evidence of ammonium urate or oxalic acid crystalluria.
   b. A venous blood sample should be obtained for a WBC count, differential, hematocrit, hemoglobin, glucose, sodium, BUN, amylase/lipase, pH, pCO_2, HCO_3, plasma osmolality, potassium, and chloride (see p. 737). Also consider measuring blood ammonia concentrations and checking for lead levels.
   c. A sample of cerebrospinal fluid should be obtained (see p. 496) and examined (see p. 646), and the cerebrospinal pressure should be determined.

Care of the Comatose Animal

Therapy should be aimed at finding and eliminating the cause of coma; however, there may be no specific therapy for some disease processes. If direct, specific therapy is not possible, supportive measures must be instituted.

Specific Forms of Therapy

Diabetic Coma. In the uncontrolled diabetic animal, disorientation, prostration, and coma can result. Evidence indicates that abnormalities in serum osmolality (hyperosmolarity) can markedly alter the level of consciousness. Plasma osmolality can be estimated by the formula:

$$\text{Plasma osmolality (mOsm/L)} = 2(NA + K) + \frac{\text{blood glucose}}{18} + \frac{\text{BUN}}{2.8}$$

Signs of hyperosmolar state can occur with serum osmolality levels over 340 mOsm per L.

Treatment of diabetic acidosis is accomplished by reducing ketoacid production, stimulating carbohydrate utilization, and impeding peripheral release of fatty acids (see p. 138). During ketosis, a marked insulin resistance may be present. IV rehydration with Ringer's solution or sodium chloride should be carried out. In severe acidosis, give sodium bicarbonate, 1 mEq per kg, given over 15 minutes, then another 1 to 2 mEq per kg given over a period of 3 hours.

Hepatic Coma (see also p. 293). The treatment of very severe cases of hepatic encephalopathy can be considered a medical emergency. The following treatment rationale can be used:

1. Prevent ammonia and other nitrogenous substances from entering the blood through the gastrointestinal tract by (a) achieving total withdrawal of dietary protein (see dietary protocols, p. 877); (b) using cleansing enemas to rid the colon of residual material; and (c) beginning antibiotic therapy to reduce the bacterial population in the gastrointestinal tract. Administer neomycin by high retention colonic enema, 15 mg per kg every 6 hours.

2. Begin general supportive care to restore fluid and electrolyte balance (see p. 591).

3. Stop administration of all drugs such as diuretics, tranquilizers, barbiturates, and others that may be extensively metabolized through the liver.

4. Administer lactulose, 1 tbs t.i.d., orally (Cephulac syrup, Merrell-National Laboratories). Do not administer to a comatose animal. Lactulose causes a decrease in blood ammonia concentration and reduces the degree of portosystemic encephalopathy. Bacterial degradation of lactulose in the colon acidifies the colonic contents, resulting in the retention of ammonia in the colon. Lactulose syrup therapy reduces blood ammonia levels by 25 to 50 per cent. Lactulose acts as a laxative; diarrhea should be expected.

Seizures (see also p. 290)

A seizure or convulsion is a transient disturbance of brain function that is sudden in onset, ceases spontaneously, and has a tendency to recur. Most seizures are generalized and involve the loss of consciousness and severe involuntary contraction of skeletal muscles, causing tonic and clonic limb activity and opisthotonos. Mastication, salivation, pupil dilation, and excretions are common. Partial seizures vary from limited limb activity, to episodic behavioral abnormalities, to brief loss of consciousness. See Table 20 for diagnostic considerations.

Immediate Measures

Most seizures are of short duration and may have subsided by the time the animal is presented for treatment. It is important, however, to prevent the patient from injuring either itself or a bystander. Confinement in a blanket may be useful in this regard.

Table 20. DIFFERENTIAL DIAGNOSIS OF SEIZURES

Acquired Seizures	
Viral encephalitis	History of previous symptoms suggestive of viral invasion (distemper complex). Hyperexcitability or depression. Electroencephalography is useful for diagnosis.
Toxoplasmosis	Previous chronic disease signs; i.e., anorexia, weakness, emaciation, pulmonary symptoms, ocular lesions, seizures progressively more frequent and occasionally of long duration. (Test: serum titer.) Electroencephalography is useful for diagnosis.
Cerebral neoplasia	Neurologic examination usually suggestive of focal abnormality, abnormal reflexes, "Jacksonian" fit. Seizures progressively more frequent. Electroencephalography and radiography (plain and contrast) are useful for diagnosis.
Trauma following electrical injuries	History of injury to skull, unconsciousness followed by incoordination. Seizures may begin soon after injury or 3 to 6 months later. Electroencephalography and radiography are useful for diagnosis.
Cryptococcosis	Variable neurologic signs, occasional seizures. Culture of cerebrospinal fluid.
Cerebral ischemia	History of cardiopulmonary arrest, airway obstruction, etc.
Familial (Congenital) Seizures	
Idiopathic epilepsy	Neurologic examination negative in young animal 6 to 18 months old with no previous illness. Aura, short seizure period (20 to 90 seconds), rapid recovery after seizure. Seizures may occur at regular intervals. Electroencephalographic findings usually negative.
Hydrocephalus	Retarded intelligence, incoordination, lethargy. May or may not have increased head size and open fontanelles. Seizures start at 3 to 9 months of age. Electroencephalography and radiography (plain and contrast) are useful for diagnosis.
Portocaval anomalies	Usually in young dogs. Characterized by rate of growth, vomiting, diarrhea, polydipsia and polyuria, drug intolerances, listlessness, depression, disorientation, changes in temperament, convulsions, and coma.

Table continued on following page

Table 20. DIFFERENTIAL DIAGNOSIS OF SEIZURES *(Continued)*

Metabolic Seizures	
Carbon monoxide poisoning	History of riding in truck or trunk of automobile prior to seizure, which occurs 5 to 15 minutes after muscular activity. Pink mucous membranes.
Parasitism	Very young puppies affected. Low blood calcium, low blood sugar, anemia. Frequent seizures of short duration.
Hypoglycemia	Muscular twitching, hunger, low blood sugar. Seizures occur 30 to 60 minutes after exercise and are related only to the exercise. (Exception: islet cell tumor.) Interseizural electroencephalogram nondiagnostic.
Hypocalcemia	Muscular twitching, anxious attitude, low blood calcium associated with pregnancy, whelping, and parasitism in puppies. Seizures of the tonic type.
Drug–Induced Seizures	
Organophosphate poisoning	Gastrointestinal hypermotility, salivation, miosis, dyspnea. Muscular twitching followed by seizures of long duration.
Chlorinated hydrocarbon poisoning	Hyperexcitability, tremors followed by tonic-clonic seizures of long duration.
Cyanide poisoning	Weakness, tremors, rapid deep respiration, seizures tonic in nature. Bright red mucous membranes.
Other Causes of Seizures	
Hypothalamic syndrome	Hypothermia or hyperthermia, polyuria, polydipsia. Occasional seizures with postseizural confusion. Electroencephalography is useful for diagnosis.
Tetanus	Muscular stiffness, hypertonus of extensor musculature, ears pulled back, nictitating membranes protruding.

Modified from Hoerlein, B. F.: Canine Neurology, 2nd ed. Philadelphia, W. B. Saunders Company, 1971, pp. 494–495.

In beginning treatment of the animal that has seizures, it is important to evaluate the possibility of coexisting systemic diseases that can predispose the animal to epileptic attacks, such as uremia, hepatic disorders, insulin-secreting tumors of the pancreas, electrolyte imbalances, hypoglycemia, lead poisoning, carbon monoxide poisoning, organophosphate poisoning, chlorinated hydrocarbon poisoning, cyanide poisoning, strychnine poisoning and thiamine deficiency in cats. Treatment of these disease entities will help to control the seizures (Table 21).

Status epilepticus, meaning continuous seizures, is an emergency situation in which there is usually no time for an extensive diagnostic work-up. The seizures must be controlled as quickly as possible.

To stop the seizures, give diazepam (Valium), 10 to 35 mg IV, and phenobarbital, 60 to 120 mg IV or IM. If this regimen fails to control the status epilepticus, anesthetize the patient with a gaseous anesthetic or IV barbiturate. Immediately begin supportive treatment with fluids and collect blood, urine, and cerebrospinal fluid samples for diagnostic work-up. Careful attention should

Table 21. DRUGS, DOSAGES, ADVANTAGES AND DISADVANTAGES OF THE MOST COMMONLY USED ANTICONVULSANT DRUGS

Drug	Indication Uses	Dose Availability	Dose Range	Advantages	Disadvantages
Phenobarbital	Generalized major motor seizures, minor motor seizures and behavioral seizures	Tablets: 15 mg 30 mg Liquid Injectable: 30–60 mg Injectable: 0.5–1 gm/ml	8 mg twice daily to 120 mg four times daily (Usually 2–6 mg/ kg q 6 to 12 h) Cats 1 mg/kg q 12 h. Therapeutic serum concentration 6 hr after oral administration. Effective serum level in dogs is >25–40 μgm/ ml. Side effects at >40 μgm/ml.	High efficacy Rapid action, few hours Low toxicity in animals Can be adminis- tered by several routes (IV, IM and orally) Generally the most effective drug in status epilepticus Low cost Worldwide availability Drug of choice in cats	Sedative effects Restricted drug Long-term prescription not honored Polyphagia, polydipsia, polyuria Reverse effects, irritability and restlessness Length of sedation precluding a neurologic examination, following IV, IM, and oral administration, is often several hours
Primidone (Mysoline), (Mylepsin)	Generalized major motor seizure, minor motor seizure Not for cats	Tablets: 50 mg scored 250 mg scored	10–15 mg/kg/day 40 BID mg/kg/day May vary both up and down	High level of efficacy Rapid action Useful in most clinical seizure disorders Not controlled by BNDD	Sedation dramatic and severe in many animals; sedation may be transient as the patient becomes accustomed to the medication

Table continued on following page

Table 21. DRUGS, DOSAGES, ADVANTAGES AND DISADVANTAGES OF THE MOST COMMONLY USED ANTICONVULSANT DRUGS (*Continued*)

Drug	Indication Uses	Dose Availability	Dose Range	Advantages	Disadvantages
				Widely available 85% of effect associated with phenobarbital	Great variability in dose tolerances Only one form available; no parenteral form Only two size tablets available (50 and 250 mg) Occasionally hepatotoxic
Diazepam (Valium)	Control of the exacerbation of seizures Control of status epilepticus Feline seizure epilepticus	Tablets: 2.5 mg 5 mg 10 mg Injectable: 5 mg/ml in 2-ml vials	2.5–100 mg IV, or IM to effect	Effectiveness in stopping status epilepticus and other generalized seizure disorders Rapid action Safety Relative brevity of action; neurologic evaluation can be done shortly afterward: few hours if further seizures do not occur Useful in cats, parenterally or orally Can be used as a tranquilizer	Relatively short action; often needs to be repeated several times in status epilepticus management Cannot control violent status epilepticus Relatively expensive Controlled by BNDD Seldom used for oral prevention and control Reverse effects sometimes seen, restlessness, viciousness

Diphenylhydantoin, Phenytoin (Dilantin)	Generalized major motor seizures, minor motor seizures and behavioral seizures / Not for cats	Capsules: 30 mg / 100 mg / 100 mg with 0.25 gm phenobarbital	20 mg/kg/day / 100 mg/kg/day (Usually 10–20 mg/kg q 8 to 12 h)	Absence of sedation / Low toxicity and absence of many side effects noted in humans / Low cost / Not a controlled substance (BNDD) / Worldwide availability / In combination with phenobarbital, is not a controlled substance	Transient ataxia / Rapid metabolism, difficulty in maintaining adequate blood levels; possibly is poorly absorbed in dogs / Some polyphagia, polydipsia, polyuria / Relatively toxic in cats; generally not desirable as an anticonvulsant in cats / Does not stop initial ictal discharge / Occasionally, liver toxicity
Valproic acid (Depakene)	In controlled seizures, used alone or in combination with other anticonvulsants		75–200 mg/kg t.i.d. lower doses if combined with other anticonvulsants*		Unknown

Modified from Kay, W., and Fenner, W. R.: Epilepsy. In Kirk, R. W. (ed.): Current Veterinary Therapy VI. Philadelphia, W. B. Saunders Company, 1977.

*Not approved by FDA for use in dogs or cats.

be given to blood sugar and calcium levels, and dextrose and/or calcium gluconate should be provided, if needed.

Seizures in cats are not as common as in dogs. They can be associated with systemic diseases such as infectious feline peritonitis, cryptococcosis, toxoplasmosis, lymphosarcoma, meningiomas, and thiamine deficiency.

Thiamine deficiency in the cat may present as a neurologic emergency characterized by dilated pupils, ataxic gait, cerebellar tremor, abnormal oculovestibular reflex, and seizures. Treatment consists of administration of thiamine, 50 mg per day for 3 days.

References and Additional Readings

Bunch, S. E., Castleman, W. L., Hornbuckle, W. E., and Tenant, B. C.: Hepatic cirrhosis associated with long-term anticonvulsant drug therapy in dogs. J.A.V.M.A., 181(4):357, 1982.

Christman, C. L.: Problems in Small Animal Neurology. Philadelphia, Lea & Febiger, 1982, pp. 155–184.

Cunningham, J. G., Haidukewych, D., and Jensen, H. A.: Therapeutic serum concentrations of primidone and its metabolites phenobarbital and phenyl ethyl malonamide in epileptic dogs. J.A.V.M.A., 132(10):1091, 1983.

deLahunta, A.: Veterinary Neuroanatomy and Clinical Neurology, 2nd ed. Philadelphia, W. B. Saunders Company, 1983.

Gulen, P. J. M., and Vonder Kleijn, E.: Rational Antiepileptic Drug Therapy. Elsevier/North Holland Biomedical Press, New York, 1978.

Kay, W. J., and Fenner, W. R.: Epilepsy. In Kirk, R. W. (ed.): Current Veterinary Therapy VI. Philadelphia, W. B. Saunders Company, 1977.

Meyer, D. J., and Noonan, N. E.: Liver tests in dogs receiving anticonvulsant therapy. J.A.A.H.A., 17:261, 1981.

Nafe, L., Parker, A., and Kay, W.: Sodium valproate: a preliminary clinical trial in epileptic dogs. J.A.A.H.A., 17(1):131, 1981.

Oliver, J. E., Jr., and Lorenz, M. D.: Handbook of Veterinary and Neurologic Diagnosis. Philadelphia, W. B. Saunders Company, 1983.

ELECTROCUTION (ELECTRIC SHOCK)

Electric shock is usually the result of a young animal chewing an electric cord. Other causes are contacting defective electrical equipment or being struck by lightning. Electric current passing through the body can produce several major abnormalities: (1) electrophysiologic abnormalities producing ventricular fibrillation. (Other electrically induced cardiac arrhythmias are ventricular tachycardia, and first- and third-degree heart block.), (2) tissue destruction by heat and electrothermal burns, and (3) acute pulmonary edema. The likelihood for ventricular fibrillation developing depends on the intensity of the current, the duration of contact, and the path of the current (whether or not the heart is in the pathway). (See p. 43 for treatment of ventricular fibrillation).

Signs include acute onset of dyspnea, with moist rales, and localized burns, with necrosis of lips and tongue. Caudal lung lobes may have alveolar infiltration (radiographs). Additional signs are muscular contractions, loss of consciousness, pulmonary edema, and ventricular fibrillation. The first 12 hours are the most critical for the patient, then the prognosis improves.

Administer oxygen (40 to 60 per cent), support respiration with positive pressure if needed, large doses of corticosteroids (as in shock therapy), diuretics (furosemide, IV); bronchodilators (aminophylline, IV), and antibiotics prophylactically for possible pneumonia. If pulmonary congestion is severe, consider performing a phlebotomy and remove up to 10 per cent of the blood volume (see Pulmonary Edema, p. 209). Sedate the animal with oxymorphone IV for anxiety only if needed.

Reference and Additional Reading

Kolata, R. J., and Burrows, C. F.: Clinical features of injury by chewing electrical cords in dogs and cats. J.A.A.H.A., 17(2):219, 1981.

POISONINGS

POISON CONTROL CENTERS *

With several hundred thousand potentially toxic substances on the market, it is impossible to remain knowledgeable of their toxicities. However, poison control centers located throughout the United States and Canada do maintain readily available information. For additional information, contact the nearest Poison Control Center.

The poison control centers have been organized to aid physicians, veterinarians, and others in health-related fields. Some are equipped to administer expert treatment to poisoned human patients, but all are centers for information on poisons and the treatment of poisoning.

All available information on the toxic ingredients in thousands of medicines, insecticides, pesticides, and other registered commercial products has been placed confidentially by the government in these poison control centers. As new products are marketed, information regarding the toxic ingredients is forwarded to the centers.

It has been conservatively estimated that over 1,000,000 different household trade-name products are currently on the market and that 1500 new items are added each month.

TELEPHONE INSTRUCTIONS

When a client calls about a poisoned animal, ask about the identity of the suspected poison: When was it ingested or contacted? How is the patient acting? Then give the following first aid instructions (as applicable):

---

*From the Directory of Poison Control Centers, U.S. Department of Health, Education and Welfare, Public Health Service, Division of Direct Health Service, National Clearinghouse for Poison Control Centers, Washington, D.C.

1. Induce vomiting (5 ml of hydrogen peroxide orally every 5 minutes) and save the vomitus. Do not induce vomiting if it appears that the animal has ingested corrosive materials, such as strong acid, alkali, or kerosene. Give milk or water to dilute the poison.
2. If the animal was in physical contact with toxic or corrosive material, wash its skin clear with profuse quantities of water.
3. For excitement or convulsions, try to protect the animal from injuring itself.
4. Bring the sample or container of suspected poison to the hospital with the patient.
5. Do not speed, but proceed without delay to the hospital.

General Approach to Management of Poisonings

Treat the patient not the poison. Treat the specific poison when possible. However, few poisons have specific antidotes. Immediate supportive care can be life-saving. (Tables 22 and 23 list equipment useful in the treatment of poisoning.)

MANAGEMENT PROCEDURES

The poisoned animal should be managed in a specific step-by-step procedure. Each step is listed below and discussed in detail in the sections that follow.
1. Emergency stabilization
2. Clinical evaluation
3. Eliminate poison from the gastrointestinal tract, skin, and eyes
4. Administer antidote, if available
5. Eliminate absorbed poisonous material
6. Observe and give supportive therapy
7. Follow-up care

Emergency Stabilization

Resuscitate the animal if necessary. Provide adequate ventilation and perfusion. Collect a blood sample (for baseline values). Start an intravenous (IV) infusion of saline (add a glucose bolus if the patient is comatose or ataxic).

Clinical Evaluation

History

An accurate patient history is very important in trying to identify poison agents. The rate of onset, development of clinical syndromes, environmental exposures such as sprays, spilled drugs or chemicals, and other regular medications used are all important. Owners should bring package labels and urine, fecal, or vomitus specimens with the animal, if possible.

Table 22. EMERGENCY KIT FOR TREATMENT OF SMALL ANIMAL
POISONING (ANTIDOTES, DRUGS, EQUIPMENT)

Parenteral Solution
Amphetamine
Apomorphine
Atropine sulfate
Barbiturates (phenobarbital,
  pentobarbital)
3% bemegride (Mikedimide)
Calcium borogluconate
Calcium disodium edetate
Calcium disodium edetate in 5%
  dextrose
5% dextrose
Diazepam (Valium)
Dimercaprol (BAL)
2% doxapram (Dopram)
20% ethanol
Glyceryl guaiacolate
Glyceryl monoacetate
Lactated Ringer's solution
10% methocarbamol (Robaxin)
Neosynephrine
Nicotinamide (nicotinic acid,
  niacin)
Normal saline
10% pentylenetetrazol (Metrazol)
Pralidoxine chloride (2-PAM,
  Protopam chloride)
Propranolol

Sedatives, tranquilizers
5% sodium bicarbonate
Vitamin K_1
Whole blood, citrated
  (fresh within 2 weeks)

Oral Medications
Activated charcoal
0.2–0.4% copper sulfate
  solution
Diphenylthiocarbazone
Egg whites, diluted
Hydrogen peroxide
Ipecac syrup
20% magnesium sulfate
  solution
Milk of magnesia
Mineral oil
D-penicillamine
Potassium chloride
1:10,000 potassium
  permanganate solution
Prussian blue
Sodium chloride
Sodium ferrocyanide
20% sodium sulfate
  solution
Tannic acid

Miscellaneous Items
Mild detergent
Oxygen
Sodium bicarbonate paste
Various wide mouth plastic
  jars and bags for collecting
  samples for toxicologic
  analysis

Equipment
Aspirator bulb
Blankets
Endotracheal tubes, several
  sizes*
Enema kit, colon tubes*
Gauze rolls and tape
IV catheters and stylets
Mechanical respirator or
  compression bag
Needles (hypodermic)
Stethoscope
Stomach tubes, several
  sizes*
Syringes
Thermometers
Urinary catheters, various
  sizes
Venostomy kit

Tube Sizes for Toxicologic Procedures

Weight of Animal	Endotracheal Tubes	Stomach Tubes	Colon Tubes
2 kg	22 French	⅛–¼ in. OD	⅛ in. OD
2– 5 kg	28 French	¼ in. OD	¼ in. OD
5–10 kg	34 French	⅜ in. OD	⅜ in. OD
10–20 kg	40 French	½ in. OD	⅜ in. OD
20–30 kg	46 French	⅝ in. OD	½ in. OD

Modified from Oehme, F. W., Manhattan, Kansas.

Table 23. SUMMARY OF DRUGS AND DOSAGES USEFUL IN THE
TREATMENT OF CHEMICAL POISONING

Purpose	Drug	Dosage and Route
Adsorption of poison	Activated charcoal	5 heaping teaspoonsful in 200 ml tap water, orally for a 15-kg dog
Emesis	Apomorphine	40 μ/kg by rapid IV injection (0.04 mg/kg)
	Hydrogen peroxide	5 ml orally; repeat every 10 min
Lavage fluid	Tap water at body temperature	200 ml per cycle, orally, and 500 ml/cycle rectally for a 15-kg dog; repeat until the washings are clear
Catharsis	Sodium sulfate	0.5–1.0 gm/kg orally
Sedation	Diazepam (Valium)	5–20 mg IV
	Thiobarbiturates followed by an inhalation anesthetic	To effect
	Phenobarbital	4.0 mg/kg orally, IM or IV, q 12h, for dogs and cats
Analgesia	Meperidine	10 mg/kg SC for dogs and 2 mg/kg cats
	Morphine	1.0 mg/kg SC, for dogs
		0.1 mg/kg SC, for cats
	Oxymorphone	0.2 mg/kg SC with atropine, for dogs and cats
Forced diuresis	Mannitol (20 percent) in isotonic sodium chloride	1.0 gm/kg IV
	Furosemide	2.0 mg/kg/ q 8h IV for dogs
Circulatory support	Isoproterenol	1.0–5.0 mg in 500 ml D5W, IV, to effect
	Propranolol	0.5–1.0 mg/kg IV, as needed
Respiratory stimulants	Doxapram	3.0–5.0 mg/kg IV only
	Bemegride	5.0–1.0 mg/kg IV only
Dehydration and acid-base imbalance	See section on fluid therapy, pp. 591–617	
Hypotension and cardiovascular shock	See section on shock, pp. 59–68	

See Table 24, Nontoxic Ingestions, and Table 25, Chemical Products Potentially Hazardous to Pets. Table 26 lists adverse drug reactions in dogs, Table 27 lists adverse drug reactions in cats, and Tables 28 to 30 list sources of poisonous plants, common poisonous plants, and plants causing mechanical injury.

Epidemiologic and frequency data of small animal poisonings has been summarized by Osweiler and may be useful to clinicians working on diagnoses. Numerical data are often unreliable, because diagnostic laboratory reports may be slanted toward severe fatal cases and hospital data cover less severe problems, many of which recover and may not have proven etiologic diagnoses. Incidence data vary with urban or rural locales and the types of toxicants that are in common use. The following general statements may be useful to indicate trends or principles to help clinicians "play the odds" with their differential diagnoses.

Table 24. NONTOXIC INGESTIONS

abrasives	fabric softeners	phenolphthalein laxatives (Ex-
antacids	fishbowl additives	Lax)
antibiotics	glues and pastes	Play-Doh
baby product cosmetics	hair dyes, sprays, tonics	Polaroid picture-coating fluid
ballpoint pen inks	hand lotions and creams	porous tip marking pens
bath oil (castor oil and perfume)	3% hydrogen peroxide,	prussian blue (ferricyanide)
bathtub floating toys	medicinal	putty (less than 2 oz.)
birth control pills	incense	rubber cement
bleach (less than 5% sodium	indelible markers	sachets (essential oils, powder)
hypochlorite)	ink (black, blue)	shampoos (liquid)
body conditioners	iodophil disinfectant	shaving creams and lotions
bubble bath soaps (detergents)	laxatives	soap and soap products
calamine lotion	lipstick	spackles
candles (beeswax or paraffin)	lubricant	suntan preparations
chalk (calcium carbonate)	Magic Markers	sweetening agents (saccharin)
colognes	makeup (eye, liquid, facial)	teething rings (water sterility)
cosmetics	matches	thermometers (mercury)
crayons marked AP, CP	mineral oil	toothpaste, with or without
dehumidifying packets (silica or	modeling clay	fluoride
charcoal)	newspaper	vitamins, with or without
deodorants	pencil (graphite lead,	fluoride
deodorizers, spray	coloring)	water colors
Elmer's Glue	perfumes	zinc oxide
Etch-A-Sketch	petroleum jelly (Vaseline)	zirconium oxide

From Mofenson, H. C., and Greensher, J.: The non-toxic ingestion. *In* Haddad, L. M., and Winchester, J. (eds.): Clinical Management of Poisoning and Drug Overdose. Philadelphia, W. B. Saunders Company, 1983.

1. Total incidence of poisoned animals may be 1 to 2 per cent of the total cases seen.
2. There is no difference in the poisoning incidence between sexes.
3. There is no general overall seasonal variation in poisonings, but specific poisons have definite seasonal peaks. These include exposure to insect stings, snake bites, ethylene glycol, insecticide, and rodenticide compounds.
4. Cats in general are less frequently poisoned than dogs, but certain agents, including lead, arsenic, poisonous plants, fungi, and ethylene glycol (which they lick off their skin), more commonly affect cats. Cats may be secondarily poisoned by ingesting poisoned insects or rodents.
5. In one study, pointers, dachshunds, and beagles had twice the incidence of poisoning compared with mixed breed dogs.
6. The overall mortality rate of poisoning cases approximates 12 per cent (only 0.1 per cent of animals at risk), but specific poison mortality rates may be high. In one report, the mortality rate from ethylene glycol was 71 per cent; from heavy metals, 18 per cent; insecticides, 11 per cent; rodenticides, 9 per cent; and ingestion of human drugs, 7 per cent. There were 43 snake bites reported, and none of the victims died.
7. Of poisonings caused by carelessness, 69 per cent were from baits or

Text continued on page 182

Table 25. CHEMICAL PRODUCTS POTENTIALLY HAZARDOUS TO PETS

Arts and Crafts Supplies

Antiquing Agents
Methyl ethyl ketone
Turpentine

Oil Paints and Tempera Paints
Pigment salts of lead, arsenic, copper, and cadmium

Pencils, Indelible
Crystal violet

Photographic Supplies

Developers
Borates
Bromides
Iodides
Thiocyanates

Fixatives
Sodium thiosulfate

Hardeners
Aluminum chloride
Formaldehyde

Automotive and Machinery Products

Antifreeze, Fuel System De-icer
Ethylene glycol
Isopropyl alcohol
Methanol
Rust inhibitors
  Borates
  Chromates
  Zinc chloride

Brake Fluids
Butyl ethers of ethylene glycol and related glycols
Ethyl ethers of ethylene glycol and related glycols
Methyl ethers of ethylene glycol and related glycols

Carburetor Cleaners
Cresol
Ethylene dichloride

Corrosion Inhibitors
Borates
Sodium chromate
Sodium nitrate

Engine and Motor Cleaners
Cresol
Ethylene dichloride
Methylene chloride

Frost Removers
Ethylene glycol
Isopropyl alcohol

Lubricants
Barium compounds
Isopropyl alcohol
Kerosene
Lead compounds
Stoddard solvent

Motor Fuel
Gasoline
Kerosene
Tetraethyl lead

Radiator Cleansers
Boric acid
Oxalic acid
Sodium chromate

Shock Absorber Fluids
Petroleum ether

Tire Repair
Benzene

Windshield Washer
Ethylene glycol
Isopropyl alcohol
Methyl alcohol

Cleaners, Disinfectants, Sanitizers

Cleaners, Bleaches, Polishes
Ammonium hydroxide
Benzene
Carbon tetrachloride
Hydrochloric acid
Methyl alcohol
Naphtha
Nitrobenzene
Oxalic acid
Phosphoric acid
Sodium fluoride
Sodium or potassium hydroxide
Sodium hypochlorite
Sodium perborate
Sulfuric acid
Trichloroethane
Turpentine

Disinfectants, Sanitizers
Acids
Alkalis

Table continued on opposite page

Table 25. CHEMICAL PRODUCTS POTENTIALLY
HAZARDOUS TO PETS *(Continued)*

Hypochlorites
Iodophors
Paradichlorobenzene
Phenol, cresols
Phenyl mercuric acetate
Pine oil
Quaternary ammonium

Health and Beauty Aids
Athlete's Foot
 Caprylic acid
 Copper
 Propionic acid
 Sodium
 Undecylenic acid
 Zinc salts
Bath Preparations
 Bath oils
 Perfume
 Sodium lauryl sulfate
 Trisodium phosphate
Corn Removers
 Phenoxyacetic acid
 Salicylic acid
Deodorants and Antiperspirants
 Alcohol
 Aluminum chloride
Diet Pills
 Amphetamines
 Diuretics
 Thyroid hormone
Eye Make-up
 Boric acid
 Peach kernel oil, qs
Hair Preparations
 Cadmium chloride
 Cupric chloride
 Dyes, tints
 Ferric chloride
 Lead acetate
 Permanent wave lotions
 Pyrogallol
 Silver nitrate
 Thioglycolic acid
Headache
 Aspirin
 Phenacetin
Suntan Lotions
 Alcohol
 Tannic acid and derivatives

Laxatives
 Irritant or stimulant laxatives
 Aloes
 Aloin
 Cascara sagrada
Liniments
 Camphor
 Chloroform
 Oil of wintergreen (methyl salicylate)
 Pine oil
 Turpentine
Nailetics
 Acetone
 Alcohol
 Benzene
 Ethyl acetate
 Nail enamel
 Nail polish
 Nail polish remover
 Toluene
 Tricresyl phosphate
Ointments
 Benzoic acid
 Borates
 Caprylic acid
 Menthol
 Mercury compounds
 Oil of wintergreen (methyl salicylate)
 Phenols
 Salicylic acid
Perfumes, Toilet Waters, and Colognes
 Alcohol
 Essential oils
 Floral oils
 Perfume essence
Shampoos
 Sodium lauryl sulfate
 Triethanolamine dodecyl sulfate
Shaving Lotions
 Alcohol
 Boric acid
Somnolents (Sleeping Pills)
 Barbiturates
 Bromides
Stimulants
 Amphetamine
 Caffeine
 NONFLAMMABLE
  Methylene chloride
  Toluene
   Table continued on following page

Table 25. CHEMICAL PRODUCTS POTENTIALLY HAZARDOUS TO PETS (Continued)

Paints and Related Products

Caulking Compounds
Barium
Chlorinated biphenyl
Chromium
Lead
Mineral spirits
Petroleum distillate
Xylene

Driers
Cobalt compounds
Iron compounds
Manganese compounds
Vanadium compounds
Zinc compounds

Lacquer Thinners
Aliphatic hydrocarbons
Butyl acetate
Butyl alcohol
Toluene

Paint
Arsenic oxide
Coal tar
Cuprous oxide
Lead chromate
Petroleum ether
Pine oil
Red lead oxide
Zinc chromate

Paint Brush Cleaners
Benzene
Kerosene
Naphthas

Paint and Varnish Cleaners
Ethylene dichloride
Kerosene
Naphthalene
Trisodium phosphate

Paint and Varnish Removers
FLAMMABLE
Benzene
Cresols
Phenols
Toluene

Preservatives
BRUSH
Kerosene
Turpentine
CANVAS
2 Chlorophenylphenol
Pentachlorophenol
FLOOR
Magnesium fluorosilicate
WOOD
Copper naphthenate
Copper oleate
Mineral spirts
Pentachlorophenol
Zinc naphthenate

Pest Control

Birds
Aminopyridine
Endrin
Toluidine

Fungicides
Captain
Copper compounds
Maneb
Mercurials
Pentachlorophenol
Thiram
Zineb

Insects and Spiders
Baygon
Carbaryl
Chlordane
Diazinon
Dichlorvos
Kelthane
Mirex
Paradichlorobenzene
Pyrethrins
Rotenone
Toxaphene

Lawn and Garden Weeds
Arsenic
Chlordane
Dacthal

Table continued on opposite page

Table 25. CHEMICAL PRODUCTS POTENTIALLY
HAZARDOUS TO PETS *Continued*

Pentachlorophenol	**Solvents**
2,4-D	*Alcohols*
Rats, Mice, Gophers, Moles	*Chlorinated Solvents*
Arsenic	Carbon tetrachloride
Barium carbonate	Methylene chloride
Dicoumarol	Orthodichlorobenzene
Phosphorus	Trichloroethylene
Sodium fluoroacetate	*Esters*
Strychnine	Amyl acetate
Thallium (rare)	Ethyl acetate
Warfarin	Isopropyl acetate
Zinc phosphide	Methyl acetate
Snails, Slugs	*Hydrocarbons*
Metaldehyde	Aromatics, chiefly benzene, toluene, and xylene
	Naphthenes
Safety Products	*Ketones*
Fire Extinguishers	Acetone
LIQUID FIRE EXTINGUISHERS	Methyl ethyl ketone
Carbon tetrachloride	*Other Common Solvents*
MISCELLANEOUS FIRE EXTINGUISHERS	Aniline
Methylbromide	Carbon disulphide
POWDER EXTINGUISHERS	Cresylic acid
Borax compounds	Kerosene
Nonskid Products	Mineral spirits
Stoddard solvent	Phenols
Methyl ethyl ketone	Turpentine

From Osweiler, G. D.: *In* Kirk, R. W. (ed.): Current Veterinary Therapy VIII: Small Animal Practice. Philadelphia, W. B. Saunders Company, 1983, p. 94.

Table 26. ADVERSE DRUG REACTIONS REPORTED IN DOGS

Drug	Clinical Signs and Lesions
Analgesics	
Aspirin	Bleeding disorders
Meclofenamic acid/ corticosteroids	Diarrhea, gastrointestinal bleeding, death
Phenylbutazone	Anemia, leukopenia, thrombocytopenia, emesis, hemorrhagic enteritis, epistaxis, elevated liver enzymes, death
CNS Depressants	
Acetyl promazine	Atypical behavior, aggression, apprehension, lameness of injected leg, prolonged effect, respiratory distress, bradycardia, pallor, seizures, syncope, weak irregular pulse, urination, defecation
Fentanyl/droperidol	Behavioral change, lameness, ataxia, hyperthermia, aggression, seizures, bradycardia, tachycardia, hyperpnea, apnea, tremors, hyperventilation, hyperexcitability, hyperkinesia, nystagmus, cardiac arrest, prolonged recovery, death
Ethylisobutrazine	Hyperexcitability
Halothane	Cardiac arrhythmia, malignant hyperthermia, nystagmus, torticollis, emesis
Ketamine	Convulsions, cyanosis
Lidocaine	Laryngeal and facial edema, respiratory arrest, seizures, ataxia, tremors
Methoxyflurane	Cardiac arrest, hepatitis after 2 weeks, death
Oxymorphone	Bradycardia
Prochlorperazine/ isopropamide	Tachycardia
Promazine	Depression, hypotension, hyperthermia, death
Thiamylal	Cardiac arrest, respiratory arrest, prolonged anesthesia, cyanosis, apnea, cardiac arrhythmias, bradycardia, temporary hearing loss, prolonged recovery, death
Thiopental	Cardiac arrest, prolonged recovery, pulmonary edema, slough at injection site, death
Xylazine	Viciousness, bradycardia, cardiac arrest, death
Anticonvulsants	
Phenytoin	Ataxia, hepatotoxicity, leukopenia, emesis, coma, death
Primidone	Liver failure, icterus, emesis, alopecia, polydipsia, polyuria, death
Antiparasitics	
Arecoline/ tetrachlorethylene	Mydriasis, ataxia, emesis, diarrhea, severe colic, inability to walk, depression, hypothermia
Bunamidine	Dyspnea, ataxia, emesis, weakness, bloat, gastroenteritis, lung hemorrhage, seizures, sudden death
Butamisole	Dyspnea, ataxia, muscle tremors, collapse, coma, depression, icterus, swelling at injection site, abscess formation, death
n-Butyl chloride	Stupor, ataxia, death

Table continued on opposite page

Table 26. ADVERSE DRUG REACTIONS REPORTED
IN DOGS *(Continued)*

Drug	Clinical Signs and Lesions
Dichlorophene/toluene	Incoordination, convulsions, emesis, disorientation, mydriasis, lethargy, anorexia, fever, death
Dichlorvos	Diarrhea, emesis, ataxia, tremors, weakness, death
Diethylcarbamazine	Pruritus, weakness, emesis, diarrhea, icterus, anaphylactoid reaction, death
Diethylcarbamazine/ styrylpyridinium	Diarrhea, emesis, sterilization, teratogenesis, death
Disophenol	Hyperthermia, hyperventilation, ataxia, collapse, dyspnea, respiratory distress, swelling at injection site, death
Dithiazine iodide	Emesis, diarrhea, depression, apprehension, hyperpyrexia, anorexia, lethargy, death
Glycobiarsol	Emesis
Levamisole	Dyspnea, pulmonary edema, emesis
Mebendazole	Icterus, emesis, anorexia, diarrhea, lethargy, abnormal liver function tests, hepatotoxicity, death
Piperazine	Paralysis, death
Metronidazole	Lethargy, rear limb weakness
Phthalofyne	Hepatitis, splenitis, ataxia, death
Pyrantel pamoate	Emesis
Ronnel	Emesis, twitching, depression
Thenium closylate	Emesis, diarrhea, enteritis, anaphylaxis, hemorrhagic enteritis and liver seizures, dyspnea, cyanosis, death
Thiacetarsamide	Emesis, icterus, bilirubinuria, elevated liver enzymes, depression, anorexia, cough, renal failure, swelling at injection site, alopecia, dermatitis, bleeding disorders, death
Toluene	Collapse
Trichlorfon	Anorexia, weakness, lethargy
Uredofos	Emesis, diarrhea, death
Hormones	
Betamethasone	Shock, polydipsia, polyuria
Dexamethasone	Polydipsia, polyuria, emesis, diarrhea, bloody diarrhea, melena, panting
Prednisolone	Anorexia, polyphagia, pica, anemia, lethargy, diarrhea, polyuria, elevated liver enzymes
Methylprednisolone	Disorientation, panting
Triamcinolone	Cushing's syndrome, emesis, depression, urticaria, dyspnea, seizures, shock
Estradiol cypionate	Pain at injection site, pyometra
Megestrol acetate	Polyphagia, hydrometra, uterine inertia, uterine rupture, anorexia, depression, death
Mibolerone	Elevated liver function tests, icterus, vaginal discharge, behavioral changes, urinary incontinence
Antimicrobials	
Amoxocillin	Skin rash, emesis
Ampicillin	Wheals, injection site inflammation, emesis, diarrhea
Bacitracin/polymyxin B/ neomycin (ophthalmic)	Eye irritation

Table continued on following page

Table 26. ADVERSE DRUG REACTIONS REPORTED
IN DOGS *(Continued)*

Drug	Clinical Signs and Lesions
Cephalexin	Panting, salivation, hyperexcitability
Chloramphenicol	Emesis, depression, ataxia, diarrhea, death
Gentamicin	Injection site inflammation, edema of lips, eyelids, and vulva; elevated BUN
Hetacillin	Emesis
Lincomycin	Emesis, soft stools, diarrhea, shock after IM injection, death
Nitrofurantoin	Emesis
Potassium penicillin G	Increased respiration and heart rate
Procaine penicillin G	Ataxia, edema, dyspnea
Procaine and benzathine penicillin G	Sterile abscess, anaphylaxis
Sulfachlorpyridazine	Ataxia, hyperirritability
Sulfaguanidine	Keratoconjunctivitis
Sulfamerazine/ sulfapyridine	Emesis, dyspnea
Tetracycline	Emesis
Trimethoprim/sulfadiazine	Emesis, diarrhea, anorexia, icterus, elevated liver function tests, bilateral keratoconjunctivitis
Trimethoprim/ sulfamethoxazole	Facial edema, depression
Miscellaneous	
Aminopropazine	Injection site necrosis
Aminophylline	Emesis, anorexia, polyphagia, polydipsia, polyuria, hyperexcitability
Asparaginase	Ataxia, muscle weakness, lethargy
Atropine	Paradoxical bradycardia, heart block
Calcium edetate	Emesis, diarrhea, anorexia, depression
Copper naphthenate (topical)	Skin burns
Dichlorphenamide	Disorientation
Dinoprost tromethamine	Panting, hypersalivation, discomfort, emesis
Digoxin	Emesis, anorexia
Epinephrine/pilocarpine (ophthalmic)	Conjunctivitis
Ibuprofen	Depression, emesis, gastric ulcers, death
Metrizamide	Seizures after myelogram
Neostigmine/ physostigmine (ophthalmic)	Emesis, diarrhea, bradycardia, pannus
Neostigmine methyl sulfate	Apnea, cardiac arrest, death
Pyridostigmine	Diarrhea, emesis
Sulfurated lime (topical)	Skin burns, edema, dehydration
Theophylline	Diarrhea

From Aronson, A. L., and Riviere, J. E.: *In* Kirk, R. W. (ed.): Current Veterinary Therapy VIII: Small Animal Practice. Philadelphia, W. B. Saunders Company, 1983, pp. 124–125.

Table 27. ADVERSE DRUG REACTIONS REPORTED IN CATS

Drug	Clinical Signs and Lesions
Analgesics	
Acetaminophen	Depression, death
Acetaminophen/codeine	Restlessness, excitement, fear, mydriasis, death
Aspirin	Depression or excitability, ataxia, nystagmus, anorexia, emesis, weight loss, hyperpnea, hepatitis, bone marrow depression, anemia, gastric lesions, death
Phenylbutazone	Inappetence, weight loss, alopecia, dehydration, emesis, severe depression, death
CNS Depressants	
Acetyl promazine	Prolonged effect, cardiac arrest, hyperactivity, convulsions, death
Ketamine, ketamine/acetyl promazine	Anoxia, apnea, hypopnea, ineffective and prolonged recovery, tremors, convulsions, excitement, hyperpyrexia, dyspnea, cardiac arrest, bladder and renal hemorrhage, nephrosis, fatty liver, lung edema, deafness, death
Halothane	Cardiac arrest, apnea, shock
Methoxyflurane	Ataxia, death
Thiamylal	Cardiac arrest, respiratory arrest, apnea, prolonged anesthesia, ataxia, shock, death
Xylazine	Prolonged anesthesia, apnea, convulsions
Proparacaine	Mydriasis
Antiparasitics	
Bunamidine	Seizures, coughing, dyspnea, pulmonary congestion, choking, lethargy, pallor, coma, hypersalivation, anorexia, fever, hypothermia, oral lesion, tongue edema, sudden death
n-Butyl chloride	Emesis
Dichlorophene/toluene	Ataxia, twitching, seizures, mydriasis, disorientation, posterior weakness, incoordination, hypersalivation, emesis, hyperpnea, tachycardia, death
Dichlorvos	Death
Glycobiarsol	Emesis, icterus, death
Levamisole	Salivation, excitement, diarrhea, mydriasis
Niclosamide	Depression, ataxia, hypothermia
Piperazine	Emesis, dementia, ataxia, hypermetria, hypersalivation
Hormones	
Megestrol acetate	Polyphagia, hydrometra, uterine rupture
Triamcinolone	Nervousness, hypersalivation, disorientation, syncope
Antimicrobials	
Ampicillin	Diarrhea
Amoxicillin	Emesis
Amphotericin B	Marked elevation of BUN and serum creatinine following single dose
Cephalexin	Emesis, fever
Chloramphenicol	Anaphylactoid-type reaction, anorexia, emesis, depression, diarrhea, neutropenia, death
Gentamicin	Pruritus, alopecia, erythema
Lincomycin	Diarrhea, emesis, collapse, and coma following IM injection
Tetracycline	Malignant hyperthermia, emesis, dehydration
Tylosin	Irritation at injection site
Hexachlorophene	Anorexia, ataxia
Miconazole	Erythema, alopecia
Sulfisoxazole	Emesis
Procaine penicillin/ dihydrostreptomycin	Ataxia
Trimethoprim/sulfadiazine	Emesis, hypersalivation, mydriasis, ataxia seizures
Miscellaneous	
Bethanechol	Emesis

From Aronson, A. L., and Riviere, J. E.: *In* Kirk, R. W. (ed.): Current Veterinary Therapy VIII: Small Animal Practice. Philadelphia, W. B. Saunders Company, 1983, p. 123.

Table 28. SOURCES OF POISONOUS PLANTS

Location	Examples
House plants	Daffodil, oleander, poinsettia, dumb cane, mistletoe, philodendron
Flower garden	Delphinium, monkshood, foxglove, iris, lily-of-the-valley
Vegetable garden	Rhubarb, spinach, tomato vine, sunburned potatoes
Ornamentals	Oleander, castor bean, daphne, golden chain, rhododendron, lantana
Trees and shrubs	Cherry, peach, oak, elderberry, black locust
Woodland plants	Jack-in-the-pulpit, moonseed, May apple, Dutchman's-breeches
Swamp plants	Water hemlock, mushrooms
Field plants	Buttercup, nightshade, poison hemlock, jimsonweed, pigweed
Range plants	Locoweed, lupine, halogeton
Grain contaminants	Crotalaria, corn cockle, ergot
Cultural changes	Nitrate, cyanide, herbicides, insecticides

From Osweiler, G. D.: In Kirk, R. W. (ed.): Current Veterinary Therapy VIII: Small Animal Practice. Philadelphia, W. B. Saunders Company, 1983, p. 93.

pesticides. Agents lying around the home, such as ethylene glycol, were the cause of 20 per cent and therapeutic human drugs were the cause of 11 per cent.

8. In urban areas, human abuse drug intoxication may be seen in dogs. One clinic reported 17 per cent of its poisoning cases were in this category.

9. Herbicide poisoning is rare, because the common organic herbicides have low acute toxicities.

10. The reported incidence of poisoning by certain compounds varies with the dates of surveys, because many severely toxic agents are being removed from the market and are being replaced by newer compounds or are released only to licensed technicians. Compounds in these groups include phenolics and chlorinated hydrocarbons, vacor, sodium fluoracetate (1080), ANTU, and thallium. Reformulation of metaldehyde snail baits and anticoagulant rodent baits is reducing the incidence of poisoning; and the preponderant use of leadfree paint and a better understanding of *old* paint as a toxicant offers hope that lead poisoning will decrease.

Physical Examination*

Poisoning may be suspected by exclusion but may also be present as a coexisting problem. Look for trauma and systemic disease and perform a careful examination to determine the extent of the poisoning.

1. *Look carefully at the patient.* Are there signs of trauma? Are vital signs evident? Fever may indicate infection but may also indicate heat stroke,

---

*Adapted from Haddad, L. M., and Winchester, J.: Clinical Management of Poisoning and Drug Overdose. Philadelphia, W. B. Saunders Company, 1983.

Table 29. COMMON POISONOUS PLANTS

Plant	Toxic Part	Comments and Syndrome
Common Lilies: amaryllis, daffodil, tulips, jonquil, narcissus, death camas, autumn crocus, star-of-Bethlehem, lily-of-the-valley, others	Bulbs mostly	Violent gastrointestinal upsets, nausea, emesis, dyspnea, CNS excitement, followed by depression, collapse, coma, and death; young and very aged most likely to be severely poisoned
Tropical Potted Ornamentals: caladium, philodendron, dumbcane (*Dieffenbachia*), elephant ear, and similar common house plants	Leaf, stem, stalk	Severe burning sensation in mouth and nasopharynx, swelling of oral passages and tissues, obstruction of air passage; asphyxia and gastroenteritis are causes of death; rich in oxalates
Spring Staggerweeds and Cultivated Ornamentals: *Dicentra* (bleeding-heart) and *Corydalis* sp	Top growth, corms	Much as above plus powerful alkaloids, which produce CNS signs; can be fatal to small pets or children
Ornamental Shrubs: often potted house, flowering, or decorative tropicals; *Daphne* sp, boxwood (*Buxus*), *Nerium oleander* sp, yew (*Taxus*), azalea, and other heath family shrubs; privet	All parts poisonous. Fruit (berries) attractive to children and pets of all kinds	Many have supertoxic cardiac principles, violent gastroenteritis, or CNS excitement or depressant active principles of complex nature
Legumes: rosary pea (*Abrus precatorius*)	All parts of seed	Supertoxic; only one pea may be fatal if eaten; abrin a supertoxic principle if given intradermally or SC
Black locust (*Robinia*)	Bark, green growth, and, likely, seeds	Robin produces intense gastroenteritis, cardiac effects, and CNS depresion in any species
Wisteria, horse beans, java beans, loco weeds, and lupines have toxic principles; crotalaria may be ornamental	Seeds, especially	Toxic beans and peas have hepatoxic, teratogenic, and other poisonous properties

Table continued on following page

Table 29. COMMON POISONOUS PLANTS (Continued)

Plant	Toxic Part	Comments and Syndrome
Spurges and Similar Plants: poinsettia, snow-on-the-mountain; castor bean, and croton seeds	All parts, especially seeds	Only one leaf may be fatal to small pets or children; hull of one castor bean may be lethal to adult human; violent gastroenteritis and CNS shock; hepatoxic and nephrotoxic
Buttercups: monkshood (*Aconitum*) Foxglove (*Digitalis*)	All parts, seed is potent	CNS effects, intense GE upset, cardiotoxic effects, depression, collapse, coma, and death
Larkspur (*Delphinium*)	Flowers and seeds	As above, and CNS effects result in early impairment of judgment and walking syndrome
Peony (*officinalis*)	All top growth	Severe GE upset
Buttercups (*Ranunculus*), most species	All parts, seed very toxic	Narcotic alkaloids, GE upsets, abnormal thirst, delirium, coma, death
Nightshades: jimsonweed (*Datura* sp.)		Contain solanins
Eggplant, tomato, potato, ground cherry	Fruit and tubers edible; green growth and sprouts toxic	
Nightshades (*Solanum* sp.) of many species	Variable, but toxic	Solanin principles
Tobacco	All parts	Alkaloid nicotine
Parsleys: poison hemlock (*Conium maculatum*)	All parts	General CNS depressant from coniine
Water hemlock (*Cicuta maculata*)	Tubers mostly	Violent CNS convulsant
Toxic Roots: may apple (*Podophyllum*), poke weed (*Phytolacca*)	Roots	Violent GE syndromes, vomiting and purging, exhaustion, coma, death
Mistletoe	Berries	Fatal to both small pets and children; loss of cattle has also been reported from mistletoe

From Case, A. A.: *In* Kirk, R. W. (ed.): Current Veterinary Therapy VIII: Small Animal Practice. Philadelphia, W. B. Saunders Company, 1983, p. 146.

Table 30. PLANTS THAT CAUSE PENETRATING (MECHANICAL)
INJURIES*

Plant	Structure	Injury
Burdock *(Arctinum lappa)*	Hooked barbs of florets	Lacerations of eye, ears, nares, trachea and bronchus, subcutis
Rose, blackberry, dewberry	Hooked barbs of stems	Punctures and lacerations of eye, mouth, skin, feet
Quince, hawthorn, osage orange	Heavy spines on stems	Stab wounds of eye, skin, feet, legs
Honey locust *(Gleditsia triacanthos)*	Pronged spines	Eye lacerations and punctures; puncture wounds of skin
Cacti of a dozen types	Sharp spines of leaf	Multiple punctures with migrating spine fragments
Nettles	Hollow hairs of stem	Hairs penetrate and break off under skin; chemical injection
Grasses—many species, (bromes, spear grasses, triple-awns, foxtails, bristle grasses, wheat, barley, rye, rice)	Awns, beards, barbs, fragmented seed heads	Barbs penetrate and migrate into ear canal, air passages, other natural body openings, into and under skin; into body cavities and internal organs

*These have been the common trauma-producing plants and plant structures seen
in our veterinary clinics during the period 1948 to 1981. We have personal knowledge
from having collected and identified the offending structures for the attending clinician,
if we were not the actual veterinarians on the case. Most of the illustrations in this article
are from our collection of artifacts.

Modified from Case, A. A.: *In* Kirk, R. W. (ed.): Current Veterinary Therapy VIII:
Small Animal Practice. Philadelphia, W. B. Saunders Company, 1983, p. 147.

poisoning with salicylates, dinitrophenols, or anticholinergics. Bradycardia
may indicate cyanide, digitalis, or beta-blocker toxicity. Tachycardia may
indicate atropine, sympathomimetics, and so on.
2. *Look at the skin.* Discolorations, sweating, extremes in temperature, and
petechiae may indicate salicylate, bocate, carbon monoxide, or organophosphate poisonings or hepatic or coagulation disorders.
3. *Smell the breath.* Odors that are fruity indicate ketoacidosis; urine, uremia;
silver polish, cyanide; and carbon tetrachloride, cleaning fluid. Insecticides,
turpentine, kerosene, and gasoline have characteristic odors.
4. *Listen to the heart and lungs.* Pulmonary edema suggests ANTU, whereas
pneumonia and pericarditis or pleuritis may be infectious in nature. Cardiac
arrhythmias suggest electrolyte disturbances or a host of toxins (see pp. 36–
59).

5. *Examine the abdomen.* It is important to determine whether there is hepatic or splenic enlargement, abdominal pain, or distention and the level of peristalsis.
6. *Examine the extremities and the nervous system.* Look for fractures, dislocations, muscle fasciculation, and so on. Assess the degree of mental acuity or coma (see pp. 293 and 410).

Assess the Major Toxic Syndromes

Coma. Be sure that the animal is stabilized. Determine the level of responsiveness. Consider trauma (hematoma, fractured skull); anoxia; metabolic causes such as ethylene glycol; diabetic ketoacidosis; uremia; overdosage of barbiturates, tranquilizers, or other sedatives or narcotics; metaldehyde; and tick paralysis.

Respirations may give diagnostic clues. Cheyne-Stokes–type breathing suggests structured lesions, whereas Kussmaul's-type breathing is more of an indication of acidosis or metabolic or pulmonary disease.

Pupils that are fixed or unilaterally dilated may be an indication of structured causes of coma, whereas pinpoint pupils are associated with organophosphate toxicity or overdosage of sedatives. Dilated pupils are not a specific indication.

Cardiac Arrhythmia. Electrocardiograms (ECGs) are indicated in all cases in which poison is suspected. Electrolyte abnormalities may be diagnosed. Toxicity from the following agents may cause arrhythmia: amphetamine, arsenic, carbon monoxide, chloral hydrate, cocaine, cyanide, digitalis, dinitrophenol, phenol, phenothiazine(s), physostigmine, propanolol, quinidine, succinylcholine, theophyline, and tricyclic antidepressants.

Metabolic Acidosis. This must be measured by laboratory determinations of blood gases, Na^+, K^+, Cl^-, CO_2, BUN, glucose, acetone, osmolality, and urine pH.

Agents that may cause metabolic acidosis include cyanide, phenol, methanol, ethanol, ethylene glycol, salicylates, iron, and carbon tetrachloride.

Factors causing high anion gap metabolic acidosis include uremia, diabetic ketoacidosis, lactic acidosis, and toxicity from salicylates, methanol, ethylene glycol, and paraldehyde.

Gastrointestinal Syndromes. Severe disturbances may be specific to each agent. In general, treatment may need to be concentrated on correcting hypovolemia and shock.

Agents that may cause these problems include arsenic, mercury, phenols and cresols, phosphorus, thallium, lead, copper, garbage, acids, alkalies, and certain plants.

Seizures or Central Nervous System Stimulation. Many seizures are self-limiting and require only supportive care. Status epilepticus (constant seizure state) is life-threatening and best handled with diazepam given IV to effect.

Agents that may cause seizures as a major effect include camphor, carbon monoxide, chlorinated hydrocarbons, cocaine, organophosphate insecticides, carbamate, phencyclidine, phenol, phenothiazines, propoxyphene hydrochloride, strychnine, tricyclic antidepressants, nicotine, rotenone, fluoroacetate (1080), and toad venom.

Eliminate Poison from the Gastrointestinal Tract, Skin, and Eyes

Although animals can be exposed to poisons by six routes of entry: injections, envenomation, inhalation, ingestion, ocular contact, and skin contact, only the last three offer hope of removal to prevent toxicity.

Aggressive washing/irrigation with copious volumes of water or saline should be accomplished within 20 to 30 minutes to be most effective. Speed is of paramount importance, especially with caustics and especially with eye contact. The small animal's heavy pelage is often a protective factor in preventing direct contact between toxins and the skin. However, once contact is established, it may be a detriment that keeps the toxin in contact with the skin. Insecticides, herbicides, paints, solvents, and so on should be washed off promptly, using repeated soap and water wash/rinse cycles. (Never use solvents such as paint removers, gasoline, and kerosene. They are toxic, too.) If necessary, clip off the coat to remove the toxin.

Compounds that are ingested present a more serious problem for removal. Immediate action is essential. *Dilution* with milk or water is indicated in conscious patients if methods for gastric emptying are not readily available. Milk may be especially useful for dilution, because it is a demulcent and its protein provides a substrate for caustics.

Gastric emptying can best be accomplished in dogs by a single IV dose of apomorphine, 40 μg per kg (0.04 mg/kg). There is little depression with this dose, and the emetic action is prompt, reliable, and transitory. A small dose of xylazine IV is an effective emetic in cats (see p. 77). Hydrogen peroxide, 3 per cent solution, given orally in 5- 10-ml doses repeated in 5 to 10 minutes is sometimes an effective emetic.

Gastric lavage, if done within 1 to 2 hours of poison ingestion, can be very effective. Several prerequisites are needed for maximum effect. The patient should be unconscious or lightly anesthetized. Pass a cuffed endotracheal tube (which extends to the incisor teeth) to prevent aspiration of gastric contents. Pass a large-bore stomach tube (same diameter as the endotracheal tube), lower the animal's head, and repeat lavages, using 5 to 10 ml per kg of water, saline, or water containing a slurry of *activated* charcoal. The lavage should be repeated 8 to 10 times, with fluid injected and removed by gravity or bulb syringe. At the last lavage, leave one quarter of the charcoal slurry in the stomach. Avoid passing the stomach tube too far and avoid using too much pressure or too high a volume of lavage solution. Otherwise, the procedure is effective and relatively safe.

Activated charcoal is probably the most effective compound to use for ingested toxins. It absorbs many toxicants and prevents absorption. It is completely safe but very messy to use. Crushed tablets are slightly less effective than the powder but are much cleaner and more handy to use. Activated charcoal is vegetable, not animal or mineral in origin. Norit, Nuchar C powders, and compressed tablets by Regua Manufacturing Company are available commercially. Activated charcoal can be used in a lavage or merely given as medication. One gm of charcoal is added to each 10 ml of water and dosed at a rate of 2 to 8 gm per kg of body weight. Following treatment with activated charcoal, a saline laxative should be given. This is a further aid in preventing absorption. Sodium sulfate is given orally at a dose of 1 gm per kg. Milk of magnesia is a less effective alternative laxative.

If lipid-soluble toxicants are ingested, *mineral oil*, which is not absorbed by the body but will mix with the toxicant, may be given instead of charcoal and followed with the saline laxative. (Vegetable oils are contraindicated, because they may be absorbed).

High-colonic enemas (irrigations), using isotonic saline or dilute soap and water solutions, may be used to hasten the removal of toxicants from the intestinal tract. It is important to be gentle, to use only mild solutions to prevent dehydration and electrolyte imbalances, and to avoid pressure or rapid injection of large volumes of solution.

Administer Antidote, if Available

Locally acting antidotes against unabsorbed poisons are listed in Table 31. Systemic antidotes for absorbed poisons are listed in Table 32.

Eliminate Absorbed Poisonous Material

If the preceding steps have been followed, it is hoped that most poisons have been removed, neutralized, or metabolized or prevented from being absorbed. It may be necessary to encourage elimination by stimulating the function of organ systems known to be active in that process.

Alkalinization, acidification, forced diuresis, and peritoneal dialysis or hemodialysis may be indicated, but the techniques are complex and are discussed elsewhere. Furosemide, 2 mg per kg q8h, and mannitol 2 gm per kg per hour, are commonly used to induce diuresis. Sodium bicarbonate, 5 mEq per kg per hour, ascorbic acid and ammonium chloride, 50 mg per kg q6h, are used to modify urine pH. In all cases, excellent hydration must be maintained to ensure high urine output.

Observe and Give Supportive Therapy

In some cases, medical support is the only or the most important factor in the management of poisoning cases.

Body temperature control is important and is accomplished by using blankets and water heating pads for hypothermia and ice packs, cold enemas, fans, oxygen chambers, and so on for hyperthermia. *Do not overcorrect for the problem.*

Respiratory support must ensure a patent airway. An endotracheal tube in unconscious patients or a tracheostomy in any patient will ensure a patent airway and/or allow use of a Bird respirator or an Ohio ventilator for support. Increased oxygenation (40 per cent) in a chamber or respirator may be useful.

Text continued on page 196

Table 31. LOCALLY ACTING ANTIDOTES AGAINT UNABSORBED
POISONS AND PRINCIPLES OF TREATMENT

Poison	Antidote and Dose or Concentration
Acids, corrosive	Internally; weak alkali–magnesium oxide solution (1:25 warm water); Milk of magnesia (1–15 ml). *Never give sodium bicarbonate!*
	Externally; flush with water. Apply paste of sodium bicarbonate.
Alkali, caustic	Weak acid—vinegar (diluted 1:4), 1% acetic acid or lemon juice given orally.
	Diluted albumin (4–6 egg whites/1 qt tepid water) followed by an emetic and then a cathartic, because some compounds are soluble in excess albumin.
	Externally; flush with copious amounts of water and apply vinegar.
Alkaloids	Potassium permanganate (1:5000 to 1:10,000) for lavage and/or oral administration.
	Tannic acid or strong tea (200–500 mg in 30–60 ml of water) except in cases of poisoning by cocaine, nicotine, physostigmine, atropine, and morphine.
	Emetic or purgative should be used for prompt removal of tannates.
Arsenic	Sodium thiosulfate–10% solution given orally (0.5–3.0 gm for small animals).
	Protein—evaporated milk, egg white, etc.
	Tannic acid or strong tea.
Barium salts	Sodium sulfate and magnesium sulfate (20% solution given orally). Dosage: 2–25 gm.
Bismuth salts	Acacia or gum arabic as mucilage.
Carbon tetrachloride	Empty stomach, give high protein and carbohydrate diet, maintain fluid and electrolyte balance.
	Hemodialysis is indicated in anuria. Epinephrine is contraindicated (ventricular fibrillation!).
Copper	Albumin (as for Alkali).
	Sodium ferrocyanide in water (0.3–3.5 gm for small animals).
	Magnesium oxide (as for Acids).
Detergents, anionic (Na, K, NH_4^+ salts)	Milk or water followed by demulcent (oils, acacia, gelatin, starch, egg white, etc.).
Detergents, cationic (chlorides, iodides, etc.)	Soap (castile, etc.) dissolved in 4 times its bulk of hot water.
	Albumin (as for Alkali).
Fluoride	Calcium (milk, lime water, or powdered chalk mixed with water) given orally.
Formaldehyde	Ammonia water (0.2% orally) or ammonium acetate (1% for lavage).
	Starch—1 part to 15 parts hot water added gradually.
	Gelatin soaked in water for one-half hour.
	Albumin (as for Alkali).
	Sodium thiosulfate (as for Arsenic).
Iron	Sodium bicarbonate—1% for lavage.

Table continued on following page

Table 31. LOCALLY ACTING ANTIDOTES AGAINST UNABSORBED
POISONS AND PRINCIPLES OF TREATMENT *(Continued)*

Poison	Antidote and Dose or Concentration
Lead	Sodium or magnesium sulfate given orally. Sodium ferrocyanide (as for Copper). Tannic acid (as for Alkaloids). Albumin (as for Alkali).
Mercury	Protein—milk, egg whites (as for Alkali). Magnesium oxide (as for Acid). Sodium formaldehyde sulfoxylate—5% solution for lavage. Starch (as for Formaldehyde). Activated charcoal—5–50 gm.
Oxalic acid	Calcium—calcium hydroxide as 0.15% solution. Other alkalis are contraindicated, because their salts are more soluble. Chalk or other calcium salts. Magnesium sulfate as cathartic. Maintain diuresis to prevent calcium oxalate deposition in kidney.
Petroleum distillates (aliphatic hydrocarbons)	Olive oil, other vegetable oils, or mineral oil given orally. After one-half hour, sodium sulfate as cathartic. Both emesis and lavage are contraindicated.
Phenol and cresols	Soap-and-water or alcohol lavage of skin. Sodium bicarbonate (0.5%) dressings. Activated charcoal and/or mineral oil given orally.
Phosphorus (white or yellow phosphides; red and black are nontoxic)	Copper sulfate (0.2–0.4% solution) or potassium permanganate (1:5000 solution) for lavage. Turpentine (preferably old oxidized) in gelatin capsules or floated on hot water. Give 2 ml four times at 15-minute intervals. Activated charcoal. Do not give vegetable oil cathartic. Remove all fat from diet.
Silver nitrate	Normal saline for lavage. Albumin (as for Alkali).
Unknown (toxic plants, etc.)	Activated charcoal (replaces universal antidote). For small animals—2–8 gm/kg in gelatin capsules or via stomach pump, as a slurry in water. Follow by emetic or cathartic, and repeat procedure.

From Bailey, E. M.: *In* Kirk, R. W. (ed.): Current Veterinary Therapy VIII: Small
Animal Practice. Philadelphia, W. B. Saunders Company, 1983, pp. 85–86.

Table 32. SYSTEMIC ANTIDOTES AND DOSAGES

Toxic Agent	Systemic Antidotes	Dosage and Method for Treatment
Acetaminophen	N-acetylcysteine (Mucomyst)	140 mg/kg orally (loading dose), then 7 mg/kg q4h for 17 additional doses.
Amphetamines	Chlorpromazine	1 mg/kg IM, IP, IV; administer only half dose if barbiturates have been given; blocks excitation.
Arsenic, mercury, and other heavy metals except silver, selenium, and thallium	Dimercaprol (BAL)	10% solution in oil; give small animals 2.5–5.0 mg/kg IM q4h for 2 days, 3 TID for the next 10 days or until recovery. NOTE: In severe acute poisoning, 5 mg/kg dosage should be given only the first day.
	D-Penicillamine (Cuprimine)	Developed for chronic mercury poisoning, now seems most promising drug; no reports on dosage in animals. Dosage for man is*250 mg orally, q6h for 10 days (3–4 mg/kg).
Atropine-belladonna alkaloids	Physostigmine salicylate	0.01–0.6 mg/kg. (Do not use neostigmine.)
Barbiturates	Pentylenetetrazol	10% solution; give small animals 10–20 mg/kg IV or IM, repeated at 15- to 30-minute intervals as needed.
	Doxapram	2% solution; give small animals 3–5 mg/kg IV only, repeated as necessary.
	Bemegride	3% solution; give small animals 5–10 mg/kg IV only, by slow infuson or in intermittent doses. NOTE: All the above are reliable only when depression is mild; in deeper levels of depression, artificial respiration (and oxygen) is preferable.
Bromides	Chlorides (sodium or ammonium salts)	0.5–1.0 gm daily for several days; hasten excretion.
Carbon monoxide	Oxygen	Pure oxygen at normal or high pressure; artificial respiration; blood transfusion.
Cholinergic agents	Atropine sulfate	0.02–0.04 mg/kg, as needed.
Cholinesterase inhibitors	Atropine sulfate	Dosage is 0.2 mg/kg, repeated as needed for atropinization. Treat cyanosis (if present) first. Blocks

Table continued on following page

Table 32. SYSTEMIC ANTIDOTES AND DOSAGES *(Continued)*

Toxic Agent	Systemic Antidotes	Dosage and Method for Treatment
		only muscarinic effects. Atropine in oil may be injected for prolonged effect during the night. *Avoid atropine intoxication!*
Cholinergic agents and cholinesterase inhibitors (organophosphates, some carbamates; but not carbaryl, dimethan, or carbam piloxime, etc.)	Pralidoxime chloride (2-PAM)	2% solution; give 20–50 mg/kg IM or by slow IV injection (maximum dose is 500 mg/min), repeated as needed. 2-PAM alleviates nicotinic effect and regenerates cholinesterase. Morphine, succinylcholine, and phenothiazine tranquilizers are contraindicated.
Copper	D-Penicillamine (Cuprimine)	Dose for animals not established. Dose for man is 1–4 gm daily in divided doses (250-mg tablets).
Coumarin-derivative anticoagulants	Vitamin K₁ (Aquamephyton)	5% stable emulsion. 1 mg/kg IV in 5% dextrose. Give 5 mg/kg IM for 5 days.
	Whole blood or plasma	Blood transfusion, 25 ml/kg.
Curare (tubocurarine)	Neostigmine methylsulfate	Solution: 1:2000 or 1:5000 (1 ml = 0.5 mg or 2 mg). Dose is 0.005 mg/5 kg, SC. Follow with IV injection of a 1% solution of atropine (0.04 mg/kg). 1% solution; give 0.05–1.0 mg/kg IV.
	Edrophonium chloride (Tensilon)	1% solution; give 0.05–1.0 mg/kg IV.
	Artificial respiration	
Cyanide	Methemoglobin (sodium nitrite is used to form methemoglobin)	1% solution of sodium nitrite, dosage is 16 mg/kg IV. Follow with:
	Sodium thiosulfate	20% solution at dosage of 30–40 mg/kg IV. If treatment is repeated, use only sodium thiosulfate. NOTE: Both of the above may be given simultaneously as follows: 0.5 ml/kg of combination consisting of 10 gm sodium nitrite, 15 gm sodium thiosulfate, distilled water qs 250 ml. Dosage may be repeated once. If further treatment is required, give only 20% solution of sodium thiosulfate at level of 1 ml/kg.

Digitalis glycosides, oleander, and Bufo toads	Potassium chloride	Dog: 0.5–2.0 gm, orally in divided doses, or in serious cases, as diluted solution given IV by slow drip (ECG control is essential).
	Phenytoin	25 mg/min IV until control is established.
	Propranolol (beta blocker)	0.5–1.0 mg/kg IV or IM as needed to control cardiac arrhythmias (ECG monitoring is essential).
Fluoride	Atropine sulfate	0.02–0.04 mg/kg as needed for cholinergic control.
	Calcium borogluconate	3–10 ml of 5–10% solution.
Fluoroacetate (compound 1080)	Glyceryl monoacetin	0.1–0.5 mg/kg IM hourly for several hours (total 2–4 mg/kg); or diluted (0.5–1.0%) IV (danger of hemolysis). Monoacetin is available only from chemical supply houses.
	Acetamide	Animal may be protected if acetamide is given prior to or simultaneously with 1080 (experimental).
	Phenobarbital or pentobarbital	May protect against lethal dose (experimental).
Hallucinogens (LSD, phencyclidine-PCP)	Diazepam (Valium)	As needed; avoid respiratory depression.
Heparin	Protamine sulfate	1% solution; give 1.0–1.5 mg to antagonize each 1 mg of heparin; slow IV injection. Reduce dose as time increases between heparin injection and start of treatment. (After 30 minutes, give only 0.5 mg.)
Iron salts	Desferoxamine (Desferal)	Dose for animals not yet established. Dose for man is 5 gm of 5% solution given orally, then 20 mg/kg IM q4h. In case of shock, dose is 40 mg/kg by IV drip over a 4-hour period; may be repeated in 6 hours, then 15 mg/kg by drip q8h.
Lead	Calcium disodium edetate (EDTA) EDTA and BAL	Dosage: Maximum safe dose is 75 mg/kg/24 hours (only for severe case). EDTA is available in 20% solution; for IV drip, dilute in 5% glucose to 0.5%; for IM, add procaine to 20% solution to give 0.5% concentration of procaine. BAL is given as 10% solution in oil.

Table continued on following page

Table 32. SYSTEMIC ANTIDOTES AND DOSAGES *(Continued)*

Toxic Agent	Systemic Antidotes	Dosage and Method for Treatment
		Treatment: (1) In severe case (CNS involvement of > 100 mg Pb/100 gm whole blood), give 4 mg/kg. BAL only as initial dose; follow after 4 hours, and q4h for 3–4 days, with BAL and EDTA (12.5 mg/kg) at separate IM sites; skip 2 or 3 days, then treat again for 3–4 days. (2) In subacute case or < 100 mg Pb/100 gm whole blood, give only 50 mg EDTA/kg/24 hours for 3–5 days.
	Penicillamine (Cuprimine)	(3) May use following either (1) or (2) with 100 mg/kg/day orally for 1–4 weeks. Experimental for nervous signs; 5 mg/kg IV, BID, for 1–2 weeks; give slowly and watch for untoward reactions.
Metaldehyde	Diazepam (Valium) Triflupromazine Pentobarbital	2–5 mg/kg IV to control tremor. 0.2–2.0 mg/kg IV. To effect.
Methanol and ethylene glycol	Ethanol	Give IV, 1.1 gm/kg of 25% solution, then give 0.5 gm/kg q4h for 4 days. To prevent or correct acidosis, use sodium bicarbonate IV. Sodium bicarbonate: 0.4 gm/kg. Activated charcoal: 5 mg/kg orally if soon after ingestion.
Methemoglobinemia-producing agents (nitrites, chlorates, etc.)	Methylene blue	1% solution (maximum concentration), given by *slow IV* injection, 8.8 mg/kg; repeat if necessary. To prevent fall in blood pressure in cases of nitrite poisoning, use a sympathomimetic drug (ephedrine, epinephrine, etc.).
Morphine and related drugs	Naloxone chloride (Narcan)	0.1 mg/kg IV. Do not repeat if respiration is not satisfactory.
	Levallorphan tartrate (Lorfan)	Give IV, 0.1–0.5 ml of solution containing 1 mg/ml. NOTE: Use either of the above antidotes only in acute poisoning. Artificial respiration may be indicated. Activated charcoal is also indicated.
Oxalates	Calcium	Treatment: 23% solution of calcium gluconate IV. Give 3–20 ml (to control hypocalcemia).

Phenothiazine derivatives	Methylamphetamine (Desoxyn)	0.1–0.2 mg/kg IV; also transfusion. Only available in tablet form.
	Diphenhydramine HCl	For CNS depression, 2–5 mg/kg IV for extrapyramidal signs.
Phytotoxins and botulin	Antitoxins (not available commercially)	As indicated for specific antitoxins. Examples of phytotoxins: ricin, abrin, robin, crotin.
Plants		Treat signs as necessary.
Red squill	Atropine sulfate, propranolol	As for Digitalis Glycosides.
Snake bite (rattlesnake, copperhead, water moccasin, coral snake)	Antivenin (Wyeth, Trivalent Crotalidae)	Caution: equine origin.
Spider bite (black widow)	Antivenin (Wyeth)	Caution: equine origin.
Strontium	Antivenin (Merck)	Caution: equine origin.
	Calcium salts	Usual dose of calcium borogluconate.
	Ammonium chloride	0.2–0.5 gm orally 3–4 times daily.
Strychnine and brucine	Pentobarbital	Give IP or IV to effect; higher dose is usually required than that required for anesthesia. Place animal in warm quiet room.
	Amobarbital	Give by slow IV injection to effect. Duration of sedation is usually 4–6 hours.
	Methocarbamol (Robaxin) (guaifenesin)	10% solution; average first dose is 150 mg/kg IV (range: 40–300 mg), repeat half dose as needed.
	Glyceryl guaiacolate, guaifenesin	110 mg/kg IV, 5% solution. Repeat as necessary.
	Diazepam (Valium)	2–5 mg/kg to control convulsions, induce emesis; then use other agents.
Thallium	Diphenylthiocarbazone	Dog: 70 mg/kg orally, TID for 6 days. Hastens elimination, but is partially toxic.
	Prussian blue	0.2 mg/kg in 3 divided doses daily.
	Potassium chloride	Give simultaneously with thiocarbazone or Prussian blue, 2–6 gm orally daily in divided doses.

From Bailey, E. M.: *In* Kirk, R. W. (ed.): Current Veterinary Therapy VIII: Small Animal Practice. Philadelphia, W. B. Saunders Company, 1983, pp. 87–89.

Analeptic agents are of doubtful value and should be used only in rare special cases.

Cardiovascular support is intended to ensure adequate tissue perfusion, normal acid-base balance, normal blood volume, and normal cardiac activity. The packed cell volume should be 75 per cent of normal levels for the species; otherwise, transfusion should be considered. Hypovolemia can be monitored by tissue perfusion tests and central venous pressure measurements. Specific details can be found in the sections entitled Shock (pp. 59–68), and Cardiac Emergencies (pp. 36–59).

Pain is rarely a major concern in poisoned animals, but veterinarians should always be aware of the need for analgesia. Dogs may be given morphine, 1 to 2 mg per kg q6h, or meperidine, 5 to 10 mg per kg, although the latter has a very short effective time. Cats can be given morphine, 0.1 to 0.2 mg per kg q8h or meperidine, 1 to 2 mg per kg q4h.

Central nervous system (CNS) disorders are difficult to manage. Analeptics are sometimes suggested for depressed patients but are difficult to dose accurately. They are short acting and may produce seizures. They are rarely used today, because respiratory support is the primary concern in offended or comatosed animals. Patients with excitement and hyperactivity may be managed by tranquilizers (for hallucinogenic drugs), whereas patients with seizures may be treated with anticonvulsants such as phenobarbital, anesthetics such as pentobarbital, or muscle relaxants and minor tranquilizers such as diazepam.

Follow-up Care

Successful management of acute poisoning cases must not stop when the immediate emergency has passed. Some antidotal medications (i.e., analeptics) may have a shorter effective life than the toxicant, and some poisons (i.e., lead, thallium) can not be eliminated completely in a short time. In addition, the animal's normal physiologic mechanisms often take days or weeks to regain homeostasis. This may be seen with exposures to cholinesterase inhibitors, anticoagulant toxins, drugs producing erythrocyte destruction, and long-term abuse of drugs such as the corticosteroids.

Because of these potentially complex problems, it is imperative that clinicians follow these guidelines:

1. Plan appropriate follow-up appointments and laboratory tests to provide guidelines for options in changing medication schedules and to critically evaluate the patient's progress.

2. Discuss with the owner the circumstances that caused the poisoning, so that the owner can take preventive measures to prevent a recurrence. Human exposure, errors of dosage, carelessness, and inappropriate use of dangerous substances should be discussed in detail.

3. Adverse drug reactions in individual animals may be rare idiosyncrasies or sensitivities, but they are still toxic reactions in that particular patient. Lists of some of the more common adverse reactions of dogs and cats are listed in Tables 26 and 27.

SNAKE BITES (NONPOISONOUS)

Identify the offending reptile, if possible.

Signs

1. Bite is usually "U"-shaped, multitoothed, and relatively painless.
2. Adjacent reaction is negligible.
3. Bites appear as superficial scratches and do not produce signs of a poisonous snake bite. See Snake Bites, Poisonous, which follows.

Treatment

Treatment for nonpoisonous snake bites involves the following steps:
1. Clip hair, clean the wound carefully with surgical soap, and apply a sterile, dry dressing.
2. Because the mouths of snakes contain a profuse bacterial flora (including Clostridia), systematically administer antibiotics (penicillin, ampicillin, or cephalosporins) and tetanus antitoxin (may cause an allergic reaction in some cases because of the horse serum component).
3. Observe the patient closely for at least 3 hours after the bite was inflicted if the type of the offending reptile is in question.
4. Modify treatment appropriately if signs of venom toxicity appear.

SNAKE BITES (POISONOUS) (See Table 33)

Source

The venomous snakes of North America are members of the phylum chordata, class Reptilia, order Squamata, suborder Serpentes, and families Crotalidae and Elapidae.

The major group of poisonous snakes native to the United States are the pit vipers. Included in this group are cottonmouth or water moccasin, copper-

Table 33. RELATIVE TOXICITY OF VENOMS

Species of Snake	Lethal Dose (Intramuscular) Per Gram of Mouse
Naja naja (common cobra)	0.38 μg
Vipera russelli (Russell's viper)	2.50 μg
Crotalus scutulatus (Mohave rattler)	2.70 μg
Crotalus terrificus (South American rattler)	2.70 μg
Crotalus adamanteus (Eastern diamondback)	11.0 μg
Crotalus atrox (Western diamondback)	11.0 μg
Bothrops atrox (fer-de-lance)	12.8 μg
Agkistrodon piscivorus (cottonmouth)	18.0 μg

head, numerous species of rattlesnakes, and the Mexican cantil. Coral snakes are found predominantly in the southern United States and Mexico and belong to a different subfamily (Elapidae) than the pit vipers.

Pit vipers are characterized by a deep pit located between the eye and nostril, their elliptical pupils, and two well-developed fangs in the jaw (Fig. 8).

All venomous snakes are dangerous; however, deadliness depends on the venom's toxicity, the size of the snake, the volume of venom injected, and the nature of the venom (neurotoxic, hematoxic, or both).

Coral snake venom *(Micrurus)* contains no common antigen with the venom of rattlesnakes. The coral snake produces a neurotoxin that must be neutralized with a specific neural endotoxin (Wyeth Laboratories) administered IV.

Signs

The signs of snake venom poisoning are dependent on several factors, including (1) age and size of the victim; (2) location, depth, and number of bites; (3) amount of venom injected; (4) species of snake involved; (5) sensitivity of the victim to the venom; (6) pathogens present in the snake's mouth; and (7) initial care received.

Local

Local signs of poisonous snake bites include the following:
1. Presence of two fang marks.

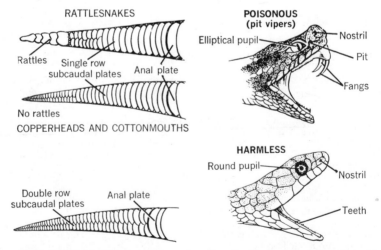

Figure 8. Characteristics of poisonous snakes. (From Parrish, H. M., and Carr, C. A.: Bites by copperheads (Ancistrodon contortrix) in the United States. JAMA, 201:927, 1967.)

2. Immediate severe pain in a specific area, so that the patient resents palpation.
3. Edema, petechiae, and ecchymosis developing rapidly in the area.
4. The area subsequently becomes anesthetic and paralytic.

General

Snake envenomation produces a multiple type of poisoning. A therapeutic program should be undertaken that takes into account all the changes produced by venom-hypovolemia, plasma protein loss, destruction of platelets, hemolysis, tissue necrosis, pulmonary edema, alterations in cardiac function, renal damage, and neurologic dysfunction.

General signs of snake envenomation include nausea, vomiting, vertigo, epistaxis, hematuria, melena, and convulsions, followed by coma, then death.

Signs of coral snake envenomation are different. There may be a 2-hour delay before signs of envenomation are evident. Coma, difficulties in swallowing, weakness, fasciculation, tremor, salivation, nausea, vomiting, pinpoint pupils, dyspnea, death associated with respiratory and cardiac failure, are signs of coral snake envenomation.

Treatment

Initiate treatment for poisonous snake bites as soon as possible after the bite has been inflicted.

Containing the Venom

1. Apply a flat tourniquet between the location of the bite and the heart, so that venous and lymphatic circulations are impeded but arterial circulation is not.
2. The tourniquet should be left intact until definitive treatment is provided or for a maximum of 2 hours.
3. Keep the patient passive; do not allow it to exercise.

Removing the Venom

1. Make a continuous linear incision through both fang marks, extending to the fascia covering the muscle.
2. Avoid severing tendons, motor nerves, and large blood vessels by making incisions parallel to these structures.
3. If possible, apply mechanical suction to the wound.
4. Where the bite wound is located in areas of muscle tissue, an elliptical excision of the fang marks and débridement of the wound, including subdermal fat, can be helpful in eliminating toxin.

Neutralizing the Venom

The antivenin is prepared from hyperimmune equine serum. It contains basic antigens common to most of the pit vipers of the Americas. Prior to antivenin administration, a horse serum hypersensitivity test should be done.

Table 34. SOME TOXINS OF ZOOLOGIC ORIGIN

Organisms	Locations	General Problems Encountered
Snakes		
Pit vipers	Terrestrial; Eastern United	Necrosis, inflammation,
Rattlesnake	States through South	anaphylaxis
Copperhead	Central, Midwest, and	
Water moccasin	Southwest	
Coral snake	Southeast United States;	Neuroparalytic, loss of
	mainly Florida	sensation
Lizards		
Gila monster	Terrestrial; primarily	Inflammation, vomition, shock
Mexican beaded	Southwest United States	
lizard		
Toads		
Bufo sp	Terrestrial-aquatic; Southern	Parotid glands exude a
	and Southwestern United	cardiotoxic and cholinergic
	States	toxin
Spiders		
Black widow	Terrestrial	Neuromuscular wound heals
Brown recluse		with difficulty, infection
Tarantula		from the bite
Insects		
Fire ant	Terrestrial; Southern and	Painful, necrotizing bite;
Wasps	Southwestern United States	inflammation, anaphylaxis
Bees		
Invertebrates		
Jellyfish	Aquatic-marine	Pain, swelling, cramps,
Coral		nausea, CNS derangement
Sea anemone		
Sea urchin		Burning sensation,
		inflammation, paralysis
Vertebrates		
Fish	Aquatic-marine	Sharp pain, inflammation
Stingray		
Catfish		
Scorpion fish		

From Osweiler, G. D.: Common potential sources of small animal poisonings. *In* Kirk, R. W. (ed.): Current Veterinary Therapy VIII: Small Animal Practice. Philadelphia, W. B. Saunders Company, 1983.

To carry out the horse serum sensitivity test, if normal horse serum is provided, make 1:100 or 1:10 saline dilution and inject it intracutaneously using a 26-gauge needle to raise a small wheal. If normal horse serum is not provided in the package, 1:10 saline dilution of the antivenin can be used. Read the skin test in 15 minutes.

Inject crotaline antivenin, polyvalent,* intra-arterially at a dosage of 1 to 5 units. Place reconstituted antivenin into 250 ml of saline or D5W and administer over a 1-hour period. An IV catheter should be in place and, because the antivenin contains horse serum, aqueous epinephrine (1:1000 dilution) should be available for hypersensitivity reactions.

Some toxins of zoologic origin are listed in Table 34.

GILA MONSTER (HELODERMA SUSPECTUM) BITE

A gila monster is a lizard of the family Helodermatidae, the only venomous lizards. It is found in Southwestern United States and Mexico and is a nocturnal reptile. Its venom glands are inferior labial glands, located on either side of the lower jaw. Its bites are usually deep, producing multiple teeth marks, pain, swelling, weakness, and shock.

There are no proven first aid measures of value. Use a stick, screwdriver, or bar to pry open the gila monster's mouth and remove it from the victim. Cleanse the wound. Start IV fluids. Observe for hypotension. Give tetanus antiserum. Soak the injured part in Burow's solution. Irrigate teeth wounds with lidocaine, and use a 30-gauge needle to probe and find any broken-off teeth. No commercial antiserum is currently available.

---

*Antivenin (Crotalidae) polyvalent; Fort Dodge Laboratories Inc., Fort Dodge, Iowa; or Wyeth Laboratories, Radnor, PA.

In cases of bites caused by snakes not indigenous to the United States, exotic antivenins can be obtained from the Oklahoma Poison Control Center, Oklahoma City, OK.

References and Additional Readings

Aronson, A. L., and Riviere, J. E.: Adverse drug reactions. *In* Kirk, R. W. (ed.): Current Veterinary Therapy VIII: Small Animal Practice. Philadelphia, W. B. Saunders Company, 1983.

Aronson, A. L.: Chemical poisonings in small animal practice. Vet. Clin. North Am., 2:379, 1972.

Bailey, E. M.: Emergency and general treatment of poisonings. *In* Kirk, R. W. (ed.): Current Veterinary Therapy VIII: Small Animal Practice. Philadelphia, W. B. Saunders Company, 1983.

Buck, W. B., Osweiler, G. D., and Van Gelder, G. A.: Clinical and Veterinary Toxicology, 2nd ed. Dubuque, Kendal/Hunt, 1976.

Case, A. A.: Poisoning and injury by plants. *In* Kirk R. W. (ed.) Current Veterinary Therapy VIII: Small Animal Practice. Philadelphia, W. B. Saunders Company, 1983.

Casarett, L. J., and Doull, J.: Toxicology, The Basic Science of Poisons. New York, Macmillan Publishing Co., Inc., 1975.

Fowler, M.: Plant Poisoning in Small Companion Animals. St. Louis, Ralston Purina Company, 1980.

Gosselin, R. E., Hodge, H. C., Smith, R. P., and Gleason, M. N.: Clinical Toxicology of Commercial Producers, 4th ed. Baltimore, Williams & Wilkins, 1976.

Haddad, L. M., and Winchester, J.: Clinical Management of Poisoning and Drug Overdose. Philadelphia, W. B. Saunders Company, 1983.

Martin, E. W.: Hazards of Medication, 2nd ed., Philadelphia, J. B. Lippincott Co., 1978.

Meerdink, G. L.: Bites and stings of venomous animals. In Kirk, R. W. (ed.): Current Veterinary Therapy VIII: Small Animal Practice. Philadelphia, W. B. Saunders Company, 1983.

Oehme, F. W. (ed.): Symposium on clinical toxicology for the small animal practitioner. Vet. Clin. North Am., 5:1975.

Osweiler, G. D.: Common poisonings of small animal practice. In Kirk, R. W. (ed.): Current Veterinary Therapy VIII: Small Animal Practice. Philadelphia, W. B. Saunders Company, 1983.

Osweiler, G. D.: Potential sources of small animal poisonings. In Kirk, R. W. (ed.): Current Veterinary Therapy VIII: Small Animal Practice. Philadelphia, W. B. Saunders Company, 1983.

Ridgeway, R. L.: Mushroom (Amanita pantherina) poisoning. J.A.V.M.A., 172:681, 1978.

Russell, F. E.: Snake Venom Poisoning. Great Neck, New York, Scholum International, Inc., 1980.

Sattler, F. P., Knowles, R. P., and Whittick, W. G.: Veterinary Critical Care. Philadelphia, Lea & Febiger, 1981.

Zaslow, I. M.: Veterinary Trauma and Critical Care. Philadelphia, Lea & Febiger, 1984.

RESPIRATORY EMERGENCIES

Respiratory emergencies threaten the life of the clinical patient by producing severe hypoxia or hypercarbia. The conditions most often encountered are obstruction to airflow in the respiratory tract, lack of pulmonary expansion or collapse, interference with alveolar gaseous exchange, and altered pulmonary circulation.

Pleural Effusions

The inside of each hemithorax is covered by parietal pleura, whereas the surface of lobes of lungs is covered by visceral pleura. These two surfaces are in close contact and are contiguous with each other at the hilum.

The general term *pleural effusion* means a collection of liquid in the pleural space between the parietal and visceral pleurae but does not indicate what kind of fluid or how much is present.

Clinical signs associated with pleural effusion depend on how much fluid accumulates and how rapidly. Severe signs are dyspnea, reluctance to lie down, cough, and lethargy. Auscultation may reveal muffled heart sounds, increased bronchial sounds, or regional dullness.

Radiographic confirmation should include films taken in right and left lateral recumbency and ventrodorsally. When large amounts of fluid are suspected, a standing lateral view is indicated so that fluid collected in the costrophrenic recess will be visualized.

When attempting to explain pleural effusions one must think of (1) an imbalance of transpleural or hydrostatic osmotic forces or protein osmotic forces, (2) changes in the permeability of membranes, (3) a decrease in the rate of reabsorption fluid, and (4) combinations of these mechanisms (see Table 35).

Pathological involvement of the pleura is almost always a secondary complication except for primary bacterial pleuritis and pleural mesotheliomas.

Inflammations of the Pleura

Inflammations of the pleura include the following:

1. Serofibrinous pleuritis may be secondary to inflammatory diseases of the lungs. The specific gravity of the fluid is greater than 1.020, and there are inflammatory cells in the exudate.
2. Suppurative pleuritis (empyema) usually implies bacterial or mycotic seeding of the pleural space. It is caused by contiguous spread from pulmonary, but occasionally from lymphatic or hematogenous infections. Masses of PMNs are present in the exudate.
3. Hemorrhagic pleuritis is usually caused by neoplastic, traumatic or inflammatory disorders.

Noninflammatory Pleural Effusions

Noninflammatory pleural effusions include the following:

1. Hydrothorax, in which the fluid is a transudate. The specific gravity of the fluid is less than 1.018. The most common cause is cardiac failure accompanied by pulmonary congestion and edema.
2. Hemothorax is commonly caused by trauma or by ruptured neoplasms.
3. Chylothorax is usually the result of trauma to the thoracic duct.
4. Fluid administration overload.

Therapy

Diagnosis of pleural effusions requires tapping the chest to obtain a fluid sample for laboratory evaluation. At the same time, as much fluid as possible should be removed (see p. 523 for technique of thoracentesis). Specific treatment depends on the diagnosis (see appropriate references).

Epistaxis

Severe epistaxis may result from trauma to the nasal area, nasal tumors, coagulation disorders, or violent sneezing. Epistaxis and resultant nasal blockage may be well tolerated for a short period of time. More prolonged epistaxis can interfere with normal respiration because of the development of anemic hypoxia and the aspiration of blood into the respiratory passageways.

Table 35. ANALYSIS OF PLEURAL EFFUSIONS

| | Transudates | | Exudates | | | | |
	Transudates	Modified Transudates	Nonseptic Exudates	Septic Exudates	Chylous Effusions	Pseudochylous Effusions	Hemorrhagic Effusions
Color	Pale yellow	Yellow-pink	Yellow-pink	Yellow	White-pink	White-pink	Red
Transparency	Clear	Clear to cloudy	Cloudy	Cloudy to flocculent	Opaque	Clear to opaque	Opaque
Protein (gm/dl)	< 2.5	> 2.5	> 3.0	> 3.0	> 2.5	> 2.5	> 3.0
RBC	Absent to rare	Variable	Variable	Variable	Variable	Variable	Acute: high number Chronic: moderate number
Nucleated cells/μl	< 500	> 200	> 2000	> 4000	> 400	> 100	> 1000
Neutrophils	Rare	Variable number Nondegenerative	Moderate number Nondegenerative	Moderate to high number Nondegenerative to degenerative	Acute: low number Chronic: moderate number Nondegenerative	Variable number Nondegenerative	Variable number Nondegenerative
Lymphocytes	Rare	Variable	Variable	Variable	Acute: high number Chronic: low number	Variable	Variable
Macrophages	Occasional	Variable	Increased number Contain ingested debris	Increased number Contain debris	Present	Present	Chronic: moderate number Contain ingested RBCs
Mesothelial cells	Occasional	Occasional	Rare	Rare	Occasional	Occasional	Chronic: present
Fibrin	Absent	Absent	Present	Present	Chronic: present	Chronic: present	Variable
Bacteria	Absent	Absent	Absent	Present intra- and extracellularly	Absent	Absent	Absent
Lipid	Absent	Absent	Absent	Absent	High triglycerides, low cholesterol, positive to lipotrophic stains	Low triglycerides, high cholesterol, negative to lipotrophic stains	Absent
Etiology	Right heart failure Hypoproteinemia	Chronic transudates Diaphragmatic hernia	Neoplasia Feline infectious peritonitis Chronic diaphragmatic hernia Lung torsions	Foreign body Penetrating wound	Ruptured thoracic duct	Neoplasia Feline cardiomyopathy	Trauma Neoplasia Bleeding disorders Lung torsions

From Kirk, R. W. (ed.): Current Veterinary Therapy VIII: Small Animal Practice. Philadelphia. W. B. Saunders Company, 1983.

In the initial treatment of epistaxis, place ice packs over the nasal passages, use tranquilizers to sedate the animal and lower blood pressure, and place tampons soaked with 1:10,000 epinephrine in the nasal passages. Protracted epistaxis requires a more complete diagnostic work-up for blood coagulation (see p. 709) and radiographs of the nasal passageways. Significant and persistent epistaxis resulting from major vessel erosion or tearing may require general anesthesia, tracheal intubation, and posterior nasal pharynx packing, as well as nasal passage packing. (In extreme cases, ligation of the external or common carotid artery has been suggested as the only hope for controlling the hemorrhage).

Obstructions of the Respiratory Passages

Obstructions from tumors, trauma, deformities, infection, and foreign bodies are found in small animals. All are serious, and those that have an acute onset require immediate care.

Foreign bodies can often be removed from the nose or pharynx with an alligator forceps. General anesthesia is usually needed, particularly if the foreign object is in the trachea or larynx. In any obstructive emergency, always be prepared to pass a small endotracheal tube (see p. 629) or perform a tracheotomy (p. 627) and administer oxygen (see p. 633).

Foreign objects lodged in the trachea are small and often act like a ball valve, causing episodic collapse or anoxia. In attempting to remove these objects, suspend the patient with the head down. The object may be situated just posterior to the larynx, and a sharp blow to the head or chest may dislodge it. If the object is firmly lodged in the lower trachea, is causing marked respiratory embarrassment, and cannot be quickly removed via forceps or bronchoscope, the object may have to be forced into a bronchus and then surgically removed via a thoracotomy.

Deformities such as prolapsed lateral ventricles; laryngeal collapse, bilateral laryngeal muscle paresis, and paralysis due to recurrent nerve injury, section, or degeneration; elongation of the soft palate; or stenotic nares may produce acute difficulties that can be corrected only by appropriate surgery.

Fractures of the hyoid bones, trauma to the larynx, tracheal collapse, edema, chemical burns, and tumors all produce obstruction and possible anoxia. Severe inspiratory stridor with cyanosis that becomes more severe with effort suggests laryngeal obstruction. A tracheotomy may have to be performed for temporary relief until definitive treatment can be accomplished. Tracheal collapse may present as an acute respiratory emergency in small breeds, particularly Chihuahuas, Pomeranians, miniature poodles, and Yorkshire terriers. The condition is exacerbated by excitement, elevated environmental temperature, and overexertion. A cool oxygen tent, humidification, and tranquilization are very beneficial. Additionally, corticosteroids and aminophylline, 4 to 8 mg per kg intravenously (IV), should be administered.

Infections and tumors rarely cause acute obstructions. Treatment should be determined only after a careful diagnostic appraisal.

Smoke Inhalation

Animals trapped in building fires may be presented with thermal burns (see p. 33), but more commonly, they are presented with signs of severe respiratory distress associated with burns of the respiratory tract and carbon monoxide and smoke toxicity.

Carbon monoxide results in hypoxia, because it combines with hemoglobin and displaces oxygen in the transport system. The percentage of carboxyhemoglobin in the blood depends on the amount of carbon monoxide in the inspired air and the time of exposure. Carboxyhemoglobin concentrations of 40 to 80 per cent in the blood result in cyanosis, nausea, collapse, respiratory failure, and death.

Smoke toxicity is caused by excessive heat severely damaging the mucous membranes of the upper respiratory tract, including the larynx, leading to laryngeal edema. Inhalation of incomplete products of combustion can enter the bronchi and bronchioles and combine with mucus to produce noxious acids and alkalis, damaging the bronchioles. Specific noxious fumes may damage lungs when plastics, rubber, or other synthetic products may burn.

Initial physical examination of an animal that has been trapped in a fire should include:

1. Examination of the mouth and pharynx to detect evidence of burns.
2. Careful examination of the respiratory system—rate and rhythm and evidence of acute pulmonary edema.
3. Evidence of respiratory acidosis, or pCO_2, pO_2, and carboxyhemoglobin levels. Caution must be used in interpreting pO_2 levels in carbon monoxide poisoning, because blood oxygen may be normal, even though carboxyhemoglobin levels may be very elevated.
4. Radiographs can be helpful, although severe lung changes do not usually develop until 16 to 24 hours after inhalation damage. Radiographs may reveal edema, atelectasis, or evidence of beginning pneumonia. Pleural effusion may develop.
5. More accurate evaluation of upper respiratory injury can be achieved by bronchoscopy (see p. 558). However, caution must be used in an already severely inflamed larynx and trachea, where bronchoscopy may worsen the condition.

Initial Treatment

The initial treatment of smoke inhalation includes the following procedures:

1. If severe laryngeal edema is present and an endotracheal tube (even a small one) cannot be inserted, a tracheostomy is indicated (see p. 627). The affected animal may require a neuroleptanalgesic and local anesthesia, and positive pressure ventilation (PPV) can be begun, if needed. The trachea should be suctioned of mucus and debris (see p. 627).
2. Treat carbon monoxide poisoning with the administration of 100 per cent oxygen. The half-life of carboxyhemoglobin is 4 hours in room air and 1/2

hour in 100 per cent oxygen. If there is no severe respiratory difficulty, the patient can be placed in an oxygen cage (see p. 633) and 40 per cent oxygen that has adequate humidity can also be placed in the cage. If more severe signs of carbon monoxide poisoning are evident or if the animal is having respiratory difficulty, it is better to use a neuroleptanalgesic agent, intubate the trachea, and use positive pressure controlled ventilation. PPV can be maintained for 30 to 50 minutes or longer, if necessary. Some cases will require 12 to 48 hours of PPV with a respirator. Use of muscle blockers by IV administration is necessary during prolonged controlled respiration (see pp. 80–87).

3. Treat fluid loss and electrolyte needs.
4. Evaluate for further injury, and begin treatment for pulmonary edema, if indicated (see p. 209).

Feline Bronchial Asthma

Airway hypersensitivity in cats can result in altered pulmonary function secondary to airway obstruction. Resistance to the passage of gases is increased, associated with bronchospasm, mucous plug formation, and reduction in bronchial lumen. This form of airway hypersensitivity and the clinical signs produced have been staged:

Stage I—asymptomatic	May have had previous asthma attack
Stage II—moderate airway obstruction	Increased bronchovesicular sound, cough, mild hyperventilation, wheezing
Stage III—severe airway obstruction	Coughing, gagging, open-mouthed breathing, marked hyperventilation, wheezing
Stage IV—hypoxemia	Open-mouthed breathing, forced expirations, aerophagia, cyanosis, anxiety, intolerance to stress
Stage V—status asthmaticus	Respiratory acidosis, marked cyanosis, gasping, marked aerophagia

Cats that are presented in Stages III to V of bronchial asthma have increasingly marked hyperventilation, open-mouthed breathing, forced expiratory effort, aerophagia, cyanosis, and marked abdominal component to the respiratory pattern. In the most severe stage, status asthmaticus may be present.

Seventy-five percent of cats with asthmatic bronchitis will have eosinophilia on complete blood count (CBC) exam. With severe respiratory problems, abnormalities in blood gases will be found. Radiographs may reveal air trapped within the lung tissue, bronchial wall thickening, collapsed alveoli, and increased vascular markings.

The stage of the asthmatic attack determines the therapy to be instituted. Cats in severe respiratory distress are given corticosteroids such as prednisolone sodium succinate, 1 to 3 mg per kg IV, aminophylline, 2 mg per kg IV by slow IV drip, epinephrine, 0.1 ml of 1:1000 subcutaneously (SC), and isoproterenol,

0.1 to 0.2 ml of 1:200 dilution SC, and are placed in an oxygen cage. Nebulization therapy in an oxygen cage during the acute period can be done with 0.5 ml of 1:200 isoproterenol or terbutaline (Brethine).

Acute emphysema secondary to bronchial spasm and bronchiolar obstruction from mucus and cellular debris is characteristic of cats with bronchial asthma. Treatment with systemic administration of antibiotics is advisable. Do not handle, exercise, or excite these patients more than is necessary. Do not depress the cough reflex.

Pulmonary Edema

Pulmonary edema refers to the accumulation of excessive amounts of fluid within the lung. The most serious form of pulmonary edema is alveolar edema.

Pulmonary edema can be associated with several underlying pathophysiologic mechanisms: increased capillary hydrostatic pressure, increased capillary permeability to proteins, insufficient lymphatic drainage, decreased colloidal osmotic pressure of plasma, increased colloidal osmotic pressure of plasma, altered alveolar surface tension, and enlarged capillary surface area.

Causes

The major causes of pulmonary edema are those associated with cardiac failure and noncardiac causes.

Causes Associated with Cardiac Failure (Hemodynamic Edema)

Such causes include congenital cardiac disease—patent ductus arteriosus, aortic stenosis, atrial septal defect, and ventricular septal defect; cardiomyopathies—hypertrophic cardiomyopathy, endomyocarditis, restrictive cardiomyopathy, and severe arrhythmias; chronic mitral valve disease; cardiac arrhythmias—bradyarrhythmia and tachyarrhythmia; and myocardial disease. Left heart failure causes elevated pulmonary venous and capillary hydrostatic pressure. Pulmonary capillary hydrostatic pressure exceeding 24 mm Hg will result in the development of pulmonary edema. Edema begins in the central perihilar area and involves peribronchial and perivascular interstitial spaces and also produces alveolar edema.

Noncardiac Causes

Noncardiac causes include diseases that decrease colloid oncotic pressure (low plasma colloid oncotic pressure lowers the threshold to pressure-induced pulmonary edema), shock, upper airway obstruction, smoke inhalation, heat stroke, electrocution, uremia, IV fluid overload, infections, thoracic neoplasia, poisonings, hypoproteinemia, thoracic trauma, anaphylaxis, inhaled irritants and toxins, acute respiratory distress, disseminated intravascular coagulation (DIC), drowning, and neurogenic causes.

Signs

The most common signs of pulmonary edema are dyspnea, tachypnea, moist rales, cyanosis, open-mouthed breathing, distress, inability to lie down without being uncomfortable, and restlessness. Acute pulmonary edema may produce gurgling, bubbling noises during breathing, foaming at the mouth and nose that is often blood tinged, extreme dyspnea, and anxiety.

Radiographs should not be taken during acute pulmonary edema, because the added stress of restraint may severely jeopardize the life of the animal. Following emergency treatment for edema, radiographs of the thorax are indicated.

Therapy

Initial treatment of pulmonary edema depends on the severity of respiratory distress of the patient when presented. Initial emergency treatment is aimed at: (a) decreasing oxygen demand, (b) decreasing the amount of excess pulmonary fluid, (c) supporting pulmonary circulation, and (d) treating the underlying hypertension of pulmonic vasculature or underlying heart disease (Table 36).

Animals with acute pulmonary edema must receive oxygen and must have the accumlating fluid removed. The clinician must quickly decide whether the

Table 36. INITIAL EMERGENCY MANAGEMENT
OF PULMONARY EDEMA

Sedate and Reduce Respiratory Effort	
Morphine sulfate	0.50–1.0 mg/IV or SC (dog)
Chlorpromazine	0.50 mg/kg IM or SC
Acepromazine	0.10–0.20 mg/kg IM or SC
Administer Oxygen (see also p. 633)	
Transtracheal—use 3–5 Fr. catheter	
Use oxygen cage—nebulize 40% ethyl alcohol	
Use nasopharyngeal catheter to give O_2	
Use positive pressure ventilation to give O_2	
Administer Bronchodilator	
Aminophylline	6–10 mg/kg IM or IV
Papavitrol 20	Cats: ¼ tab q 12 h
Begin Diuresis (depending on cause)	
Furosemide	2–3 mg/kg IV q 6–8 h (dog)
	2–3 mg/kg IV or IM q 12 h (cat)

For more specific treatment of pulmonary edema associated with congestive heart disease and other cardiovascular disease, see pp. 36–59.

major underlying problem is: (a) increased hydrostatic pressure, as with cardiovascular disease, or (b) altered lung vascular permeability, with increased protein leakage.

The quickest way to get oxygen to the lungs is via a transtracheal catheter (see p. 633) connected to an oxygen source. The oxygen must be humidified (90 per cent) with warm water. Suction at 15 cm of water can be used with the same catheter to remove bronchial fluids. The content of these fluids should be evaluated for cells and protein. If lung fluids contain a protein content of 50 per cent or greater than the blood protein level, severe vascular permeability problems exist in the lungs, and water-soluble steroids should be started immediately.

If there is altered hydrostatic pressure, as evidenced by pulse rate and tone, evaluation of mucous membranes, evaluation of jugular pulse, heart rate, and electrocardiogram (ECG), begin appropriate therapy immediately (see Cardiac Failure and Use of Vasodilators, pp. 51–56).

Pulmonary Thromboembolism

Thrombogenesis of major veins and/or arteries has usually been a post-mortem finding in small animals. However, preclinical diagnosis of thrombogenesis, especially in dogs, is being made on a more frequent basis.

Hypercoagulable states of the blood and vessels may be associated with blood vessel endothelial injury, alterations in blood flow with increased blood stasis, and altered blood coagulability.

Clinical conditions in the dog that may predispose to thrombogenesis are: (1) catheterization of blood vessels, (2) DIC, (3) bacterial endocarditis, (4) dysproteinemias, (5) Cushing's disease, and (6) nephrotic syndrome.

Diagnosis of pulmonary thromboembolism is difficult but is predicated on a high degree of suspicion, based on clinical signs coupled with radiographic findings. Clinical signs of pulmonary thrombosis include dyspnea, pleural effusion, restlessness, orthopnea, cough, cyanosis, and syncope. Cardiovascular changes are acute right-sided heart failure (cor pulmonale), jugular pulse, pleural effusion, hepatic congestion, and increased peripheral venous pressure.

Diagnostic radiology is based on the use of a nonselective angiogram to demonstrate obstructive abnormalities in pulmonary arteries.

The nephrotic syndrome in the dog can produce a hypercoagulable state that in its severe form may produce pulmonary thrombosis. In the nephrotic syndrome, particularly those associated with renal amyloidosis, there is marked proteinuria, with selective loss of low–molecular weight proteins. A hypercoagulable state is associated with the renal loss of antithrombin III and the increase of fibrinogen and factor VIII concentrations in the blood. Use an ACT test to screen for coagulation abnormality (see p. 709).

Dogs with antithromboplastin III activity less than 70 per cent of normal and fibrinogen values greater than 300 mg per dl should be treated with anticoagulation therapy (see p. 63). Heparin is likely to be less effective than

Coumadin in controlling the hypercoagulable state. Corticosteroids should be avoided, if possible.

Severe thrombosis can develop in a wide variety of disease processes, including consumptive coagulopathies, renal disease, Cushing's disease, and following IV catheter use. When IV catheters are used, thrombi usually develop at the area of valves in the veins.

In treating cases in which thrombosis is suspected, the following principles are suggested:

1. Use heparin low-dose therapy IV (see DIC, pp. 63–65)
2. Use cyclo-oxygenase inhibitors to reduce prostaglandin production and to reduce platelet aggregation. Aspirin can be given to dogs, 15 to 25 mg per kg q 12 h and to cats 10 to 15 mg per kg q 24 h. More potent agents such as Banamine have been used 0.5 to 1.0 mg per kg IV q 24 h in dogs (not approved).
3. Use colloids administered as fluids; low molecular weight dextran (Dextran 40) to maintain fluid volume.
4. In the longer term management of thromboembolic disease, racemic warfarin sodium should be used, and the prothrombin time should be maintained at 1 1/2 to 2 times normal. The initial loading dose is 10 mg per day for 1 to 3 days for a 15- to 18-kg dog. The initial maintenance dose can be started on a daily basis at 0.2 to 0.4 mg per kg per day and then tapered to administration that may require dosage 2 to 3 times a week to maintain the prothrombin time at 1 1/2 to 2 times normal. The antidote to racemic warfarin is vitamin K, administered IV (see p. 928).

Adult Respiratory Distress Syndrome
(Shock Lung)

Adult respiratory disease (ARD) can follow numerous systemic diseases or trauma. Adult respiratory distress syndrome (ARDS) has been called "shock lung," "traumatic wet lung," and a variety of other names. The onset of severe respiratory symptoms and radiologically observable lung signs is usually delayed 24 to 48 hours following injury.

ARDS is secondary to injury of pulmonary capillary membrane, with leakage of both water and protein into pulmonary interstitium. When the leaking exceeds the lymphatic clearance ability, fluid will enter the alveolus and produce an inhibition or washout of surfactant, with eventual alveolar collapse. This produces perfusion of ventilated alveoli, and blood passes through the lung unoxygenated.

The major clinical manifestations of ARDS are tachypnea, hyperpnea, and harsh bronchial sounds with no tracheobronchial secretions. Blood gas determinations reveal a falling pO_2 and pCO_2 and, if hyperpnea exists, a respiratory alkalosis. Respiratory vital capacity becomes markedly reduced. Functional residual capacity decreases, physiologic dead space increases, and there is a decreased V/Q with ventilation/perfusion mismatching.

Radiographic indications of lung abnormalities are progressive and usually develop 12 to 24 hours after the initial onset of signs. Initial indications are perivascular cuffing and interstitial edema that progress to intra-alveolar edema, hemorrhage, and lung consolidation. Heart size remains normal; lung vascular markings are normal; and there is no marked fluid accumulation in the alveoli of the lung, a characteristic that differentiates ARDS from severe pulmonary edema.

Changes in the normal physiologic integrity of the lungs lead to a decrease in functional residual capacity and an increase in venous admixture.

The prevention of and initial treatment of ARDS are based on the maintenance of good cardiovascular function and the institution of ventilatory support. The control of sepsis and looking for causes and organisms involved in clinical, post-traumatic infection are also very important. In administering fluids, the animal should be kept rehydrated and adequate urine output should be maintained; however, excessive fluids may increase pulmonary capillary wedge pressure and lung permeability. Central venous pressure (CVP) can be monitored during fluid administration.

Although the lungs contain edema fluid in ARDS, the use of diuretics is indicated only if there is severe hypervolemia from fluid administration overload. In normovolemic or hypovolemic states, diuretic therapy can decrease extracellular fluid volume, thus producing an even more marked hypovolemia, which compounds the shock syndrome.

Drug therapy in cases of established ARDS is controversial and, in general, has been shown not to be helpful. Drugs evaluated include steroids, heparin, and vasodilators.

The timing of the use of steroids such as methylprednisolone appears to be critical in its effectiveness in ARDS. The steroid has a preventative effect only when administered during the initial 2 to 3 hours of ARDS, and most patients are recognized later than this.

Other forms of treatment that may help in ARDS syndrome are: (1) tracheobronchial toiletry, including periodic hyperventilation of the lungs, humidification of inspired air, postural drainage, and percussion thorax; (2) mobilizing the patient into sternal recumbency and encouraging ambulation; and (3) maintaining adequate hydration of the patient to maintain open airways for the secretion of fluids.

Pneumothorax

The presence of air within the pleural cavity is called *pneumothorax*. It is classified as: (1) open pneumothorax—an open chest wound; (2) closed pneumothorax—tears in the visceral pleura; (3) valvular pneumothorax—air entering the pleural cavity during inspiration leading to (4) tension pneumothorax; (5) traumatic pneumothorax—frequently associated with rib fractures and possible hemothorax; and (6) bilateral pneumothorax—from extensive unilateral injuries to the pleura and lung. Not all pneumothorax cases are traumatic in origin, and spontaneous pneumothorax can be seen in the dog and cat. Emphysematous bullae, lung granulomas, and cystic lung lesions are associated with *Paragonimus kellicotti* infestation.

Severe ventilatory and circulatory insufficiency following traumatic injury to the chest could be associated with several conditions: (1) open pneumothorax, (2) airway obstruction, (3) flail chest, (4) tension pneumothorax, (5) hemothorax, and (6) cardiac tamponade. Treat all penetrating wounds of the chest wall as open or sucking wounds until careful inspection proves otherwise. Wounds should be immediately closed with a pressure dressing while the animal is stabilized. Never administer PPV to a dyspneic animal until it has been ascertained that a pneumothorax is or is not present. In pneumothorax, the abnormal accumulations of air in the thorax must first be removed. A thoracentesis (see p. 523) should be done immediately using the technique described, and air should be aspirated.

Air entering one hemithorax will produce a bilateral pneumothorax because of weakness of the mediastinum. Tension pneumothorax occurs because the pulmonary tissue develops a valvelike leak or a valvelike sucking chest wound; air continues to enter the thoracic cavity on inspiration but cannot escape.

Cystic pulmonary lesions may be seen in the lungs and may be associated with blebs, bullae, pneumatoceles, cystic bronchiectasis, congenital cysts, and infections. Acquired bullae are cystic air spaces within the lung parenchyma that form because of the confluence of alveoli following the breakdown of alveolar septa. Intrapulmonary cavitary lesions in dogs and cats are most commonly associated with destruction of pulmonary parenchyma and its replacement with air, congenital cyst formation, paragonimus infestations in dogs and cats, and traumatic lesions. Cystic pulmonary lesions may rupture and lead to spontaneous development of tension pneumothorax. Congenital intrapulmonary cysts usually have a smooth thin wall and often present as spontaneous pneumothorax cases. Radiographs of the chest taken with a horizontally directed beam are advantageous in establishing a diagnosis.

Esophagobronchial fistulas can be associated with bony foreign bodies of the esophagus and can result in pneumothorax, atelectasis, and foreign body pneumonia. Radiographic evaluation of the anterior mediastinum and thorax may show a foreign body pneumonia. Radiographic evaluation of the anterior mediastinum and thorax may show a foreign body pneumonia, mediastinitis, or pleural effusion. In demonstrating the foreign body using contrast media, aqueous iodine (Gastrografin, 66 per cent diatrizoate meglumine with 10 per cent diatrizoate solution is mixed equally with sterile water. *(Barium should not be used.)*

Pneumothorax results in dyspnea, diminished breath sounds, and hyperresonance to percussion. Confirmatory diagnosis of pneumothorax is based on radiography or thoracentesis. Radiographs should not be taken until dyspnea is corrected via aspiration and/or chest tube placement. Radiographs should be taken in the standing lateral position, if possible. If spontaneous pneumothorax resulting from ruptured lung bullae are suspected, radiographs taken from the decubital position may reveal surface bullae of the lungs. Radiography may reveal: (1) elevation of the cardiac silhouette in radiographs taken in the recumbent position, (2) increased density of the pulmonary tissue, (3) free air between the parietal and visceral pleura, and (4) absence of vascular shadows in the peripheral portion of the thorax.

Treatment

Treatment should be aimed at re-establishing negative pressure in the thorax. In mild cases, cage rest and avoidance of heavy exertion may be curative within several days.

Thoracentesis (see p. 523) should be performed and air should be removed until dyspnea is relieved. Small, visceral pleural tears will often seal following removal of air from the thorax. If thoracentesis has to be repeated more than twice in 24 hours or if tension pneumothorax develops, a thoracic drainage tube must be inserted (see p. 215) and attached to an underwater seal and suction system.

Severe drainage to the thorax may indicate that an exploratory thoracotomy may have to be performed. The following are indications for performing a thoracotomy in cases of thoracic trauma:

1. Extensive and apparently uncontrollable intrapleural hemorrhage.
2. Cardiac tamponade that cannot be relieved by pericardiocentesis.
3. Ruptured esophagus.
4. Foreign body present in the thorax.
5. Massive pleural air leak, with failure to respond to tube thoracostomy and underwater suction and drainage, subcutaneous emphysema, or complete atelectasis of a lung lobe, with possible ruptured bronchus, evidence of pulmonary cavitation, and/or bullae formation.

Pneumomediastinum refers to the presence of free air in the mediastinum. Causes of air within the mediastinum include: (1) deep wounds of the neck, (2) lacerations or rupture of the trachea or esophagus, (3) bronchial rupture, (4) rupture of lung alveoli, and (5) lumbar and retroperitoneal wounds with free gas accumulation.

Tracheobronchial injuries can result in rapid and severe respiratory distress. There may develop marked subcutaneous emphysema involving the neck and thoracic inlet area and tension pneumothorax. The chest must be drained of air, and emergency measures for pneumothorax must be started (see p. 212) while surgical repair of the trachea is attempted.

Hemothorax

Extensive bleeding into the thoracic cavity can lead to severe respiratory embarrassment. Hemothorax can be associated with: (1) eroding lesions in the thorax, (2) lung lacerations, (3) rupture of intercostal vessels, and (4) diaphragmatic hernias. Hemothorax is associated with reduced tidal volume, dullness to percussion, and lung atelectasis. Standing lateral radiographs are very helpful in making a diagnosis of fluid in the chest cavity. Initial treatment of hemothorax should include treating shock and stabilizing the patient (see pp. 57–68).

Thoracentesis can be helpful in confirming the diagnosis of hemothorax. Each side of the chest should be aspirated (see p. 523). If a large amount of blood is present, a chest tube should be inserted. The chest tube is placed at dorsal one-third to mid-third junction of the ribs and is advanced to mid third to ventral third. For small animals (up to 11.3 kg [25 lb]), a No. 14–18 French red rubber urethral or feeding catheter (Brunswick) can be used. Argyle catheters or homemade Silastic silicone catheters of various diameters work well as chest tubes.

Pull the clipped and surgically prepared skin forward 1 to 2 inches, and block the area locally with 2 to 5 ml of lidocaine into the 7th intercostal space at the junction of the dorsal third and mid third. Make a small incision in the skin and subcutaneous tissue over the 7th intercostal space, and use a Kelly clamp to make a tract down into the pleura of the 7th intercostal space. The clamp and catheter enter the pleura by exerting a quick thrust of the clamp. The clamp is then removed. The skin is let go; it moves caudally back to its natural position creating a skin/subcutaneous tunnel over the tube. The skin is closed around the catheter with heavy silk or nylon suture. The end of the chest tube can be attached to: (1) a Heimlich valve with or without suction, (2) a three-way stopcock for aspiration, or (3) an underwater seal and suction drainage system.

Contusion

Contusion of the lung can be a frequent finding in trauma to the chest, especially when rib fractures are present. The radiologic pattern of lung contusion can be quite variable. It may appear as diffuse or localized mottled densities or, in more severe cases, as a complete density of an entire lung lobe. This produces signs of an air bronchogram because of fluid in the lung lobe, with air trapped in the bronchial tree. Free air or blood may be trapped in the pleural space.

General supportive care is the treatment of choice in lung contusion. The use of water-soluble steroids such as dexamethasone phosphate or hydrocortisone hemisuccinate should be used as early as possible following lung contusion and should be continued for 48 to 72 hours. Animals with lung contusions are very susceptible to fluid overload and lung edema; therefore, IV fluids should be limited, especially in cats, and should not be administered at rates over 20 ml per kg per hr. Administer antibiotics systemically, and institute cage rest; the use of an oxygen cage may prove beneficial. Use diuretics systemically to control edema formation (see p. 209). Use narcotics to control pain when indicated. If pulmonary edema develops, see p. 209.

Chylothorax

Chylothorax refers to the abnormal accumulation of chylous fluid (lymphatic drainage fluid) into the chest cavity because of damage to the thoracic duct, resulting from trauma, tumor invasion, or spontaneous, unknown leakage.

The cisterna chyli is the dilated collecting pool of the lymphatics located ventrodextrad from the first to the fourth lumbar vertebrae and leads into the thoracic duct cranially. More complete descriptions of the thoracic duct are given by Quick and Berg. The thoracic duct enters the chest through the aortic hiatus; however, numerous collateral ducts extend craniad from the cisterna chyli.

Signs of chylothorax are related to accumulations of chylous fluid in the anterior mediastinal and thoracic spaces, producing dyspnea, cachexia, weight loss, cyanosis, coughing, atelectasis, pneumonitis, and fever. Chyle contains 60 to 70 per cent of ingested fats, especially long–chain fatty acids, 1 to 6 gm of protein per 100 ml of chyle, and approximately 22,000 lymphocytes per ml of chyle. Loss of chylous fluid may result in hypoproteinemia and peripheral edema or ascites.

Diagnosis is based on thoracentesis and the removal of a milky, often blood-tinged, chylous fluid. Shaking of a true chylous fluid with ether after alkalinization usually clears the fluid. Chylous fluid is usually bacteriologically negative, and has a specific gravity greater than 1.012 and a protein content greater than 3 gm per 100 ml.

Cases of chylothorax in the dog and cat may be secondary to trauma, either surgical or nonsurgical. In one study, all dogs that developed lung lobe torsion developed chylothorax as a postoperative complication.

Nontraumatic chylothorax may indicate invasive neoplastic disease in the thorax. In cats, mediastinal lymphosarcoma is common.

The exact localization of the damaged thoracic duct is difficult.

Lymphangiography of the thoracic duct in the dog, using aqueous contrast media, may locate the damaged thoracic duct. For further discussion of lymphangiography and surgical treatment of chylothorax, see the reference articles by Quick and Berg.

Cardiovascular Changes Associated with Thoracic Trauma

Cardiac injury is a frequent complication of nonpenetrating thoracic trauma. It is difficult to suspect thoracic trauma if there is no external evidence of chest trauma, such as rib fractures or contusions. Severe cardiac trauma may produce rupture of the intraventricular septum, valvular damage, atrial tears, and pericardial hemorrhage, leading to cardiac tamponade. (See Pericardial Effusion, p. 56.)

More common cardiac abnormalities result from myocardial injury leading to supraventricular arrhythmias that can be characterized by: (1) multiple premature systoles, (2) ventricular tachycardia, (3) abnormal S-T segment elevation or depression, (4) atrial fibrillation, and (5) evidence of myocardial infarction and cardiac failure.

It is advisable that all cases of thoracic trauma be evaluated with an ECG. If changes occur in rhythm or form characterized by elevation of the S-T segment or depression and slurring, repeated ECGs should be performed. Severe weakness, depression, and pulse deficits associated with cardiac arrhythmias such as paroxysmal ventricular tachycardia and multifocal ventricular ectopic beats should be treated as emergencies (see p. 57).

Rib Fractures (See also p. 102)

Rib fractures are characterized by localized pain, possible subcutaneous and bone crepitus, and painful respiratory movements. Radiographs are helpful in confirming the diagnosis; however, careful and gentle palpation may reveal crepitus and instability of the ribs. Depending on which ribs are fractured and the level of damage, other associated complicating problems can be lung contusions, pericardial laceration, contusion heart, diaphragmatic hernia, and splenic rupture. Radiographs and a thoracic tap are indicated for pneumothorax evaluation (see p. 212). Radiographs should not be done in the severely dyspneic animal until dyspnea is relieved. Always evaluate the heart for traumatic myocarditis in chest injuries. An ECG may reveal arrhythmias that can be treated medically (see pp. 36–59).

Severe chest injuries can result in multiple rib fractures and produce a "floating" segment of the thorax. This floating area of the chest wall moves in and out with respirations and can result in poor aeration of the underlying lung—a condition called *flail chest*.

The animal should be placed on its side, with the flail chest down, thus putting the "good lung" up and stabilizing the flail from moving outward. PPV can help stabilize the respirations of an animal with flail chest but requires general anesthesia. If PPV is used, adequate pleural decompression must be maintained; otherwise, a tension pneumothorax can be produced. The flail chest must be stabilized surgically. If PPV is not immediately available, the chest wall can be stabilized by passing a towel clamp around the central portion of the flailing segment and applying traction to it until surgical stabilization can be effected. Stabilization of flail ribs can be done by the use of a large piece of orthoplast. The orthoplast is "anchored" to the fractured ribs and the adjacent normal ribs using nonabsorbable sutures.

In managing rib fractures, reduction of pain can be accomplished with intercostal nerve blocks, using 0.5 per cent bupivacaine HCl and repeated as needed. Small doses of narcotics, that is, oxymorphone, 0.02 to 0.04 mg per kg IV or IM, may be helpful in allowing the animal to obtain relief from pain and to help its breathing. Bandaging of the chest is not particularly effective and may *reduce* already compromised pulmonary function.

Diaphragmatic Hernia

A diaphragmatic hernia is a protrusion of abdominal viscera through the diaphragm. The most common type of diaphragmatic hernia in small animals is produced by rupture of the diaphragm secondary to trauma. Associated traumatic lesions may be rib fractures, pneumothorax, lung contusions, and shock. Most tears penetrate diaphragmatic muscle; the position of the tear depends on the position of the animal and abdominal viscera when a sudden force is applied to the abdomen. The tear or tears in the diaphragm may be unilateral or bilateral and may vary in shape. In addition, tears may occur costally or transsternally. In dogs, diaphragmatic hernias are more common on the left side; whereas in cats, hernias are more prevalent on the right side.

The contents of the hernia may vary with the size and location of the tear and the activity of the animal. Changes in the condition of an animal with a diaphragmatic hernia may occur very rapidly. After initial presentation, the amount of tissue herniated through the diaphragm may increase, producing acute respiratory distress. Many hernias go undiagnosed for months before clinical signs make the diagnosis apparent. The chief sign associated with diaphragmatic hernia is dyspnea, although this may be masked by shock in acute trauma cases. The degree of dyspnea depends on the extent of displacement of lung tissue. Auscultation of the thorax reveals that normal respiratory sounds are muffled, and peristaltic sounds may be heard. Frequently there is pleural effusion. The patient prefers to sit or keep its front end elevated.

Auscultation of the chest reveals respiratory sounds as muffled and the heart as being displaced by abdominal organs. Peristaltic sounds may be heard from prolapsed abdominal organs, and percussion of the chest may reveal resonant sounds if a hollow viscus distended with gas is in the thorax. Often, however, no abnormalities can be detected on auscultation or percussion.

The diagnosis of diaphragmatic hernia is based on history (especially that of trauma), clinical signs, and radiographs (see p. 365). Contrast radiographs made following the administration of barium may occasionally be needed to localize a portion of alimentary tract in the chest; however, the characteristic radiographic finding of an alteration in the diaphragmatic line can be visualized on plain films.

Treatment of acute diaphragmatic hernias is designed to stabilize normal patterns of respiration, control shock, and prepare the patient for surgery. Draining fluid from the chest and relieving an existing pneumothorax can assist in establishing normal respirations. Elevation of the forequarters may also be helpful. Correction of fluid and electrolyte disturbances prior to surgery is necessary. With acute injuries, shock should be treated (see p. 63) and the pleural space decompressed with chest tube placement (see p. 215). Anesthetic management is critical, and anoxia can rapidly develop. Always keep the side of animal with the diaphragmatic hernia down so that the opposite pulmonary tissue does not become compromised.

Preoperatively, the animal should be treated for septic shock, especially if the liver is entrapped within the chest cavity (see p. 59). The ventral abdominal approach will provide exposure for hernias on either side of the chest.

Malignant Hyperthermia Syndrome

Malignant hyperthermia syndrome is a pharmacogenetic disease involving the uninhibited flow of calcium into the muscle substance. Unfortunately, the disease entity is usually diagnosed only when an animal is placed under general anesthesia. The signs of malignant hyperthermia are massive muscle fasciculations or spasms, tachycardia, unstable blood pressure, metabolic and respiratory acidosis, and very elevated temperature (108–110° F). If malignant hyperthermia is not immediately controlled, cellular death results.

The current theory of malignant hyperthermia suggests that there is an abnormality in sarcoplasmic membrane permeability. Abnormalities in the release of calcium ions result in accentuation of the actin-myosin interaction and muscle contractures. Calcium is not resorbed into the sarcoplasmic reticulum. Continued release of calcium poisons the muscle cells and causes uncoupling of exudative phosphorylation at the mitochondrial level.

Predisposing and aggravating factors in malignant hyperthermia include hypercarbia or hypoxia; hyperthermia caused by infections; high ambient temperatures; high sympathetic activity; muscle trauma; and the use of depolarizing muscle blocking agents, that is, succinylcholine hydrochloride.

Treatment

Malignant hyperthermia syndrome is treated using the following procedures:

1. Surgery must be immediately stopped—discontinue all anesthetic gases and muscle blocking agents.
2. Hyperventilate the patient with 100 per cent oxygen.
3. Begin cooling with cold packs, give an ice bath, but stop cooling when the animal's temperature is down to 102° F.
4. Administer Dantrolone sodium, 1 to 5 mg per kg IV—decreases the permeability of the sarcoplasmic membrane to calcium ion.
5. Give procainamide, 1 gm in 500 ml of D5W—if needed for cardiac arrhythmia or IV lidocaine (see p. 36).
6. Administer IV solutions—fluids can be 0.9 per cent NaCl, lactated Ringer's solution, or D5W. Add 10 to 50 ml of 50 per cent dextrose (depending on size) because of the increased metabolic demands during hyperthermia. Correct the base deficit with sodium bicarbonate (see p. 608).
7. Following an acute episode, Dantrolone, 2.2 mg per kg q 8h for 24 hours can be used.

References and Additional Readings

Aron, D. M., Kornegay, J. N.: Clinical significance of traumatic lung cysts and associated pulmonary abnormalities in the dog and cat. J.A.A.H.A., 19(6):903.
Bauer, T. G., and Thomas, W. P.: Pulmonary edema. In Kirk, R. W. (ed.): Current Veterinary Therapy VIII: Small Animal Practice. Philadelphia, W. B. Saunders Company, 1983.
Berg, J.: Chylothorax in the dog and cat. Compendium on Continuing Education, 4(12):986, 1982.
Burns, M. G., Kelly, A. B., Hornof, W. J., and Howorth, E.: Pulmonary artery thrombosis in three dogs with hyperadrenocorticism. J.A.V.M.A., 178(4):388, 1981.
Cantwell, H. D., Rebar, A. H., and Aller, A. R.: Pleural effusion in the dog. J.A.A.H.A., 19(2):227, 1983.

Carb, A.: Diaphragmatic hernia in the dog and cat. Vet. Clin. North Am., 5:477, 1975.

Caywood, D. D., and Feeney, D. A.: Acquired esophagobronchial fistula in a dog. J.A.A.H.A., 18(4):590, 1982.

Gilroy, B.: Effect of intercostal nerve blocks on post thoracotomy ventilation and oxygenation in the canine. J. Vet. Crit. Care Soc., March, 1983, pp. 1–9.

Green, R. A., and Kabel, A. L.: Hypercoagulable state in three dogs with nephrotic syndrome: role of acquired antithrombin III deficiency. J.A.V.M.A., 181(9):914.

Harvey, C. E., and O'Brien, J. A.: Management of respiratory emergencies in small animals. Vet. Clin. North Am., 2:243, 1972.

Haskins, S.: Management of pulmonary disease in the critical patient. In Zaslow, I. M. (ed.): Veterinary Trauma and Critical Care. Philadelphia, Lea & Febiger, 1984, pp. 339–383.

Hunt, C. A.: Chest trauma: the approach to the patient with chest injuries. Compendium on Continuing Education, 1:537, 1979.

Moise, N. S., and Spaulding, G. L.: Feline bronchial asthma. Compendium on Continuing Education, 3(12): 1091, 1981.

Quick, C. B.: Chylothorax—A review. J.A.A.H.A., 16(1):23, 1980.

Silverman, S., et al.: Cavitary pulmonary lesions in animals. J. Am. Vet. Radiol. Soc., 18(4):134, 1976.

Suter, P. F., and Ettinger, S. J.: Pulmonary edema. In Ettinger, S. (ed.): Textbook of Veterinary Internal Medicine, Philadelphia, 2nd ed. W. B. Saunders Company, 1982, pp. 747–759.

Tams, T. R., and Sherding, R. G.: Smoke inhalation injury. Compendium on Continuing Education, 3(11):986, 1981.

Tranbaugh, R. F., and Lewis, F. R.: Respiratory insufficiency. Surg. Clin. North Am., 62(1):121, 1982.

Yoshioka, M. M.: Management of spontaneous pneumothorax in twelve dogs. J.A.A.H.A., 18(1):57, 1982.

ACUTE SOFT–TISSUE INJURIES

ASSESSMENT OF THE INJURED ANIMAL

Acute soft-tissue injuries in small animals are a common occurrence. When the animal is first presented, a quick initial survey should be made of the state of consciousness, respiratory function, heart action, and the presence of bleeding or shock. The comatose animal may be suffering from acute central nervous system (CNS) injury, acute blood loss, or hypoxia, all of which predispose to shock (see pp. 57–68). The animal should be handled gently to avoid further injury. The fractured limbs should be immobilized before the animal is moved; and, if a spinal cord injury is suspected, the animal is moved on a flat board.

Preliminary treatment must include measures to keep the animal alive, for example, ensure an adequate airway, assist ventilation if necessary, control hemorrhage, and replace any deficit in circulatory volume (see p. 591).

ANESTHESIA

Carefully evaluate the patient's general condition before deciding on whether to administer a general anesthetic. Establish a patent airway, and stabilize the animal's cardiovascular system. If the animal's stomach is full, the animal should be intubated immediately after anesthesia is induced. Remove any blood, secretions, or vomitus from the mouth and pharynx. Intubation of the trachea may be accomplished under sedation with neuroleptanalgesia if the oropharynx is anesthetized topically with lidocaine, 4 per cent. When small dose of narcotics such as Numorphan are given, they should be injected intravenously (IV), because absorption by other routes is unpredictable in shock.

EARLY WOUND MANAGEMENT

The early time period following the creation of a wound with contamination, debris, and bacteria and when infection is considered to begin is called *the golden period.* The length of this period is generally considered 6 hours, during which time the wounds can be decontaminated by washing and débridement. After this time, bacteria invade wounds from the wound margin.

In general, wounds can be categorized into classes, depending on the progression of infection:
1. 0 to 6 hours old—little bacterial multiplication
2. 6 to 12 hours old—bacteria multiplying
3. 12 hours or more—infected wound (greater than 10^6 bacteria)

On initial examination of a wound older than 6 hours, a bacterial culture should be obtained and a sensitivity test should be taken. A rapid slide test can be done by smearing exudate on a slide and performing a Gram stain and examining cell content and type. For severely infected wounds, a smear that is gram stained can be helpful in evaluating the predominant bacterial population.

When examining the wound, further contamination should be avoided. Rubber gloves and sterile instruments should be used and unnecessary manipulation of the wound must be avoided. The following factors should be evaluated:
1. Condition of the tissues. Is the local blood supply intact?
2. Location of the wound. Wounds around the face and mucous membranes usually heal well provided that the tissues are viable.
3. Contamination of the wound with soil. Components of soil, especially clay and organic fractions, contain infection-producing factors. These factors provide for physical alterations in the wound, promoting greater infection.
4. Presence of foreign bodies.

A wide area around the wound should be clipped, and the hair should be removed with a vacuum system. Hair at the wound margins is clipped with a scissors, with blades coated with K-Y jelly to cause hairs to adhere. The skin around the wound should be scrubbed with a povidone-iodine scrub solution or a 2 per cent chlorhexidine diacetate (Nolvasan Surgical Scrub) solution. If the animal is severely soiled with urine, feces, or road dirt, it should be placed on a wire grill, suspended over a tub, and washed with warm water.

Wounds can be initially lavaged with a 2 per cent lidocaine solution to make animals more comfortable if neuroleptanalgesia is used. The use of continuous or pulsating high–pressure lavage of the wound with sterile irrigating fluids can be very helpful in the removal of detritus and debris. Low concentrations of sodium hypochlorite can be used as a wound irrigant; this solution promotes resolution of inflammation and edema, early separation of eschar with no putrefaction, good healing with healthy granulation tissue, and minimal scarring. Sources of available sodium hypochlorite are Chlorox, 5.25 per cent available as chlorine; add 9 gm of sodium chloride to each L of 1 per cent solution. To make a 1 per cent solution, add one part Chlorox to four parts tap water (not sterile water). This is 1 per cent stock solution. For initial toilet of wounds, use one part stock solution to four parts water (98°F); for additional irrigations, use one part stock solution to 19 parts water (98°F). Numerous irrigation devices can be used. The Water Pik system is acceptable. Antibiotics can be added to saline or lactated Ringer's solution. Detergent substances, including most surgical soaps, should not be used in open wounds with exposed tissue and muscle, because they may cause chemical irrigation.

IV prophylactic systemic antibiotic therapy should be started prior to initiating operative procedures on wounds. Antibiotics should then be continued for further treatments. The choice of antibiotics in severely infected wounds can be aided by initial gram staining of the exudate. Culture and sensitivity results may later alter the treatment regimen. Wounds can also be irrigated with topically applied antibiotics or 0.5 per cent Betadine solution. Solutions of bacitracin (50 units/ml) and polymyxin B (0.05 mg/ml) can be used. (Rehydrate 1-50,000-unit vial of bacitracin with 1 L of saline and 1-50-mg vial of polymyxin B with 1 L of saline.) The two drugs can be mixed to form an effective lavage solution.

Layered débridement involves removing devitalized tissues, beginning at the surface of the wound, and progressing to the wound depths. Wound débridement involves the removal of devitalized, contaminated, and dead tissue.

Drains should be placed in wounds in which the following conditions apply:
1. Débridement has not removed all diseased tissue, and foreign material is still present.
2. Massive contamination of wounds is present.
3. Accumulations of tissue fluid or blood clots will build up in "dead spaces," creating pockets for infection.
4. There is tissue of questionable viability in a wound.
The wound is not closed but is allowed to undergo delayed closure for at least 3 days while treatment is begun.

Various types of drains can be used, but the penrose or tube drains are those most commonly in use. Suction-type drains may also be very helpful, more so than the penrose.

The following factors influence whether primary wound closure should be undertaken: (1) time lapse since injury, (2) extent of tissue damage and status of blood supply, and (3) ability to close wound without excessive tension.

Animals presented for wound treatment several days following injury with grossly contaminated wounds, necrotic tissue, and poorly generalized physical state are not good candidates for surgery. These animals should have secondary closures performed following control of infection and development of granulation tissue. This usually takes at least 5 days.

In considering whether or not a wound should be bandaged or dressed, one should remember the four functions of dressings: (1) protection, (2) absorption of drainage material, (3) compression to prevent hematomas and eliminate dead space, and (4) stabilization.

Nonadherent sterile material such as a Telfa pad is placed on a wound surface to prevent disruption when the dressing is being changed. On limbs, a modified Robert Jones or a Schanz dressing works well where immobilization for protection is needed. With extensive wound discharge, the bandage dressing (which is very absorbent) should be changed at least once a day in the early stages of wound healing.

For further information on wound management, see Swaim in the reference list at the end of this article.

Bite Wounds

Although only a single puncture wound may be evident following an animal bite, extensive traumatic injury to underlying muscles, fascial planes, tendons, arteries, veins, and nerves may take place. All bite wounds should be opened, and the underlying tissues should be exposed and examined. A dorsoventral excision is preferred to allow for ventral drainage, if required. Flush bite wound with quantities of sterile saline containing antibiotics or a dilute solution of Betadine (10 per cent) or of chlorhexidine (0.05 per cent), which is a 1:40 dilution of a 2 per cent stock solution.

Muscle, Tendon, and Joint Injuries

Muscle injuries include contusions, lacerations, and ischemic necrosis. Before repairing muscle injuries, damage to the bones, joints, nerves, and tendons should be assessed. Injured nonviable muscle should be removed from open wounds. If possible, sutures should be placed in lacerated muscles through the overlying fascia.

Tendons may be repaired with double-armed, nonabsorbable sutures of monofilament stainless steel, nylon, or polyprolene. Tendons may be sutured by the technique of Mason or Bunnell. Following reapposition of the tendon, immobilize the part in a position so that the tendon is relaxed.

Open wounds of joints can be caused by traumatic lacerations or by penetration of a fractured bone (see p. 102). Treatment of these wounds includes performing aseptic cleaning and wound débridement, taking radiographs to delineate bone fractures, suturing tendons when necessary, and administering antibiotics. Under strict aseptic conditions, surgically explore the joint and remove any foreign bodies, bone chips, blood clots, or devitalized tissue. Close the synovial sac with fine absorbable suture material. If the synovial membrane is extensively damaged, closure can be performed using full thickness or split thickness skin flaps as temporary coverage. Immobilize the joint. The aminoglycosides and synthetic penicillins such as the cephalosporins are the initial antibiotics of choice.

Penetrating and Nonpenetrating Injuries

Abdominal (See pp. 29–30)
Chest (See pp. 212–215)

References and Additional Readings

Jennings, P. B., Jr., and Geggers, J. P.: General principles in the care of open wounds. *In* Zaslow, I. M., (ed.): Veterinary Trauma and Critical Care, Philadelphia, Lea & Febiger, 1984, pp. 155–168.
Swaim, S.: Surgery of Traumatized Skin. Philadelphia, W. B. Saunders Company, 1981.

VASCULAR EMERGENCIES

Arterial Injuries

ARTERIAL LACERATION

Laceration of an artery, if open, can result in the loss of large quantities of blood or, if closed, in the development of a hematoma.

Hemorrhage may be controlled by any one or a combination of the following methods:
1. Application of a pressure bandage.
2. Location of the bleeding vessel, clamping it with a hemostat, and ligating it.
3. Applying digital pressure to the femoral or brachial artery. Applying a pneumatic cuffed tourniquet to an extremity proximal to the injury. The pressure of the tourniquet must be higher than the systolic blood pressure.

When bleeding is stanched, treat the animal for shock (see pp. 57–68) and soft-tissue injury.

Intracranial Bleeding (See p. 149)

SECTION 2

Interpreting Signs of Disease

THE DIAGNOSTIC CHALLENGE

Each time the clinician faces a new patient, he deals with the challenge of making a correct diagnosis. In many cases, the challenge is small and the answer is provided easily. Occasionally, patients present with questions of great complexity. This section does not attempt to give detailed diagnostic methods; rather, it has taken a group of common *signs*, which often are *presenting complaints*, and attempted to define and explain them. Fundamental causes are outlined, and conditions for differential or diagnostic consideration are discussed. These steps should give the clinician further insights into possible diagnoses, but specific details about each entity must be found by consulting other references.

FLUCTUATIONS IN BODY WEIGHT

WEIGHT LOSS

Physiologic Considerations

Decreased food intake results in metabolic changes within the body designed to conserve energy. These changes influence the activity, temperature, temperament, and overall health of the animal. Increased environmental temperature and activity (physical and emotional) create greater energy demands that must be met by an increased caloric intake.

Diagnosis and Tests

It may be difficult to confirm an owner's complaint about an animal's weight loss, especially if the diet varies, if an animal was overweight to begin with, or if previous weight records are unavailable. The two major considerations in weight loss are changes in appetite or food consumption and evidence of disordered gastrointestinal function such as vomiting or diarrhea. The magnitude of the weight loss and the time during which it has taken place are important considerations. Anorexia can occur in such a wide variety of conditions that this sign in itself is not helpful in reaching a diagnosis. However, decreased absorption of food may occur in pancreatic or hepatic disease, enteritis, or malabsorption syndromes. Weight loss with gastrointestinal disorders may accompany general illness such as distemper, hepatitis, renal disease, and neoplasms of the alimentary tract. Fever, itself a sign of disease, increases the caloric requirements of the animal and may result in severe weight loss. Weight loss accompanied by polyuria suggests diabetes mellitus, diabetes insipidus, or chronic renal disease.

Weight loss without a significant change in food consumption may suggest a hypermetabolic state such as hyperthyroidism or a psychogenic state such as extreme nervousness, created by a new environment or the introduction of ～ots into the household.

Weight loss without a significant change in food consumption may suggest a hypermetabolic state such as hyperthyroidism or a psychogenic state such as extreme nervousness, created by a new environment or the introduction of new pets into the household.

Weight loss may frequently occur because of underfeeding. Although an animal may be receiving large quantities of food, the caloric density of the food and the total calories may not be enough to fulfill the animal's need. An animal's caloric requirements fluctuate with its activity, the environmental temperature and humidity, body temperature, environmental and emotional stress, and such specific conditions as pregnancy (see Nutrition, p. 847).

Diagnosing the cause of weight loss demands a careful investigation of the animal's diet, when and how much the animal is fed, how much it eats, its environment, and its general health. Carefully kept weight records are necessary to follow the course of a patient who is losing weight.

WEIGHT GAIN

A gain in weight reflects excessive accumulation of fat tissue or of fluid and may be either local or general.

Tests and Diagnostic Considerations

A normal caloric intake accompanied by a reduced energy expenditure may result in weight gain. Underactivity resulting from hypothyroidism, hypoestrogenism, diseases such as osteoarthritis that limit physical activity, or advancing age may produce weight gain. Older animals with a reduced basal metabolic rate and reduced physical activity tend to put on excessive weight.

Excessive caloric intake results in the deposition of fat. Occasionally, compulsive eating may be caused by damage to the hypothalamus, with attendant loss of control over appetite. Hypoglycemia is a potent stimulus to the ingestion of food, and excessive food intake may be a compensatory mechanism to hyperinsulinism and pancreatic tumor. Most instances of weight gain due to excessive caloric intake are caused by the animal's being fed too much or having access to outside sources (such as garbage cans). Weight gain may also be associated with Cushing's syndrome, exogenous steroid administration, and hypogonadism.

A sudden increase in weight suggests the accumulation of fluid in the body (ascites) and is commonly indicative of underlying renal, cardiac, or hepatic disease (see p. 242). Alterations in daily weight can be used as a guideline in the management of animals being administered fluid therapy or in those cases being given diuretic drugs because of ascites.

References and Additional Readings

Ettinger, S. J.: Textbook of Veterinary Internal Medicine, 2nd ed. Philadelphia, W.B. Saunders Company, 1983.

Harrison, T. R. (ed.): Principles of Internal Medicine, 10th ed. New York, Blakiston Division, McGraw-Hill, 1983.

Kirk, R. W. (ed.): Current Veterinary Therapy VIII. Philadelphia, W..B. Saunders Co., 1983.

FEVER

In the normal animal, body temperature is maintained within a narrow range, despite extremes of environmental temperature and physical exertion. Animals are thus homeothermic. The control of body temperature by integrating physical and chemical processes is a function of cerebral centers in the hypothalamus.

Fever or pyrexia is an abnormally high body temperature. It is thought to be caused by the action of exogenous or endogenous pyrogens or toxins on the hypothalamus. In fever, the thermoregulatory mechanisms behave as though the body thermostat were adjusted to a higher level. Temperatures above 41°C (106°F) for prolonged periods result in permanent brain damage. Temperatures above 43°C (109°F) are associated with a high mortality.

Cause

In evaluating hyperthermic states in animals, one must distinguish between true fever associated with endogenous or exogenous pyrogens and mechanisms producing hyperthermia because of increased body activity or inadequate heat loss.

Excessive heat production by muscular activity, convulsions, excitement, and hyperthyroidism causes increased temperatures.

Impairment of heat loss by interference with transpiration from the skin (coating with oils or grease) or by interference with cooling by panting are important. Stenosis (brachycephalic breeds), paralysis, or tracheal intubation may cause the latter problem. Confinement in a hot, humid, or poorly ventilated environment may inhibit heat loss too (heat stroke; see p. 101).

Abnormal alteration in body temperature, namely fever, is associated with many diverse disease processes. The common mechanism in most of these disease processes is tissue injury, with resultant pyrogens causing abnormalities in thermoregulation. Among the agents producing pyrogens are bacteria; bacterial products, including staphylococcal exotoxin, staphylococcal endotoxin, lipopolysaccharides, fungi, and fungal polysaccharides and proteins; antigen-antibody complexes, a variety of drug agents; viral agents; tumors; tissue inflammation; and necrosis.

Physical Signs

The obvious criterion for fever is a body temperature above 39.5°C (103°F). Subjects are commonly depressed and anorexic, and have a languid eye or expression. Some may act as though they are cold and shiver, but they usually feel hot and seek a cool place in which to lie down. Feverish dogs may have either a wet, cool nose or a dry, warm one. Usually attendant on the fever is an increase in cardiac and respiratory rates. By recording temperature 2 to 4 times a day and considering etiology, fevers can be categorized into: sustained, ̄ͦmittent, intermittent, relapsing, septic, and hyperthermic.

Tests

In addition to the rectal temperature and a daily temperature graph, a total and differential white blood cell (WBC) count and an erythrocyte sedimentation rate are useful in initial tests. Most fevers can be explained after a careful physical examination and a complete history have been obtained. Heat, swelling, localization of pain, and disturbed locomotion as revealed by the physical examination and radiographic studies that show accumulations of pus may be diagnostic. Specific organ changes may dictate a need for special tests such as the following: blood cultures (see p. 500), FeLV (p. 698) or FIP tests (see p. 705), toxoplasmosis or *Brucella* titres, immunologic screen—Coombs', ANA, and LE prep (see p. 728), aspiration of body fluids (see pp. 522–524), CSF tap (see p. 496), and fiberoptic examination of the abdomen or the tracheobronchial tree (see p. 598).

Diagnostic Considerations

Consideration should be given to infectious diseases, chronic endocarditis and myocarditis, urinary infections, metritis, abscesses (accumulated pus under tension), subperiosteal hemorrhage (osteodystrophy), extensive tissue necrosis (emboli and infarction, neoplastic necrosis), postsurgical infection, osteomyelitis, encapsulated foreign bodies, leukemia, traumatic or neoplastic brain damage, severe dehydration, and pyrogen reactions.

Bacterial endocarditis is characterized by bacterial infection of one or more heart valves. Sources of bacteria may be other systemic infections such as abscesses, pyelonephritis, oral infections, perianal fistulas, cystitis, and prostatitis. Bacterial endocarditis should be considered as a possible diagnosis in all dogs with the following symptoms: (1) fever of unknown origin; (2) unexplained cardiac murmur; (3) lameness, usually shifting; (4) unexplained anemia; (5) embolic disease; (6) marked leukocytosis or monocytosis; and (7) myalgia, weight loss.

The mitral valves are most commonly involved, and a systolic murmur is most frequent. Diastolic murmurs indicate involvement of the aortic valve. Approximately 30 per cent of dogs with bacterial endocarditis will not have a fever, but the other signs may mimic autoimmune disease. Large male dogs and possibly the German Shepherd breed in particular appear to have a higher prevalence of bacterial endocarditis.

Diagnosis should be confirmed by blood cultures (see p. 500). The timing of blood cultures is important, as is obtaining more than one culture. In the dog, 90 per cent of bacterial isolates consist of beta streptococcus, coagulase positive staphylococci, or *Escherichia coli*.

Many of the forenamed entities are obscure conditions, but they may be the cause of a so-called fever of unknown origin. A fever of unknown origin (FUO) is defined as a temperature exceeding 39.5°C (103°F) of 2-weeks' duration and for which no established diagnosis can be made after 1 week of hospital investigation (Table 37).

Table 37. PROPOSED CLASSIFICATION OF FEVER OF
UNDETERMINED ORIGIN IN DOGS AND CATS

Infections
  I. Systemic
     A. Subacute bacterial endocarditis (SEB)/secondary septicemia
        1. Staphylococcus
        2. Streptococcus
        3. Enteric bacteria
        4. Unusual organism, i.e., Salmonella, Erythecia
     B. Early atypical manifestations of common systemic diseases
        1. Canine distemper with secondary immunosuppression
        2. Canine infectious hepatitis
        3. Feline panleukopenia
        4. Feline infectious peritonitis
        5. Feline upper respiratory disease complex
        6. Ectopic helminth migration
        7. Hemobartonellosis
     C. Miscellaneous less commonly diagnosed diseases
        1. Toxoplasmosis
        2. Brucellosis
        3. Leptospirosis
        4. Disseminated mycoses
        5. Rickettsia (ehrlichiosis)
        6. Babesiasis
 II. Localized
     A. Urogenital tract
        1. Pyelonephritis/perirenal abscess
        2. Prostatic abscess
        3. Endometritis/pyometra
        4. Atypical cystitis emphysematous)
     B. Liver
        1. Abscess
        2. Cholangitis
     C. Other organ systems
        1. Pancreatitis
        2. Pericarditis
        3. Meningitis
        4. Pulmonic abscess
        5. Polyarthritis
     D. Retroperitoneal, peritoneal, pleural infections
Neoplasms
     A. Lymphoma
     B. Leukemia
     C. Plasma cell myeloma
     D. Pancreatic carcinoma
     E. Retroperitoneal sarcoma
     F. Metastatic neoplasia (usually to liver)
     G. Intracranial tumors

Table continued on opposite page

Table 37. PROPOSED CLASSIFICATION OF FEVER OF
UNDETERMINED ORIGIN IN DOGS AND CATS *(Continued)*

Immune–Mediated Disease
  A. Systemic lupus erythematosus
  B. Rheumatoid arthritis
  C. Polyarteritis nodosa
  D. Autoimmune hemolytic anemia
  E. Immune-mediated thrombocytopenia
Miscellaneous
  A. Drug fever
    1. Sulfonamides
    2. Tetracyclines
    3. Penicillins
    4. Amphotericin B
    5. Novobiocin
    6. Quinidine
  B. Pulmonary emboli due to dirofilariasis, or other causes
  C. Hepatic cirrhosis/active hepatocellular necrosis
  D. Hyperthyroidism
  E. Undiagnosed

From Drazner, F.: Diagnostic approach to patients with prolonged febrile illness.
Compendium on Continuing Education—Small Animal, *1*:754, 1979.

In considering causes, geographic factors are important, because diseases
common in Africa, Asia, or certain regions of the United States would be
different from those seen in urban America. In man, infection causes 40 per
cent of FUOs, neoplastic disease 20 per cent, and collagen-vascular disease 15
per cent.

References and Additional Readings

Calvert, C. A.: Valvular bacterial endocarditis in the dog. J.A.V.M.A., *180*(9):1080, 1982.
Drazner, F. H.: Prolonged febrile illness. Compendium on Continuing Education, *1*:753,
  1979.
Greene, C. E.: Clinical Microbiology and Infectious Diseases of the Dog and Cat.
  Philadelphia, W. B. Saunders Company, 1984.
Greene, C. E.: Fever. Proc. Am. Anim. Hosp. Assoc., 49th meeting, pp. 111–113, 1982.

PAIN

Pain is a relatively localized sensation of discomfort, distress, or urgency, resulting from the stimulation of specialized nerve endings. In animals, pain is not a subjective manifestation, but rather a condition that can be measured only by the observer with the aid of signs evidenced by the animal. Important clues in recognizing the cause of pain are finding what precipitates the pain and what relieves it. In addition, the following considerations are very important.

Physiologic Considerations

Pain is one of the earliest signs of disease. The sensation of pain depends on receptors located in the skin and deeper structures. Adequate stimuli for visceral pain are different from those that cause cutaneous pain. The skin is sensitive to pricking, cutting, and burning, whereas visceral pain is caused by local trauma of an engorged or inflamed mucosa, distention or spasm of smooth muscle, and traction upon mesenteric attachments. Local ischemia and prolonged contraction of muscles may also be a cause of pain.

Physical Signs

Animals in pain may become listless, move constantly, continually get up and lie down, refuse to stay in one place, groan, and whimper. Some animals become phlegmatic when in pain; others have a stark or frightened expression, resent any handling or forced movement, and will "favor" the painful part (carrying an injured leg, holding the neck stiffly and moving the head as little as possible in a cervical disc protrusion, or keeping the abdominal musculature tensed when suffering from visceral pain). Acute abdominal pain may cause the animal to assume a "praying position"—the hind legs are normally upright while the patient lies down with the forequarters.

Tests and Diagnostic Considerations

Pain may not be noticed until some normal physiologic act is provoked. Thus, swallowing, coughing, chewing, defecating, or any bodily movement can induce pain. It should be determined whether the pain is associated with a normal physiologic act or seems to be constant, even in the absence of a provoking act. The mode of onset may be helpful in making a diagnosis. Sudden acute pain is usually associated with fractures, rupture, or torsion of hollow visceral organs, acute inflammation, or the sudden loss of blood from an organ. Male cryptorchid dogs may develop an intra-abdominal testicular torsion and severe sudden abdominal pain. Slowly developing pain is associated with osteoarthritis, slowly developing tumors, and chronic inflammation. In any given disease, as well as among different breeds of animals, there is a wide variation in tolerance and in response to pain. One should not judge the severity of a disease process by the pain response of the animal.

Palpation is an important procedure in trying to localize pain, but may be confusing, as when pain referred from a visceral injury simulates musculoskeletal injury over the lumbar area.

Pain is a way of following the course of a disease process, and its complete alleviation may not always be desirable. For example, alleviation of pain in osteochondritis dissecans would allow an animal full utilization of a diseased part that should ordinarily be kept inactive. However, pain that causes the animal to mutilate itself or to suffer great discomfort must be immediately ameliorated.

References and Additional Readings

Breazile, J. E., and Kitchell, R. L.: Pain perception in animals. Fed. Proc., 28:1379, 1969.

Harrison, T. R. (ed.): Principles of Internal Medicine, 10th ed. New York, Blakiston Division, McGraw-Hill, 1983.

Sodeman, W. A., Jr., and Sodeman, W.T. M.: Pathologic Physiology, 7th ed. Philadelphia, W. B. Saunders Company, 1984.

VISUAL LOSS

Impairment of vision in animals may be difficult to assess, especially if the visual loss involves only one eye. Assessment of visual function in animals depends mainly on objective signs. Interpretation of field defects or uniocular visual loss is difficult except for the very acute observer. Important considerations in assessing visual dysfunction are the following:

1. Observing the inequality of the animal's pupillary responses to direct and consensual light stimulation.

2. Finding the animal bumping into objects on one side.

3. Patching first one eye of the animal, then the other eye, and observing how the animal behaves.

4. Putting the affected animal through an obstacle course.

5. Establishing the presence of ocular pain in the animal—characterized by blepharospasm, photophobia, redness, and lacrimation.

The sudden loss of vision or marked visual impairment may involve one or both eyes. The following differential diagnosis should be considered:

1. Massive vitreous or retinal hemorrhages from any cause (no pain).

2. Bilateral optic neuritis or retrobulbar optic neuritis (painful).

3. Retinal detachment (no pain).

4. Severe anterior and/or posterior uveitis (painful).

5. Severe keratitis with blepharospasm (painful).

6. Acute congestive glaucoma (painful).

Other forms of ocular disease may predispose the animal to gradual loss or impairment of vision in one or both eyes. Included in these types of disease are (see also Fig. 9):

SUDDEN ACQUIRED BLINDNESS

Fundic Reflection → Present → Pupillary Response to Light → Hyporeflexic or Areflexic → Position of Iris → Mydriatic → Funduscopic Examination

1. ABSENT	2. NORMAL	3. MIOTIC	4. NORMAL	5. ABNORMAL
A. Abnormal opaque substance in aqueous or vitreous humor 1. Hemorrhage 2. Exudate B. Opacity of cornea 1. Edema C. Opacity of lens 1. Cataract D. Absence of pupil 1. Inflammation 2. Neoplasia	A. Lesions of lateral geniculate nucleus, optic radiations and occipital cortex 1. Trauma 2. Necrosis 3. Hydrocephalus 4. Toxicity 5. Infection 6. Mass 7. Degeneration 8. Biochemical	A. Iritis B. Cerebral edema	A. Lesions optic nerves, optic chiasm and optic tracts 1. Trauma 2. Mass 3. Infection 4. Degeneration 5. Inflammation B. Cortex and oculomotor nerve 1. Severe increased intracranial pressure	A. Papillitis 1. Optic nerve same as 4A B. Cupping of disc 1. Glaucoma C. Retinal detachment 1. Secondary to colobomas, ectasia 2. Trauma 3. Neovascularization 4. Inflammation 5. Infection 6. Toxicity 7. Idiopathic 8. Neoplasia

Figure 9. *Legend below.*

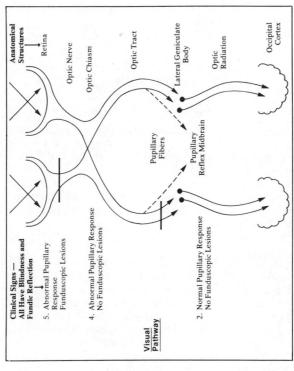

Figure 9. Algorithm for sudden acquired blindness. Developed by Gretchen Schmidt. (From Hoerlein, B. F.: Canine Neurology, 2nd ed. Philadelphia, W. B. Saunders Company, 1971.)

1. Various forms of keratitis.
2. Severe corneal dystrophies.
3. Marked corneal edema.
4. Opacification of the lens from any cause.
5. Uveal tract inflammation.·
6. Hemorrhage in the anterior chamber.
7. Developing glaucoma.
8. Opacities developing within the vitreous, including asteroid hyalosis and organized vitreal exudates.
9. Developing retinopathies, including inflammatory lesions and degenerative retinopathies.
10. Optic nerve atrophy.

POLYDIPSIA–POLYURIA

POLYDIPSIA

Fluid intake in animals is variable, depending on environment, type of food, water content of the feces, and other considerations. Water consumption of 100 ml per kg of body weight per day is considered as the upper limit of the normal range in the dog and cat.

Polydipsia refers to a condition of excessive thirst, especially one that persists for long periods of time. An average dog's total oral water input in approximately 50 ml per kg per day and an average cat's is 80 ml per kg per day; however, these figures are unreliable.

Physiologic Considerations

Water intake is controlled by the thirst center in the hypothalamus. Osmoreceptors, which are cells in the hypothalamus, are stimulated to initiate thirst and drinking by increases in the osmotic pressure of the body fluids. Decreases in extracellular fluid volume also stimulate thirst. Extracellular fluid osmoreceptors are regulated by fluid intake and urine production. Urine volume is determined largely by the action of antidiuretic hormone (ADH). Concentration of urine results from active transport of sodium mainly in the loop of Henle, and a concentration gradient is established in the medullary tissue as urine passes from the corticomedullary junction to the calyx.

Cat or dog owners who substitute dry products (8 per cent water) for moist foods (70 per cent water) may report physiologic thirst in their animals. Because a normal animal has a fairly constant water intake, it will drink more water if less is ingested in the food. This is particularly noticeable when animals have fasted. Most dogs drink a large share of their daily water ration shortly after eating; most cats drink very little water unless they are on a dry food diet.

Animals with excessive water loss will ingest more fluid to balance this loss. Conditions such as fever, diarrhea, vomiting, draining wounds, nervousness (diarrhea and panting), and urinary losses—namely, osmotic diuresis (diabetes mellitus, high-salt diet), lack of ADH (diabetes insipidus), or any renal damage that precludes water conservation—are of major concern.

Corticosteroids in high doses, gastritis, pharyngitis, ascites, toxemias (e.g., pyometra), and psychogenic water drinking are miscellaneous causes of polydipsia.

Physical Signs

The history of polydipsia is often vague. Animals drink from other sources (such as ponds, streams, or toilet bowls) in addition to their water bowls, so the owner's description of the problem may be incorrect. In the initial physical examination, attempt to determine the patient's state of hydration and whether there is an abnormal fluid loss or fluid consumption. The most accurate information is obtained by confining the animal and actually measuring its water consumption for several days.

Tests and Diagnostic Considerations

Because water intake and output are closely related, several days' data should be used in evaluating these parameters. Water measurements should be made with the patient in a metabolic cage; a few days of acclimation are desirable before the test period begins (see p. 812).

Serious polydipsia usually involves the urinary system, and examinations should emphasize kidney function tests (see p. 828).

POLYURIA

Polyuria is the passage of a greater than normal volume of urine during a given period of time. One can estimate an average dog's urine output to be 25 ml per kg per day and an average cat's to be 45 ml per kg per day. Urine production in the dog and cat should not exceed 50 ml per kg per day.

Urine volume ordinarily is influenced by water and nutritional intake, excretory load, and renal and hypothalamic regulation. The kidney performs the most critical regulation of urine volume; consequently, renal disease has a marked effect on urine volume.

The most spectacular urine volume changes, however, are mediated by ADH secretion. This hormone increases the permeability of the collecting tubules and allows reabsorption (and conservation) of water. ADH is stored in the posterior pituitary gland and released by neural control from the hypothalamus. Osmoreceptors in the hypothalamus are stimulated by increased plasma osmotic pressures to release ADH (see p. 655). (It is not known whether these are the same receptors that control thirst; however, much larger increases in plasma osmolality are needed to stimulate thirst.)

Lowered extracellular fluid volume also stimulates ADH release and water retention. This stimulus overrides the osmotic mechanism and is important as a possible cause of postsurgical retention and hyponatremia and as a cause of water (and salt) retention in congestive heart failure, cirrhosis of the liver, and nephrosis. Pain, trauma, emotions, and drugs (such as morphine and barbiturates) also cause ADH secretion. Cold and alcohol decrease ADH secretion.

Polyuria can be caused by factors that increase the water intake—such as gastritis, nervousness, and psychogenic water drinking. Most cases of polyuria reveal underlying renal or metabolic disease. Differential diagnosis of polydipsia-polyuria (PD-PU) should include renal disease, diabetes mellitus, liver disease, hyperthyroidism, hypercalcemia associated with pseudohyperparathyroidism, hyperadrenocorticism, abnormalities in ADH production (diabetes insipidus), excessive water consumption (psychogenic polydipsia), pyometra-endometritis complex, and high level administration of corticosteroids. (See Table 38 and Fig. 10.)

The history of polyuria often begins with the owner's recognition of nocturia or "accidental" urination in the house, resulting from the animal's need to urinate frequently. An appreciation of concomitant polydipsia may be an early sign of input-output abnormalities. The passage of a large volume of light-colored urine of low specific gravity is often present. Confirmation of PD-PU often depends on observing the patient's pattern of fluid intake and urine output under controlled conditions.

1. Observe the patient's pattern of fluid intake and urine output under controlled conditions.

2. Establish the existing urine specific gravity or osmolality, the urine tonicity, and the glucose level. For the initial evaluation of urine specific gravity, divide the causes of PD-PU into two groups: those with water diuresis and those with solute diuresis (Hardy).

Table 38. DIFFERENTIATING COMMON CAUSES OF POLYURIA

	Chronic Renal Disease	Diabetes Insipidus	Diabetes Mellitus	Excessive Water Consumption
Urine volume	Increased	Increased	Increased	Increased
Urine specific gravity	Decreased	Decreased	Variable (normal)	Decreased
Urine glucose	Negative	Negative	Positive	Negative
Blood urea nitrogen	Increased	Normal	Normal	Normal
Effect of water deprivation on specific gravity of urine	None	None	Increased	Increased
Effect of ADH on specific gravity of urine following water deprivation	None	Increased	—	—
Mechanism	Tubular damage / End organ resistance to ADH / Impaired conc. ability: Ca ↑ or K ↓	Decreased ADH secretion	Osmotic diuresis	Obsessive water drinking / Excessive adrenocorticosteroid hormone

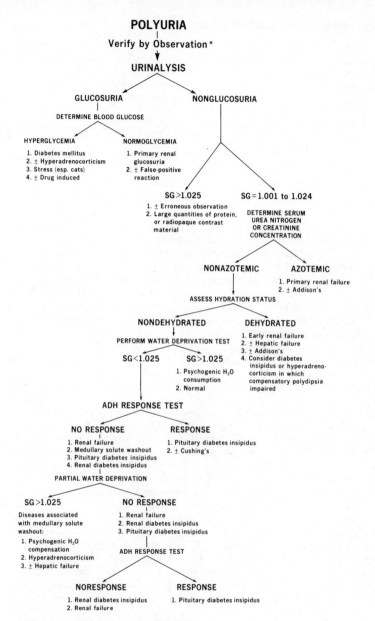

POLYURIA
Verify by Observation *
URINALYSIS

GLUCOSURIA

DETERMINE BLOOD GLUCOSE

HYPERGLYCEMIA
1. Diabetes mellitus
2. ± Hyperadrenocorticism
3. Stress (esp. cats)
4. ± Drug induced

NORMOGLYCEMIA
1. Primary renal glucosuria
2. ± False-positive reaction

NONGLUCOSURIA

SG >1.025
1. ± Erroneous observation
2. Large quantities of protein, or radiopaque contrast material

SG = 1.001 to 1.024

DETERMINE SERUM UREA NITROGEN OR CREATININE CONCENTRATION

NONAZOTEMIC

AZOTEMIC
1. Primary renal failure
2. ± Addison's

ASSESS HYDRATION STATUS

NONDEHYDRATED

PERFORM WATER DEPRIVATION TEST

SG <1.025

SG >1.025
1. Psychogenic H_2O consumption
2. Normal

DEHYDRATED
1. Early renal failure
2. ± Hepatic failure
3. ± Addison's
4. Consider diabetes insipidus or hyperadreno-corticism in which compensatory polydipsia impaired

ADH RESPONSE TEST

NO RESPONSE
1. Renal failure
2. Medullary solute washout
3. Pituitary diabetes insipidus
4. Renal diabetes insipidus

RESPONSE
1. Pituitary diabetes insipidus
2. ± Cushing's

PARTIAL WATER DEPRIVATION

SG >1.025
Diseases associated with medullary solute washout:
1. Psychogenic H_2O compensation
2. Hyperadrenocorticism
3. ± Hepatic failure

NO RESPONSE
1. Renal failure
2. Renal diabetes insipidus
3. Pituitary diabetes insipidus

ADH RESPONSE TEST

NORESPONSE
1. Renal diabetes insipidus
2. Renal failure

RESPONSE
1. Pituitary diabetes insipidus

* Measurement of 24 hour urine volume is recommended

Figure 10. Diagnostic algorithm for patients with polyuria. (From Hardy, R. M., and Osborne, C. A. *In* Kirk, R. W. (ed.): Current Veterinary Therapy VII. Philadelphia, W. B. Saunders Company, 1980, p. 1081.)

Water Diuresis	**Solute Diuresis**
Urine specific gravity = 1.001–1.007	Urine specific gravity = 1.008–1.024
Pituitary diabetes insipidus	Primary renal failure
Nephrogenic diabetes insipidus	Pyelonephritis
Psychogenic polydipsia	Diabetes mellitus
Pyometra	Renal glycosuria
Hepatic failure	Hepatic failure
Hyperadrenocorticism (solute	Hyperadrenocorticism
medullary washout)	Hypoadrenocorticism
	Hypercalcemia
	Hypokalemia
	Hyperthyroidism

3. If the urine is hypotonic, evaluate the patient's state of hydration and determine serum urea nitrogen and creatinine concentration. Animals that are dehydrated and have hypotonic urine should be carefully evaluated for primary renal disease. Obtain the following diagnostic information on polyuric patients prior to beginning water deprivation or vasopressin concentration tests: complete blood count (CBC), urinalysis, serum urea nitrogen, creatinine, potassium and calcium, total plasma protein, SGPT, and alkaline phosphatase. If the initial renal and liver screens are normal and the animal is not dehydrated, initiate a water dehydration test to detect the patient's concentrating ability.

4. If the patient is not markedly dehydrated and the urine is hypotonic, perform a water deprivation test, weigh the patient, and collect urine either by catch or catheterization. Fast the dog for 12 hours prior to testing, but provide water until the beginning of the test. At the start of the test, empty the bladder and obtain urine and plasma osmolality. Continue water deprivation until there is a decrease of no more than 5 per cent body weight or until the decrease in body weight reaches 3 per cent and there is a marked increase in urine osmolality or plateau of osmolality or even with less than 3 per cent body weight loss, urine osmolality reaches 1000 mOsm per kg. Obtain urine samples every 2 to 3 hours during the test. If total body weight is reduced by 3 to 5 per cent and urine osmolality is not above 300 mOsm per kg, begin a vasopressin response test (see p. 239) by administering 2 to 3 IU of lysine vasopressin subcutaneously (SC) and collecting urine 45 to 60 minutes later.

Extreme caution must be used when subjecting severely polyuric dogs to extended periods of water deprivation (longer than 12 hours). Dogs with pituitary diabetes insipidus, renal diabetes insipidus, or medullary solute washout can become clinically dehydrated very rapidly, so the water deprivation test should not exceed 12 hours. Re-evaluate urine specific gravity (and/or osmolality) and serum osmolality. Normal dogs with a slight degree of dehydration following water deprivation should have a urine specific gravity of at least 1.048, a Uosm of at least 1787 mOsm per kg, and a Uosm/Sosm ratio of at least 5.7 to 1. It is not necessary, however, to deprive dogs of water until the urine specific gravity reaches 1.048. When urine specific gravity reaches 1.025, this indicates renal concentrating ability; the test may then be terminated. Water deprivation can also be used in cats; however, cats appear to have the ability to concentrate urine in the range of 1.040 to 1.080 under normal conditions.

5. The results of a water deprivation test are not always clear-cut. If an animal cannot concentrate its urine to a level greater than 1.008 to 1.018, despite the fact that the animal becomes clinically dehydrated or its SUN elevates, this may indicate generalized renal disease or partial pituitary diabetes insipidus. If the patient's urine is persistently dilute (1.007–1.010) following water deprivation, the animal most likely has pituitary diabetes insipidus, renal diabetes insipidus, or severe renal medullary solute washout. A vasopressin concentration test should be done on these animals (see p. 240).

6. If spontaneous pituitary diabetes insipidus is present, a significant response to ADH should be evident. Hyposthenuric animals with no response to intravenous (IV) ADH have either renal diabetes insipidus or severe medullary washout. Animals having isosthenuric or mildly hypertonic urine and no response to ADH most likely have generalized renal disease.

7. Some dogs may have persistent hyposthenuria after both water deprivation and ADH administration. These animals may have renal diabetes insipidus; pituitary diabetes insipidus with severe medullary solute washout; or medullary solute washout associated with hyperadrenocorticism, hepatic failure, or primary polydipsia. Beginning a partial water deprivation test may allow these dogs to concentrate their urine. In this test, water is gradually reduced over 3 to 5 days by 10 per cent per day, while renal concentrating ability is monitored daily. Animals that have medullary solute washout at normal ADH production will gradually increase their urine concentration with restricted water consumption. Animals with renal diabetes insipidus have no response to gradual water restriction and may become rapidly dehydrated.

8. *Modified Water Deprivation Test.* This test is used to help establish a differential diagnosis between nephrogenic diabetes insipidus, psychogenic polydipsia, and PD-PU resulting from washout of Na^+ from the renal medullary interstitium.

Weigh the animal. Withhold food for at least 12 hours, but provide water ad libitum. Collect urine at 2- to 3-hour intervals, and empty the bladder at each collection, recording volume and urine osmolality. Remove the animal from all water intake. Collect urine until there is less than 5 per cent change in osmolality between two successive collections and the body weight has not decreased more than 3 per cent. When this plateau has been reached, obtain a blood sample and remove plasma for measurement of osmolality. Inject 3 to 5 units of lysine vasopressin SC. Obtain a final urine sample in 45 to 60 minutes. If an osmometer is not available, urine osmolality can be calculated from the urine specific gravity (using a refractometer) by multiplying the refractometer reading by 36—that is, if the specific gravity is 1.020, the urine osmolality is 20 × 36, or 720 mOsm per kg.

In central diabetes insipidus, dehydration develops rapidly over 4 to 6 hours. There is little change in urine osmolality associated with dehydration, and urine osmolality dramatically increases with ADH administration. In nephrogenic diabetes insipidus, initial Uosm may be between 200 and 600 mOsm; however, there is little change during dehydration, and little or no response to lysine vasopressin. In psychogenic polydipsia, during water deprivation, there is gradual restoration of ADH, a rise in urine osmolality (to 1000 mOsm over 12 to 16 hours), and usually no change in plasma osmolality. Once a plateau is reached, there is no response following lysine vasopressin administration.

9. *Additional Diagnostic Tests.* A complete urinalysis and blood chemistry profile are indicated. Important laboratory findings may include hyperglycemia; hypercalcemia; elevated T_3 or T_4; elevated blood cortisol, either baseline or in response to ACTH stimulation; azotemia, and an abnormal liver profile.

An interesting but not common cause of PD-PU is renal tubular acidosis in the dog. In this condition, PD-PU is present, as is hyperchloremic metabolic acidosis, with a normal anion gap; glucosuria, even though there is a normal blood glucose; hyposthenuria; normal glomerular filtration; and defective tubular transport of sodium, potassium, phosphate, urates, and multiple amino acids. The disease has been found in a variety of dog breeds but is inherited in a line of adult Basenji dogs and is compared to idiopathic adult Fanconi's syndrome in man.

In the distal tubular acidosis disease, the urine pH remains alkaline, despite the presence of metabolic acidosis, and the urine cannot be acidified by oral loading doses of ammonium chloride.

References and Additional Readings

Dibartola, S. P.: Renal tubular acidosis in a dog. J.A.V.M.A., *180*(1):70, 1982.

Graver, G. F.: Differential diagnosis of polyuric-polydipsic diseases. Compendium on Continuing Education, 3(12):1079, 1981.

Hardy, R. M.: Disorders of water metabolism. Vet. Clin. North Am., *12*(3):353, 1982.

Joles, J. A., and Mulnix, J. A.: Polyuria and polydipsia. *In* Kirk, R. W. (ed.): Current Veterinary Therapy VI. Philadelphia, W. B. Saunders Company, 1978.

ASCITES

Ascites is the abnormal accumulation of fluid within the peritoneal cavity. The fluid may be bile, chyle, urine or blood, or may be exudative or transudative in nature. It is a sign of disease, not a diagnosis.

Physiologic Considerations

Ascites is the result of two or more interacting forces—namely, portal hypertension, a lowered plasma colloid osmotic pressure, hypoalbuminemia, excessive sodium retention, and aldosteronemia.

Physical Signs

In most instances, the first recognizable sign of ascites is abdominal enlargement. On percussion, a fluid thrill can be felt. Movement of the animal may result in a change in position of the fluid and therefore a change in body contour. Considerable abdominal enlargement may go unnoticed for some time because of the insidious accumulation of fluid, which has not caused any discomfort to the animal. Localized pain, anorexia, depression, vomiting, and either diarrhea or constipation may become evident as the fluid mass begins to interfere with normal body function. A concomitant dyspnea may exist if the fluid exerts pressure on the diaphragm and leads to pleural effusion.

Inspection of the abdomen is an important part of every examination. In generalized ascites, the abdomen may be tensely distended, with tightly stretched skin, and the flanks may bulge. The venous channels on the ventral abdomen may become quite pronounced. Ballottement of the abdomen will reveal a fluid thrill. A fluid wave that changes in position as the animal moves is associated with accumulation of fluid in the peritoneal cavity. Small amounts of fluid accumulation may be very difficult to detect, especially in the obese animal. A carefully performed abdominal paracentesis is indicated as part of the routine examination in every patient with ascites (see p. 522). Dyspnea may be present if the fluid exerts pressure on the diaphragm. Concomitant signs of heart disease (see p. 335), liver disease (see p. 755), and anemia (see p. 677) may be present.

Besides ascites, other causes of abdominal distention can include obesity, neoplasia, pyometra, pregnancy, splenomegaly, gastric torsion, urethral obstruction with bladder enlargement, hyperadrenocorticism, and bowel distention.

Diagnosis and Tests

Right-sided congestive heart failure with resultant increased venous pressure is a common cause of massive liver congestion and ascites in the dog. Both primary liver disease, such as hepatitis, lymphosarcoma, and carcinoma, and secondary liver disease, such as cirrhosis secondary to the ingestion of liver toxins, can result in ascites; disturbances in hepatic venous circulation and a lowering of the plasma albumin level contribute to its development. Part of the transudate that characterizes the ascites of liver disease leaks into the peritoneal cavity from the splanchnic capillary bed and part weeps from the liver itself.

Hypoproteinemia with total serum albumin below 1.0 gm per dl may also result in ascites, but this situation is seen infrequently. Hypoalbuminemia is usually accompanied with expansion of plasma volume, reduction of glomerular filtration rate (GFR) and reduction in effective circulating blood volume; pooling of blood in the splanchnic circulation, along with portal hypertension, is also seen. Hypoproteinemia can be caused by liver disease, chronic fever, infection, parasitism, inadequate intake of protein, nephritis, and nephrosis. Obstructions

Table 39. ASCITIC FLUID COMPOSITION DEPENDING ON SITE OF
OBSTRUCTION AND
PLASMA PROTEIN CONCENTRATION

	Normal Plasma Protein	Hypopro-teinemia
Normal dog	Not present	Transudate*
Hepatic venousa hypertension (postsinusoidal)	Modified transudate	Transudate
Acute or uncomplicated portal venous obstruction (pre-sinusoidal)	Not present	Transudate
Abdominal neoplasia	Modified transudate†	Transudate
Hepatic arteriovenous fistulas; cirrhosis	Modified transudate or transudate	Transudate

Generalized edema is often present.

†Transudate if portal venous obstruction is present.

Modified from Greene, C. F.: Ascites: diagnostic and therapeutic considerations. Compendium on Continuing Education, *1*:712, 1979.

Table 40. COMMON CAUSES OF ABDOMINAL EFFUSION

Transudate
  Hypoproteinemia
    Intestinal malabsorption
    Intestinal protein loss
    Glomerular disease
  Lymphangiectasia
  Neoplasia
  Obstructing lymph drainage

Modified Transudate
  Congestive heart failure
  Portal venous obstruction
  Hepatopathies
    Postnecrotic cirrhosis
    Hepatoma
    Bile-duct carcinoma
  Abdominal neoplasia
    Obstructing lymphatics and
      blood vessels
    Carcinomas
    Sarcomas

Serosanguineous Exudate
  Feline infectious peritonitis
  Urine peritonitis
  Bile peritonitis
  Pancreatic peritonitis
  Gastric peritonitis
  Steatitis

Hepatopathies
  Chronic active hepatitis
Diaphragmatic hernia
Abdominal neoplasia
  Carcinoma
  Sarcoma
  Lymphosarcoma

Purulent Exudate
  Intestinal perforation
  Penetrating wounds
  Ruptured pyometra
  Ruptured abscess
  Extension of infection

Hemorrhagic Effusion
  Traumatic injury to major vessel, spleen, liver
  Neoplasm
    Hemangiosarcoma
    Vascular
  Bleeding disorders
    Warfarin toxicity
  Thrombocytopenia

Thrombosis
  Torsion
    Stomach
    Spleen
  Tumor eroding a vessel
    Pheochromocytoma

From Ettinger, S. J. (ed.): Textbook of Veterinary Internal Medicine, 2nd ed. Philadelphia, W. B. Saunders Company, 1983, p. 123.

to normal lymph flow or venous drainage, such as those produced by abdominal or thoracic tumors, can also result in ascites.

The radiographic signs of ascites are independent of the cause and include the following:

1. Overall abdominal haziness
2. Poor visualization of abdominal visceral silhouettes
3. Increased distance between segments of bowel loops
4. Floating of gas-containing bowel loops
5. Distention of abdominal wall

In many instances, the cause of ascites will be apparent. The characteristics of the ascitic fluid are very helpful in reaching a diagnosis (see Table 39). Exudates reveal that an inflammatory process such as peritonitis is responsible for the ascites. Feline infectious peritonitis frequently produces large quantities of ascitic fluid. Transudates indicate disease of the heart, liver, or other organ that interferes with normal circulatory or osmotic mechanisms in the body (see Table 40). Other tests that can be helpful in establishing a data base are total protein and A/G ratio, an abdominal radiograph, and an ECG.

References and Additional Readings

Ettinger, S. J.: Textbook of Veterinary Internal Medicine, 2nd ed. Philadelphia, W. B. Saunders Company, 1983.

Greene, C. E.: Ascites: diagnostic and therapeutic considerations. Compendium on Continuing Education, 1:712, 1979.

Sodeman, W. A., Jr., and Sodeman, T. M.: Pathologic Physiology, 7th ed. Philadelphia, W. B. Saunders Company, 1984.

Strombeck, D. R.: Small Animal Gastroenterology. Davis, California, Stonegate Publishing Company, 1979.

CONSTIPATION

Constipation can be defined as infrequent or difficult evacuation of the bowel. When constipation becomes so severe that no feces can be passed, obstipation has occurred. Constipation may be accompanied by rectal tenesmus and dyschezia. If megacolon has developed, straining and the urge to defecate are absent. In severe cases of constipation or obstipation, anorexia and retention toxemia can develop.

Physiologic Considerations

Colon function is regulated by the stomach through the gastrocolic reflex. Altered gastric motility can cause reflex inhibition of colonic motility.

Two principal forms of constipation are recognized: one form is caused by impaired motility of the colon; the second is due to rectal insensibility or a change in the natural mechanism involved in defecation. These two types may frequently be combined in the constipated animal. Diminished gastric and intestinal motility from many causes may lead to constipation.

Tests and Diagnosis

Constipation may result from the following conditions: a disturbance in the neural or vascular supply of the large bowel and colon, mechanical obstruction of the small intestine, fecal impaction, or the presence of painful anal lesions.

Constipation may be acute or chronic. The acute form is usually associated with fecal impactions resulting from the ingestion of excessive roughage in the diet, faulty bile production, or acute intestinal obstructions, as well as from pelvic and lumbar vertebral fractures. Protrusion or herniation of an intervertebral disc, with resulting paresis or paralysis, can produce constipation. Male cats with urethral blockage strain excessively to urinate and may appear to be constipated.

Chronic and progressive constipation may be associated with prostatic hypertrophy, perineal hernias, developing tumors in the large bowel and anus, megacolon (as in Hirschsprung's disease), large masses of internal parasites, abscessed anal sacs, or perianal fistulas; it also may be a sign of old age. Animals that are placed in strange surroundings such as veterinary hospitals or animals who do not get enough exercise may become constipated.

Diagnosis of the cause of constipation depends on results obtained from the history of the animal, palpation of the large intestine and colon, digital examination, barium enemas, and gastrointestinal x-rays of the upper tract.

Causes for Increased Diameter of Large Bowel*

Nutritional hyperparathyroidism
Megacolon (Hirschsprung's disease)
Pelvic or spinal trauma
Congenital spinal, rectal, or anal abnormality
Stricture of the rectum or lower colon
Severe, chronic abdominal inflammation
Severe canine histiocytic ulcerative colitis

References and Additional Readings

O'Brien, T. R.: Radiographic Diagnosis of Abdominal Disorders in the Dog and Cat. Philadelphia, W. B. Saunders Company, 1978.
Sodeman, W. A., Jr., and Sodeman, T. M.: Pathologic Physiology, 7th ed. Philadelphia, W. B. Saunders Company, 1984.

---

*Adapted from O'Brien, T. R.: Radiographic Diagnosis of Abdominal Disorders in the Dog and Cat. Philadelphia, W. B. Saunders Company, 1978.

DIARRHEA

Diarrhea refers to an alteration in the normal pattern of defecation resulting in the frequent passage of unformed stools. It should not be regarded in terms of a diagnosis but only as a sign of an underlying disease process (see Tables 41–43 and Fig. 11).

Physiologic Considerations

The consistency of the stool is determined largely by dietary intake, fluid intake, and fecal water content. In normal bowel movements, water content is 60 to 80 per cent. More than 98 per cent of all fluid entering the intestine is normally absorbed.

In diarrhea, there is often an increase in fecal fluid content that overwhelms the ability of the colon to absorb it. Causes of fluid overloading may be: (1) hypersecretion into the intestinal tract, (2) altered motility of the intestinal tract (hypomotility is usually a consequence of inflammation), (3) altered permeability of the intestinal tract, (4) malabsorption, including both structural and biochemical abnormalities, (5) altered osmotic constituents in the intestinal tract, and (6) altered bacterial flora.

Tests and Diagnostic Considerations

The initial step in the diagnosis of chronic or problem diarrhea in the dog is the anatomic localization of the lesion to large or small bowel, using the

Table 41. CLINICAL SIGNS ASSOCIATED WITH THE SITE OF ORIGIN OF CHRONIC DIARRHEA

| | Disease Involving | |
Clinical Signs	*Small Intestine*	*Large Intestine*
Appetite	May be ravenous or decreased	Usually normal
Weight loss	May be prominent	Minimal
Vomiting	Occasional to often	Occasional
Belching	Occasional	Rare
Flatulence	Common	Rare
Bloated abdomen	Common	Rare
Stool quantity	Large	Small
Number of stools per day	Near normal	Many
Tenesmus	Rare	Common
Gross examination of stool		
Blood	Dark, black	Fresh, red
Mucus	Absent	Present
Fat	May be present	Absent
Rectal examination	Normal	Blood, mucus, pain

From Zimmer, J. F.: Examination of the gastrointestinal system. Vet. Clin. North Am., *11*:569, 1981.

Table 42. DIFFERENTIAL DIAGNOSIS OF PANCREATIC
INSUFFICIENCY AND MALABSORPTION

Test	Normal Value	Pancreatic Insufficiency	Malabsorption Syndrome
Stool exam			
Fat droplets	2/3/LPF	Numerous of large size	Absent to fewer in number May be smaller in size Severe cases— numerous
Fatty acid crystals	Absent	Absent	May be present
Muscle fibers	Occasional	Numerous	Occasional
Starch granules	Absent to occasional	Numerous	Absent to occasional
Trypsin gel test	Liquefication of gelatin	Absent	Present
24-hour fat excretion	4–7 gm/24 hr	>7 gm, may be as high as 20–50 gm	>7 gm/24 hr
D-Xylose test	9–12 gm/5 hr in urine	Normal	Decreased in most cases (Tests jejunal function in man)
Glucose tolerance test	↑ blood glucose by 30–35 mg/100 ml (minimum)	Normal or diabetic response	Flat curve, false normals occur
Gross fat absorption	Gross lipemia 2 hr after feeding	Absent	Absent
^{131}I-Triolein	8–15% absorption (11%)	Low uptake	Low uptake
^{131}I-Oleic acid	10–15% absorption (13%)	Normal uptake	Low uptake
Intestinal biopsy	Normal histology	Normal	Clubbing and flattening of villi; thickening of mucosa, dilation of lymphatics

Courtesy of M. D. Lorenz, D.V.M.

Table 43. DETERMINATION OF DEPTH OF COLON LESIONS

	Mucosal	Transmural
Depth of lesion	Epithelium, colon glands, lamina propria, and muscularis mucosae	Lamina propria, submucosa and lymphatics, blood vessels, muscle layers, and subserosa
Lymph node involvement	None	Frequently affected
Proctoscopic appearance	Glistening surface, friable epithelium, and small ulcers with smooth edges. Colon distends evenly with air. No shortening or strictures evident.	Firm corrugated mucosal surface; deep or large rough-edged ulcers. May not distend easily with air. Strictures often present.
Barium enema	Serration and spiculation of profile. No strictures, fistulae, or shortening of colon.	Strictures, fistulae, and short-ended colon. Decrease in lumen diameter.
Direct smear of feces	Erythrocytes and often numerous leukocytes	Erythrocytes and rarely leukocytes
Response to treatment	Usually good	Poor—a stormy course is to be expected
Diseases	Trichuris colitis, amebic colitis, allergic colitis, and spastic colon syndrome	Granulomatous colitis, protothecal enterocolitis, lymphosarcoma, and adenocarcinoma

Courtesy of M. D. Lorenz, D.V.M.

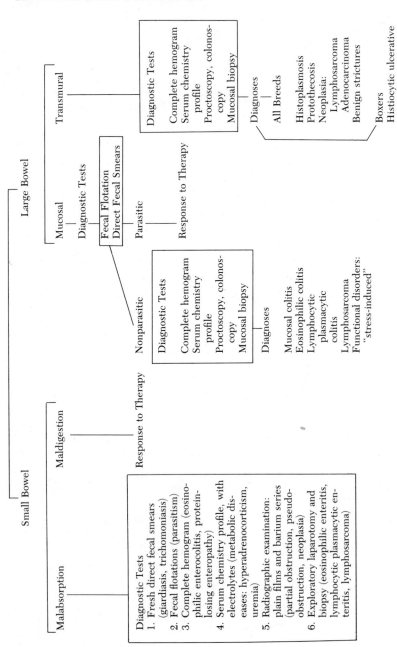

Figure 11. Chronic Diarrhea

history, physical examination, and stool characteristics (see p. 798 and Table 41). Diarrhea of large bowel origin, which has been estimated to comprise 50 per cent of the cases of chronic diarrhea in the dog, is caused by diseases of the cecum and ascending, transverse, or descending portions of the colon. Small bowel diarrhea is associated with diseases of the small intestines or the accessory digestive glands whose secretions function within the small intestinal lumen (pancreas—enzymes; liver—bile salts). This distinction is an important one, because it determines the direction of further work-up. Large bowel diseases are accessible to diagnosis by direct sampling of luminal examination (proctoscopy, colonoscopy), and biopsy through an endoscopic instrument without requiring surgical intervention. Diagnosis of small bowel disease requires studies into factors such as infection, parasitisms, and malabsorption (see p. 798).

There are four major mechanisms that can produce excess fecal water resulting in diarrhea:
1. Osmotic retention of water within the intestinal lumen.
2. Secretion of solute into the bowel lumen—inflammation.
3. Exudation of blood and tissue into the bowel.
4. Disordered motility of the bowel.

Osmotic diarrheas are common in animals that are garbage eaters and those that have had a sudden change in diet, eaten spoiled food, developed acute or chronic enteritis, had their absorptive villus surface damaged, or developed pancreatic exocrine insufficiency.

Secretory diarrheas are associated with acute enteritis such as *Escherichia coli* infections or campylobacter infections. Malabsorptive syndromes may also lead to secretory diarrheas. Exudative diarrheas are associated with intestinal inflammation resulting from parasitic infestation or bacterial inflammation.

The diagnosis of the cause of diarrhea depends on (1) careful history taking, which should include dietary history, appetite, duration of current illness, and previous illness, environmental changes, vaccination history, past treatment for diarrhea, and the daily number of bowel movements and (2) physical examination, which should include a careful examination of the feces in which consistency, color, odor, and the presence of blood or mucus are noted. An assessment of the animal's general health should be made, and the alimentary system should be carefully examined (see p. 319).

Diarrhea may be acute or chronic. Acute diarrhea is manifested by the appearance of a watery, sometimes bloody stool in an animal who has previously been healthy. Diarrhea accompanied by fever, depression, anorexia, increased peristalsis, or gastric pain suggests an inflammation of the gastrointestinal tract.

Etiologic factors of diarrhea can be divided into three groups:
1. Functional disorders—food or drug allergy, defective digestion, defective absorption, and psychogenic aspects.
2. Generalized or metabolic disease affecting the intestines secondarily—uremia, congestive heart failure, liver cirrhosis, hypoadrenocorticism, and heavy metal poisoning.
3. Intrinsic disease of the intestine—bacterial, fungal, protozoan, or metazoan parasites, and viral and nonspecific inflammatory disease.

Diarrhea may be caused by localized diseases of the intestinal tract such as bacterial (proteus, salmonella, campylobacter, staphylococcus) and viral infections (parvo, coronavirus, distemper, hepatitis) together with protozoan infections (coccidiosis, giardiasis, trichomoniasis, amebiasis) and spirochetal organisms (Borrelia and Spirillum species).

Parasites such as ascarids, hookworms, strongyloides, whipworms, and tapeworms and intestinal neoplasms and obstructive lesions such as incomplete intussusception may also produce diarrhea. It may be a manifestation of a generalized systemic disease such as hepatitis, distemper, leptospirosis, uremia, or poisoning. Diarrhea can be caused by specific inflammatory diseases such as eosinophilic enteritis and granulomatous colitis. Overeating, food allergies, ingestion of spoiled foods, and sudden dietary changes may produce diarrhea. Defective pancreatic secretions, uremia, chronic liver disease, abdominal neoplasia, and nervousness may produce chronic diarrhea.

INFECTIOUS DIARRHEAS

Evidence indicates that *Campylobacter fetus* subspecies *jejuni* is increasing as a source of infectious diarrhea in dogs and has public health significance for man. The incidence of campylobacter infection is higher in "pound"-obtained dogs and in dogs younger than 6 months old. Campylobacter enteritis is spread by the fecal and oral routes. Dogs may harbor more than one species of pathogenic campylobacter organisms.

When submitting fecal samples for campylobacter isolation, Cary-Blair transport medium can be used for *C. fetus* subspecies *jejuni* isolation or feces may be placed in semisolid Mueller Hinton broth. In both cases, the specimens should be kept chilled on ice. A stool sample that is kept in a tightly sealed plastic cup and chilled on ice to 4°C may yield campylobacter sp for up to 3 days.

Specialized bacteriologic media (Campy blood agar plate growth medium and Campy Pak* atmosphere envelope) or gaspak jars are needed. Most commercial laboratories doing bacteriologic work can attempt to isolate campylobacter sp.

Campy-BAP plates are placed in a 5 per cent oxygen atmosphere and incubated at 42 and 43°C and examined after 48 to 72 hours. Positive colonies are composed of gram-negative rods, and further biochemical testing is needed for positive identification.

Canine parvovirus (CPV) is a small DNA virus of the family parvoviridae. CPV infections are most frequently seen in puppies younger than 5 months of age. Many of the infections are asymptomatic. When severe clinical signs are evident, two forms of the disease are seen: enteritis and myocarditis. Enteritis is the most common form; however, it is often impossible to distinguish parvovirus infection from other clinical diseases causing gastroenteritis using only clinical signs.

---

*BBL Microbiology Systems, P.O. Box 243, Cockeysville, MD

In the enteric form, there is usually a history of depression and inappetence. Severe vomiting may develop as early as 2 days before the onset of diarrhea. Diarrhea is of variable severity and contains blood in about 50 per cent of the cases. The animal may be acutely febrile, with temperatures ranging from 104° to 106°F. Leukopenia is observed in about one third of the cases and is characterized by lymphopenia, neutropenia, degenerative left shift, and toxic neutrophils. The more severe the leukopenia, the poorer the prognosis. Rapid dehydration and debilitation may develop, and peracute death may appear, especially in young puppies. CPV has an affinity for rapidly dividing cells such as the crypt cells in the intestinal mucosa.

(Acute parvoviral myocarditis has been reported only in puppies younger than 12 weeks of age. Affected puppies die acutely and may only exhibit signs of dyspnea, crying, and retching. Mortality may be as high as 50 per cent. Parvoviral myocarditis usually occurs without concurrent enteritis.)

Parvovirus antibody is transmitted to puppies from their dams through the placenta and colostrum. This passively acquired antibody is lost with a half-life of approximately 9 days. Effective maternal immunity may last 16 weeks, however. Puppies vaccinated while sufficient maternal antibody persists will produce no active reaction from the vaccination.

Feces of infected dogs are an important source of virus and may excrete as much as one billion infectious virions per gram of stool on the fifth or sixth day after oral exposure. Virus cannot be recovered in tissue culture from feces collected 2 weeks following oral exposure (5 to 8 days after clinical signs). Dogs recovered from infection for 3 weeks or more were not contagious to other dogs. Recovered dogs may retain very high antibody titers and remain immune throughout life.

The clinical signs of canine coronavirus can be confused with CPV. Acute diarrhea is also evident in coronavirus infection, as is lethargy and anorexia. The feces often have an orange color. Affected dogs are usually afebrile and become rapidly debilitated. Unlike parvovirus infection, there is usually no change in white blood cell (WBC) count. The disease runs an untreated course of 7 to 10 days, and the mortality is low. Coronavirus reproduces in and destroys villus absorptive cells, causing villus atrophy and resultant malabsorption of ingesta. Normal intestinal function is resumed as villae resume their normal function.

Colostral transfer of maternally derived antibody to parvovirus accounts for 90 per cent of the levels in puppies and the half-life is 9.7 days. Puppies with hemagglutination-inhibition titers greater than or equal to 1:80 are immune to oronasal challenge with virulent CPV. The outcome of vaccination with CPV prior to 16 weeks of age may be questionable because of maternally derived immunoglobulins.

CANINE VIRAL ENTERITIS SCREENING TESTS

Canine Parvovirus Hemagglutination Test (CPV-HA)

This is the test of choice to confirm acute CPV infection. CPV-HA titers of 1:10 or less indicate that CPV is not currently being shed in the feces. Titers of 1:10 to 1:80 are nonspecific. Titers of 1:80 or greater demonstrate that CPV is present in the feces. The patient is typically symptomatic and contagious at this time. Fresh stool should be used for the CPV-HA test.

Canine Parvovirus Serologic Antibody Titer Test (CPV-IFA)

The CPV-IFA test is an indirect immunofluorescent procedure to detect the presence of circulating antibodies to canine parvovirus. (The test does not measure the presence of antigen or virus.) It is the test of choice when the immune status of the patient to CPV is desired. Paired serum samples are necessary to demonstrate a stable or nonrising titer over a 3- to 4-week period, indicating previous exposure and immunity to subsequent reinfection. Titers range from 1:25 to 1:10,000. The higher titers indicate severity or length of infection. The CPV-IFA test is considered an excellent adjunct procedure when the results are interpreted in conjunction with the patient's history and clinical findings.

Canine Coronavirus Serologic Antibody Titer Test (CCV-IFA)

This test is identical to the CPV-IFA test in indication, technique, and submission. However, interpretation differs in that the titers tend to be lower, ranging from 1:25 to 1:400, because the disease tends to be more mild than CPV.

MALABSORPTION SYNDROMES AS CAUSES OF CHRONIC DIARRHEAS

The term *maldigestion* should be distinguished from *malabsorption,* although in both cases the affected animal may develop osmotic diarrhea with loss of electrolytes and nutrients and/or wasting disease. Maldigestion refers to abnormalities in the secretion of digestive enzymes, bile, or other gastrointestinal products contributing to the breakdown of nutrients. The most common disease in this category is pancreatic insufficiency.

Malabsorption is any disorder of the small intestine in which dietary nutrients are not absorbed following digestion.

In both cases, chronic diarrhea with increased fecal volume (see p. 801) and increased fecal fat (see p. 803) are present. Inadequate absorption of calories results in weight loss, loss of fluids in dehydration, and loss of nutrients in dry, brittle hair coat, general unthriftiness, hypoproteinemia, and anemia.

In chronic diarrhea states, if nutrients are being broken down adequately yet diarrhea persists and hypoproteinemia is evident, a protein-losing enteropathy may be present (see p. 255).

Causes of Maldigestion

1. Pancreatic exocrine insufficiency: acquired, juvenile pancreatic atrophy, and iatrogenic
2. Biliary obstruction

3. Gastric disease
4. Bacterial overgrowth intestinal tract

Causes of Intestinal Malabsorption

1. Lymphangiectasia
2. Villous atrophy
3. Chronic inflammatory bowel disease: eosinophilic gastroenteritis, lymphocytic—plasmacytic enteritis, histoplasmosis, and salmonellosis
4. Acute inflammatory bowel disease with chronic structural changes: parvoviral enteritis and coronaviral enteritis
5. Lymphosarcoma
6. Lactase deficiency

Protein–Losing Enteropathies—Etiology

1. Inflammatory disease of the gastrointestinal tract—structural damage: acute bacterial infections, parasitic, chronic regional enteritis, gastrointestinal ulceration (carcinoma, lymphosarcoma, parasitic), and histoplasmosis
2. Circulatory diseases: lymphangiectasia; lymphosarcoma, and congestive heart disease
3. Immune-mediated diseases: eosinophilic enteritis, gluten enteropathy, and food allergy

Animals presented with chronic diarrheas, loss of weight, hypoalbuminemia, and hypoglobulinemia should be suspected of having a protein-losing gastroenteropathy. Both albumin and globulin will be lost at equal rates. The kidneys must be evaluated to ensure that protein loss is not associated with a glomerulopathy, and liver function tests will indicate that albumin is being produced normally. Differential laboratory tests, namely, D-xylose absorption (see p. 804) and fat absorption (see p. 803), should be done. Endoscopy and intestinal biopsy can be helpful in confirming the diagnosis.

Diagnostic aids may include fecal examination for parasites (see p. 798), wet smears of the feces to look for protozoa, spirochetes, and undigested food particles, fecal cultures (see p. 499), enzyme function tests (see p. 801), fat and glucose absorption tests (see p. 803), radiologic examinations (see p. 567), hematology and blood chemistries (see pp.671 and 737), liver function tests (see p. 755), proctoscopy (see p. 561), and exploratory laparotomy.

Diseases of the large bowel are common causes of chronic diarrhea in the dog. Tenesmus and urgency—with passage of frequent, small volumes of bloody, mucoid feces—are characteristic signs of large bowel diarrhea. The diagnosis of large bowel diarrhea includes (1) fecal examinations, including flotations, saline smears, and cytology; (2) colonoscopy combined with colon biopsy; (3) barium enema radiography; and (4) microbiologic-serologic testing. The results of these tests are used to differentiate (1) parasitic colitis (whipworms, hookworms, and protozoa); (2) chronic colitis (idiopathic histiocytic and eosinophilic); (3) infectious colitis (bacterial, histoplasmosis, and protothecosis); (4) colonic tumors and polyps; (5) cecal inversion; and (6) functional diarrhea.

References and Additional Readings

Anderson, N. V.: Veterinary Gastroenterology. Philadelphia, Lea & Febiger, 1980.

Burns, M. G.: Intestinal lymphangiectasia. J.A.A.H.A., 18(1):97, 1982.

Burrows, C. F.: The assessment of canine gastrointestinal function. 31st Gaines Symposium Proceedings, 1981, pp. 1–8.

Burrows, C. F.: Chronic diarrhea in the dog. Vet. Clin. North Am., 13(3): 521, 1983.

Dillon, A. R., and Wilt, G. R.: Campylobacter species in dog and cat. Vet. Clin. North Am., 13(3): 647, 1983.

Fox, J. G., Moore, R., and Ackerman, J. I.: *Campylobacter jejuni*-associated diarrhea in dogs. J.A.V.M.A., 183(12): 1430, 1983.

Hayden, D. W., and VanKruiningen, H. J.: Lymphocytic-plasmacytic enteritis in German Shepard dogs. J.A.A.H.A., 18(1): 89, 1982.

Johnson, G. F.: Gastrointestinal fiberoptic endoscopy in small animal medicine. 28th Gaines Veterinary Symposium, 1978, pp. 27–31.

Jones, B. D.: Medical problem of small intestinal diarrhea. Proc. A.A.H.A., pp. 207–222, 1983.

Lorenz, M. D.: A diagnostic approach to chronic diarrhea. In Kirk, R. W. (ed.): Current Veterinary Therapy VI. Philadelphia, W. B. Saunders Company, 1977.

O'Brien, T.: Radiographic Diagnosis of Abdominal Disorders in the Dog and Cat. Philadelphia, W. B. Saunders Company, 1979.

Pollack, R. V. H., and Carmichael, L. E.: Canine viral enteritis. Vet. Clin. North Am., 13(3): 551, 1980.

Sherding, R. G.: Canine large bowel diarrhea. Compendium on Continuing Education, 2:279, 1980.

Strombeck, D. R.: Small Animal Gastroenterology, Davis, California, Stonegate Publishing Company, 1979.

Zimmer, J. F.: Gastrointestinal fiberoptic endoscopy. In Kirk, R. W. (ed.): Current Veterinary Therapy VII. Philadelphia, W. B. Saunders Company, 1980, pp. 954–961.

DYSPHAGIA

Dysphagia refers to difficulty in swallowing; it may be associated with localized diseases of the oropharynx or with central nervous system (CNS) disease. Disorders of swallowing can produce a variety of clinical signs, including anorexia, oral and nasal regurgitation, hypersalivation, coughing, dyspnea, inhalation pneumonia, and malnutrition.

Physiologic Considerations

Cranial nerves IX, X, and XI (the glossopharyngeal, vagus, and accessory) are associated with the normal swallowing reflexes and have their origin within the nucleus ambiguus of the medulla.

The clinical signs frequently associated with dysphagia are the drooling of saliva, choking, gagging, nasal discharge caused by the regurgitation of food through the nares, cough associated with food blocking the trachea, and possible aspiration pneumonia.

Swallowing is a complex, neuromuscular function that is initiated by voluntary action and becomes involuntary. Cranial nerves V, IX, X, XI, and XII supply motor impulses necessary for normal swallowing.

Tests and Diagnostic Considerations

Dysphagia associated with motility disturbances may be accompanied by neurologic, muscular or neuromuscular disease. Disorders of the pharyngeal area can result in dysphagia. In addition to complete visual inspection of the mouth and anterior pharyngeal area, radiographic examination using both flat plates and barium swallows are indicated. Radiographic signs of pharyngeal disorders are characterized by change in the size or shape of the anatomic area of the pharynx, displacement of the larynx, and altered radiographic contrast of the pharynx. Changes in size of the pharynx characterized by decreased size can be associated with inflammation, neoplasia, laryngeal edema, and elongation of the soft palate. Increased size of the pharynx can be seen with cricopharyngeal dysphagia, neurologic disorders of the pharyngeal musculature, chronic respiratory disease, megaesophagus, and interruption of the hyoid apparatus.

Foreign bodies such as bones, needles, and woodchips may lodge in the posterior nasopharynx or oropharynx. The major lymph node in the pharyngeal region of the dog is the medial retropharyngeal node, which drains the deeper structures of the head, larynx, and esophagus. Enlargement of this lymph node can result in displacement of the larynx and pharyngeal area, evident radiographically. Neoplasms of the pharyngeal area can be squamous cell carcinoma, lymphosarcoma, thyroid carcinoma, and squamous cell carcinoma of the tonsils. Traumatic injury to the pharyngeal area may lead to dysphagia; the hyoid apparatus should be carefully evaluated radiographically. Accurate localization of swallowing problems usually require specialized contrast studies using video fluorography to visualize the swallowing process.

Oral dysphagias may be associated with hypoglossal nerve dysfunction and loss of normal tongue mobility. Animals that cannot manipulate the tongue cannot grasp food or drink liquids in a normal manner. They may place the head deeply into the bowl of liquid, throw the head back to swallow, lose food and fluid from the mouth, and chew and salivate excessively. They cannot normally lick their nose.

Pharyngeal dysphagias are associated with weakened pharyngeal contracture. Food material is retained in the pharynx and may be regurgitated through the nose. These disorders can resemble cricopharyngeal sphincter disease; however, swallowing of liquids and soft foods can eventually take place with much effort.

CNS lesions can be associated with dysphagia. Lesions of the rostral two thirds of the nucleus ambiguus or the somatic visceral efferent axons in the glossopharyngeal and vagal nerves can cause difficulty in swallowing. In considering the diseases that may affect the CNS, refer to the following differential diagnosis:

1. *Botulism.* Rarely seen in small animals, this disorder affects all neuromuscular junctions.

2. *Myasthenia gravis.* In this disease, there is episodic weakness associated with exercise and physical exertion. Clinical signs are weakness in all four limbs, collapse, dysphagia, regurgitation, and dilated esophagus (see p. 262).
3. *Rabies* should always be considered when an animal shows dysphagia and paralysis of the muscles of mastication, with a characteristic dropped jaw.
4. *CNS neoplasms involving the brain stem* can lead to abnormalities of nerves V, VII, VIII, IX, X, and XI.
5. *Traumatic injuries to the pharyngeal area* could produce fracture of the hyoid bone and injury to the hypoglossal nerve.
6. *Chronic polyneuritis and damage to vagal nerves during the course of intervertebral disk surgery* can lead to laryngeal paresis, paralysis, and esophageal dysfunction with regurgitation.

Cricopharyngeal dysphagia refers to an inability to open (achalasia) or failure to coordinate the opening and closure of the cricopharyngeal passageway or failure of the passageway to close (chalasia). Cricopharyngeal achalasia is observed in the dog, and there may be pharyngeal muscle hyperplasia, inflammation, or atrophy. Young dogs are frequently affected and have the following symptoms: nasal reflux, coughing, pneumonia, loss of weight, and debilitation.

Severe inflammation of the pharyngeal area, including the palate, pharynx, and tonsils can cause difficulty in swallowing. Cats with upper respiratory diseases associated with herpesvirus, picorna virus, or calice virus frequently have a pharyngitis and ulcerative glossitis producing difficulty in swallowing. Marked inflammation of the oral mucosa in dogs can be associated with embedded foreign bodies, epithelial erosions associated with infection of bacterial or fungal organisms, and epithelial disease that may be associated with bullous pemphigoid.

References and Additional Readings

Hoffer, R. E.: Diseases of the esophagus. *In* Kirk, R. W. (ed.): Current Veterinary Therapy VI. Philadelphia, W. B. Saunders Company, 1977.

Ridgway, R. L., and Suter, P. F.: Clinical radiographic signs in primary and metastatic esophageal neoplasms of the dog. J.A.V.M.A., *174*:700, 1979.

Shelton, G. D.: Swallowing disorders in the dog. Compendium on Continuing Education, *4*(7):607, 1982.

Strombeck, D. R.: Small Animal Gastroenterology. Davis, California, Stonegate Publishing Co., 1979.

Suter, P. F., and Watrous, B. J.: Oropharyngeal dysphagias in the dog. A cinefluorographic analysis of experimentally induced and spontaneously occurring swallowing disorders. Vet. Radiol., *21*:24, 1980.

Watrous, B. J.: Clinical presentation and diagnosis of dysphagia. Vet. Clin. North Am., *13*(3): 437, 1983.

VOMITING

Vomiting is a coordinated visceral and somatic muscular reflex controlled by a vomiting center in the medulla. It starts with salivation and nausea, followed by repeated swallowing movements that lead to relaxation of the gastroesophageal sphincter. The glottis closes, the patient holds his breath (ribs fixed), the abdominal muscles contract (to raise intra-abdominal pressure), the cardia relaxes, and the gastric contents are ejected. Dogs may initiate this reflex easily.

Projectile vomiting is the violent ejection of stomach contents without nausea or retching.

Regurgitation is the expulsion from the esophagus of undigested food. It is caused by esophageal (and sometimes gastric) action without retching and forceful contraction of the abdominal muscles.

Gagging, or a "reverse sneeze," is often mistaken by owners for vomiting, because a small amount of mucus is expelled.

Physiologic Considerations

Although the central vomiting center initiates vomiting, it must first be stimulated. Even when it is drug induced, this stimulation is not accomplished directly, but by stimulation of a medullary chemoreceptor trigger zone that forwards impulses to the vomiting center; vomiting can occur only if the center is intact. Emetic impulses can be mediated by many sensory nerves; therefore, intense pain (especially abdominal), nervous (psychic) stimuli, disagreeable odors, tastes, and smells, sensations from the labyrinth and pharyngeal areas, toxins, drugs, and presumably metabolic retention products can all initiate vomiting. Numerous receptors for vomiting are located in the abdominal viscera, especially the duodenum. Afferent nerve fibers are found in the vagal and sympathetic nerves.

The reasons for projectile vomiting are unknown. It is seen with increased intracranial pressure and high intestinal obstructions or foreign bodies.

The physical appearance of the vomitus and the time it occurs in relationship to the ingestion of food can be helpful in formulating a differential diagnosis. Material vomited from the stomach usually contains a frothy fluid and partially digested food. Material vomited from the intestinal tract is bile stained with digested or putrefied food material. Mechanical or functional bowel obstruction can lead to protracted vomiting. The higher the obstruction, the more profuse the vomiting and the more undigested the food material.

Vomiting is very debilitating. When excessive, it causes severe extracellular fluid deficits, particularly of sodium, potassium and chloride ions, and water. Loss of mainly gastric contents results in loss of hydrochloric acid, a high serum bicarbonate concentration, and metabolic alkalosis. Vomiting of material from the high intestinal tract (duodenum) contains large amounts of bicarbonate, resulting in metabolic acidosis.

Classifying the causes of vomiting is difficult, and this abbreviated list only serves to emphasize the complexity of this sign of disease. In the initial evaluation of the vomiting animal, it is important to:

1. Determine whether the vomiting is acute or chronic.
2. If acute, determine whether there is evidence of shock, acute abdominal pain, convulsions, severe electrolyte and fluid abnormalities, elevated temperature, or life-threatening physiological imbalances that require an immediate work-up and treatment.

determine whether the etiology of the vomiting can be placed in the *primary* category, caused by a gastrointestinal disease, or in the *secondary* category, caused by metabolic disease.

Causes

Causes of vomiting may include the following:

1. Infectious disease—panleukopenia, hepatitis, parvovirus, and distemper.
2. Acute abdomen—acute pancreatitis, peritonitis (from myriad causes), intestinal obstruction, penetrating wounds and ruptured visceral organs (see pp. 10–15), toxic ingestion, and neoplastic disease.
3. Indigestion—chronic pancreatitis, overeating, spoiled foods, poisons, and esophageal or gastrointestinal deformities.
4. Metabolic disorders—acidosis, alkalosis, uremia and hypoadrenocorticism, and hepatic disease.
5. Drugs—digitalis, morphine, xanthines, and certain antibiotics.
6. Neurologic problems—motion sickness, cranial and vestibular lesions, and nervousness (see p. 422).
7. Pharyngeal or laryngeal irritations caused by enlarged tonsils or, in cats, by a piece of string with one end caught around the base of the tongue and the other end in the esophagus, stomach, or small intestine.

Diseases That Often Cause Persistent Vomiting

1. Esophageal origin: (a) cricopharyngeal achalasia; (b) persistent vascular ring around the esophagus (ligamentum arteriosum or left subclavian artery); (c) esophageal achalasia, megaesophagus, and aperistalsis; (d) foreign body obstruction; (3) congenital or traumatic stenosis; (f) diverticula; and (g) hiatus hernia.
2. Gastric origin: (a) pyloric stenosis; (b) pylorospasm; (c) achlorhydria; (d) inflammation; (e) foreign body; (f) tumor; and (g) ulcer.
3. Intestinal origin: (a) obstruction—foreign body, tumor, intussusception, and adhesions; (b) inflammation; and (c) neoplasia—adenocarcinoma, leiomyoma, lymphosarcoma, and pancreatic carcinoma.
4. Visceral diseases: (a) peritonitis; (b) inflammation of the pancreas, liver, and biliary system; (c) distention of the uterus; and (d) ulcer, tumors of the bowel.
5. Miscellaneous causes: (a) systemic disorders such as uremia; (b) endocrine disorders—hypoadrenal; (c) CNS disorders; (d) drugs and toxic agents; and (e) psychogenic causes.

Physical Signs

Nausea in dogs and cats is evidenced by frequent swallowing and licking of the lips, as well as by restlessness, salivation, and a worried expression. A few spasmodic contractions of the abdomen usually precede the actual vomiting. Some animals vomit quickly without much apparent nausea. A large quantity of vomitus may be presented first, with smaller amounts at subsequent episodes. After much vomiting by the animal, reverse peristalsis will have delivered intestinal fluids into the stomach, and the vomitus may be stained with bile.

Tests and Diagnostic Considerations

The character of the vomitus and its relationship to the time of feeding may be important. A large quantity of partially digested vomitus suggests obstruction of the pylorus. Much blood suggests a tumor or ulcer (rare in dogs), and a few streaks of blood are not significant. A highly acid pH indicates that gastric juice is present; whereas, a less acid or alkaline reaction suggests that the food may have remained in the esophagus. In general, the longer the interval between feeding and vomiting, the lower the lesion is located in the gastrointestinal tract. Vomiting immediately after swallowing usually implicates the esophagus; vomiting shortly after eating (30 to 60 minutes) usually implicates the stomach; and vomiting 3 to 4 hours after eating usually implicates the ileum. Colonic lesions rarely cause vomiting. Vomiting unrelated to feeding may be associated with toxic, systemic, metabolic, or neurologic lesions.

Functional lesions tend to produce intermittent vomiting; organic lesions cause constant signs.

Radiographic examinations, usually with contrast media (air or barium), are often key procedures in a differential diagnosis (see p. 564).

Diet and eating habits are important, because changes in foods, hot or cold food, spoiled food (garbage), overeating, and allergic tendencies all may produce vomiting.

Diarrhea as a concurrent sign implies a more generalized gastrointestinal involvement, such as infection (parvovirus; see pp. 252–253).

Involvement of other systems may indicate that the vomiting is secondary to metabolic causes, infections, or neurologic diseases.

Gastroscopic examination and exploratory surgery are often helpful in difficult cases.

References and Additional Readings

Ettinger, S. J.: Textbook of Veterinary Internal Medicine, 2nd ed. Philadelphia, W. B. Saunders Company, 1983.

O'Brien, T.: Radiographic Diagnosis of Abdominal Disorders in the Dog and Cat. Philadelphia, W. B. Saunders Company, 1978.

Schaer, M.: A general diagnostic approach to vomiting in the cat. Proc. A.A.H.A., 48th meeting, pp. 127–133, 1981.

Strombeck, D. R.: Small Animal Gastroenterology. Davis, California, Stonegate Publishing Co., 1979.

Thayer, G. W.: Vomiting: a clinical approach. Compendium on Continuing Education, 3(6):522, 1981.

Twedt, D. C.: Differential diagnosis and therapy of vomiting. Vet. Clin. North Am. 13(3):503, 1983.

HEMATEMESIS

Hematemesis is the vomiting of blood. Frank blood is usually associated with acute lesions in the esophagus or mouth. Blood that has remained in the stomach for any appreciable time is presented as brownish-black flakes resembling coffee grounds.

Causes

Lacerations of the mucosa from foreign objects; erosion of neoplasms; ulcers caused by uremia; stress; chronic histamine produced by mastocytomas; and drugs such as aspirin, arsenicals, and corticosteroids may be common causes of bloody vomiting.

Tests and Diagnostic Considerations

The patient's history of chewing on foreign objects or of being exposed to poisons or drugs should be followed by a careful inspection of the mouth and throat. Endoscopic evaluation of the esophagus and stomach is now readily performed. If these steps are not diagnostic, radiographs of these organs and biopsy of tissue masses are usually necessary.

REGURGITATION

Regurgitation refers to the bringing up of undigested food and should be distinguished from the act of vomition, which is the forcible expulsion of contents of the stomach through the mouth. Regurgitation usually reflects a disorder of the esophagus or stomach.

Physiologic Considerations

In the dog, the esophagus is a musculomembranous tube that extends from the level of the second cervical to the eleventh thoracic segment (see p. 329). The muscular coat of the esophagus in the dog has two oblique layers of striated muscle. In the cat, there is striated muscle in the anterior two thirds, with smooth muscle in the distal third. The esophagus cannot be identified on plain film radiographic examination, because it is normally collapsed except during the swallowing process. Disorders of the esophagus resulting in regurgitation are considered to be intraluminal, intramural, or periesophageal.

Signs of regurgitation associated with esophageal disease are regurgitation through the mouth or nares, dysphagia, repeated swallowing movements, increased salivation, drooling, dyspnea, moist cough (inhalation pneumonia), weight loss, tonsillitis, halitosis, and persistent nasal discharge.

Tests and Diagnostic Considerations

Persistent regurgitation in the dog and cat is an indication for careful evaluation of the pharynx and esophagus. Persistent regurgitation causes undigested or partially digested food to be expelled, usually immediately or very soon after eating. The act of regurgitation does not involve the forcible expulsive events present in vomiting. Persistent regurgitation can be associated with the following: cricopharyngeal achalasia, esophageal foreign body, esophageal stenosis, esophagitis, reflux esophagitis, hiatal hernias, esophageal neoplasms, vascular ring anomaly, megaesophagus, esophageal diverticulum, gastroesophageal herniation, peritoneopericardial diaphragmatic hernia, pyloric stenosis, and spasm.

Routine laboratory screens should include a blood chemistry profile (see pp.671 and 737), complete blood count (CBC), BUN, and fecal, for parasite check. Radiologic procedures should include survey thoracic films to look for megaesophagus, radiopaque esophageal foreign bodies, vascular rings, and diverticula. Thoracic films following positive contrast studies should be examined. Endoscopy may be extremely helpful in visualizing strictures, foreign bodies, neoplasms, or esophagitis.

References and Additional Readings

Jones, B. D.: Medical aspects of esophageal disease—regurgitation. 50th Proc. A.A.H.A., pp. 193–198, 1983.

MELENA

Melena is the passage of dark, pitchy, and lumpy stools stained with blood pigments or altered blood. This color of dog and cat feces varies greatly, depending on the diet. Because of high meat diets, the tests for occult blood may be mildly positive. Extra bile pigments in the stool may also cause a change in its color. This may occur in diarrhea, in the newborn receiving milk, or when bacterial action is suppressed.

In most cases of melena, the blood comes from the upper gastrointestinal tract, and the color change is a result of action by the digestive juices on blood.

When lost from the colon and rectum, blood is fresh, bright red, and accompanied by clotted masses (hematochezia). This or the production of fecal discoloration from excess bile is not melena.

Cause

Melena may result from chronic rather than continuous bleeding from the upper gastrointestinal tract (pharynx to colon). Neoplasms, ulcers, and non-healing lacerations or erosions commonly are found in older patients. Hookworms and other bloodsucking parasites are probably common causes in young or poorly housed patients. Histoplasmosis may cause chronic diarrhea and melena.

Physical Signs

The appearance of dark, black, or pitch-colored stool, either lumpy or soft in consistency, is a typical sign of melena.

Tests and Diagnostic Considerations

Melena is a serious finding. Confirmation by tests for occult blood—by producing hemolysis in water or by finding numerous erythrocytes in saline smears—is necessary for diagnosis.

The history is important to eliminate factors causing ulcers, such as stress, uremia, and the presence of mastocytomas and corticosteroids, aspirin, and other medications.

Fecal examination for endoparasites should be repeated several times as an early test.

The cause may need to be determined by endoscopic examination of the esophagus, stomach, and duodenum, and/or by plain and contrast radiographic examination of the entire gastrointestinal tract.

RECTAL PAIN, DYSCHEZIA, AND ANORECTAL DISEASE

Dyschezia is defined as pain on defecation.

Physiologic Considerations

The rectum is the passageway for feces, whereas the anus is the muscular orifice of the alimentary canal, controlling the passage of fecal material. The anus is under both voluntary and involuntary control; the rectum and internal anal sphincter are supplied by autonomic nerve fibers. Parasympathetic fibers are motor to the rectum and inhibitory to the internal sphincter. Sympathetic fibers are inhibitory to the rectum and motor to the internal anal sphincter. The external anal sphincter is innervated by somatic nerve fibers in the pudendal nerve. The pudendal nerve is formed from the first three sacral nerves. The internal anal sphincter and rectum receive nerves from the pelvic plexus.

The anal sphincter canal is normally closed by tonic contraction of the external anal sphincter produced by proprioceptive nervous feedback, with afferent nerves extending through the second sacral nerves and efferents through the pudendal nerve. The cord centers for the motor pathway are caudal to the fourth lumbar nerves (see p. 437). Fecal continence depends on sphincter continence and reservoir continence. Defecation occurs when fecal material passes into the rectum and nerve fibers are stimulated and the internal anal sphincter dilates. Sphincter continence is lost when the external anal sphincter is divided or loses neurologic function.

The basic signs associated with diseases of the anorectal area can be classified into: pruritus, dyschezia, bleeding, tenesmus, diarrhea, constipation, and flatulence. These signs can be associated with disease of the colon, rectum, and anus or a combination of these. Rectal pain is most frequently associated with one or more of the following problems: (1) prolonged treatment of chronic diarrheas, (2) tenesmus or straining to defecate, and (3) dyschezia.

Tests and Diagnostic Considerations

When carrying out the initial history and physical examination on patients with rectoanal disease, the following are important to remember:

1. Always examine the perianal area by elevating the tail and looking for the presence of neoplasms, anal gland fistulas, abnormal swellings, perineal hernia, imperforate anus, anus closed with matted fecal material, rectal prolapse, blood, or perineal fistulas. A benign tumor found in the rectum can be a leiomyoma, adenoma, or fibroma. A malignant tumor can be an adenocarcinoma, a lymphosarcoma, or a hemangiosarcoma.

2. Digital rectal examination can be helpful in achieving a diagnosis. If the procedure is very painful to the animal, sedation or anesthesia may be necessary. Note abnormal prostatic size or pain in males, rectal foreign bodies, rectal strictures, and abnormal size of the pelvic inlet. The rectal sphincter tone and rectal diverticula should be evaluated. A fecal sample should be obtained during digital examination and a wet mount should be done. One should look for occult blood.

3. When external visual inspection and digital palpation fail to reveal any abnormalities, an internal visual examination, using an anoscope or proctoscope, is indicated. This form of examination must be performed under short-acting general anesthesia (see p. 78).

4. Radiographic studies using a barium enema may be indicated to visualize abnormalities (see p. 567).

References and Additional Readings

Greiner, T. P., Johnson, R. G., and Betts, W. C.: Diseases of the rectum and anus. *In* Ettinger, S. J. (ed.): Textbook of Veterinary Internal Medicine, 2nd ed. Philadelphia, W. B. Saunders Company, 1983, Chap. 64, pp. 1493–1521.

Palminteri, A.: Symposium on gastrointestinal medicine and surgery. Vet. Clin. North Am. 2:1, 1972.

Strombeck, D.: Small Animal Gastroenterology. Davis, California, Stonegate Publishing Co., 1979.

ICTERUS (See p. 755)

Icterus or jaundice is the abnormal accumulation of bile pigments in the blood or tissues.

Physiologic Considerations

The degree of icterus (tissue staining with bile pigments) depends on the type and level of bilirubin present in the serum and is influenced by the type of tissue and duration of the disease. Unconjugated bilirubin is transported bound to albumin. Albumin-bound pigment is distributed only in the vascular compartment and interstitial space. Conjugated bilirubin is water soluble and is distributed to most body water. Conjugated bilirubin stains the tissues much more readily than does free bilirubin.

Hyperbilirubinemia that exceeds 1 to 5 mg per dl and is mainly conjugated bilirubin will produce clinical icterus.

Physical Signs

Careful examination of the mucous membranes will reveal clinical icterus. Signs in hemolytic diseases may include weakness, increased respiratory and heart rates, anemic cardiac bruits, and petechial or ecchymotic hemorrhaging. Liver disease may produce ascites, hepatomegaly, abdominal pain, weakness, vomiting, diarrhea, and bleeding tendencies. Increased hemolysis may result in dark brown or black stools, whereas simple biliary obstruction produces clay-colored stools.

Tests and Diagnostic Considerations

Abnormalities of bilirubin metabolism can occur through any of four mechanisms: (1) overproduction, (2) decreased hepatic uptake, (3) decreased hepatic conjugation, and (4) decreased excretion of bilirubin into bile (associated with both intrahepatic and extrahepatic factors). For the metabolism of bile pigments, see p. 756.

Classification of icterus is based on the underlying alteration of pigment metabolism, namely those types in which conjugated bilirubin is found (direct reacting) in the blood and those types in which unconjugated (indirect reacting) bilirubin is found (Tables 44 and 45).

Excess unconjugated or indirect reacting bilirubin may be produced by an increased destruction of circulating red blood cells as occurs in lymphosarcoma, sepsis, parasitism, or with the production of hemolysins. Increased destruction of sequestered red blood cells can occur in the absorption of hematomas or intraperitoneal blood, the absorption of blood in massive infarctions, following burns, in autoimmune hemolytic anemia, and in transfusion reactions.

Elevated levels of conjugated or direct-reacting bilirubin can be produced by the impaired transport and excretion of bilirubin conjugates as happens in hepatitis, toxemias, cirrhosis, fatty degeneration, and dysfunction of the liver. Obstruction to biliary drainage, either extrahepatic or intrahepatic, will also cause elevated levels of conjugated bilirubin.

Signs of Jaundice in Cats

The most common cause of icterus in cats is hepatocellular and partial intrahepatic obstruction. When evaluating cats for liver disease, certain species'

Table 44. RULE-OUTS FOR ICTERUS IN DOGS

Hemolytic
    Autoimmune hemolytic anemia
    Heartworm disease—postcaval syndrome
    Hemolytic bacteremia/septicemia
    Incompatible blood transfusion
Hepatocellular
    Idiopathic hepatic necrosis (toxin?)
    Hepatic neoplasia, primary or metastatic
    Cholangitis/cholangiohepatitis
    Chronic active hepatitis
    Hepatic fibrosis ("cirrhosis")
    Drugs or toxins
        Thiacetarsamide
        Aflatoxins (moldy grains)
        Mebendazole
    Bacteremia/septicemia (usually gram negative)
    Leptospirosis
    Hepatic copper accumulation (Bedlington terrier)
    Infectious canine hepatitis
Obstructive
    Intrahepatic
        Cholangitis/cholangiohepatitis
        Neoplasia
        Hepatic fibrosis/cirrhosis
    Extrahepatic
        Acute pancreatitis—bile duct compression
        Neoplasm compressing bile duct
        Traumatic rupture of bile duct or gallbladder
        Cholelithiasis

From Cornelius, L. M.: Proc. A.A.H.A., 1982.

Table 45. RULE-OUTS FOR ICTERUS IN CATS

Hemolytic
  Hemobartonellosis
  Drugs
    Acetaminophen
    Methylene blue
  Bacteremia/septicemia
Hepatocellular
  Feline leukemia virus-associated diseases (lymphosarcoma,
      myeloproliferative disorders such as reticuloendotheliosis,
      immunosuppression and subsequent bacterial infection)
  Cholangitis/cholangiohepatitis
  Idiopathic hepatic lipidosis
  Feline infectious peritonitis
  Bacteremia/septicemia (usually gram negative)
  Drugs or toxins
    Acetaminophen
  Neoplasia
    Feline leukemia, virus related (lymphosarcoma,
      reticuloendotheliosis)
Obstructive
  Intrahepatic
    Cholangitis/cholangiohepatitis
    Neoplasia (primary or metastatic)
  Extrahepatic
    Neoplasm compressing bile duct
    Trauma—ruptured gallbladder or bile duct
    Cholelithiasis (usually secondary to chronic cholestasis and bile
      inspissation associated with cholangiohepatitis)

From Cornelius, L. M.: Proc. A.A.H.A., 1982.

differences must be considered. For example, normal serum alkaline phosphatase (SAP) values in cats are one third those of dogs, and the serum half-life of SAP in cats is 6 hours, whereas it is 72 hours in dogs. Even slight increases in SAP in cats is significant as an indication of biliary stasis.

Common diagnoses involving the liver in cats with resultant icterus are: cholangiohepatitis, liver neoplasia, hepatic lipidosis, and feline infectious peritonitis.

Classification of Jaundice Based on Abnormalities in Bilirubin Metabolism

1. Predominantly unconjugated hyperbilirubinemia
   a. Overproduction
      1. Hemolysis
      2. Ineffective erythropoiesis
   b. Impaired hepatic uptake
   c. Impaired bilirubin conjugation

2. Predominantly conjugated hyperbilirubinemia
   a. Impaired hepatic excretion
   b. Extrahepatic biliary obstruction

The type of icterus can usually be determined by a clinical examination for the presence of anemia, color of the feces and urine, bleeding tendencies, changes in liver size, and the presence of pain over the liver. A total white blood cell (WBC) count, differential, hematocrit, hemoglobin, and Van Den Bergh test will aid in correctly classifying the type of icterus.

For further discussion of the interpretation of icterus, see p. 755.

References and Additional Readings

Cornelius, L. M., and Denovo, R. C.: Icterus in cats. *In* Kirk, R. W. (ed.): Current Veterinary Therapy VIII: Small Animal Practice. Philadelphia, W. B. Saunders Company, 1983, pp. 822–829.

Lees, G. E.: Clinical implications of feline bilirubinuria. J.A.A.HA. 20:765, 1984.

POLYPHAGIA

Polyphagia is a condition of excessive or voracious eating. (Its opposite, anorexia, is so common and found in so many different disease states that it cannot be covered in a brief outline.)

Physiologic Considerations

Hunger is controlled by the interaction of two centers in the hypothalamus. The feeding center, which stimulates appetite, is thought to be chronically active, but its activity is transiently inhibited by activity of the satiety center after ingestion of food. Probably, the activity of the satiety center is directly related to its cellular utilization of glucose (and to the blood glucose level).

A cold environment and contractions of the empty stomach stimulate appetite, whereas a hot environment and distention of the gastrointestinal tract depress appetite. The act of chewing and swallowing has a vague satiety effect, whereas environment, habit, sight, smell, and taste all stimulate food intake. Usually these regulatory mechanisms adjust food intake so that the animal's caloric intake equals its energy needs.

Polyphagia can be ascribed to conditions preventing receipt, absorption, or utilization of nutritional elements or to factors increasing requirements or losses. In the first category are inadequate or imbalanced diet, malabsorption syndromes, chronic pancreatitis, enteritis or colitis, diabetes mellitus, brain lesions, and anatomic abnormalities of the gastrointestinal tract.

Factors that increase losses or intake requirements are pregnancy and lactation, heavy work, extreme parasite loads, nervous diarrhea, anxiety, chronic bleeding or wound drainage, a cold environment, renal or ascitic losses of protein, and hyperthyroidism. Several drugs such as megesterol acetate, glucocorticoids, and anticonvulsants such as phenytoin and primidone are appetite stimulants.

Physical Signs

A ravenous appetite and pica, which is eating foods unusual for the species (lettuce or fruit, for example, in carnivores), are obvious signs. These should be evaluated in conjunction with water intake and with the patient's general physical condition.

Tests and Diagnostic Considerations

The differential diagnosis of polyphagia involve the following procedures:
1. Establish baseline weights, and record weight gain or loss with dates, if possible. Polyphagia with weight loss can be seen in diabetes mellitus, hyperthyroidism (especially in cats), and maldigestion/malabsorption syndromes.
2. Determine the average diet and daily food intake together with housing and exercise data.
3. Perform fecal tests (see p. 798) to determine the parasite load and the degree of digestion and absorption of key nutrients.
4. Evaluate the patient for anemia and renal (see p. 677) and liver function by appropriate laboratory screening tests (see p. 755).

DYSPNEA (See p. 447)

Dyspnea is difficult or labored breathing.

Causes

The causes for dyspnea can be separated into two major categories: (1) stimulus for increased ventilation, which could be created by arterial hypoxemia, arterial hypercapnia, arterial acidemia, muscular exercise, fever, increased metabolic rate, and heart disease; and (2) reduction of ventilatory capacity, which could be caused by low total lung volume, weakened respiratory muscles, or increased resistance to air flow.

Differential Diagnosis of Dyspnea

1. Airway obstruction—characterized by forcible attempts on inspiration and ineffective expiration; (a) inflammatory—infectious, allergic, foreign body; (b) neoplastic; (c) traumatic; and (d) laryngeal paralysis or collapse—everted lateral ventricles.

2. Nonpulmonary diseases impairing lung expansion: (a) hydrothorax; (b) pneumothorax; (c) diaphragmatic hernia; (d) cardiomegaly; (e) trauma (pain); (f) diseases displacing the diaphragm (ascites, hepatomegaly); and (g) neoplasia.

3. Primary pulmonary disease: (a) pneumonia; (b) bronchiectasis/bronchitis; (c) emphysema; (d) neoplasia; (e) pulmonary vascular disease; and (f) trauma.

4. Cardiovascular and hemic abnormalities: (a) cardiac failure and heart worm disease; (b) aortic and pulmonary emboli; (c) anemia; (d) shock; (e) electric shock; (f) hemoglobin disorders; and (g) heat stroke.

5. Metabolic disorders: (a) acidosis (renal failure, diabetic ketoacidosis); and (b) hepatic coma (respiratory alkalosis).

6. Nervous or emotional disorders: (a) primary CNS disease—medullary center depression; (b) fear; (c) pain; (d) heat stroke; and (e) fever.

Physical Signs

Signs of severe dyspnea include a rapid respiratory rate with the mouth open. The subject may salivate, its tongue thrust out, and its head extended. Many subjects sit or stand but refuse to lie down. The intense effort to breathe is evidenced by "heaving activity" of the respiratory muscles. Cyanosis, pallor, or injection may be observed in the skin and mucous membranes.

Tests and Diagnostic Considerations

Be certain that the airway is open. Look for tumors, foreign bodies, tight collars, laryngeal edema, stenosis, or pulmonary exudates. Hold a mirror or a wisp of cotton in front of each nostril to determine the relative patency.

A history and physical examination will be useful in determining the most probable causes of dyspnea. It is especially helpful to determine the type of dyspnea, that is, inspiratory, expiratory, or mixed (see p. 447). In performing an examination of a dyspneic animal, it is important to try to localize the disease to the upper or lower respiratory tract. Signs associated with upper respiratory disease are sneezing, nasal discharge, facial swellings, sonorous breathing, voice changes, inspiratory dyspnea, and loud upper respiratory sounds. Careful examination of the laryngeal area is also indicated when looking for laryngeal paralysis, which, if bilateral, can cause severe inspiratory dyspnea characterized by the following clinical findings:

1. Arytenoid cartilages displaced ventromedially.
2. Aryepiglottic folds assume a more medial position.
3. Vocal folds are flaccid and create stenosis of the glottis.
4. Voice changes may be present.

A good physical examination is important to rule out multisystemic disorders such as the following:

1. Lameness, which can be associated with hypertrophic pulmonary osteoarthropathy.
2. Skin lesions associated with deep mycotic infections.
3. Cyanosis of the mucous membranes, indicating reduced hemoglobin, is

associated with airway obstruction, small airway collapse, barrier to diffusion (as seen in pulmonary edema associated with congestive heart failure), abnormal pulmonary perfusion or shunting, and cyanotic heart disease.

4. Severe anemia.
5. Neoplasia metastasizing to lungs.

Disease of the lungs and thorax should be eliminated as causes. Usually auscultation and radiographic examinations of the chest are most helpful, but thoracentesis, percussion, palpation, and the presence or absence of pain offer additional clues to the cause. The following conditions should also be considered: pneumothorax, hydrothorax, hemothorax, pyothorax, pulmonary edema or thrombosis, pneumonia, thoracic tumors, fractured ribs, diaphragmatic hernia, pulmonary emphysema, bronchitis, and asthma. More details about these conditions can be found in the section explaining examination of the respiratory system (see p. 447).

Diseases of the heart should be investigated. Very often dyspnea, as a consequence of heart disease, is slowly progressive in its course and directly proportional to the amount of physical exertion. Ascites, hydrothorax, and hydropericardium may be obvious in advanced congestive heart failure. Circulation time, ECG, auscultation, and radiographs may be useful in establishing a diagnosis (see p. 335). In addition to congestive heart failure and the conditions producing it, one should consider the following factors in a differential diagnosis; heart base tumors (hydropericardium), chronic myocarditis or degeneration, aortic thrombosis (cats), congenital defects, and dirofilariasis.

Certain laboratory tests are useful in evaluating anemia, shock, acidosis, hypocalcemia, and other metabolic disorders that may produce dyspnea. The data base should include a CBC, microfilaria test, and thoracic radiographs. More advanced data base may include aspiration of thoracic cavity, transtracheal aspiration, bronchoscopy, and specialized radiographic techniques.

COUGH

A cough is a reflex response to irritation of the respiratory mucosa. It begins with a deep inspiration and is followed by forced expiration against the closed glottis. The glottis is suddenly opened, producing an explosive outflow of air at high velocity. (Sneezing is a similar reflex, with a continuously open glottis.)

Physiologic Considerations

Cough is an important clinical sign, a warning that disease is present. In general, it has a protective function, but excessive coughing may be harmful and cause bronchial trauma or force bronchial secretions deeper into the lungs. Persistent coughing may be physically exhausting, and the repeated episodes of high intrathoracic pressure during coughing interfere with venous return to the heart and result in reduced cardiac output.

Cough may be caused by conditions listed in Table 46.

There are two general types of cough:

1. A soft, moist, or productive cough is associated with exudates or transudates. It is found in bronchiectasis, pulmonary edema, and some types of pneumonia.
2. A harsh, dry, nonproductive cough is associated with congestive heart failure, bronchitis, bronchial asthma, tonsillitis, neoplasia, some allergic conditions, tracheitis, tracheal collapse, emphysema, pulmonary fibrosis, and some types of pneumonia.

Physical Signs

A cough is a noisy, hacking sound that (if productive) may be mistaken by owners for vomiting. The animal gasps, puts its head down, and retches, but

Table 46. CAUSES OF COUGHING IN DOGS AND CATS

Inflammation	**Allergic**
Pharyngitis	Bronchial asthma
Tonsillitis	Eosinophilic pneumonitis
Tracheobronchitis	Pulmonary infiltrate with eosinophilia (PIE)
Chronic bronchitis	Other immune states
Bronchiectasis	**Trauma and Physical**
Pneumonia (bacterial, viral, fungal)	Foreign body (esophageal, tracheal)
Granuloma	Irritating gases
Abscess	Trauma
Chronic pulmonary fibrosis	Collapsed trachea
Collasped trachea	Hypoplastic trachea
Hilar lymph node enlargement	Hepatomegaly
Secondary to achalasia	Inhalation (liquid, solid)
Inhalation	**Parasites**
Neoplasia	Visceral Larval Migrans
Primary	*Filaroides oslieri* (lungworm)
Mediastinal	*Aelurostrongylus* (feline lungworm)
Metastatic	*Paragonimus kellicotti* (lung fluke; dog, cat)
Tracheal	*Dirofilaria immitis* (dog, cat)
Laryngeal	Pneumocystis
Ribs, sternum, muscle	*Capillaria aerophilia* (dog, cat)
Lymphoma	*Crensoma-vulpis* (dog)
Cardiovascular	*Filaroides milksi* (dog)
Left-sided heart failure	
Enlarged heart, especially left atrium	
Heart failure—pulmonary signs	
Pulmonary emboli	
Pulmonary edema of vascular origin	

From Ettinger, S. J. (ed.): Textbook of Veterinary Internal Medicine. 2nd ed. Philadelphia, W. B. Saunders Company, 1983, p. 96.

ejects only a few ml of mucus. This is a productive cough and may be associated with the production of fluid, mucus, purulent material, or hemorrhage. It may be either intermittent or progressive.

A dry cough is usually repeated rapidly as a harsh, grating, short sound. The dog often extends its head and neck while coughing. This type of cough is often aggravated by exercise or cold air. It may progress to the productive type or may remain chronic, persistent, and nonproductive.

Inflammatory stimuli that activate the cough reflex are associated with edema and hyperemia in either the tracheobronchial tree or the alveoli of the lungs (e.g., pneumonia). Lesions that produce airway compression may lead to coughing, for example, mediastinal tumors, pulmonary neoplasms, intramural lesions (including bronchiogenic carcinoma), foreign bodies, tracheal collapse, and bronchial asthma.

Hemoptysis is a sign of serious pulmonary disease and refers to the expectoration of blood from the respiratory passages. Because animals usually swallow their sputum, hemoptysis is not commonly recognized; it may be observed through the animal's sneezing. Hemoptysis is commonly caused by thoracic trauma, pulmonary edema (pink froth), or pulmonary infarction due to heart worms or to lung worms. Other causes are neoplasms, foreign bodies, abscesses, fungal infections, chronic bronchitis or pneumonia, disseminated intravascular coagulation (DIC), and any of the clotting or hemorrhagic diseases. Before evaluating hemoptysis, it is important to be sure that blood is coming from the respiratory tract and not from the nasopharynx or gastrointestinal tract.

Tests and Diagnostic Considerations

The differential diagnosis of a cough depends on many of the following factors:

1. In the history, the type of onset, duration, persistence and periodicity, exposure to other animals, and vaccination history are all important.

2. In the physical examination, determination of the type of cough (i.e., productive vs. nonproductive) and careful auscultation of the lungs are useful in determining the presence of exudation, strictures, consolidation, and other changes affecting sound transmission. Carefully observe the coughing sequence. Try to determine whether the cough is associated with an upper or lower respiratory disease process. Is the cough easily elicited by tracheal palpation? Inspiratory stridor is typical of obstructions from tracheal collapse or palatal or laryngeal lesions. Cough associated with mechanical obstruction, chronic bronchitis, or pneumonia may be worsened by exercise or excitement.

3. Chest radiographs in two planes are most helpful in delineating consolidation, fluid or air, foreign bodies, and other abnormalities.

4. Culture of bronchial washings and routine hemograms, ECG, and microfilaria examinations should be carried out. Fecal analysis should be done in cases of chronic cough to detect the presence of lungworms (see p. 787).

5. Special tests of the cardiopulmonary system (see p. 335) such as special contrast radiograms, circulation time, bronchoscopy, tracheal smears, and exploratory thoracotomy may be needed in certain cases.

References and Additional Readings

Bonagura, J.: Approach to the patient with chronic cough and dyspnea. 46th Proc. A.A.H.A., *14*:31, 1979.
Cornelius, L.: Coughing. 49th Proc. A.A.H.A., 147, 1982.
Ettinger, S. J. (ed.): Textbook of Veterinary Internal Medicine, 2nd ed. Philadelphia, W. B. Saunders Company, 1983.
Hardie, E. M., Kolata, R. J., Stone, E., and Steiss, J. E.: Laryngeal paralysis in three cats. J.A.V.M.A., *179*(9):879, 1981.
Harvey, C. E., and O'Brien, J. A.: Upper airway obstruction surgery. J.A.A.H.A., *18*(4):535, 1982.
Wheeldon, E. B., Suter, P. F., and Jenkins, T.: Neoplasia of the larynx in the dog. J.A.V.M.A., *180*(6): 642, 1982.

CYANOSIS

Cyanosis results in a bluish discoloration of the mucous membranes (and skin) resulting from excessive concentration of reduced blood hemoglobin in the capillaries. Cyanosis is most obvious in the mucous membranes and in thin, unpigmented skin with a sparse hair covering. The reduced hemoglobin concentration of the blood must exceed 5 gm per dl to be recognized. In general, cyanosis is a late sign of pulmonary disease, occurring when arterial oxygen saturation is less than 80 per cent. Animals that are severely anemic will not show clinical signs of cyanosis.

Cyanosis is not synonymous with hypoxia, although it may be one of its clinical signs.

CAUSES

Cyanosis can result from cardiovascular, respiratory, or blood abnormalities. When cyanosis is associated with cardiovascular or respiratory causes, the dark color of the blood will lighten when the sample is shaken in the air. The hemoglobin molecule in the blood in the ferric form (Fe^{3+}) is called *methemoglobin* and, in this form, is unable to bind oxygen. The severity of the cyanosis and the physiologic anemia in an animal is proportional to the percentage of methemoglobin in the blood. In the red blood cell, nonenzymatic and enzymatic reducing mechanisms are constantly maintaining a conversion from methemoglobin back to hemoglobin. Chemical abnormalities of hemoglobin resulting in increased concentrations of methemoglobin can be produced when: (1) the blood has been exposed to an oxidizing substance (nitrates, nitrites, phenacetin, sulfonamides, benzocaine, aniline dyes in laundry markers and crayons, and dapsone; (2) an abnormal hemoglobin structure is present; and (3) a deficiency of reduced nicotinamide-adenine dinucleotide (NADH) methemoglobin reductase exists.

Central cyanosis results in delivery of cyanotic blood to the tissues. It may be caused by a reduced airway, depression of rate or depth of breathing, reduction of the effective size of the lungs (tidal volume), reduction in alveolar membrane permeability, and reduction of oxygen pressure in the inhaled air. Administration of oxygen may be beneficial in these cases of cyanosis. Central cyanosis can also be caused by arteriovenous shunts (blood passing through unventilated areas of the lung) or by arteriovenous blood being mixed within the heart (congenital cardiac and vascular anomalies). Oxygen therapy is rarely beneficial in these conditions.

Peripheral cyanosis results when normally oxygenated blood is delivered to the tissues but is delayed in passage through the capillaries, or when too little blood is delivered so that excess oxygen is extracted (shock, congestive heart failure, thrombosis, tourniquets, or external pressure on veins).

NADH-MR deficiency (Atkins, 1981) is a rare disease of dogs in which levels of 10 to 40 per cent methemoglobinemia may develop, although clinical signs associated with this problem are usually not severe unless the animal undergoes physical exertion. Differential diagnosis in NADH-MR involves determining the cardiopulmonary cause and the presence of hemoglobin M, sulfhemoglobinemia, or toxic hemoglobinemia. NADH-MR deficiency has been treated using oral new methylene blue (1 mg/lb BID initially, followed by dosage as needed). Methylene blue reduces the Fe^{3+} in methemoglobin to ferrous iron (Fe^{2+}).

Cats may develop severe methemoglobinemia and cyanosis, with acetaminophen toxicosis (see p. 191).

Physical Signs

The dark blue pigmentation of cyanosis is most apparent in mucous membranes or unpigmented skin. Examination must be made in daylight or under strong artificial light. Color changes in the blood can often be noted directly during surgery. Because the pigment of cyanosis is inside the vessels, finger pressure to "blanch" an area of mucous membrane by driving out the blood also decreases the cyanosis. Pigment in tissue outside vessels cannot be removed in this way.

Diagnostic Considerations

When cyanosis is a prominent sign, examination of the blood can indicate whether the cyanosis is associated with reduced hemoglobin, methemoglobin, or other blood abnormalities. When the blood sample is shaken in the air for 15 minutes, reduced hemoglobin becomes bright red in color, whereas methemoglobin remains chocolate brown in color.

Other conditions that may cause cyanosis include foreign bodies; laryngeal edema; pulmonary edema or exudates; tight collars; tumors or hematomas;

drug depressions; air; fluid, pus or blood in the thorax; pneumonia; asthma; diaphragmatic hernia; high altitude; and those listed in the section entitled Dyspnea (see p. 270).

References and Additional Readings

Atkins, C. E., Kaneko, J. J., and Congdon, L. L.: Methemoglobin reductase deficiency and methemoglobinemia in a dog. J.A.A.H.A., *17*(5):829, 1981.

Gaunt, S. D., Baker, D. C., and Green, R. A.: Clinicopathologic evaluation of N-acetylcysteine therapy in acetaminophen toxicosis in the cat. Am. J. Vet. Res., *42*(11):1982, 1981.

Letchworth, G., et al.: Cyanosis and methemoglobinemia in two dogs due to a NADH-methemoglobin reductase deficiency. J.A.A.H.A., 13:75, 1977.

SYNCOPE

Syncope (or fainting) is a transient, sudden loss of consciousness. It is much more common in man than in animals, because, in man, psychic, orthostatic, and vasodepressor mechanisms are etiologic. The usual cause is a temporary decrease in cerebral blood flow, but brief disturbances in consciousness may also be due to changes in the chemical composition of the blood, as in hypoglycemia, anoxia, or hypocapnia caused by hyperventilation. Atrioventricular heart block, mediastinal pressure from a dilated esophagus or bloating, severe organic heart disease, and paroxysms of severe coughing may be etiologic in animals.

Syncope may be confused with asthenia or with akinetic epileptic seizures such as petit mal attacks (see pp. 290–293) with narcolepsy.

Syncope	Asthenia
Sudden onset	Chronic weakness
Normal between attacks	Constant fatigue
Usually rapid recovery	Slow recovery
Loss of consciousness	Consciousness often intact

Physical Examination and Special Tests

The following procedures should be carried out in determining the presence and extent of syncope:

1. Carefully examine the cardiovascular system; include auscultation, pulse, and ECG, with special emphasis on detecting possible heart block (see p. 335).

2. Look for evidence of diffuse neurologic damage (possible referral for EEG).

3. Determine fasting blood sugar level.

4. Determine serum calcium levels.

EDEMA

Edema is the presence of abnormally large amounts of fluid in the intercellular spaces of the body. The term is usually applied to demonstrable amounts of fluid in the subcutaneous tissues. Edema is produced by a complex process that may involve any of the factors causing hypoproteinemia or sodium retention; it may also be the result of cardiovascular, renal, or hepatic disorders. Generalized subcutaneous edema is called *anasarca*.

Physiologic Considerations

Edema constitutes an expansion of one portion of the extracellular volume, the interstitial fluid. This may be accomplished with the extracellular volume remaining the same (i.e., the plasma volume decreases as the interstitial fluid increases), or the kidneys may retain salt and water; thus, both compartments increase in volume. Edema exists if the interstitial fluid pressure is above the atmospheric pressure. It does not exist if the fluid pressure is less than the atmospheric pressure. The interstitial space is really a small area for fluid, because most of the area is filled by collagen fibers and a gel matrix composed mainly of hyaluronic acid. These structures keep the fluid from "sloshing" freely from one area to another. If kinins or hyaluronidase (produced in allergy or by bacteria) upsets the integrity of the gel, fluid collects in the area easily (as in edema of urticaria and infection). When the fluid volume increases, the first 30 per cent of new water expands the gel matrix, which is not easily movable. The amount that accumulates over this percentage is free fluid and can be moved by pressure—hence, "pitting" edema.

Interstitial fluid protein, pressure, and volume work together to control the dynamic equilibrium of capillary exchange. Four major changes can lead to edema formation: increased capillary pressure, decreased plasma colloidal oncotic pressure, increased capillary permeability, and blockage of lymphatic flow. These changes may develop individually or concurrently. A schematic chart of the balance of osmotic and hydrostatic forces and the lymphatic pump can be found on page 279. Normally, there is a net filtration pressure of 0.5 mm Hg at the capillary membrane, which causes a trickle of fluid from the capillaries through the tissues and into the lymphatics. Changes in any of the factors shown on the chart will cause appropriate movement of fluid.

Physical Signs

Edema in superficial tissues has the appearance of slightly swollen or tense skin, which may or may not pit on pressure. Fluid may accumulate in dependent areas. If edema is generalized, the patient may have increased weight and show other signs of fluid accumulation such as ascites or pulmonary edema (with coughing or dyspnea). This usually signifies heart failure or pericardial disease, and ascites will develop before peripheral edema develops. Hypoproteinemia can also produce generalized peripheral edema with ascites.

Edema of a limb that is focal and not generalized may be associated with: (a) inflammation and infection, (b) venous or lymphatic obstruction, (c) arteriovenous fistula, and (d) trauma. Bilateral forelimb edema without hindlimb edema is associated with cranial vena cava obstruction, whereas hind limb edema is associated with caudal vena caval obstruction or chronic portal hypertension, which can also produce ascites. Sublumbar iliac venous obstruction can produce hind limb edema and cold extremities without ascites. Sudden edema of the head and neck is usually angioneurotic edema and is allergic in etiology.

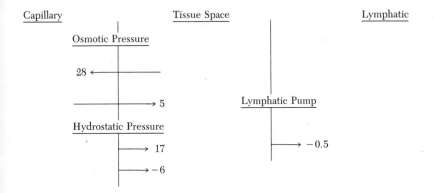

Tests and Diagnostic Considerations

Edema is a grave sign; it must be carefully investigated and its cause defined. Abnormalities of protein absorption (decreases), metabolism, or excretion (losses) should be documented. Diet and thyroid, pancreatic, renal, hepatic, and intestinal function should be checked. Sodium retention and cardiovascular dysfunction are especially important in the pathogenesis of edema.

In addition to a complete history and physical examination, the following tests are particularly useful: water input/output; urinalysis (especially quantitative protein); serum and urinary electrolytes; serum protein; albumin/globulin ratio; serum electrophoresis; sodium sulfobromophthalein (BSP) retention; fecal examinations for parasites, undigested protein, and fecal fat; intestinal absorption tests; and intestinal biopsy. The ECG, thoracic radiographs, and measurement of circulation time are also helpful.

Major syndromes to check in the differential diagnosis include congestive heart failure (with its many causes), renal failure, the nephrotic syndrome, nutritional deficiency, pancreatic insufficiency, malabsorption syndromes, hepatic cirrhosis, and angioneurotic edema. Additional focal edema of the forelegs, hindlegs, or one limb generally requires angiographic study or lymphangiography.

Reference and Additional Reading

Bolton, G. R.: Peripheral edema. *In* Ettinger, S. J. (ed.): Textbook of Veterinary Internal Medicine, 2nd ed. Philadelphia, W. B. Saunders Company, 1983, Chap. 7, pp. 67–73.

DYSURIA

Dysuria denotes difficulty or pain associated with voiding (Fig. 12). Under the term *dysuria* the following abnormalities in urine voiding may be grouped: increased urgency, stranguria, increased frequency, and painful emission of urine. A wide variety of pathologic conditions can lead to dysuria; inflammatory lesions in the bladder, prostate, or urethra are common causes of dysuria. Increased urgency in voiding is associated with urethral inflammation or stone

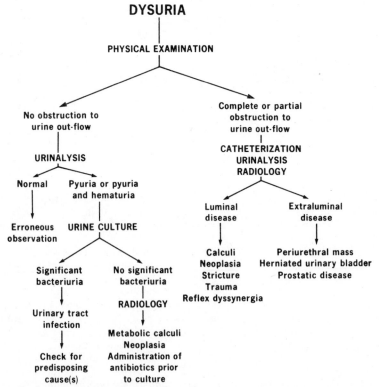

Figure 12. From Osborne, C. A., and Klausner, J.: A problem-specific data base for urinary tract infections. Vet. Clin. North Am., 9:788, 1979.

formation. The pain and irritation that induces urgency may be so severe that all voluntary control over urination is lost, and the animal voids involuntarily. The increased frequency of urination associated with lesions of the bladder occurs with decreased bladder capacity or pain on distention of the bladder. With chronic inflammation of the bladder wall, loss of normal elasticity of the bladder will cause pain or distention and increased frequency of urination.

Pollakiuria refers to unduly frequent passage of urine, commonly seen in cystitis, urethritis, and vaginitis.

URINARY INCONTINENCE

The normal micturition reflex is a result of the complex interaction of the autonomic and somatic nervous systems. Normal control of micturition can be divided into a series of nervous pathways: (1) The first circuit is a series of pathways to and from the frontal lobes to the pontine-mesencephalic reticular formation. Neurons in the pontine-mesencephalic reticular area respond to impulses from the frontal cortex and subcortical nuclei, which in turn respond to stretching of the detrusor muscle. (2) The second pathway is from the brain stem reticular formation to detrusor motor neurons in the sacral spinal cord. (3) The third pathway involves the detrusor nuclei and pudendal nuclei in the gray matter of the sacral spinal cord. These neurons permit coordination between detrusor muscle contraction and relaxation of the periurethral striated muscle during micturition. (4) The willful voiding of urine is normally prevented by contraction of the striated urethral muscle innervated by nerves from general somatic efferent neurons in the first two sacral segments of the spinal cord. Sensory neurons that are part of the general visceral afferent and general proprioception systems have stretch receptors located in the bladder wall.

Urinary incontinence may be classified as neurogenic, nonneurogenic, paradoxical, and miscellaneous. Initial examination of the animal with incontinence should be aimed at determining whether the problem corresponds to the major categories of neurologic and nonneurologic. Careful history may enable determining whether the incontinence is continuous or intermittent. Observation of the urinating patterns of the animal may reveal evidence of pain, straining, and dribbling or of intermittent voiding of spurts of urine. It is important to know whether the animal can empty the bladder satisfactorily or whether abnormally large amounts of urine remain in the bladder after the animal micturates. Residual urine volume can be measured by catheterization and should be about 0.2 to 0.4 ml per kg in the dog and cat. Catheterization may also indicate any urethral obstruction that may be present. Bladder capacity is decreased in upper motor neuron neurologic lesions and increased in lower motor neuron lesions. Lower motor neuron lesions produce an anatomic bladder.

Urine entering the bladder is accommodated by relaxation of the detrusor muscles of the bladder, resulting from central inhibition of parasympathetic fibers. There is little increase in intravesical pressure until a critical volume is reached. Central recognition of this increased pressure initiates an integrated contractile system, which stimulates contraction of the detrusor muscle via the parasympathetic system (pelvic nerves) and relaxation of the external sphincter via the pudendal nerves. These stimuli must be maintained to ensure complete evacuation of the bladder.

Abnormal voiding of urine can be caused by lesions of nervous tissue anywhere along the pathways described. Abnormalities in the normal neurogenic control of bladder function have been classified into four major categories:
1. Loss or alteration of voluntary detrusor reflex control.
2. Disordered spread of excitation in the detrusor and urethral sphincter.
3. Loss of normal contractility of the detrusor muscle.
4. Loss of urethral resistance and involuntary expulsion of urine.

Neurogenic bladder may be caused by nerve damage, resulting from trauma, neoplasia, or congenital anomalies of the vertebrae or the spinal cord. A paralytic bladder usually results in overdistention and dribbling. Urine can be easily expressed by manual compression of the bladder. A "cord bladder" is caused by a lesion between the brain and the spinal reflex center of micturition. There is usually temporary bladder paralysis; later, increased vesical pressure causes reflex, but involuntary, micturition.

Nonneurogenic urinary incontinence may be due to anomalies (ectopic ureter, patent urachus) or to endocrine imbalance in spayed females. Because the nerve supply is intact, there is no overdistention of the bladder, and the animal urinates normally.

Paradoxical incontinence occurs in patients with partial urethral obstructions (calculi, strictures, neoplasms). In these patients, the bladder is overdistended; there is dribbling and difficulty in expressing urine or in passing a catheter. Severe diseases of the bladder itself due to neoplasia, severe cystitis, or fibrosis may cause the bladder to become indistensible and insensitive to normal pressure stimuli.

Tests and Diagnostic Considerations

A complete neurologic examination should be performed in an attempt to detect abnormalities of the spinal cord and sacral nerves. The bulbourethral and perineal reflexes should be checked. These responses are controlled through the pudendal nerve and sacral segments one and two. Abdominal palpation of the bladder is very helpful in determining the presence of a large, overdistended bladder or a small contracted bladder. The bladder should be catheterized immediately after voiding to determine whether any residual urine is present (Table 47). Quantities in excess of 5 to 10 ml are abnormal.

The following may be helpful in arriving at a correct evaluation of the problem: careful palpation of the bladder, passage of a catheter or sound, a pneumocystogram or urethrogram, intravenous pyelography, radiographs of the pelvis and spine, urinalysis and cultures, and possibly cystometry.

Patients with retention of urine are highly susceptible to urinary infection. Instrumentation should be avoided, if possible, and antibacterial prophylaxis is

Table 47. ALGORITHM FOR DIAGNOSIS OF URINARY INCONTINENCE

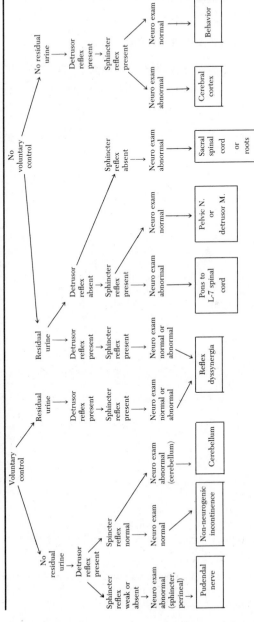

From Oliver, J. E., Jr., and Osborne, C. A.: Neurogenic urinary incontinence. *In* Kirk, R. W. (ed.): Current Veterinary Therapy VI. Philadelphia, W. B. Saunders Company, 1977, p. 1163.

always indicated. The bladder should be emptied with assistance as needed (at least every 6 hours).

References and Additional Readings

deLahunta, A.: Veterinary Neuroanatomy and Clinical Neurology, 2nd ed. Philadelphia, W. B. Saunders Company, 1983.

Moreau, P. M.: Neurogenic disorders of micturition in the dog and cat. Compendium on Continuing Education, 4(1):12, 1982.

Oliver, J. E. (ed.): Symposium on neurology of visceral function. Vet. Clin. North Am., 4:517, 1974.

Osborne, C. A., Low, D. G., and Finco, D. R.: Canine and Feline Urology. Philadelphia, W. B. Saunders Company, 1972.

OLIGURIA

Anuria is failure to form urine, whereas oliguria is failure to form urine in amounts adequate to meet metabolic demands. The daily urine volume at which oliguria begins is a function of solute load and renal concentrating power, but an estimate might be approximately 25 per cent of the patient's usual volume. Production of 0.5 to 1.0 ml of urine per kg per hour is used to indicate adequate perfusion of the kidney of the dog. Anuria either begins or terminates with oliguria, so the two are closely related.

Physical Signs

By definition, oliguric patients will be uremic; therefore, the clinical signs of uremia should be expected. Oliguria can be determined only by measuring urine output; in animals, this is best done in a metabolism cage. Owners, however, may be well aware of a pet's reduced or lack of urine output.

Causes

Prerenal Azotemia

Causes of prerenal azotemia include volume depletion, hemorrhage, diarrhea and vomiting, urinary loss—diuretics, peritonitis, and peripheral vasodilation—shock.

Reduced cardiac output, congestive heart failure, pericardial tamponade, acute pulmonary embolism, and shock may also be causes. Vascular obstruction and thrombosis of the renal arteries may also lead to this state.

Postrenal Azotemia

Causes of postrenal azotemia include bladder obstruction, urethral obstruction, and bladder neck obstruction (prostatitis, tumor, calculus). Bilateral ureteral obstruction, stones, and trauma may also be factors.

Renal (Parenchymal) Azotemia (See also p. 122)

Causes of renal azotemia include glomerular disease, glomerulonephritis, and vasculitides. Tubular lesions, with accompanying postischemic insult—hypotension; nephrotoxins—antibiotics, heavy metals, radiocontrast dye, poisons (i.e., ethylene glycol, methanol, carbon tetrachloride); pigment release—myoglobin, hemoglobin; and tubular obstruction (uric acid, sulfonamide, hypercalcemia, and Bence Jones protein) may also result in renal azotemia.

Tests and Diagnostic Considerations

The first step in the evaluation of a patient with oliguria and potential acute renal failure is to determine the degree of hydration and eliminate potentially reversible causes of acute azotemia. A complete urinalysis, including, if possible, urine osmolality, urine sodium, and blood chemistry profile (see p. 812) should be done.

Oliguria associated with prerenal causes will produce a urine with high specific gravity, high osmolality, elevated urine/plasma/osmolar ratio, elevated urine/plasma/urea ratio, and low serum sodium concentration. The urine of animals with oliguria associated with intrinsic acute renal failure is diluted, reflecting degrees of inability of the diseased kidney to concentrate, and urinary sodium levels are increased.

Following initial urinalysis and blood chemistries, selected radiographic studies are very helpful in establishing a differential diagnosis. Flat plates of the abdomen should be obtained to visualize kidney size and to look for calculi. Patients with chronic renal failure and oliguria often have reduced renal size (see p. 407).

Intravenous (IV) pyelography should be reserved for those critical cases in which a diagnosis cannot be established without its aid, for example, traumatic injuries or ruptures of the kidneys or ureters. IV pyelography in the oliguric renal patient may precipitate further renal damage.

Prerenal problems can usually be eliminated by promoting normal hydration, cardiac function, and adequate peripheral circulation. In prerenal oliguria, the urine specific gravity is usually elevated (above 1.030 in the dog and 1.035 in the cat).

Postrenal problems can be evaluated by palpation, radiographs, or catheterization to determine a patent and intact bladder and urethra. The ureters are more difficult to delineate.

Acute primary renal failure may be associated with acute renal tubular necrosis from vascular ischemia or nephrotoxins. Other causes may be hypercalcemia, pyelonephritis, immune disorders, drug reaction, leptospirosis, and glomerulonephropathy.

References and Additional Readings

Lucas, C. E.: Renal considerations in the injured patient. Surg. Clin. North Am., 62(1):133, 1982.

Osborne, C. A., Finco, D. R., and Low, D. G.: Pathophysiology of renal disease, renal failure, and uremia. *In* Ettinger, S. J. (ed.): Textbook of Veterinary Internal Medicine, 2nd ed. Philadelphia, W. B. Saunders Company, 1983, Chap. 73, pp. 1733–1792.

NOCTURIA

Nocturia refers to the nocturnal formation of a large volume of urine. Nocturia is indicated by the animal's need to go outdoors or by the appearance of multiple urine pool "accidents" in the house. The animal disregards house-breaking training, because it cannot maintain itself over relatively long periods of time without the need to urinate.

Causes

The basic problem is commonly hyposthenuria and/or polydipsia and polyuria. It may by an early sign of diabetes mellitus or insipidus, psychogenic water drinking, or renal insufficiency.

Physical Signs

Common signs are increased urine output, the frequent desire to urinate and/or accidents in the house. There is usually concurrent polydipsia.

Tests and Diagnostic Considerations

See Polydipsia and Polyuria (pp. 236–242).

HEMATURIA-HEMOGLOBINURIA

Hematuria is the gross or microscopic presence of erythrocytes in the urine. A few red blood cells (RBC) per high power field in a specimen of urine may be normal. An excess of 5 RBCs per high power field in urine is abnormal. Large numbers of RBCs indicate hemorrhage, inflammation, trauma, necrosis, ulceration, or neoplasia of the urinary tract. Hematuria found uniformly throughout a urine sample suggests a lesion high in the urinary system. Blood found primarily at the beginning of micturition suggests a lesion of the genital or distal urinary tract. Hematuria most obvious at the end of micturition suggests a bladder lesion, because RBCs tend to collect in the bottom of the bladder.

Gross hematuria is not always red. The color of urine containing blood depends on the amount of blood present and the pH of the urine. In acid urine, the color may be brown or smoky, where as in alkaline urine, the color is red. Not all red urine contains blood, because cell-free hemoglobin or myoglobin can stain urine red. Red cells can be centrifuged in the urine sample while hemoglobin and myoglobin remain in the supernatant. See p. 812 for additional information on color changes of the urine.

Causes

The following conditions may be causes of hematuria:
1. Systemic —hemophilia, thrombocytopenia, gammopathies, and coagulation defects.
2. Renal—polycystic renal disease, renal infarction, glomerulonephritis, acute pyelonephritis, renal tumor, renal calculi, and renal vascular anomalies such as arteriovenous fistula and ruptured aneurysm.
3. Bladder—calculi, tumors, chronic infection, and obstruction.
4. Prostatic—infection, tumor, and hyperplasia.

In addition to these general causes, hematuria is often found with urinary calculi, iatrogenic trauma, infection (especially viral infection, in cats), renal infarcts, parasites (*Dictophyma renale, Capillaria plica*), and systemic diseases involving hemorrhagic tendencies and platelet deficiencies. These include leptospirosis, warfarin poisoning, lupus, and hemophilia. Normal estrus or genital trauma may, at times, give the appearance of "urinary bleeding."

Hemoglobinuria is the presence of free hemoglobin in the urine. It usually occurs as a result of high levels of plasma hemoglobin. Unlike man, dogs usually pass large quantities of hemoglobin freely into the urine. Tubular blockage is not usually a serious problem following severe hemolytic crises in dogs. Hemoglobinuria can be differentiated from hematuria by centrifuging a sample of the urine. In the former, the entire sample of urine will retain its deep red color. Intravascular hemolysis, such as is caused by autoimmune hemolytic anemia, snake venom, babesiasis, bacterial toxins, hemolytic diseases of the young and transfusion reactions will cause gross hemoglobinuria. Low specific gravity or highly alkaline urine may cause hemolysis of excess erythrocytes in the urine sediment.

Red-colored urine can be produced following medication with certain drugs (neoprontosil) or test dyes such as phenolsulfonphthalein (PSP).

Tests and Diagnostic Considerations

Blood or hemoglobin in the urine is a very serious sign. Procedures to determine the cause should be both promptly instituted and thorough. Careful palpation, endoscopic examination, and radiographic evaluations are useful. Urinalysis, cultures, and exfoliative cytology of urinary sediment may be diagnostic (see p. 822). In those cases in which gross hematuria is not associated with trauma or lower urinary tract disease, exploratory laparotomy to visualize the kidneys, ventral cystotomy, and catheterization of the ureters may be necessary to demonstrate the source of bleeding. These examinations may indicate that nephrectomy must be performed.

Hematologic tests that may be helpful are (1) complete blood count and platelet count (thrombocytopenias; see p. 671), (2) bleeding time, prothrombin time, and PTT (coagulopathies); and (3) antinuclear antibody (lupus erythematosus; see p. 731).

Radiologic examinations that may be helpful include (1) pneumocystography (see p. 573); (2) double contrast cystography (see p. 573); and (3) intravenous (IV) pyelography (see p. 570).

References and Additional Readings

Osborne, C. A., Low, D. G., and Finco, D. R.: Canine and Feline Urology. Philadelphia, W. B. Saunders Company, 1972.

Stone, E. A., DeNovo, R.C., and Rawlings, C. A.: Massive hematuria of nontraumatic renal origin in dogs. J.A.V.M.A., *183*(8):868, 1983.

PYURIA

Pyuria refers to the abnormal presence of leukocytes in the urine. A few white blood cells (WBCs) are normally found in the urine. Pyuria, with clumping of WBCs, indicates the presence of an inflammatory process in the urinary tract and usually signifies the need for bacteriologic studies of the urine and studies to localize the site of infection.

Bacteriuria may be present with gross pyuria, especially in chronic pyelonephritis. Pyuria and alkaline urine suggest a urea-splitting, ammonia-producing organism such as *Proteus vulgaris* or staphylococci.

The presence of urinary tract infection has been associated with the formation of phosphate, oxalate-cystine, urate, and silica calculi. In urine samples taken (as aseptically as possible) by cystocentesis, the isolation of bacteria at a proportion greater than 10^3 ml suggests urinary tract infection. The isolation of 10^4 to 10^5 bacteria per ml in catheterized or midstream samples also suggests the presence of infection.

Factors Predisposing to Urinary Tract Infection

1. Retention of urine
   Mechanical obstruction to outflow: urethral calculi, strictures, neoplasms; herniated urinary bladder; and prostatic disease (uncommon).
   Incomplete emptying of urinary bladder: damaged innervation (vertebral fractures, luxations, subluxations; invertebral disc disease; vertebral osteomyelitis; neoplasia; vertebral or spinal cord anomalies; reflex dyssynergia) and anatomic defects (vesicoureteral reflux, diverticula).
2. Damage to epithelial barrier
   Trauma: external force, palpation, catheterization, and calculi.
   Neoplasia.
   Excretion of cytotoxic drugs.
3. Altered urine volume or composition
   Decreased urine volume: decreased water consumption and oliguric renal failure.
   Glucosuria(?).

4. Retrograde migration of bacteria
   Congenital: ectopic ureters, urethral anomalies, and primary vesicoureteral reflux.
   Acquired: urethral disease and secondary vesicoureteral reflux.
5. Immunodeficiency
   Disease: congenital and acquired.
   Immunosuppressant drugs.

Reference and Additional Reading

Osborne, C. A., and Klausner, J.: Urinary tract infections. Vet. Clin. North Am., 9:585, 1979.

VULVAR DISCHARGE

The normal vulva is soft, sparsely covered by clean hair, and free of discharges. Licking by the bitch or queen will keep it clean; in fact, small amounts of discharging fluids may be so carefully removed by a fastidious animal that minor flows may be missed.

Causes

Small amounts of clear mucus or a few drops of urine may appear in normal females. During estrus, the queen will have an increased flow of clear fluid, so the vulva may appear moist. The bitch in estrus has an edematous vulva and a bloody, tan-mucoid or viscid discharge, depending on the stage of estrus or proestrus.

Frank blood can appear in the following ways: at proestrus; pathologically, due to trauma, foreign bodies, or tumors; and postpartum, due to subinvolution of the placental sites. The latter cause produces prolonged bloody discharge.

Fetid bloody to brownish discharge usually indicates acute metritis (postpartum) or a necrotic tumor mass.

Purulent exudates of variable color, odor, and viscosity may result from vulvitis, vaginitis, cervicitis, endometritis, or cystic endometrial hyperplasia. These inflammations may be associated with bacterial infection, trauma, cysts, and neoplasms; they may also be a sequela of abortion or retained placentas.

Clear or yellow fluid discharging from the vulva may be incontinent urine. Obese bitches may have extra folds of skin in the perivulvar area that "overhang" the vulva. The moisture, heat, and skin maceration produces a perivulvar dermatitis associated with purulent material, which may falsely appear to be a vulvar discharge.

Physical Signs

Physical signs of vulvar discharge include accumulation of fluid, blood, or pus at the vulvar opening; spotting of these materials on the bedding and floor; and constant licking of the perineal area.

Tests

It is necessary to determine the source and cause of the discharge. In addition to the history and physical examination, vaginal smears for cytology, culture, speculum examination, temperature, complete blood count (CBC), urinalysis, and perhaps radiographs or surgical exploration of the abdomen may be indicated.

Diagnostic Considerations

Diagnostic considerations are outlined under Causes. In addition, concurrent anal sac infections and tonsillitis or pharyngitis may be associated with vulvar discharge.

SEIZURES (CONVULSIONS)

The terms *seizure, convulsion, epileptic attack*, and *fit* all describe a disorder of the brain, producing spontaneous depolarization and excitation of brain nerves. The seizure or ictus may result in involuntary contraction of a series of voluntary muscles, either localized or general. Severe seizures are accompanied by disturbances of consciousness and autonomic hyperactivity. Disturbances in brain function can arise extracranially from metabolic or toxic diseases or intracranially from alterations in brain function associated with organic brain disease. Idiopathic epilepsy occurs in animals with no apparent organic or metabolic central nervous system (CNS) abnormalities.

History and Examination

Careful history and examination can be helpful in attempting to arrive at an etiology for convulsion:

Age of the Animal. Seizures in young animals (less than 1 year old) are commonly caused by developmental abnormalities, hydrocephalus (age 3 to 9 months), idiopathic epilepsy (normal until 6 to 18 months), encephalitis (distemper), toxoplasmosis, lead poisoning, severe intestinal parasitism, portacaval shunt abnormalities, and lissencephaly. Idiopathic epilepsy usually begins when animals are 1 to 3 years of age. Animals over 5 years of age may suffer from CNS tumors or hypoglycemia from insulin-secreting beta-cell pancreatic neoplasms.

Breed Predisposition. Some basic knowledge about breed predisposition to seizure disorders may be helpful in establishing a differential diagnosis. Idiopathic epilepsy has been seen in numerous dog breeds, including German Shepherds, Belgian Turveren, Keeshond, St. Bernards, standard and miniature Poodles, Beagles, Irish Setters, Cocker Spaniels, Alaskan malamutes, Siberian huskies, and Labrador and Golden retrievers. Hypoglycemia is most prevalent in toy breeds. Hydrocephalus is common in the toy and brachycephalic breeds. Neoplastic diseases are seen in brachycephalic breeds over 5 years of age.

Concerning disorders of the CNS metabolism, leukodystrophy is most common in Cairn and West Highland Whites; lipodystrophy, in German Short-Haired Pointers and English Setters; lissencephaly in the Lhasa Apso; and portocaval shunts and hyperlipoproteinemia in miniature Schnauzers.

Environment. Exposure to infectious agents or other sick animals may be important, as is exposure to sources of intoxicants such as lead in paints, linoleum, tar, batteries, or roofing material; hexachlorophene soap; ethylene glycol antifreeze; metaldehyde snail bait; and various other insecticides, including chlorinated hydrocarbons, organophosphates, and rodenticides. Dogs and cats on the same premises with swine may be exposed to *Herpesvirus suis* (pseudorabies, or Aujesky's disease). In affected cats and dogs, the mortality rate of pseudorabies approaches 100 per cent. In cats, clinical signs are hypersalivation, intense pruritus, labored respiration, anisocoria, convulsions, and death. In dogs, pseudorabies has an incubation period of 2 to 10 days and a rapidly fatal course involving encephalitis, convulsions, coma, and death.

Past Medical History. The following information can prove helpful in establishing an etiology: history of previous traumatic injury; past febrile illness possibly associated with a systemic illness; diagnosis of a neoplastic mass growing elsewhere in the body; progressive neurologic deficit; and behavioral changes such as polydipsia, polyuria, appetite changes, and skin abnormalities.

Complete Neurologic Examination. Abnormalities detected during the interictal period can indicate intracranial structural brain disease. Careful neurologic examination can be used to distinguish possible focal vs. diffuse disease. The most common extracranial diseases causing neurologic abnormalities are hypoglycemia and hepatoencephalopathy (see pp. 94–96 and 144). Uremic encephalopathy can lead to neurologic dysfunction not unlike that seen with hypexemia, hyperosmolality, hepatic encephalopathy, and water intoxication. Suggested mechanisms include depressed cerebral oxygenation, cerebral acidosis, increased brain calcium levels, accumulation of toxic organic acids, and increased cerebrospinal fluid (CSF) phosphorus levels.

Careful Description of the Type of Seizure. The signs seen in focal seizures can indicate the possible location in the brain. Seizure focus in the motor area of the cerebrum can produce clonus of the limbs, head turning, or flexion of the body initially on the side contralateral to the lesion. Focus of activity in the visual centers can lead to snapping at invisible objects (fly biting) and light-induced seizures. Increased activity in the limbic system can lead to altered behavior patterns (such as changes in temperament, screaming, barking, somnolence, confusion, changes in appetite, chewing, and licking).

More generalized seizures associated with "idiopathic epilepsy" are usually preceded by an aura. Examples of the preictal aura can be licking of lips, twitching of muscle groups, restlessness, nervousness, salivation, wandering, hiding, and seeking of affection. The duration of the aura can be a few seconds to hours. It may be hard to detect the presence of an aura. The seizure can begin with clonic twitches or tonic muscle contractions. It can continue with the animal losing apparent consciousness and falling to the ground. There can be violent spasms of muscles with running motions, with frothing of saliva, and clamping motions of the jaws. The signs seen with seizures depend on where the initial abnormal electrical discharge begins and how the discharge spreads to other areas of the brain.

The ictus (fit) can last from a few to several seconds or may be continuous, developing into status epilepticus. Immediately following the seizure, there is a period of confusion, disorientation, pacing, salivation, unresponsiveness to external stimuli, and temporary visual impairment.

Seizures may be repeated frequently in groups of two or three or may occur singly. If a series of convulsions occurs without the patient's regaining consciousness in between them, the condition is called *status epilepticus*. It is a rare but ominous development (see p. 164).

Although many seizures in dogs are classified as major or generalized (grand mal), there are partial seizures of a focal motor type that may go unrecognized.

A complete neurologic examination should be performed in all seizure cases (see p. 422).

It is important that the patient be examined during the interictal period. The finding of neurologic deficits in the interictal period usually indicates a structural brain lesion. A normal interictal neurologic examination can occur with structural brain lesions in "quiet" areas of the brain, which do not produce detectable neurologic signs. Most patients with metabolic diseases, some patients with toxic diseases, and all patients with idiopathic epilepsy have a normal interictal examination.

A seizure work-up should include ophthalmoscopic examination, complete hemogram, blood chemistry, and urine and fecal examination. This should be followed by CSF evaluation. Further studies will depend on the availability of equipment and will include radiography, pneumoventriculography, electroencephalography (EEG), scintigraphy, and computerized tomography.

References and Additional Readings

Chrisman, C. L.: Symposium on advances in veterinary neurology. Vet. Clin. North Am., *10*:1, 1980.

Chrisman, C. L.: Problems in Small Animal Neurology. Philadelphia, Lea & Febiger, 1982.

deLahunta, A.: Veterinary Neuroanatomy and Clinical Neurology, 2nd ed. Philadelphia, W. B. Saunders Company, 1983.

Farnbach, G. C.: Serum concentrations and efficacy of phenytoin, phenobarbital, and primidone in canine epilepsy. J.A.V.M.A., *184*(9): 1117, 1984.

Hoerlein, B. F.: Canine Neurology, 3rd ed. Philadelphia, W. B. Saunders Company, 1978.

Kay, W. J., and Fenner, W. R.: Epilepsy. *In* Kirk, R. W. (ed.): Current Veterinary Therapy VI. Philadelphia, W. B. Saunders Company, 1977.

Kornegay, J. N.: Feline neurology. Compendium on Continuing Education, 3(3):203, 1981.

Oliver, J. E., and Lorenz, M.: Handbook of Veterinary Neurologic Diagnosis. Philadelphia, W. B. Saunders Company, 1983.

Oliver, J. E.: Seizure disorders in companion animals. Compendium on Continuing Education, 2(1):77, 1980.

Shepherd, D. E., and deLahunta, A.: Central nervous system disease in the cat. Compendium on Continuing Education, 2(4):306, 1980.
Whitebey, D. R., and Nelson, S.: Pseudorabies in the canine. J.A.A.H.A., 16(1):69, 1980.
Wolf, A. M.: Canine uremic encephalopathy. J.A.A.H.A., 16(5):735, 1980.

COMA

Coma is a state in which the patient appears to be asleep but is unable to respond to external stimuli or to inner needs. It is not an independent disease entity, but rather a symptomatic expression of disease.

Clinically, sleep and coma resemble each other, but sleep can be interrupted by adequate stimulation.

Consciousness implies the ability of an animal to be aware of its surroundings, to perceive environmental stimuli and to respond appropriately to them. *Wakefulness* implies the ability to respond immediately, fully and effectively. *Lethargy* means a state of drowsiness, inaction, and indifference in which the patient responds in an incomplete and delayed manner. A further degree of dulled indifference while still awake is *obtundation*. *Stupor*, or semi-coma, is a condition in which the patient is not wakeful. He can be aroused with vigorous stimulation; but upon cessation of the stimuli, he returns to a state of unawareness.

The ascending reticular activating system (ARAS) is primarily responsible for maintenance of consciousness and is composed of a network of neurons that run from the medulla of the brain stem, through the pons and midbrain, into the diencephalon. Hemorrhages in the midbrain and pons are relatively frequent in dogs following severe head injury. These dogs usually are comatose and exhibit decerebrate rigidity (extensor hypertonus of all limbs). The pupils are usually dilated and not responsive to light.

Physiologic and Etiologic Considerations

Coma is usually the result of abnormalities causing diffuse or widespread multifocal lesions in the cerebral hemispheres or lesions involving the ARAS of the rostral brain stem. Most cases of coma are associated with brain stem lesions.

Causes

Causes of coma include diseases that cause no focal neurologic signs or changes in cerebrospinal fluid (CSF), such as drug intoxications, metabolic disturbances (uremia, diabetic acidosis, hepatic coma, hypoglycemia, hypoxia, hypocalcemia and hypoadrenocortical crisis), systemic infections, shock, epilepsy, hypothermia, and hyperthermia.

Other causes may involve diseases that *do* cause focal neurologic signs, with or without CSF changes, such as brain hemorrhage, abscess, contusion, tumor, thrombosis, and subdural hemorrhage, and diseases that cause meningeal irritation with the presence of either blood or leukocytes in the CSF, usually without focal signs, such as meningitis and subarachnoid hemorrhage.

Types of Abnormalities Causing Coma

Primary Brain Disease
1. Space-occupying lesions (neoplasm, hemorrhage, abscess).
2. Injury (concussion, epidural or subdural hematoma, cerebral edema, brain stem contusion).
3. Infarction (diffuse cerebral or brain stem lesion).
4. Infection (meningitis and/or encephalitis).
5. Degenerative disease (lipodystrophy, terminally).
6. Hydrocephalus.
Secondary Encephalopathy
1. Renal disease (uremia, acidosis).
2. Liver disease (hypoglycemia, hyperammonemia).
3. Pancreatic disease (beta-cell neoplasm hypoglycemia, diabetes mellitus hyperglycemia).
4. Myocardial disease (ischemic anoxia).
5. Pulmonary disease (anoxic anoxia, acidosis).
6. Nutritional deficiency (thiamin).
7. Anemia (carbon monoxide poisoning, hemorrhage).
8. Endocrine disease (hypoadrenocorticoidism, hypothyroidism).
9. Postictal depression.
10. Exogenous toxicity (hexachlorophene, cyanide, barbiturates, ethylene glycol, benzene hexachloride, carbon tetrachloride, lead salts, dinitrophenol (DNP), kerosene, nitrobenzene, turpentine, arsenic, zinc, phosphide).
Abnormal Osmotic States
1. Hyperosmolar states: hyperglycemia, diabetes mellitus; hypernatremia, diarrhea, diabetes insipidus, severe water loss.
2. Hyposmolar states, such as water intoxication.

Hepatic Coma—Canine Hepatic Encephalopathy
(See pp. 160 and 422)

Neurologic abnormalities involving generalized transient disturbances of brain function have been associated with congenital and developmental hepatic disease. Neurologic signs have been seen most commonly in congenital portacaval shunts in dogs, predominantly patent ductus venosus, with a breed predilection for miniature schnauzers. They also may occur in advanced liver disease, and a few cases of urea cycle enzyme deficiency have been recognized.

The colon is the major source of ammonia (NH_3) formation in the body because of the high population of coliform bacteria. The kidneys excrete NH_3 and are an endogenous source of ammonium ion (NH_4+). The liver receives NH_3 via the portal circulation and converts NH_3 to urea. Seventy-five per cent of the urea produced by the liver is excreted by the kidneys, and the remaining 25 per cent undergoes enterohepatic recirculation.

Developmental hepatic coma has been seen in animals with chronic hepatic failure associated with increased levels of NH_3 in the blood. Respiratory alkalosis and hypokalemia can influence the effect of NH_3 on the central nervous system (CNS). Alkalosis increases the ease of entry of ammonia into CSF fluid, and hypokalemia causes increased renal NH_3 production. Animals with elevated blood NH_3 levels have an increased sensitivity to other known cerebral intoxicants such as barbiturates and sedatives.

The biochemical abnormalities resulting in CNS alterations in hyperammonemia may be related to the presence of short-chain fatty acids; mescaptans from sulphur containing amino acids; production of false neurotransmitters; increased levels of aromatic blood amino acids, including tyrosine, tryptophan, and phenylalanine; increased blood levels of indoles, and skatoles from bacterial deamination of tryptophan (Table 48).

The neurologic signs most frequently observed in canine hepatic encephalopathy are listlessness and depression, compulsive circling and pacing, head pressing, ataxia, blindness, convulsions, disorientation, changes in temperament, grand mal seizures, hypermetria, and severe stupor progressing to coma. Young dogs with congenital portocaval shunts are often stunted in their growth.

Table 48. CAUSES OF CANINE HEPATIC ENCEPHALOPATHY

Congenital Portosystemic Shunts (Usually Younger Dogs)
  Patent ductus venosus
  Anomalous connection of portal vein to vena cava
    caudal to liver
  Anomalous connection to portal vein to azygous vein
  Anomalous connection of portal vein and vena cava to azygous vein
  Atresia of portal vein with collateral portosystemic shunts
Endstage Liver Disease (Cirrhosis, Usually Older Dogs)
  Parenchymal failure
  Acquired portosystemic shunts
    Splenorenal collaterals
    Gastroesophageal collaterals
    Mesenteric to renal collaterals
    Mesenteric to deep circumflex iliac collaterals
    Mesenteric to rectal collaterals
Extensive Parenchymal Destruction
  Fatty liver (e.g., diabetes mellitus)
  Hepatotoxicity
  Hepatitis
  Extensive hepatic neoplasia
Hyperammonemia Due to Congenital Urea Cycle Enzyme Deficiency
  Arginosuccinate synthetase
  Carbamyl phosphate synthetase I and others (not yet described in the dog)

Modified from Sherding R. G.: Hepatic encephalopathy. Compendium on Continuing Education, *1*:55, 1979.

The neurologic signs associated with hepatic encephalopathy are most severe a few hours after feeding, because many of the toxins are derived from dietary proteins.

Clinical pathologic tests that may be of value in diagnosing hepatic encephalopathy are BSP (sulfobromophthalein dye test; see p. 760); BUN (see p. 743); blood ammonia and ammonia tolerance test (see p. 741); urinalysis—presence of ammonium biurate crystals (see p. 822); and splenoportogram.

Physical Signs

Signs observed in hepatic encephalopathy are chronic weight loss and unthriftiness, low serum albumin and low serum urea nitrogen, prolonged BSP test, abnormal ammonia tolerance test and presence of ammonium biurate crystals in the urine.

There is much variation in the depth of depression. The animal may appear to be sleeping, yet may be responsive to stimulation of some reflexes. At other times, no reaction of any kind can be elicited. The history and type of onset are important in evaluating the physical signs.

Tests and Diagnostic Considerations

The following procedures must be followed in order to diagnose coma:

1. Ensure the patient has a *patent airway*; establish that the patient is not in shock and is not bleeding. Check for head injuries or spinal trauma.
2. Test for *normal visual function*; this can be difficult. A positive menace reaction indicates that the central visual pathway to the visual cerebral cortex is intact; however, if the menace response is absent—pupillary response to light and facial muscle function are normal—a lesion may be present in the cerebral hemispheres. Functional vision in a semicomatose, recumbent animal would indicate a severe brain stem lesion.
3. *Pupillary response.* Severe brain stem disease that produces coma usually leads to fixed, dilated pupils. Diffuse, cerebrocortical disease often produces very small pupils. In tentorial herniation, pupils first appear fixed and small, then become dilated.
4. The *pattern of motor function* may also be helpful in localizing lesions, that is, metabolic deficits produce symmetric motor abnormalities, whereas neurogenic deficits produce asymmetric abnormalities and are usually associated with structural defects. Acute cerebral lesions produce contralateral motor abnormalities, whereas brain stem lesions tend to produce ipsilateral abnormalities.
5. *If poisoning is suspected*, lavage the stomach and save the contents. Collect urine for urinalysis. Check glucose, acetone, specific gravity, and albumin levels (Table 49).
6. Take *radiographs* of the skull or spine, if indicated.
7. If indicated, *collect blood or CSF* for analysis (see pp. 496 and 888).

Table 49. DIAGNOSIS OF GLUCOSE ABNORMALITIES IN COMA

	Hypoglycemia	Hyperglycemia and Ketoacidosis
Onset	Sudden	Gradual
Cause	Excess insulin	Too little insulin
	Excess exercise	Infection
	Delayed meal	Stress
Respiration	Normal	Kussmaul
Skin	Pale	Flushed
	Cool and moist	Hot and dry
Hydration	Normal	Dehydrated
Pulse	Firm and bounding	Weak and thready
Urine sugar	Negative	Positive
Urine ketone	Negative	Positive
Blood sugar	Low	High
Plasma ketone	Negative	Positive
Response to treatment	Rapid	Slow
Neurologic signs	Ataxia, seizures, or depression	Depression variable

References and Additional Readings

Christman, C.: Problems in Small Animal Neurology. Philadelphia, Lea & Febiger, 1982.

deLahunta, A.: Veterinary Neuroanatomy and Clinical Neurology, 2nd ed. Philadelphia, W.B. Saunders Company, 1983.

Drazner, F.H.: Hepatic encephalopathy in the dog. In Kirk, R.W. (ed.): Current Veterinary Therapy VIII: Small Animal Practice. Philadelphia, W.B. Saunders Company, 1983, pp. 829–834.

Harrison, T.R. (ed.): Principles of Internal Medicine, 9th ed. New York, Blakiston Division, McGraw-Hill, Inc., 1980.

Levesque, D.C., et al.: Congenital portocaval shunts in two cats. Diagnosis and surgical correction. J.A.V.M.A., 181(2): 143, 1982.

Sherding, R.G.: Hepatic encephalopathy in the dog. Compendium on Continuing Education, 1:55, 1979.

NARCOLEPSY

Narcolepsy is a central nervous system (CNS) disorder in which the affected animal has episodes of uncontrollable sleep. The most obvious clinical sign is cataplexy, which is a recurrent episode in which there is sudden loss of function of some or all of the voluntary muscles (excluding respiratory and extraocular). This causes brief periods of collapse. Recovery is as sudden as the onset. Episodes of narcolepsy in dogs may be associated with eating or physical exertion and excitement. Characteristic electroencephalographic (EEG) features are seen, and signs are present in REM sleep. The disease, usually idiopathic, has been seen in a variety of dog breeds, including poodles, Doberman pinschers, dachshunds, and St. Bernards. In the Doberman and Labrador retriever, the disease is inherited as an autosomal recessive trait.

Differential diagnosis of those entities causing profound weakness must be considered (see p. 299). The response to neostigmine administered intravenously (IV) is used in the differential diagnosis of a myasthenia-like syndrome. Diagnosis of narcolepsy is aided by a positive response to the IV administration of imipramine (Tofranil), 0.5 to 1.0 mg per kg IV. Further treatment of narcolepsy involves long-term treatment with imipramine at varying dosage levels, starting at 0.5 mg per kg q8h. It is important to titrate the dose to the patient's response.

In cases in which the clinical signs are infrequent, they can be provoked with physostigmine IV at a dosage of 0.05 to 0.1 mg per kg.

References and Additional Readings

Baker, T. L., et al.: Diagnosis and treatment of narcolepsy in animals. *In* Kirk, R.W. (ed.): Current Veterinary Therapy VIII: Small Animal Practice. Philadelphia, W. B. Saunders Company, 1983.

deLahunta, A.: Veterinary Neuroanatomy and Clinical Neurology, 2nd ed. Philadelphia, W. B. Saunders Company, 1983.

LASSITUDE AND ASTHENIA

The term *weakness* can be used to describe generalized loss of energy and listlessness associated with a wide variety of systemic diseases. Weakness can also appear with loss of strength, paresis, or paralysis. These neurologic symptoms may be persistent or episodic and may involve individual muscles or muscle groups.

Numerous systemic diseases can result in episodic weakness: (a) metabolic diseases—hypoglycemia, adrenal insufficiency, hypokalemia, and hypocalcemia; (b) cardiovascular causes—arrhythmias such as atrial fibrillation, heart block, congestive heart disease, heartworm infestation, ventricular tachycardia, sinus arrest and atrial standstill; and (c) neuromuscular diseases—myasthenia gravis, polymyositis, narcolepsy, hepatic encephalopathy, and peripheral neuropathies.

History

A carefully taken history is important in formulating a diagnostic plan for animals with episodic weakness (Table 50). The following factors should be considered:

1. Determine whether the weakness occurs at any specific time of day and whether there is any relationship to feeding or exercise. The glycogen storage diseases are seen primarily in puppies of the toy breeds, and functional hypoglycemia is seen in working dogs.
2. Weakness and lassitude accompanied by hypotension, shocklike signs, and chronic vomiting and diarrhea may be indicative of adrenal cortical insufficiency (see p. 147).
3. Determine whether the weakness is accompanied by signs of cardiovascular

disease such as hypotension, coughing, syncope, and cyanosis. In brachycephalic breeds of dogs, stertorous respiration may constantly irritate the pharynx, causing reflex hypertonia of the vagus nerve, which can lead to increased vagal tone, cardiac slowing, and syncope. The following cardiac arrythmias may predispose to periodic weakness: sinus arrest, sick sinus syndrome, atrial fibrillation, ventricular tachycardia, atrial standstill, and third-degree heart block.

4. Exercise intolerance, associated with weakness, is characteristic of a myasthenia gravis–like syndrome. Weakness accompanied by pain on motion, lameness, and stiffness can be associated with a polymyositis problem.

5. Hypocalcemia or eclampsia can produce marked weakness, nervousness, and excitability. Other electrolyte abnormalities, including those of potas-

Table 50. A DIAGNOSTIC PLAN FOR PATIENTS WITH EPISODIC
WEAKNESS

Disease	Diagnostic Test	Positive Result
Hypoglycemia	Fasting blood glucose	50 mg/100 ml or less
Adrenal insufficiency	Serum electrolytes	Potassium > 5.2 mEq Sodium < 135 mEq Na:K ratio < 25:1
	ECG	Tall spiked T waves Wide QRS; absence of P waves Bradycardia
Hypokalemia	Electrolytes	Potassium < 2.4 mEq
	ECG	Prolonged QT interval
Cardiac arrhythmias		
Ventricular tachycardia	ECG	Series of PVCs
Atrial fibrillation	ECG	No P waves; presence of "f" waves; rapid irregular rates
Heart block (third degree)	ECG	P waves unassociated with QRS complexes; atrial rate normal; ventricular rate very slow
Heartworm	Modified Knott's ECG Thoracic radiograph	Microfilaria of *D. immitis* Right heart enlargement, enlarged pulmonary arteries; enlarged pulmonary outflow tract; right ventricular enlargement
Myasthenia gravis	Response to neostigmine testing	Improvement in weakness and greater exercise tolerance
Polymyositis	Muscle enzymes Muscle biopsy	Increase in LDH, GOT and CPK; inflammation and necrosis of muscle

From Lorenz, M. D.: Episodic weakness in the dog. *In* Kirk, R. W. (ed.): Current Veterinary Therapy VI. Philadelphia, W. B. Saunders Company, 1977, p. 822.

sium (see p. 748), sodium (see p. 747), and chloride (see p. 747) may manifest as weakness. Blood chemistry profiles and an ECG are indicated when electrolyte abnormalities are suspected (see p. 602).

6. A variety of peripheral neuropathies must be included in the differential diagnosis of weakness. When one refers to the peripheral nervous system, one is referring to the lower motor neuron system; however, one should really include all parts of the nervous system associated with Schwann's cells, including dorsal and ventral roots, dorsal root ganglia, plexuses, peripheral nerves, and the peripheral autonomic nervous system.

   Clinical signs in peripheral neuropathies are weakness, which may be progressive, limb ataxia, and loss of limb muscle mass. Neurologic examination should attempt to evaluate the integrity of the lower motor neuron system. Movement, muscle mass, loss of muscle tone, and patellar reflex should be evaluated. In lower motor neuron disease, a change in voice may also take place. In evaluating sensory perception associated with lower motor neuron function, normal proprioceptive positioning, touch sensitivity, and pain sensitivity should be evaluated. Pain can be evaluated by skin prick with a needle and squeezing the digits.

   The rate of onset of peripheral neuropathies may be acute or chronic, may involve motor and sensory nerves or primarily sensory nerves, and may be a polyneuropathy or a mononeuropathy.

   Confirmation of peripheral neuropathies is based on use of the electromyogram (EMG) to study nerve conduction, electromyography, and peripheral nerve biopsies.

   Two major types of pathologic processes affect peripheral nerves: axonal degeneration and segmental demyelination. Axonal degeneration may result from diseases of the nerve cell body or the axon itself. Segmental demyelination is a result of disease of the Schwann's cell or myelin sheath.

7. Severe malnutrition associated with dietary abnormalities or systemic diseases can lead to profound weakness.

Physical Examination and Diagnostic Considerations

The following recommendations are suggested for conducting the physical examination and obtaining the data base:

1. Complete physical examination, with special emphasis on the cardiovascular system. Evaluate the animal's ability to bark properly and to swallow normally.

2. Also include a complete blood count (CBC) microfilaria check, urine analysis, blood electrolytes, and fasting blood glucose taken before and after vigorous exercise. Additional ancillary tests should include an ECG and thoracic radiographs.

3. Evaluate serum enzymes such as LCD and CPK if polymyositis is suspected.

4. If a myasthenia gravis–like syndrome is suspected, edrophonium chloride (Tensilon) can be given intravenously (IV) in a dosage of 0.1 to 1.0 mg, depending on the size of the patient. A marked improvement in the clinical condition should occur in 15 minutes (see p. 729).

5. Periodic weakness has also been observed in dogs with bleeding hemangiosarcomas where intra-abdominal bleeding may occur. Physical examination reveals a palpable abdominal mass, ascites due to bleeding, and markedly pale mucous membranes.
6. Hepatic insufficiency, coupled with increased blood ammonia levels, can lead to marked weakness (see p. 94).

References and Additional Readings

Bolton, G. R.: Handbook of Canine Electrocardiography. Philadelphia, W. B. Saunders Company, 1975.
Chrisman, C. L.: Differential diagnosis of stroke and vestibular disease in aging dogs. Proc. A.A.H.A., 241, 1979.
Duncan, I.: Peripheral nerve disease in the dog and cat. Vet. Clin. North Am. 10(1):177, 1980.
Kelly, M. J.:Periodic weakness. Proc. A.A.H.A., pp. 159–162, 1982.
Palmer, A. C.:Myasthenia gravis. Vet. Clin. North Am., 10:213, 1980.
Sherding, R. G., Meuten, D. J., Chew, D. J., et al.: Primary hypoparathyroidism in the dog. J.A.V.M.A., 176:439, 1980.

JOINT STIFFNESS, PAIN, AND SWELLING

Arthritis refers to inflammation of a joint. Diseases of joints not associated with true inflammation can be grouped under the general heading of degenerative joint disease. The following classification has been used for the canine arthropathies:

Noninflammatory Joint Disease
1. Degenerative joint disease (osteoarthrosis, osteoarthritis)
   a. Primary
   b. Secondary
2. Miscellaneous conditions (secondary degenerative joint disease)
   a. Osteochondrosis
   b. Ununited anconeal and coronoid processes
   c. Hip dysplasia
   d. Aseptic necrosis
   e. Hemarthrosis
3. Traumatic
4. Neoplastic
Inflammatory Joint Disease (Arthritis)
1. Infectious
2. Noninfectious (immunologic)
   a. Erosive
   b. Nonerosive

Physical Signs and Diagnostic Considerations

Osteoarthrosis refers to degenerative joint diseases, with the primary lesion being in the articular cartilage. The changes in the soft tissue are secondary. Most of the occurrences of osteoarthrosis seen in the dog are usually secondary to previous injury or insult to the joint tissue. The initial injury can be congenital in origin, for example, osteochondrosis of the shoulder, elbow, stifle, and back; failure of ossification centers to fuse, such as an ununited anconeal process; abnormal development of joints, as seen in hip dysplasia and patellar luxations; and deformities in conformation, placing undue pressure on joint surfaces such as coxa vara and valgus. Osteoarthrosis can result from a ligamentous injury, such as a ruptured anterior cruciate ligament, or secondary to an intra-articular fracture. The clinical signs associated with osteoarthrosis usually develop slowly and become progressively more severe with time. As the osteoarthrosis condition progresses, stiffness and lameness often appear after exercise. As the degree of degeneration becomes worse, stiffness and lameness are most prevalent following rest, and the animal may "warm out" of the joint pain. Cold weather may make the condition worse.

Radiographically, one or more of the following changes may be manifested: (1) narrowing of the joint space, (2) increased density of subchondral bone (sclerosis), (3) formation of spurs or lipping of the joint margins, (4) subluxation, (5) wearing away of subchondral bone, (6) remodeling of adjacent bone, and (7) intra- or periarticular calcification.

The diagnosis of degenerative joint disease (osteoarthrosis) is dependent on physical signs, palpation, radiography, and examination of synovial fluid. The degree of pain and discomfort of the affected animal is variable and does not always parallel the radiographic findings. Joints should be flexed and extended over their full range of motion to elicit pain, and muscles should be palpated to detect any evidence of atrophy. In the more chronic cases, an enlarged joint may be associated with increased synovial fluid, thickening of joint capsules, and osteophyte formation. Synovial fluid examination may be helpful in the prognosis (see p. 810).

Inflammatory joint disease is characterized by inflammation of the synovial membrane and changes in the synovial fluid along with signs of systemic illness such as fever, leukocytosis, depression, and increases in fibrinogen and gamma globulins.

Infectious arthritis can be associated with exogenous or endogenous infections. The presence of pus within the joint cavity is characteristic of suppurative arthritis. Nonsuppurative infectious arthritis can be associated with viral organisms, pleuropneumonia-like organisms (PPLO), and fungal organisms. Infectious arthritis results in thickening of the synovial membrane, distention of the joint capsule, and accumulation of exudate with widening of the joint space. Septic arthritis leads to the destruction of the articular cartilage, joint destruction, irregular joint surfaces, periarticular rarefaction, and fibrous or bony ankylosis.

In septic or infectious arthritis, the characteristics are pain; a warm, tender, swollen joint; and usually associated systemic signs, including fever. Synovial fluid examination is commonly diagnostic. Cellular examination of synovial fluid may indicate a large polymorphonuclear count of 80,000 to 200,000 per mm.

The noninfectious arthritides of dogs have been grouped into those disease entities that cause erosions on joint surfaces and those entities that are nonerosive. The erosive arthritides have been seen mainly in the small breeds of dogs, and the changes resemble rheumatoid arthritis as seen in man. Dogs with rheumatoid disease have multiple leg lameness and stiffness of the joints, especially in the morning. There is often generalized joint swelling and pain, intermittent fever, and peripheral lymphadenopathy. The diagnostic criteria for canine rheumatoid arthritis include: (1) morning stiffness, (2) pain on moving a joint, (3) soft-tissue swelling, (4) swelling of at least one other joint within a 3-month period, (5) symmetric joint swelling, (6) radiographic findings consistent with rheumatoid arthritis, (7) presence of rheumatoid factor (see p. 731), and (8) characteristic synovial histology. To make a confirmatory diagnosis of rheumatoid arthritis, any five of the just mentioned criteria must be present, and one of the first five signs in the list must be present for 5 or more weeks. The antinuclear antibody (ANA) and lupus erythematosus (LE) tests must be negative.

Rheumatoid arthritis in the dog can range, radiographically, from soft-tissue changes to marked bone changes involving the joints. Signs may include periarticular rarefaction and the appearance of coarse epiphyseal trabeculae; rarefaction of the subchondral bone plate and cancellous bone of the epiphysis, producing a rough irregular joint; and, in advanced cases, fibrous ankylosing of joints.

Confirmatory diagnosis is based on immunologic tests, radiography, and synovial fluid cytologic examination. Cytologic examination of synovial fluid may reveal an increase in nucleated cells, ranging from 3,000 to 38,000 per mm, with 20 to 80 per cent mononuclear cells and 20 to 80 per cent neutrophils.

Rheumatoid arthritis is associated with the deposition of immune complexes in the synovia of the joints. Development of autoantibodies to gamma globulin (IgG) is characteristic of the disease. These autoantibodies are called *rheumatoid factors* and are of the maternal gamma globulin (IgM) class. Rheumatoid factors can also be formed in other conditions in which extensive immune complex formation develops. (See p. 731 for the test to determine the rheumatoid factor.)

Lameness associated with arthritis can be a component in many systemic LE cases in the dog (see also p. 730). Dogs with systemic LE will exhibit multiple systemic signs, including lethargy, depression, fever, skin lesions, lymphadenopathy, hemolytic anemia, and thrombocytopenia.

A Coombs' test, ANA test, and LE prep should be carried out as part of the immunologic profile. The ANA test should be strongly positive.

Nonerosive arthritis has been seen with increasing frequency in dogs. The disease appears to be mediated by immunopathologic mechanisms. Joint inflammation usually involves the smaller, distal joints, particularly the carpus and tarsus. Systemic signs of illness may also be present and include cyclic fever, depression, generalized stiffness, and muscle atrophy. During periods of active arthritis, the joints are swollen and hot, fever is present, and leukocytosis is evident. Abnormalities in serum proteins may also be apparent. In most of these cases, no etiologic diagnosis can be established. During acute exacerbations of this disease, swelling and heat in the distal joints as well as generalized lymphadenopathy, are frequently seen. The results of routinely performed tests for immunologically mediated disease (e.g., LE test, ANA, or rheumatoid factor) are negative.

FELINE CHRONIC PROGRESSIVE POLYARTHRITIS

This proliferative periosteal polyarthritis occurs exclusively in male cats, and the common age of onset is 4.5 years. The disease is characterized by high fever, severe joint pain, stiffness in the carpal and tarsal joints, and regional lymphadenopathy. Radiographically, there is osteoporosis, and periosteal new bone formation, with joint enlargement and ankylosis. Feline syncytia–forming virus (FeSFV) is isolated from all cats with the disease, and feline leukemia virus (FeLV) is found in 70 per cent of affected cats. The incidence of FeSFV is two to four times greater in cats with chronic progressive polyarthritis than in the normal feline population, whereas the incidence of FeLV is 6 to 10 times greater than in the normal feline population. The joint disease has been described as being immunologically mediated. Aspiration of joint fluid reveals high numbers of PMNs and protein.

References and Additional Readings

Berzon, J.L.: A review of canine joint disease. Calif. Vet., 2:17, 1980.

Morgan, J. P.: Radiology of Skeletal Disease. Davis, California, Veterinary Radiologic Association, 1981.

Pederson, N. C.; Pool, R. R., and Morgan, J. P.: Joint diseases of dogs and cats. In Ettinger, S. J. (ed.): Textbook of Veterinary Internal Medicine, 2nd ed. Philadelphia, W. B. Saunders Company, 1983, Chap. 84, pp. 2187–2235.

Pederson, N. C., and Pool, R. R.: Canine joint disease. Vet. Clin. North Am., 8:465, 1978.

Pedersen, N. C., Pool, R. R., and O'Brien, T.: Feline progressive polyarthritis. Am. J. Vet. Res., 41:522, 1980.

Siemering, B.: Painful joints: a review of rheumatoid arthritis, systemic lupus erythematosus, infectious arthritis, and degenerative joint disease. Compendium on Continuing Education, 1:213, 1979.

ENLARGEMENT OF LYMPH NODES

The immune system includes lymphoid organs—namely, the thymus, lymph nodes, spleen, portions of the liver and bone marrow, and areas within the intestinal and respiratory tracts.

The primary role of the lymph node is to respond to a variety of antigenic stimuli. Lymph node hyperplasia can be associated with an increase in the number and size of lymphoid follicles, with proliferation of lymphocytes and reticuloendothelial cells or with infiltration of nodes by cells not normally present (e.g., tumor cells).

The lymphatic system can be involved in a variety of conditions, including: (1) metastatic spread of tumor growths, (2) infectious adenopathy, (3) infiltration by foreign substances, (4) primary hematopoietic disease, and (5) disturbance of metabolism.

Peripheral lymph nodes, such as anterior cervicals, precapsular, axillary, and popliteal, can be easily examined by palpation. The tonsils can be inspected. Difficulty arises when lymphadenopathy develops in those lymph nodes that cannot be routinely palpated, for example, intrathoracic, such as anterior mediastinal and hilar lymph nodes. Clinical signs such as dyspnea, cough, pleuritis, pleural effusion, and tracheal elevation may develop. Intra-abdominal lymph node enlargement may include mesenteric and iliac lymph nodes. The rapidity of enlargement and the consistency of the nodes, as well as associated systemic signs, are important in determining etiology.

Lymphadenopathy may result from neoplastic proliferation of abnormal lymphoid cells, spread of neoplastic tissue from a primary site to regional lymph node, or reactive lymphadenopathy secondary to bacterial, fungal, viral, or immunologically mediated diseases. Among those diseases resulting in lymphadenopathy *not* associated with lymphoid tumor formation are toxoplasmosis, ehrlichiosis, salmon poisoning, brucellosis, deep pyodermas with a

Table 51. DRAINAGE SITES OF THE PERIPHERAL LYMPH NODES OF THE DOG

Lymph Node	Drainage Site
Parotid	Cutaneous area of the posterior half of the dorsum of the muzzle, side of the cranium, external ears, temporomandibular joint, and parotid salivary gland.
Mandibular	The parts of the head not drained by the parotid. There is overlap with many of the areas drained by the parotid node.
Medial retropharyngeal	All deep structures of the head that have lymphatics (tongue and the walls of the various passages, salivary glands, and deep parts of external ear), larynx and esophagus, parotid and mandibular nodes.
Superficial cervical	Skin of the posterior part of the head, lateral surface of the neck, much of the front leg, shoulder and anterior part of the thoracic wall.
Axillary	Thoracic wall and deep structures of the thoracic limb, anterior mammary glands. There is often an anastomosis between the afferent lymphatics of this node and those of the superficial inguinal node.
Popliteal	All parts of the rear leg distal to the location of the node.
Superficial inguinal	Ventral half of the abdominal wall, posterior mammary glands. The penis, skin of the prepuce and scrotum, ventral part of the pelvis, tail, medial side of the thigh, stifle joint and popliteal node.

From Zinkl, H. G., and Keeton, K. S.: Lymph node cytology II. Calif. Vet., 33:6, 1979.

Table 52. CYTOLOGIC CLASSIFICATION OF
LYMPH NODE ASPIRATES

Classification	Cell Type
Normal	Predominantly mature pale and basophilic lymphocytes. Some lymphoblasts, plasma cells, macrophages. A few inflammatory cells.
Reactive	Mainly mature lymphocytes. A marked increase in basophilic lymphocytes and/or plasma cells. There may be an increase in macrophages. Often neutrophils, eosinophils, mast cells, and basophils will be increased.
Purulent	Many neutrophils that may be in various stages of degeneration. Macrophages are often increased. Mature lymphocytes may be prominent or markedly reduced, depending on the nature and extent of the neutrophilic reaction. Other inflammatory cells are usually present.
Mixed	Elements of both reactive and purulent nodes.
Neoplastic	
Primary	Blast cells of lymphocytic origin. Usually a pattern of large monomorphic, basophilic lymphoblast. Marked reduction in mature lymphocytes.
Metastatic	Tumor cells may be very rare or extremely abundant depending on the tumor type and the extent of the nodal involvement. The nodal cells will also vary in numbers. Often, metastatic tumors will elicit a reactive-type change in lymph nodes.

From Zinkl, H. G., and Keeton, K. S.: Lymph node cytology II. Calif. Vet., 33:6, 1979.

variety of bacterial organisms, systemic mycotic diseases, systemic lupus erythematosus (SLE), and immune mediated follicular hyperplasia—etiology unknown.

In active infections, enlarged lymph nodes are often firm and tender to the touch and the overlying skin may be warm, edematous, and erythematous. Enlarged lymph nodes associated with lymphoma are usually symmetrically enlarged, firm, immovable, and not painful.

Lymph nodes containing metastatic tumor tissues such as carcinoma are usually very hard, immovable, and well localized—being bound down to the surrounding tissue.

Primary hematopoietic disease may involve the lymphatic, the leukocytic, or the erythrocytic divisions of the hematopoietic system. Primary tumors of the lymph nodes are all malignant. Tumors may arise from the lymphoid and reticuloendothelial elements of the nodes or their derivatives.

Generalized Approach to the Animal with Lymphadenopathy

It is important to determine whether the lymphadenopathy is regional or generalized and associated with systemic disease. Physical examination, history, hematologic examination, lymph node biopsy, and radiographic examination will assist in making a diagnosis (Tables 51 and 52). Careful cytologic study of lymph node aspirate and toxoplasmosis or systemic fungal diseases or ehrlichiosis may be necessary (see p. 525). Bone marrow and liver biopsy may be needed.

Cats may develop lymphadenopathy secondary to abscesses induced by bite and fight wounds. Recently, lymphadenopathy, fever, and depression have been seen in cats infested with *Yersinia pestis*. This form of feline plaque was originally reported in New Mexico, and diagnosis was made by aspiration of lymph nodes and isolation of the organism. Sylvatic plaque is endemic in areas of the southwestern United States and cats with lymphadenopathy, high fever, and flea infestation are suspects. These cats should be immediately treated for flea infestation and isolated from contact with people until definitive diagnosis can be made. This can be a serious public health problem.

References and Additional Readings

Feldman, B., and Zinkl, J. G.: Diseases of the lymph nodes and spleen. *In* Ettinger, S. J. (ed.): Textbook of Veterinary Internal Medicine. 2nd ed., Philadelphia, W. B. Saunders Company, 1983, Chap. 79, pp. 2045–2076.

Weniger, B. G., et al.: Human bubonic plague transmitted by a domestic cat scratch. JAMA 251,(7):927, 1984.

PRURITUS

Pruritus, or itching, of the skin is an unpleasant or uneasy sensation that provokes the desire to scratch. Itch sensitivity is distributed to pinpoint spots on the skin, and their density correlates with similar numbers of pain spots. There are regional and individual differences in itch sensitivity. Both itch and pain sensation are thought to use a common nerve pathway. Itching is only elicited from the epidermis, dermis, and conjunctiva. Scratching may reduce itching by interrupting the rhythm of afferent impulses or by locally depleting kinins. Heat, cold, pain, and pressure may act in a similar manner or may affect spinal or higher centers.

Iggo reported that cutaneous pain receptors with nonmyelinated afferent fibers may be "itch" receptors. Stimulation of mechanoreceptors by rubbing affected skin may lower the animal's awareness of itching. This may occur by interaction in the lower spinal cord between excitation of pain receptors and inhibition of mechanoreceptors.

Itching is triggered by physical and clinical stimuli that generate polypeptide kinins through the activation of proteases.

Causes

Exogenous Factors

1. Allergic or irritant contactants (plants, soaps)
2. Ectoparasites, foreign bodies (awns, fiberglass)
3. Environmental factors (drying, matted hair, dirt)

Endogenous Factors

1. Drug reactions
2. Allergic (atopy, inhalants)
3. Psychogenic (from boredom or depression)
4. In man, many metabolic disorders, such as diabetes, jaundice, renal insufficiency, mastocytosis, leukemia, lymphoma malignancies, and thyroid abnormalities, produce itching; however, these disorders usually do not have a similar effect in animals.

Physical Signs

Excoriations, broken hair, worn nails, wheals, crusts, and bleeding may be seen with pruritus. In chronic pruritus, there may be areas of skin lichenification. Patients may rub, lick, and/or scratch at localized or general areas of the skin.

Diagnostic Considerations

Primary considerations in diagnosing pruritus are determining the date and nature of onset and establishing whether the itching is seasonal or nonseasonal. A careful inspection and skin test should be completed to eliminate exogenous factors such as parasites and fungi. The most common nonparasitic cause of pruritus in small animals is allergy, and attention should be directed toward a differential diagnosis of this entity.

References and Additional Readings

Iggo, A.: Itch receptors, and itch. Br. Vet. Derm. Newsletter, 8(2):3, 1983.

Moschella, S. L., Pillsbury, D. M., and Hurley, H. J., Jr.: Dermatology. Philadelphia, W. B. Saunders Company, 1975.

Muller, G. H., Kirk, R. W., and Scott, D. W.: Small Animal Dermatology. 3rd ed. Philadelphia, W. B. Saunders Company, 1983.

Medical Records and Special Systems Examination

Medical Records

MAKING THE DIAGNOSIS

Every new case is a challenge for diagnosis. Everything is keyed to the proper and complete answer of the question: What is wrong with the patient? Only when the question is answered can one plan the proper treatment and forecast the results with reasonable accuracy. Experienced clinicians often "eyeball" the patient, or arrive at possible diagnoses almost by intuition, but this approach to medicine is dangerous. Important, even vital, information is almost always missed.

One must collect and analyze clinical evidence methodically and accurately so that no diagnostic possibility is overlooked. Diagnosis necessitates two basic steps: (1) collecting the facts and (2) analyzing the facts.

The problem-oriented system of record keeping is based on a logical and systemized approach to history taking, physical examination and the recording of clinical data. The Problem-Oriented Medical Record (POMR) system involves four basic elements:

1. *The Data Base* may include chief complaint, patient profile, past history and systems review, physical examination, and initial laboratory results.
2. *The Problem List* itemizes each of the patient's problems in a numbered list.
3. *The Initial Plan* lists diagnostic and therapeutic orders for each problem. Information is keyed by a number corresponding to the original problem list.
4. *Progress Notes* are narrative notes, indicating how the patient is responding to treatment formulated under the initial plan. Progress notes are organized by numbers that correspond to the problems identified in the initial problem list. S-O-A-P is a mnemonic for the kinds of information that should be included in progress notes:
   S—Subjective data
   O—Objective data
   A—Assessment
   P—Plans

The POMR system allows for the replication of a medical record and enables more than one veterinarian to examine a medical record and make valid interpretations from it. One advantage in following a single, repeatable outline when performing a physical examination is that the clinician is less likely to omit a system from examination. When the clinician formulates the problem list at the level of refinement that he or she understands, there is less risk of missing a significant clinical problem; in addition, the clinician may begin to discern a disease profile for the animal.

Various levels of sophistication of the POMR system can be used depending on factors such as professional goals, economic factors, and size of practice. The POMR system provides a mechanism of thinking systematically about cases. Using the system requires some additional time, which must be equated with the economic necessities of the clinician's practice.

Data Base

Collecting the facts involves four steps: (1) obtaining a complete clinical history, (2) performing a thorough physical examination, (3) using ancillary methods for further evaluation (radiographs, laboratory data, endoscopy, etc.) and (4) observing the course of the illness.

The first three points will be discussed in the following pages. The fourth point, however, deserves comment here. In many cases, a diagnosis is not immediately evident, even after a careful case work-up. Patients may be hospitalized "for observation" or the patient may be seen at appropriate intervals, serial tests performed, and consultation with special colleagues arranged. As a disease progresses, more evidence becomes available, and eventually the diagnosis becomes a reality. There should be no stigma attached to delay in reaching a definitive diagnosis, but many veterinarians feel that there is; thus, they fail to use one of the most important aids to diagnosis: observing the course of the illness.

CLINICAL HISTORY

It requires skill to elicit an unbiased history of their pet's illness from most owners. Some owners are good observers and can supply important information, whereas others either do not notice things or may purposely withhold information. It is important to impress upon the owner how important it is that he or she help you help his or her pet. When talking to the pet owner, one should use a vocabulary commensurate with his or her intelligence, background, and formal education. Ask neutral questions—ones that will not prejudice his or her answers—such as, "Tell me about your dog's water consumption." Direct or leading questions can be asked provided that one realizes that bias may be introduced. Comments such as "Anything else?" "How do you mean?" or "Tell me about that" are helpful in inducing the owner to elaborate. Do not belittle the owner's opinion of the illness or its cause.

If the same sequence of history taking and physical examination is followed each time, the procedure gradually requires less time and important facts will not be glossed over or omitted.

The Chief Complaint (CC)

This is the reason the patient is being presented. What should be recorded is a sign (diarrhea), not a diagnosis (enteritis), that may have been made by the owner or another clinician. It is important to record the duration of the sign, for example, diarrhea for 3 months.

Present Illness (PI)

No exact description can be given because of the variety of presenting complaints. It is important, however, to record data in chronological sequence *by date*. Record the type of onset and possible exposure to other sick animals.

Determine whether other persons or animals have become infected by contact with the patient.

If the PI has progressed in attacks separated by intervals of good health, obtain a history of a typical attack (onset, duration, signs, and treatment). Both positive and negative data about disturbances to organic and systemic functions are important.

Past History (PH)

The past history of the animal should include whether it has experienced any of the following:
1. Infectious diseases: distemper, hepatitis, leptospirosis, panleukopenia, and pneumonitis.
2. Major illnesses: dates of infections or severe illness, treatment, complications, and sequelae.
3. Allergies: contact, atopy, and food and drug reactions.
4. Accidents.
5. Operations.
6. Pregnancies: number of offspring whelped and weaned from each delivery.
7. Immunizations: panleukopenia, pneumonitis, distemper, hepatitis, leptospirosis, rabies, and dates of immunization and the products used.

Kennel History

The animal's kennel history may be obscure, but information about the present health of the parents, siblings, and offspring may be of interest. Find out when and where the animal was born and raised; the environments it has been exposed to during travel and with different owners; whether it is a working animal or a house pet; and the kind of shelter, care, diet, grooming, and medications it routinely receives. Consider the person presenting the animal and providing the history; data obtained from very young or very old owners or by a nonowner may be unreliable.

Review of Systems (RS)

Questions pertaining to major regions of the body should be asked in order to detect illness in areas other than those covered in the PI and to ensure that certain unusual manifestations of the PI have not been omitted. Review the following structures and systems from front to rear:
1. *Head, eyes, ears, nose:* Look for signs of head tilt or shaking of the head, signs of blindness or deafness; a discharge from the eyes, ears, or nose; pain in the area.
2. *Mouth and throat:* Look for signs of abnormal salivation, dental problems, difficulty in swallowing, or change in voice.
3. *Skin and coat:* Look for evidence of scratching, loss of hair, types of skin lesions, patterns of affected skin involvement, seasonal incidence, and progression of severity.

4. *Cardiopulmonary:* Look for evidence of dyspnea at rest or upon exertion, cough, wheezing, gagging, cyanosis, edema, ascites, or fainting.
5. *Gastrointestinal:* Determine whether the animal's appetite, digestion, and bowel movements are normal. Question the owner about the incidence of vomiting, diarrhea, type of stool, constipation, abdominal pain, and food idiosyncrasies or allergies.
6. *Genitourinary:* Examine the animal for, or ask the owner about, urinary frequency, water consumption, presence of dysuria, hematuria, and incontinence, regularity of the estrous cycle, and breeding dates and results. Find out whether the animal has been neutered and, if so, when.
7. *Neurologic:* Look for indications of nervousness, seizures, dispositional change, changes in sensory or motor functions, neurologic reflexes, or paralysis.
8. *Locomotor:* Look for evidence of bone or joint swelling, joint pain, stiffness or restricted joint motion, or weakness.
9. *Endocrine:* Check for previous evidence of abnormal functioning of the thyroid, adrenal, gonadal, pituitary, and pancreatic glands. Determine loss of hair and appetite, and polyuria.

ROUTINE PHYSICAL EXAMINATION

Record pertinent findings, both normal and abnormal, in a systematic manner (Figs. 13 and 14). Small animals are usually placed on a table in a well-lighted, quiet room, and the examination is carried out with care and gentleness. The owner should be present to calm and restrain the animal and to answer questions (Tables 53 and 54).

A routine physical examination should include determining the state of the following:
1. *Vital signs:* temperature, pulse, respiration, and weight.
2. *General appearance:* conformity, state of nutrition, apparent age, degree of grooming care, type of disposition, mental alertness, gross deformities, striking findings (e.g., severe dyspnea, weakness, and depression).
3. *Skin:* Inspect and palpate. Note the color, texture, degree of moisture or oil present, amount, texture and distribution of hair, pattern of alopecias, ease of epilation, presence of parasites, and types and distribution of primary and secondry skin lesions.
4. *Lymph nodes:* Palpate all superficial nodes and the spleen. Note enlargement, consistency, mobility, and pain.
5. *Eyes:* Examine the conjunctiva and sclera for injection, exudation, and petechia. Elicit the pupillary reflex. Perform an ophthalmoscopic examination (cornea, iris, lens, and retina).
6. *Ears:* Look for discharge and perform an otoscopic examination for exudates or parasites. Note the appearance of the tympanic membranes.
7. *Nose:* Look for evidence of discharge and patency.
8. *Mouth and throat:* Smell the breath, note any discharges or excess saliva, and observe the color and appearance of mucous membranes, the pharynx, and the tonsils.

PEDIATRIC DEFINED MINIMUM DATA BASE

Owner_____ Breed_____ Name_____ Sex_____ Age_____ Date_____

Well Animal Care_____ Acute Illness_____ Other_____

Chief Complaint_____

PATIENT PROFILE—In House_____ % Outside_____ % Fenced_____ Chained_____ Loose_____

HISTORY_____

PHYSICAL EXAMINATION—Temperature_____   DESCRIBE THE ABNORMAL

(1) GENERAL APPEARANCE	☐ Normal ☐ Abnormal	Weight _____pounds _____ounces Body condition N Thin Fat Breed conformation
(2) INTEGU-MENTARY	☐ Normal ☐ Abnormal	Hair coat condition N Alopecia Ectoparasites Dehydration
(3) MUSCULO-SKELETAL	☐ Normal ☐ Abnormal	Gait N Abn Position of head and neck Observe Walking N Abn
(4) CIRCULATORY	☐ Normal ☐ Abnormal	Auscultate heart N Abn Palpate heart N Abn Pulse N Abn
(5) RESPIRATORY	☐ Normal ☐ Abnormal	Auscultate lung fields R L Presence of cough Yes No
(6) DIGESTIVE	☐ Normal ☐ Abnormal	Appetite Diet Vomiting Mouth Teeth Tonsils Tongue Palpate abd Liver Bladder Spleen Intestines Anal area
(7) GENITO-URINARY	☐ Normal ☐ Abnormal	Drinking water Dysuria Housebreaking Female: Vulva Perineal area Nipples Male: Sheath Penis Scrotum Testicles R L Hernias Umbilical Inguinal
(8) EYES	☐ Normal ☐ Abnormal	Eyelids: Entropion Ectropion Distichiasis Epiphora Cornea: Color Laceration Ulceration Pigment Lens: N Abn
(9) EARS	☐ Normal ☐ Abnormal	Pinna wounds Canal open Ear mites
(10) NEURAL SYSTEM	☐ Normal ☐ Abnormal	Disposition N Aggressive Shy Biter Reflexes: Seizures Loss of consciousness
(11) LYMPH NODES	☐ Normal ☐ Abnormal	Cervical N Abn
(12) MUCOUS MEMBRANES	☐ Normal ☐ Abnormal	Color N Pale Icteric Injected Cyanotic

PROBLEM LIST (TEMPORARY) PLAN	DIAGNOSTIC PLANS	THERAPEUTIC PLANS	CLIENT ED.
(1)_____			
(2)_____			
(3)_____			
(4)_____			

Figure 13. Pediatric-defined minimum data base. (From Saidla, J. E.: The problem-oriented veterinary medical record. *In* Ettinger, S. J. (ed.): Textbook of Veterinary Internal Medicine, 2nd ed. Philadelphia, W. B. Saunders Company, 1983.)

ADULT DEFINED MINIMUM DATA BASE

Date_____

OWNER_____ Breed_____ Name_____ Sex_____ Age_____

Annual Physical Exam_____ Routine PE_____ Chronic Condition_____ Acute Illness_____

CHIEF COMPLAINT_____

PATIENT PROFILE—In house_____ % Outside_____ % Fenced_____ Chained_____ Loose_____

HISTORY_____

PHYSICAL EXAMINATION		T_____ WT_____	DESCRIBE THE ABNORMAL
(1) GENERAL APPEARANCE	☐ Normal ☐ Abnormal	Body condition N Thin Overweight Weight change Inc Dec Observe walking N Abn	
(2) INTEGU-MENTARY	☐ Normal ☐ Abnormal	Hair coat condition Alopecia Dehydration Skin Lesions Tumors Ectoparasites Toe nails Dewclaws Anal glands	
(3) MUSCULO-SKELETAL	☐ Normal ☐ Abnormal	Gait N Abn Position of head and neck N Abn Joint palpation Neck-head RF LF RR LR Tail	
(4) CIRCULATORY	☐ Normal ☐ Abnormal	Pulse /min Character Heart Palpable thrill Arrhythmia Sounds N Abn Murmur Cough Nocturnal	
(5) RESPIRATORY	☐ Normal ☐ Abnormal	Respirations /min Nasal discharge Cough Dyspnea Insp. Expir. R lung field Dry Moist L lung field Dry Moist	
(6) DIGESTIVE	☐ Normal ☐ Abnormal	Halitosis Appetite Mouth Teeth Tonsils Salivary glands Vomiting Diarrhea Abdominal palpation: Colon Small Intestine Spleen Liver Stools Freq Color Consistency Parasites Hooks Rounds Whips Tapes Protoz.	
(7) GENITO-URINARY	☐ Normal ☐ Abnormal	Water intake inc dec N Urine production inc dec N Dysuria Palpate Bladder Kidneys R L Male Penis Sheath Scrotum Testicles Prostate Female Vulva Vag. secretions Pseudocyesis Last estrus Last litter Difficulty whelping Breasts Swollen Masses Nipple disch	
(8) EYES	☐ Normal ☐ Abnormal	Eye lids N Distichiasis Epiphora Harderian gland Sclera N Injection Icterus Cornea N Ulcer Laceration Keratitis Pupils N Equal Unequal Light reactive Lens N Cataract Lenticular sclerosis	
(9) EARS	☐ Normal ☐ Abnormal	Pinna N Carriage Hairloss Wounds Lesions Canal N Wax Infection Mites Hair Hears sound Deaf	
(10) NEURAL SYSTEM	☐ Normal ☐ Abnormal	Disposition History of head trauma Hx back pain Disc syndrome Seizures Loss of consciousness	
(11) LYMPH NODES	☐ Normal ☐ Abnormal	Cervical N Abn Axillary N Abn Popliteal N Abn Mesenteric N Abn	
(12) MUCOUS MEMBRANES	☐ Normal ☐ Abnormal	Color Pink Pale Cyanotic Icteric Injected Oral Conjuctival	

PROBLEM LIST (TEMPORARY) PLAN	DIAGNOSTIC PLANS	THERAPEUTIC PLANS	CLIENT ED.
(1)_____			
(2)_____			
(3)_____			
(4)_____			

Figure 14. This is an example of an adult minimum data base and can be modified to suit the individual practitioner's needs. (From Saidla, J. E.: The problem-oriented veterinary medical record. *In* Ettinger, S. J. (ed.): Textbook of Veterinary Internal Medicine, 2nd. ed. Philadelphia, W. B. Saunders Company, 1983.)

Table 53. GENERAL PRIORITIES FOR CLINICAL EVALUATION

Collect Information
   Define data to be collected.
   Follow written protocol on all patients.
Define Problem
   Refine to highest degree of refinement.
   Do not overstate problems.
Formulate Diagnostic Plans
   Verification of problem.
      Especially important for historical problems such as hematuria, polyuria, and
         dysuria.
      Of significance for transient or intermittent problems.
   Localization of problem to body systems or organs.
   Consider probable causes.
      Pathophysiology (D-A-M-N I-T; see Table 54)
      Specific causes.
Formulate Prognosis
Formulate Therapeutic Plans
   Specific
   Supportive
   Symptomatic
   Palliative
Formulate Follow-Up Plans

From Osborne, C. A., and Finco, D. R.: Diagnostic procedures in urology: use and misuse. Proc. A.A.H.A, 1978.

Table 54. D-A-M-N I-T ACRONYM OF PATHOPHYSIOLOGY

        D— Degenerative disorders
        A — Anomalies
           — Auto immunity
        M— Metabolic disorders
        N — Neoplasia
           — Nutritional disorders
        I — Inflammation (infectious or noninfectious)
           — Immune disorders
           — Iatrogenic disorders
           — Idiopathic disorders
        T — Toxicity (endogenous or exogenous)
           — Trauma (external or internal)

Modified from Osborne, C. A.: The transition of quality patient care from an art to a science; the problem-oriented concept. J.A.A.H.A., *11*:250, 1975.

9. *Neck and back:* Assess the extent of rigidity or limitation of motion, deformities, and pain.

10. *Thorax:* Evaluate for conformity, symmetry, and free respiratory movements. Percuss and auscultate systematically from the dorsal to the ventral aspects.

11. *Heart:* Palpate, noting the intensity of apex beat and the presence of thrills. Evaluate rate, rhythm, quality of sounds, bruits, or rubs. Record auscultated heart rate and femoral pulse rate if they are different. Carefully auscultate all four valvular areas.

12. *Abdomen:* Determine the conformity, symmetry, masses, gases, fluids, rigidity, or "splinting." Auscultate for peristalsis and palpate deeply.

13. *Genitalia:* In the male, palpate and inspect the testes and penis; in the female, palpate and inspect the vulva and the mammary glands.

14. *Rectum:* Palpate the confines of the pelvic canal; check the prostate for size, conformity, and consistency.

15. *Extremities:* Watch the animal walk. Inspect and palpate the legs and joints. Note the presence of pain, heat, swelling, deformities, or limitation of motion.

16. *Neurologic:* Watch the animal walk. From dorsal recumbency, allow it to right itself and perform coordinated tasks. Palpate muscles and compare tonus and balance with opposite numbers. Check tendon reflexes and sensory responses.

ROUTINE LABORATORY PROCEDURES

Although more testing may be needed in many cases, the screening tests described here are usually done as part of a complete physical examination.

Blood (See p. 671)

Erythrocyte sedimentation rate, packed cell volume, and occasionally a complete blood count (CBC) are done. In older patients, a BUN is routine.

Urine (See p. 812)

Routine urinalysis, including a specific gravity, pH, protein, glucose, and sediment examination are routinely carried out.

Feces (See p. 798)

Analyze for the presence of parasites and for occult blood if indicated. The latter may be misleading, because animals on high meat diets may have mild positive test results.

Problem List

The problem list can be considered as a table of contents listing all the animal's problems, past as well as present. Many problem lists in veterinary medicine are being organized to also include a vaccination history. The problem statements should be formulated according to the level of the clinician describing the problem. Problems may include a diagnosis, a physiologic finding, a sign that may correlate with a physiologic finding, or an abnormal laboratory finding. Single problems that turn out to be manifestations of a particular disease may be grouped together. There are four levels of problem refinement: (1) unqualified clinical finding, (2) reproducible diagnostic finding, (3) pathophysiologic finding, and (4) diagnostic entity. Problems should be defined to their highest state and diagnostic entities should be identified where evidence exists.

Initial Plan

The initial plan is arranged so that information concerning the possible diagnosis and management of a particular problem is keyed to the problem list by number. For each problem, there should be: (1) plans for the collection of further data in order to establish a diagnosis or facilitate management, (2) plans for treatment with specific drugs, and (3) plans to educate the owner of the animal about existing problems. The plans should be dated when initiated, and the goals of therapeutic plans should be stated briefly.

Progress Notes

The progress notes are the follow-up mechanism for a problem. It is necessary to carefully evaluate each aspect of the treatment plan and to note this assessment in the record. Progress notes should reflect the problem list, and each progress note should be numbered to correspond to the problem list. The following information should be included in the progress notes:

1. *Subjective data* should include all the information regarding signs manifested by the animal as observed by the clinician or other people who have contact with the animal. (Because animals cannot talk, much of this data is objective.)
2. *Objective data* should include all the ancillary testing procedures being used in the management of the animal.
3. *Assessment* should include an analysis by the clinician of the present status of the animal based on subjective and objective data and the animal's response to the treatment plan.
4. *Immediate plans* should include notes that establish a treatment plan for the individual problems. Plans for further diagnostic and laboratory work are also recorded here.

References and Additional Readings

Osborne, C. A.: The problem-oriented medical system. Symposium on practice management. Vet. Clin. North Am., *13*(4):745, 1983.

Saidla, J. E.: Problem-oriented veterinary medical record. *In* Ettinger, S. J. (ed.): Textbook of Veterinary Internal Medicine, 2nd ed, Philadelphia, W. B. Saunders Company, 1983.

Saidla, J. E., Jeffrey, K. L., Lorenz, M. D., et al: Medical Records Manual. South Bend, Indiana, American Animal Hospital Association, 1978.

Special Systems Examination ─────────

ALIMENTARY SYSTEM

Diseases of the gastrointestinal tract are common afflictions of small animals. Careful examination with a systematic approach is necessary in order to evaluate the alimentary system completely. History taking and acquiring answers to the following questions are extremely important:

1. What is the duration of the clinical illness?
2. What is the dog's vaccination history?
3. Where did the dog come from and what is its travel history?
4. Is vomiting part of the syndrome, and what is the relationship to eating? Is it projectile?
5. What is the diet? Is the appetite affected? What is the sequential relationship of the gastrointestinal abnormality to the dog's eating pattern?
6. Has the dog been examined for endoparasites?
7. Have any treatments already been instituted?
8. Has the animal had previous illness or surgery? Is the animal losing weight?

If diarrhea is present, eliciting answers to the following questions may be helpful in localizing the cause (see pp. 247–256):

1. How many stools are there each day?
2. What is the quantity of each stool?
3. Is blood or mucus present in the stool?
4. Is there flatulence?
5. Does the stool smell peculiar or offensive?
6. Is tenesmus present?
7. Is the diarrhea projectile?

Before proceeding to examination of specific areas of the alimentary system, carefully observe the general physical status of the animal, particularly noting any evidence of emaciation, abdominal enlargement or asymmetry, the position of the animal at rest, and body carriage while moving (tucked up abdomen, stiffness, and so forth).

ORAL EXAMINATION

In most animals, a routine examination of the mouth can be done without anesthesia or tranquilization. Gently retract the lips and examine the teeth and gums (see also pp. 323–327).

Dentition in the Dog (Habel)

Formula for deciduous dentition: $2 \left(\text{Di} \frac{3}{3} \text{ Dc} \frac{1}{1} \text{ Dm} \frac{3}{2} \right) = 26$

Formula for permanent dentition: $2 \left(\text{I} \frac{3}{3} \text{ C} \frac{1}{1} \text{ PM} \frac{4}{4} \text{ M} \frac{2}{3} \right) = 42$

(See Table 55 and Fig. 15.)

It is possible to estimate the age of dogs up to 10 years of age by examining their teeth. Remember that dogs with over- or undershot jaws or dogs that chew excessively on rocks or bones will not reflect a normal dental wear pattern.

At 5 months, permanent incisors have erupted. Third incisor is not yet in wear.

At 6 months, permanent canines have erupted.

At 1½ years, cusp has been worn off lower first incisor.

At 2½ years, cusp has been worn off lower second incisor.

At 3½ years, cusp has been worn off upper first incisor.

At 4½ years, cusp has been worn off upper second incisor.

At 5 years, cusp of lower third incisor is slightly worn; wearing surface of lower first and second incisors is rectangular. Canines are slightly worn.

At 6 years, cusp has been worn off lower third incisor. Canines are now blunt. Lower canines show impression of upper third incisor.

Table 55. ERUPTION DATES OF DECIDUOUS AND PERMANENT TEETH (DOG)

Deciduous		Permanent	
Di1	4–5 weeks	I1	4–5 months
Di2	4–5 weeks	I2	4–5 months
Di3	5–6 weeks	I3	4–5 months
Dc	3–4 weeks	C	5–6 months
Dm2	4–6 weeks	PM1	4–5 months
Dm3	4–6 weeks	PM2	5–6 months
Dm4	6–8 weeks	PM3	5–6 months
		PM4	5–6 months
		M1	4–5 months
		M2	5–6 months
		M3	6–7 months

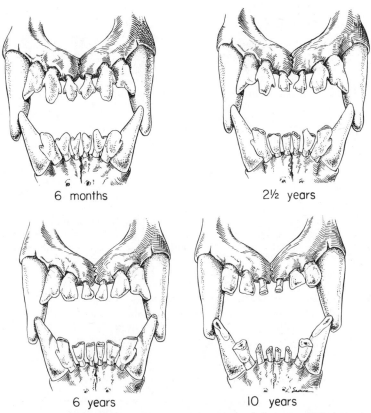

6 months

2½ years

6 years

10 years

Figure 15. Canine dentition at various ages. (From Habel, R. E.: Applied Veterinary Anatomy. Ithaca, New York, published by the author, 1973.)

At 7 years, lower first incisor has been abraded to the root, so that wearing surface is elliptical and the long axis is in a sagittal plane.

At 8 years, wearing surface of lower first incisor is inclined forward.

At 10 years, lower second and upper first incisors have elliptical wearing surfaces.

At 16 years, incisors are gone.

At 20 years, canines are gone.

Dentition in the Cat

Formula for deciduous dentition: $2 \left(\text{Di} \frac{3}{3} \text{ Dc} \frac{1}{1} \text{ Dm} \frac{3}{2} \right) = 26$

Formula for permanent dentition: $2 \left(\text{I} \frac{3}{3} \text{ C} \frac{1}{1} \text{ PM} \frac{3}{2} \text{ M} \frac{1}{1} \right) = 30$

(See Table 56.)

Examine the teeth for caries, faulty enamel, exposure of roots, deposition of tartar, periodontitis, and loose, crooked, or sharp-edged teeth. Determine the apposition of the upper and lower jaws for prognathism (undershot jaw) or brachygnathism (overshot jaw).

The normal oral mucosa is pink or partially pigmented, depending on the breed of animal. Discharge from the mouth is usually not evident.

Examine the gums for color; petechiae or gross hemorrhage; hypertrophy or recession of the gums; any discharge around the base of the teeth; or any inflammation, swelling, or growth. Examine the hard palate for the presence of foreign bodies, an oronasal fistula, or palatoschisis. Inflammation of the mucous membranes of the mouth is referred to as stomatitis and can be associated with a variety of primary pathogens, as well as being secondary to systemic diseases. Stomatitis may be associated with plant foreign bodies; uremia; diabetes mellitus; heavy metal poisoning (such as thallium); viral infections (especially those of the respiratory system in the cat); mycotic infections associated with *Candida albicans (Monilia)*; and chemical, thermal, or electrical burns.

Table 56. ERUPTION DATES OF DECIDUOUS AND
PERMANENT TEETH (CAT)

Deciduous		Permanent	
Di1	2–3 weeks	I1	3½–4 months
Di2	2–4 weeks	I2	3½–4 months
Di3	3–4 weeks	I3	4–4½ months
Dc	3–4 weeks	C	5 months
Dm2 (upper)	8 weeks	PM2 (upper)	4½–5 months
Dm3	4–5 weeks	PM3	5–6 months
Dm4	4–6 weeks	PM4	5–6 months
		M1	4–5 months

Tooth Terminology

Crown— Portion above the gum line and covered by enamel.

Neck— Constriction of the tooth located at the gum line where the enamel ends and the dentin covered by cementum begins.

Root— Portion below the gum line.

Apex— Most terminal portion of the root.

Apical delta— Very small openings found at the apex allowing the nerves and vessels of the tooth to enter.

Enamel— Outer covering of the crown; very shiny, hard substance. It is the hardest substance in the body and is made up of less than 5 per cent of organic material.

Dentin— Dense, bony-like material underlying the enamel and making up the substance of the tooth. It can be sensitive to heat and cold and is made up of 26 to 28 per cent of organic material.

Cementum—Layer of bony tissue that covers the root of the tooth and is attached to the alveolar bone by the periodontal ligament fibers.

Pulp— The soft tissues of the tooth: the nerves, which contain sensory fibers only, and the vessels coming in through the apical delta extending through the length of the tooth in the root canals.

Record Forms

As all medical disciplines, dentistry has its special forms. Diagnostic and therapeutic procedures should be carefully recorded. Figure 16 is an example of an appropriate dental record form.

Formation of Teeth

Each tooth has four surfaces: the labial surface is next to the lips; the lingual surface is next to the tongue, the occlusal surface or masticatory surface is the surface that meets the opposite tooth during mastication; and the contact surface is the surface between the teeth.

The teeth of small animals are fully developed (erupted) into their adult form by the time that the animal is 6 to 7 months of age. Teeth have both an epithelial and a mesenchymal precursor. Cells that produce the enamel of the tooth are called *ameloblasts*. The enamel organ of the developing tooth is in the shape of a crown, and the columnar cells lying next to the ameloblast are the odontoblast cells that produce the dentin of the tooth. The nerves and vessels are in the center of the tooth.

The deciduous teeth are replaced with permanent teeth starting between 2 and 3 months of age. If the deciduous teeth are not replaced by permanent teeth, the retained deciduous teeth cause crowding and displacement of the permanent canines. Basically, no two teeth can reside in one location at the same time. When looking at canine incisors, the deciduous teeth are to the outside of the permanent teeth; in the upper canine, the deciduous tooth is

DENTAL RECORD

Date _____

Owners Name	Breed	Patients Name	Age	Sex

Chief Complaint: _____

Patient Profile _____

Previous
Dental Treatment _____

History _____

Diet _____

Physical Examination

1. Skull Type   A. Brachycephalic   2. Malocclusion   A. Dental   3. Halitosis
               B. Mesaticephalic   B. Brachyonathia
               C. Dolichocephalic   C. Prognathia

4. Salivary Flow   A. Norm   5. Tonsils   A. R   6. Submaxillary LN   A. R
                B. Dry   B. L   B. L

7. Gingivitis   8. Plaque   9. Calculus   A. Supragingival   10. Periodontal Disease
                                           B. Subgingival

11. Exposed Roots   12. Loose Teeth   13. Fractured Teeth   14. Deep Periodontal Sulci

15. Gingival Recession   16. Osseous Recession   17. Caries   18. Heart   19. Kidneys

Anatomical Location

R   UPPER   L   L   LOWER   R   R   UPPER   L   L   LOWER   R
              FELINE   CANINE

Treatment

	Date	Comments	Date	Comments	Date	Comments
Scaling						
Polishing						
Root Planning						
Subgingival Curettage						
Gingivectomy						
Medication						
Extraction						
Oral Hygiene						
Brushing						
Oral Rinse						
Antibiotics						
Diet Alteration						

Figure 16. Dental record form. (From John E. Saidla, D.V.M.; Auburn, Alabama. Used with permission.)

caudal, and in the lower canine it is lateral to the permanent tooth. Deciduous premolars are found lateral to the permanent teeth. Retained deciduous teeth should be surgically removed if they are not loose and ready to come out.

Defects of Teeth

The major malocclusion defects that are inherited are brachygnathism and prognathism. In brachygnathism, the upper jaw is longer than the lower. In prognathism, the mandible is longer than the maxilla. This condition is normal for brachycephalic breeds, including boxers, bulldogs, and Pekingese. The problem in nonbrachycephalic breeds results when the lower canines are in front of the upper incisors, resulting in improper mastication and trauma to the teeth.

Supernumerary teeth in the maxilla are usually located behind the permanent teeth and result in crowding of the dental arcade. These supernumerary teeth should be extracted.

Staining of deciduous teeth can occur when tetracyclines are administered to pregnant female dogs during gestation. The deciduous teeth are stained yellow. Tetracyclines administered to young dogs during the development and eruption of permanent teeth will result in staining of permanent teeth. The use of tetracyclines should be avoided in pregnant bitches and young puppies.

Enamel hypoplasia develops when the ameloblasts are affected during the formation of the teeth. Systemic diseases associated with an epithiliotropic virus such as distemper can result in this condition. The enamel is easily broken in these cases, and the underlying dentin becomes stained. If focal areas of enamel are damaged, the areas can be acid etched and sealed with acrylics. More severe lesions may require dental caps to cover the diseased teeth and to protect them from further decay.

Dental calculus and associated periodontal disease are the most common conditions for which small animals are presented with oral disease. These animals have halitosis, loose teeth, and oral pain and are unable to chew food properly.

Calculus formation begins as plaque, which is an accumulation of soft-tissue debris, bacteria, and bacterial by-products mixed with salivary secretions. The build-up of plaque results in dental calculus. Small breeds of dogs and animals on soft diets tend to develop excessive dental calculus. Calculus is a yellowish brown, hard mineral material that adheres to the tooth surface. The progressive build-up of calculus along with other factors such as calcium/phosphorus balance and bacterial infection leads to periodontal disease. In periodontal disease, there is gum recession, loosening of the periodontal ligament, loosening of the teeth, and loss of alveolar bone. Foul mouth odor, pain, and inability to properly chew result.

Abscessed Teeth

Abscessed teeth are usually associated with advanced periodontal disease. The following signs may indicate a tooth abscess: (1) a loose tooth, (2) pain on chewing or manipulation of the tooth, (3) purulent discharge in periodontal pockets around the tooth, (4) radiographic evidence of lucency around the tooth root, and (5) recession of alveolar bone away from the neck of the tooth.

Abscess of a tooth may produce an oronasal fistula when the maxillary canines are involved or a fistula draining tract below the eye when the root of the carnassial tooth is involved (upper fourth premolar). Carnassial teeth are used to chew on hard objects, resulting in chipping of the crown and pulp exposure, periodontal disease, or root damage.

Treatment for abscessed teeth is surgical extraction, flushing of the sockets, and systemic antibiotics.

Extractions

Teeth should be extracted when they are loose, split below the gum, or abscessed, secondary to periodontal disease; when there is severe root exposure; or when there are retained deciduous or supernumerary teeth. Dental extractions should be carried out under general anesthesia or sedation with neuroleptanalgesia. The following items are needed:

1. Sterile pan with saline, gauze sponges, cotton tips, and 5 per cent iodine tincture.
2. Several sizes of root elevators.
3. A dental crown extractor with one size whose tips meet to extract the incisors.
4. A molar splitter or cutting disc.

The basic technique in dental extraction is that the tooth is pushed from the dental socket by means of a dental elevator. The following procedures should be used.

1. Separate the collar of gingival tissue or gum from around the tooth by using a scalpel; then insert an appropriate-sized dental elevator between the surface of the tooth and the adjacent bone. Keep the shaft of the dental elevator parallel with the long axis of the tooth. Loosen the periodontal ligament fibers around the entire tooth. The tooth should be made loose in the dental socket. When the tooth is completely loose, it can be elevated by a crown extractor.
2. The root tip of the tooth should not be left behind in the bony socket. *Do not* twist the dental extractors in an attempt to remove the tooth; this may result in fracturing the jaw.
3. When teeth have multiple roots, such as the fourth upper premolar, the crown should be split between the roots. This can be done with either a molar splitter (if sharp) or a rotating cutting disc. Each root is then elevated and extracted separately.
4. Extraction of the canine tooth presents special problems. Incise the gum tissue on the labial side down to the alveolar bone and gently move the gum away from the side wall of the alveolar bone with a periosteal elevator. Use a dental cutting bar to cut the buccal cortical plate. Cut out a plate of bone about two thirds the depth of the root. Place an elevator in the grooves on both sides of the tooth, and break the periodontal fibers. Extract the

loosened tooth using forceps. Suture the flap of gum closed using polyglycolic acid suture. *Do not* lever the canine tooth laterally, because this rotates the tip of the root medially, forcing the root through the bone into the nasal cavity.
5. Following extraction, the exposed dental socket should be irrigated with sterile saline and wiped out with iodine and sterile cotton–tipped pledgets.

Prophylaxis

Dental prophylaxis is necessary to control calculus formation and periodontal disease. The following points are important in dental prophylaxis:
1. Removal of dental calculus requires general anesthesia or neuroleptanalgesia. The animal should be intubated and the head placed in a downward position so that water drains away from the pharynx.
2. Heavy dental calculus can be initially "chipped" off the tooth surface carefully with a dental crown extractor.
3. The mouth should then be cleansed using a physiologic saline solution.
4. The mouth is held open with a moveable mouth gag attached to the canine teeth.
5. Additional dental plaque and calculus can be removed with an ultrasonic scaler whose tip is water cooled. The tip of the scaler is moved along the tooth and not concentrated in one location; the latter may produce etching of the tooth. Do not concentrate the scaler on any tooth for more than 10 to 15 seconds at a time.
6. Wear rubber gloves and a face mask during ultrasonic scaling.
7. The scaler can be used to carefully débride affected root surfaces below the gingiva.
8. Hand scaling can be used to supplement ultrasonic scaling and to reach periodontal pockets. The following hand scalers and curettes have been found to work well in veterinary dentistry: Goldman Fox Universal Scaler, Gracey 11–12, and Gracey 13–14 Curettes.
9. When the teeth have been cleaned, they can be polished using a power-driven dental drill, a prophylactic attachment with rubber prophylactic cups, and dental pumice. The prophylactic cup should be moved rapidly along the tooth to avoid heat build-up. Polishing eliminates dental defects and surface roughness, which cause rapid reformation of plaque and accumulation of calculus.

The Tongue

Examine the tongue for the presence of any abnormal discoloration, membrane or pseudomembrane, foreign bodies, inflammation, ulcers, or growth. Note whether the tongue protrudes normally and whether both halves are bilaterally symmetrical. The underside of the tongue should be examined for ulcers, foreign bodies such as string wrapped around the base of the tongue (in cats), and swelling of the lingual frenulum.

Palate, Pharynx, and Buccal Mucosae

The ability of the animal to swallow effectively should be tested by stimulating the pharyngeal area. Dysphagia refers to difficulty in swallowing and can be associated with localized diseases of the oropharynx or central nervous system diseases (CNS) (see pp. 256–258).

Careful examination of the palate, pharynx, and cheeks requires sedation or a short-acting anesthetic. A focal source of illumination and a tongue depressor or laryngoscope are also needed. Culturing material (see p. 499) and a biopsy of tissue may be done to obtain useful information.

Retropharyngeal tumors or abscesses may produce a ventral displacement of the pharynx and larynx. Careful digital exploration of the retropharyngeal area may reveal an undiagnosed mass. Fractures of the hyoid bone may occasionally occur, leading to difficulty in swallowing. Palpation of the posterior pharyngeal area may reveal crepitus and swelling. Inspiratory stridor in brachycephalic breeds of dogs is often associated with an elongated soft palate, weakened laryngeal cartilages, and evagination of the laryngeal ventricles.

Squamous cell carcinoma, malignant melanoma, and fibrosarcoma are the most common oral and pharyngeal neoplasms. Thoracic radiographs should always be taken to check for lung metastases. Todoroff and Brodey (1979) have reported a necropsy study in which 81 per cent of malignant melanomas, 77 per cent of tonsillar squamous cell carcinomas, and 35 per cent of fibrosarcomas had metastasized to or beyond regional lymph nodes.

Tonsils

Inspect the oral mucous membranes for changes in color, hemorrhage, inflammation, abrasions, ulceration, abnormal discharges, membranes or pseudomembranes, and abnormal growths. The tonsils should be examined for size, color, and consistency; the surrounding tissue should be examined for any abnormality. Conclusive diagnosis of the cause of tonsillar enlargement may depend on the results of a biopsy. Examine the uvula and note its length. Foreign bodies may lodge at the opening of the posterior nares, and the uvula must be pulled down and forward and the posterior nares visualized. Examine the hard and soft palate with a dental mirror for the presence of tumors or foreign bodies. Fractures of the hard palate are frequently seen in cats that fall from high elevations.

Odors

Smell the breath. Mouth odors may be caused by bad teeth, ulcerations of the lip folds or the mucous membranes, and tonsillitis. Uremia produces an ammoniacal odor; diabetic ketosis, a smell of acetone; and suppurative conditions of the lungs, a putrid odor.

EXAMINATION OF THE ESOPHAGUS

The esophagus starts in the posterior pharynx dorsal to the cranial portion of the trachea and continues in a caudal direction slightly dorsal and to the left of the trachea to the thoracic inlet. Just caudal to the thoracic inlet, the esophagus becomes more ventral in position and further to the left of the trachea. At the base of the heart, the esophagus is dorsal to the bifurcation of the trachea. The esophagus then continues caudally to the diaphragm and empties into the fundus of the stomach.

Examination of the esophagus depends on the use of either a gastroscope or radiographic techniques. It is important, however, to know whether the animal can swallow normally. The signs of esophageal disease are general and include regurgitation, abnormal or painful deglutition, and weight loss associated with a caloric deficit. Regurgitation is the act of ejecting undigested food through the mouth; vomiting indicates the expulsion of gastric contents. Physical findings in esophageal disease may include distention of the cervical esophagus by food, liquid, foreign body, or tumor and the possible filling of the esophagus with air when the hind legs are elevated. Dogs with regurgitation problems associated with an esophageal lesion frequently have aspiration pneumonia and pharyngitis.

Disorders of the esophagus can be divided into the following categories:
1. Impaired function—dilatation, constriction or obstruction, abnormal peristalsis, gastric reflux.
2. Irregular contour—mucosal and submucosal disease, intramural disease with secondary mucosal alteration.
3. Abnormal position—diphragmatic or hiatal hernia, periesophageal mass, pneumothorax.

EXAMINATION OF THE ABDOMEN

Observation

Stand the animal on a table, its head facing away from you. Step back and inspect the abdomen as to general contour and for swelling or retraction. Swelling can be either localized or general. The most common cause of localized swelling is a neoplasm. General swelling can be caused by fat, fluid, flatus, or fetus.

Note whether the abdominal walls move normally during respiration. Abnormal movement may reflect pain from peritonitis. Decide whether the abdominal musculature seems tense, the abdomen "tucked up." The animal will frequently stand with the hind legs drawn forward well under the body, giving an arched back appearance. When in severe abdominal pain, some animals will assume a "praying position" (lie down with front legs, stand up on hind legs). Look for soft-tissue edema as well as abnormal venous distention of the abdominal wall, indicating circulatory interference.

Palpation

Following visual inspection, palpate the abdomen. Stand behind the animal while an assistant gently restrains the animal's head. In order to gain the animal's confidence, move the hands lightly over its entire abdomen. When performing palpation, avoid using the fingertips; instead, use the metacarpophalangeal joints, with the hand placed flat on the abdominal wall. Begin with a very light, systematic palpation of the entire abdomen, and note any localized or general rigidity and tenderness. Next, palpate the deeper structures. Palpate the liver by pressing the fingers inward and forward around the costal arches on either side. The liver of the dog is composed of the left lobes (medial and lateral), right lobes (medial and lateral), caudate lobe, and quadrate lobe. The normal dog liver is not easy to palpate. Enlargement, however, causes it to protrude beyond the costal margins and facilitates palpation. Note the amount of distention beyond the costal margins, and determine whether the edge of the liver is sharp or rounded. The spleen can be palpated in the upper left lateral region of the abdomen.

The spleen is a tongue-shaped organ resting against the left rib cage at the level of the eleventh to twelfth ribs. In the normal dog or cat with an empty stomach, the nonengorged spleen is entirely within the intrathoracic portion of the abdominal cavity. The degree of distention of the stomach and engorgement of the spleen with blood must be known in order to evaluate the position of the spleen. Abnormal position of the spleen is present if the proximal extremity and body of the spleen are not in contact with the left lateral abdominal wall or are caudal and lateral to the fundus of the stomach. Abnormal position of the spleen may be seen in diaphragmatic herniation, gastric torsion, splenic enlargement, and intra-abdominal tumors.

The kidneys are palpable in certain dogs. The right kidney lies ventral to the first to third lumbar vertebrae; the left kidney is ventral to the second to fourth lumbar vertebrae. In the normal cat, the liver and kidneys can be palpated. Do not confuse the kidneys of a cat with a fetus or tumor.

The fundus of the dog's stomach is on the left side; the pylorus, on the right. When moderately filled, the stomach expands to the left; and the greater curvature parallels the twelfth rib. The filled stomach is distended caudoventrally, so that the greater curvature lies transversely on the floor of the abdomen midway between the xiphoid cartilage and the pubis.

The small bowel is located in the midventral portion of the central abdomen. In the dog, the small intestine is approximately 3.5 times the body length.

The duodenum passes caudad from the pylorus on the right side, lateral to the ascending colon and cecum. The jejunum occupies the right ventral quadrant of the abdomen. The ileum approaches the cecum from the left and joins it at the cecocolic junction. The cecum is usually ventral to the second and third lumbar vertebrae and is in the middle of the right half of the abdomen. Palpate the descending duodenum and the ileocecocolic junction on the right by pressing them dorsally against the sublumbar muscles and rolling them from medial to lateral.

The large bowel of the dog and cat includes the cecum, colon, rectum, and anus. The cecum is a diverticulum of the colon near the ileocolic junction. It is located to the right of the midline, approximately at the level of the third lumbar vertebrae. The transverse colon passes from right to left in front of the root of the mesentery. The descending portion extends from the splenic flexure to the level of the fifth or sixth lumbar vertebrae, parallels the left lateral abdominal wall, then enters the pelvic canal to become the rectum. The descending colon can be palpated on the left and is more prominent when the dog is constipated. Intussusceptions often begin at the ileocecocolic junction. The bladder is located within the posterior portion of the abdomen and is capable of distention as far craniad as the umbilicus (Habel).

If an abnormal mass is felt while palpation is being carried out, note its position, associated pain, degree of mobility, and consistency, if possible (see Table 57). Masses such as lipomas may seem to be in the abdomen upon palpation when they are actually in the abdominal musculature.

As an aid in helping to differentiate abnormalities in size, shape, and position of abdominal organs, O'Brien has described a scheme for classifying the abdomen into five arbitrary regions based on lateral radiographs (Fig. 17).

The major abdominal organs found within each region are:

1. Dorsocranial region: right lateral and caudate liver lobes, spleen, left part of stomach, kidneys, adrenals, right ovary, dorsal limb pancreas, and hepatic and splenic lymph nodes.
2. Ventrocranial region: right and left liver lobes, body and pyloric portions of stomach, pancreas, gallbladder and bile duct, right hepatic, duodenal, and gastric lymph nodes.
3. Central abdomen: spleen, pancreas, connecting peritoneum, mesenteric lymph nodes, intestinal tract, ovaries, left kidney and uterus.
4. Dorsocaudal region: sublumbar lymph nodes, terminal rectum or colon, and terminal ureters.
5. Ventrocaudal region: urinary bladder, prostate, and uterus and vagina, (enlargement associated with retained testicle).

Figure 17. Radiographic evaluation of an abdominal mass can be facilitated by dividing the abdomen into arbitrary regions and determining those organs that are located in each region. The lateral radiographic projection of the abdomen can be divided into the dorsocranial (1), ventrocranial (II), central (III), dorsocaudal (IV), and ventrocaudal (V) regions for the purpose of assessing an abdominal mass. (From O'Brien, T. R.: Radiographic Diagnosis of Abdominal Disorders in the Dog and Cat. Philadelphia, W. B. Saunders Company, 1978, p. 86.)

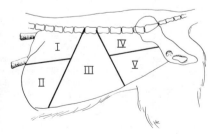

Table 57. MASS-LIKE LESIONS OF THE ABDOMEN*

	Right Dorsocranial	Right Ventrocranial	Left Dorsocranial	Left Ventrocranial
Frequency → More common of Lesion ↓ Uncommon	*Liver* Neoplasia Inflammation Cyst (rare)	*Liver* Neoplasia Inflammation Cyst (rare)	*Liver* Neoplasia Inflammation Cyst (rare)	*Liver* Neoplasia Inflammation Hyperplasia Cyst (rare)
	Kidney Neoplasia Hydronephrosis Inflammation Cystic hypertrophy	*Stomach* Neoplasia Obstruction	*Stomach* Neoplasia Obstruction	
	Adrenal Neoplasia (rare)	*Pancreas* Inflammation Neoplasia	*Adrenal* Neoplasia	

	Ovary and Oviduct
	Neoplasia
	Cystic
	  inflammation
	Oviduct
	  obstruction
		Bile duct and Gallbladder
		Neoplasia
		Rupture		

Table continued on opposite page

Based on ventrodorsal radiographs, the abdomen can be divided into four regions (Fig. 18).

1. Right cranial region: pyloric portion of stomach; right liver lobes; gallbladder and bile duct; pancreas; right kidney; and adrenal, duodenal, gastric, and right hepatic lymph nodes.

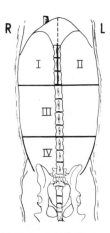

Figure 18. After the lateral radiographic projection has been evaluated, the dorsoventral (or ventrodorsal) radiograph should be evaluated in a similar manner. The illustration shows a method of dividing the abdomen into the right cranial (I), left cranial (II), central (III), and caudal (IV) regions. (From O'Brien, T. R.: Radiographic Diagnosis of Abdominal Disorders in the Dog and Cat. Philadelphia, W. B. Saunders Company, 1978, p. 98.)

Table 57. MASS-LIKE LESIONS OF THE ABDOMEN* *(Continued)*

	Central	Dorsocaudal	Ventrocaudal
		Lymph Nodes of Sublumbar Region	
	Spleen	*Uterus*	
	Neoplasia	Neoplasia	Inflammation
	Torsion	Inflammation	Physiologic enlargement (pregnancy)
	Connecting Peritoneum and Mesenteric Lymph Nodes	*Large Intestine (mesorectum)*	Neoplasia Torsion
	Neoplasia	Neoplasia	
	Inflammation (chronic)	*Ureter*	*Prostate*
	Intestinal Tract	Obstruction	Neoplasia
	Neoplasia	Inflammation	Inflammation
	Obstruction		Cystic hypertrophy
	Torsion		
	Uterus and Pancreas		*Urinary Bladder*
	Inflammation		Obstruction
	Ovaries		Neoplasia
	Neoplasia		Inflammation
	Cystic inflammation (Stump abscess)		Calculus
	Left Kidney		*Retained Testicle or Enlargement of Rudimentary Genital Tract* (rare)
	Neoplasia		
	Hydronephrosis		
	Inflammation		
	Cystic hypertrophy		
	Traumatic rupture		

(left margin, vertical) Uncommon ← Frequency → More Common
of Lesion

*This classification, based on frequency of lesions, was a subjective clinical impression without documentation.

From O'Brien, T. R.: Radiographic Diagnosis of Abdominal Disorders in the Dog and Cat. Philadelphia, W. B. Saunders Company, 1978, p. 1086.

2. Left cranial: left liver lobe, stomach, spleen, and left adrenal.
3. Central region: spleen, pancreas, mesenteric lymph nodes, intestinal tract, ovaries, left kidney, and uterus.
4. Caudal: urinary bladder, prostate, uterus and vagina, large bowel, iliac lymph nodes, mesorectum, and related lymph nodes.

Percussion

Following palpation, percuss the abdomen. The normal abdomen yields a tympanitic-like note throughout except over a solid viscus such as the liver, spleen, or a full bladder. Increased accumulations of air in the stomach or abdomen will give a larger area of tympanitic sound.

Free fluid in the peritoneum (ascites) may shift as the patient is moved. When ascites is suspected, place one hand on one side of the abdomen over the lumbar area and, with the other hand, "flick" or tap the opposite abdominal wall. A distinct impact is felt from one hand to the other if fluid under tension is present.

Auscultation

Carry out the auscultation in a quiet room and determine whether the peristaltic sounds are normal, increased, decreased, or absent.

RECTAL EXAMINATION

The rectum is an elongated tube, 5 to 6 cm in length. Its diameter varies with the breed and size of the animal. The rectum traverses the pelvic canal and ends at the anal canal. Innervation to the anorectal area is supplied by the pudenal nerve (formed by S1, S2, and S3), which also provides motor nerves to the external anal sphincter and to the skin of the anus and perianal region. The rectum and internal anal sphincter are supplied by nerves from the pelvic plexus.

Tenesmus and dyschezia are the primary signs in anorectal diseases. Carefully examine the external anal area and perineum for evidence of inflammation, swelling, neoplasms, and crypts at the mucocutaneous line.

Conclude the examination of the intestinal tract by performing a rectal examination. Use a rubber glove or a finger cot lubricated with a water-soluble gel or petroleum jelly. Digital examination will reveal the color and consistency of the stool in the rectum, any narrowing of the rectum, the possibility of a fractured pelvis, the size of the pelvic canal, impaction or tumors of the anal glands, and the presence of rectal polyps. In male subjects, always check the size of the prostate gland. Little discomfort should accompany this examination. Following digital examination of the rectum, direct visualization of the rectal canal can be accomplished by use of a proctoscope (see pp. 561–563) or an anoscope. This procedure may be performed under sedation or a light plane of anesthesia.

A careful examination of the alimentary tract and abdomen may indicate that further diagnostic work is needed. Passage of a stomach tube (see p. 582), esophagoscopy, radiography (see pp. 567–578), test meals, proctoscopy (see pp. 561–563), or clinical pathologic tests may be required. Do not hesitate to perform those tests that may help in arriving at a definitive diagnosis.

References and Additional Readings

Colmery, B. H.: Dentistry. *In* Bojrab, M. J. (ed.): Pathophysiology in Small Animal Surgery. Philadelphia, Lea & Febiger, 1981.

Dubelzieg, R.: Proliferation of dental and gingival diseases in dogs and cats. J.A.A.H.A., 18:577, 1982.

Eisenmenger, E., Zetner, K.: Tierärztliche Zahnheilkunde. Berlin, Paul Parey, 1982.

Ettinger, S. J. (ed.): Textbook of Veterinary Internal Medicine, 2nd ed. Philadelphia, W. B. Saunders Company, 1983.

Evans, H. E., and Christensen, G. C.: Miller's Anatomy of the Dog, 2nd ed. Philadelphia, W. B. Saunders Company, 1979.

Frost, P.: Canine Dentistry. Day Communications/Nabisco Brands, Inc., 1982.

Habel, R. E.: Applied Anatomy, 6th ed. Ithaca, N. Y., published by author, 1973.

O'Brien, T. R.: Radiographic Diagnosis of Abdominal Disorders in the Dog and Cat. Philadelphia, W. B. Saunders Company, 1978.

Palminteri, A. (ed.): Gastrointestinal medicine and surgery. Vet. Clin. North Am., 2:1972.

Richardson, K. C., Jones, M. S., and Elliot, G. S.: Oral neoplasms in the dog: a diagnostic and therapeutic dilemma. Compendium on Continuing Education, 5:441, 1983.

Strombeck, D. R.: Small Animal Gastroenterology, Davis, California, Stonegate Publishing Co., 1979.

Thalen, M.: Concepts in Veterinary Dentistry. Edwardsville, Kansas, Veterinary Medical Publishing Co., 1982.

Thrall, D. E.: Orthovoltage radiation of acanthomatous epulides in 39 dogs. J.A.V.M.A., 184(7):826, 1984.

Todoroff, R. J., and Brodey, R. S.: Oral and pharyngeal neoplasia in the dog: a retrospective study of 361 cases. J.A.V.M.A., 175:567, 1979.

CARDIOVASCULAR SYSTEM

N. Joel Edwards*

HISTORY

Age

The age of the patient is an important clue in the diagnosis of cardiac diseases. Congenital heart disease is most often diagnosed before the age of 2 years. Canine idiopathic cardiomyopathy is generally seen between the ages of 2 and 7 years. Mitral insufficiency is generally asymptomatic until 7 to 9 years of age. Myocarditis and other acquired cardiac diseases generally increase in frequency with age. Feline cardiomyopathies are usually diagnosed between 1 and 5 years of age. Canine hypertrophic cardiomyopathy is generally seen before 5 years of age.

Breed

There are breed predispositions toward many congenital and acquired cardiac abnormalities.

*This section contributed by N. J. Edwards, D.V.M., Diplomate A.C.V.I.M., Adjunct Associate Professor of Medicine, New York State College of Veterinary Medicine, Cornell University, Ithaca, New York and Gary R. Bolton, D.V.M., deceased.

Congenital Cardiac Anomalies

Patent ductus arteriosus—poodle, collie, Pomeranian, and German shepherd.

Pulmonic stenosis—English bulldog, Old English sheepdog, fox terrier, Chihuahua, beagle, schnauzer, pointer, and Siberian husky.

Aortic stenosis—German shepherd, boxer, Newfoundland, and Golden retriever.

Tetralogy of Fallot—keeshond, fox terrier, and Siberian husky.

Aortic arch abnormalities—German shepherd, Irish setter, and Weimaraner.

Congenital mitral insufficiency—Great Dane.

Acquired Cardiac Abnormalities

Mitral and/or tricuspid insufficiency—cocker spaniel, poodle, schnauzer, dachshund, Chihuahua, Pomeranian, and miniature pinscher.

Myocarditis—boxer, St. Bernard, German shorthair pointer, and Afghan hound.

Idiopathic cardiomyopathy—large breeds of dogs.

Collapsed trachea—toy breeds.

Heart base tumors—Boston terrier, boxer, and English bulldog.

Sex

Female: patent ductus arteriosus and sick sinus syndrome.

Male: mitral and tricuspid insufficiency, feline hypertrophic cardiomyopathy, canine idiopathic cardiomyopathy, aortic stenosis, and canine hypertrophic cardiomyopathy.

Pertinent Questions

1. *Is the animal excessively weak or tired?* An animal with a clinically significant cardiac abnormality has less cardiac reserve and loses strength and stamina. The owner reports that the pet is unable to exercise as strenuously as it once could.

2. *Is there coughing or dyspnea?* The most frequent presenting complaint associated with heart disease is a cough, which is first noticed mainly at night or is aggravated by exercise or excitement. As pulmonary congestion or edema advances, breathing may become labored. The owner notices that the pet cannot catch its breath or that a small amount of exercise causes the pet to pant or breathe heavily for longer than would be expected.

3. *How long has the problem been present?* In most cases, cardiac disease is a slowly progressive problem. It usually does not begin acutely, and it may become gradually worse over a period of months or even years. Occasionally, the development of an arrhythmia such as atrial fibrillation or ventricular tachycardia may result in an "apparent" acute onset.

4. *Is the problem getting worse?* Cardiac disease is usually progressive, with symptoms that gradually get worse.

5. *Is the cough worse during the day or at night?* The cough caused by chronic mitral valvular fibrosis is first noticed at night because of the gravitational shift of blood from the lower portions of the body toward the heart when the animal lies down to sleep. This increase in venous return (preload) causes an increased cardiac workload resulting in increased pulmonary vascular volume with resultant congestion.

6. *Does the animal sleep well or is it restless at night?* The gravitational shift of blood just mentioned causes discomfort to the animal when pulmonary congestion increases. The animal may get up to move; when it does, breathing becomes easier. Consequently, it gets up and moves often, whenever breathing becomes difficult. Recurring bouts of pulmonary edema may develop (cardiac asthma). Most of these subside within a few minutes after the animal has gotten up. When this becomes severe, the animal may not be able to lie down; it then attempts to sleep standing up or sitting down with its head and neck outstretched.

7. *Does the animal expectorate material after the cough?* The cardiac cough is a productive cough. The animal may expectorate a small amount of frothy white or, occasionally, blood-tinged fluid. The owner sometimes reports this as gagging or vomiting. Clinical signs of hemoptysis are often associated with ruptured chordae tendineae or eosinophilic pneumonitis.

8. *Has the animal had any syncopal attacks?* Cardiac syncope (fainting) may occur when cardiac output falls and cerebral hypoxia occurs. This is usually caused by atrial or ventricular arrhythmias or sinus tachycardia. Third-degree atrioventricular (A-V) block can also cause exertional syncope. It may occur when an animal that has cardiac disease exercises too hard or becomes too excited. Electrocardiographic (ECG) evidence of sick sinus syndrome is often associated with the female minature schnauzer, the breed most prone to fainting from cardiac disease. Pugs are prone to stenosis of the His bundle, which is often associated with fainting episodes and sudden death.

9. *Describe the cough.* The cardiac cough is a low pitched, resonant cough occurring in paroxysms, followed by gagging or coughing up of a white frothy phlegm, which is occasionally blood tinged.

10. *If medication was given, did it help?* If the dog has been treated with digitalis, diuretics, aminophylline, or low-sodium diet and rest and has responded well, this suggests that the problem was cardiac oriented.

11. *Are there other problems?* Cardinal signs of illness should be investigated in the cardiac patient as in any other patient. These signs include anorexia, polydipsia, polyuria, vomiting, diarrhea, previous illnesses, and so on. It is well known that cardiac disease may affect the kidney and the liver; thus, dysfunctions of these organs must always be investigated in the medical evaluation of the cardiac patient.

PHYSICAL EXAMINATION

In the evaluation of the cardiovascular competence of an animal, the clinician uses inspection, palpation, percussion, and auscultation to make a tentative diagnosis. Specialized examinations are used as an aid to determine the diagnosis, prognosis, and treatment (Figs. 19 and 20). Physical examination is especially important in cats. Most cats minimize their clinical signs by curtailing their movements. The owner may not even realize that the cat has heart disease. Even the smallest murmur or subtlest gallop rhythm should be evaluated thoroughly.

Inspection

Careful inspection of the animal may reveal many signs indicative of cardiac disease.

1. *Physical condition.* The cardiac patient in the terminal stages is usually thin. The owner may think that the pet is fat when it really is severely ascitic. Most cardiac patients remain in fairly good physical condition until Class III or IV congestive heart failure is present.

2. *Dyspnea.* The dyspnea may be very subtle and easily missed, or it may be very obvious. The dyspnea may occur only during exercise. Inspiration and expiration should be evaluated individually.

3. *Postural abnormalities.* An animal with severe respiratory embarrassment may stand with the elbows abducted in an effort to expand its vital capacity. Animals with pulmonary edema may sit on their haunches with their forelegs and head and neck extended.

4. *Abdominal distention.* A distended abdomen may be caused by ascites. Palpation, percussion, and laboratory examination of the fluid are helpful in making a differential diagnosis.

5. *Color of mucous membranes.* Some cardiac diseases, such as Tetralogy of Fallot, Eisenmenger's syndrome, or other defects resulting in right-to-left shunting of blood may cause cyanosis of the mucous membranes without exercise. The is not a feature of chronic mitral valvular fibrosis. Capillary refill time may be checked by blanching the gums with the finger and observing how quickly the color returns when the finger is removed. Diseases that lower cardiac output may delay the capillary refill time (shock, pericardial effusion, severe mitral insufficiency, or primary myocardial diseases).

6. *Venous distention.* Right heart failure causes increased venous pressure. This is best judged by examining the jugular vein or the superficial mammary veins. If both are distended or engorged, right heart failure or pericardial effusion is likely to be present.

7. *Jugular pulse.* Normally, a pulse in the jugular vein can be seen only as high as one third of the way up the neck. When such a pulse is visible higher than that, it signifies right ventricular failure, pericardial effusion, or a severe arrhythmia (atrioventricular heart block, frequent ectopic beats, and ventricular tachycardia).

8. *Subcutaneous edema.* This is not a common feature of cardiac disease in small animals. It rarely occurs unless ascites is present. In the male dog, the scrotum is often the first area to become edematous.

N.Y.S. VETERINARY COLLEGE — CORNELL UNIVERSITY — VETERINARY HOSPITALS

DATE_____ C A R D I O V A S C U L A R   E X A M I N A T I O N   R E C O R D

Ward _____

Present Illness and Medications Received:

ACO # _____ PHONE _____
OWNER _____
STREET _____
CITY _____ STATE ____ ZIP ____
BORN _____ SEX ____ COLOR ____
SPEC. _____ BREED ____ ID ____

REF. DVM _____
CLINICIAN _____
SECONDARY # _____

CARDIAC EXAMINATION

Inspection:
1. General Attitude   □ Alert   □ Depressed   □ Prostrate
2. General Condition   □ Normal   □ Thin   □ Emaciated   □ Obese
3. Respiration   □ Normal   □ Dyspnea   □ Cough
4. Mucous Membranes   □ Normal   □ Pale   □ Cyanotic   □ Jaundice   □ Injected
5. Posture   □ Normal   □ Pot Bellied   □ Abducted Elbows   □ Head Ext.
6. Capillary Refill Time □ Normal   □ Delayed

Palpation:
1. Cardiac Region:
   □ Normal   □ Precordial Thrill   □ Arrhythmia   □ Other _____

   Point of Maximal Intensity _____

2. Abdominal Abnormalities: _____

3. Pulse:
   Venous: □ Jugular Pulse   □ Venous Distention   □ Other _____
   Arterial: □ Strong   □ Weak   □ B-B Shot   □ Rapid   □ Slow   □ Arrhythmic   □ Other _____

Auscultation:

1. *Heart Sounds:* □ Normal □ Abnormal □ Murmur
   Timing of Murmur: □ Systolic □ Diastolic □ Continuous
   Duration: □ Early systolic □ Late systolic □ Early diastolic □ Late diastolic
   Frequency: □ High frequency □ Low frequency □ Mixed frequency
   Loudness: □ Grade 1, 2(Soft) □ Grade 3, 4(Medium) □ Grade 5, 6(Loud)
   Valve Area: □ Pulmonic □ Aortic □ Left A-V □ Right A-V □ Radiation _____

   Other Heart Sounds _____

2. *Lung Sounds:* □ Normal □ Abnormal

   Describe _____

Signature: _____

C A R D I O V A S C U L A R   E X A M I N A T I O N   R E C O R D

Figure 19. Cardiovascular examination record.

NYS VETERINARY COLLEGE — CORNELL UNIVERSITY — VETERINARY HOSPITAL
CARDIOVASCULAR EXAMINATION SHEET

REF. DVM
CLINICIAN

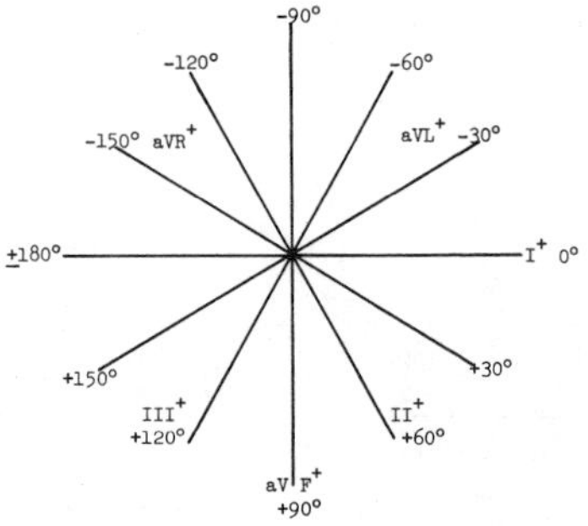

Heart Rate

Heart Rhythm

Heart Axis

P Wave

P-R Interval

QRS Complex

ST-T

Q-T Interval

Other

ECG Diagnosis

HISTORY

PHYSICAL EXAMINATION

ROENTGENOGRAPHIC FINDINGS:

CARDIAC DIAGNOSIS:

RECOMMENDATIONS:

SERVICE: STUDENT SIGNATURE: CARDIOLOGIST SIGNATURE:

Figure 20. Cardiovascular examination sheet.

9. *Strength and stamina.* A clinical cardiac problem may cause signs that vary from lack of stamina to severe weakness, collapse, and sudden death.

Palpation

Palpation provides additional clues in the examination for cardiac disease.

Palpation of the Neck Area

It may be possible to stimulate a cough by tracheal palpation. Palpation may reveal a collapsing trachea or other structural abnormalities. Masses in the area of the carotid bifurcation may cause bradycardia via the carotid sinus reflex or through direct vagal stimulation.

Thoracic Palpation

Palpate fractures, deformities, or abnormal chest and abdominal wall movement. The normal point of maximal intensity (PMI) is the left intercostal space 4 to 6 at the sternal border (mitral valve area). The PMI may shift or be diminished owing to thoracic masses, diaphragmatic hernias, precordial thrills, pericardial or pleural effusions.

Precordial thrill is caused by loud murmurs that cause enough fremitus to be palpated (see Classification of Cardiac Murmurs, pp. 344–346).

In the cat, the heart size can be palpated through the chest wall. In cats with hypertrophic cardiomyopathy, prominent apical impulses can often be detected by placing both hands over the precordia with the animal facing away.

Abdominal Palpation

Abdominal distention may be caused by masses (may be asymmetrical) that become evident on palpation. Fluid may be palpated by the hands on each side of the abdomen. One hand pushes in quickly, and a "fluid wave" may be felt against the opposite hand.

Try the hepatojugular reflex. Gentle compression of the abdomen increases blood flow through the liver and thus through the vena cavae. In animals with chronic hepatic congestion caused by right heart failure, pressure applied to the abdomen will cause the jugular vein to distend. This positive hepatojugular reflex confirms the presence of right heart failure. In animals with persistent aortic ring abnormalities, compressing the abdomen while holding the animal's nares closed will cause the dilated esophagus to bulge, usually in the left thoracic inlet.

Palpation of the Femoral Pulse

Palpation of the femoral pulse requires constant practice in order to become proficient. Palpate healthy animals until you are confident in your ability to recognize the normal pulse wave. Animals that have short stubby legs or that are trembling may be difficult to evaluate.

Correlation of Classic Murmur with Classic Pulse

1. A jerky or "b-b shot" pulse is seen with mitral insufficiency, ventricular

septal defect, patent ductus arteriosus, and anemias. This is a strong pulse, easily felt, but it rises and falls rapidly.

2. A normal pulse is seen with normal dogs, in pulmonic stenosis, and in pure tricuspid insufficiency. This is strong, easily felt, with an even rise and fall.

3. A small, slow rising pulse is seen with aortic stenosis. This pulse is not strong. It rises late and falls off normally. It is difficult to evaluate.

4. A weak, thready pulse is seen in shock, in pericardial effusion, or in diminished cardiac contractility.

Pulse Rate and Rhythm

1. Normal pulse rate is 70 to 160 beats per minute (up to 180 in toy breeds and 220 in puppies). For cats, a pulse rate of 110 to 240 beats per minute is normal. A marked sinus bradycardia (90 beats/min or less) in the cat usually indicates that the animal is seriously ill. Sinus bradycardia in the cat is often associated with dilated cardiomyopathy.

2. There should be one pulse for each heart beat. A pulse deficit is present when there are more heart beats than there are femoral pulses. Pulse deficits occur when arrhythmias are present. In general, the greater the pulse deficit the more serious the arrhythmia. Generally, the left hand is placed over the heart area, and the right hand is placed on the femoral pulse.

3. Sinus arrhythmia is characterized by an irregular pulse rate. It is correlated with respiration. When the animal breathes in, the pulse rate increases; when it breathes out, the pulse rate decreases. With sinus arrhythmia, the pulse is usually regularly irregular (because of respiration).

4. Other pulse irregularities that cannot be correlated with respiration require an ECG to diagnose the arrhythmia.

Percussion

Thoracic percussion is often useful. Decreased resonance may be caused by thoracic masses, diaphragmatic hernia, cardiac enlargement, thoracic effusion, or obesity. Increased resonance may be caused by emphysema or pneumothorax.

Abdominal percussion may delineate masses or determine the presence of fluid. Percussion techniques should be carried out routinely on every cardiac patient.

AUSCULTATION

The last procedure during the cardiac examination is auscultation of the thorax. This should be accomplished with the patient standing up, with the head facing away from the clinician. Auscultation of the heart is done in a systematic manner, by valve area (Fig. 21). The diaphragm head of the stethoscope allows better hearing of high frequency sounds, whereas the bell allows one to hear low frequency sounds more clearly. When using the bell portion of the stethoscope, it should be placed very lightly on the thorax.

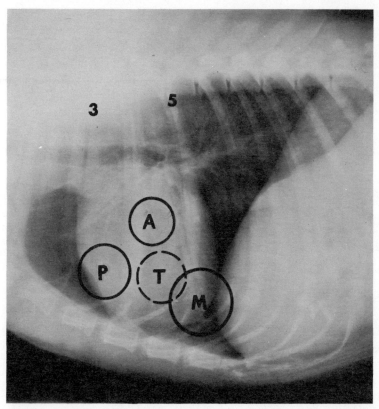

Figure 21. Left lateral radiograph of the canine thorax. Circles identify the valve areas: M, mitral valve area; P, pulmonic valve area; A, aortic valve area; T, tricuspid valve area. Because the tricuspid valve area is located on the right side of the thorax, it is indicated by a broken circle. (From Ettinger, S. J., and Suter, P. F.: Canine Cardiology. Philadelphia, W. B. Saunders Company, 1970.)

Pulmonic valve area—left intercostal space 2 to 4, just above the sternal border.

Aortic valve area—left intercostal space 3 to 5, mid thorax.

Mitral valve area—left intercostal space 4 to 6, just above the sternal border.

Tricuspid valve area—right intercostal space 3 to 5, mid thorax.

In the cat, only two areas are identified on the left: the base (aortic-pulmonic area), and the apex (left AV valve area). The tricuspid valve is usually best heard over the right 3rd to 4th intercostal spaces in the lower third of the thorax.

Heart Sounds

Characteristics

1. Frequency—pitch.
2. Intensity—loudness: increased—thin chested, young, athletic, anemia, fever, or severe tachycardias; decreased—pericardial effusion, pleural effusion, intrathoracic masses, or extreme obesity.

Normal

Normal heart sounds are caused by the abrupt acceleration or deceleration of blood and associated heart vibrations:

1. S_1–A-V valve closure (mitral and tricuspid).
   a. Normally loudest at apex beat (L mitral area; R tricuspid area).
   b. Longer, louder, lower pitched than S_2.
   c. Arterial pulse occurs just after S_1.
   d. Four parts: early ventricular contraction, deceleration of blood when A-V valves close, oscillation of blood between major arteries and ventricles, and vibrations associated with ejection of blood into the great arteries.
2. S_2–Aortic and pulmonic valve closure

Artifacts

1. Respiration.
2. Shivering and twitches (rumble).
3. Movement.
4. Rubbing of hair (static or crackling).

Abnormal

Abnormal heart sounds are usually transient (sounds of short duration, including S_1 and S_2)

Split S_1—asynchronous closure of mitral and tricuspid valves.
1. Occasionally occurs in normal, large, or giant breeds.
2. Certain arrhythmias (ventricular premature contractions, VPCs; left bundle branch block, LBBB; and right bundle branch block, RBBB).

Split S_2—asynchronous closure of aortic and pulmonic valves.
1. Occurs in normal dogs (physiologic); on inspiration only.
2. Pathologic: (a) delayed pulmonic valve closure (inspiration) associated with pulmonary hypertension (heartworms), increased pulmonary outflow resistance (pulmonic stenosis), cor pulmonale (chronic lung disease), and RBBB; and (b) delayed aortic valve closure (paradoxical split S_2; splits more on expiration associated with increased aortic outflow resistance (aortic stenosis), increased left ventricular load (PDA), and LBBB.

S_3—protodiastolic gallop or ventricular gallop.
1. Caused by rapid ventricular diastolic filling.
2. Usually inaudible.
3. Low frequency (use bell) loudest at L apex and follows S_2.
4. Associated with congestive heart failure: dog—chronic valvular disease and heartworm disease; dog and cat—congestive cardiomyopathy.

S_4—presystolic or atrial gallop.
1. Caused by atrial contraction.
2. Usually inaudible.
3. Low frequency loudest at L base and occurs just prior to S_1.
4. Associated with severely dilated atria (hypertrophic cardiomyopathy) and tertiary heart block.

S_3 *and* S_4—summation gallop.
1. May be loudest sound heard.
2. Feline cardiomyopathies.

Systolic clicks
1. High frequency occurring during systole (between S_1 and S_2).
2. Usually associated with parachuting of the mitral valve.
3. Prolonged audible vibrations occurring during a normally silent period of the cardiac cycle.

Cardiac Murmurs

The auscultation of a cardiac murmur is usually a reliable sign that there is a cardiac abnormality that might or might not be clinically significant. Certain defects cause characteristic murmurs. Each murmur is classified for diagnostic purposes by the following characteristics.

Timing. Is the murmur systolic, diastolic, or both? In general, A-V insufficiency and semilunar valve stenosis cause systolic murmurs. These constitute 95 per cent of the murmurs heard. Diastolic murmurs are often caused by A-V stenosis or semilunar insufficiency. Pure diastolic murmurs are rare in small animals. In continuous murmurs, both systolic and diastolic phases are present. The classic example of this continuous or "machinery murmur" is the murmur heard in patients with a patent ductus arteriosus.

Duration. Is the murmur early systolic, midsystolic, late systolic, or holosystolic (throughout systole) or when during diastole does it occur? Mitral insufficiency and ventricular septal defect have holosystolic murmurs. Aortic and pulmonic stenosis have midsystolic murmurs. Anemic and physiologic murmurs are early systolic. Patent ductus arteriosus is holosystolic, holodiastolic.

Frequency (Pitch). Certain murmurs may be high, low, or mixed in pitch. Low frequency is 30 to 80 cps, mid frequency is 80 to 120 cps, and high frequency is 120 cps and higher. Ventricular septal defect and mitral insufficiency are classic mixed frequency murmurs. Patent ductus arteriosus usually has a low rumbling quality. Pulmonic and aortic stenosis have many high frequency components. Anemic and physiologic murmurs are generally of high frequency.

Intensity (Loudness). Loudness is graded by the ability to hear and/or feel the murmur.

Soft	Grade I—soft, nearly imperceptible
	Grade II—soft but definite
Medium	Grade III—easily heard, but not palpable
	Grade IV—loud with no precordial thrill

Table 58. SUMMARY CHARACTERIZATION OF COMMON MURMURS

	Mitral Insufficiency	Patent Ductus Arteriosus	Aortic Stenosis
Timing	Systolic	Continuous	Systolic
Duration	Holosystolic	Holosystolic, holodiastolic	Midsystolic (crescendo-decrescendo or diamond-shaped murmur)
Pitch	Early—high frequency Later—mixed frequency	Mixed frequency with low frequency components	Harsh mixed frequency, with some high frequency components
Intensity	Usually moderate to loud	Usually loud	Usually loud
Valve Area	Mitral valve area	Anterior on chest in area of pulmonic and aortic valve areas; may have PMI on ventral sternum cranial to left foreleg	Aortic valve area
Radiation	Rightward, cranioventral, or dorsal	Craniodorsal	Cranial and rightward; even heard over cervical vessels

Pulmonic Stenosis	Ventricular Septal Defect	Anemic Murmur	Physiologic (Functional) Murmur
Systolic	Systolic	Systolic	Systolic
Midsystolic (crescendo-decrescendo or diamond-shaped murmur	Holosystolic	Early systolic	Early systolic
High frequency	Mixed frequency	High frequency	High frequency
Usually loud	Usually loud	Usually very soft; may wax and wane	Very soft; may wax and wane; usually disappears by 8 weeks of age
Pulmonic area on left	Mitral area on left; anterior midthorax on right	Mitral area	Mitral area
Tends not to radiate beyond thoracic inlet	Heard on both sides of chest, but PMI is on right side	None	None

Loud   Grade V—loud, palpable thrill present
              Grade VI—loudest murmur, palpable thrill, and radia-
              tion detectable without stethoscope

There is not necessarily any correlation between loudness of murmur auscultated and the severity of the disease. Some small defects create loud murmurs;
very large defects may not produce a murmur.

       Valve Area. Generally, the point of maximal intensity will be located in
the area of the valve that is affected.

       Radiation. Certain murmurs tend to radiate their sound over the chest in
characteristic directions. Mitral insufficiency murmurs tend to radiate rightward, cranioventral or dorsal. Aortic stenosis tends to radiate rightward and
cranially, even up to the cervical vessels. Ventricular septal defect is heard on
both sides of the chest in the mitral area on the left and at the cranial midthorax
on the right, with the murmur being loudest on the right. The murmur of
pulmonic stenosis tends not to radiate beyond the thoracic inlet (Table 58).

INDIRECT BLOOD PRESSURE MONITORING

       The following definitions are pertinent to blood pressure monitoring:

       Diastolic—minimal pressure prior to next ejection cycle.

       Mean pressure—average pressure (one third the difference between
systolic and diastolic).

       Pulse pressure—the difference between systolic and diastolic.

       Systolic—maximal pressure obtained with each cardiac ejection.

       It is possible to have a weak pulse in a normotensive patient if the heart
rate is fast and stroke volumes are small.

       Indirect blood pressure monitoring can be accomplished in the dog and
cat by using ultrasonography and the Doppler principle of arterial wall motion
detection. The Arteriosonde 1010* sphygmomanometer is used in indirect
blood pressure monitoring. The Doppler cuff is placed on top of a shaved skin
area over the cranial tibial artery. A small amount of gel is applied between
the skin and transducer. The 4.0-cm neonatal cuff is used for medium to large
dogs, and the 2.5-cm premature infant cuff, for cats and smaller dogs. When
an occlusive cuff is placed around the distal tibia and inflated to a pressure
greater than the systolic blood pressure, the cranial tibial artery is compressed
and no motion of the arterial wall occurs, and there is no sound. When the
cuff pressure is reduced to a level just below systolic pressure but above
diastolic pressure, the artery rapidly opens during the peak of the pulse
pressure wave and an ultrasound frequency is produced. When the cuff pressure
drops below diastolic pressure, the artery rhythmically expands and collapses
with the passing pulse waves. This expansion produces a slow velocity to the
arterial wall, and there is a marked change in the intensity of the Doppler
sound. The systolic pressure is interpreted as the point at which Doppler
sounds are first heard; diastolic pressure is the point at which the Doppler
sounds change in character and/or intensity.

       Even newer devices, such as the Critikon Dinamap Blood pressure

---

*Roche Medical Electronics Division,

recorder,† enable continuous, noninvasive systolic and diastolic blood pressure on a digital display. With this device, blood pressure is recorded by indirect automatic inflating and deflating sphygmomanometry.

Normal blood pressures in the dog as recorded with indirect Doppler technique and sphygmomanometry have been estimated to be 155 ± 27 mm Hg for systolic and 73 ± 14 mm Hg for diastolic, and 147 ± 15 mm Hg systolic, 87 ± 8 mm Hg diastolic, and 102 ± 9 mm Hg mean.

Hypertension in the dog is defined as a systolic blood pressure greater than 180 mm Hg or a diastolic pressure greater than 95 mm Hg. The major diseases that alter pressure are renal disease and hyperadrenocorticism. In one study of dogs with glomerular disease, 80 per cent were hypertensive (Kallet and Cowgill).

Blood pressure monitoring during surgical procedures and in evaluating vasodilator efficiency during congestive heart failure therapy is a valuable aid.

Specialized Examinations

The diagnosis or list of rule-outs is generally determined from the history and physical examination. ECG and radiography are useful tools that assist in confirming the diagnosis and in determining treatment and prognosis.

ELECTROCARDIOGRAPHY

The ECG provides the clinician with a fast, efficient way to obtain considerable data about a patient's cardiovascular status. The ECG is a clinical test and must be correlated with clinical findings (Tables 59–62). It should be kept in mind that an ECG measures only electrical activity of the heart as seen on the body surface at any one instant.

Uses

The ECG is used for the following purposes:
1. It detects enlargement of any of the cardiac chambers.
2. It is useful in the diagnosis of cardiac arrhythmias.
3. It detects electrolyte imbalances.
4. It monitors response to therapy (digitalis therapy for heart failure; antiarrhythmic therapy; treatment of metabolic diseases that cause electrolyte imbalances; and pericardiocentesis).
5. It is useful in the diagnosis of nonspecific diseases (myocarditis; endocarditis; metabolic diseases; and neoplasia).
6. It is useful for permanent records.
7. It helps to establish prognosis (estimated severity of enlargement and of arrhythmia; serial ECGs are helpful in determining the rate of change).

---

†Critikon Corporation, 1410 N. Westshore Blvd., Tampa, Florida.

Table 59. NORMAL CANINE ELECTROCARDIOGRAPHIC VALUES (LANNEK)

Lead	Amplitudes (mv)						Intervals (sec)		
	P	Q	R	S	S-Tj	T	P–R	QRS	Q–T
I	0.070 ± 0.064	0.522 ± 0.388	0.778 ± 0.480	0.184 ± 0.180	0.016 ± 0.036	− 0.072 ± 0.140	0.096 ± 0.019	0.035 ± 0.007	0.167 ± 0.018
II	0.242 ± 0.116	0.682 ± 0.454	2.406 ± 0.876	0.318 ± 0.258	− 0.036 ± 0.052	− 0.146 ± 0.336	0.098 ± 0.016	0.041 ± 0.008	0.176 ± 0.018
III	0.180 ± 0.112	0.428 ± 0.268	1.890 ± 0.760	0.432 ± 0.330	− 0.036 ± 0.048	− 0.030 ± 0.310	0.099 ± 0.017	0.041 ± 0.008	0.177 ± 0.018
(V4)	0.350 ± 0.114	0.570 ± .370	4.246 ± 1.438	0.528 ± 0.406	− 0.062 ± 0.092	0.370 ± 0.554	0.100 ± 0.018	0.047 ± 0.009	0.194 ± 0.022
(V2)	0.334 ± 0.100	0.406 ± 0.276	4.766 ± 1.348	0.726 ± 0.540	− 0.022 ± 0.108	0.588 ± 0.570	0.102 ± 0.019	0.045 ± 0.007	0.192 ± 0.021
(rV2)	0.164 ± 0.100	—	2.598 ± 1.206	1.236 ± 0.766	0.006 ± 0.086	0.724 ± 0.480	0.104 ± 0.021	0.038 ± 0.007	0.191 ± 0.019

Lannek, N.: A Clinical and Experimental Study on the Electrocardiogram in Dogs. Thesis, Stockholm, 1949. Reported by Detweiler, D. K.: Cardiovascular disease in animals. *In* Luisada, A. A. (ed.): Cardiology: An Encyclopedia of the Cardiovascular System, Vol. V. New York, McGraw-Hill Inc., 1961, 27–10.

Table 60. NORMAL CANINE ELECTROCARDIOGRAPHIC VALUES

Wave		Leads (mm)					
		I	**II**	**III**	**aVR**	**aVL**	**aVF**
P	Mean	0.44	+ 3.0	+ 2.5	− 1.6	− 1.01	+ 2.91
	S.D.*	0.10	0.10	0.09	0.09	0.15	0.12
Q	Mean	0.27	1.2	1.3	12.6	8.5	1.7
	S.D.	0.10	0.15	0.10	0.46	0.48	0.09
R	Mean	2.2	16.5	14.8	1.10	2.10	16.2
	S.D.	0.50	0.44	0.43	0.30	0.30	0.34
S	Mean	0.88	1.4	1.30	10.2	0.75	1.95
	S.D.	0.09	0.22	0.15	0.33	0.50	0.20
T	Mean	− 0.10	− 1.10	− 1.00	+ 1.10	+ 1.12	− 0.95
	S.D.	0.20	0.11	0.18	0.23	0.23	0.17

Interval	Lead (sec)		
	I	**II**	**III**
P–R	0.096 ± 0.024	0.098 ± 0.024	0.099 ± 0.024
QRS	0.037 ± 0.021	0.045 ± 0.024	0.044 ± 0.024
Q–T	0.167 ± 0.054	0.176 ± 0.054	0.177 ± 0.054

*Standard deviation.

Burman, S. O., Panagopoulos, P., and Kahn, S.: J. Thorac. Cardiovasc. Surg., 51:379, 1966.

Table 61. DURATION OF P, P–R QRS, AND Q–T IN NORMAL CATS (LEAD II); NORMAL ELECTRICAL AXIS (RANGE, MEAN); AND NORMAL HEART RATE (RANGE, MEAN)*

	P (sec)	**P–R** (sec)	**QRS** (sec)	**Q–T** (sec)
Mean	0.03	0.071	0.026	0.148
		[0.074]	[0.036]	[0.210]
Standard deviation		0.010	0.010	0.020
		[0.011]	[0.010]	[0.040]

*Values from The Animal Medical Center are compared with Rogers' values; Rogers' values are bracketed. From Tilley, L. P.: Feline cardiology. Vet. Clin. North Am., 7:263, 1977.

Electrical axis (frontal plane): 6° to 180° (46 cats); mean = 79° [30° to 170°, 24 cats] Heart rate: 160 to 240 beats/min; mean = 195 beats/min [90 to 240 beats/min, mean = 159 beats/min].

Table 62. AMPLITUDES (MILLIVOLTS) OF ELECTROCARDIOGRAPHIC WAVES IN NORMAL CATS. COMPARISON OF STUDIES WITH (ROGERS) AND WITHOUT (THE ANIMAL MEDICAL CENTER) ANESTHESIA*

Lead	Right Lateral Recumbency With Anesthesia (Rogers)							Right Lateral Recumbency Without Anesthesia (AMC)							Sternal Position Without Anesthesia (AMC)
	I	II	III	aVR	aVL	aVF	V_{10}	I	II	III	aVR	aVL	aVF	V_{10}	II
P wave positive															
No. of cats	16	25	24	—	4	25	—	22	39	26	—	—	32	—	38
Mean	0.04	0.12	0.11	—	0.08	0.15	—	0.11	0.16	0.15	—	—	0.12	—	0.17
SD†	—	—	—	—	—	—	—	0.05	0.07	0.07	—	—	0.06	—	0.04
P wave negative															
No. of cats	—	—	—	24	18	—	20	—	—	—	23	3	—	10	—
Mean	—	—	—	0.07	0.05	—	0.04	—	—	—	0.09	0.03	—	0.02	—
SD	—	—	—	—	—	—	—	—	—	—	0.07	0.08	—	0.08	—
Q wave															
No. of cats	16	20	15	15	16	13	26	24	13	13	35	36	11	45	9
Mean	0.13	0.08	0.15	0.16	0.22	0.10	0.32	0.22	0.24	0.14	0.28	0.21	0.16	0.38	0.16
SD	—	—	—	—	—	—	—	0.13	0.18	0.08	0.13	0.10	0.11	0.15	0.11
R wave															
No. of cats	22	25	24	19	22	25	23	39	46	46	20	24	45	38	46
Mean	0.18	0.43	0.36	0.10	0.16	0.38	0.16	0.30	0.50	0.42	0.22	0.19	0.35	0.27	0.53
SD	—	—	—	—	—	—	—	0.20	0.25	0.23	0.15	0.12	0.18	0.11	0.31
S wave															
No. of cats	5	10	9	13	11	9	—	11	11	12	40	24	10	7	15
Mean	0.11	0.20	0.26	0.26	0.11	0.17	—	0.29	0.23	0.22	0.33	0.22	0.15	0.27	0.26
SD	—	—	—	—	—	—	—	0.21	0.12	0.09	0.19	0.11	0.07	0.12	0.10
T wave positive															
No. of cats	2	22	21	4	9	23	—	14	30	17	—	2	16	—	31
Mean	0.05	0.11	0.10	0.05	0.06	0.10	—	0.15	0.19	—	—	0.30	0.13	—	0.21
SD	—	—	—	—	—	—	—	0.07	0.07	0.11	—	0.04	0.05	—	0.07
T wave negative															
No. of cats	—	4	4	19	9	2	24	—	—	—	13	—	—	15	—
Mean	—	0.10	0.12	0.08	0.05	0.12	0.09	—	—	—	0.06	—	—	0.04	—
SD	—	—	—	—	—	—	—	—	—	—	0.10	—	—	0.14	—

*Right lateral recumbency and sternal positions.
†Standard deviation.
From Tilley, L. P.: Feline cardiology. Vet. Clin. North Am., 7:264, 1977.

Production

1. Place the animal in right lateral recumbency (Fig. 22). Use a rubber sheet or cloth towel to insulate it from the table surface. Cats may be placed in right lateral or sternal recumbency.
2. In general, light sedation will have little effect on the ECG. Preferably, the ECG is taken with no chemical sedation.
3. Limbs are held perpendicular to the body and parallel to each other.
4. Attach leads to forelimbs on the elbows and to hindlimbs on the stifles. Alligator clips are not painful if bent slightly. It is helpful to pad the clips with a little cotton for cats and thin-skinned dogs.
5. Clips are moistened with alcohol, pHisoHex, or electrode jelly.
6. Standardize the machine so that needle deflection of 1 mv goes up 10 small boxes on the ECG paper (1 mv = 1 cm). Run the paper speed at 50 mm per sec (Fig. 23).
7. Record 5 to 10 complexes of leads I, II, III, aVR, aVL, and aVF, then return to lead II and run 12 to 24 inches of paper for use as a rhythm strip.
8. Specialized unipolar exploring leads (V_{10}, CV_6LL, CV_6LU, and CV_5RL) are run by placing the exploring lead (usually marked V or C) in various locations and recording with the V setting on the ECG machine. For $CV_6LL(V_2)$, the electrode is placed on intercostal space 6 near the left edge of the sternum. For $CV_6LU(V_4)$, use intercostal space 6 at the costochondral junction. For $CV_5RL(V_2R)$, use intercostal space 5 near the right edge of the sternum. For V_{10}, place the lead on the dorsal midline over the dorsal process of the seventh thoracic vertebra.

Interpretation

Each ECG should be read using a definite system. Begin by examining the lead II rhythm strip: Is there a P for every QRS? Is there a QRS for every P? Do all the P waves look alike? Do all the QRS complexes look alike? Are the P and QRS consistently related to each other?

If the answer to any of these questions is "NO," proceed to identify the abnormality. Next, determine, the rate, rhythm, and measurements of the P wave, P-R interval, and QRS complex. Evaluate the S-T segment and T wave, and Q-T interval. Use all leads to determine axis and any miscellaneous criteria.

Heart Rate

Normal heart rate is 70 to 160 beats per minute, up to 180 beats in toy breeds, and 220 in puppies. The normal heart rate for the awake cat is 90 to 240 beats per minute (mean = 195 beats/min).

Determination of Heart Rate

There are small liner marks at the top of the ECG paper. At 50 mm per seconds paper speed, the time between each mark is 1.5 seconds. By counting

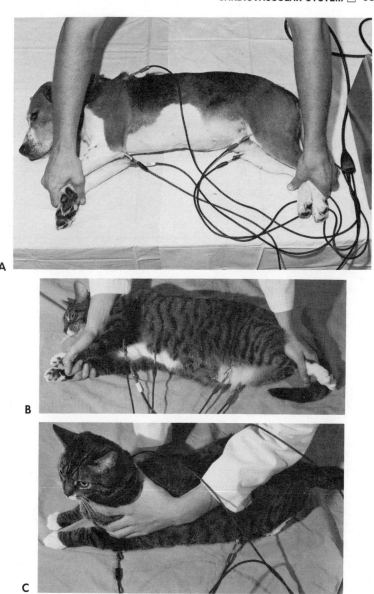

Figure 22. A, Dog in right lateral recumbency with ECG leads attached by alligator clips. Cats may be recorded in either right lateral or sternal recumbency. B, Cat in lateral recumbency. C, Cat in sternal recumbency.

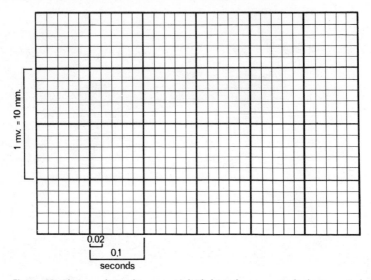

Figure 23. Electrocardiographic paper is divided into large squares by heavy vertical and horizontal lines at 5-mm intervals. Within each large square are 25 1-mm² boxes. At the standard amplitude of 1 mv and a paper speed of 50 mm/sec each box is equal to 0.1 mv on the vertical axis and 0.02 sec on the horizontal axis; five boxes equal 0.1 sec. (From Ettinger, S. J., and Suter, P. F.: Canine Cardiology. Philadelphia, W. B. Saunders Company, 1970.)

two of those divisions and multiplying by 20, the heart rate is calculated (Fig. 24). Heart rate may also be determined by counting the number of small squares between R waves and dividing into 3000 at 50 mm per second paper speed (Fig. 25).

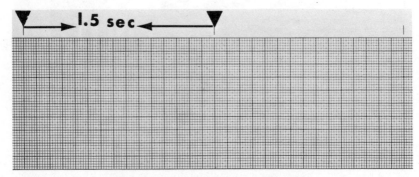

Figure 24. Normal ECG paper run at 50 mm/sec.

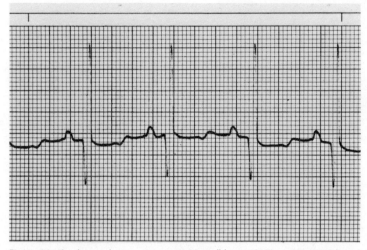

Figure 25. The distance between R waves is 20 small boxes, 3000 ÷ 20 = 150 beats/min. Paper speed is 50 mm/sec.

Heart Rhythm

The normal heart rhythm is sinus in origin. There is a P wave for every QRS complex (Fig. 26). The P waves are related to QRS complexes (P-R interval is constant). Sinus arrhythmia, sinus arrest, and wandering pacemaker are all normal variations of rhythm. In sinus arrhythmia, the P-P interval is irregular. The pauses are never longer than twice the usual P-P interval (Fig. 27). A wandering pacemaker means that the P waves vary in height and may even temporarily be negative (Figs. 28 and 29). Sinus arrest is defined as a prolongation of the P-P interval longer than twice the usual P-P interval.

Normal Electrocardiogram Measurements

P Wave

Normal P wave is 0.04 seconds by 0.4 mv (2 boxes wide by 4 boxes tall) for the dog and 0.04 seconds by 0.2 mv for the cat. In P mitrale (left atrial enlargement), the P wave is wider than 0.04 seconds (Fig. 30). In P pulmonale (right atrial enlargement), the P wave is taller than 0.4 mv for the dog and 0.2 mv for the cat.

P–R Interval

The P-R interval is measured from the beginning of the P wave to the beginning of the QRS complex. Normal is 0.06 to 0.13 seconds (3 to 6.5 boxes wide) for the dog and 0.06 to 0.08 seconds for the cat. In first degree A-V

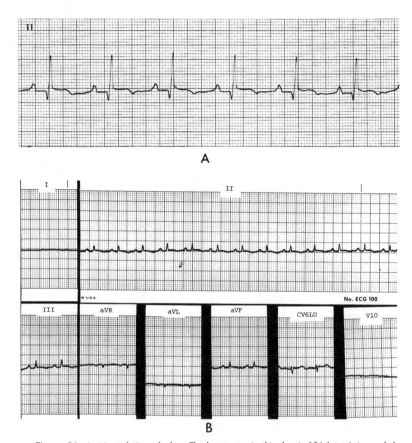

Figure 26. *A,* Normal sinus rhythm. The heart rate in this dog is 136 beats/min, and the rhythm is regular. The complexes are equidistant. *B,* Normal sinus rhythm. The heart rate in this cat is 230 beats/min. Note the regular R-R interval. This 8-lead ECG recording is typical and normal for a healthy cat. (From Ettinger, S. J., and Suter, P. F.: Canine Cardiology. Philadelphia, W. B. Saunders Company, 1970.)

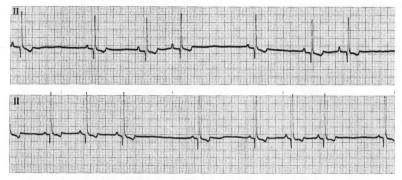

Figure 27. Sinus arrhythmia. Notice the marked fluctuation in heart rate resulting from respiratory sinus arrhythmia in recordings from two normal dogs. The rate may be described as regularly irregular. (From Ettinger, S. J., and Suter, P. F.: Canine Cardiology. Philadelphia, W. B. Saunders Company, 1970.)

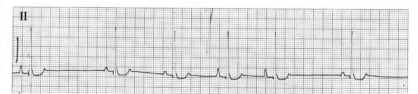

Figure 28. Wandering pacemaker. As the heart rate increases owing to decreased vagal tone, the amplitude of the P waves is increased, and the P waves originate from the sinoatrial node. As the heart rate diminishes when vagal tone increases, the form of the P waves changes, in this case becoming smaller as they arise from a pacemaker other than the sinoatrial node. The duration of the P-R interval is constant at 0.10 sec. (From Ettinger, S. J., and Suter, P. F.: Canine Cardiology. Philadelphia, W. B. Saunders Company, 1970.)

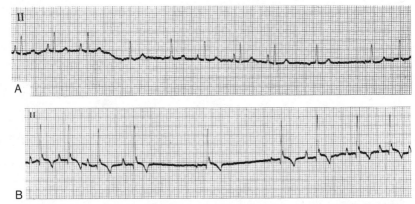

Figure 29. *A,* The wandering pacemaker in this recording is suggested by the slightly negative P waves in some of the complexes. Negative P waves of this nature result from vagal depression of the sinoatrial node and the development of a junctional atrioventricular nodal rhythm. *B,* Marked sinus arrhythmia and a wandering pacemaker result in a decreased heart rate (increased R-R interval) and negative P waves in the fifth complex. As the pacemaker returns to the sinoatrial node, the rate increases, and positive P waves of varying amplitude result in the sixth and seventh complexes.

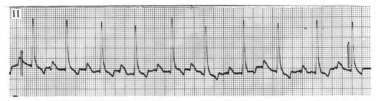

Figure 30. P mitrale. Enlarged left atria are recognized electrocardiographically by prolongation of the atrial conduction time if the P wave is greater than 0.04 sec. The P waves in this dog with chronic mitral valvular fibrosis and mitral valvular insufficiency are prolonged to 0.08 sec. Such extreme prolongation is unusual, even in dogs with severe mitral valvular insufficiency. The amplitude and duration of the QRS complex are consistent with left ventricular hypertrophy. (From Ettinger, S. J., and Suter, P. F.: Canine Cardiology. Philadelphia, W. B. Saunders Company, 1970.)

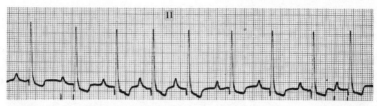

Figure 31. First degree atrioventricular block (incomplete block) is characterized by a normal rhythm in which the duration of the P-R interval is greater than 0.13 sec. Here, the P-R interval is 0.14 sec and is easily seen. (From Ettinger, S. J., and Suter, P. F.: Canine Cardiology. Philadelphia, W. B. Saunders Company, 1970.)

heart block, the P-R interval is prolonged (Fig. 31). The P-R interval is sometimes useful in monitoring the effects of digitalis therapy.

QRS Complex

The QRS complex duration is measured from the beginning of the Q wave to the end of the S wave. Normal is up to 0.04 seconds in cats, 0.05 seconds in small dogs, and 0.06 seconds in large dogs. If the QRS complex is too wide, it indicates left ventricular enlargement (Fig. 32). If the R wave is too tall, it indiates left ventricular enlargement. It is measured from the baseline to the top of the R wave (Fig. 33). The R wave can be up to 0.8 mv tall in cats, 2.5 mv in small dogs, and 3.0 mv in large dogs.

S–T Segment

The S–T segment is between the end of the S wave and the beginning of the T wave. Normally it lies on the baseline and then dips into the T wave. S–T slurring indicates left ventricular enlargement and is seen when the S

II

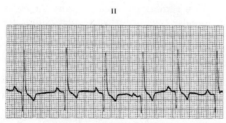

Figure 32. Left ventricular hypertrophy. ECG of a dog with chronic mitral valvular fibrosis and mitral valvular insufficiency. The QRS complex is prolonged to 0.07 sec. S-T repolarization changes are present, and P mitrale is seen. (From Ettinger, S. J., and Suter, P. F.: Canine Cardiology. Philadelphia, W. B. Saunders Company, 1970.)

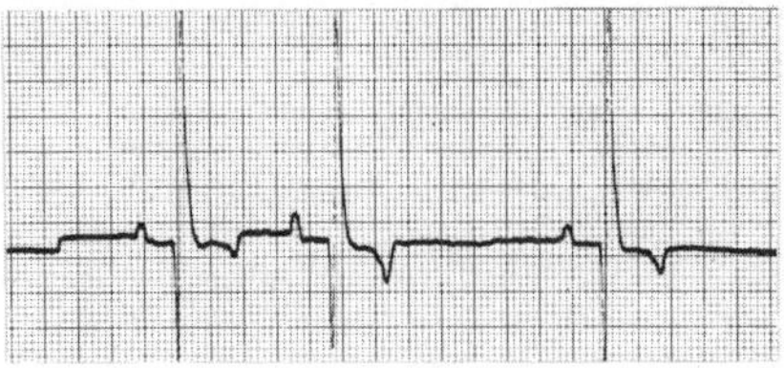

II

Figure 33. Left ventricular hypertrophy. This dog had markedly enlarged ventricles owing to insufficiency of the mitral and tricuspid valves. The amplitude and duration of the QRS complexes are increased. The amplitude of the R waves is greater than 25 mm (35 mm here), and the QRS complex is prolonged to 0.07 sec. The deep Q waves suggest that biventricular enlargement has occurred. (From Ettinger, S. J., and Suter, P. F.: Canine Cardiology. Philadelphia, W. B. Saunders Company, 1970.)

wave slurs into the T wave and no S–T segment is discernible (Fig. 34). The S–T segment is elevated if it lies greater than 0.1 mv (1 box) above the baseline (>0.2 mv in CV_6LL and CV_6LU). This may happen with hypercalcemia or myocardial hypoxia. The S–T segment is depressed if it lies more than 0.1 mv (1 box;) (> 0.2 mv in CV_6LL and CV_6LU) below the baseline. This may be seen with myocardial ischemia, hypoxia, or hypocalcemia.

Q–T Internal

The Q–T interval is measured from the beginning of the Q wave to the end of the T wave. Normal is 0.14 to 0.22 seconds (7–11 boxes wide) in dogs and up to 0.16 seconds in cats. A lengthened Q–T interval may be seen with hypokalemia or hypocalcemia. It varies with heart rate, and it tends to be prolonged when bradycardia occurs. A decreased Q–T interval may be seen with hypercalcemia.

Axis Determination

The mean electrical cardiac axis measures the direction (vector) that the cardiac ventricular impulse travels during depolarization. Therefore, the QRS complex is examined in leads I, II, III, aVR, aVL, and aVF. These six leads determine the axis. They are arranged in a manner known as Bailey's Hexaxial Lead System (Fig. 35). The procedure is as follows:

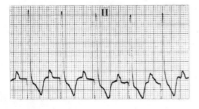

Figure 34. S-T slurring is characterized by the slurring of the downstroke of the R wave into the T wave, with no discernible S-T segment. This occurs because of ischemia secondary to wall strain in cardiac enlargement.

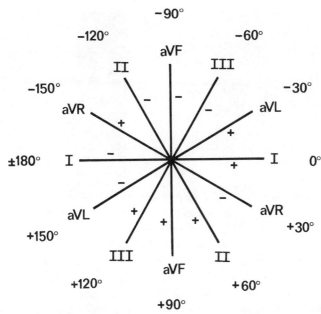

Figure 35. Bailey six-axis reference system. The lead axes are marked in 30° increments from 0° to 180° and from 0° to −180°. The six leads are marked with a + at the positive electrode and a − at the negative electrode. Notice that for leads I, II, III, and aVF the polarity and angle of the leads are positive or negative simultaneously. Leads aVR and aVL are positive at the positions of −150° and −30°, respectively, since the positive electrodes for those leads lie in the negative 0° to −180° zone. (From Ettinger, S. J., and Suter, P. F.: Canine Cardiology. Philadelphia, W. B. Saunders Company, 1970.)

1. Find an isoelectric lead. This is a lead whose number of positive (upward) and negative (downward) deflections of the QRS complex are equal to zero (Fig. 36). There will not always be a perfectly isoelectric lead. When this happens, the one that comes the closest is used.
2. Find the lead that is perpendicular to the isoelectric lead: lead I is perpendicular to aVF; lead II is perpendicular to aVL; and lead III is perpendicular to aVR (see Fig. 35).
3. Determine whether that perpendicular lead is positive or negative on the patient's ECG. If it were negative, the axis is at the negative end of that lead (each lead has a + and − pole marked; Fig. 35). If it were positive, the mean electrical axis is at the positive end of the perpendicular lead. For example, if aVL were isoelectric (normally it is), lead II is its perpendicular. If lead II were + on the ECG, the axis is +60 degrees. If lead II were − on the ECG, then the axis would be —120 degrees.

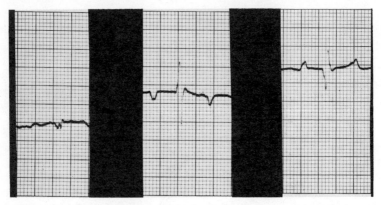

Figure 36. In each of these three leads, the total positive and negative deflections equal zero. Each is considered an isoelectric lead.

Significance of Changes

Normal axis in the dog is +40 to +100 degrees; for the cat it is more variable at ±0 to ±180 degrees. Right axis deviation (axis is over +100) indicates right ventricular enlargement in the dog (Fig. 37). Left axis deviation (axis is less than +40°) indicates left ventricular enlargement in the dog (Fig. 38). When there is biventricular enlargement, the axis usually remains normal.

Axis determinations are of less value in the cat, because the normal range is so wide.

Miscellaneous Criteria for Ventricular Enlargement

Summary of Criteria for Left Ventricular Enlargement

1. Left axis deviation (dog).
2. QRS complex too wide.
3. R wave too tall.
4. S–T slurring.
5. May be associated with P mitrale, because left atrium and ventricle tend to be stressed together.

Summary of Criteria for Right Ventricular Enlargement

1. Right axis deviation (dog and cat).
2. Presence of an S wave in leads I, II, and III (S_1—S_2—S_3 pattern; dog only; Fig. 39).
3. S wave deeper than 0.7 mv in lead CV_6LU (V_4) in the dog.
4. May be associated with P pulmonale, because the right atrium and ventricle tend to be stressed together.

Summary of Criteria for Biventricular Enlargement

1. Tall R wave.
2. Wide QRS complex.

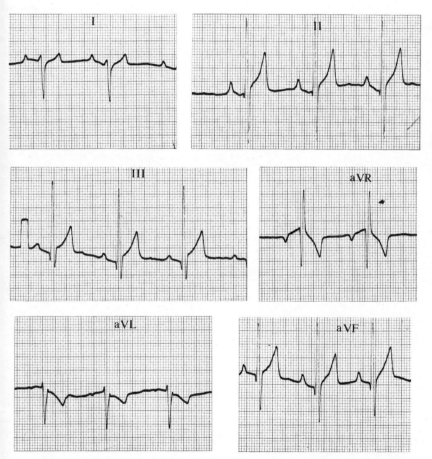

Figure 37. Notice the + 120° axis. (From Ettinger, S. J., and Suter, P. F.: Canine Cardiology. Philadelphia, W. B. Saunders Company, 1970.)

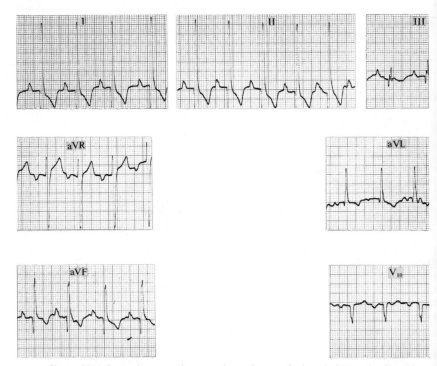

Figure 38. Left axis deviation. The mean electrical axis in the frontal plane in this dog with mitral valvular fibrosis is 35°. Notice that the R wave in lead I is tall and positive, as would be expected in left axis deviation. Also present in this tracing are P mitrale, tall and prolonged QRS complexes, and S-T repolarization changes, all of which are consistent with left atrial and left ventricular hypertrophy. (From Ettinger, S. J., and Suter, P. F.: Canine Cardiology, Philadelphia, W. B. Saunders Company, 1970.)

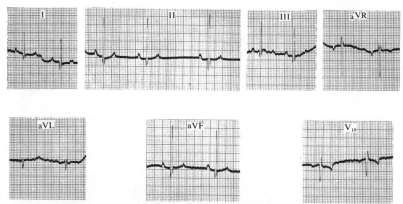

Figure 39. S_1-S_2-S_3 pattern. This tracing was made from a dog with heartworm disease. The S_1-S_2-S_3 pattern is unusual in normal dogs, and the finding can suggest right ventricular hypertrophy. Such findings warrant further study, especially in areas where heartworms are endemic. (From Ettinger, S. J., and Suter, P. F.: Canine Cardiology. Philadelphia, W. B. Saunders Company, 1970.)

3. S–T segment slurring.
4. Deep Q waves in lead II; deeper than 0.3 mv for the cat and 0.5 mv for the dog (see Fig. 33).
5. Normal mean electrical axis.
6. P mitrale and/or P pulmonale.

RADIOGRAPHIC PROCEDURES

Lateral and dorsoventral radiographs are valuable in assessing both cardiac enlargement and pulmonary changes that may have occurred (Figs. 40–44), thus assisting in diagnosis, treatment, and prognosis.

Changes in lung vasculature may be evident on radiographs. With pulmonary congestion, the pulmonary veins are engorged with blood. With pulmonary overcirculation, the pulmonary arteries are engorged. On lateral radiographic films, the veins appear indistinct and tortuous and are seen emanating from the area of the left atrium. On the other hand, the pulmonary arteries appear straight and branching, like a tree. On the dorsoventral view, veins are medial and arteries are lateral to each bronchus. Mitral insufficiency causes pulmonary venous congestion; heartworm disease, chronic lung disease, and congenital left-to-right shunt anomalies cause pulmonary artery enlargement. It is also important to thoroughly evaluate the mediastinum.

The mediastinum is a compartment of the thorax between the medial aspects of the two pleural sacs. The mediastinal pleural layers are thin and disease processes such as pneumothorax and hydrothorax seldom remain unilateral.

Text continued on page 370

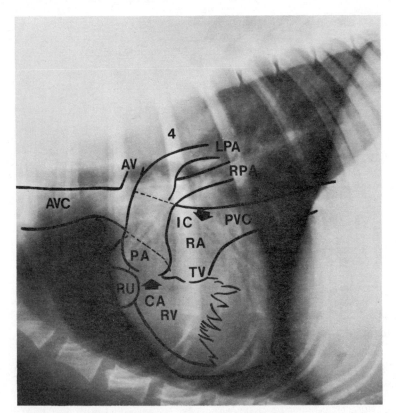

Figure 40. Left lateral radiograph of dog. Tracing delineates the structures of the right heart. The details for the tracing were obtained from angiocardiograms.

AVC—cranial vena cava; AV—junction of the azygos vein with the AVC; RU—right auricle; RV—right ventricle; CA—conus arteriosus, or right ventricular outflow tract, extending to the tricuspid valve (arrow); PA—main pulmonary artery; LPA—left pulmonary artery; RPA—right pulmonary artery; RA—right atrium, divided dorsally by the intervenous crest, IC; arrow caudal to IC points at foramen ovale; PVC—caudal vena cava; 4—fourth rib. (From Ettinger, S. J., and Suter, P. F.: Canine Cardiology. Philadelphia, W. B. Saunders Company, 1970.)

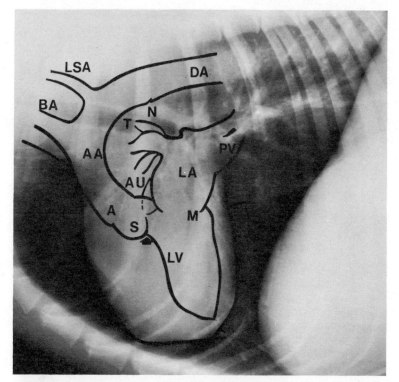

Figure 41. Lateral radiograph of dog in Figure 39. Tracing delineates the structures of the left heart. The details for the tracing were obtained from angiocardiograms.

BA—brachiocephalic artery; LSA—left subclavian artery; AA—aortic arch; A—ascending aorta; S—sinus of Valsalva (arrow points at aortic valve); AU—small portion of the left auricle; T—tracheal bifurcation; N—notch in the descending aorta, DA, indicating the area of the ligamentum arteriosum; LV—left ventricle; M—mitral valve; LA—left atrium; PV—pulmonary veins. (From Ettinger, S. J., and Suter, P. F.: Canine Cardiology. Philadelphia, W. B. Saunders Company, 1970.)

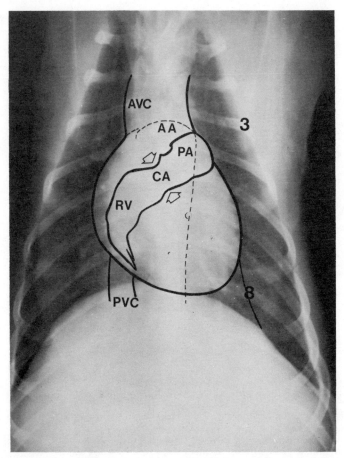

Figure 42. Dorsoventral radiograph of dog in Figure 39. Tracing delineates the right ventricle. Details for the tracing were obtained from angiocardiograms.

AVC—cranial vena cava; AA—aortic arch; PA—main pulmonary artery, so-called pulmonary artery segment; CA—conus arteriosus, or right ventricular outflow tract; RV—right ventricle; PVC—caudal vena cava; numbers 3 and 8 indicate the respective ribs. (From Ettinger, S. J., and Suter, P. F.: Canine Cardiology. Philadelphia, W. B. Saunders Company, 1970.)

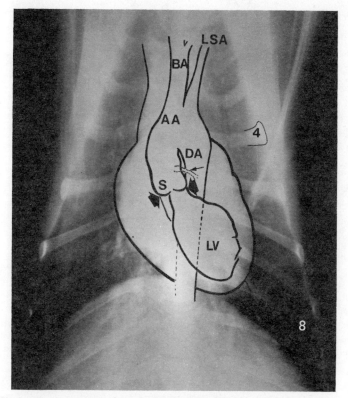

Figure 43. Dorsoventral radiograph of dog in Figure 39. Tracing delineates the structures of the left ventricle and aorta. Details for the tracing were obtained from angiocardiograms.

LSA—left subclavian artery; BA—brachial artery; AA—aortic arch; DA—descending aorta; S—sinus of Valsalva; large arrows point to the muscular lining of the left ventricular outflow tract; small arrow indicates the origin of the left coronary artery, which is indicated by broken lines; LV—left ventricle; numbers 4 and 8 indicate the respective ribs. (From Ettinger, S. J., and Suter, P. F.: Canine Cardiology. Philadelphia, W. B. Saunders Company, 1970.)

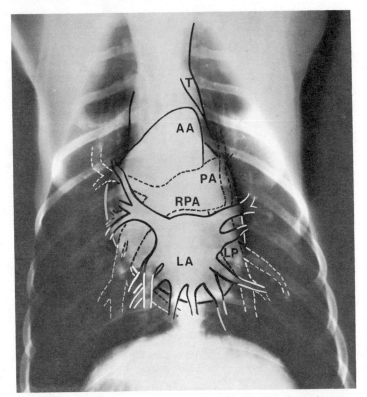

Figure 44. Dorsoventral radiograph of dog in Figure 39. Tracing outlines pulmonary arteries and the confluence of the pulmonary veins at the left atrium. Solid lines represent veins and left atrium; broken lines indicate the pulmonary arteries. Details for the tracings were obtained from angiocardiograms.

T—thymus, seen only in growing dogs; AA—aortic arch; PA—pulmonary artery; RPA—right pulmonary artery; LP—left pulmonary artery; LA—left atrium. (From Ettinger, S. J., and Suter, P. F.: Canine Cardiology. Philadelphia, W. B. Saunders Company, 1970.)

Signs related to abnormalities in the mediastinal area may be dysphagia, regurgitation, coughing and dyspnea, syncope, head and neck edema, thoracic pain, abdominal breathing, Horner's syndrome, and emphysema.

Disease Processes that Alter Mediastinal Position

1. Unilateral pleural or pulmonary masses.
2. Unilateral pneumothorax or hydrothorax.
3. Lung lobe collapse, agenesis, hypoplasia, or resection.
4. Pleural adhesions.
5. Hypostatic congestion of a lung.

Diseases that Result in Mediastinal Widening

1. Accumulation of medistinal fat or fluid.
2. Inflammation secondary to tracheal or esophageal puncture.
3. Hemorrhage.
4. Tumor formation (lymphosarcoma, thymoma).
5. Heart base tumors.
6. Enlargement of tracheobronchial lymph nodes.

The intrathoracic trachea is about 3 times the width of the proximal third rib but increases in diameter on inspiration and decreases on expiration. Normal trachea enters the thoracic inlet in the dorsal third of the inlet. The intrathoracic trachea may collapse on expiration which may extend to the carina and main stem bronchi.

Congenital tracheal hypoplasia is seen in the English bulldog.

Tracheal compression and/or left main stem bronchus compression may be associated with enlargements of tracheobronchial lymph nodes or of the left atrium.

Survey Radiographs of the Heart

1. The normal canine heart is on a 45-degree angle with the sternum.
2. The heart extends from the third to eighth thoracic vertebrae.
3. Breed variation can greatly affect the appearance of the cardiac silhouette, as can respiratory and cardiac cycle.
4. Thoracic radiographs should be taken at the height of inspiration.
5. The heart of the cat assumes a more elongated and elliptical position than the dog; it occupies 2 to 2.5 intercostal spaces, and the caudal border is separated from the diaphragm by one or two intercostal spaces.
6. In ventrodorsal (V-D) and dorsoventral (D-V) positions, the canine heart has a curved right border, straight left border with the long axis oriented at a 30-degree angle to the spine and to the left of the midline.
7. The feline heart is more oval in appearance on V-D; D-V view, cardiac apex is just to the left midline; the ratio of the longitudinal axis to the transverse axis is 1.4:1.

Radiographic evaluation of the cardiovascular system and lungs is an important differential diagnostic feature in cardiovascular disease. It is especially important to evaluate: (1) enlargement of cardiac chambers; (2) dilatation of great vessels; (3) increased or decreased pulmonary circulation; (4) venous congestion, pulmonary edema, and pleural effusion; and (5) mediastinal space.

When viewing thoracic radiographs to determine whether there is evidence of cardiovascular disease concomitant with clinical findings, the following questions should be asked:

1. Is the cardiac silhouette larger or smaller than normal?
2. Is the cardiac apex pointing to the right or left?
3. Are cardiac chamber shapes normal or abnormal?
4. Are there changes in size, shape, or position of cardiac or intrathoracic vessels or of trachea and bronchi?

5. Is there evidence of pleural fluid accumulation?
6. If there evidence of pulmonary edema?
7. Is there evidence of intrathoracic disease other than cardiovascular in origin?
8. Is the mediastinum normal or abnormal?

When interpreting changes in cardiac size and shape, consistency of radiographic technique is important. Short radiographic exposure times one sixtieth to one one hundred twentieth of a second with radiographs taken at full inspiration give the best results.

Enlargement of Right Atrium (usually associated with right ventricular enlargement)

1. Bulging cranial heart border on lateral view.
2. Bulging at 9 to 11 o'clock position of V-D (D-V) view.

Right Ventricle

1. Cranial border of heart is more rounded with increased sternal contact; (>3 sternebrae) and the heart may be elevated dorsally on lateral view.
2. Overall width of heart is increased.
3. Elevation of trachea cranial to tracheal bifurcation.
4. V-D (D-V) view; heart rounded from 6 to 11 o'clock position.
5. Distance between right heart border and thoracic wall is decreased.

Left Atrium

1. Bulging caudal dorsal heart border on lateral view.
2. Loss of caudal waist on lateral view.
3. Elevation of trachea, compression of main stem bronchi.
4. Bulging at 2 to 3 o'clock position on V-D (D-V) view.
5. Increased size of pulmonary veins.

Left Ventricle

1. Elongation cardiac silhouette on either lateral or V-D (D-V) view.
2. Elevation of trachea.
3. Rounded caudal border of the heart.
4. Distance between left heart border and thoracic wall is decreased on V-D (D-V) view.

Biventricular Enlargement

1. Heart appears rounded on both views.
2. Increased sternal contact on lateral view, with elongation and widening of the heart shadow.
3. May mimic pericardial effusion if uniform and severe.

Decrease in Size of Cardiac Silhouette

1. Heart elevated off the sternum.
2. Increase in ratio of longitudinal axis to transverse axis is greater than 1.4:1.
3. Shifting of heart away from midline.
4. Small caudal vena cava.
5. Seen in Addison's disease, hypothyroidism, shock, and pneumothorax.

Differential Diagnosis of Diseases Based on Survey Radiographs
See Table 63.

A severe degree of cardiomegaly with evidence of right heart failure suggests advanced mitral and tricuspid valvular fibrosis, congestive cardiomyopathy, or pericardial effusion. Nonselective angiocardiography can be helpful

Table 63. TYPICAL RADIOGRAPHIC FINDINGS IN HEART DISEASE

Lesion	RA	RV	LA	LV	Aorta	MPA	Circ	PV	VC	Other Features
Mitral insufficiency	N	N↑	↑	↑	N	N	N	↑	N	Can be secondary to cardiomyopathy, endocarditis, or left-to-right shunt.
Aortic stenosis	N	N↑	N↑	↑	↑	N	N	N↑	N	Widened mediastinum is common.
Aortic insufficiency	N	N↑	↑	↑	N↑	N	N	N↑	N	Caused by endocarditis or congenital disease.
Tricuspid insufficiency	↑	↑	N	N	N	N	N	N	↑	Can be secondary to cardiomyopathy, heartworm disease, or pulmonary stenosis.
Pulmonary stenosis	↑	↑	N↓	N↓	N	↑	N↓	N↓	↑	Apex displacement mimics LVH.
Tetralogy of Fallot	N↑	↑	N↓	N↓	N	N↑	↓	↓	N	Aortic position is cranial and may widen the mediastinum. Apex shift is common.
Atrial septal defect	↑	↑	N↑	N	N	N↑	N↑	N	N↑	Generalized cardiomegaly if VSD is present.
Dirofilariasis	↑	↑	N	N	N	↑	↑	N	↑	Enlarged pulmonary arteries, pulmonary infiltrates.
Patent ductus arteriosus	N	↑	↑	↑	N	↑	↑	↑	N↑	Pulmonary edema is common.
Ventricular septal defect (VSD)	N	↑	↑	↑	N	N↑	↑	N↑	N↑	Findings vary. May be part of endocardial cushion defect in cats.
Hypertrophic cardiomyopathy	↑	↑	↑	N↑	N	N	N	↑	N↑	Valentine-shaped heart, apex shift, pulmonary edema, or pleural effusion.
Congestive (dilated) cardiomyopathy	↑	↑	↑	↑	N↓	N	N↓	↑	↑	Pleural effusion, pulmonary edema are common.
Pericardial disease	↑	↑	↑	↑	N↓	N	N↓	↑	↑	Globoid silhouette.

RA = right atrium, RV = right ventricle, LA = left atrium, LV = left ventricle, MPA = main pulmonary artery, Circ = pulmonary vascular, PV = pulmonary veins, VC = caudal vena cava, N = normal, ↑ = enlarged or increased, ↓ = smaller or decreased, and LVH = left ventricular hypertrophy.

From Myer, et al.: Survey radiography of the heart. Vet. Clin. North Am., *12(2)*:223, 1982.

in distinguishing between cardiomyopathy, congenital cardiac abnormalities, and pericardial effusion.

Radiographic Appearance of the Lungs in Left-Sided Heart Failure

1. *Pulmonary congestion*—engorgement and distention of pulmonary veins, especially at the junction of the veins with the left atrium. Pulmonary radiodensity is unchanged.
2. *Pulmonary interstitial lung edema phase*—pulmonary radiodensity is increased, and lungs appear hazy. Accumulated fluid in perivascular spaces makes the vascular markings appear hazy.
3. *Alveolar edema*—fluid enters the alveoli and peripheral bronchioles, creating alveolar radiodensity and air bronchograms. Alveolar radiodensity is most severe in the perihilar area.

The lung fields should also be carefully reviewed for evidence of vascular changes compatible with heartworm disease or pulmonary embolism.

Ancillary Radiographic Signs Associated with Heart Disease

1. Ascites.
2. Liver enlargement.
3. Increased size of portal venous circulation.
4. Decreased pulmonary circulation.
5. Increased venous congestion of the intestines.
6. Pleural effusion, pericardial effusion.
7. Increased size of cranial and caudal vena cava.
8. Splenic enlargement.

Cardiac Catheterization

Cardiac catheterization may be either selective or nonselective in type. Selective catheterization consists of passing a catheter into the right side of the heart, through either the femoral or jugular veins, and into the left-sided cardiac chambers, through the femoral or carotid arteries, under fluoroscopic guidance. Injections of contrast media either by hand or mechanical pressure injector will selectively outline individual chambers and major vessels. Individual chamber and vessel pressures may be obtained (Tables 64 and 65). Blood gas analysis can be performed on blood withdrawn from selected cardiac chambers.

Nonselective catheterization is limited to angiographic evaluation of cardiac chambers and major vessels. A bolus of contrast medium is hand injected through a large-bore (16- to 18-gauge) catheter placed in one of the jugular

Table 64. NORMAL CARDIAC CHAMBER PRESSURES (mm Hg)

	PA	RV	RA	AO	LV	Wedge (LA)
Systolic	15–30	15–30	3–5	100–180	100–180	6–10
Diastolic	10	0–5	3–5	60–90	0–10	6–10

Table 65. INTRACARDIAC PHYSIOLOGIC VALUES OF DOGS

| Condition | Pressures (mm Hg) | | | Diastolic Heart Vol ml/kg BW | Total Heart Weight gm/kg BW | Blood Volume ml/kg BW | Heart Rate (Untreated) |
	JVP	PAP	FAP				
Normal	0–6	20–30	140–180	15–20	6–10	75–90	70–120
Mitral insufficiency							
Mild	0	35	120–180	20	8	90	100–190
	to	to		to	to	to	
Severe	20	55	100–165	60	15	120	120–240
Heartworms							
Mild	0	30	120–200	20	8	90	70–120
	to	to		to	to	to	
Severe	25	125	140–200	60	15	125	90–190
Pulmonic stenosis	25	115	100	36	12	122	170
Patent ductus arteriosus	5	60	190	—	10	—	150
	(not in congestive failure)						
Ventricular septal defect	20	150	150	56	15	—	140

JVP = jugular venous pressure, PAP = pulmonary arterial pressure, systolic; FAP = femoral arterial pressure, systolic; and BW = body weight.

Values obtained in dogs studied by the Department of Physiology, Medical College of Georgia, Augusta, Ga., under United States Public Health Service Grants HTS 5044, H 240 and AHA.

From Wallace, C. R.: Cardiac catheterization to aid in diagnosis of cardiovascular disease. Small Anim. Clin., 2:324, 1962.

Table 66. CONTRAST MEDIA FOR ANGIOCARDIOGRAPHY

Brand Name	Active Agent	Iodine (mg/ml)	Sodium (mg/ml)	Viscosity 25° C	Viscosity 37° C
Renografin-76 (Squibb)	60% diatrizaoate meglumine 10% diatrizoate sodium	370	4.48	13.9	9.1
Conray (Mallinckrodt)	60% iothalamate meglumine	282	0	6	4
Angio-Conray (Mallinckrodt)	80% iothalamate sodium	480	28.9	14	9
Hypaque-M 75% (Winthrop)	50% diatrizoate meglumine 25% diatrizoate sodium	385	9	8.3	—
Conray 400 (Squibb)	66.8% iothalamate sodium	400	23.1	—	4.5
Vascoray (Mallinckrodt)	52% iothalamate meglumine 26% iothalamate sodium	400	—	—	—

From Fox, P. R.: Vet. Clin. North Am., *13*(2): 1983.

veins. Because of the length of time needed to make the bolus injection, this technique is best accomplished in patients who weigh less than 15 kg (33 lb). Sequential radiographs can be obtained by using the "tunnel technique" for multiple radiographic exposures. (See Owens and Twedt, 1977 and Fox and Bond, 1983). Various types of contrast agents are available (Table 66). The dosage for the cat is 0.8 to 1.8 ml per kg, and for the dog, it is 1.0 to 2.0 ml per kg. Four exposures are made as rapidly as possible following the injection.

Time	Structures Opacified
1–3 sec postinjection	precava, right atrium, right ventricle, and pulmonary arteries
4–8 sec postinjection	pulmonary veins, left atrium, left ventricle, and aorta

In the cat the radiographic film should be large enough so that emboli can be detected in the renal arteries, distal aorta, and femoral arteries.

Other Tests

CBC, BUN, creatinine, SGPT, urinalysis, and microfilaria examination are ancillary tests that may be helpful in evaluating cardiovascular abnormalities.

Abdominal centesis fluid may also be useful. Fluid resulting from congestive heart failure has the following characteristics: (1) specific gravity is less than 1.018; (2) clear, straw colored, or slightly blood-tinged; (3) protein content is less than 3.0 gm per dl, and (4) absence of significant numbers of inflammatory cells.

ECHOCARDIOGRAPHY

Echocardiography is the technique of displaying the image of the heart and its structure by transmitting and receiving ultrasound waves as they are reflected from cardiac structures. Both unidimensional ("M mode") and two-dimensional real time echocardiography ("2 D") methods have been used.

M-mode echocardiography uses a narrow beam to produce unidimensional images of cardiac structures moving toward or away from the transducer and parallel to the beam. Two-dimensional echocardiography uses a thin wedge-shaped ultrasonic beam producing a two-dimensional tomographic image of the heart and its structures.

Using either of these techniques and coordinating the image with the ECG, measurements can be made of diastolic and systolic chamber sizes and motion, valve shapes and motion, interventricular septal thickness and motion, free wall thickness and motion, chordae tendineae, papillary muscles, pericardium, and the pericardial space.

Because it is noninvasive, most patients will tolerate this procedure with little or no sedation. The transducer frequencies used are:

Cat:	5.0–7.5 MHz
Dog:	3.5–5.0 MHz
Horse	1.5–2.25 MHz
Cow:	1.5–2.25 MHz

The most consistent position for recording the echocardiogram is left lateral recumbency, placing the transducer between the right intercostal spaces, 3 and 5, 1 to 8 cm above the sternum. Other positions that are sometimes helpful are sitting or standing or in right lateral recumbency through a hole cut in the table surface to allow placement of the transducer over the right thorax. Ultrasound coupling gel should be applied to both the thoracic echo area and the transducer head. The two-dimensional technique uses both long-axis (longitudinal) and short-axis (cross section) views (Figs. 45–47).

Indications for echocardiography include the following:
1. Unexplained cardiomegaly.
2. Murmurs of questionable origin.
3. Diagnoses and monitoring of congenital and acquired heart disease.
4. Monitoring of the effects of drugs on cardiac function.
5. Monitoring of the effects of noncardiac diseases on cardiac function (i.e., hyperthyroidism, Addison's disease, etc.).
6. Identification of intracardiac masses, heartworms, or vegetative valvular lesions.
7. Evaluation of the pericardium and the pericardial space.

ECHOCARDIOGRAPHY NORMAL VALUES

	Horse	Cow	Pig	Cat	Dog
Ao diameter (cm)	5.8 – 9.2	5.2 – 6.8	1.6 – 2.5	0.4 – 1.18	Ao:LA = 1:1
LA size (cm)	3.5 – 5.5	3.7 – 5.8	1.4 – 2.0	0.45– 1.12	–
RV dim (cm)	2.1 – 4.3	2.5 – 4.8	–	–	–
Septal th (cm)	2.0 – 4.3	1.9 – 2.8	0.5 – 0.92	0.28– 0.60	0.5 – 0.9
LVD (diast) (cm)	7.0 – 1.8	5.5 – 8.7	2.7 – 3.8	1.12–2.18	3.0 – 4.7
LV wall th (cm)	2.1 – 4.5	1.8 – 2.5	0.4 – 0.8	0.33– 0.50	0.5 – 0.8
% △ D	26–42	34–51	34–59	23–56	>25
Vcf (cm/sec)	0.45– 0.99	0.67– 1.20	0.7 – 1.4	1.27– 4.55	–
PEP (sec)	0.13– 0.36	0.06– 0.17	0.05– 0.12	–	0.06– 0.08
LVET (sec)	0.43– 0.62	0.39– 0.67	0.16– 0.27	0.11– 0.19	0.11– 0.17
Q-S$_2$ (sec)	0.62– 0.83	0.50– 0.78	0.25– 0.37	–	–

Ao = aorta, LA = left atrium, RV = right ventricle, LVD = left ventricular diameter, PEP = positive expiratory pressure, L:VET = left ventricular ejection time, and Q = S$_2$ = electromechanic systole.

From Pipers, F. S., University of Florida. School of Veterinary Medicine, Gainesville, Florida.

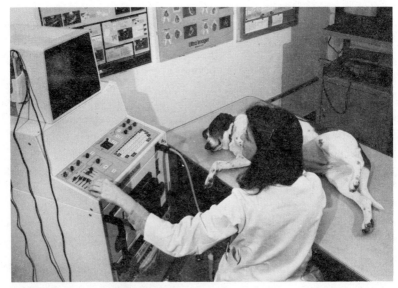

Figure 45. Two-dimensional echocardiography being performed. Note outline of wedge-shaped image of heart on monitor screen.

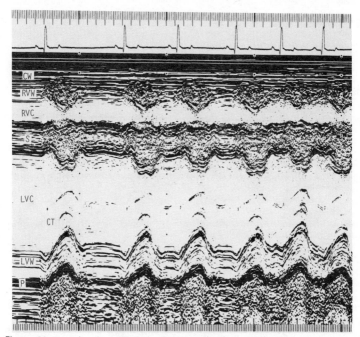

Figure 46. M-mode echocardiogram, with ECG visible at the top.

P, pericardium; LVW, left ventricular wall; CT, chordae tendineae; LVC, left ventricular chamber; S, interventricular septum; RVC, right ventricular chamber; RVW, right ventricular wall; CW, chest wall.

Figure 47. An 11-year-old castrated male setter-cross-breed suspected of having bacterial endocarditis. Long axis view of the left ventricle and left atrium in diastole via two-dimensional echocardiography. The left ventricular lumen is the dark area to the left. The enlarged left atrial lumen is the dark area to the right. The anterior mitral leaflet with a vegetative lesion attached is seen within the box. The posterior leaflet can be seen outside the lower left corner of the box.

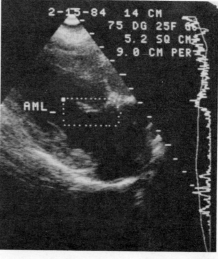

References and Additional Readings

Academy of Veterinary Cardiology. Report of the Committee on Echocardiography. Annual Meeting, San Antonio, Texas, 1983.

Bolton, G. R.: Handbook of Canine Electrocardiography. Philadelphia, W. B. Saunders Company, 1975.

Ettinger, S. J., and Suter, P. F.: Canine Cardiology. Philadelphia, W. B. Saunders Company, 1970.

Feigenbaum, H.: Echocardiography, 3rd ed. Philadelphia, Lea & Febiger, 1981.

Fox, P. R., and Bond, B. R.: Nonselective and selective angiocardiography. Vet. Clin. North Am., *13* (2):259, 1983.

Garner, H. E., Hahn, A. W., Hartley, J. W., et al.: Indirect blood pressure measurement in the dog. Lab. Anim. Sci. *25*:197, 1975.

Kallet, A., and Cowgill, L. D.: Hypertensive states in dogs: Proc. Am. Coll. Vet. Intern. Med. 79, 1982.

Kittleson, M. D. and Oliver, B. N.: Measurement of systemic arterial blood pressure. Vet. Clin. North Am., *13*(2):321, 1983.

McGrath, C. J., Nichols, M. F., and Hartley, J.: Indirect arterial blood pressure monitoring in dogs during anesthesia. Proceedings of the 24th Gaines Veterinary Symposium, 1974, pp. 29–33.

Myer, W., and Bonagura, J. D.: Survey radiographs of the heart. Vet. Clin. North Am., *12*(2):213, 1982.

Owens, J. M.: Radiographic Interpretation for Small Animal Clinician. Ralston Purina Co., 1982.

Owens, J. M., and Twedt, D. C.: Nonselective angiography in the cat. Vet. Clin. North Am., 7:309, 1977.

Suter, P. F.: Radiographic diagnosis canine and feline heart disease. Compendium on Continuing Education, 3(5):441, 1981.

Tilley, L. P.: Essentials of Canine and Feline Electrocardiography. 2nd ed. Philadelphia, Lea & Febiger, 1984.

Tilley, L. P. (ed.): Symposium on feline cardiology. Vet. Clin. North Am., 7:1977.

Weisser, M. G., Spangler, W. L., and Gribble, D. H.: Blood pressure measurement in the dog. J.A.V.M.A., *171*:364, 1977.

EYE, EAR, NOSE, AND THROAT

Examination of the Eye

An example of an eye examination record is shown in Figure 48.

EXTERNAL EXAMINATION

Inspection of the Globe and Neuromuscular Examination

A general inspection of the globe and external ocular structures should be conducted before any detailed examination of the eye is undertaken. Inspect the globe in normal daylight or roomlight and observe the relationship of the globe to the orbit and the eyelids. Note whether the eyes are in the same

N.Y.S. COL. OF VET. MEDICINE — CORNELL UNIVERSITY — TEACHING HOSPITALS

DATE_____ O P H T H A L M O L O G Y   E X A M I N A T I O N

HISTORY:_____

IRIS_____

PUPILLARY REFLEX_____
OCULAR PRESSURE_____

LENS_____

REF. DVM_____

CLINICIAN_____

GLOBE/ORBIT_____

LIDS_____

A ( ) ( ) P

O.D.   O.S.   O.D.   O.S.

PALPEBRAL REFLEX_____
MENACE REFLEX_____
NASAL-LACRIMAL_____ FUNDUS:_____

NICTITANS_____

CONJUNCTIVA_____

CORNEA_____

CORNEAL REFLEX   O.D.   O.S.
ANTERIOR CHAMBER_____

O.D.   O.S.

ASSESSMENT:_____ PLAN:_____

_____
_____
_____

CLIENT. ED._____

(Teaching   Kowa   Donaldson   2X2   Pathology   Culture   Cytology   Surgery)

O P H T H A L M O L O G Y   E X A M I N A T I O N

Figure 48. Eye examination record chart.

visual axis or whether a tropia is present. Note any undue prominence of either or both eyes. Note the presence of any other facial lesions (e.g., facial paralysis) that may affect the symmetry of the orbit. Inspect the external ocular structures (lids, conjunctiva, cornea, sclera, and lacrimal apparatus). Note the position of the eyelids, the size of the palpebral aperture, the position of the membrana nictitans, and the presence of nystagmus, unequal pupils, blepharospasm, lagophthalmos, or ocular discharges.

The tonic eye reflexes are used in the determination of extraocular muscle function and localization of lesions in the central nervous system (CNS). Cranial nerves III (oculomotorius), IV (trochlearis), and VI (abducens) innervate the extraocular striated muscles and are examined together. Nerve IV innervates the m. obliquus dorsalis, nerve VI innervates the m. rectus lateralis and part of the m. retractor bulbi, and nerve III innervates the m. rectus medialis and m. rectus ventralis, m. obliquus ventralis, and m. levator palpebral superioris. Pupillary dilatation is controlled by preganglionic neurons in the first three thoracic spinal cord segments, the cranial thoracic and cervical sympathetic trunks, and by postganglionic neurons in the cranial thoracic and cervical trunks and in the cranial cervical and sympathetic nerves that course through the middle ear to reach the orbit and m. dilator pupillae. Parasympathetic fibers in nerve III innervate the sphincter pupillae muscle.

The integrity of cranial nerve III may be evaluated by examining: (1) the size of the pupil; (2) the reaction of the pupil to light; (3) the presence or absence of ptosis or drooping of the upper eyelid because of paralysis of the levator palpebrae superioris muscle; and (4) the medial deviation of the eye, which occurs in oculomotor nerve palsy (different than in man), possibly because the m. obliquus dorsalis muscle is stronger than the m. rectus lateralis. In oculomotor nerve palsy with a normal pupillary response, if all the extraocular muscles innervated by nerve III are affected, an intracranial lesion should be suspected. If individual extraocular muscles are involved, a peripheral nerve lesion may exist. If an oculomotor nerve palsy exists in association with a dilated pupil, an intraorbital and/or intracranial lesion should be suspected.

Paralysis of the trochlear nerve produces a transient strabismus, resulting in a slight upward deviation of the eye (rarely seen). The affected animal may compensate for this by developing a head tilt.

Paralysis of the abducens nerve results in a medial deviation of the affected eye with inability to gaze laterally.

It is important to check tonic neck and eye reflexes when evaluating the extraocular muscle. When the nose is elevated, the forelimbs extend and the hindlimbs flex. As the nose is elevated, the eye should remain focused within the center of the palpebral fissure. Deviating the head to one side results in increased extensor tonus on that side. Normally, nystagmus should be observed on lateral deviation of the head (with the quick phase toward the side of the deviation). Normal tonic eye reflexes signify a heathly brain stem and peripheral vestibular system and motor efferent pathways to the eyes. Tonic eye reflexes are not dependent on vision.

Cranial nerve II (opticus) has its origin in the retina at the optic disk. In the cat, about 66 per cent of the optic nerve fibers, and in the dog, about 75 per cent, decussate at the optic chiasm. The optic nerve has two components: one is composed of those fibers that pass to the pupillary centers within the brain stem; the other is composed of those fibers that synapse in the thalamus, which in turn project the impulses to the visual cortex of the brain. The pupillary fibers leave the optic tract and synapse in the midbrain, where crossing occurs. Impulses reach the parasympathetic portion of the oculomotor nucleus. From here, parasympathetic preganglionic fibers exit in cranial nerve III to synapse in the ciliary ganglion caudal to the globe. The postganglionic fibers go to the iridic sphincter and ciliary muscles. Always note and record the direct and consensual pupillary reflexes. Shine a light in the temporal portion of each eye. Note the pupillary response. Test the consensual pupillary response by shining a focal source of light in one eye and noting the effects in the opposite eye. The normal pupillary response requires that nerves II and III be intact and involves only brain stem connections.

Assessment of Visual Function

Veterinarians must depend on objective signs and reflexes to estimate vision. A common test often used to assess vision is the "menace reaction." This involves passing the hand or an object in front of the animal's eyes and noticing the presence or absence of a blink reflex. The possibility of stimulating the corneal reflex during the menace response test can be abolished by placing a clear piece of Plexiglass in front of the eye and then menacing the dog.

The response of the pupil to light can also be used to evaluate function of the visual system. Each pupil should be tested individually using a bright focal source of illumination, and the opposite eye should be covered. Normal pupillary responses require only brain stem connections; therefore, cortical lesions can result in blindness with normal pupillary response to light. An obstacle course can also be valuable in assessing visual function. Styrofoam cylinders mounted on a platform can be used to create the course. The light intensity in the examining room can be varied, and alternate patching of the eyes can be helpful in detecting lesions.

Examination of the Orbit

Observe the orbits for size. Look for swelling, depression, fistula, or laceration of the orbital margin. If the orbit is enlarged, note whether the swelling is hard or soft, painful or nonpainful. Retrobulbar abscesses produce exophthalmos accompanied by pain, immobility of the eye, chemosis, edema of the eyelids, and pain on opening of the mouth. Orbital tumors may not be painful. Orbital retrobulbar hemorrhage or orbital fracture may occur following severe head trauma from automobile accidents. Enophthalmos may result from shrinkage of orbital contents (as in pthisis bulbi following ocular injury), from paralysis of the sympathetic nerve in Horner's syndrome, or from loss of retrobulbar fat in emaciation and dehydration.

Examination of the Eyelids

Note any inflammation along the margins of the eyelids and any inability to close the lids (lagophthalmos). The eyelids should touch the globe, thus preventing an accumulation of tears and debris. The cilia or eyelashes on the dog's upper eyelids are arranged in three irregular rows. The lower eyelids of dogs and both eyelids of cats are devoid of cilia. When examining the lids for the presence of entropion or ectropion, it is best not to manipulate the head, because this may distort the normal lid–globe relationship. The lids of dogs and cats have a very poorly developed tarsal plate, making manipulation relatively easy. Observe the edges of the lids for signs of entropion, ectropion, trichiasis, or distichiasis. Observe the eyelids for symblepharon or for swelling, edema, redness, or a localized inflammation, which may indicate an internal or external hordeolum. Examine the lid margins for indication of any growths.

Examination of the Eye Using Focal Illumination

In examining the anterior segment of the eye, the use of a simple optical system combining a focal source of illumination and condensing lens with an ophthalmic loupe or magnifying glass enables the observer to illuminate and examine various structures of the eye. A halogen, illuminated Finoff transilluminator on a rechargeable 3.5 volt hand* works well.

Examination of the Conjunctiva

Note whether the conjunctiva is pale, injected, pigmented, hemorrhagic, or jaundiced. The inferior or ventral conjunctiva is usually more hyperemic than the upper. Pigmentation is occasionally present, especially on the superior bulbar conjunctiva. Usually a few follicles are present on the conjunctival surface, especially that of the third eyelid.

Note whether the conjunctiva is relatively smooth and dry or excessively moist. Note any lacerations or erosions of the conjunctiva. These may be demonstrated using fluorescein. After initial inspection of the conjunctiva, additional tests may be required, such as Schirmer's tear test, culture, cytologic examination, or the use of stains.

It is important to recognize pathologic congestion of the bulbar conjunctiva. There are two forms: superficial and deep. Superficial congestion is usually characteristic of external ocular irritation from foreign bodies, bacteria, trauma, or allergic reactions. Deep congestion indicates an involvement of the cornea or the deeper structures within the eye. Normally, the deeper vessels around the limbus are difficult to see; however, when congested, they produce a distinctive "red flush" around the eye.

When presented with a "red eye" due to conjunctival vascularization, the clinician must decide whether it is a superficial ocular condition with conjunctival congestion or a problem deeper within the eye, producing ciliary congestion. Tables 67 and 68 may be helpful in differential diagnosis.

---

*Welch Allyn, Inc., Skaneateles Falls, New York.

Table 67. DIFFERENTIATION OF DEEP AND
SUPERFICIAL CONGESTION

Signs	Ciliary Congestion	Conjunctival Congestion
Pain	Usually present	Usually absent
Photophobia	Usually marked	Usually absent
Location of congested area	More intense circumcorneally	More marked in fornices and tarsal conjunctiva
Course of vessels	Straight, radiating limbus	Irregular and tortuous
Mobility of vessels	Cannot be moved	Easily moved
Blanching by vasoconstriction	Not blanched	May be blanched
Discharge	Absent	May or may not be present
Pupil size	Usually contracted	Unaffected
Iris	Usually congested	Unaffected

Table 68. DIFFERENTIAL DIAGNOSIS OF ACUTE CONJUNCTIVITIS,
ACUTE IRITIS, AND ACUTE GLAUCOMA

	Acute Conjunctivitis	Acute Iritis	Acute Glaucoma
Onset	Gradual	Gradual	Sudden
Pain	None to mild irritation	Fairly severe	Fairly severe
Discharge	Mucopurulent or purulent	Tearing	None
Vision	Unaffected	Slightly reduced	May be markedly reduced
Conjunctiva	Superficial congestion	Deep circumcorneal and ciliary congestion	Deep conjunctival, episcleral, and ciliary congestion
Cornea	Clear	Keratic precipitates may be present	Steamy and insensitive
Iris	Unaffected	Muddy and congested; posterior synechiae may be present	Congested and displaced forward
Pupil	Normal	Contracted	Dilated
Anterior chamber	Unaffected	May contain cells, opacities, and exudates	Shallow
Tenderness	Absent	Present over ciliary body	Usually absent
Tension	Unaffected	Lower than normal	Increased
Constitutional signs	Absent	Slight	Slight to moderate

The palpebral (outer) and bulbar (inner) surfaces of the nictitating membrane should be inspected. The anterior surface of the membrane is normally smooth, and the leading edge is frequently pigmented. The bulbar surface can be examined by placing a few drops of topical anesthetic (proparacaine hydrochloride) in the eye and gently using a small, atraumatic thumb forceps to evert the third eyelid. The bulbar surface usually contains a few small follicles. The following are frequently found abnormalities that may be associated with the third eyelid: eversion of the cartilage, hypertrophy, protrusion, inflammation and hypertrophy of the gland of the third eyelid, foreign bodies, and neoplasia.

Conjunctival Smears, Scrapings, and Cultures

Conjunctival scrapings and cytologic examination can be very helpful in establishing an etiology and outlining an effective treatment regimen in conjunctivitis. In performing conjunctival scrapings, use a platinum spatula (Kimura spatula) whose tip has previously been sterilized in the flame of an alcohol lamp. Scrape the inferior conjunctival cul-de-sac, preferably without prior topical anesthesia, because anesthetics may distort the cells. Place the material on two glass slides, and fix one in acetone-free 95 per cent methanol for 5 to 10 minutes; then stain with Giemsa stain. Heat fix the other slide, and apply Gram's stain.

Culturing the conjunctiva also can be a valuable aid, especially in chronic conjuntivitis. Sterile cotton applicators, fluid thioglycollate media, and blood agar media are needed to perform cultures. Evert the palpebral conjunctiva of the lower lid, and pass one side of a sterile cotton applicator, previously moistened with sterile broth or thioglycollate media, over the palpebral conjunctival surface. Streak the swab onto a sterile blood agar plate; then place it into a tube of thioglycollate broth. No topical anesthesia is used prior to culturing, because preservatives present in anesthetics can inhibit the growth of bacteria.

Examination of the Lacrimal System

Look for excessive tearing or a hypofunction of tear secretion. Note any swelling, redness, or pain in the area of the lacrimal puncta and the lacrimal sac. The nasolacrimal system can be evaluated by several basic tests. When excessive tearing exists, it must be determined whether the tearing is due to: (1) partial or complete obstruction of the excretory mechanism; (2) increased lacrimal secretion from chronic ocular irritation, as in distichiasis or trichiasis; or (3) physiologic increase in tear production, as may occur with uveitis. The first diagnostic step is the use of the primary dye test. To perform this test, place a drop of fluorescein dye from a sterile fluoro-strip into the eye. After 2 to 5 minutes, examine the external nares with the aid of a cobalt blue filter or Wood's light for the presence or absence of fluorescein dye. If dye is present, one can conclude that the lacrimal excretory system is patent and functioning. If epiphora exists yet the primary dye test indicates that the lacrimal excretory system is patent, hypersecretion of tear fluid may be implicated as the cause of the epiphora.

If no stain appears at the external nares, the primary dye test is negative, demonstrating an obstruction to normal tear flow in the excretory mechanism. Irrigation of the nasolacrimal system is then indicated. In the dog, the nasolacrimal puncta are located 1 to 3 mm from the medial canthus on the mucocutaneous border of the upper and lower lid. In the dog, a 20- to 22-gauge nasolacrimal cannula (in the cat a 23-gauge) should be used. A 2-ml syringe is filled with saline, and the lacrimal cannula is attached and passed into the lacrimal puncta of the upper lid. In most dogs, this can be done with the aid of topical anesthesia and local restraint. Some animals require additional sedation. The saline is injected and should exit through the lower puncta, if this "arc" is patent. If the lower puncta is patent, it is held closed by digital pressure on the lower lid, and the system is again irrigated. If fluid comes out of the nose and is dye stained, an obstruction existed somewhere in the nasolacrimal duct and the canaliculi were patent enough to get dye part way into the excretory system. If no dye comes out the nose, a complete obstruction of the nasolacrimal system existed.

Dacryocystorhinography involves the use of radiopaque contrast material to outline the nasolacrimal system. The upper lacrimal punctum is cannulated, and the system is flushed with 0.25 to 0.5 ml of 40 per cent Lipiodol solution. The lateral and ventrodorsal portions are used for radiography.

Several points should be made about evaluating the nasolacrimal system: First, brachycephalic breeds of dogs may occasionally have a negative primary dye test, although no blockage in the nasolacrimal system exists. In flushing the nasolacrimal system of some animals, fluid may not appear at the nose; however, the animal may gag and exhibit swallowing movements, indicating that the fluid has entered the mouth and the system is patent.

Basic tear secretion comes mainly from the tarsal and conjunctival glands and the accessory tarsal glands. The reflex tear secretors are the main lacrimal gland and accessory lacrimal glands. The production of normal lacrimal secretion can be tested by using Schirmer's tear test. The amount of wetting is measured in mm after a period of 1 minute. No topical anesthesia or drops of any kind should be used prior to conducting the test. The tear flow response in the dog as measured with Schirmer's tear test paper is a measure of corneal sensitivity and the animal's ability to produce tears. In normal dogs, wetting of Schirmer's test papers ranges from 10 to 25 mm in 1 minute. Variation in the relative humidity can alter Schirmer's test values. Values less than 10 mm wetting in 1 minute when combined with the clinical signs of keratoconjunctivitis are usually indicative of keratoconjunctivitis sicca or "dye eyes."

Examination of the Sclera

Note the color of the sclera, and look for nodules, hemorrhage, lacerations, cysts, and tumors. Normal sclera is white to blue-white. The sclera may appear blue, because it is abnormally thinned, and the uveal tract shows through.

Look for staphylomas, and for any injection of the scleral vessels and accompanying edema. Episcleritis can produce local scleral inflammation, whereas deep-seated ocular diseases such as glaucoma and uveitis produce generalized scleral vessel injection.

Examination of the Cornea

The cornea should be smooth, moist, free of blood vessels, and transparent. Note any ulceration or opacity of the cornea. Slight opacities are termed nebulae; dense ones, leukomas. The canine cornea is oval, with a diameter of 12.5 to 17 mm. The horizontal measurement is 1 to 2 mm greater than the vertical axis. Measurement of the corneal diameter with calipers may prove valuable when evaluating glaucoma and buphthalmia. In puppies, the cornea tends to be hazy, thus restricting ophthalmoscopic examination until the animals are 4 to 6 weeks of age. Such diseases of the cornea as corneal inflammation, pigmentation, degeneration, trauma, and neoplasia frequently may alter its transparency.

Test the corneal sensitivity by touching the cornea with a wisp of dry cotton. Instill a topical anesthetic, proparacaine hydochloride, 0.5 per cent (Ophthanine), into the conjunctival sac of each eye. Use a small forceps to pull the third eyelid gently away from the corneal surface, and examine its inner surface for foreign bodies, hyperplastic tissue, inflammation, follicle formation, or parasites (*Thelazia*). Observe the corneal surface for the presence of foreign bodies.

External ophthalmic stains can be very helpful in diagnosing lesions of the cornea. Fluorescein does not actually stain tissues. The intact corneal epithelium, having a high lipid content, resists penetration of water-soluble fluorescein and is not colored by it. Any break in the epithelial barrier permits rapid fluorescein penetration into the stroma or even into the anterior chamber. When the epithelial surface has regenerated, the green color disappears, regardless of whether the underlying stroma is thickened, thinned, scarred, or irregular.

Unlike fluorescein, rose bengal actually stains cells and their nuclei. It selectively stains devitalized corneal and conjunctival epithelium a readily visible red. Its main use has been in the identification of corneal and conjunctival lesions caused by keratitis sicca.

If an ulcer is present, note whether the borders are regular or irregular and whether the ulcer is superficial or deep. Ulcers that are progressive and deep present a guarded prognosis. It is advisable to culture deep ulcers and to make a scraping of their borders. The scrapings should be stained with Giemsa, and the type of cells should be determined. If the ulcer appears to be deep, look for evidence of anterior synechia, prolapsed iris, iridocyclitis, cataract, extrusion of the lens, fistula, or hemorrhage.

Note the presence of blood vessels in the cornea. It is important to determine the depth at which vascularization is taking place, because it is usually directly related to the cause of the vascularization. Superficial vascularization is commonly associated with superficial keratitis, superficial ulcers, or pannus. Deep vascularization usually indicates a deep corneal stromal lesion, uveitis, or glaucoma.

Look for deposits on the posterior surface of the cornea (keratic precipitates). These precipitates vary in size and shape, but they usually are indicative of a disease of the uveal tract.

EXTERNAL EXAMINATION

Examination of the Anterior Chamber

Examine the anterior chamber, and observe its depth; note changes in the transparency of the ocular media, such as hypopyon, hyphema, fibrin, or foreign bodies. Look for anterior synechiae.

The anterior drainage angle cannot be visualized readily in the dog without the use of a contact lens. Large tumors and some anterior synechiae can be visualized with a loupe and a focal light source.

Examination of the Iris

The color of the iris in each eye may vary. Observe the shape or size of the iris. An iris that is thickened and muddy in color indicates an infiltration of the uveal tract. Look for the presence of atrophy, tears, synechiae, persistent pupillary membranes, iridodonesis, iridodialysis, nodules, tumors, cysts, or colobomas. Examine the pupillary border of the iris for signs of atrophy or posterior synechiae to the anterior lens capsule. Complete posterior synechia results in iris bombe and secondary glaucoma.

Examine the pupil of each eye by diffuse and focal illumination. Note the pupil size and shape and its direct and consensual response to light. Note any inequalities between the two pupils. Check to see whether the pupils are dilated. Find out from the owner whether the subject has had a mydriatic placed in its eye. Determine whether the pupils, when dilated, constrict when light is applied. The pupil may be dilated because of trauma, a mydriatic, fear, stimulation of the cervical sympathetic nerve, glaucoma, paralysis of the third cranial nerve, or retinal atrophy. The pupil may be contracted (miosis) because of a miotic, from synechiae, stimulation by light, in acute iritis, following the use of a narcotic, in paralysis of the sympathetic nerve, or from irritation of the third cranial nerve.

Note whether the pupil of one eye is equal in size to the pupil of the other and whether it remains so with changes in the degree of illumination. Inequality of pupil size (anisocoria) may be caused by physiologic or pathologic factors.

Examination of the Lens

It is easier to examine the lens when the pupil is dilated. The lens may be examined with a focal source of illumination, with an ophthalmoscope, or with a biomicroscope. Examine the lens for the presence of pigment, adhesions, opacities, the position of the lens (subluxation or luxation), or the absence of the lens (aphakia). Normal aging changes of the lens can be observed in dogs over 7 years and in cats 8 years of age. This is called *nuclear sclerosis*. True opacities of the lens are called *cataracts*.

Ophthalmoscopy

Examination of the Retina

Examination of the retina with an ophthalmoscope is an essential part of every complete eye examination. For adequate visualization of the fundus, dilate the iris with tropicamide solution, 1 per cent.

Examine each patient's eye grounds in a dark room. To examine the right fundus, hold the ophthalmoscope in the right hand and view the fundus with the right eye. Keep both eyes open when using the ophthalmoscope; it causes less strain to accommodation. Starting with the ophthalmoscope at 0 setting, hold the ophthalmoscope about 20 inches from the patient's eye. Observe the pupil and the tapetal reflex. Bring the ophthalmoscope to within 1 inch of the patient's eye, and placing the setting on −1 to 3 to view the optic disk and retina. If the disk is not immediately seen, follow the retinal vessels back to the disk. Find the setting at which the retina can be seen most clearly. Inserting more plus lenses into the ophthalmoscope focuses the lens on more anterior structures within the eye.

Direct ophthalmoscopy provides a highly magnified view of the fundus in which the image is real and upright. The magnification is 15× in an emmetropic eye, less in hyperopia, and more in myopia. The area of visualization is usually about 2 disk diameters. The extent to which the peripheral retina may be examined in dogs varies with the degree of dilatation of the pupil and the length of the muzzle. In dolicocephalic breeds, the peripheral, medial aspect of the fundus can be examined in greater detail using direct ophthalmoscopy. Indirect ophthalmoscopy permits good visualization of all areas of the fundus.

The fundus is that portion of the inner eye that includes the optic disk or papilla, the retinal vessels, tapetum lucidum, and nigrum.

SPECIALIZED DIAGNOSTIC TECHNIQUES IN OPHTHALMOLOGY

Tonometry

Glaucoma is an increase in intraocular pressure incompatible with normal ocular and visual functions. Therefore, it is important to be able to record changes in ocular tension in order to diagnose and treat glaucoma.

The method used clinically is tonometry, in which the tension of the outer coat of the eye is assessed by measuring the impressibility or applanability of the cornea. Because the measurements based on tonometry involve calculations that have a wide base of variations, tonometry readings are always approximations and are referred to as "ocular tension" readings, as opposed to intraocular pressure readings obtained by manometry. Ocular tension can be recorded in several ways.

Digital Tonometry

This method involves estimating ocular tension by judging the impressibility of the ocular coats when pressure is applied to the globe by the index fingers, which are placed on the upper eyelids of the animal. The sensation of ocular fluxation from the normal eye is learned with practice, and variations can be detected as experience is gained. This method requires much practice and is inaccurate, and usually, it is impossible to detect less than 5 mm Hg change in intraocular tension.

Schiötz Tonometry

This tonometer has been widely used in veterinary medicine to determine ocular tension in small animals. The instrument consists of a corneal footplate, plunger, holding bracket, recording scale, and 5.5-, 7.5-, 10.0-, and 15.0-gm weights. The principle of the Schiötz tonometer is that the amount that the plunger protrudes from the footplate is related to the indentability of the cornea, which in turn is related to the intraocular pressure. The plunger is connected to a scale so that 0.05 mm protrusion of the plunger equals one scale unit (Table 69).

The technique of Schiötz tonometry in dogs and cats is not difficult. The dog is placed in the sitting or dorsal recumbent position. Topical anesthesia is instilled, and the eyelids are held open by the fingers, which are placed quite far away from the lid margins. The footplate must be placed vertically on the central aspect of the cornea. Three readings are taken in each eye and then averaged. Normal intraocular tension with the Schiötz tonometers in dogs is 15 to 25 mm Hg.

Applanation Tonometry

In applanation tonometry, a known, very small area of the cornea is flattened by a known force. The advantage of this technique over the indentation method (Schiötz) is that the errors resulting from ocular rigidity and corneal curvature are greatly reduced.

Gonioscopy

Glaucoma is an increase in intraocular pressure incompatible with normal ocular visual functions. Glaucoma can be caused by many different disorders, all elevating intraocular pressure. In many types of glaucoma, there is an abnormality in the anterior angle of the eye (filtration angle). Gonioscopy permits one to visualize and examine the iridocorneal angle, which cannot be seen without the use of a contact lens.

The Koeppe gonioscopic lens seems to be well suited to dogs and cats. It is available in 17-, 19-, and 21-mm sizes. The lens can be inserted into the eye following the application of topical anesthesia. In fractious animals, a tranquilizer may be needed. The lens can be filled with 1 per cent methylcellulose or saline. Avoid having air bubbles present; this distorts the view. The inside of the lens is illuminated with a Barkan lamp, otoscope head, or binocular indirect ophthalmoscope. Magnification suitable to visualize the angle can be provided by an otoscope head, indirect ophthalmoscope, or with a Haag-Streit goniomicroscope.

Table 69. SCHIÖTZ TONOMETER–CALIBRATION TABLE
FOR THE CANINE EYE

Schiötz Scale Reading	Intraocular Pressure (mm Hg) 5.5 gm weight	Intraocular Pressure (mm Hg) 7.5 gm weight	Intraocular Pressure (mm Hg) 10.0 gm weight
0.5	52.6	71.2	93.6
1.0	49.3	67.0	88.3
1.5	46.3	63.1	83.3
2.0	43.4	59.4	78.6
2.5	40.8	55.9	74.1
3.0	38.3	52.6	69.9
3.5	36.0	49.6	66.0
4.0	33.9	46.7	62.2
4.5	31.9	44.0	58.7
5.0	30.1	41.6	55.4
5.5	28.4	39.2	52.3
6.0	26.9	37.1	49.4
6.5	25.5	35.1	46.7
7.0	24.2	33.2	44.2
7.5	23.0	31.5	41.8
8.0	21.9	29.9	39.6
8.5	21.0	28.5	37.5
9.0	20.1	27.1	35.6
9.5	19.3	25.9	33.8
10.0	18.6	24.8	32.1
10.5	18.0	23.8	30.6
11.0	17.4	22.8	29.1
11.5	17.0	22.0	27.8
12.0	16.6	21.3	26.6
12.5	16.3	20.6	25.5
13.0	16.0	20.0	24.5
13.5	15.8	19.5	23.6
14.0	15.7	19.1	22.8
14.5	15.7	18.8	22.0
15.0	15.7	18.5	21.4
15.5	15.8	18.3	20.8
16.0	15.9	· 18.1	20.3
16.5	16.1	18.0	19.9
17.0	16.4	18.0	19.5
17.5	16.8	18.1	19.2
18.0	17.2	18.2	19.0
18.5	17.7	18.4	18.8
19.0	18.3	18.7	18.7
19.5	19.0	19.0	18.6
20.0	19.7	19.4	18.7

After R. L. Peiffer, Jr., D.V.M.

Transillumination of the Eye

If an intense light (Finoff ocular transilluminator) is placed on the sclera behind the ciliary body, the light will be transmitted to the interior of the eye and will produce a tapetal reflex in the pupil. If the light is placed over a solid mass in the eye, the light will not be scattered, and a light reflex will not be produced in the pupil. If the light is placed over a cystic area in the eye, the rays of light will not be interfered with, and the light will diffuse throughout the eye. Thus, transillumination can be used to aid in differentiating solid tumor masses in the eye as opposed to cystic lesions. Transillumination may also be used to diagnose atrophy of the pigment layer of the iris. This layer normally prevents transilluminated light from going through the iris. In iris atrophy, the transilluminated light will appear in the areas of iris atrophy. To use the principles of transillumination, the examining room should be completely dark and the observer should be partially dark adapted.

Electroretinography

It is beyond the scope of this discussion to enter into the details of the mechanism and interpretation of electroretinography.

The retina, like other nervous tissue, generates electrical currents. An electrical potential exists between the retina and the cornea, with the cornea being more positive. When a flash of light strikes the retina, rapid changes in retinal potentials occur and are recorded as the electroretinogram.

The electroretinogram represents the mass response of the retina to a stimulus. The pattern of the electroretinogram can vary among different species of animals, depending on whether retinal photoreceptors are predominantly rods or cones.

References and Additional Readings

Acland, G. M.: Developmental anomalies of the eye. *In* Blogg, R. J. (ed.): The Eye in Veterinary Practice, Vol. 1. Philadelphia, W. B. Saunders Company, 1980.

Bistner, S., and Shaw, D.: Examination of the eye. Vet. Clin. North Am., *11*(3):595, 1981.

Bistner, S.: Clinical diagnosis and treatment of infectious keratitis. Compendium on Continuing Education, *3*(12):1056, 1981.

Blogg, R. J. (ed.): The Eye in Veterinary Practice, Vol. 1. Philadelphia, W. B. Saunders Company, 1980.

deLaHunta, A.: Veterinary Clinical Neuroanatomy, 2nd ed. Philadelphia, W. B. Saunders Company, 1983.

Gelatt, K. N.: Textbook of Veterinary Ophthalmology. Philadelphia, Lea & Febiger, 1981.

Martin, C. L.: The eye and systemic disease. *In* Kirk, R. W. (ed.): Current Veterinary Therapy VII. Philadephia, W. B. Saunders Company, 1980.

Peiffer, R. L. (ed.): Symposium on Ophthalmology. Vet. Clin. North Am., *10*:239, 1980.

Peiffer, R. L.: Ophthalmic disorders of proven or suspected genetic etiology in dogs and cats. *In* Kirk, R. W. (ed.): Current Veterinary Therapy VII. Philadelphia, W. B. Saunders Company, 1980.

Riis, R. C.: Diseases of the lens. *In* Kirk, R. W. (ed.): Current Veterinary Therapy VII. Philadelphia, W. B. Saunders Company, 1980.

Scagliotti, R.: Current concepts in veterinary neuro-ophthalmology. Vet. Clin. North Am., *10*:417, 1980.

Schmidt, G.: Algorithms for ophthalmologic problems. *In* Kirk, R. W. (ed.): Current Veterinary Therapy VII. Philadelphia, W. B. Saunders Company, 1980.

Slater, D.: Fundamentals of Veterinary Ophthalmology. Philadelphia, W. B. Saunders Company, 1981.

Examination of the Ear

General Examination

Note any unusual appearance of the external ear. Compare one ear with the other. Observe the skin for signs of inflammation (swelling, redness, or desquamation of the epithelium). Movement and handling of the normal pinna should not produce pain. Look for pus or blood emanating from the external meatus.

Otoscopic Examination

An otoscope is required to examine the auditory canal. Use a clean, preferably sterile, otoscope head. Do not examine a noninfected ear with the head that was used for an infected ear, and always examine the noninfected or normal member first.

To examine the right ear, hold the otoscope in the right hand and the pinna between the thumb and first two fingers of the left hand. Reverse the procedure for the left ear. Draw the ear flap caudally. Insert the otoscope cone carefully in a rostroventral direction, but always watch the progress of the tip by looking through the otoscope. When the angle of the meatus is encountered, draw the ear laterally and turn the tip of the instrument medially to straighten the meatus. Otoscopes are usually provided with several specula, and visualization of the ear canal is easier if the largest one that will fit the canal is used.

The ear drum is a thin membrane with a white curved bone running from the dorsal margin postventrally. The bone is the handle of the malleus (Fig. 49). The tympanic membrane consists of a small upper portion, the pars flaccida, and a large lower part, the pars tensa. The membrane separates the horizontal portion of the external auditory canal from the tympanic cavity. The posterior portion of the pars tensa is the part that is usually visualized to the greatest extent with the otoscope. The tense part of the tympanic membrane is dark, because the dark cavity of the middle ear is seen through it. The flaccid part is opaque white with red blood vessels.

The ear drum can usually be seen in normal dogs younger than 1 year of age. It may be difficult to visualize the eardrum in older dogs, because the meatus is narrowed, the tense part of the eardrum is obscured by the flaccid part, the lining of the meatus obscures the eardrum, or the eardrum is

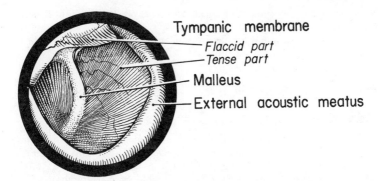

Tympanic membrane
— Flaccid part
— Tense part
— Malleus
— External acoustic meatus

Figure 49. Canine tympanic membrane. (From Habel, R. E.: Applied Veterinary Anatomy. Ithaca, N.Y., published by the author, 1973.)

ruptured. Chronic otitis externa is a common problem in dogs, and in more than 50 per cent of the chronic cases, the tympanic membrane is ruptured.

Any abnormal changes in the tympanic membrane, such as swelling, redness, loss of translucency, or absence of the membrane, should be recorded. If the tympanic membrane has recently ruptured, a small amount of blood-stained discharge may be seen around the membrane.

Cleaning the Ear Canal

In otitis externa, the external canal is frequently blocked with cerumen, exudate, and tissue debris. In many breeds, but especially poodles, Bedlington terriers, and Kerry Blue terriers, the canal contains hair that frequently obscures the view. If the canal is plugged with wax, the hair must be removed first. Instill warm olive oil or a ceruminolytic agent (Ceruminex) to soften the wax. Cotton applicators may be used to wipe the wax gently from the outer part of the external meatus. If the animal resents the cleaning, administer a short-acting general anesthetic or tranquilizer. Any deep cleaning of the ear canal should be done very cautiously and gently, and the patient should be adequately restrained or, preferably, anesthetized. For all but very simple external cleaning, it is best to use gentle irrigation with warm water solutions to thoroughly clean the canal and enable a complete otoscopic examination. Cotton applicators can be dangerous and may pack debris into the canal.

If the canal contains pus or other exudates, a culture should be taken to determine antibacterial sensitivity. Before the canal can be visually examined, the discharges must be removed. The recent advent of the pulsating water dental hygienic apparatus has made irrigation and careful cleansing of the ear canal a much easier process. Five ml of Betadine or Nolvosan is added to each 8 to 12 ounces of warm water. The irrigation stream is kept parallel to the external ear canal and is applied in a rotating motion. The excess water and debris can be caught in a sink or basin. The canal can then be reinspected and carefully dried with cotton or by using an aspirator (Venker-van Haagen).

This technique should not be used in cases of acute otitis media or if the tympanic membrane has been ruptured.

Examination of the Larynx and Pharynx

General Examination

Thorough examination of the larynx and pharynx in the dog and cat requires the use of a short-acting general anesthetic. Extreme caution should be exercised when anesthetizing brachycephalic dogs that may have laryngeal problems. In these cases, it may be preferable to use a tranquilizer or a combination narcotic/tranquilizer.

Tonsils, Pharynx, Soft Palate, and Posterior Nares

Common signs associated with diseases of the oropharynx are inappetence, excessive salivation, halitosis, pawing at mouth, and retching. Examination of the oropharynx in the awake animal can reveal the presence or absence of cranial nerve reflexes such as the normal gag reflex (see pp. 431–443).

Smell the breath of the animal. Alterations in odor may indicate disease, e.g., halitosis, in dental and gum disease; sweet smell (fruity), in ketoacidosis and ethylene glycol; and necrotic odor, in uremia, foreign bodies, and necrotic respiratory disease.

Open the mouth with a mouth gag, and gently pull the tongue forward with a tongue forceps. Examine the tonsils for size, color, and consistency. Gently wipe away any discharge in the pharynx or larynx. Observe the mucous membranes of the pharynx for color, swelling, inflammation, or follicle formation. Place the index finger on the soft palate, apply dorsal pressure, and feel for abnormal swellings. This may be the site of visually concealed retropharyngeal tumors. Examine the oral mucous membranes for any evidence of stomatitis. Stomatitis, or inflammation of the oral mucous membranes, may be associated with trauma such as chewing on plant material, uremia, diabetes mellitus, deficiency diseases, viral lesions (especially in cats with viral rhinotracheitis and calici virus infection), mycotic infections, hematologic and reticuloendothelial diseases (especially in cats with FeLV), and chemical and electrical burns.

Inspect the oral mucous membranes for any evidence of tumor formation—for example, oral papillomatosis, transmissible venereal tumor, melanomas, squamous cell carcinoma, and fibrosarcoma.

Inspect the posterior nares for a foreign body or tumor. Gently grasp the end of the soft palate with a tissue forceps and pull it forward. Use a dental mirror and focal illumination to view the posterior nares. Note any changes in the normally pink, moist epithelium. Insert a finger behind the soft palate and palpate the pharynx for masses or a foreign body. In cases in which a nasal foreign body is suspected, a soft No. 5 French feeding tube can be passed through the mouth and the end placed in the posterior nares. Forceful saline flushes may be used to dislodge foreign material. The collected discharge can also be examined via exfoliative cytology for cell content.

Problems of the soft palate are confined largely to the brachycephalic breeds. Examine the soft palate for length. Elongation of the soft palate leads to respiratory distress, gagging, and expectoration. Look for an incomplete soft palate, a cause of chronic nasal discharge.

Larynx

The dog has a valvular glottis with well-developed aryepiglottic folds. The ventricular bands are minimally developed, and there is a distinct laryngeal ventricle with a large saccule. The cat has a dome-shaped aditus and no well-developed aryepiglottic fold. The ventricular bands are well developed and the laryngeal saccules are not prominent.

Laryngeal disorders resulting in loss of function can produce the following signs: change in the quality of sound produced by the patient, difficulty in swallowing food, changes in respiration with stertorous breathing on inspiration, stridor on inspiration, coughing, cyanosis, and decreased exercise tolerance. Spontaneous laryngeal paralysis has been described in the Bouvier breed of dog and laryngeal paralysis can be seen as a result of trauma, congenital defect, or iatrogenesis.

The larynx should be palpated for signs of pain, fractures, abnormality in position, and size. Auscultation over the area of the larynx is also important. The larynx can be inspected most effectively with a large laryngoscope of appropriate size. Pulling the tongue too far forward will simulate collapse of the larynx. Collapse of the larynx is seen most frequently in brachycephalic dogs and is characterized by severe inspiratory distress. Examine the corniculate cartilages. Displacement ventromedially can cause collapse of the laryngeal opening. Collapse of the larynx may involve the epiglottis, the corniculate or the cuneiform process of the arytenoid cartilage, or any combination of defects in these structures. Severe inspiratory dyspnea accentuates the anatomic problem. Collapse of the corniculate cartilages permits them to be displaced ventromedially, causing a marked reduction in the size of the lumen of the larynx. Examine the epiglottis for length and for collapse over the laryngeal opening.

Examine the lateral ventricles of the larynx for eversion. This condition is seen in brachycephalic breeds and results from negative pressure leading to inspiratory dyspnea. Note any signs of inflammation or swelling in the laryngeal area. A more detailed examination of the trachea may be carried out with a bronchoscope (see pp. 558–559).

Examination of the Nose

General Examination

Observe the muzzle and nasal area, and compare both sides for any disproportion in size. Examine the external nares for changes in pigmentation or size or abnormal discharge. If a discharge is present, note whether it is bloodstained, mucopurulent, or watery and whether it flows from one or both nostrils. Hold the mouth closed, place a wisp of cotton in front of each nostril, and compare the movement of the cotton on expiration. Note any deviation of the nasal septum. Stenotic nares are characterized by partial or complete occlusion of the nasal orifice and are commonly seen in brachycephalic dogs. The lateral wings of the nostril collapse upon inhalation, forcing the dog to breathe through its mouth.

Nasal Passages

Rhinoscopy in the dog and cat must be performed under general anesthesia with tracheal intubation. Part of the nasal passages can be inspected with an

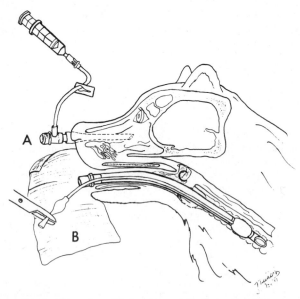

Figure 50. Illustration of nasal flush techique. Stiff plastic tubing (A) is measured to a length corresponding from external nares to medial canthus of the eye. Gauze sponges are placed on table near the nares (B) and behind the soft palate (C) to trap dislodged tissue. Intermittent positive and negative pressure is applied with saline via the syringe while the catheter is pushed in and out of the turbinates to cut or dislodge cores of tissue. (From Withrow, S. J., and Lowes, N.: Biopsy techniques in small animal oncology. JAAHA, 14(6):889, 1981.)

otoscope and a small otoscope cone. Note any signs of inflammation, ulceration, hemorrhage, or foreign bodies in the nasal passages. The parasite *Pneumonyssoides caninum* can produce chronic rhinitis and nasal discharge. Hyperemia of the mucosa and pus indicate infection. A unilateral foreign body in the passage frequently produces an offensive odor from the affected nasal passage. Hemorrhage from the nostrils may occur in blood dyscrasias, idiopathic thrombocytopenia, autoimmune hemolytic anemia, tumors, foreign bodies, and trauma. A small, rigid fiberoptic endoscope can be used to examine the nose. Biopsy forceps and brush catheters can be used to obtain biopsy material. A flushing technique can also be used to obtain culture and tissue samples (Fig. 50). The major complication of rhinoscopy is epistaxis obscuring the visual field. A history of chronic partial or complete nasal obstruction and respiratory difficulty, persistent unilateral or bilateral nasal discharge, and frequent episodes of sneezing and snorting could be signs of a nasal tumor. Examine the muzzle for any evidence of increase in size or pain on palpation.

Further examination of the nasal passages can be accomplished radiographically.

The hard palate should be inspected for any signs of cleft palate or oronasal fistulae. The nasopharynx is examined with a nasopharynx illuminator* and a dental mirror. An Allis tissue forceps can be used to pull the soft palate forward.

Diseases of the sinuses that communicate with the nasal passages may produce discharge from the nares.

---

*Nasopharynx Illuminator, Welch Allyn Inc., Skaneateles Falls, New York.

References and Additional Readings

Habel, R. E.: Applied Anatomy, 6th ed. Ithaca, N. Y., published by the author, 1973.

O'Brien, J. A., and Harvey, C. E.: Diseases of the upper airway. *In* Ettinger, S. J.: Textbook of Veterinary Internal Medicine, 2nd ed. Philadelphia, W. B. Saunders Company, 1983, pp. 692–722.

Rosin, E., Greenwood, K.: Bilateral arytenoid cartilage lateralization for laryngeal paralysis in the dog. J.A.V.M.A., *180*(5):515, 1982.

Venker-van Haagen, A. J.: Managing diseases of the ear. *In* Kirk, R. W. (ed.): Current Veterinary Therapy VIII: Small Animal Practice. Philadelphia, W. B. Saunders Company, 1983.

Venker-van Haagen, A. J.: Laryngeal paralysis in young Bouviers. *In* Kirk, R. W. (ed.): Current Veterinary Therapy VII. Philadelphia, W. B. Saunders Company, 1980.

GENITOURINARY SYSTEM

Reproductive Organs

EVALUATION OF THE MALE BREEDER

History and General Examination

General data should include age, breed, general demeanor, psychologic problems, body condition, vaccination, and comments on specific disease problems. Also determine the environmental setting, feeding, management practices, fertility, and breeding data about related animals. The degree of inbreeding may be important in evaluating sexual function. Previous information relating to reproduction is particularly important and should include dates and results of all matings (especially for the last year). Data should include comments about libido, breeding techniques, previous fertility studies and therapy, number of pups born, number weaned, and the cause of any abortions or deaths.

Special Examinations Related to Reproduction

Inspection and palpation of the genital organs is the first procedure. A thickened scrotal wall may produce testicular degeneration from increased temperature. Check the spermatic cord for varicocele and the testes for size, asymmetry, cryptorchidism, and consistency. There should be firm resiliency. Small, soft testes indicate degeneration or hypoplasia; firm masses may be the result of inflammation, fibrosis, or tumors. Tumors are relatively common in dogs and may produce estrogens or testosterone, with a severe impact on reproductive function. The epididymis, dorsal to the testes, may be congenital aplasia or fibrosis from ascending infections or from brucellosis.

The penis and sheath should be checked for congenital malformations involving, for example, the urethra, penis, or opening of the sheath. Look for phimosis, balanoposthitis, and transmissible venereal tumors (TVTs).

Naturally occurring canine TVTs can be found on the external genitalia of dogs of both sexes. The exfoliated tumor cells are transplanted into vaginal or penile tissue during coitus. Contact of infected genital discharge into the eye, mouth, or skin wounds may produce tumors at the sites. In the male, TVTs are usually located around the glans penis and result in preputial discharge. In the female, TVTs are often located in the vagina, where they assume a cauliflower appearance. The tumors may ulcerate, and bleeding from the vagina may develop. Spread of tumor tissue may be from the vagina to the fallopian tubes and uterus and then to the internal iliac lymph node. Treatment for TVT can be found in the suggested reading by Richardson.

The prostate is the only accessory gland that can be examined easily. Examine the prostate by rectal palpation. It should be smooth, bilaterally symmetrical, nonpainful, and usually smaller than 3 cm in size. Nodules, fixation, and pain are found in carcinomas; nonpainful symmetrical enlargements (often so large as to pull the organ into the abdomen) are seen with cysts or hyperplasia. The four major causes of prostatomegaly are benign hyperplasia; prostatitis, including abscessation of the prostate; prostatic cysts; and primary or secondary prostatic tumors. The radiographic appearance of an enlarged prostate on survey radiographs combined with positive contrast retrograde urethrography can be helpful in the differential diagnosis. Hyperplastic and inflammatory prostatic disease result in more symmetrical prostatomegaly than do cystic, neoplastic, or prostatic abscesses. Signs of acute bacterial prostatitis may be urethral discharge, constipation, tenesmus, stilted gait, fever, depression, abdominal pain, dysuria, and leukocytosis. Chronic bacterial prostatitis may involve signs associated with recurrent urinary tract infection, and the use of radiographic, prostatic fluid evelution, cultures, and biopsy may be necessary in order to establish a diagnosis.

There are numerous additional testing procedures that can be used in evaluating the animal with prostatic disease: ejaculation and microscopic evaluation (see pp. 538–541); prostatic biopsy (see p. 534); and prostatic aspiration and massage (see p. 503).

Testicular biopsy is a most important procedure that provides karyotypic and histologic evidence of infertility. While the patient is under general anesthesia, make a small incision over the lateral wall of the scrotum. Using a No. 11 Bard-Parker blade, cut the tunica albuginea with three connecting incisions. With compression of the testis, a small triangular plug of tissue will protrude from the incision. It is sliced off with a razor-sharp blade and placed in Bouin's solution (*not* formalin) for prompt transportation to the laboratory. If testicular abnormalities are palpated, it is best to open the scrotum more liberally, so that the entire testis can be examined carefully.

Semen collection and evaluation are described on pages 538–541. This is the most important aspect in evaluating male breeders. Semen volume, concentration, motility, and morphology should be within normal ranges for good fertility. If a dog has not ejaculated for a long period of time, it may be necessary to collect semen for a few days to make evaluation more reliable. Abnormal semen samples may indicate testicular hypoplasia or degeneration, hypothyroidism, other hormonal interferences, and senility or may be caused by toxic agents, nutritional factors, obstructive lesions in the efferent tubules, severe stress, acute immune disease, or even extreme cold. If infection in the reproductive tract is present, the pH of one of the three semen fractions may be abnormally high. Culture and sensitivity studies of semen fractions, prostatic fluid, urethra washings, or preputial swabs may be necessary for proper microbiologic evaluation. All male dogs should be blood tested for evidence of *Brucella canis*, because it produces acute or chronic orchitis and epididymitis. Positive rapid-slide-test sera should be confirmed by laboratory tube tests and/or blood culture. Using the tube agglutination test (TAT), canine sera usually screened at 1:50 dilution and positive sera should be retested with the 2-mercaptoethanol tube agglutination test (2ME-TAT). Animals that test positive in the TAT test but negative in the 2ME-TAT test are considered suspicious. A titer of 1:200 with the 2ME-TAT test is considered presumptive evidence of canine brucellosis infection. Other bacterial organisms that may cause genital infection in males include *Escherichia coli; Proteus vulgaris; Streptococcus, Staphylococcus,* and *Mycoplasma* species; and fungi. Distemper infection causes epididymitis; and ascending urine via the vas deferens following trauma, may cause a sterile epididymitis.

EVALUATION OF THE FEMALE BREEDER

History and General Examination

With breeding problems, the history is particularly important and is often neither detailed nor reliable. General data should include age, breed, general demeanor, psychologic problems, body condition, vaccination, and comments on specific disease problems. Highly nervous or shy bitches frequently have reproductive behavior and cycling problems. Determine the environmental setting, feeding, breeding, and other management practices concerning the animal and the fertility and breeding data about related animals. The stud dog's records should also be examined. Pedigrees should be examined to determine inbreeding or possible genetic defects. Obtain information on the initiation of first estrus; number and frequency of estrous cycles; breedings; pregnancies; parturitions; urogenital problems; litters whelped; and numbers of pups born and weaned, with causes for abortions or deaths, if known. Treatments and prophylactic measures, especially if they involve sex hormones, should be investigated.

Special Examinations Related to Reproduction

Inspection and palpation of the genital organs furnishes much valuable information. The vulva is usually small and wrinkled, with good tone and almost no discharge. Note the size and condition of the clitoris. The vulva swells during estrus and has a normal odorless bloody or mucoid discharge. Exudates at other times, especially if fetid, may be suggestive of infections, tumors, or endocrine problems (pyometra). External palpation of the vulva and vagina and abdominal palpations of the ovaries and uterus may complement radiography and hysterography. More details about examination of the vagina and evaluation of vaginal smears are found on pages 552–557. Cytologic studies of vaginal smears are very important in evaluating female breeders.

The mammary glands should be palpated and inspected for mastitis and tumors. Acute infections are hot, painful, and swollen; usually involve only one gland; and produce a purulent secretion. Chronic mastitis involves several glands; they are enlarged, firm, and nodular on palpation.

Mammary gland tumors constitute 52 per cent of all neoplasms in the bitch. Forty-five per cent of mammary gland tumors in the dog are malignant. The median age of affected bitches is 10.5 years, and mammary gland tumors are multicentric in 50 per cent of bitches. Of the benign tumor forms, the most frequently recognized histologic patterns are fibroadenomas (benign mixed tumors), 45 per cent, simple adenomas, and benign mesenchymal tumors. Of the malignant tumors in the dog, the most common histologic types are solid carcinomas, tubular adenocarcinomas, papillary adenocarcinomas, anaplastic carcinomas, and sarcomas.

In malignant tumors that metastasize, metastasis from glands 4 and 5 drain to the inguinal lymph nodes and via thoracic duct to the lungs. The iliac lymph nodes may also be involved with metastasis. Metastasis from glands 1 and 2 drain to the axillary lymph nodes and to the lungs and may involve the intrathoracic lymph nodes. Gland 3 appears to drain more commonly to the axillary lymph nodes. There is also the possibility for hematogenous spread of mammary tumors with no lymph node involvement.

When mammary gland tumors are examined, they should be staged, if possible, with a routine scheme. Fine needle biopsy and cytologic examination may be helpful in distinguishing benign from malignant cell types. Multiple mammary gland tumors, which are present in 50 per cent of dogs, may have different tumor types; thus, all tissues and regional lymph nodes should be sectioned.

Mammary gland neoplasia in the bitch is *almost 100 per cent preventable* if ovariectomy is performed prior to the first estrous cycle. The incidence of mammary gland neoplasia can be *markedly reduced* if ovariectomy is done before the animal is 2.5 years old or prior to the first four estrous periods. Pharmacologic doses of progestational compounds have been associated with the development of mixed mammary gland tumors.

Mammary tumors in cats occur more frequently than in any other domestic animal except the dog. Eighty per cent of those observed are usually malignant. They are usually adenocarcinomas and present most commonly in cats 7 years of age or older. The tumors usually ulcerate early in their development. The cat usually has four pairs of mammary glands. The cranial two glands on each side have a common lymphatic system and drain into the axillary lymph nodes. The caudal two mammary glands also have a common lymphatic system and drain into the superficial inguinal lymph nodes.

Cats that have mammary gland tumors should be evaluated according to the classification system of the World Health Organization (TNM classification scheme: T = extent of primary tumor; N = condition of regional lymph nodes, and M = presence or absence of distant metastases).

Bacteriologic examination of mammary secretion, vaginal smear or culture, and intrauterine culture (collected at laparotomy) is very important if infectious processes are suspected. All breeding bitches should be tested for brucellosis; if the rapid-slide-test plate is positive, it should be confirmed by laboratory tube tests and/or blood cultures.

Infertility, abortion, premature births, stillbirths, or neonatal deaths can be caused by many infectious agents, such as beta hemolytic *Streptococcus, E. coli; Staphylococcus, Proteus, Pseudomonas,* and *Mycoplasma* species; canine distemper; adenovirus; and herpesvirus. Fetal resorption, mummification, and abortion may be caused by any of the infectious agents just listed or by genetic lethals, lack of uterine space, trauma, placental hemorrhage, hormone deficiency (progesterone), exogenous estrogen, myometrial cysts, hyperplasia, and endometritis. In evaluating these problems, supplement the bacteriologic examination with hormone analysis, pedigree studies, and, particularly, with careful consideration of the history and physical examination.

Radiographic examination of the uterus can be performed easily if the organ is enlarged (pyometra, pregnancy, tumors). Radiopaque dye injected through the cervix via a metal catheter (not always easy to perform) will help delineate problems that involve little change in organ size (cystic hyperplasia, myometrial cysts). Pneumoperitoneal contrast radiography or ultrasonic examination may also reveal pathologic changes. *Peritoneal laparoscopy* is a new technique that may be useful for directly observing abdominal organs such as the uterus. The ovaries are embedded in fatty bursae and, thus, are difficult to visualize. *Exploratory laparotomy* is sometimes necessary to complete examination of the genital organs. One can directly view and palpate the uterus, oviducts, and ovaries for malformations and pathologic changes that cannot be delineated in other ways. Placental sites or corpora lutea can be counted to determine embryonic death, and microbiologic samples and biopsy material can be obtained for laboratory evaluation. At the same time, surgical or medical measures may be performed for treatment of abnormalities. A dye solution such as Mercurochrome can be injected into the uterus and milked forward to determine the patency of the oviducts. With patency, the dye can be expressed from the uterus and appears at the fimbria.

Pregnancy Examination

Palpation of the uterus through the abdominal wall is the most practical method for pregnancy examination. Twenty to 22 days postbreeding, the uterus has distinct swellings 2 cm in diameter. After 28 days, these swellings have increased to about 3 cm in diameter, and this is the optimum time for diagnosis. (Diagnosis in the queen is easiest within 18 to 24 days, difficult after 30 days.) By 35 days, the uterine swellings become confluent and diagnosis becomes more difficult. As pregnancy continues, individual fetuses may be palpated per rectum or through the abdominal wall.

Mammary glands enlarge at about 35 days, and the teats become enlarged and turgid. The nipples of a primipara bitch are often quite red in color. Milk can be expressed from the teats during the last week of pregnancy.

Radiographs delineate portions of the fetal skeletons after about 43 days' gestation. Radiographs may be especially helpful if only one or two fetuses are present.

Other methods of diagnosis include ultrasonography (bitches 30 to 35 days pregnant produce characteristic reflected sounds from uterine and fetal structures).

NORMAL BREEDING—PHYSIOLOGY AND BEHAVIOR

Canine Female

Puberty in the bitch usually occurs between the ages of 6 and 12 months; reproductive life of the female dog is 8 to 10 years. The canine female is seasonally monestrus and ovulates spontaneously. The interval between estrus cycles is from 4 to 18 months, depending on the size and breed of the animal (e.g., Basenji, once/yr; small breeds, 2 or 3 times/yr; and large breeds, one or more times/yr). For cellular characteristics of vaginal smears, see pages 552–557.

Proestrus lasts for 7 to 10 days, during which pheromones increase. Other characteristics are a bloody discharge from the vagina and a swollen vulva. The bitch attracts males but is antisexual. Plasma estrogens reach a maximum level at the end of proestrus, then decrease.

Estrus lasts for 7 to 10 days. Proestrus and estrus periods combined are called the "heat" period. The character of the discharge changes from bloody (during proestrus) to mucoid. The vulva is less turgid. The bitch is receptive and courts the male through foreplay, jumping, and trying to mount the male. The canine female presents the perineum in a lordosis-like posture and reflexively deviates the tail to one side. After estrus, the antisexual attitude of the bitch returns. Ovulation occurs early in estrus (usually within the first 3 days). The ovum is not ready for fertilization until 24 hours later, after the second polar body has been extruded. The ovum lives 4 days—the transit time to the uterus being from 4 to 10 days. Implantation occurs in 18 to 20 days, and an endotheliochorial deciduate zonary placenta forms. The gestation cycle is from 58 to 65 days (usually 63).

Luteinizing hormone (LH) surges within 24 hours of estrogen peak and causes ovulation. Progesterone increases gradually during estrus and is the cause of "behavioral" estrus. Progesterone reaches maximum 25 to 30 days after the LH surge, then gradually decreases to less than 1 mg per ml at parturition in the pregnant bitch. The progesterone decline is the cause of the temperature drop just before parturition. After ovum implantation, the hematocrit falls from 40 to 45 per cent to 30 per cent (may help in differential diagnosis of pseudopregnancy).

Metestrus (4 months) is the period when the corpus luteum is forming and functional.

During *anestrus* (1 to 6 months), the genital organs are relatively quiescent.

Canine Male

Puberty in the canine male occurs between 6 and 12 months of age. (See pp. 538–541 for data about normal sperm.)

Follicle-stimulating hormone (FSH) initiates spermatogenesis; LH increases testosterone secretion of Leydig cells needed to complete spermatogenesis and to maintain accessory sex glands, secondary sex characteristics, and libido. Testosterone has a negative feedback on pituitary gonadotrophins. Oxytocin and prostaglandins are important in the transport of sperm during ejaculation. Prostaglandins increase LH output and testosterone production, and they are the reason that sexual foreplay increases ejaculatory output and total number of sperm.

Testosterone is of little value in the treatment of infertility except to increase libido for 2 to 3 days following administration of low doses. Prolonged use causes testicular degeneration and negative feedback on LH release.

Weekly injections of FSH for 5 weeks have been of some benefit for selected cases of aspermia.

In copulation, the male responds to the female in estrus by biting and nuzzling her neck and licking her flanks and perineal region. The male mounts early and clasps the female's hind quarters at the rear flank with his forelegs. After pelvic copulatory movement, intromission takes place. It ceases within 2 to 3 minutes, and the pair are joined for 5 to 30 minutes. Most males will rebreed within 2 hours of separation.

Feline Female

Puberty in the feline female occurs at 4 to 12 months of age. The reproductive life lasts 8 to 10 years. The feline female is seasonally polyestrus (January–September in the northern hemisphere; continuous if 14 hours of light are available daily). Ovulation is induced by coitus or simulated coitus. The estrus cycle is of 14 to 30 days' duration. For cellular characteristics of the vagina, see page 557. Proestrus lasts 1 or 2 days, during which pheromones increase and a very slight mucoid discharge from the Bartholin glands occurs. The feline female attracts the male but is antisexual.

Estrus lasts 3 to 5 days if the cat is bred; 10 to 20 days if there is no coitus. Estrus can be terminated by LH (25 IU human chorionic gonadotropin, intramuscularly, IM) or by simulated coitus. Following pseudocopulation, the corpora lutea last 30 to 40 days and the cycle averages 6 weeks. The feline female has a characteristic call, rubs the head against objects in affection, purrs, crouches with forelegs, elevates rear quarters and treads, and deflects tail laterally. Ovulation is 24 to 50 hours after copulation (sensory nerves stimulate hypothalamus to release gonadotrophic-releasing hormone, which acts on anterior pituitary release surge of LH, causing ovulation). Sperm requires 24-hour capacitation in the uterus to be fertile; and fertilization may occur up to 48 hours after ovulation.

Fertilized ova are in the oviduct for 4 days. Implantation is 14 days after breeding, and an endotheliochorial zonary placenta forms. The gestation cycle is 61 to 69 days (usually 65).

Metestrus is 7 to 21 days long; the ova degenerate, and the queen returns to estrus. It is not a true metestrus, because ovulation has not been stimulated. The feline female is antisexual.

Anestrus is 1 to 6 months, during which time the queen is antisexual.

Feline Male

Puberty occurs in 6 months (depends on age at beginning of breeding season). See page 544 for data about artificial insemination and feline sperm. The tom has depressed sexual activity in the fall. He has rigid territorial and behavioral habits regarding the breeding ritual, and the feline male does much calling and fighting to retain his harem and home territory.

The male approaches the female, makes chattering sounds, and rubs his face over her shoulder and body. Foreplay is limited; the tom grasps the queen's neck skin in his teeth and mounts. Rapid intromission and ejaculation occur. The queen shrieks, twists aside, rolls over and over, and licks the vulva. The male cat will rebreed in 20 to 60 minutes, either with the same partner or with another queen. The female cat will accept breeding for 1 to 3 days.

References and Additional Readings

Barsanti, J. A., Shotts, E. B., Prasse, K., and Crowell, W.: Evaluation of diagnostic techniques for canine prostatic disease. J.A.V.M.A., 177(2):160, 1980.

Brodey, R. S., Goldschmidt, M. H., and Roszel, J. R.: Canine mammary gland neoplasms. J.A.A.H.A., 19(1):61, 1983.

Carmichael, L. E.: Canine brucellosis: an annotated review with selected cautionary comments. Theriogenology, 6:105, 1976.

Concannon, P. W., Powers, W. H., and Hansel, W.: Pregnancy and parturition in the bitch. Biol. Reprod., 16:517, 1977.

Herron, M. A.: Tumors of canine genital system: J.A.A.H.A., 196:981, 1983.

Hornbuckle, W. E., MacCoy, D. M., Allan, G. S., and Gunther, R.: Prostatic disease in the dog. Cornell Vet., 68:284, 1978.

Johnston, S. D.: Diagnostic and therapeutic approach to infertility in the bitch. J.A.V.M.A., 176(12):1335, 1980.

Klausner, J. S., and Osborne, C. A.: Management of canine bacterial prostatitis. J.A.V.M.A., 182(3):292, 1983.

Lein, D. H.: Reproductive disorders. In Kirk, R. W. (ed.): Current Veterinary Therapy, 8: Small Animal Practice. Philadelphia, W. B. Saunders Company, 1983.

Oglive, G. K.: Feline mammary neoplasis. Compendium on Continuing Education, 5(5):384, 1983.

Pollack, R. V. H.: Canine brucellosis: current status. Compendium on Continuing Education, 1:255, 1979.

Richardson, R. C.: Canine transmissible venereal tumor. Compendium on Continuing Education, 3(11):951, 1981.

Rosenthal, R. C.: Infertility in the male dog. Compendium on Continuing Education, 5(12):983, 1983.

Thrall, D.: Radiographic aspects of prostatic disease in the dog. Compendium on Continuing Education, 3(8):418, 1981.

Wykes, P. M., and Soderberg, S. F.: Congenital abnormalities of the canine vagina and vulva. J.A.A.H.A., 19(6):995, 1983.

Urinary Organs (See also pp. 812)

History

Complete the general physical examination and history. Some findings, such as weight loss, dehydration, ascites, injected or ulcerated mucosa, fetid breath, and softened membranous bones of the face and jaw, may suggest renal or urinary abnormalities.

The onset of urinary disease is often insidious, so that a careful detailed history is imperative. In particular, inquire about *changes* in the following:

pattern of urination, drinking habits, volume of water ingested, volumes of urine formed, and appearance and odor of urine. If it is not accompanied with increased urine volume, nocturia is often a sign of lower urinary tract disease and infection; it may be the result of polyuria, too. When polyuria is present, implying a prolonged total urine volume increase, it usually indicates chronic renal failure, diabetes mellitus or insipidus, or hyperaldosteronism. Polyuria exists when urine volume is more than two times the normal volume (on an unchanged diet).

Normal daily urine volume can be estimated at 20 to 30 ml per kg body weight. Anuria may be defined as daily urine volume of less than 7 ml per kg body weight. In these cases, one should be suspicious of urine retention or obstruction, and catheterization is indicated. Hematuria suggests infection, trauma, calculi, or neoplasm. The degree of bleeding and appearance in the urine stream, whether it is present uniformly in the urine stream or appearing just at the beginning (distal urethral lesion) or just at the end (proximal urethra or bladder), are important diagnostic features. Painful micturition or dysuria is often associated with inflammation and neoplasm, and it must be differentiated from difficult defecation, especially in cats.

Related signs of a more general nature include vomiting, defecation, and anemia, which may reflect chronic uremia or marginal renal function. Abnormal losses or retention of water, electrolytes, and other metabolites may produce signs of dehydration, ascites, cardiac arrhythmias, muscle tremors, and convulsions. It is important to determine possible exposure to potentially toxic agents (such as ethylene glycol), trauma, surgery, and drugs (such as certain antibiotics, sulfonamides, sedatives) that may cause or be influenced by reduced renal function. Previous diagnoses and results of other tests and therapeutic measures are especially important, because many urinary problems are chronic, recurrent, and recalcitrant.

Physical Examination

It is desirable to collect a voided urine sample prior to detailed palpation and inspection of the urinary tract. With the animal standing, note its posture and the conformation of its abdomen. Palpate the abdomen deeply by pressing the hands from beneath the costal margins dorsally and anteriorly. The left kidney is more pendulous and posterior and is more readily palpated. The right kidney may be inaccessible, especially if the dog is obese and/or tense. Sedation or anesthesia can be used as an aid in palpation if it is not contraindicated. Unless it is empty, the bladder can also be assessed by abdominal palpation. Pain, abnormal masses, and firmness or elasticity of organs are noted in these procedures. The palpation process can be aided by elevating the animal's front legs while palpating the abdomen bimanually with one hand at the rear flank and the index finger of the other hand placed in the rectum. This maneuver is especially useful when evaluating bladder, uterus, cervix, prostate, and pelvic urethra. Following gentle digital prostatic massage, one can obtain prostatic fluid from a urethral catheter placed so as to aspirate material from the prostatic urethra.

Palpate the penis and lower urethra, and inspect them for tumors, adhesions, or balanoposthitis. Use a catheter to determine obstruction (such as stenosis and calculi), to collect urine, and to inject air or contrast media (if needed for other procedures). This technique is particularly indicated when trauma is suspected and when one is trying to determine the integrity of the bladder wall. It is also useful in determining bladder capacity and neurogenic bladder problems or in measuring residual urine (see pp. 281–284).

In the female, examination of the vagina (see pp. 552–557) is part of the physical evaluation. Inspect the urethral orifice with the aid of a vaginal speculum, and pass a flexible catheter to determine patency and to obtain a urine sample. Ectopic ureters in the female may enter the vagina and cause constant dribbling. (In the male, ureters entering the proximal urethra do not cause incontinence.) It may be possible to identify urine in the vagina or to even visualize the aberrant opening, especially if urinary dyes are used. The external urinary openings (prepuce, penis, vulva) are inspected for ulceration or irritation (as occurs with incontinence).

Laboratory Evaluation

The following tests are useful in evaluating renal function.

1. Daily water intake and urine output over several days with free access to water.
2. Urinalysis (at admission and again during free water access). See page 812. Urinalysis should include as routine procedures: pH, specific gravity, glucose, ketones, bilirubin, occult blood, and proteinuria.
   a. If proteinuria is elevated, an electrophoretic pattern should be done and further tests scheduled to evaluate possible neoplasms, nephrosis, nephrotic syndrome, or glomerular disease.
   b. Positive glucose and ketonuria suggest diabetes.
   c. The presence of blood suggests infection, trauma, calculi, or tumors.
   d. Microscopic examination of the urine sediment (p. 822) is especially useful, because cell types, casts, bacteria, parasite eggs, and crystals are strong leads for specific diagnoses.
3. Tests for urine cultures and sensitivities (p. 501) must be anticipated so that aseptically acquired urine can be collected using one of the following techniques (listed according to increasing likelihood of successful results):
   a. Midstream catch of voided urine obtained in a sterile container after gentle cleansing of the external urinary openings.
   b. Catheterization (see pp. 545–551).
   c. Suprapubic cystocentesis performed through a surgically prepped ventral abdominal wall using a 1.5- to 2-inch, 22-gauge needle (p. 552).
4. Chemistry tests: BUN (p. 743), PCV (p. 671), CBC (p. 671), chloride, potassium, and sodium (p. 748).
   a. Acid-base studies (pp. 593–597): Blood pH, pCO_2, HCO_3, and base excess.
5. Special function tests.
   a. Urine concentration test, page 240 (ADH and tubular function).

    b. Phenolsulfonphthalein test, page 829 (tubular function).

    c. Creatinine clearance test, page 828 (glomerular function).

6. Radiographic examination.

    a. Flat plates of the abdomen give basic impressions and may diagnose tumors, calculi, and traumatic injury.

    b. Pneumocystogram or opaque contrast studies further delineate calculi, tumors, and discontinuity of organs (ruptures, see pp. 573–574).

    c. Intravenous pyelograms are useful to determine obstructions to urine flow or formation and to outline the kidneys and ureters. They may also show the bladder and urethra with contrast studies not suitable to retrograde injections.

7. Exploratory laparotomy—surgical exploration of the abdomen permits inspection, palpation, culture, and biopsy of intra-abdominal urinary organs as well as allowing for diagnosis and immediate treatment of calculi, tumors, stenosis, and traumatic injuries of the deep abdominal organs.

References and Additional Readings

Osborne, C. A., Low, D. G., and Finco, D. R.: Canine and Feline Urology. Philadelphia, W. B. Saunders Company, 1972.

Osborne, C. A.: Genitourinary disorders. *In* Kirk, R. W. (ed.): Current Veterinary Therapy 8: Small Animal Practice. Philadelphia, W. B. Saunders Company, 1983.

LOCOMOTOR SYSTEM

The locomotor system includes the muscles, bones, and joints. Diseases involving the locomotor system can be produced by alterations in muscles, bones, or joints, together with the vessels and nerves that supply these structures.

History

Question the owner as to the time sequence involved in the development of lameness: Was it an acute onset? Is the lameness continuous or intermittent? Is more than one limb involved? Is the lameness static? Examine the member that the owner believes to be abnormal, and determine the time sequence in the development of the abnormality. Traumatic injuries to bone, muscle, or tendon cause a sudden development of lameness; osteoarthosis causes slowly progressive gait changes. The history may indicate that a shifting leg or multiple lameness is present. This frequently occurs in enostosis (eosinophilic panosteitis). Determine whether the gait abnormality improves or becomes worse after exercise by climbing stairs or jumping. Is it worse first thing in the morning or later in the day? Is it a lameness that the animal "warms out of?" Is there any history of traumatic injury?

Physical Examination

Examine the "posture" of the standing animal. Does the animal carry the limb? Is the foot placed on the floor? Does the animal have difficulty in getting up? lying down? sitting? Observe the stance for the following: rotation of limb (inward–outward), stance (wide or narrow), position of neck (flexed or extended). Determine where there is dorsal flexion of the back and whether the rear quarters are tucked under the abdomen. Also observe whether the animal is leaning forward, supporting its weight on its front limbs, or leaning to one side.

Evaluate the range of motion (ROM), using a goniometer. The following table summarizes measurements based on large breed normal dogs in the standing position. The values can vary ±5 degrees.

	Flexion (degrees)	Extension (degrees)	Standing (degrees)	Total ROM (degrees)
Shoulder	45	150	105	105
Elbow	20	165	140	145
Radiocarpal	30	210	160	180
Hip	40	150	75	110
Stifle	40	180	115	140
Tibotarsal	30	165	150	135

Contributed by Dr. James Toombs and Dr. Larry Wallace, University of Minnesota School of Veterinary Medicine.

Gait

Observe for changes in the animal's gait. Notice which limb is favored by the animal. Determine whether there is pain upon movement. Note whether the animal pursues a relatively straight course or deviates from side to side as it walks. Notice whether the head is carried in an abnormal position. Normally, the dogs bears 60 per cent of its weight on its front limbs. This can be detected by putting your hands under the dog's feet so that he stands on them. The dog can shift more weight forward by extending its head and neck and placing its forelegs further back under the center of gravity. In severe disease of the hind limbs, 90 per cent of the weight may be carried by the forelimbs. Examine the stance and gait from the lateral and caudal aspects. A base-wide stance usually indicates rear limb lameness and pain but may indicate neurologic disease, too. Proprioceptive deficits must be ruled out. Neurologic and musculoskeletal disease are not always mutually exclusive; they frequently occur simultaneously in older dogs and cats.

Observe the posture in a standing position. Determine whether there is (1) a base-wide or base-narrow stance; (2) internal or external rotation of the limb; (3) hyperflexion, hyperextension, or recurvation of any joint; (4) valgus (away from the midline) or varus (inward deviation of the distal component toward the midline) deformity; (5) one limb shorter than another; and (6) muscular swelling or muscular dystrophy.

Palpation and Observation. Examine the soft tissue and long bones of the extremities. Look for deviation from the normal shape and outline of the limb as well as swelling, pain and crepitation, increased heat, and sites of tenderness. Determine whether there is abnormal joint laxity or abnormal motion in the limb. Measure the range of motion of involved joints. Examine the digits and pads for cuts, foreign bodies, ingrown nails, thorns, foxtails, or chemical burns. Look for penetrating soft-tissue injuries (such as muscle swelling, pain, heat, tenderness, or a developing abscess). Check for abnormal enlargement in the diameter of long bones, with attendant pain. Hypertrophic osteoarthropathy produces bone enlargement without pain; hypertrophic osteodystrophy produces bony enlargement with pain and frequently fever and anorexia. Palpation of the periosteum of the long bones may produce pain in cases of eosinophilic panosteitis and osteomyelitis as well as draining tracts in the latter.

Several skeletal abnormalities may be associated with characteristic changes of weight bearing and gait. In animals with chronic medial luxation of the patellae, the femur is rotated laterally and the tibia medially resulting in a "toe-in" and "bow-legged" (genu varum) appearance. These dogs walk with a shuffling gait because it is impossible for them to fully extend the stifle. If there is genu valgum, the patella will luxate laterally with contraction of the quadriceps group. In animals with osteochondrosis dissecans of the shoulder, the stride is short and choppy because of apparent pain when the foreleg is extended and/or flexed. In ununited anconeal process of ulna and radius-ulna growth dissymmetries resulting from premature physeal closures, there is often pain when the elbow joint is flexed or extended. The animal may compensate by keeping the elbow joint in a semiflexed position, abducting the limb when moving. In traumatic luxation of the elbow (rare), the radius and ulna dislocate laterally. Tension and spasm of the brachial muscles cause abduction of the antebrachium and foot. Flexion and extension are impossible. Ligamentous injuries to the elbow joint are more common. For forelimb lameness in immature dogs, the following differential diagnosis should be considered: ununited anconeal process of ulna, osteochondrosis dissecans in various locations, hypertrophic osteodystrophy, panosteitis, and fragmented coronoid process. Multiple conditions may exist simultaneously.

Other pertinent findings in specific musculoskeletal diseases include the following:

1. Hip dysplasia—adductor contracture, Ortolani's sign, Barlow's sign, Barden's sign, and pain on abduction and extension of the hip.
2. Legg-Calvé-Perthes disease—pain and lameness on extreme abduction of the hip, often *bilateral.*
3. Hypertrophic osteodystrophy—firm bilateral swelling of distal radial and/or distal tibia metaphyses.

Lameness—Osteochondrosis

Osteochondrosis dissecans is a disease of the immature joint with localized fractures of the articular cartilage. In large and giant breeds of dogs, the syndrome is seen most frequently in the chondral and subchondral tissues of the proximal end of the humerus. The condition also occurs in the medial condyle of the distal humerus, lateral condyle of the femur, articular processes of the cervical spine and the distal radius and medial trochlear ridge of the talus.

Osteochondrosis of the elbow develops on the medial humeral condyle and may occur singly or in combination with fragmented medial coronoid process. It may be bilateral. Animals are presented because of lameness and pain on flexion or extension of the elbow. The diagnosis may be confirmed radiographically by finding a concave radiolucent defect in the articular aspect of the medial humeral condyle or by identifying a fragmented coronoid process. More often it is diagnosed by a raised index of suspicion for certain breeds, by finding osteophytes on the anconeal process, lipping on the cranial aspect of the radial head, and mixed lytic and productive changes on the medial epicondyle of the humerus.

Osteochondrosis of the stifle occurs most frequently on the medial, weight-bearing surface of the lateral femoral condyle. This condition usually affects the large or giant breeds between the ages of 3 and 9 months.

Osteochondrosis of the hock affects primarily the medial ridge of the trochlea and may occur bilaterally. Swelling of the hock joint develops, and pain and crepitus may be evident on flexion.

Careful examination of the stifle joint for ligamentous injuries often requires general anesthesia. Rupture of the cranial cruciate ligament allows cranial displacement of the tibia (cranial drawer sign) and excessive internal rotation. Caudal cruciate rupture, which usually does not occur unless there is extensive damage to the stifle joint, permits excessive caudal tibial movement and outward rotation. Excessive outward rotation of the tibia with partially flexed limb may indicate rupture of the medial collateral ligament. Palpation that opens the medial or lateral compartment of the joint indicates damage to the respective collateral ligament. Excessive outward rotation of the tibia and abduction of the stifle joint can be produced by rupture of the medial collateral ligament. Inward rotation of the tibia and adduction of the stifle joint can be produced by lateral collateral ligament rupture.

Coxofemoral luxations may produce a variety of abnormal conditions. The most common abnormality is a craniodorsal luxation of the femoral head, in which the limb is rotated outward, adducted, and held in a flexed position. If the femoral head is displaced caudally, the limb is rotated inward.

Inspection and Palpation of the Joints

Examine the joints by inspection and palpation and determine their range of motion. Look for enlargements or irregularities of the joint. Determine whether the enlarged joint is warm and tender, or firm and hard to the touch. Look for the presence of a traumatic wound in the soft tissue over the joint or a sinus tract leading from the joint (see Signs, pp. 301–304). Palpate the joint to check for the presence of bony growths or for grating (crepitation) within the joint.

Move the joint and decide whether the range of motion is normal. Limitation of movement within a joint may result from pain, muscle spasm, contractures of muscle, inflammation, thickening fibrosis of the periarticular structures, effusion within the joint, bony or cartilaginous overgrowths, or ankylosis. Degenerative osteoarthrosis may be characterized by pain, joint deformity, progressive lameness, and stiffness upon rising; however, symptoms become less severe during exercise. However, pain and lameness return shortly after exercise. They frequently are exaggerated by strenuous exercise, such as jumping in obedience training. Bony proliferation and crepitation within the joint occur in the hip, stifle, elbow, and tarsus. Rheumatoid arthritis is a severe, usually progressive polyarthritis, with an apparent immunologically mediated pathogenesis (see p. 301).

Muscular Diseases and Locomotor Changes

Muscular diseases can also produce locomotor changes. Myopathies may be inflammatory (either infectious or noninfectious) or degenerative (inherited or acquired). Inflammatory myopathies are characterized by muscle pain, weakness, fever, elevated serum muscle enzymes, evidence of inflammation, or muscle biopsy. Electromyographic changes include polyphasic motor potentials, fibrillation potentials, and positive waves. An immune profile should be performed in cases of polymyositis (see p. 730). Serum enzyme measurements include CPK, serum aspartate animo-transferase, serum alanine aminotransferase. Polymyositis, which has been observed mostly in German shepherds, can result in a mild to moderate paresis of the limbs. Polymyositis can also affect vocalizing, chewing, and swallowing. Toxoplasmosis can result in a severe necrotizing myositis. Autoimmune myositis has been seen associated with systemic lupus erythematosus (LE). Muscular atrophy can result from disease of the affected limb (as in fractures) or from loss of nervous innervation to the limb (as in radial paralysis). Muscular atrophy may also occur because of primary muscle disease resulting from vascular insults, leading to muscle necrosis and atrophy. "Scotty cramp" is a condition produced in Scottish and Cairn terriers during periods of forced exercise. When forced to move, these dogs demonstrate hypertonicity of the pelvic limb musculature, so that the hind legs take short, jerky steps. The muscle spasm may eventually involve the forelimbs and the neck muscles, and the dog can no longer move. The attack usually subsides within minutes. This is an autosomal recessive disease that may be a disorder of serotonergic spinal cord neurons. Diazepam and vitamin E may decrease the incidence and severity. Racing greyhounds may suffer from acute muscle spasm of the hindlimbs while racing; the condition appears more frequently in poorly conditioned animals.

Myotonia is the continued active contraction of a muscle that persists after the stimulation or voluntary effort has stopped. Clinical signs are muscle stiffness and gait abnormalities that improve upon exercise; other findings are electromyographic abnormalities. Congenital myotonia has been observed in chow dogs in Australia, New Zealand, and Europe; the disorder may have a genetic basis. Other breeds reported as having congenital myotonia are young male Irish terriers and Golden retrievers. Muscle-induced gait change myopathy in male Irish terrier puppies has been reported as a possible recessive x-linked inheritance pattern. The affected puppies were found to have a stiff gait, difficulty in swallowing, an enlarged tongue, and atrophic muscles.

An acquired myotonic myopathy may accompany chronic hyperadrenocorticoidism in older dogs and, rarely, chronic hyperthyroidism.

Canine Myopathies

Canine myopathies can be categorized under inflammatory and degenerative. See the following subcategories:*

Inflammatory
1. Infectious: (a) *Toxoplasma gondii,* (b) *Leptospira icterohaemorrhagiae,* and (c) *Clostridium* sp.
2. Noninfectious: (a) idiopathic polymyositis, (b) systemic LE-associated polymyositis, and (c) eosinophilic myositis

Degenerative
1. Inherited: (a) Irish terrier myopathy, (b) hip dysplasia-associated myopathy, (c) Labrador retriever myopathy, and (d) greyhound cramp (questionable origin).
2. Acquired: (a) atrophic (idiopathic atrophic myositis, denervation, and disuse); (b) ischemic (bacterial endocarditis and dirofilariasis); (c) nutritional (vitamin E deficiency and selenium deficiency); (d) metabolic (hyperadrenocorticism); and (e) miscellaneous (muscular dystrophy, myotonia, and muscle neoplasia).

Neuromuscular Diseases Affecting Gait and Posture

Neuromuscular diseases that affect gait and posture include the following:
1. Congenital and familial disorders: (a) globoid cell leukodystrophy, (b) giant axonal neuropathy, (c) myotonia (chows, Labrador retrievers, Irish terriers), (d) central—peripheral neuropathy, (e) myasthenia gravis, and (f) progressive spinal muscular atrophy (Brittany spaniels, Swedish Lapland dogs).
2. Inflammatory and immune mediated disorders: (a) acute polyradiculoneuritis, (b) brachial plexus neuritis, (c) polymyositis, and (d) toxoplasmic polymyositis.
3. Toxicity: (a) tick paralysis, and (b) botulism.
4. Metabolic: (a) hypoglycemia, (b) diabetes mellitus polyneuropathy, (c) hyperadrenocortical- and corticosteroid-induced polyneuropathy.
5. Neoplastic: lymphosarcoma.

---

*Adapted from Kornegay, J. N., et al.: Polymyositis in dogs. J.A.V.M.A., *176*(5):431, 1980.

Neurologic Defects and Locomotor Changes

Diseases of the lower motor neuron (LMN) innervation of muscles cause signs most easily confused with signs of muscle disease. Loss of reflexes and denervation atrophy help implicate the peripheral nerves and/or spinal cord segments or roots.

The locomotor signs of neurologic deficits are summarized in the section entitled Nervous System (pp. 422–447).

SIGNS OF LESIONS IN FUNCTIONAL SYSTEMS

Lower motor neuron— short stiff strides or flaccid paralysis in complete injuries, buckling, difficulty supporting weight, often looks like a lame gait.

Upper motor neuron— spasticity, decreased to absent voluntary movements; paresis to paralysis.

General proprioception—ataxia, lack of knowledge of where the limbs are located, crossing limb under body, swinging it wide on turns; circumduction, hypermetria, standing on the dorsal surface of the paw.

Vestibular system— loss of balance, head tilt, stumbling, falling, rolling usually to one side. With peripheral lesions (cranial nerve VIII), this is toward the side of the lesion.

Cerebellum— spasticity, dysmetria, hypermetria, loss of balance, falling or lurching movements.

Neurologic defects may produce a variety of changes in gait. Consider the etiology on the basis of: (1) skeletal abnormalities, (2) muscular abnormality, (3) central nervous abnormality, (4) spinal cord abnormality, and (5) peripheral nerve disease. A cerebellar gait is characterized by a wide base stance, unsteadiness, and falling or lurching to one side or the other. Sensory ataxia is characterized by the animal's lack of knowledge about how the limbs are positioned. Animals with this deficit will move their legs with great uncertainty, frequently cross their legs when walking, keep a wide stance, and show hypermetria. Inherited degenerations of motor neurons have been reported in various breeds of dogs. These degenerations lead to progressive muscle loss and weakness, with atrophy of the paraspinal and proximal appendicular muscles. Among these hereditary neurologic diseases are hereditary spinal muscular atrophy in Brittany spaniels, Swedish Lapland dog abiotrophy, and Stockard's paralysis.

Spinal Lesions

Ataxia, paraparesis, paraplegia, quadriparesis, or quadriplegia unaccompanied by cranial nerve disease is indicative of spinal cord or neuromuscular disease.

A wide variety of spinal cord lesions can result in neurologic disease that is manifested by locomotor changes. Below the spinal lesion, paresis, paralysis, alterations in muscle tone, and segmental spinal reflexes may be seen. A more complete discussion of neurologic examination can be found on page 424.

The following outline may be helpful in evaluating the level at which spinal cord disease is present:

1. Low thoracic-high lumbar—partial or complete UMN (upper motor neuron) and GP (general proprioceptive) lesion.
   a. Paraparesis to paraplegia.
   b. Normal or hyperreflexic flexor and patellar reflexes.
   c. Muscle tone normal, hypertonic, hypotonic.
   d. Crossed extensor reflex ($\pm$).
   e. Postural reactions poorly performed or absent in hind limbs.
   f. Schiff-Sherrington phenomenon ($\pm$).
   g. Hypalgesia to analgesia or eugesia.
2. Low lumbar (L_4-L_5-L_6-L_7)—partial or complete UMN/LMN and GP lesion.
   a. Neurologic signs identical to those that occur with injury to the roots of the spinal nerves of these segments.
   b. Analgesia, atonia, or areflexia of areas innervated by those segments with complete lesions.
   c. Direct injury to the spinal cord segments is much more serious than injury to the roots.
3. High cervical (C_1-C_2)—partial or complete UMN and GP lesion.
   a. Quadriparesis to quadriplegia.
   b. Normal or hyperreflexic segmental reflexes (fore *and* hind).
   c. Muscle tone normal or hypertonic.
   d. Postural reactions absent or poorly performed (fore *and* hind).
   e. Hypalgesia-analgesia-eugesia.

Lesions of the spinal cord involving cell bodies of the general somatic efferent LMN, can produce LMN disease: (1) compression of the spinal cord associated with extruded intervertebral disks or vertebral fractures; (2) ischemic myelopathy associated with fibrocartilaginous emboli in arteries and veins in the parenchyma and leptomeninges of the spinal cord; and (3) diffuse myelomalacia associated with acute intervertebral disk extrusion.

In many spinal cord diseases, abnormalities of gait are indicative of damage to the ascending general proprioceptive tracts, producing ataxia, and to the descending UMN tracts, causing paresis. The gait should be evaluated on a firm, nonslippery surface.

Evaluate the degree of paresis associated with spinal cord disease according to the animal's ability to stand and walk. In severe, UMN–associated paresis with spasticity, the animal may not be able to stand; however, when physically placed in position, the animal may be able to support itself, although it may not be able to move voluntarily. Ataxia in the gait is displayed by the animal's crossing the limbs, walking on the dorsal surface of a paw, and appearing hypermetric. For severe weakness of the pelvic limbs, evaluate the affected animal by supporting it at the base of the tail and observing its movement and gait. Table 70 may be used to evaluate the degree of paresis in the pelvic limbs associated with spinal cord disease.

Etiology of spinal cord disease can involve trauma, inflammation, degen-

Table 70. CLINICAL GRADING SYSTEM USED TO EVALUATE
PELVIC LIMB PARESIS

Grade	Characteristics	Degree of Paresis
0	Shows absence of purposeful movement	Paraplegia
1	Unable to stand to support; slight movement when supported by tail	Severe paraparesis
2	Unable to stand to support; can move legs when assisted, but stumbles and falls frequently	Moderate paresis
3	Can stand to support	Mild paresis and ataxia
4	Can stand to support	Minimal paresis and ataxia
5	Shows normal strength and coordination	None

From Trotter, E.: Canine intervertebral disk disease. *In* Kirk, R. W. (ed.): Current
Veterinary Therapy VI. Philadelphia, W. B. Saunders Company, 1977.

eration, neoplasia, or malformation. The resultant neurologic abnormalities, characterized by changes of gait, postural reactions, and spinal reflexes, are dependent on the level of the spinal cord lesion (see Nervous System, pp. 422–447).

Diseases Resulting in Spinal Cord Disorders

1. Congenital and familial—degenerative: (a) cervical vertebral malformations of Great Danes and Doberman pinschers, which may cause spinal cord contusion, compression, or stretching; (b) Afghan myelopathy; (c) multiple cartilaginous exostoses; (d) lysosomal storage disease; (e) hereditary ataxia in Jack Russell terriers, smooth-haired fox terriers; (f) atlanto-axial subluxation (miscellaneous vertebral malformations); and (g) Cauda equina syndrome, which may result from inflammation, trauma, neoplasia, or vascular changes.
2. Inflammatory: (a) meningitis; (b) discospondylitis; (c) myelitis—viral, bacterial, protozoal, fungal; and (d) reticulosis.
3. Traumatic: (a) intervertebral disc disease and (b) spinal cord fractures, contusions.
4. Vascular: (a) fibrocartilaginous embolization; (b) spinal cord hemorrhage; and (c) vascular malformation.
5. Neoplastic: (a) extramedullary (meningiomas, neurofibrosarcomas, neurinoma); (b) intramedullary (astrocytoma, ependymoma, gliomas); and (c) bone (vertebral) neoplasia.

Of particular importance in evaluating the animal with signs of spinal cord disorder is the age and breed of the animal, the onset and course of clinical signs, exposure to chemicals, trauma, evidence of accompanying systemic illness, and generalized neurologic signs. Multifocal or diffuse neurologic disease can be characterized by the presence of seizures; changes in behavior, coordination, and head posture; and cranial nerve deficits.

The acuteness of onset of paraplegia or quadriplegia may be significant in establishing a differential diagnosis. Acute quadriplegia can be associated with acute polyradiculoneuritis, tick paralysis, botulism, spinal cord trauma, herniated intervertebral disc, spinal cord hemorrhage, fibrocartilaginous emboli, and acute meningitis. Slower in onset with progressive paresis, ataxia progressing to paraplegia could be degenerative myelopathy in German shepherds and Afghans, lysosomal storage diseases, cervical vertebral malformation, slowly protruding intervertebral discs, spinal cord tumors, discospondylitis, and cauda equina syndrome.

For young dogs (under 9 months of age) presenting with ataxia, quadriparesis, or paraparesis associated with spinal cord disease, the differential diagnosis should include the following: congenital spinal cord disease (spinal dysraphia, lipid storage diseases, globoid cell leukodystrophy, and Afghan leukodystrophy); inflammatory disease (distemper myelitis); spinal cord trauma; and vertebral malformations, including those seen in the cervical area of Great Danes and Doberman pinschers.

For adult dogs presenting with ataxia, quadriparesis, or paraplegia, the differential diagnosis should include disc disease, spinal cord hemorrhage, meningitis, fibrocartilaginous infarct, distemper myelitis, reticulosis, discospondylitis, cauda equina syndrome, and spinal cord neoplasia.

Cervical disc disease is associated with neck pain and neck and leg pain (root signature indicated by pain radiating down the front legs, which is involved with entrapment of nerve roots in C_4-C_8, T_1-T_2). Extrusion of disc material into the dorsomedian, paramedian, or dorsolateral plane results in myelopathies and cervical cord compression. Intraforaminal, lateral, and ventral disc extrusions cause compression of nerve roots, and myelopathy is not a distinct clinical sign. Demonstration of nerve root compression requires myelography and dorsal recumbency oblique cervical spine radiographs taken at a 45- to 60-degree angle with the table.

Discospondylitis refers to intervertebral disc infection with concurrent osteomyelitis of the bordering vertebrae. The condition primarily affects larger breeds of dogs. Male dogs predominate, and the condition has a breed predilection for Great Danes and German shepherds. The midthoracic spine C_{6-7} and L_7-S_1 are the sites that are most involved. Etiology may involve foreign bodies or bacterial or fungal infections. Diagnosis is based on radiographic examination, with variable degrees of vertebral lysis, sclerosis, and spondylosis. Of significance is the possible role of *Brucella canis* infection causing infection. Blood cultures, urine cultures, and serodiagnosis should be performed for this organism in acute discospondylitis. Another bacteria frequently isolated in these cases is *Staphylococcus aureus*.

A wide range of abnormalities in peripheral nerves can lead to changes in gait and alter the range of motion of limbs (see Fig. 51, *A* and *B*). Lesions at any point of the LMN can produce similar clinical signs, and it may be difficult to separate diseases of the peripheral nerve and ventral root from disorders of the ventral horn cell. The following signs may indicate peripheral nerve disorder: paresis, ataxia, hypotonia of muscles, altered peripheral pain sensa-

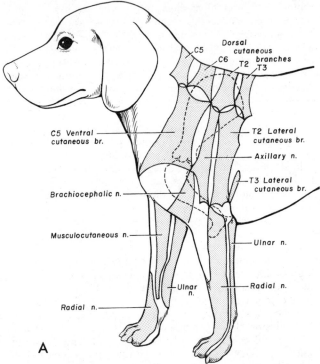

Figure 51. A, Autonomous zone of the cutaneous innervation of the thoracic limb. B, Autonomous zones of the cutaneous innervation of the canine pelvic limb. Caudal cutaneous femora (CCF), genitofemoral (GF), lateral cutaneous femoral (LCF), peroneal (Per), Saphenous (Sa), sciatic (Sci), tibial (Tib). Asterisks indicate palpable bony landmarks—medial and lateral tibial condyles, greater trochanter, and lateral end of tuber ischiadicum. The sciatic nerve autonomous zone is for lesions proximal to the greater trochanter and includes the zones for the peroneal and tibial nerves. For sciatic nerve lesions caudal to the femur, the autonomous zone varies depending upon how many of its cutaneous branches are affected. (From deLahunta, A.: Veterinary Neuroanatomy and Clinical Neurology, 2nd ed. Philadelphia, W. B. Saunders Company, 1983.)

Illustration continued on opposite page.

tion, loss of bladder tone, loss of perianal reflexes, change in voice. Additional studies such as nerve conduction studies using EMG and nerve biopsy may be needed to confirm peripheral nerve disease. A more complete discussion of peripheral nerve disease can be found in the article by Duncan (1978).

Acute inflammation of LMNs can be seen in acute idiopathic polyradiculoneuritis (coonhound paralysis) and brachial plexus neuropathy. Chronic canine polyneuritis can involve LMN innervation to limbs, facial musculature, and voice. There is no joint pain, no joint abnormalities, no ataxia, a presence of

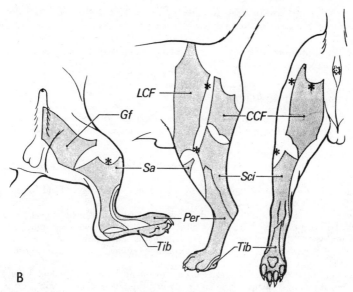

Figure 51. *(Continued)*

neurogenic atrophy of muscle tissue, and paresis on postural reaction. Difficulty may be encountered in the early stages of this disease with primary musculoskeletal disease and electromyography, and biopsy of nerve tissue may be needed for confirmatory diagnosis.

Brachial plexus neuritis has been seen in dogs with allergic reactions to a foreign protein such as horsemeat. Additional signs included vomiting, facial edema, and generalized urticaria.

Abnormalities of the general somatic efferent LMN can cause signs of muscle weakness (paresis) or paralysis, hyporeflexia or areflexia, hypotonia or atonia, and neurogenic-induced atrophy. Ataxia generally is not observed in peripheral nerve disorders.

Injuries to the peripheral nerves can result in alterations in segmental spinal reflexes.

	Affected Reflex	Peripheral Nerve	Spinal Cord Segments	Level in Vertebral Canal
Thoracic limb	Biceps	Musculocutaneous	C_6–C_8	C_5–C_7
	Triceps	Radial	C_7–T_2	C_6–T_1
	Flexor	All peripheral nerves of thoracic	C_6–T_2	C_5–T_1
Pelvic limb	Patellar	Femoral	L_3–L_5	L_4–L_6
	Flexor	Sciatic	L_6–S_1	L_4–L_5
	Perineal	Pudendal	S_1–S_3	L_5

Trauma can also severely damage spinal roots, resulting in LMN disease. Avulsion of the roots of the brachial plexus can result in thoracic limb paralysis. Extensive damage to the brachial plexus involves nerves C_6-T_1 resulting in paralysis of all muscles and the limb being dragged on the ground, unable to support weight.

References and Additional Readings

Averill, D. R., Jr.: Diagnosis and treatment of diffuse disorders of peripheral nerves and muscle. Proc. of September 23–24 Kal Kan Symposium, 1978, pp. 36–38.

Chrisman, C. L. (ed.): Symposium on advances in veterinary neurology. Vet. Clin. North Am., *10*:1980.

Chrisman, C. L.: Disorders of the spinal cord—not involving vertebrae or discs. Proc. A.A.H.A., Annual Meeting, 1979, p. 243.

deLahunta, A.: Veterinary Neuroanatomy and Clinical Neurology. Philadelphia, W. B. Saunders Company, 1983.

Duncan, I. D.: Some aspects of the diagnosis and treatment of small animal neuromuscular disease. Proc. of September 23–24 Kal Kan Symposium, 1978, pp. 31–35.

Hollenbeck, L.: The Dynamics of Canine Gait. Akron, N.Y., published by author, 1971.

Roy, W. G.: Examination of the canine locomotor system. Vet. Clin. North Am., *1*:53, 1971.

Siemering, B.: A review of the diagnosis and treatment of common forelimb lameness in immature dogs. Compendium on Continuing Education, *1*:357, 1979.

Trotter, E. J.: Canine intervertebral disk disease. *In* Kirk, R. W. (ed.): Current Veterinary Therapy VI. Philadelphia, W. B. Saunders Company, 1977.

VanSickle, D. C.: Selected orthopedic problems in the growing dog. Special Report, Am. Anim. Hosp. Assoc., 1975, pp. 20–35.

Whittick, W. G.: Canine Orthopedics. Philadelphia, Lea & Febiger, 1974.

NERVOUS SYSTEM

by A. deLahunta, D.V.M.*

The nervous system is examined to ascertain the site and nature of the lesion responsible for signs of nervous disease. In examining the animal with a neurologic disorder, three basic questions should be answered: (1) Where is the lesion in the nervous system? (2) What type of lesion is present? (inflammation, degeneration, neoplasm, malformation, or injury) (3) What causes the lesion?

Follow an outline (Fig. 52) in performing an examination of the nervous system. Examine the animal in quiet surroundings. The following equipment is helpful in performing a neurologic examination: reflex hammer, penlight, and hemostat.

---

*Professor of Anatomy, Chairman, Department of Clinical Sciences, New York State College Veterinary Medicine, Cornell University, Ithaca, New York.

N.Y.S. VETERINARY COLLEGE — CORNELL UNIVERSITY — VETERINARY HOSPITALS

NEUROLOGIC EXAMINATION

History:

REF. DVM
CLINICIAN
SECONDARY #

Mental Status:

Gait & Posture:

Cranial Nerves:

II—Menace

III—Pupils

  Strabismus

V—Motor: Mand.

  Sensory: Ophth. Max. Mand.

VI—Strabismus

VII—

VIII—Cochlear

  Vestibular—Head tilt

  Nystagmus—Resting

    Positional

    Vestibular

IX, X—   XII

Muscle Tone:

  Atrophy

Spinal Reflexes:

  Patellar LH   RH

  Biceps L R Triceps L R

  Perineal   Tail

  Flexor LF   RF   Crossed

    LH   RH   Extensor:

  Pain Perception

Postural Reactions:

  Wheelbarrowing

  Hopping LF   RF

    LH   RH

  Extensor Postural Thrust

  Hemistand

  Hemiwalk

  Proprioceptive LF RF   LH RH

  Positioning

  Placing—Optic   Tactile

Anatomic DX:

Differential DX:

Ancillary Studies:

NEUROLOGIC EXAMINATION

Figure 52. Nervous system examination record chart.

SIGNALMENT AND HISTORY

The breed, sex, and age of the animal should be noted, because considered together with the chief complaint, they may help direct the line of questioning in the historical review. Certain breeds are predisposed to specific neurologic ailments, and the age of the animal may tend to eliminate certain neurologic diseases (see Table 75).

The history should include a summary of all past medical and surgical illnesses and the facts surrounding the present complaint. The line of questioning will be influenced by the chief complaint.

Injury
1. When did it occur? Was it observed?
2. Describe the animal's condition.
3. How has this changed since the accident?

Seizures
1. Describe completely. How do they start? How does the animal act during the seizure? Is the animal conscious? How long does the seizure last? How does the animal act during the recovery? Is the patient normal between seizures? What are the intervals between seizures? Is there a period of abnormal behavior associated with the seizure?
2. Is there a past history of an injury?
3. When does the animal eat, and what does it eat?
4. Is there any source of intoxication, especially lead?
5. Has the animal been ill recently?
6. What is the vaccination history?

Weakness or ataxia
1. Describe the first appearance of these signs. Was the onset sudden or gradual?
2. When did the signs begin? How have the signs changed since? Have the signs been progressively getting worse, or have they been intermittent?
3. Has the animal had periods of being normal since the first onset of the signs?
4. Have there been any seizures or periods of abnormal behavior or other signs of disturbed cerebral function?

Puppy with neurologic signs
1. Were the signs present at birth or at least as soon as the pup could walk?
2. How have the signs changed since then?

Neurologic Examination

The neurologic examination can be divided into five parts: mental attitude-behavior, gait, postural reactions, spinal nerves, and cranial nerves. In this description, an intact reflex only requires the function of the peripheral nerves being tested and the segments of the spinal cord or brain stem in which the afferent axon enters and the cell bodies and axons of the efferent neurons are located. A reaction depends on the same components as the reflex, plus the ascending pathways through the white matter of the spinal cord and brain stem to the cerebellum and sensorimotor cortex of the cerebrum, and the descending pathways that return from the cerebrum by way of its internal capsule and the white matter of the brain stem and spinal cord. The lower motor neuron (LMN) has its cell body and dendritic zone in the ventral grey column of the spinal cord or specific cranial nerve nucleus in the brain stem. Its axon leaves the central nervous system (CNS) and courses through peripheral nerves to its telodendron in the group of muscle fibers it innervates. The upper motor neurons (UMNs) have cell bodies and dendritic zones in collections of grey matter in the cerebrum (motor cerebral cortex) or brain stem (red nucleus, reticular nuclei). Their axons descend in tracts through the white matter in the brain and spinal cord to end in telodendria in the vicinity of the LMN that they ultimately influence (Fig. 53).

The precise order in which the parts of a neurologic examination are performed varies with the preference of the examiner and the attitude of the patient. An initial assessment should be made of the patient's mental attitude and behavior. If the animal is resting quietly in a cage at the time of examination, the cranial nerve examination may be done first. If the animal is excited or apprehensive, it may be more convenient to perform the cranial nerve examination after the animal has been handled during the examinations of gait, postural reactions, and reflexes.

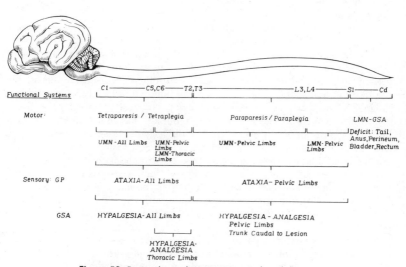

Figure 53. Regional neurologic signs in spinal cord disease.

Mental Attitude-Behavior

An assessment should be made of the patient's mental attitude, sensorium, or behavior. The owner is usually the best judge of the subtle changes in the patient's behavior and should be questioned about this. Is the animal bright, alert, and responsive on your first approach and throughout the examination? The various terms that characterize alterations of this attitude and behavior are depression, lethargy, unresponsiveness, stupor, coma, anxiety, disorientation, hyperactivity, hysteria, propulsion, and aggression.

As a rule, these alterations in the animal's normal sensorium reflect disturbances in the diencephalon and telencephalon and often implicate some portion of the limbic system. It is especially important to evaluate these carefully in the recumbent animal. Cervical spinal cord disease that produces recumbency will not alter the animal's mental attitude except that some animals may become frantic and hyperexcitable if they are unable to get up. The same degree of tetraplegia can occur with a brain stem lesion that severely alters the animal's responsiveness to its environment.

Gait

Examination of the gait should be done in a place where the animal may be allowed to move freely, unleashed, and where the ground surface is not slippery. The floor of many examining rooms is too slippery for adequate evaluation of the animal's gait. In some patients with vertebral column injury with spinal cord contusion resulting in paresis and ataxia, moving the patient on a slippery floor may cause a fall, and further injury may result. A carpeted room is ideal.

The degree of functional deficit dictates the necessity for further examination of strength and coordination. A patient that is tetraplegic—unable to support its weight or move its limbs when the weight is borne on them—need not have further tests performed for the postural reactions. A grade 0 paraplegic patient need not be examined for postural reactions in the pelvic limbs, but the thoracic limbs should be examined carefully. Occasionally, a patient with progressive myelitis may present as paraplegic because of an extensive thoracolumbar spinal cord location of the lesion but also has an asymmetric thoracic limb gait because of a less severe focus of the lesion in the cervical spinal cord. An early sign in dogs with ascending myelomalacia associated with an acute intervertebral disc extrusion may be a hesitant, stumbling, awkward gait in the thoracic limbs. The severity of advanced pelvic limb weakness is evaluated best by holding the animal suspended at the base of the tail and observing its gait. The degree of pelvic limb strength and coordination present following a thoracolumbar spinal cord lesion may be graded according to the following scheme:

5—normal strength and coordination.

4—can stand to support; *minimal paraparesis and ataxia.*

3—can stand to support but frequently stumbles and falls; *mild paraparesis and ataxia.*

2—Unable to stand to support; when assisted, moves limbs readily but stumbles and falls frequently; *moderate paraparesis and ataxia.*

1—unable to stand to support; slight movement when supported by the tail; *severe paraparesis.*

0—absence of purposeful movement; *paraplegia.*

Postural Reactions

Following observation of the gait for strength and coordination, the postural reactions can be tested especially to determine whether there are less obvious deficits in strength and coordination when the gait appears to be normal. Each of these requires that all major components of the peripheral and CNSs be intact. They are not of localizing value by themselves.

Wheelbarrowing. The thoracic limbs may be tested by supporting the animal under the abdomen so that the pelvic limbs are off the ground surface and forcing the animal to walk on its thoracic limbs. The normal animal walks with symmetric movements of both thoracic limbs and the head extended in normal position. Animals with lesions of the peripheral nerves of the thoracic limbs, cervical spinal cord, or brain stem may have asymmetric movements, with stumbling or knuckling over on the dorsum of the paw of the affected limb. Hypermetria is occasionally observed. With more severe lesions in this area, there is a tendency to carry the head flexed with the nose close to and occasionally reaching the ground surface for support. If no deficit is observed, extend the neck while the animal is wheelbarrowed. This sometimes reveals a mild deficit, a tendency to knuckle over on the dorsum of the paw, which was not observed previously. This may be helpful to confirm a cervical spinal cord lesion in Great Danes or Doberman pinchers that have a cervical vertebral malformation and show mild pelvic limb paresis and ataxia, but no overt thoracic limb signs.

Hopping—Thoracic Limb. While still supporting the pelvic limbs, hop the animal on one thoracic limb while holding the other off the ground surface so that the entire weight of the body is supported by the limb to be tested. Move the dog forward and to each side but especially laterally, and observe the strength and coordination of the limb. Repeat this on the other thoracic limb and compare the response. Asymmetry occurs with paresis or ataxia. Hypermetria may be seen with general proprioceptive or cerebellar deficits. This is an effective way of determining minor deficits when the gait appears to be normal, as occurs with contralateral cerebral sensorimotor cortex lesions.

Extensor Postural Thrust. The same sequence of tests can be done on the pelvic limbs. The extensor postural thrust reaction is performed by holding the animal off the ground surface by supporting it caudal to the scapulae, lowering it to the ground surface, and observing the animal extend its pelvic limbs to support its weight. Moving the animal forward and backward in this position tests the symmetry of pelvic limb function, strength, and coordination.

Hopping—Pelvic Limb. Continuing to support the animal by the thorax so that the thoracic limbs are not in contact with the ground surface, one pelvic limb can be held up and the animal forced to hop laterally or forward on the supporting limb. Both pelvic limbs should be tested this way and the responses compared. It is important to compare the pelvic limb hopping responses with each other and not the ipsilateral thoracic limb. Normally, the hopping response of the pelvic limb seems more stiff or hypertonic, with a slightly larger excursion than that of the thoracic limb.

Hemistanding and Hemiwalking. The animal's ability to stand and walk with the thoracic and pelvic limbs on one side can be tested by holding the opposite thoracic and pelvic limbs off the ground surface and forcing the animal to walk forward or to the side. These are referred to as the hemistanding and hemiwalking reactions. With a large dog or uncooperative patient that resists hopping, you may be able to evaluate the hopping responses by observing the responses of the limbs during hemiwalking.

An animal with a unilateral lesion of the sensorimotor cortex or internal capsule may have a normal gait but show deficits in its postural reactions on the side opposite the lesion. Attempts to hemiwalk on the contralateral side are delayed and/or exaggerated (hypermetric) and spastic, and stumbling may occur. With unilateral cervical spinal cord lesions, the limbs on the same side as the lesion show a deficiency in the gait and are unresponsive on postural reaction testing, including inability to support the animal in the hemiwalking reaction.

Placing. Other postural reactions that can be tested include placing with the thoracic limbs. The animal is supported off the ground surface and its thoracic limbs are brought to the edge of a table or similar surface so that the dorsal surface of the paws makes contact. This test should be performed on both thoracic limbs simultaneously and individually, with and without blindfolding the animal. Vision can compensate for the sense of position when the general proprioceptive system is abnormal.

Tonic Neck Reaction. The tonic neck reaction involves extension of the head and neck so that the nose is directed dorsally. The normal patient responds by extension of all the joints of both thoracic limbs. An animal with disease of the general proprioceptive system in the cervical spinal nerves, cervical spinal cord, or medulla fails to extend its carpus or digits or both, and these joints passively flex so that the weight is borne on the dorsal surface of the paw. The same response may occur if an animal is paretic either as a result of disease of the motor neurons that innervate the thoracic limb or in the white matter of the spinal cord that influences these motor neurons.

Proprioceptive Positioning. Proprioceptive positioning tests this afferent system by determining the animal's ability to recognize when the paw has been flexed so that the weight is borne on its dorsal surface. The normal animal returns the paw to its usual position. In patients with severe paresis, this test may also be deficient.

SPINAL NERVES

Spinal nerve evaluation includes assessment of muscle tone and size, spinal reflexes, and cutaneous sensation. Muscle tone and spinal reflexes are evaluated best when the animal is in lateral recumbency and as relaxed as possible. It is important to test muscle tone, tendon reflexes, and the flexor reflex to noxious stimuli, in that order, to maintain the cooperation of the animal.

Muscle Tone. Muscle tone is evaluated by passive manipulation of the limbs individually. The degree of resistance is determined to be less than normal (hypotonic), normal, or more than normal (hypertonic). The latter may be referred to as spasticity. The degree of spasticity varies from a mild increased resistance to passive manipulation, to a marked increase that may be "clasp knife" in character. It is referred to as "clasp knife" because, as attempts are made to flex a limb, the degree of extension of the limb increases, until suddenly it gives way to complete flexion without resistance.

Hypotonia usually occurs with LMN disease, whereas UMN disease is characterized by hypertonia or spasticity. The functional integrity of the LMN is necessary to cause muscle cell contraction in order to maintain muscle tone. It is also necessary to maintain the normal health of the muscle cell it innervates. When denervated, these cells degenerate. This is observed clinically as neurogenic atrophy and can be detected electromyographically by the production of abnormal potentials in resting muscle. The UMN influences the activity of the LMN to produce voluntary motor activity and to maintain muscle tone for support of the body against gravity. Although the UMN includes both facilitatory and inhibitory functions on the activity of the LMN, when the UMN is diseased, the result usually observed is a release of the LMN from inhibition and overactivity of the facilitatory mechanism. This release is seen as hypertonia or spasticity.

Dogs that are tetraplegic should be held in a supporting position to observe the muscle tone in the limbs and any voluntary responses. Usually dogs with cervical spinal cord disease will have rigidly extending limbs, and the entire trunk and limbs will feel stiff when you hold the dog up and move the limbs along the ground surface. The hypertonia may be severe enough to permit the animal to stand unsupported. Tetraplegic dogs with diffuse neuromuscular diseases such as polyradiculoneuritis are hypotonic or atonic and appear and feel limp when you attempt to hold them in a supporting position. There is no reflex tension of the limb and no support elicited by placing the paws on the ground. Instead, the limbs buckle under the weight of the body.

Patellar Reflexes. The most reliable tendon reflex is the patellar reflex. It is the only tendon reflex that is present in all normal animals. It is obtained by lightly tapping the patellar tendon with the animal in lateral recumbency and as relaxed as possible for proper evaluation. A pediatric neurologic hammer is the most useful instrument, but any hard object such as scissor handles can be used. The reflex can be elicited in all normal dogs and is mediated by the femoral nerve through the fourth to sixth lumbar spinal cord segments. The degree of normal response varies with the breed. Large breeds of dogs have a brisker reflex than the short-limbed breeds such as the dachshund. The response should be evaluated as absent (0), hyporeflexic (+1), normal (+2), hyperreflexic (+3), or clonic (+4). This reflex should be tested with the animal lying on each side. An absent reflex or hyporeflexia occurs when there is disease of a portion of the reflex arc. Hyperreflexia or clonus is often present in UMN disease.

Biceps and Triceps Reflex. In the thoracic limb, the biceps and triceps reflexes can be elicited in many dogs that are relaxed and in lateral recumbency. Lightly tapping the tendon of insertion of the triceps proximal to the olecranon elicits a slight extension of the elbow. The reflex is mediated by the radial nerve through the seventh and eighth cervical and first and second thoracic spinal cord segments. The biceps reflex is elicited by placing a finger on the distal ends of the biceps and brachialis muscles at the level of the elbow. Tapping this finger with the hammer elicits a slight flexion of the elbow. The muscle contraction can be palpated in some instances when no movement of the joint is seen. The musculocutaneous nerve mediates this reflex through the sixth, seventh, and eighth cervical spinal cord segments. The normal animal has a mild reflex response to these stimuli. In a few normal animals, they are difficult to elicit. They are absent when there is disease of some portion of the reflex arc. They may be hyperactive in some animals with disease of the UMN.

Flexor Reflex—Pelvic Limb. The flexor reflexes to painful stimuli determine the integrity of the reflex arc as well as the pathway in the CNS that is concerned with the animal's response to painful stimuli. The most reliable stimulus is pressure exerted on the base of the toenail with hemostats. Many normal animals do not respond to the stimulus of a pin. In the pelvic limb, the flexor reflex is mediated by the sciatic nerve through the sixth and seventh lumbar spinal cord segments and the first sacral segment. Abnormality of the motor portion of the sciatic nerve distal to the pelvis causes paralysis, hypotonia, and atrophy of the flexors of the stifle, tarsus, and digits as well as of the extensors of the hip, tarsus, and digits. There is no resistance to flexion or extension of the tarsus. On walking with a sciatic nerve paralysis, the tarsus is lower on the affected side and the paw may be placed on its dorsal surface; however, the limb is able to support weight as long as the femoral nerve is intact.

Sensory branches of the peroneal nerves supply the dorsal surface of the paw. The plantar surface is supplied by tibial nerve sensory branches. The medial side of the paw is supplied by the saphenous nerve, a branch of the femoral nerve at the femoral triangle. This enters the spinal cord through the fourth to sixth lumbar segments. A patient may have a contused sciatic nerve from a pelvic fracture and have no function of the muscles innervated by this nerve and analgesia of the lateral, dorsal, and plantar surfaces of the paw. However, the intact saphenous nerve provides sensation to the medial surface of the paw. If this area is stimulated, the animal will flex the hip with the intact innervation of the iliopsoas muscle, but the stifle, tarsus, and digits fail to flex. For this reason, both the medial and lateral surfaces of the paw should be tested for reflex responses as well as pain perception.

Pain Perception. The animal shows signs of pain when the impulses generated by a noxious stimulus have entered the spinal cord over the peripheral nerves and dorsal roots and are relayed to tracts in the lateral funiculi of the spinal cord bilaterally. These tracts ascend the spinal cord in the lateral funiculi, and continue through the medulla, pons, and mesencephalon to specific nuclei in the thalamus for relay to the somatic sensory cerebral cortex. Pain may be evidenced when the impulses reach the thalamus or cerebrum.

Flexor Reflex—Thoracic Limb. In the thoracic limb, the thoracodorsal, axillary, musculocutaneous, median, ulnar, and radial nerves are responsible for flexion of the shoulder, elbow, carpus, and digits when a painful stimulus is applied to the paw. These arise from the sixth cervical to the second thoracic spinal cord segments. The specific sensory nerve stimulated depends on the location of the stimulus. The median and ulnar nerves innervate the skin of the palmar surface of the paw; the radial nerve supplies the dorsal surface. In the forearm, the radial nerve supplies the skin on the cranial and lateral surfaces. The ulnar nerve supplies the caudal surface, and the musculocutaneous nerve supplies the medial surface. Be aware of the amount of overlap of the cutaneous innervation by these nerves.

Crossed Extensor Reflex. In animals with UMN disease and release of the LMN, a crossed extensor reflex may be elicited in the recumbent animal when the flexor reflex is stimulated. This occurs in the limb opposite the one being tested for a flexor reflex. To avoid voluntary extension of the contralateral limb as a response to pain, the flexor reflex first should be elicited with as mild a stimulus as is necessary and the opposite limb observed for extension. When elicited in an animal in lateral recumbency, this is an abnormal reflex, indicative of UMN disease.

Perineal Reflex. The perineal reflex is elicited by stimulating the anus with a noxious stimulus and observing contraction of the anal sphincter and flexion of the tail. It is mediated by branches of the sacral and caudal nerves through the sacral and caudal segments of the spinal cord.

Cutaneous Reflex. The cutaneous reflex is the contraction of the cutaneous trunci in response to mild stimulation of the skin of the trunk. It can be elicited from the thoracic and most of the lumbar region. The regional segmental spinal nerves contain the sensory neurons that are stimulated. The impulses are carried into the related spinal cord segments and then relayed through the white matter of the spinal cord cranially to the eighth cervical spinal cord segment. Here synapse occurs on LMNs of the lateral thoracic nerve that innervate the cutaneous trunci. This reflex may require multiple stimulation to elicit, and occasionally normal dogs resist this stimulation and show no reflex. This reflex may be useful in diagnosing the level of a complete transverse thoracolumbar spinal cord lesion (see Fig. 51 A, B, page 436).

CRANIAL NERVES

The cranial nerve examination should be performed at the time that the animal is in the most cooperative attitude. The procedure for examining the cranial nerves is described here, with the specific cranial nerves being examined indicated in parentheses.

Observe the head for any evidence of a head tilt (vestibular VIII), facial muscle asymmetry from weakness or contracture-hemifacial spasm (VII), or atrophy of the muscles of mastication (motor V). Palpate these muscles for tone and atrophy. With one eye of the patient covered, menace the opposite eye with threatening gestures of the hand, being careful to avoid striking the patient or stimulating the hair with air currents (II–VII). Repeat this on the opposite side. If the response is absent, check the eyelids for ability to close (VII). Observe the symmetry of the pupils and their reaction to light in either eyeball (II–III). Observe the eyes for evidence of abnormal position, strabismus (III, IV, VI, vestibular VIII), or abnormal nystagmus (vestibular VIII). Move the head from side to side to generate normal vestibular nystagmus. This stimulates the vestibular nerve (VIII), and impulses pass through the vestibular nuclei (medulla) and medial longitudinal fasciculus (medulla-pons-midbrain) to abducent neurons in the medulla for abduction and oculomotor neurons in the midbrain for adduction. Test the corneal and palpebral reflexes (sensory V–VII), ear movement (VII), and the position of the philtrum (VII). Examine the commissure of the lips for hypotonia that exposes mucosa and allows saliva to escape (VII). Check the skin sensation to blunt forceps from the corners of the eyelids (lateral angle-maxillary nerve V; medial angle-ophthalmic nerve VI; and the mucosa of the nasal septum (ophthalmic nerve V). If further evaluation is necessary, a pin can be used over the entire surface of the head. If evaluation is difficult and a deficit is suspected, the most sensitive area to test with a blunt object is the mucosa of the nasal septum inside each naris. Observe the jaws for normal closure (motor V). Open the mouth and observe whether resistance is normal (motor V). Observe the position of the tongue, its movements and size (atrophy), and pull on it to test its strength (XII). Check the gag reflex by probing the pharynx with finger (IX, X).

Additional Tests: Visual. Additional tests may be performed for certain of the cranial nerves if an abnormality is suspected. If a visual deficit is suspected from the menace test, the animal should be walked through a maze once with the lights on and again with the lights off. After observing the animal without a blindfold, cover one eye and repeat the maneuver through the maze. Observe this for each eye. These tests for vision test not only the eyeball and second cranial nerve, but also the central visual pathway to the visual cerebral cortex. Because approximately 65 per cent (cat) to 75 per cent (dog) of the optic nerve axons cross in the optic chiasm, clinically an animal will show a unilateral blindness with an ipsilateral optic nerve lesion or a contralateral lesion in the optic tract, lateral geniculate nucleus, optic radiation, or visual cerebral cortex. The deficit is more complete with optic nerve lesions, and the pupil on the affected side may be more dilated than the pupil in the normal eyeball and unresponsive to light directed to the affected eyeball. The pupil in the blind eyeball will respond to light directed to the normal eyeball as long as the oculomotor nerve (III) is intact. With unilateral lesions in the central visual pathway from the optic tract to the visual cerebral cortex, pupillary function is normal. This occurs becuse some of the optic nerve axons concerned with pupillary control cross in the optic chiasm as well as in the pretectal area, so that impulses stimulated by light in one retina reach both oculomotor nuclei. Lesions in the central visual pathway from the optic tract caudally may only produce a deficient menace response in the eye on the opposite side and may not be detected when the animal walks around objects in a room, even with the normal eye covered. This is because there are optic nerve axons from the eyeball with the menace deficit that do not cross in the optic chiasm.

Disease of one optic nerve causes blindness in that eye, with a dilated pupil and no response to light directed into that eye. Both pupils constrict to light placed in the opposite eye.

Disease of one oculomotor nerve causes a widely dilated pupil on that side that is unresponsive to light directed into either eyeball.

Cerebellar lesions may cause a failure of the menace response, but visual function and facial muscle function are normal in all other tests. These animals will have significant evidence of cerebellar disease in their posture and gait.

Additional Tests: Vestibular. For further examination of the vestibular system (vestibular VIII), the head should be held laterally over each shoulder with the exposed eyeball covered except for the limbus. Observe the eyeball for the development of a positional nystagmus. Make a similar observation with the head and neck extended and both eyeballs covered with the lower eyelids except for the limbus at the superior portion of the eyeball. In the normal patient, no nystagmus develops and the corneas remain in the center of the palpebral fissure. In patients with unilateral disease of the vestibular system, the eye on the affected side is depressed and does not elevate into the center of the fissure, and nystagmus may be observed. The head should be moved from side to side, and the normal vestibular nystagmus elicited should be observed. In bilateral peripheral vestibular disease or severe lesions in the brain stem, this response may be absent. This lack of normal eye movement offers a poor prognosis in animals with intracranial injury. In unilateral vestibular lesions, the rapidity of the response may not be equal in both directions of head movement.

The nystagmus elicited by spinning the patient should be observed, and the rapidity and duration compared following spinning both to the left and the right. An assistant is needed to hold the animal in a normal standing position and to spin it rapidly six or seven times. The postrotatory nystagmus elicited is observed immediately upon stopping the spin.

The presence of a spontaneous or positional nystagmus or a postrotatory nystagmus that is markedly different on each side is evidence of disturbance of the vestibular system. With disturbance of the peripheral portion of this system (the eighth cranial nerve), the abnormal spontaneous or positional nystagmus is either horizontal or rotatory, with the quick phase directed toward the side opposite the lesion. The postrotatory nystagmus developed after spinning the animal to the opposite side from the lesion is depressed when compared with the response observed on spinning the animal toward the side of the lesion. With extensive bilateral peripheral vestibular disease, the examiner may not be able to elicit nystagmus.

A horizontal, rotatory, or vertical spontaneous or positional nystagmus occurs with disturbance of the central portion of the vestibular system. In addition, with central vestibular lesions the direction of the nystagmus may vary with changes in the position of the head. A rapid pendular congenital nystagmus may occur in puppies with or without abnormalities of the visual system.

Vestibular system disease is characterized by loss of balance. Disease on one side produces ipsilateral head tilt, and the patient will lean, fall, or roll toward the side of the lesion. Strength and postural reactions are normal. Abnormal nystagmus may occur and may be spontaneous or positional. Peripheral vestibular system lesions cause a jerk nystagmus directed away from the side of the lesion (quick phase).

Peripheral Vestibular System Disease
  Seldom roll
  Nystagmus: quick phase always to opposite side
  Other signs: facial paresis-paralysis
            Horner's syndrome (cat, dog)
Central Vestibular System Disease
  More tendency to roll
  Nystagmus: quick phase may change directions with different head positions
            vertical
  Other signs: ipsilateral hemiparesis-ataxia
            slow postural reactions
            depression
            head tremor, hypermetria
            dysphagia
            medial strabismus
            weak jaw, atrophy of masticatory muscles
            facial hypalgesia

The sense of smell (I) and hearing (cochlear VIII) are difficult to evaluate unless the deficit is complete. Usually the owner's observations of the patient in its natural environment are more reliable for determination of these sensations.

Figure 52 is a copy of the neurologic examination form routinely used at the New York State College of Veterinary Medicine.

Summary of Signs with Lesions at Specific Locations in the Spinal Cord (Table 71)

Lumbosacral: Fourth Lumbar to Fifth Caudal Segment

  Complete malacia from fourth lumbar through fifth caudal segments:
    Flaccid paraplegia: no support, gait, or movement of pelvic limbs and tail. Normal thoracic limbs.
    No postural reactions in pelvic limbs.
    Areflexia: flexor, patellar, perineal reflexes.

Table 71. SIGNS OF COMPLETE SPINAL CORD TRANSECTION

Spinal Cord Segments	Signs Caudal to Lesion		
	Motor	Sensory	Autonomic
C1–4*	Tetraplegic with hyperreflexia	Anesthesia	Apnea, no micturition
C5–6	Tetraplegia with hyperreflexia LMN suprascapular nerve	Hypalgesia, hyperesthesia midcervical	Apnea, phrenic nerve LMN, no micturition
C7–T1	Tetraplegia or paraplegia with hyperreflexia, LMN brachial plexus	Anesthesia, hyperesthesia brachial plexus	Diaphragmatic breathing only, no micturition
T2–L3	Paraplegia with hyperreflexia, Schiff-Sherrington syndrome	Anesthesia, hyperesthesia segmental	Diaphragmatic, some intercostal and abdominal respiration depending on level, no micturition
L4–S1	Paraplegia with LMN lumbosacral plexus	Anesthesia, hyperesthesia segmental	No micturition, S1-anal sphincter may be atonic
S1–S3	Knuckling hind foot, paralysis of tail	Anesthesia, hyperesthesia segmental	No micturition, sphincters atonic
Cy1–Cy	Paralysis of tail	Anesthesia, hyperesthesia segmental	None

*Note: Complete transection at C1–4 (and possibly at C5–6) will cause respiratory paralysis and death.
C—cervical; T—thoracic; L—lumbar; S—sacral; Cy—coccygeal; LMN—lower motor neuron.
From Oliver, J. E.: Neurologic emergencies in small animals. Vet. Clin. North Am., 2:346, 1972.

Atonia: soft muscles, no resistance to manipulation of pelvic limbs or tail.

Neurogenic atrophy: in chronic lesions.

Dilated anus.

Analgesia from pelvic limbs, tail, and perineum.

Partial malacia of gray and white matter between the fourth lumbar and fifth caudal segments:

Flaccid paraparesis and ataxia of pelvic limbs with normal thoracic limbs.

Postural reactions of pelvic limbs attempted, but poorly accomplished.

Hyporeflexia or areflexia: flexor and patellar reflexes.

Hypotonia: normal or weak resistance to manipulation of pelvic limbs.

Slight neurogenic atrophy: in chronic lesions.

Normal or depressed pain perception (hypalgesia) from pelvic limbs, tail, and perineum.

Thoracolumbar: Third Thoracic to Third Lumbar Segment

Complete malacia—focal site between third thoracic and third lumbar segments.

Spastic paraplegia: no voluntary support, gait, or movement of pelvic limbs; normal thoracic limbs. With acute lesions, the thoracic limbs may be spastic (Schiff-Sherrington syndrome). With cranial thoracic lesions, there may be more difficulty in standing up on the thoracic limbs from a recumbent position, and loss of trunk support may also be observed when the animal is walked on the thoracic limbs with the pelvic limbs supported by the tail. The trunk may sway to the side abnormally.

No postural reactions in pelvic limbs.

Reflexes normal or hyperactive: flexor and patellar.

Crossed extensor reflex may occur.

Muscle tone normal or hypertonic, no atrophy.

Analgesia from area caudal to the lesion.

Partial malacia—focal site between third thoracic and third lumbar segments.

Spastic paraparesis and ataxia of pelvic limbs with normal thoracic limbs.

All postural reactions poorly performed in pelvic limbs.

Reflexes normal or hyperactive: flexor and patellar.

Crossed extensor reflex may occur.

Muscle tone normal or hypertonic, no atrophy.

Pain perception normal or depressed from area caudal to the lesion.

Note: Lesions confined to the white matter from L_4 to L_6 or L_7 may produce the same signs.

Caudal Cervical: Fifth Cervical to Second Thoracic Segment

Partial malacia of gray and white matter between fifth cervical and second
thoracic segments:

Tetraparesis and ataxia of all four limbs, with the thoracic limb deficit
sometimes worse than that of the pelvic limb, or tetraplegia, with
the patient in lateral recumbency. Lesions confined to the white
matter at this level usually cause more abnormality in the pelvic
limbs than thoracic limbs.

Thoracic limbs: hyporeflexic or areflexic; normal tone or hypotonic;
neurogenic atrophy if a chronic lesion. Lesions confined to the
white matter at this level cause hypertonia, hyperreflexia, and no
atrophy.

Pelvic limbs: normal reflexes or hyperreflexia; normal tone or hypertonia; no atrophy.

Pain perception: normal or depressed from all four limbs, or depressed
from thoracic limbs only.

All postural reactions poorly performed with the thoracic limb function
sometimes worse than that of the pelvic limb.

Miosis, protruded third eyelid, ptosis, and enophthalmos (T_1–T_3
lesion).

Cranial Cervical: First Cervical to Fifth Cervical Segment

Partial malacia—focal site between first and fifth cervical segments:
Spastic tetraplegia with patient in lateral recumbency: (1) no postural
reactions present; (2) reflexes normal or hyperactive in all four limbs; (3) crossed
extensor reflexes may occur; (4) muscle tone is usually hypertonic, occasionally
normal; and (5) hypalgesia from area caudal to the lesion.

Spastic tetraparesis and ataxia of all four limbs. The deficit in the pelvic
limbs is often worse than in the thoracic limbs. Occasionally, the opposite is
found. (1) Postural reactions are poorly performed. (2) Reflexes are normal or
hyperactive. (3) Crossed extensor reflexes may occur. (4) Muscle tone is usually
hypertonic, occasionally normal. (5) Pain perception is normal or depressed
from area caudal to the lesion.

Dogs with cervical spinal cord disease that have a significantly worse
abnormality in the forelimbs compared to the hind limbs usually have two
possible locations for lesions. Extensive lesions in the cervical intumescence
with grey matter involvement cause hypotonic hyporeflexic thoracic limbs and
more severe thoracic limb deficit. An extramedullary lesion that compresses
the central region of any segment of the cervical spinal cord from a ventral
midline site has also been observed with this disparity in limb abnormality.
Most commonly these are midline intervertebral disk extrusions, less commonly
atlantoaxial subluxations or neoplasms. The spinal cord is "tented" over the

Table 72. EVALUATION OF CRANIAL NERVES

Nerve	Sign of Dysfunction	Test/Responses
I Olfactory	Anosmia	Observe response to smell of food or some mild volatile oils
II Optic	Visual deficit bumping objects	No menace response—failure to close eyelids, or retract head when affected eye is menaced
	Unilateral disease	Light in affected eye—no pupillary response from either eye
	Mild mydriasis in affected eye (slight anisocoria)	
	Bilateral disease	Light in either eye—no pupillary constriction
III Oculomotor	Marked mydriasis bilateral	Examine with ophthalmoscope
	Marked mydriasis	Light in affected eye—only pupil of normal eye constricts
	Severe anisocoria	Light in normal eye—only pupil of normal eye constricts
	Ventrolateral strabismus	Incomplete adduction of affected eyeball on moving head side to side
	Ptosis	Inability to completely elevate upper eyelid
IV Trochlear	Slight extorsion of eyeball, which may only be visualized in the dog by ophthalmoscope examination of the position of the retinal veins	
V Trigeminal	Dropped jaw, unable to close mouth if bilateral disease	
	No motor deficit if unilateral disease	
	Atrophy of muscles of mastication	
	Hypalgesia or analgesia of face	Hypalgesia can be determined by patient's lack of response to touching nasal septum with forcep
VI Abducent	Medial strabismus	Incomplete abduction of affected eyeball on moving head side to side

VII Facial	Paresis/paralysis of facial muscles—inability to close palpebral fissure, drooped hypotonic lip with drooling of saliva, inability to move ear but the ears will not droop in all patients—(cats and some prick-eared dogs), incomplete dilation of naris on inspiration
VIII Vestibulocochlear	
Cochlear	Lack of response to commands or any noise
Vestibular-Unilateral disease	Deafness (unilateral is difficult to determine) Head tilt and ataxic toward side of lesion—lean, fall, circle toward side of lesion Unequal response or postrotatory testing—spin away from side of lesion causes depressed response. Extended neck and eyeball on affected side does not elevate completely (vestibular strabismus). Abnormal resting or positional nystagmus with quick phase away from side of lesion Hold head to side or dorsally and observe for positional nystagmus
Bilateral disease	Crouched gait, stumble to either side No abnormal nystagmus, wide excursions of head Inability to generate nystagmus on moving head side to side or spinning—no postrotatory response
IX Glossopharyngeal	Dysphagia, gagging on eating
X Vagus	Dysphagia, gagging on eating Inspiratory dyspnea
XI Accessory	Atrophy of affected side of tongue
XII Hypoglossal	May deviate toward affected side on protrusion

compressing mass, which apparently interferes more with the medially situated UMNs to the cervical intumescence.

Bladder dysfunction often accompanies severe spinal cord disease. Total LMN paralysis occurs with sacral spinal cord lesions. Severe or total focal thoracolumbar spinal cord lesions produce a UMN type of paralysis. Paralysis is less common with cervical spinal cord lesions unless the lesion is severe. With both LMN and UMN paralysis, retention of urine occurs. Overflow takes place with both, but is more constant with LMN disease. It is less frequent in UMN disease, because greater intraluminal pressure is required to overcome the tone in the striated urethral muscle. If the integrity of the bladder wall is retained, reflex urination may follow within a variable period of time. Reflex urination is more efficient in UMN disease, using the intact peripheral nerves and sacral spinal cord segments. In LMN disease, this must be mediated within the wall of the bladder and is very inefficient. (See Table 71).

Summary of Signs with Lesions in Specific Segments of the Brain (See Table 72)

MEDULLA AND PONS

Lesions in the medulla and pons result in spastic tetraparesis and ataxia of all four limbs or tetraplegia, ipsilateral spastic hemiparesis and ataxia (unilateral lesions), central vestibular signs, depression and irregular respirations, and hypalgesia of the trunk and limbs.

Signs of cranial nerve deficit are as follows: facial hypalgesia or analgesia (sensory V), paresis or paralysis of masticatory muscles (motor V), medial strabismus (VI), facial paresis or paralysis (VII), pharyngeal paresis (IX, X), tongue paresis (XII), and loss of balance, head tilt, abnormal nystagmus (VIII).

CEREBELLUM

With diffuse lesions, the signs are symmetric ataxia with preservation of strength, dysmetric gait (hypometria or hypermetria), truncal ataxia, head tremor, muscle hypertonia, occasional abnormal nystagmus, and bilateral menace deficit.

With unilateral lesions, the signs are usually ipsilateral, occasionally contralateral. The body and the head tilt toward the side of the lesion, occasionally away from side of lesion, and there may be ipsilateral menace deficit.

With severe rostral lesions, there may be opisthotonos and rigidly extended forelimbs, and the pelvic limbs will be extended forward by hip flexion.

MESENCEPHALON (MIDBRAIN)

With lesions in this area, the following signs occur: opisthotonus with rigid extension of all limbs (decerebration), spastic tetraparesis and ataxia of all four

Text continued on page 446

Table 73. LEVEL OF LESION IN THE BRAIN*

Cerebral Cortex
Deficiency of placing and hopping reactions (contralateral)
Alteration of mental function (recognition of owner, house training)
Vision impaired
Seizures
Hypertonia or hypotonia in extensors (contralateral)
Deficiency in voluntary movements

Basal Nuclei
Deficiency of nonvisual placing and hopping reactions
Adverse turning movements
Hyperkinesias (unilateral or bilateral)
Hypertonia in contralateral limb

Diencephalon
Pain, generalized or contralateral; may be intermittent
Hypothalamic disorders. Changes in eating, drinking, sleeping, or sexual behavior; cardiovascular and temperature regulation; endocrine activity
Visual field defects—optic tract or chiasm

Midbrain
Cranial nerve III or IV
Spasticity, deficiency in voluntary movement

Decreased sensation (contralateral)

Cerebellum
Ataxia—incoordination of body movements, station, and gait
Extensor hypertonus, acute opisthotonos
Chronic muscle weakness
Dysmetria—tremor with movements and other disturbances of phasic movements in chronic disorder
Cerebellar nystagmus

Pons
Cranial nerves V, VI, and VII
Decreased sensation (contralateral)
Deficiency of voluntary movements, spasticity (may be hypotonia if caudal pons, vestibular nucleus, or fastigial nucleus involved)

Medulla Oblongata
Cranial nerves VIII, IX, X, XI, and XII
Vestibular signs
Decreased sensation
Hemiparesis or tetraplegia, usually decreased tonus
Cardiovascular or respiratory abnormalities or both

*Best evidence of level of brain stem lesion is cranial nerve involvement. Cranial nerves listed with level signify possible involvement in a lesion, not necessarily the anatomic origin of the nerve. One or more of the signs listed may not be present in a particular lesion. Losses may be total or partial.

From Hoerlein, B. F.: Canine Neurology: Diagnosis and Treatment, 3rd ed. Philadelphia, W. B. Saunders Company, 1978.

Table 74. RELATIONSHIP OF CLINICAL SIGNS TO ANATOMIC SITE OF LESION

Clinical Signs	Functional System	Anatomic Location
Inability to prehend	Masticatory and tongue muscles	Cranial nerves V, XII, pons-medulla
Dysphagia	Tongue, palatal, pharyngeal, and esophageal	Cranial nerves IX, X, XI, XII, medulla
Drooling	Facial paralysis, dysphagia	Cranial nerve VII, middle ear, medulla
		Cranial nerves IX, X, medulla
Head tilt	Vestibular system	Inner ear, medulla, cerebellum
Nystagmus		
Loss of balance		
Rolling	Vestibular system	Medulla, cerebellum (inner ear)
Strabismus	Cranial nerves to extraocuular muscles, vestibular system	Cranial nerves III, IV, VI, midbrain-medulla
Circling		
With loss of balance	Vestibular system	Inner ear, medulla, cerebellum
Without loss of balance	Limbic system(?)	Frontal lobe, rostral thalamus
Head and eye deviation—turning to one side	Limbic system (?)	Frontal lobe, rostral thalamus
Pacing, head pressing	Limbic system	Frontal lobe, rostral thalamus
Opisthotonos	UMN	Rostral cerebellum, midbrain

Sign	System	Location
Blindness	Visual System	
Dilated, unresponsive pupils		Eyeball, optic nerves
Normal pupils		Visual cortex-cerebrum, (midbrain)
Depression, semicoma, coma	Ascending reticular activating system	Pons to thalamus-cerebral cortex
Seizures		Cerebrum, thalamus-hypothalamus
Hyperesthesia, hyperactivity to external stimuli	Ascending reticular activating system	Thalamus, cerebrum
Aggressive behavior, mania-hysteria, odontoprisis	Limbic system	Thalamus, cerebrum
Tremor		
Associated with movements, head and neck	Cerebellar system	Cerebellum
Associated with movements, head, trunk, and limbs	Multiple systems	Diffuse CNS
Episodic, not associated with movements, head, trunk, and limbs		Thalamus, cerebrum
Bradycardia, hypothermia, hyperthermia	UMN for general visceral efferent system	Hypothalamus
Irregular-ataxic respirations	UMN for respiratory muscle LMN	Pons-medulla

From deLahunta, A.: Veterinary neuroanatomy and clinical neurology, 2nd ed. W. B. Saunders, Philadelphia, 1983.

Table 75. INHERITED METABOLIC DISORDERS OF THE NERVOUS SYSTEM IN DOGS AND CATS*

Diseases	Breeds Affected	Lesions
Canine globoid cell leukodystrophy (Krabbe's disease)	Cairn terriers; West Highland white terriers; beagles; mixed breeds	Demyelination; globoid cells
Feline globoid cell leukodystrophy	Domestic cat	Same as canine GLD
Feline sphingomyelin lipidosis (Niemann-Pick disease)	Siamese cat, domestic cat	Vacuolation of neurons and macrophages in liver, spleen, etc.
Feline metachromatic leukodystrophy	Domestic cat	Demyelination; gliosis
Feline CNS glycogenosis (Pompe's disease)	Domestic cat	Neuronal accumulation of glycogen
Canine GM$_2$ gangliosidosis (Tay-Sachs disease)	German short-hair pointers	Vacuolation of neurons
Feline GM$_2$ gangliosidosis (Sandhoff's disease)	Domestic cat	Vacuolation of neurons and hepatocytes
Feline GM$_1$ gangliosidosis	Siamese cat, domestic cat	Vacuolaton of neurons and hepatocytes
Canine GM$_1$ gangliosidosis	Mongrel	Vacuolation of neurons, cells in liver, spleen kidney
Canine sphingomyelin lipidosis	Poodle	Vacuolation of neurons, cells in other organs
Canine ceroid lipofuscinosis (Batten-Spielmeyer-Vogt disease; Kufs' disease)	English setter	Vacuolation of neurons
	Wire-haired dachshund (Chihuanua, Cocker spaniel, Border collie, Saluki, Yugoslavian shepherd)	
Canine glucocerebrosidosis (Gaucher's disease)	Australian Silkie	Vacuolation of RE cells of liver, spleen, lymph nodes, neuronal atrophy
Feline glucocerebrosidosis	Abyssinian	Vacuolation of neurons, RE cells
Canine glycosphingolipidosis	English springer spaniel	Vacuolation of neurons, RE cells, epithelial cells of many organs, enlarged nerves
Feline mannosidosis	Persian	Vacuolation of neurons, hepatocytes
Feline lipofuscinosis	Siamese	Vacuolation of neurons
Canine glycogenosis Type II (Pompe's disease)	Bichon Frise	Vacuolation of muscle cells, hepatocytes
Type III (Cori's disease)	German Shepherd	Glycogen in neurons, hepatocytes, muscle
Canine glycoproteinosis (Lafora's disease)	Bassett, poodle	Neuronal inclusions

*Terms in parentheses refer to eponyms used for analogous human disorders.

Modified from Baker, H. J.: Inherited metabolic disorders of the nervous system in dogs and cats. *In* Kirk, R. W. (ed.): Current Veterinary Therapy 6. Philadelphia, W. B. Saunders Company, 1977.

Table 75. INHERITED METABOLIC DISORDERS OF THE NERVOUS
SYSTEM IN DOGS AND CATS* *(Continued)*

Age of Onset	Signs	Biochemical Leson
4–5 months	Progressive motor disability	Cerebroside accumulates; β-galactosidase deficiency
5–6 weeks	Same	Unknown
2–4 months	Same	Sphingomyelin accumulates; sphingomyelinase deficiency?
2 weeks	Same; rapidly progressing to convulsions; opisthotonos	Sulfatid accumulates; arylsulfatase deficiency?
Young adult	Unknown	Glycogen accumulates; α-glucosidase deficiency?
9–12 months	Ataxia; blindness; seizures	GM$_2$ ganglioside accumulates; hexosaminidase deficiency?
8–10 weeks	Tremors; incoordination; paraplegia	GM$_2$ ganglioside accumulates; hexosaminidase deficiency?
10–16 weeks	Tremors; incoordination; paraplegia	GM$_1$ ganglioside accumulates; β-galactosidase deficiency?
4–5 months	Ataxia; tremor; blindness	β-galactosidase
Few months	Cerebellar ataxia	Sphingomyelinase
1 year	Depression; ataxia; seizures; blindness	P-phenylene-diamine–mediated peroxidase
2–3 years	Cerebellar ataxia	—
4 months	Cerebellar ataxia, tremor	β-glucocerebrosidase
8–12 weeks	Cerebellar ataxia, seizures	β-glucocerebrosidase
12–19 months	Weight loss, dysphagia, ataxia	α-L-fucosidase
2 months	Depression, ataxia, tremor, paresis	α-mannosidase
20 months	Seizures, abnormal behavior	—
3–4 months	Hypotonia, paresis	α-glucosidase
2 months	Ataxia, paresis	amylo-1, 6-glucosidase
Young adults	Seizures	—

limbs, spastic hemiparesis if the lesion is unilateral (usually contralateral), depression, stupor (semicoma), or coma, and hypalgesia of the head, trunk, and limbs. Signs of cranial nerve deficit are ventrolateral strabismus (III) and mydriasis and nonreactive pupil (III). There is deviation of the eyeballs in certain positions of the head, and the head and neck are flexed laterally, with the nose directed toward the shoulder with severe midline or unilateral lesions in the tegmentum. Visual deficits may be observed in acute lesions.

DIENCEPHALON (THALAMUS AND HYPOTHALAMUS)

Bilateral lesions of the diencephalon produce the following signs: slow postural reactions bilaterally, mild ataxia, bilateral visual deficit with dilated unresponsive pupils (optic tracts), and bilateral hypalgesia (ventral caudal lateral and medial nuclei).

Unilateral lesions are indicated by contralateral deficient postural reactions, contralateral visual deficit with normal pupils, contralateral hypalgesia (most noticeable in the head), and the adversive syndrome—propulsive circling, and head and eye deviation toward the side of lesion.

With lesions that are either bilateral or unilateral, the manifestations are: depression, stupor (semicoma), or coma, behavioral changes, seizures, and the following hypothalamo-hypophyseal disorders: body temperature, glucose metabolism, appetite control, autonomic nervous system, water balance, gonadal function, and thyroid and adrenal function.

TELENCEPHALON (CEREBRUM)

Lesions in this area are evidenced by changes in several ways. Changes in behavior or temperament include depression (lethargy, obtundation), stupor (semicoma), lack of recognition of owner or environment and bewilderment, loss of trained habits, and irritable, hysterical, maniacal, or aggressive behavior. In propulsion, the animal often paces and circles in one direction, and turns the head and eyes in one direction; this direction is usually toward a unilateral lesion, called the *adversive syndrome* (turn to). This may require a rostral thalamic involvement in the lesion. Seizures are partial (contralateral face or limbs or both) or generalized (grand mal, psychomotor). The gait is usually normal, but contralateral postural reactions are deficient. Bilateral lesions produce blindness. Unilateral lesions produce contralateral visual deficit with normal pupil responses to light. Occasionally, contralateral facial hypalgesia occurs. Rarely, the hypalgesia is observed in the contralateral trunk and limbs. Acute diffuse lesions may produce bilateral miosis. Pseudobulbar paresis rarely may be observed on voluntary movement: contralateral lower facial paralysis (lip and nose), pharyngeal paresis, and tongue paresis. (See Tables 73–74.)

References and Additional Readings

Averill, D. R., Jr.: Diagnosis and treatment of diffuse disorders of peripheral nerves and muscle. Proc. of September 23–24 Kal Kan Symposium, 1978, pp. 36–38.

Berzon, J. L., and Dueland, R.: Cauda equina syndrome. J.A.A.H.A., *15*(5):635, 1979.
Boudrieau, R. J., Hohn, R. B., and Bardet, J. F.: Osteochondritis diseases of the elbow in the dog. J.A.A.H.A., *19*(5):627, 1983.
Chrisman, C. L.: Problems in Small Animal Neurology. Philadelphia, Lea & Febiger, 1982.
deLahunta, A.: Veterinary Neuroanatomy and Clinical Neurology, 2nd ed. Philadelphia, W. B. Saunders Company, 1983.
Duncan, I. D., and Griffiths, I. R.: Myotonia in the Dog. Current Veterinary Therapy 8: Small Animal Practice. Philadelphia, W. B. Saunders Company, 1983, pp. 686–691.
Duncan, I. D.: Some aspects of the diagnosis and treatment of small animal neuromuscular disease. Proc. of September 23–24 Kal Kan Symposium, 1978, pp. 31–35.
Felts, J. F., and Prata, R. G.: Cervical disk disease in the dog: intraforaminal and lateral extrusions. J.A.A.H.A., *19*(5):755, 1983.
Kornegay, J. N., and Barber, D. L.: Diskospondylitis in dogs. J.A.V.M.A., *177*(4):337, 1980.
Kornegay, J. N., et al.: Polymyositis in dogs. J.A.V.M.A., *176*(5):431, 1980.
Olsson, Sten-Terik: The early diagnosis of fragmented coronoid process and osteochondritis diseases of the canine elbow joint. J.A.A.H.A., *19*(5):616, 1983.
Shores, A.: The differential diagnosis of ataxia paresis or paralysis in large-breed dogs. J.A.A.H.A., *20*(2):265, 1984.
Siemering, B.: A review of the diagnosis and treatment of common forelimb lameness in immature dogs. Compendium on Continuing Education, *1*:357, 1979.
Trotter, E. J.: Canine intervertebral disk disease. *In* Kirk, R. W. (ed.): Current Veterinary Therapy VI. Philadelphia, W. B. Saunders Company, 1977.
Wadsworth, P. L.: Biomechanics of the luxation of joints. *In* Bojorab M. J. (ed.): Pathophysiology in Small Animal Surgery. Philadelphia, Lea & Febiger, 1981, pp. 804–809.
Whittick, W. G.: Canine Orthopedics. Philadelphia, Lea & Febiger, 1974.

RESPIRATORY SYSTEM

History

The cardinal signs of respiratory disease are cough, dyspnea, production of abnormal secretions, noisy breathing, sneezing, and change in the characteristics of the sounds the animal makes.

Determine the presence or absence of:

Nasal Discharge. The discharge may be unilateral or bilateral.

Sneezing. Note the frequency and accompanying discharge, if any.

Coughing (See pp. 272–275). A *true cough* (sudden forced expulsion of air through a closed glottis) is characterized by the animal's lowering its head and opening its mouth during expiration. The cough itself may be moist and productive or dry, nonproductive, and paroxysmal and can be accentuated by collar pressure, exercise, or cold air. It should be noted whether the cough is productive or nonproductive. *Caution*—most dogs swallow their coughed-up secretions so that the cough may appear to be nonproductive. Examine the coughed-up material as to amount, color, and consistency and for cell content, foreign bodies, parasites, and so on. Hemoptysis is rare but may indicate tumor, or paragonimus or heartworm infestations.

Postnasal drip or *"reverse cough"* is characterized by the animal's extending its head parallel to the ground and closing its mouth during inspiration. The cough itself commonly ends with the animal's gagging, gulping, choking, or expectorating.

Dyspnea (see pp. 270–272). In the susceptible animal, dyspnea occurs readily after exercise—abating gradually, however, as the animal rests. During the distress, the subject's mouth may be open or closed. While resting, the subject commonly prefers sitting to lying down. Dyspneic animals usually exhibit an increased respiratory rate (polypnea) and depth (hyperpnea).

In considering the history of an animal with a respiratory problem, evaluate the following: associated signs of systemic illness, loss of stamina on physical exertion, activities that precipitate respiratory distress or coughing, geographic history of the animal, immunization status, and past history of respiratory disease.

Consider specific breed predilection to respiratory problems. Laryngeal problems are seen in brachycephalic breeds. Airway obstructions and marked inspiratory dyspnea in the brachycephalic breed of dog is usually associated with multiple coexisting anomalies—namely, stenotic nares, elongated soft palates, laryngeal saccule eversion, laryngeal collapse, and possible tracheal stenosis. Careful evaluation of these dogs is necessary to provide an adequate prognosis, to describe all abnormalities, and to develop a plan of treatment. Examination should include auscultation of the trachea and chest, cervical and thoracic radiographs, pharyngoscopy, and laryngoscopy performed under neuroleptanalgesia or anesthesia.

The degrees of complications in these cases is related to the extent to which multiple surgeries on the posterior pharynx and larynx are carried out in an attempt to alleviate airway obstruction. Unilateral and bilateral laryngeal surgery to relieve laryngeal collapse has a high degree of complication (60 per cent), with airway obstruction and aspiration pneumonia predominating.

Inspiratory Dyspnea

Breathing is through the mouth; the head and neck are extended, the ribs elevated and rolled forward, and the elbows abducted. The skin over the thoracic inlet sinks during inspiration. Dyspnea associated with noisy breathing suggests airway obstruction. Short, shallow, rapid breathing can indicate inability to completely expand the lungs as in rib fractures, pneumonia, pleural effusions, and pleuritis.

Nasal Discharge. Note the type and amount of nasal discharge (Table 76). Exfoliative cytology may be helpful. Discharges that contain various quantities of blood can indicate a foreign body, a destructive lesion associated with a tumor, or a possible fungal infection. Inspiratory dyspnea may be caused by tumor, obstruction, or stenosis of the respiratory tract.

Table 76. DIFFERENTIAL DIAGNOSIS OF CHRONIC NASAL DISEASES OF THE DOG

	Intranasal Neoplasia	Chronic Hyperplastic Rhinitis*	Aspergillus Fumigatus Infection	Dys-phagia	Post-Traumatic Sequestrum	Dental Periapical Abscess	Intranasal Parasitism
Nature of discharge							
Purulent	†	X	X	X	X	X	X
Epistaxis	XX		†				†
Food material				X			
Unilateral	X→	†	X→		X	X	X
Bilateral	†	X	†	X			†
Facial deformity	†		†				
Pain on nasal bone		†	†				
Obstructed air flow	†						
Radiography							
Bone trabecular destruction	X		X				
Increased soft-tissue density	X	X					
Periapical rarefaction						X	
Sequestrum					X		
Serology			X				
Culture			X				
Exploratory rhinotomy	X	X	X				
Histopathology	X	X	X				

*This includes the Irish wolfhound rhinitis syndrome.
†—occasional positive finding.
X—frequent positive finding.
From Lane, J. G.: Rhinitis and sinusitis in the dog. *In* Kirk, R. W. (ed.): Current Veterinary Therapy 6. Philadelphia, W. B. Saunders Company, 1977, p. 224.

Expiratory Dyspnea

Inspiration is normal, but expiration is prolonged and forced, the abdomen is actively lifted, and the anus protrudes. It may be caused by chronic emphysema, bronchitis, and pleural adhesions.

MIXED DYSPNEA

Mixed dyspnea, most commonly seen, in a combination of the inspiratory and expiratory forms and is caused by severe respiratory diseases such as pneumonia, pneumothorax, and hydrothorax.

Cyanosis

Cyanosis is most readily observed in the oral mucosa. Etiology may be respiratory or circulatory (see pp. 275–277).

Helpful Anatomic Landmarks

Thorax. The thorax is a laterally compressed oval, the diameter of which is greater dorsoventrally than it is either laterally or craniocaudally.

Diaphragm. The diaphragm attaches dorsocaudally at the thirteenth rib and is slanted forward to attach anteroventrally at the costal cartilage of the eighth, ninth, and tenth ribs. It bells forward as far as the sixth rib, a quarter of the way up from the sternum. In normal respiration, the diaphragm moves one and one half vertebral spaces forward and back.

Lungs. Both lungs extend anterior to the first rib. The right lung consists of diaphragmatic, intermediate, cardiac, and apical lobes. A cardiac notch is situated between the cardiac and apical lobes at ribs four and five. The apical lobe ends at roughly the fourth rib; the diaphramatic lobe begins at about the sixth rib. The intermediate lobe lies medially between the diaphragmatic lobe and the mediastinum.

Diaphragmatic, cardiac, and apical lobes constitute the left lung. A cardiac notch is absent. The apical lobe ends at about the fourth rib, and the diaphragmatic lobe originates at the intercostal space between ribs five and six.

Tracheal Bifurcation. It is situated dorsal to the cranial border of the heart at the fifth rib.

Inspection

Note the presence, consistency, color, and quantity of any nasal discharge. The exudate may originate in the nose, chest, sinus, throat, or stomach. In the early stage of an infection, the discharge is watery; in the chronic stage, the discharge becomes thick, mucoid, or purulent. A rust-colored discharge indicates blood from the lung or old blood from the nose. Pulmonary hemorrhage is red and frothy; clear froth implies pulmonary edema. If hemorrhage is present, look for petechiae in the skin and mucosa. Determine whether both nostrils are patent. Hold a mirror in front of the nose and see whether both nostrils cause fogging. In the brachycephalic breeds, examine the lateral wings of the nose for signs of collapse that might produce inspiratory difficulty. Nasal discharge may also be examined microscopically for the presence of *Lingatula serrata* or pneumonyssus mites.

Observe the general conformation of the thorax. Check for kyphosis, scoliosis, ricketic rosary, and fracture callus.

Chest Movements

Rate of respiration is normally 10 to 30 breaths per minute (20 at rest). Panting may go to 200 breaths per minute, but tidal volume is reduced drastically to prevent hypocapnia. Cats pant as fast as 300 breaths per minute but do not compensate for carbon dioxide very effectively. An increased respiratory rate may be caused by heat, exercise, pain, anoxemia, nervous excitement, or structural changes in the lungs. A decreased respiratory rate may result from narcotic poisoning or metabolic alkalosis.

The *rhythm of respiration* may be varied voluntarily or involuntarily (as with nervous excitement). Prolonged expiration may be caused by bronchial or pulmonary disease. Note carefully the degree of effort being expended in respiration.

In Cheyne-Stokes respiration, successive respirations reach a maximum, fall off slowly to apnea, and repeat the cycle. It is a serious sign of toxemia. Kussmaul's respiration is a distressing type of dyspnea in which respiration occurs in paroxysms. It usually indicates acidosis, especially in diabetics.

Types of breathing include thoracic, resulting from paralysis of the diaphragm or abdominal pressure (ascites); abdominal, caused by pain in the thorax (pleuritis); and thoracoabdominal, characteristic of normal dogs and cats.

Palpation

Palpate bones of the maxillary and frontal sinus for any indication of fractures. Palpate the trachea for deformities and to induce coughing. Regional lymph nodes in the neck should be palpated.

Percussion

This form of examination is of limited value in examining the respiratory tract. However, in addition to examining the thoracic cavity, one can percuss over the maxillary bones and sinuses and frontal sinuses, listening for changes in resonance.

Method

Using the middle finger of the left hand as a pleximeter, place it firmly on the chest. Rap the distal phalanx abruptly with the middle finger of the right hand. Three rules must be applied in percussion:

1. In defining boundaries, always move from the more to the less resonant areas.

2. The long axis of the pleximeter (finger) must be parallel to the boundary of the edge of the organ being percussed.
3. The progression of the line of percussion should be at right angles to the edge of the organ.

Application and interpretation of percussion are more difficult in small animals than in large animals. Differences in sounds are slight, and it is helpful to percuss the thorax systematically by tapping the ribs while a stethoscope is held firmly against the opposite chest wall. The percussion tones are thus greatly magnified by the instrument and differences are more obvious.

Interpretation (See Table 77)

Chest radiographs are accurate in outlining anatomic structures, but changes in resonance also offer additional helpful information.

Resonance is increased when the pleural cavity contains air and the lung is collapsed. In this case, the musical "bell sound" may also be heard. A coin is held flat against the chest wall and firmly tapped by a second coin. The observer listens to the transmitted sound through a stethoscope held against the opposite thoracic wall. Resonance may also be increased by emphysema (rare).

Resonance is decreased when the lung is more solid than usual, as with edema, pneumonia, or tumor, when the pleura is thickened, when the pleural cavity contains fluid, or when an abdominal viscus is displaced into the thoracic space.

Auscultation

The Stethoscope

Some stethoscopes are better designed acoustically than others. The Littman is lightweight, moderately priced, well designed, and has a reversible two-sided head. The bell transmits low-pitched sounds, for example, heart sounds, accurately. The diaphragm, which should be infant size, transmits soft, high-pitched sound best. For best results:
1. Be sure the stethoscope is seated firmly in the ear.
2. Perform the auscultation in a room as free of noise as possible.
3. Hold the stethoscope firmly against the chest.
4. Do not breathe on the tubing.
5. Avoid hair friction and muscle noises. Wetting the subject's hair will help.
6. Listen with the animal breathing quietly, if possible.
7. Close the mouth of a panting animal; stop the subject from shivering or trembling.
8. Stop cats from purring. Shake them gently, or bring a dog into their view.
9. Concentrate on each part of the respiratory or cardiac cycle separately. Listen intently!

Table 77. SUMMARY OF THE FINDINGS OF AUSCULTATION AND PERCUSSION IN VARIOUS PLEURAL AND PARENCHYMAL DISEASES*

Disease Condition	Findings on Auscultation	Findings on Percussion
Hydrothorax (normally similar findings bilaterally)	"Fluid line" detectable where lung sounds are decreased or absent ventrally (V), and normal (N) to bronchovesicular (BV) dorsally (D). Heart sounds may be muffled.	"Fluid line" detectable where resonance is decreased below the line and normal to slightly increased above the line.
Pneumothorax (normally similar findings bilaterally)	Line of demarcation noted with N lung sounds V, and decreased intensity (or absent) sounds D. Heart sounds N.	Line of demarcation noted with N resonance V, and a noticeably increased resonance D.
Diaphragmatic hernia (normally unilateral findings)	Increased BV and heart sounds on the N side, with absent or decreased heart and lung sounds on the hernia side.	Decreased resonance on side of hernia. (Exception: when stomach herniates it may fill with gas and an increased resonance may be detected.)
Lung consolidation (normally unilateral findings)	Increased BV to (usually) bronchial lung sounds over affected area. Absence of all sound if bronchus is occluded.	Localized area of decreased resonance over affected area.
Parenchymal mass (normally unilateral findings)	Small size: no change. Large size: shifting of the location of heart sounds (depending on mass location), with an absence of lung sounds.	Small size: no change. Large size: localized area of decreased resonance.

*Animal should be in sternal recumbency or standing when examined.
From Ettinger, S. J. (ed.): Textbook of Veterinary Internal Medicine, 2nd ed. Philadelphia, W. B. Saunders Company, 1983, p. 771.

Character of Respiratory Sounds

Normal Breath Sounds

Normal breath sounds are of two kinds: vesicular and bronchial or tubular. Vesicular sounds are heard as air passes through small bronchi and alveoli. The inspiratory phase is louder and twice as long in normal animals. These sounds are only heard over normal lung tissue, but in dogs and cats with shallow, quiet respirations, they may be inaudible.

Bronchial sounds are caused by air passing through the larger bronchi and trachea. Auscultate over the trachea of a normal dog to recognize these sounds. They are usually more pronounced on expiration, and local variations may be important signs of disease (consolidation, exudation, and effusion). The smaller the diameter of the bronchi, the softer the bronchial sounds and the higher the pitch.

Added Breath Sounds

Added breath sounds are also of two kinds: rhonchi and crepitations.

Rhonchi are prolonged noises produced by the partial obstruction of bronchi by mucosal edema or viscid secretions. In larger bronchi, they are low-pitched, sonorous, and almost continuous. In small bronchi, they are high-pitched, sibilant or squeaky, and may be more prevalent at the end of inspiration. Rhonchi are heard in bronchitis and asthma. Coarse rhonchi may be associated with bronchiectasis.

Rhonchi or rales may be separated into dry rales, moist rales, and crepitant rales. Dry rales are heard throughout both inspiration and expiration and are associated with inflammation of the mucous membranes of the bronchi and tenacious mucus occluding the bronchi. Moist rales are associated with fluid in the bronchi and produce short, discontinuous crackling sounds. Crepitant rales occur on inspiration only and are produced by the passage of air into alveoli containing fluid. They are suggestive of inflammation or pulmonary edema.

Crepitations are fine or coarse interrupted crackling noises that may be obvious during inspiration. They are caused by the opening of alveoli that are collapsed or stopped up with fluid. They are heard in early pneumonia and bronchitis. Crepitations occasionally heard in normal lungs are abolished by coughing. Crepitation sounds can be imitated by rolling hair between the fingers in front of the ear.

Another adventitious sound in the pleural cavity is the pleuritic friction sound (rare). It is heard only when the pleura is dry and inflamed and resembles a crepitation. However, it occurs at similar times during inspiration and expiration when the roughened surfaces rub together, and it is not abolished by coughing.

It is important to recognize that there are changes in breathing associated with abnormalities other than those primarily involving the respiratory system, such as heart disease, anemia, ascites, gastric dilatation, physical exertion, muscular spasms, heat, and pain.

Tracheal Smears

Tracheal smears may be useful for preparing cultures for cell studies and for identifying parasite ova. A fecal examination should also be done (see p. 798).

Transtracheal Aspiration (See pp. 527–529)

Radiographic Study

In a radiographic study, lateral and dorsoventral views should be taken. Bronchography, using iodized oil (Dionosil), can also be used. Other specialized radiographic techniques may include pulmonary angiography, tomography, and fluoroscopy.

Bronchoscopy

The trachea and main bronchi can be visualized or cultured while the animal is under thiamylal sodium anesthesia. A biopsied sample can also be taken.

Rhinoscopy

Critical examination of the external nares and nasal turbinates requires general anesthesia. Very critical visualization of the nasal turbinate bones in the dog is severely limited by the numerous convolutions present. The anterior nares can be inspected with a small otoscope head. Material can be obtained for exfoliative cytology and culture.

Complete Cardiovascular Study (See pp. 335–380)

Thoracentesis

See page 523 for technique for interpretation.

Exploratory Thoracotomy

This procedure should be carried out if required. A diagnosis can be confirmed, and in many cases (hernia, cyst, tumor, laceration of the lung, foreign body), therapy can be provided in one step.

References and Additional Readings

Bauer, T., and Thomas, W. P.: Pulmonary diagnostic techniques. Vet. Clin. North Am., 13(2):273, 1983.

Harvey, C. F., and O'Brien, J. A.: Nasal aspergillosis-penicillosis. *In* Kirk, R. W. (ed.): Current Veterinary Therapy, 8: Small Animal Practice. Philadelphia, W. B. Saunders Company, 1983. pp. 236–241.

Harvey, C. F., and O'Brien, J. A.: Upper airway obstruction surgery. Parts 1–8, J.A.A.H.A., *18*(4):535, 1982.

Hayes, H. M., Wilson, G. P., and Fraumeni, J., Jr.: Carcinoma of nasal cavity and paranasal sinuses in dogs. Cornell Vet., *72*(2):168, 1982.

Roudebush, P.: Diagnostics for respiratory diseases. *In* Kirk, R. W. (ed.): Current Veterinary Therapy 8: Small Animal Practice. Philadelphia, W. B. Saunders Company, 1983, pp. 222–241.

Schaer, M., and Ackerman, N.: Diagnostic approach to patient with respiratory disease. *In* Ettinger, S. J. (ed.): Textbook of Veterinary Internal Medicine, 2nd ed. Philadelphia, W. B. Saunders Company, 1982, Chap. 37, pp. 655–672.

Suter, P. F., and Zinkl, J. G.: Mediastinal, pleural and extrapleural thoracic diseases. *In* Ettinger, S. J. (ed.): Textbook of Veterinary Internal Medicine, 2nd ed. Philadelphia, W. B. Saunders Company, 1982, Chap. 44, pp. 840–883.

Whealson, E. B., Suter, P. F., and Jenkins, T.: Neoplasia of larynx in the dog. J.A.V.M.A., *180*(6):642, 1982.

Withrow, S. J.: Cryosurgical therapy for nasal tumors in the dog. J.A.A.H.A., *18*(4):585, 1982.

THE SKIN*

THE SYSTEMATIC APPROACH

If the veterinarian examines animals with skin disease in a cursory manner and attempts to make snap judgments, confusion and incorrect diagnoses will often result. In no other system of the body is a careful plan of examination and evaluation more important. Ideally, a thorough examination and appropriate diagnostic procedures should be accomplished the first time the animal is seen and before any masking treatments have been initiated. The following procedures should be systematically considered and correlated for a rational accurate dermatologic diagnosis.

Clinical Examination. Record the age, gender, breed, and general medical and dermatologic history of the animal. The inquiry should determine the chief complaint and data about the original lesion's location, appearance, onset, and rate of progression. Also determine the presence and degree of pruritus, contagion to other animals or people, and possible seasonal incidence. Relationship to diet and environmental factors and the response to previous medications are also important.

Physical Examination. Determine the distribution pattern and the regional location of affected areas. Closely examine the skin to identify primary and secondary lesions. Evaluate alopecias or hair abnormalities. Observe the configurations of specific skin lesions and their relationship to each other; certain patterns are diagnostically significant.

---

*Modified from Muller, G. H., Kirk, R. W., and Scott, D. W.: Small Animal Dermatology, 3rd ed. Philadelphia, W. B. Saunders Company, 1983.

Diagnostic and Laboratory Aids. Diagnostic aids such as skin scrapings, Wood's light examination, impression smears, and fungal or bacterial cultures should be done routinely. Biopsies, hormonal assays, and chemistry panels are also performed when indicated by clinical findings.

Correlate the Data. Make a list of differential diagnoses.

Narrow the List of Differential Diagnoses. Plan additional tests, observations of therapeutic trials, and so on to narrow the list and provide a definitive diagnosis.

CLINICAL EXAMINATION

Records

Recording historical facts, physical findings, and laboratory data in a systematic way is particularly important in animals with skin disease. Many dermatoses are chronic, and skin lesions are slow to change. For this reason, outline sketches of the patient enable the clinician to draw in the location and extent of lesions. One sketch is worth many words, and comparison of sketches made at different intervals graphically portrays changes in the lesions over time.

Figure 54 illustrates a satisfactory record form for noting physical and laboratory findings for dermatology cases. The special form enables one to circle pertinent descriptive terms, saves time, and ensures that no important information is omitted. This form only details dermatologic data and should be used as a supplement to the general history and physical examination record. A special dermatologic history form is also useful, especially for allergic and chronic cases (Fig. 55).

General Medical History

The clinician should obtain a complete medical history in all cases. Some dermatologists prefer to examine the skin quickly at first, so that pertinent questions can be emphasized in taking the history, while inappropriate items can be omitted. However, it is vital to use a systematic, detailed method of examination and history taking so that important information is not overlooked.

Age

Some dermatologic disorders are age related; thus, age is important in the dermatology history. For example, demodicosis usually begins in young dogs before sexual maturity. Allergies tend to appear in more mature animals, probably because repeated exposure to the antigen must occur before clinical signs develop. Hormonal disorders tend to occur in animals between 6 and 10 years of age, and most neoplasms develop in mature to older patients. Most of the ages listed in Table 78 refer to the usual age at which the disease begins.

NEW YORK STATE COLLEGE OF VETERINARY MEDICINE—VETERINARY TEACHING HOSPITAL

DERMATOLOGY

DATE: _____

REF. DVM _____

CLINICIAN _____

SECONDARY # _____

DISTRIBUTION OF LESIONS

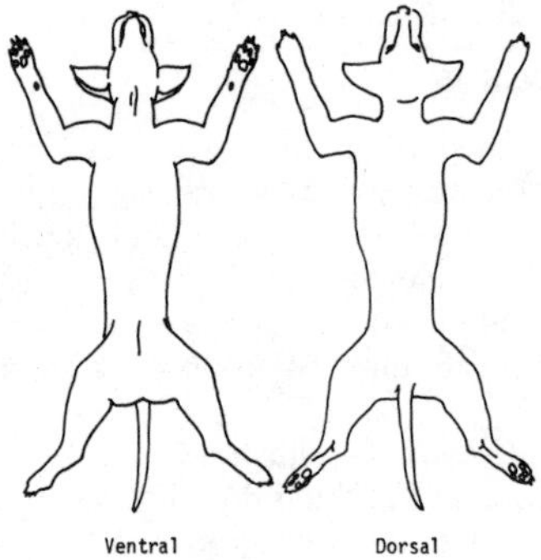

Ventral   Dorsal

PRIMARY LESIONS (Circle)

Macule	Patch	Papule	Plaque
Vesicle	Bulla	Pustule	Wheal
Nodule	Tumor		

SECONDARY LESIONS (Circle)

Scale   Epidermal collarette   Scar
Ulcer   Erosion   Crust   Excoriation
Fissure   Comedone   Cyst   Abscess
Hypopigmentation   Hyperpigmentation   Erythema
Hyperkeratosis   Callus   Alopecia

Pruritus:

Parasites:

SKIN CHANGES

Elasticity   + −   Extensibility + −
Thickness   + −

QUALITY OF HAIR COAT   OTHER FACTORS

Epilation: + −   Footpads
Pelage is: Dry,   Nails
  Brittle, Dull, Oily   Hyperhidrosis

CONFIGURATION OF LESIONS

Linear   Annular (Target)   Grouped

DIFFERENTIAL DIAGNOSIS

LABORATORY TESTS

Scotch Tape: _____Wood's Light + −
Skin Scraping: _____
KOH Digestion: _____
Direct Smear: _____
Fungal Culture: _____
Bacterial Culture: _____
Sensitivity: _____
Allergy: _____
_____
Endocrine: _____
Immune:
  D.I.T.: _____
  I.I.T.: _____
  ANA: _____
  Other: _____
Biopsy:

Figure 54. Dermatology examination sheet.

NEW YORK STATE COLLEGE OF VETERINARY MEDICINE—VETERINARY TEACHING HOSPITAL

DATE: _____

DERMATOLOGY HISTORY SHEET

CHIEF COMPLAINT(S) _____

_____

_____

_____

_____

AGE PURCHASED _____

REF. DVM _____

CLINICIAN _____

SECONDARY # _____

KENNEL ____PET SHOP ____PRIVATE ____WHERE ___

HAS ANIMAL BEEN OUT OF AREA? YES ____NO _____

IF YES—WHERE _____

Date Problem First Noticed _____ Age _____ Is It Year Round? Yes _____ No _____

If Seasonal, Is It Worse: Spring _____ Summer _____ Fall _____ Winter _____

Where Did Problem Begin? _____

What Did It Look Like Then? _____

How Has It Changed or Spread? _____

Are Other Animals or People Affected? Yes _____ No _____ If So Describe _____

When Did You Last See Fleas? _____

Describe Animal's Indoor Environment _____

Time Indoors _____% _____

Describe Animal's Outdoor Environment _____

Time Outdoors _____% _____

Does Animal Itch? Yes _____ No _____ When? Constantly _____ Sporadically _____ Night _____

Animal's Diet _____

What Medications Have Been Used? List Effects and Dates Used _____

_____

_____

Other Illnesses of Animal _____

What Other Facts Do You Think Would Be Helpful? _____

_____

_____

_____

(Use Reverse Side If Needed)

Figure 55. Dermatology history sheet.

Table 78. SKIN DISEASE WITH FREQUENT AGE-RELATED ONSET

Age	Disease
Less than 4 months	Alopecia universalis Black hair follicle dysplasia Cutaneous asthenia Epidermolysis bullosa Ectodermal defect Hypotrichosis Ichthyosis Infantile pyoderma Juvenile cellulitis Mucopolysaccharidosis Other congenital defects Pituitary dwarfism
3–6 months	Demodicosis, localized Color mutant alopecia
3–12 months	Acanthosis nigricans Canine acne Demodicosis, generalized Dermatomycoses Superficial pustular pyoderma (impetigo) Viral papillomatosis (oral) Zinc responsive dermatosis
1–3 years	Adult-onset growth hormone responsive alopecia Atopy Seborrhea
Over 6 years	Endocrine imbalances
Older dog	Lip fold pyoderma Neoplasms Vulvar fold pyoderma
Senile dogs	Alopecia Decubital ulcer Thin, fragile skin

From Muller, G. H., Kirk, R. W., and Scott, D. W.: Small Animal Dermatology, 3rd ed. Philadelphia, W. B. Saunders Company, 1983, p. 95.

Gender

The gender of the patient obviously limits the incidence of certain problems, but it is especially important in gender-hormonal imbalances. Perianal adenomas are seen almost exclusively in male dogs. One should determine whether the patient is sexually intact, and if so, whether the skin problem bears any relationship to the estral cycle.

Breed

Breed predilection determines the incidence of some skin disorders. For example, seborrhea is common in cocker and springer spaniels; acanthosis nigricans usually occurs in dachshunds; anal adenomas are often found in male wire-haired fox terriers. Many of the wire-coated terrier breeds (Scotties, Cairns, Sealyhams, West Highland whites, Irish terriers, and Welsh terriers) seem to be particularly predisposed to allergic skin disease (Table 79). As part of the history, it is important to determine whether animals related to the patient are or were affected with similar problems.

Owner's Complaint and Dermatologic History

The owner's complaint or chief cause of concern is often the major source used in compiling a differential diagnosis. The clinician who can "draw out" a complete history in an unbiased form has indeed a valuable skill. It is important that the questions presented to the client do not suggest answers or tend to shut off discussion. A friendly "Let's help this patient together" attitude often stimulates the client to reveal more information. Some owners purposely or unconsciously withhold pertinent facts, especially about neglect, diet, previous medication, or other procedures they feel may not be well received by the examining veterinarian. The skillful clinician is always tuned to listen for side comments by the client or by the children.

Next, the following information should be obtained from the owner: date of onset, original locations of the lesions, description of the initial lesions, tendency to progression or regression, factors affecting the course, and previous treatment (home, proprietary, or pet shop remedies used, as well as veterinary treatment). Notes about response to therapy, especially corticosteroids, is especially important.

Almost all animals with skin disorders have been bathed, dipped, sprayed, or larded with one or more medications, and the owner may be reluctant to disclose a complete and honest list of previous treatment. It is important that the types of medication and dates of application be completely divulged, because a modification of pertinent signs may have resulted.

Although the animal cannot relate subjective findings (symptoms), it is possible to determine the degree of hyperesthesia, pruritus, and pain reasonably well.

Pruritus is one of the most common presenting complaints and in many cases is a hallmark of cutaneous allergy. The presence and degree of itching is a most important criterion in the differential diagnosis of many skin diseases. One should note whether itching is present in the absence of morphologic skin lesions (often seen in atopy) or whether skin lesions or the itching developed first. Note whether the patient scratches while in the examination room. This is usually so with severe pruritus such as that found with scabies or pediculosis, but rarely with itching caused by dry skin or psychosomatic problems. Pyodermas may also be a major cause of itching. The owner's idea of the intensity of itching may vary considerably from the veterinarian's. Consequently, it is

Text continued on page 466

Table 79. BREED PREDILECTION FOR SKIN DISEASES

Breed	Disease
Abyssinian cat	Psychogenic dermatitis/alopecia
Beagle	Atopy Demodicosis
Boston terrier	Atopy Demodicosis Hyperadrenocorticism Mastocytoma Sebaceous gland tumor Tail fold pyoderma
Boxer	Acne, canine Demodicosis Dermoid cyst Hemangiopericytoma Histiocytoma Hyperadrenocorticism Interdigital pyoderma Mastocytoma Sertoli cell tumor
Cats (general)	Abscess Acne Dermatophytosis Otodectic otitis Endocrine alopecia Eosinophilic plaque, linear granuloma, indolent ulcer Flea allergy dermatitis Miliary dermatitis Plasma cell pododermatitis Psychogenic dermatitis/alopecia Scabies Solar dermatitis Stud tail
Chihuahua	Demodicosis
Collie	Bullous pemphigoid Discoid lupus erythematosus Epidermolysis bullosa Fibrous histiocytoma Nasal pyoderma Nasal solar dermatitis Systemic lupus erythematosus
Dachshund	Acanthosis nigricans Demodicosis Folliculitis and pododermatitis Histiocytoma Hyperadrenocorticism

Table continued on opposite page

Table 79. BREED PREDILECTION FOR SKIN DISEASES *(Continued)*

Breed	Disease
	Hypothyroidism
	Juvenile cellulitis
	Nodular panniculitis
	Pattern alopecia (ears)
	Pattern alopecia (ventrum)
	Sternal callus
Dalmatian	Atopy
	Bronzing syndrome
	Demodicosis
	Folliculitis
Doberman pinscher	Acne
	Acral lick dermatitis
	Color mutant alopecia
	Demodicosis
	Flank sucking
	Folliculitis and pododermatitis
	Hypopigmentation (lip, nose)
	Hypothyroidism
English bulldog	Acne
	Demodicosis
	Facial fold pyoderma
	Folliculitis and pododermatitis
	Hypothyroidism
	Mastocytoma
	Tail fold pyoderma
German shepherd	Calcinosis circumscripta
	Discoid lupus erythematosus
	Fly dermatitis of ear tips
	Hemangioma-hemangiosarcoma
	Hemangiopericytoma
	Nasal pyoderma
	Otitis externa
	Perianal fistula
	Pituitary dwarfism
	Pyoderma
	Seborrhea
Golden retriever	Acral lick dermatitis
	Acute moist dermatitis
	Allergic inhalant dermatitis
	Folliculitis
	Hypothyroidism
Great Dane	Acne
	Acral lick dermatitis
	Callus formation
	Demodicosis
	Dermoid cyst

Table continued on following page

Table 79. BREED PREDILECTION FOR SKIN DISEASES *(Continued)*

Breed	Disease
	Histiocytoma Hygroma Hypothyroidism Pododermatitis-folliculitis Pyoderma
Great Pyrenees	Acute moist dermatitis Demodicosis
Irish setter	Atopy Acral lick dermatitis Color mutant alopecia Hypothyroidism Seborrhea
Irish wolfhound	Hygroma Hypothyroidism
Keeshond	Keratoacanthoma Hyposomatotropism
Labrador retriever	Acral lick dermatitis Acute moist dermatitis Folliculitis Seborrhea
Malamute	Zinc-responsive dermatosis
Newfoundland	Hypothyroidism
Norwegian elkhound	Keratoacanthoma
Old English sheepdog	Demodicosis Folliculitis-pododermatitis
Pekingese	Facial fold pyoderma
Persian cat	Facial fold pyoderma Dermatophytosis Hair mats
Pointers	Acral mutilation Contact dermatitis Demodicosis Juvenile cellulitis
Poodle	Ectodermal defect Epiphora Hyperadrenocorticism Otitis externa Hyposomatotropism
Pug	Atopy Facial fold and tail fold pyoderma

Table continued on opposite page

Table 79. BREED PREDILECTION FOR SKIN DISEASES *(Continued)*

Breed	Disease
Rhodesian ridgeback	Dermoid sinus in midline of back
Shar Pei	Demodicosis Fold dermatitis Folliculitis
Siamese cat	Hypotrichosis Psychogenic dermatitis/alopecia Pinnal alopecia
Schnauzer	Atopy Hypothyroidism Schnauzer comedo syndrome Subcorneal pustular dermatosis
Shetland sheepdog	Discoid lupus erythematosus Epidermolysis bullosa Nasal solar dermatitis Systemic lupus erythematosus
Siberian husky	Zinc-responsive dermatosis
Spaniels (cocker and springer)	Cutaneous asthenia Epidermoid cyst Hypothyroidism Lip fold pyoderma Otitis externa Seborrhea

Terriers
   Cairn
   Kerry blue
	Atopy
	 Dermoid cyst
	 Pilomatrixoma
	 Footpad keratoses (corns)
	 Otitis externa

Scottish
   West Highland
     white
   White-haired fox
	Atopy
	 Demodicosis
	 Atopy
	 Atopy
	 Sebaceous gland tumor
	 Neurofibroma

Modified from Muller, G. H., Kirk, R. W., and Scott, D. W.: Small Animal Dermatology, 3rd ed. Philadelphia, W. B. Saunders Company, 1983, pp. 95–98.

helpful to phrase the question: "How many times daily do you see your dog scratch?" "Does he itch in many sites or just a few?" "Does he shake his head?" "Does he lick his paws?"

The same type of specific question is helpful when discussing diets, because the owner often remembers the atypical feedings. A more representative answer is often attained when one asks, "What did your pet eat yesterday (or over the past 48 hours)?"

Because contact irritants or allergens are important, it is necessary to inquire about the dog's external environment. Does he live in an apartment or is he outdoors in the fields and forests? Does he sleep in a dog house or in the owner's bed? Is the bedding straw, shavings, wool blankets, or silk sheets?

In determining contagion, one should inquire about the skin health of other animals on the premises. The presence of skin disease in the people associated with the patient may also be highly significant in some disorders (scabies and ringworm).

At this point, the clinician usually has a general idea of the problem and is ready to proceed with a careful physical examination. In some cases, the clinician may want to come back to the general medical history if further developments indicate a more serious or underlying systemic disease. Table 80 lists some systemic diseases with cutaneous lesions.

PHYSICAL EXAMINATION

In dermatology, the clinician can observe the pathologic lesions directly and need not rely on vague shadows or referred sounds to determine abnormality; skin lesions are clearly visible. By careful, systematic inspection alone, the diagnosis of many dermatoses becomes apparent.

The examination should be performed with good lighting. Normal daylight without glare is best, but any artificial light of adequate candle power is sufficient if it produces bright, uniform lighting. The lamp should be adjustable to illuminate all body areas. A combination loupe and light provides magnification of the field as well as good illumination.

Before concentrating on the individual lesions, the entire animal should be observed from a distance of several feet for a general impression of abnormalities.

Does the animal appear to be in good health? Is he fat or thin, unkempt or well groomed? Is the problem generalized or localized? What is the distribution of the lesions? Are they bilaterally symmetric or unilaterally irregular?

To answer some of these questions, the animal must be examined more closely. One should inspect the dorsal aspect of the body, and then carefully observe the lateral surfaces. Next, the clinician should turn the animal over for a careful examination of the ventral region.

Close Examination of the Skin

After an impression is obtained from a distance, the skin should be examined more closely. Palpation now becomes important. What is the texture

Table 80. SYSTEMIC DISEASES WITH CUTANEOUS LESIONS

Disease	Skin Lesions or Symptoms
Atopy	Pruritus
Cold agglutinin disease	Erythema, purpura, necrosis, ulceration
Diabetes mellitus	Atrophy, ulceration, pyoderma, seborrhea
Dirofilariasis	Erythema, alopecia, pruritus, nodules
Feline leukemia virus infection	Pyoderma, seborrhea, poor healing
Hyperadrenocorticism	Alopecia, hyperpigmentation, calcinosis cutis, pyoderma, seborrhea, telangiectases
Hypothyrodism	Alopecia, hypothermia, seborrhea, pyoderma, hyperpigmentation, myxedema
Leishmaniasis	Erythema, nodules, ulceration, fistulas
Male-feminizing syndrome	Alopecia, seborrhea, hyperpigmentation, gynecomastia
Mycoses, deep	Nodules, ulceration, fistulas
Mycosis fungoides	Erythroderma, plaques, nodules, ulceration
Ovarian imbalances	Alopecia, hyperpigmentation, seborrhea
Pemphigus	Purulent exudate, crusting, vesiculation, ulceration/erosion
Pituitary dwarfism	Alopecia, cutaneous degeneration, hyperpigmentation
Sertoli cell tumor	Alopecia, gynecomastia, hyperpigmentation
Systemic lupus erythematosus	Pyoderma, seborrhea, ulceration, pruritus, erythema
Thallium toxicosis	Alopecia, erythema, ulceration
Toxic epidermal necrolysis	Ulceration, blisters, pain
Tuberculosis	Nodules, ulceration, fistulas

From Muller, G. H., Kirk, R. W., and Scott, D. W.: Small Animal Dermatology, 3rd ed. Philadelphia, W. B. Saunders Company, 1983, p. 100.

of the hair? Is it coarse or fine, dry or oily, and does it epilate easily? A change in the amount of hair present is often a dramatic finding. Alopecia is a complete lack of hair in areas where it is normally present. Hypotrichosis implies a partial alopecia that may be developmental, hormonal, neoplastic, inflammatory, or idiopathic. Hypertrichosis is excess hair and, although very rare in animals, is usually hormonal or developmental in nature.

The texture, elasticity, and thickness of the skin should be determined and impressions of heat or coolness recorded. It is important to examine every inch of skin and mucous membranes. It is easier to find important skin lesions in some breeds than in others, depending on the thickness of the coat. There is a variation in density of an individual's coat in different body areas. Lesions can be discerned more easily in sparsely haired regions. However, the clinician must part the hair in many areas to observe and palpate lesions that are partially covered. When abnormalities are discovered, it is important to establish their general distribution as well as their configuration within an area. Are they single, multiple, discrete, diffuse, grouped, or confluent? With sharp observation, linear or annular configuration of the lesions may be noted.

Two special techniques of close examination of the skin are noteworthy: diascopy and Nikolsky's sign.

Diascopy is a technique that involves pressing a clear piece of plastic or glass over an erythematous lesion. If the lesion blanches on pressure, the reddish color is due to vascular engorgement. If it does not, there is hemorrhage into the skin (petechia or ecchymosis).

Nikolsky's sign is elicited by applying pressure on a vesicle at the edge of an ulcer or erosion or even on normal skin. It is positive when the outer layer of the skin is easily rubbed off or pushed away. It indicates poor cellular cohesion, as found in the pemphigus complex.

At this point, one should focus on individual lesions and examine them minutely with good light and a hand lens or a head loupe with 4- to 6-power magnification.

Lesional Changes

The evolution of lesions should be determined either by history or by finding different stages of lesions on the same patient. Thus, papules often develop into vesicles and pustules, which may rupture to leave erosions or ulcers and finally crusts. An understanding of these processes helps in the diagnostic process. As lesions develop in special patterns, they involute in characteristic ways too. Acute lesions often appear suddenly and disappear quickly and completely. Chronic lesions may leave diagnostically important pigmentation or scars that persist for months or permanently (i.e., chronic generalized demodicosis and juvenile pyoderma, respectively).

Morphology of Skin Lesions

Morphology of skin lesions is the essential feature of canine dermatologic diagnosis and sometimes the *only* guide if laboratory procedures yield no useful information. The clinician must learn to recognize primary and secondary lesions. A primary lesion is one that develops spontaneously as a direct reflection of underlying disease. Secondary lesions evolve from primary lesions or are artifacts induced by the patient or by external factors such as trauma or medications. Careful inspection of the diseased skin will frequently reveal a primary lesion pathognomonic of a specific dermatosis. In many cases, however, the significant lesion must be differentiated from the mass of secondary debris. The ability to discover a characteristic lesion and understand its significance is the first step toward mastering dermatologic diagnosis. Variations are common, because early as well as advanced stages exist in most skin diseases. In addition, the appearance of skin lesions may change with medication, self-inflicted trauma, and secondary infection.

Most skin diseases, however, are chracterized by a single type of lesion. This primary lesion varies slightly from its initial appearance to its full development. Later, through regression, degeneration, or traumatization, it changes in appearance and in its new, altered form becomes a secondary lesion.

The definitions that follow explain the importance and relationship of skin lesions to canine and feline dermatoses.

Definitions

Primary Lesions

Bulla—vesicle greater than 1 cm in diameter.

Cyst—an epithelium-lined cavity containing fluid or a solid material. A cyst is a smooth, well-circumscribed fluctuant-to-solid mass. Skin cysts are usually lined by adnexal epithelium (hair follicle, sebaceous, or apocrine) and filled with cornified cellular debris or sebaceous or apocrine secretions.

Ecchymoses—hemorrhagic patches greater than 1 cm in diameter.

Macule—a circumscribed, flat spot up to 1 cm in size characterized by change in color of the skin. The discoloration can result from several processes: an increase in melanin pigmentation, depigmentation, and erythema or local hemorrhage. Examples are the hyperpigmented patches in the axillae of dogs with acanthosis nigricans, erythematous macules in many types of acute dermatitis, lentigo, and pigmented nevi.

Nodule—a small, circumscribed, solid elevation greater than 1 cm in diameter that usually extends into the deeper layers of the skin. Nodules usually result from massive infiltration of inflammatory or neoplastic cells into the dermis or subcutis. Deposition of fibrin or crystalline material also produces nodules.

Papule—a small, solid elevation of the skin up to 1 cm in diameter. A papule can always be palpated as a solid mass. Many papules are pink or red swellings produced by tissue infiltration of inflammatory cells, by intraepidermal and subepidermal edema, or by epidermal hypertrophy. Papules may or may not involve hair follicles. Examples are the erythematous papules seen in chronic allergic contact dermatitis of dogs after exposure to plants.

Patch—a macule over 1 cm in size.

Petechiae—pinpoint hemorrhagic macules that are much less than 1 cm in diameter.

Plaque—a larger, flat-topped elevation formed by the extension or coalition of papules. A plaque composed of closely packed projecting elevations often covered by crusts is called a *vegetation*.

Purpura—a type of macule caused by bleeding into the skin. It is usually dark red but changes to purple as absorption proceeds.

Pustule—a small, circumscribed elevation of the skin filled with pus. It is technically a small abscess (occasionally sterile) that may be intraepidermal or follicular in location. The color is usually yellow but may be pink or red. Examples are acne, folliculitis, and the pustules seen on the abdomen of puppies with superficial pustular pyoderma (impetigo).

Tumor—a neoplastic enlargement that may involve any structure of the skin or subcutaneous tissue. Examples are fibromas, mastocytomas, melanomas, and carcinomas.

Vesicle—a sharply circumscribed elevation of the skin filled with clear, free fluid. Vesicles are rarely seen in dogs and cats, because they are fragile and transient. Lesions up to 1 cm in diameter are called *vesicles* and are seen in viral or autoimmune dermatoses, or dermatitis caused by irritants. They may be intraepidermal or subepidermal in location.

Wheal—a sharply circumscribed, raised lesion consisting of edema that appears and disappears within minutes or hours. Wheals are characteristically white-to-pink elevated ridges or round edematous swellings that often have pseudopods at their periphery. They blanch upon diascopy (viewing the skin through a glass slide that is pressed firmly against the lesion). A huge hive of a distensible region such as the lips or eyelids is called *angioedema.* Urticarial lesions persist for days and consist of mixed cell infiltrate as well as edema. In dogs, they produce characteristic raised areas of the hair coat that are especially prominent on the back. Examples of wheals are hives, insect bites, and positive reactions to allergy skin tests.

Secondary Lesions

Abnormal pigmentation—skin coloration caused by a variety of pigments, but most commonly melanin. Melanin is responsible for a variety of skin colors:

Black—melanin present throughout the epidermis (lentigo).

Blue—melanin within melanocytes and melanophages in the mid and deep dermis (blue nevus).

Gray—diffuse dermal melanosis (metastatic melanoma).

Tan, Brown, Black— various shades of normal skin color in breeds are due to melanin.

Brown—hemochromatosis is due primarily to melanin, not hemosiderin.

Red-Purple—hemorrhage in the skin is red at first, becoming dark purple with time (bruises).

Yellow-Green—accumulations of bile pigments (icterus).

Comedo—a dilated hair follicle filled with cornified cells, sebaceous material, and microorganisms. It is the primary lesion of acne and may predispose to bacterial folliculitis. A comedo is produced secondary to seborrheic skin disease and seborrhea or to occlusion with greasy medications or by systemic or topical corticosteroids.

Crust—a dried exudate on the surface of a lesion formed when dried exudate, serum, pus, blood, cells, scales, or medications adhere to the surface and often mingle with hair. Unusually thick crusts are found in hairy areas, because the dried material tends to adhere more tightly than in glabrous skin. Hemorrhagic crusts in staphylodemodicosis are brown or dark red; yellowish-green crusts appear in some cases of pyoderma; tan, lightly adhering crusts are found in superficial pustular pyoderma (impetigo).

Epidermal collarette—a special type of scale arranged in a circular rim of loose keratin flakes. It represents the remnants of the epidermal tissue layers that once formed the "roof" of a vesicle, bulla, or pustule.

Erosion—a shallow ulcer that does not penetrate the basal cell layers and consequently heals without scarring.

Excoriation—a superficial removal of epidermis caused by scratching, biting, or rubbing. Most excoriations are self-produced and caused by pruritus; they invite secondary bacterial infection. Acute moist dermatitis caused by self-inflicted trauma is such an example.

Fissure—a linear cleavage into the epidermis or through the epidermis into the dermis caused by disease or injury. Fissures may be single or multiple tiny cracks or large clefts several centimeters long. They have sharply defined margins and may be dry or moist, and straight, curved, or branching. They occur when the skin is thick and inelastic and then subjected to sudden swelling from inflammation or trauma, especially in regions of frequent movement. Examples are found at ear margins and at ocular, nasal, oral, and anal mucocutaneous borders.

Hyperkeratosis—an increase in thickness of the horny layer of the skin. This condition occurs in normal skin and also on specialized areas such as the digital pads and planum nasale. Examples are callus formation and nasodigital hyperkeratosis (hardpad). The keratogenic hyperplasia can occur in plaques, ridges, circular areas, or even "feathered" projections of digital pads.

Hyperpigmentation (*hypermelanosis, melanoderma*)—increased epidermal and occasionally dermal melanin. Melanophages may be found in the superficial dermis. (Postinflammatory, chronic, traumatic, and endocrine skin lesions.) Excess pigment in hair is called *melanotrichia.*

Hypopigmentation (*hypomelanosis*)—loss of epidermal melanin (postinflammatory lesions). *Leukoderma* is a general term for white skin, whereas *vitiligo* refers to a specific disease. Lack of pigment in hair is called *leukotrichia* or *achromotrichia.*

Lichenification—a thickening and hardening of the skin characterized by an exaggeration of the superficial skin markings. Lichenified areas frequently result from friction. They may be normally colored but more often are hyperpigmented. Examples are the hyperpigmented, lichenified flanks in the male-feminizing syndrome and the axillae in acanthosis nigricans.

Scale—an accumulation of loose fragments of the horny layer of the skin (cornified cells). The scale is the final product of epidermal keratinization. In seborrhea, for example, scales are the result of an increased rate of keratinization. The consistency of flakes varies greatly, and they can appear branny, fine, powdery, flaky, platelike, greasy, dry, loose, adhering, or "nitlike." The color varies from white, silver, yellow, or brown to gray. Scales are seen in seborrhea, generalized demodicosis, and chronic allergic dermatitis.

Scar—an area of fibrous tissue that has replaced the damaged dermis or subcutaneous tissue. Scars are the remnants of trauma or dermatologic lesions. Most scars in dogs and cats are alopecic, atrophic, and depigmented. Proliferative scars do occur and in dark-skinned dogs scars can be alopecic and hyperpigmented. Scars are observed following severe burns and in deep pyoderma.

Sinus—an epithelium-lined channel from a suppurative cavity to the skin surface.

Ulcer—a break in the continuity of the epidermis, with exposure of the underlying dermis. A severe pathologic process is required to form an ulcer; therefore, a search for the cause is always indicated. It is important to note the structure of the edge, the firmness of the ulcer, and the type of exudate in the crater. A scar is always left after healing of ulcers. Examples are feline eosinophilic ulcer syndrome and chronic solar dermatitis.

Vegetations—heaped-up crusts seen in pemphigus vegetans.

Distribution Patterns of Skin Lesions

A dramatic change becomes apparent when a skin disorder affects an animal whose body is covered with a dense hair coat. Even the most casual observer is aware of the loss of hair in certain areas. The alopecic pattern, which is often sharply demarcated, assumes a new meaning when it is accurately interpreted. When alopecia and other hair changes are evaluated according to their distribution pattern over the entire body, significant diagnostic clues appear. Comparatively speaking, only on the human scalp is alopecia as striking and meaningful.

In animals, the primary or secondary skin lesions are often hidden under the hair coat; in fact, it requires painstaking observation to see them. In short-coated animals, if you stand behind the animal and use both hands to roll the skin into a horizontal fold, it is possible to see between the erected hair shafts to the skin surface. By rolling the fold backward, you can see progressively new areas of skin surface and get "an impression" of the distribution of lesions. Only when the animal is clipped can the distribution pattern of such lesions be seen with ease and accuracy. Consequently, in animals there are two distinctly different patterns that aid in diagnosis: (1) the changes in external hair coat, and (2) the definition and distribution of primary and secondary skin lesions. These two factors do not necessarily have a reciprocal relationship.

Different Stages

As a skin disease progresses from its earliest appearance to its final fully developed state, the pattern must necessarily change. A small patch of alopecia can enlarge into almost total hair loss in some cases. Obviously, if all intermediate stages of such a disease were drawn diagrammatically, the result would be more confusing than helpful. Therefore, it is necessary to select for each skin disorder the single distribution pattern that is of greatest diagnostic value. Different stages of each disease exist, and the total impact of the diagram should be interpreted with that fact always in mind. In addition, note that the distribution pattern represents alopecia or changes of the skin surface or both.

Figure 56 shows many typical patterns.

Regional Diagnosis

When a dermatosis is confined to a specific region, several diagnoses are often possible. Table 81 lists areas or parts of the body and the skin diseases that are commonly localized or especially severe in those areas. This table should be useful in suggesting several differential diagnosis.

Text continued on page 483

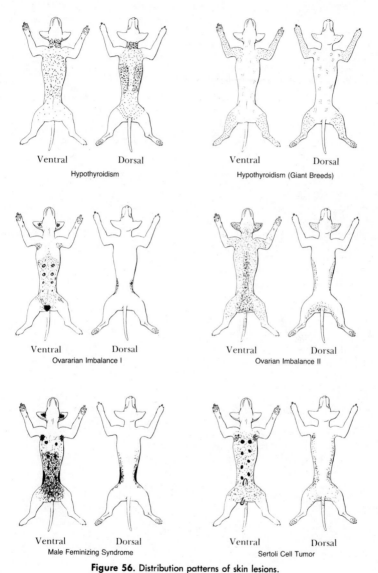

Figure 56. Distribution patterns of skin lesions.

Illustration continued on following page

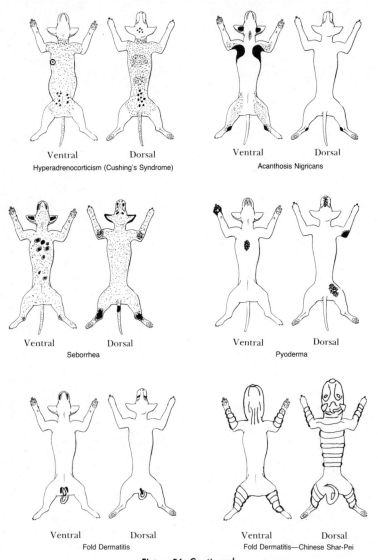

Ventral Dorsal
Hyperadrenocorticism (Cushing's Syndrome)

Ventral Dorsal
Acanthosis Nigricans

Ventral Dorsal
Seborrhea

Ventral Dorsal
Pyoderma

Ventral Dorsal
Fold Dermatitis

Ventral Dorsal
Fold Dermatitis—Chinese Shar-Pei

Figure 56. Continued.

Illustration continued on opposite page

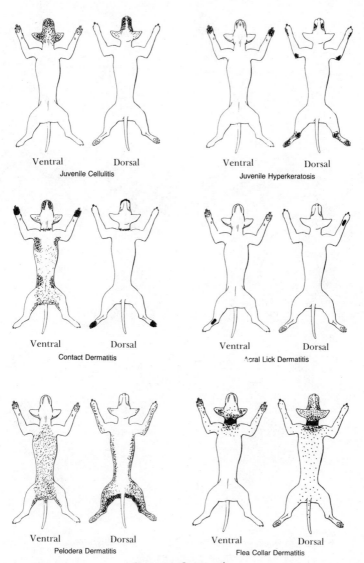

Ventral   Dorsal
Juvenile Cellulitis

Ventral   Dorsal
Juvenile Hyperkeratosis

Ventral   Dorsal
Contact Dermatitis

Ventral   Dorsal
Acral Lick Dermatitis

Ventral   Dorsal
Pelodera Dermatitis

Ventral   Dorsal
Flea Collar Dermatitis

Figure 56. Continued.
Illustration continued on following page

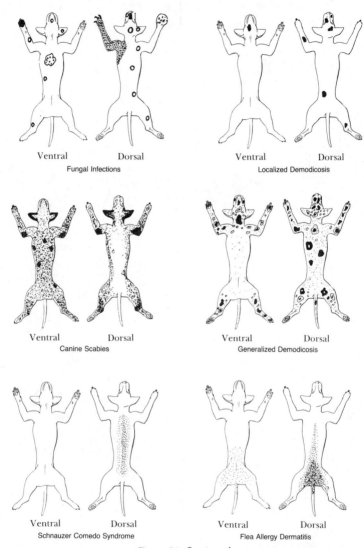

Ventral   Dorsal

Fungal Infections

Ventral   Dorsal

Localized Demodicosis

Ventral   Dorsal

Canine Scabies

Ventral   Dorsal

Generalized Demodicosis

Ventral   Dorsal

Schnauzer Comedo Syndrome

Ventral   Dorsal

Flea Allergy Dermatitis

Figure 56. Continued.

Illustration continued on opposite page

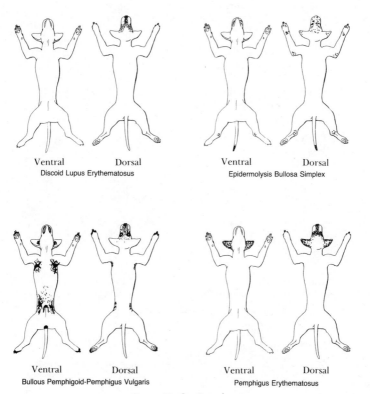

Ventral   Dorsal
Discoid Lupus Erythematosus

Ventral   Dorsal
Epidermolysis Bullosa Simplex

Ventral   Dorsal
Bullous Pemphigoid-Pemphigus Vulgaris

Ventral   Dorsal
Pemphigus Erythematosus

Figure 56. Continued.

Illustration continued on following page

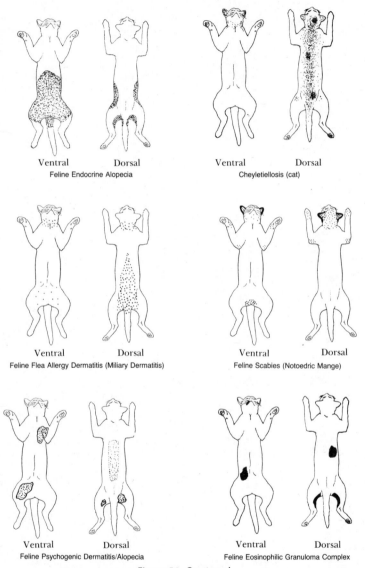

Ventral   Dorsal
Feline Endocrine Alopecia

Ventral   Dorsal
Cheyletiellosis (cat)

Ventral   Dorsal
Feline Flea Allergy Dermatitis (Miliary Dermatitis)

Ventral   Dorsal
Feline Scabies (Notoedric Mange)

Ventral   Dorsal
Feline Psychogenic Dermatitis/Alopecia

Ventral   Dorsal
Feline Eosinophilic Granuloma Complex

Figure 56. Continued.

Table 81. REGIONAL DIAGNOSIS

Area	Disease
Head	Atopy Demodicosis Dermatophytosis Facial fold dermatitis Feline food allergy Juvenile cellulitis Miliary dermatitis, feline Pemphigus erythematosus Pemphigus foliaceus Scabies, feline Sporotrichosis Systemic lupus erythematosus Zinc-responsive dermatosis

Ear	Alopecia, pattern
	Ceruminal gland tumor
	Demodicosis
	Fly dermatitis
	Frostbite
	Otitis externa
	   Malassezia (yeast)
	   Bacterial
	   Candidiasis
	   Otodectes cynotis
	   Ceruminous
	Scabies, canine and feline
	Seborrhea, marginal (pinna)
	Solar dermatitis, feline

Eyelid	Chalazion Demodicosis Dermatophytosis Distichiasis Entropion Hordeolum Seborrheic blepharitis Trichiasis
Nasal area	Contact dermatitis (plastic, rubber) Demodicosis Dermatophytosis Discoid lupus erythematosus Facial fold dermatitis Nasal pyoderma Nasal solar dermatitis Nasodigital hyperkeratosis Pemphigus erythematous Pemphigus foliaceus

Table continued on following page

Table 81. REGIONAL DIAGNOSIS *(Continued)*

Area	Disease
	Sporotrichosis
	Squamous cell carcinoma
	Systemic lupus erythematosus
	Vitiligo-like lesions
	Vogt-Koyanagi-Harada–like syndrome
Lip	Acne, canine and feline
	Candidiasis
	Contact dermatitis (plastic, rubber)
	Demodicosis
	Indolent ulcer, feline
	Juvenile cellulitis
	Lip fold dermatitis
	Oral papillomatosis, canine
	Vitiligo-like lesions
	Vogt-Koyanagi-Harada–like syndrome
Oral cavity (mucosal lesions)	Bullous pemphigoid
	Candidiasis
	Cryptococcosis
	Discoid lupus erythematosus
	Eosinophilic granuloma, canine
	Eosinophilic plaque
	Erosions, chemical
	Erosions, viral, feline
	Fibrosarcoma
	Fusospirochoetal stomatitis
	Gingival hypertrophy
	Indolent ulcer, feline
	Linear granuloma
	Malignant melanoma
	Marginal gingivitis, ulcerative, dental
	Mycosis fungoides
	Oral papillomatosis
	Pemphigus vulgaris
	Squamous cell carcinoma
	Systemic lupus erythematosus
	Thallium toxicosis
	Vegetative glossitis (foreign body)
Mucocutaneous margins	Bullous pemphigoid
	Candidiasis
	Mycosis fungoides
	Pemphigus vulgaris
	Systemic lupus erythematosus
	Thallium toxicosis
	Toxic epidermolysis necrosis
Chin	Acne, canine and feline
	Demodicosis
	Juvenile cellulitis
	Linear granuloma

Table continued on opposite page

Table 81. REGIONAL DIAGNOSIS *(Continued)*

Area	Disease
Neck	Contact dermatitis (collars) Dermoid sinus Flea allergy dermatitis, feline Flea collar dermatitis Miliary dermatitis, feline
Lower chest	Contact dermatitis Sternal callus
Axilla	Acanthosis nigricans Atopy Bullous pemphigoid Contact dermatitis Pemphigus vulgaris
Back	Calcinosis cutis Cheyletiellosis Comedo syndrome, schnauzers Flea allergy dermatitis Hypothyroidism Miliary dermatitis, feline Pediculosis Psychogenic dermatitis/alopecia, feline
Trunk	Demodicosis, generalized Eosinophilic plaque Folliculitis Hyperadrenocorticism Hypothyroidism Male-feminizing syndrome Ovarian imbalance Sertoli cell tumor Subcorneal pustular dermatosis
Abdomen	Bullous pemphigoid Calcinosis cutis Contact dermatitis (ventral abdomen) Endocrine alopecia, feline Eosinophilic plaque Folliculitis Hookworm dermatitis Hyperadrenocorticism Pelodera dermatitis Psychogenic dermatitis/alopecia, feline Subcorneal pustular dermatitis Superficial pustular pyoderma (impetigo)
Flanks	Bullous pemphigoid Mechanical irritation (flank suckers)
Tail	Acute moist dermatitis Endocrine alopecia, feline Flea allergy dermatitis

Table continued on following page

Table 81. REGIONAL DIAGNOSIS *(Continued)*

Area	Disease
	Frostbite
	Hyperplasia of tail gland, stud tail
	Mechanical irritation (tail suckers)
	Miliary dermatitis, feline
	Psychogenic dermatitis/alopecia, feline
	Tip of tail trauma
Anus	Anal sac dermatitis
	Perianal gland hyperplasia
	Perianal adenoma
	Perianal fistulas
Legs	Acral lick dermatitis
	Calcinosis circumscripta
	Contact dermatitis
	Decubital ulcers
	Demodicosis
	Elbow callus
	Elbow callus pyoderma
	Hygroma
	Linear granuloma
	Lymphangitis, bacterial, fungal
	Lymphedema
	Pelodera dermatitis
	Scabies, canine
Feet	Acral mutilation
	Atopy
	Contact dermatitis
	Demodicosis
	Dermatophytosis
	Digital pad hyperkeratosis
	Hookworm dermatitis
	Interdigital foreign bodies
	(foxtails, thorns)
	Pelodera dermatitis
	Pemphigus foliaceus
	Pododermatitis
	Idiopathic
	Plasma cell, feline
	Traumatic
	Sterile pyogranuloma
Nails	Nail deformities
	Onychogryphosis
	Onychomadesis
	Bullous pemphigoid
	Pemphigus vulgaris
	Systemic lupus erythematosus

Table continued on opposite page

Table 81. REGIONAL DIAGNOSIS *(Continued)*

Area	Disease
	Onychomycosis
	Onychorrhexis
	Paronychia
	Arteriovenous shunt
	Bacterial
	Feline leukemia
	Trauma
	Traumatic injury

From Muller, G. H., Kirk, R. W., and Scott, D. W.: Small Animal Dermatology, 3rd ed. Philadelphia, W. B. Saunders Company, 1983, pp. 130–133.

DIAGNOSTIC AND LABORATORY PROCEDURES

Diagnostic tests and laboratory procedures are valuable aids in almost every dermatologic case. Most tests are simple, quick, and inexpensive to perform. Some tests should be done "routinely," because many dermatoses are, in fact, complex problems with more than one cause. It would be embarrassing to miss a case of demodectic mange or dermatomycosis because a simple test was not run to check for a secondary problem in what superficially looked like a single primary disease.

Detailed discussions of dermatologic tests are presented in Section 4, pp. 517–523.

References and Additional Readings

Muller, G. H., Kirk, R. W., Scott, D. W.: Small Animal Dermatology, 3rd ed. Philadelphia, W. B. Saunders Company, 1983.

Clinical
Procedures

Diagnostic Procedures ━━━━━━━━━━━━━━

COLLECTION OF BLOOD

Venipuncture of the dog or cat may be accomplished by using the cephalic, jugular, femoral, or recurrent tarsal veins. In large dogs, the cephalic vein is preferred. In cats and smaller dogs, the jugular vein is frequently used. A peripheral blood sample can be obtained by deep clipping of a toenail, but this method is often undesirable.

It is essential to perform the venipuncture with as little trauma as possible so as to preserve the vein's integrity. This is vital when repeated taps must be performed. With show animals or for aesthetic reasons, it is undesirable to clip the hair over the site, but in long-haired animals, careful clipping aids in identifying the vein. The skin should be cleansed and an effective topical antiseptic applied. The hair (if not clipped) should be parted so that the sterile needle can be placed directly on the skin.

Proper restraint of the animal is of paramount importance to successful venipuncture. Details of restraint for tapping specific veins will be discussed in a later section. However, it is necessary for the animal to be restrained yet comfortable. The area of the vein must be held motionless, the skin stretched firmly to help anchor the vein, and the pressure applied proximal to the site of puncture to occlude blood flow.

The sterile, disposable Vacutainer* system has greatly facilitated the collection and processing of blood samples. In most instances, a 2- to 5-ml blood sample is adequate for routine hematology, clinical chemistry, or enzyme determinations. The Vacutainer small volume tube holder with a 22-gauge by 1-inch needle is used. In small dogs and in cats, jugular vein samples are collected (Table 82). A discussion of the type of blood sample that should be submitted for a particular clinical pathologic test can be found on page 888.

If the Vacutainer system is not used, a dry, sterile syringe and needle are used. The syringe should be held lightly between the thumb and fingers. Some clinicians place the index finger near the tip of the syringe to help guide it. Under no circumstances, however, should the finger touch the needle.

In most cases, it is best to pierce the skin just lateral to the vein. The needle is further advanced to puncture the vein from the side. Blood usually enters the syringe spontaneously but can be encouraged to do so by applying gentle suction. Some clinicians maintain continuous suction in the syringe (after the skin and fascia have been punctured) while probing for the vein so that penetration of the vein is indicated by the appearance of blood. An inadequate flow into the syringe may be caused by too much suction, which collapses the vein; partial occlusion of the needle; circulatory failure; hematoma formation; or piercing the vein wall without entering its lumen. Occasionally, the tip of the needle becomes snagged in the opposite wall of the vein. Slight retraction

---

*Becton-Dickinson Co., Rutherford, New Jersey.

Table 82. EVACUATED TUBES FOR BLOOD SAMPLES

Color of Rubber Stopper	Anti-coagulant	Purpose
Red	None	Electrolytes
		Enzymes
		Serologic studies
Lavender	EDTA	Blood counts
Blue	Citrate	Prothrombin time
		Partial thromboplastin time
Gray	Oxalate	Blood sugar
Green	Heparin	Serologic studies
		Blood gases
Yellow	ACD	Acid citric dextrose*
	AD	Acid dextrose*
	PBS	Physiologic saline*

*All tubes for blood storage are sterile.

and rotation of the needle correct the problem. When obtaining blood, the flow is often improved by alternating occlusion and release of the vein combined with slight passive motion of the leg drained by the vein.

The use of Vacutainers has simplified obtaining blood samples from small animals, especially when larger-sized veins are tapped to collect blood. Do not use large-volume Vacutainer containers in small veins, because the wall of the vein will collapse and samples will not be obtained. To ensure the proper anticoagulant/blood ratio, all tubes with anticoagulants should be filled until the vacuum is exhausted.

When a needle is placed in a vein to administer fluids for long-term infusion, it must be free in the vein but firmly fixed to the leg. After venipuncture, always inject several ml of fluid to be certain of the needle's location. Remove the syringe and attach the previously assembled intravenous (IV) tubing. Fluid is allowed to run into the circulation (see pp. 610–617).

HANDLING BLOOD SAMPLES (See p. 490)

Use syringe and needle or evacuated blood collection tubes (e.g., Vacutainer) when handling blood samples. All equipment must be chemically clean and *dry*.

Hemolysis is avoided by use of clean, dry equipment and also by avoiding trauma to the red cells. This is often the result of application of excessive or fluctuating suction during the aspiration procedure, excessive force in expelling blood from syringe to container, or excessive agitation of blood after collection. Whole blood should never be shipped, because trauma to red cells during shipment renders the specimen virtually useless.

Hemolysis may interfere with the following tests:
Serum lipase—With 0.5 gm of hemoglobin per dl, a 50% inhibition occurs.

Serum bilirubin—Large negative errors in the presence of hemoglobin may be due to the conversion of hemoglobin to methemoglobin by nitrous acid in the test and not in the control.

Icterus index—Abnormally increased by hemoglobin.

Urea nitrogen—Falsely elevated by the color in the protein-free filtrate.

Bromsulphalein—Altered in some procedures.

Inorganic phosphate—Increases rapidly in hemolyzed serum, because erythrocytes contain a high concentration of inorganic phosphate esters, which are hydrolyzed by serum phosphatases.

Serum potassium—Greatly increased in hemolyzed serum, because the potassium ratio between erythrocytes and plasma is 23:1 in man, but potassium is low in canine erythrocytes. Potassium will increase in serum in contact with the clot in the absence of visible hemolysis by diffusing into the serum. This increase is less at room temperature than at 4°C.

Alkaline phosphatase—Increased.

Acid phosphatase—May diffuse from the erythrocytes in unseparated serum and appears to be released into the serum during the clotting process, because it is present in the thrombocytes.

Transaminase—Hemolysis will have less influence on dog serum than on serum of human origin because of the variation in the ratio of transaminase between erythrocytes and serum.

   SGOT—The ratio is 2:70 in the dog and 40:1 in man.

   SGPT—The ratio is 1:38 in the dog and 6.7:1 in man.

Lactic dehydrogenase (LDH)—The ratio between erythrocytes and serum may vary from 160:1 in man to 1:38 in the dog.

Arginase—The ratio in the erythrocytes to that in plasma is 1000:1.

Blood pH—Decreased slightly by hemolysis.

Chloride—Decreased by hemolysis.

Prothrombin—Hemolysis has a negligible effect on prothrombin by the one-stage technique, but it causes interference in prothrombin consumption tests.*

   An effort should be made to fast the animal 12 hours prior to the collection of blood specimens to avoid postprandial lipemia. Lipemia, attributed to metabolic disorders as well as recent meals, is a common cause of factitious test results. Total protein, albumin, glucose, calcium, phosphorus, and bilirubin are examples of tests that can be markedly affected by lipemia. The clinician should become familiar with the testing procedures performed by the clinical laboratory handling the blood specimens to become aware of those tests affected by lipemia as well as hemolysis and various anticoagulants.

Blood for Hematology

   EDTA is the anticoagulant of choice for hematology. Heparin is especially to be avoided if blood films are to be made from blood mixed with anticoagulant.

---

*From Benjamin, M.: Outline of Veterinary Clinical Pathology, 3rd ed. Ames, Iowa, Iowa State University Press, 1979.

Heparin is acceptable for most routine procedures using blood plasma. It should be remembered that the anticoagulant effect of heparin is transitory. Specimens may clot after 1 to 3 days.

Blood films should be made immediately following blood collection. Cell morphology deteriorates progressively following collection. Although blood films made immediately following addition of blood to EDTA are acceptable, a better practice is to make films from blood remaining in the blood collection needle, because this blood has not been exposed to anticoagulant. *Blood exposed to heparin should never be used for making blood films.*

Incorrect proportions of blood to anticoagulant may result in water shifts between plasma and red cells. This may alter the packed cell volume, especially when small volumes of blood are added to tubes prepared with sufficient anticoagulant for much larger volumes of blood.

Erroneous laboratory results may also be obtained when small volumes of blood are placed in a relatively large container, causing evaporation of plasma water and adherence of cells to the surface of the container.

Liquid blood mixed with anticoagulant should be refrigerated after collection if there is to be a delay in making the laboratory determinations. White and red cell counts, packed cell volume, and hemoglobin can be done up to 24 hours after blood collection. Platelet counts, however, should be done within 1 hour after collection of blood.

Dried, unfixed blood films can be stained satisfactorily with most conventional stains 24 to 48 hours or even longer after being made. If a considerable delay before staining is unavoidable, blood films should be fixed by immersion in absolute methanol for at least 5 minutes. Such fixed films are stable indefinitely. Unfixed blood films must never be placed in a refrigerator, because condensation forming after removal from the refrigerator will ruin the film. Care should be taken to leave unfixed blood films face down on a counter top or in a closed box to avoid damage by insects. Special stains, such as peroxidase, may require fresh blood films.

Blood for Clinical Chemistry Procedures (See also p. 737).

Most clinical chemistry procedures are done on serum. This is obtained by collecting blood without any anticoagulant and allowing it to clot in a clean, dry tube. Serum should be separated from cells within 45 minutes of venipuncture. Special vacuum tube vials are available (Corvac vials*) that produce a strong barrier between the clot and the serum and eliminate having to draw off the serum into a separate vial. Clotting of the blood and retraction of the clot occurs best and achieves maximum yields of serum at room temperature or at body temperature. Refrigeration of the specimen impairs clot retraction. When firmly clotted, free the clot from the walls of the container by "rimming" with an applicator stick or by sharp taps on the outside of the tube. After the clot is freed, allow clot retraction to occur, then centrifuge and draw off the

---

*Corvac vials—Corning Glass, Corning, New York.

clear supernatant serum using a pipet and suction bulb. Serum yield is usually approximately one third of the whole blood volume.

Many clinical chemistry procedures can be done on plasma as well as serum. The advantage of using plasma is that separation of cells can be accomplished immediately without waiting for clot formation and retraction. The disadvantage of plasma is the presence of the anticoagulant, which interferes with many chemistry procedures. Plasma is often somewhat less clear than serum, which may be an additional disadvantage. Plasma and serum are virtually identical in chemical composition except that plasma has fibrinogen and the anticoagulant. For many chemical procedures in which plasma or whole blood is to be used, heparin is the anticoagulant of choice. Heparinized blood is the only acceptable specimen for pH and blood gas studies. Although EDTA blood is acceptable for certain chemical procedures, it cannot be used for determinations of plasma electrolytes, because it both contributes electrolytes to and sequesters them from the specimen. Additionally, EDTA can interfere with alkaline phosphatase levels, decrease the carbon dioxide–combining power of blood, and elevate blood nonprotein nitrogen (see p. 743).

Serum or plasma should be separated and removed from the cells as soon as possible after blood is collected, because many constituents of plasma exist in a higher concentration in the blood cells. With time, these substances leak into the plasma and cause spurious elevations in plasma values obtained. Magnesium, potassium, phosphorus, and transaminase are a few examples in which this may be a serious problem. Under no circumstances should whole blood be sent through the mail, because serum derived from such specimens is usually visibly hemolyzed and results are often inaccurate. The serum should be separated and transferred to a clean, dry tube for shipment.

Lipemia can interfere with a variety of testing procedures based on colorimetric methods, including tests for total protein, transaminase, hemoglobin, icterus index, and amylase.

Venipuncture of Dogs

To restrain a dog for a venipuncture of the cephalic vein, place him on the table in sternal recumbency. If the right vein is to be tapped, the assistant stands on the left side of the dog, places his left arm under the subject's chin to immobilize the head and neck, and reaches across and grasps the right foreleg just distal to the elbow joint (Fig. 57). The thumb rotates the vein laterally while the hand immobilizes the leg in slight extension. It is important to keep the dog pressed down on the table if a struggle ensues. The person making the venipuncture grasps the leg at the metacarpals and begins the skin puncture at the medial side of the vein slightly above the carpus.

For a recurrent tarsal vein tap, restrain the dog in lateral recumbency. The assistant holds the under foreleg and presses the dog's neck to the table with his forearm. Hold the upper rear leg above the knee joint and in extension.

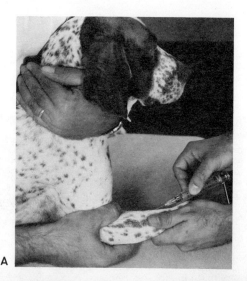

A

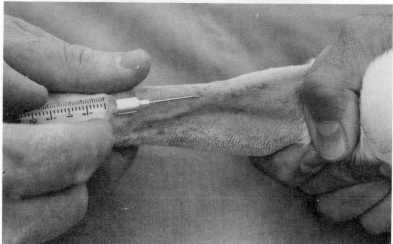

B

Figure 57. A, Cephalic venipuncture in right foreleg. A restraining arm is placed under the dog's chin, his neck and chest are held close to the assistant's body, and the cephalic vein is rolled laterally by thumb pressure. Proper restraint to prevent struggling is important. (Person doing venapuncture should hold the leg in the region of the metacarpals and start the venipuncture just proximal to the carpus.) B, Medial view of technique for cephalic venipuncture.

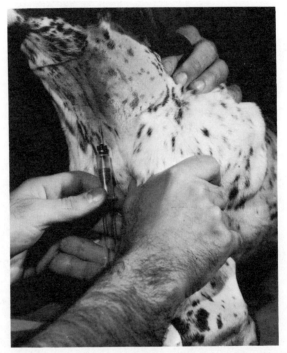

Figure 58. Jugular puncture in the dog. The hair on the neck has been clipped and the skin has been prepared with alcohol. The head and neck are extended, and the thumb is placed in the jugular furrow to distend the vein. A Vacutainer is being used to collect blood.

The vein is not easily visualized in some animals unless the hair is clipped. It is also very mobile subcutaneously, which may cause difficulty in inserting the needle.

The jugular vein is easily visualized in short-coated, long-necked breeds. Neophytes searching for the vein are often surprised at its extreme lateral location. If the dog has a heavy coat, it is probably better to clip the hair. Positioning is most important to make the vein "pop out" into view, especially for puppies and kittens less than 1 week old. Small breeds or puppies, feet hanging free, are held by an assistant who places his right arm under the dog's chest and holds it at his side. His right hand grasps one or both the pup's forelegs below the elbows. The assistant's left hand is used to lift the dog's chin up and back, thus extending the neck. If the head is rotated slightly, the veins will be seen more easily. The person making the tap places his left thumb in the jugular furrow at the thoracic inlet. The right hand manipulates the Vacutainer or syringe to make the venipuncture. Larger dogs are restrained in sternal recumbency on a table, their necks in extreme dorsal extension (Fig. 58).

Venipuncture of Cats

Jugular puncture in the cat or kitten is accomplished in a manner that is basically similar to that used for dogs. The cat bag or the wooden stocks,

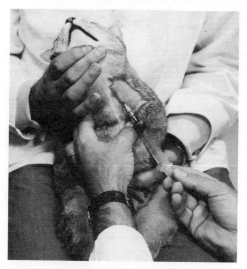

Figure 59. Jugular puncture in the cat. The legs are taped (not visible here) with the claws covered to prevent scratching. The cat is positioned comfortably on the restrainer's lap, and the head and neck are extended to make the jugular vein protrude.

however, are more efficient in restraining the cat and protecting the operator. We have found that taping first the front legs together and then the hind legs, makes jugular punctures a much easier procedure (Fig. 59). The tape should be placed low enough on the leg to cover the claws.

Puncture of the femoral vein of a cat is an effective way to obtain blood or to give medications. Because of its loose subcutaneous support, however, this vein is very mobile, and after puncture, almost always develops a hematoma. The quiet or depressed cat can be held gently on its side, the medial surface of the thigh clipped of hair, and the venipuncture made with minimal restraint. The refractory animal requires more stringent measures. We prefer rolling it in a blanket and pulling out one hind leg. The medial aspect is clipped, and the tap is performed as described previously.

Small amounts of blood can be collected easily from the marginal ear vein. Pluck hair from an area of skin about half an inch in diameter at the medial dorsal edge of the ear over the vein. Wipe the skin with alcohol, and apply pressure at the base of the ear to make the vein protrude. Coat the skin with a thin film of petrolatum, which makes the blood well up in large droplets on the skin following venipuncture. Incise the vein with a lancet or No. 11 Bard-Parker blade. Blood can be aspirated from the surface of the skin directly into a pipette. Hemorrhage stops quickly with gentle finger pressure. The whole procedure is quite painless and rarely upsets the animal.

COLLECTION OF BONE MARROW

Collection of bone marrow may prove valuable in those diseases of the blood in which examination of the peripheral blood reveals abnormal cells or cell counts. Conditions such as leukopenia, thrombocytopenia, nonregenerative anemias, agranulocytosis, pancytopenia, and leukemias may be present because of pathologic factors within the bone marrow.

Bone marrow in the young animal is very cellular and exists in the flat bones (sternum, ribs, pelvic bones, and vertebrae) and in the long bones (humerus and femur).

As the animal ages, the cellular content of the marrow decreases, especially in the long bones. In older animals, bone marrow cells still exist in the flat bones; however, in conditions of stress in which new blood cells must be produced in large numbers, primitive cells in the bone marrow of the long bones again become active.

Interpretation of the bone marrow smear may be limited by:
1. The technique used to obtain a bone marrow specimen. Technique is important because contamination with peripheral blood should be avoided.
2. The specialized knowledge necessary to interpret bone marrow cells.

Bone Marrow Collection (Dog)

The biopsy techniques that may be used in the examination of bone marrow are aspiration, core, and incisional. The most frequently used technique is that of aspiration biopsy. When aspiration biopsy fails to produce bone marrow cells (as in advanced myelofibrosis, neoplasia, or marrow aplasia), a core biopsy of bone marrow is indicated. Core biopsy samples of bone marrow can be obtained using modified versions of the Vim-Silverman or Jamshidi biopsy needles.

Equipment. (All equipment should be sterile.) Rubber gloves; Xylocaine, 0.5 per cent; skin disinfectant; clean glass slides; one 12-ml syringe; one scalpel; and sponges.

The selection of needles for aspiration biopsy of bone marrow is based on the site of the biopsy, the depth of the biopsy site from the skin, and the density of cortical bone. For bone marrow aspiration, the Kormed* modified disposable Illinois Sternal-Iliac bone marrow aspiration needle works well. For a core biopsy of bone marrow, the Jamshidi bone marrow Biopsy-Aspiration needle* (pediatric, 3.5 inch, 13 gauge) can be used.

The iliac crest is the site of choice for marrow aspiration and the only suitable site for core biopsy in the dog. To aspirate marrow, enter the widest part of the iliac crest, stopping the needle just after penetration of the bone. Remove the stylet and place a 12-ml syringe on the needle and aspirate 0.2 ml of marrow.

A short-acting anesthetic (thiamylal sodium) may occasionally be needed, but tranquilization together with local anesthesia is usually sufficient. Place the animal in lateral recumbency and clip the hair over the area of the trochanter major and the trochanteric fossa. Surgically prepare the site.

Contamination of the bone marrow with peripheral blood results if (1) the marrow is not aspirated immediately after the needle enters the marrow cavity, or (2) too much negative pressure is placed on the syringe, thus rupturing small sinusoids in the bone marrow.

Marrow can also be obtained from the proximal end of the femur via the trochanteric fossa.

Make a small skin incision over the trochanteric fossa just medial to the summit of the trochanter major. The bone marrow aspiration needle is inserted medial to the trochanter major, and the long axis of the needle is placed parallel to the long axis of the femur. Using firm pressure and an alternating rotary motion, insert the bone marrow needle 0.5 inch into the femoral canal. Remove the stylet from the needle and aspirate with a 12- or 20-ml syringe (Fig. 60).

Bone Marrow Collection (Cat)

Accessible sites for bone marrow sampling in the cat are the iliac crest and the proximal end of the femur via the trochanteric fossa. The latter is generally the most useful site. The same techniques as were previously described can be used; however, caution is advised against using vigorous restraint in a severely anemic cat. This may precipitate severe cyanosis, apnea, and cardiac arrest. Adequate sedation with supplemental oxygen administration and local anesthesia usually suffices.

*Kormed, Inc., 2510 Northland Drive, St. Paul, Minnesota 55120.

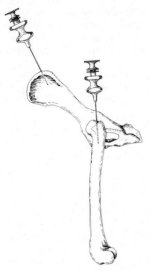

Figure 60. A diagram of the ilium and femur, illustrating the sites for bone marrow biopsy. The angle of the needle is variable for the ilial site. The needle may approach a more vertical position in larger bones, in which case the needle is started more caudally on the wing of the ilium. (From Bojarab, M. J. (ed.): Current Techniques in Small Animal Surgery, 2nd ed. Philadelphia, Lea & Febiger, 1983, p. 492.)

Smears of bone marrow should be made immediately after aspiration of material. Extrinsic thromboplastin present in bone marrow tissue will cause the marrow to clot within 30 seconds. Additionally, small pieces of marrow can be fixed in formalin for histologic preparation. Staining procedures such as new methylene blue, Wright's, May-Grünwald's or Giemsa may be used. A peroxidase stain may be helpful in differentiating granulocytic elements from lymphocytes.

References and Additional Readings

Lewis, H. B., and Rebar, A. H.: Bone Marrow Evaluation in Veterinary Practice. St. Louis, Missouri, Ralston Purina Co., 1979.

Meyer, D. J.: Bone marrow. In Bojrab, M. J. (ed.): Current Techniques in Small Animal Surgery, 2nd ed. Philadelphia, Lea & Febiger, 1983.

Perman, V., Osborne, C. A., and Stevens, J. B.: Bone marrow biopsy. Vet. Clin. North Am., 4:293, 1974.

Schalm, O. W., Jain, N. C., and Carrol, E. J.: Veterinary Hematology, 3rd ed. Philadelphia, Lea & Febiger, 1975.

COLLECTION OF CEREBROSPINAL FLUID

In the dog, the preferred site for obtaining cerebrospinal (CSF) fluid is the cerebellomedullary cistern (cisterna magna) at the atlanto-occipital articulation.

Equipment needed consists of sterile test tubes for fluid collection, an 18-

to 20-gauge, 1.5- to 3.5-inch Pitkin spinal needle with a short bevel and stylet, a spinal fluid manometer for pressure readings, a three-way stopcock, two sterile 5-ml syringes, and sterile sponges.

In order to perform an adequate cisternal puncture and not injure the animal, a short-acting, general anesthetic such as thiamylal sodium is required. Place the animal in either ventral or lateral recumbency. Clip and surgically prepare the area of skin from the external occipital protuberance to the wings of the atlas. The dog should be positioned in left lateral recumbency for right-handed personnel and in right lateral recumbency for left-handed personnel. Position the animal with the prepared area at the edge of the table. The head should be flexed ventrally and maintained at a right angle to the long axis of the neck. The flexion of the neck will serve to separate the occipital bone from the atlas.

To find the site of entrance for the needle into the cistern, an imaginary line is drawn across the neck from the prominent cranial lateral portion of the wings of the atlas. At a point where this line bisects a line drawn craniocaudally from the external occipital protuberance, the needle is passed inward at a right angle to the dorsal line of the neck (Fig. 61). As the needle is advanced, the stylet is removed periodically to see whether CSF appears in the hub. During

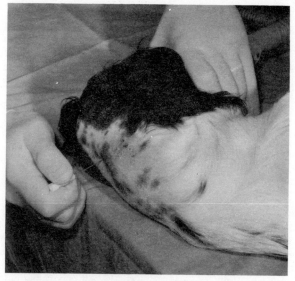

Figure 61. Collection of CSF fluid. The dog is in left lateral recumbency. The area from the external occipital protuberance to the wings of the atlas has been clipped and surgically prepared. The head is flexed ventrally. The needle is inserted at the junction of a line that bisects the cranial wings of the atlas and the external occipital protuberance. One person should hold the dog's head carefully and firmly in a flexed position while a second person makes the tap, measures opening pressure (see Figure 62), and collects a CSF sample.

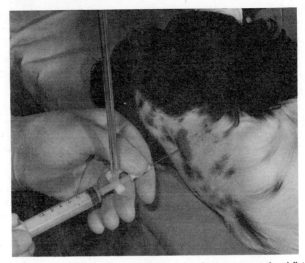

Figure 62. Recording CSF pressure. When the cisternal space is entered and fluid is seen at the needle hub, the spinal fluid pressure manometer is attached and opening and closing CSF pressure is recorded.

this procedure, the hub of the needle must be held tightly to prevent any movement of the needle. Occasionally, resistance is felt just prior to when the needle passes through the dura, but this cannot be depended upon; therefore, frequent removal of the stylet will avoid injury to the spinal cord. If bone is felt with the tip of the needle, the needle can be walked caudally (occipital bone) or cranially (atlas) to the atlanto-occipital space. Occasionally, blood without CSF is obtained. This is a result of puncture of a branch of the vertebral venous plexus. Obtain another clean sterile needle and repeat the procedure. This has not contaminated the CSF with blood. If fresh blood appears in the CSF, this may be associated with rupture of small blood vessels during the tap or with blood in the CSF as part of the disease process.

Upon entering the cisternal space and seeing fluid at the needle hub, attach the spinal fluid pressure manometer immediately and note the pressure (Fig. 62). Use a three-way valve on the manometer and record opening pressure. Next, remove 2 ml of CSF and place it in a sterile vial. More fluid may be removed if necessary, but it should be removed slowly. Record closing CSF manometric pressure. Initial CSF examination should include inspection for color and turbidity, total cell count, differential, and protein determination. Further tests such as glucose levels, differential cell count, and cultures may be indicated, depending on the clinical situation.

All animals on whom a cisternal tap was performed should be closely observed for the next 5 to 7 days for signs of adverse effects such as infection.

See Table 185 (p. 908) for normal CSF values.

BACTERIAL CULTURES

Principles of Collection

Collect a representative sample of bacteria and examine the material promptly.
1. Specimens should be collected from areas where organisms are most likely to be found, such as the edge of a spreading skin lesion, from incised pustules, or from contaminated cavities.
2. Specimens should be collected prior to the use of antibiotics, when possible.
3. Avoid accidental contamination of the specimen.
4. Label all specimens clearly and carefully.
5. Inoculate culture material into appropriate media *promptly*.

ROUTINE PROCEDURE FOR BACTERIOLOGIC CULTURE

Routine Smear

Prepare a smear by collecting material on a sterile cotton swab and rolling it onto a clear glass slide. Heat fix, and stain the slide with Quik stain or Gram stain. Fluids should be centrifuged and the sediment examined and cultured.

Routine Culture

Culture material on blood agar plates or in CLED (cystine, lactose, electrolyte–deficient) medium as an acceptable alternate; it stimulates growth, detects lactose fermentation, and prevents spreading of proteus. These media serve as a basis for the isolation of most aerobic microorganisms. Selective media may be necessary for the isolation and identification of specific microorganisms. Biopsy material may be ground in sterile sand and placed in sterile broth.

Bacterial Cultures

Recently, multiple media plates have been developed commercially* to facilitate direct antibiotic sensitivity and tentative identification of common pathogenic bacteria. These prepackaged, relatively inexpensive plates help the small laboratory identify pathogenic bacteria by their characteristic behavior on selective media. Some companies have different kits for different suspected infections. In general, they are most useful in evaluating conjunctivitis, otitis, pyoderma, wound infections, uterine or anterior vaginal infections, fresh necropsy material, and urinary infections. They are not recommended for culturing areas having a large population of normal microbial organisms, such as the respiratory tract, throat, and vulva, nor for fecal samples or for blood cultures to determine bacteremia.

---

*Bactossav Plate, Pitman-Moore Co., Washington Crossing, New Jersey; Bacti Lab Plate, Mt. View, California.

SPECIFIC CULTURE AND SMEAR METHODS

Blood Culture

Bacteria can enter the blood from extravascular sites by way of lymphatic circulation. Direct entry of bacteria into the blood stream can be observed in endocarditis, suppurative phlebitis, infected intravenous (IV) catheters, dialysis cannulas, osteomyelitis, and so on. Bacteremias can be transient, intermittent, or continuous. Transient bacteremia is produced by manipulating an abscess, dental procedures, urethral catheterization, or surgery on contaminated areas. Intermittent bacteremia is associated with undetected and undrained abscesses. Most dogs with bacteremia, especially those with gram-negative bacteremia, are febrile and have an abnormal peripheral blood picture with increased white blood cell (WBC) count, increased band and segmented neutrophils, increased monocytes, and lymphopenia. An exception to this is osteomyelitis in which bacteremia associated with staphylococci have basically normal hemograms.

The material for culture must be collected under aseptic conditions. Clip and surgically prepare the skin over the cephalic, recurrent tarsal, or jugular vein. Blood for culture should not be drawn through an indwelling IV or intra-arterial catheter. Use a Becton-Dickinson Vacutainer blood culture bottle, which can be used for both aerobic and anaerobic blood cultures. Add 10 ml of blood to the culture media. Becton-Dickinson SPB media (50-ml bottle) contains the anticoagulant sodium polyanetholesulfonate (SPS) in addition to penicillinase. The blood culture Vacutainer accepts 10 ml of blood giving a 1:5 dilution. For anaerobic blood cultures, an Analok clip is available from Becton-Dickinson for the SPB media Vacutainer. Immediately after collection, mix the contents of bottles or tubes to prevent clotting.

Blood cultures should be taken 1 hour before temperature spikes if intermittent fevers are present. Two or three separate blood culture specimens may be needed over a 24-hour period. With a 1:10 dilution of blood in broth, the normal bactericidal properties of antibiotics that may have been adminis-tered systemically are usually diluted to noninhibitory concentrations. The addition of SPS to commercial culture media inactivates clinical concentrations of aminoglycosides.

Other media that may be used as selective agents include MacConkey's agar, brain-heart infusion agar, mannitol salt agar, Streptosel agar, urea agar, blood agar, and eosin methylene blue (EMB) agar. Special techniques make it possible to determine total bacteria counts and whether an organism is coagulase positive or negative.

Anaerobe Culture

Because there is reason to believe that anaerobes may be present in significant numbers in positive cultures from blood, abscesses, wounds, and urine, it may be advisable to make these special examinations. Anaerobes are in the normal flora in fecal, throat, and bronchial swabs, so the anaerobic culture of these samples may be difficult to evaluate.

Specimens for anaerobic examination should be protected from air and held at room temperature. They should be cultured as soon as possible. They should not be used with transport or enrichment media but inoculated directly from the specimen. Specimens for anaerobic culture can be placed in modified Cary Blair media,* Vacutainer anaerobic specimen collector,† or BBL Port-A-Cul Transport System.‡ Specimens can be held for short periods in sterile, carbon dioxide–filled, tightly stoppered tubes or bottles. The sample should be inoculated onto prereduced anaerobically sterilized media under oxygen-free gas. Specimens can be inoculated deep into thioglycollate media for transfer and subculture.

With anaerobic organisms, it is especially important to make a smear and a Gram stain and to record all morphotypes present and the relative numbers of each. (See Tables 83 and 84.)

Urine Culture

Urine, as it is secreted by the kidneys, is sterile unless the kidney is infected. Most urinary tract infections result from ascending infection by organisms introduced through the urethra. The most common site of infection in female animals is the urethra and urinary bladder. Chronic prostatitis is common in male dogs and is often associated with relapsing urinary tract infections.

Urine specimens can be collected by catheterization, collecting a clean voided midstream sample, or by cystocentesis. To calibrate bacterial counts in urinary cultures, use a standard platinum milk dilution loop calibrated to deliver 0.001 ml urine to one half of a blood agar plate. The initial loop of urine is streaked onto the plate. One hundred colonies or more signifies a bacterial count in the original specimen of greater than or equal to 10^5 per ml. The number of bacteria that are significant varies with the method of collection. Cystocentesis greater than 10^3 bacteria per ml of urine is significant, and catheterization greater than 10^5 bacteria per ml is significant. Cystocentesis samples collected from animals having been treated with antimicrobial therapy should have 5 ml of urine centrifuged at 2500R for 5 minutes and the sediment streaked onto blood agar and MacConkey's agar.

MacConkey's and EMB agar are selective and differential media, which are used to identify urinary tract organisms. MacConkey's agar prevents early growth of proteus, inhibits growth of gram-positive bacteria, and allows separation of gram-negative bacteria in lactose positive and lactose negative subgroups.

Several commercial methods for urinary culture are available for screening

---

*Carr Scarborough Microbiologicals, P.O. Box 581, 1095 Delores Way, Forest Park, Georgia 30050.

†Vacutainer Anaerobic Specimen Collector, Becton-Dickinson, Rutherford, New Jersey 07070.

‡BD Co., P.O. Box 243, Cockeysville, Maryland 21030.

Table 83. GENERA OF ANAEROBIC BACTERIA COMMONLY OCCURRING IN THE DOG AND CAT

Genus Name	Familiar Synonyms
Gram-Positive Cocci	
Peptococcus	Anaerobic *Staphylococcus*
Peptostreptococcus	Anaerobic *Streptococcus*
Gram Positive	
Spore-forming rods	
Clostridium	
Gram Positive	
Non–spore-forming rods	
Actinomyces	
Bifidobacterium	
Eubacterium	
Lactobacillus	
Propionibacterium	Anaerobic *corynebacterium*
Gram Negative	
Non–spore-forming rods	
Bacteroides	*Fusiformis*
Fusobacterium	*Sphaerophorus; Fusiformis*
Spirochetes	
Treponema	

From Berg, J. N., and Fales, W. H.: Canine and feline anaerobic bacterial infections. Vet. Scope, *21*:2, 1977.

Table 84. SIGNS INDICATIVE OF ANAEROBIC INFECTIONS IN THE DOG AND CAT

Fight wounds (claw and bite wounds)
Abscesses
Foul-smelling discharges
Presence of gas in tissues or discharges
Necrotic tissues
Septic pleuritis and peritonitis
Fractures associated with trauma to soft tissues
Aspiration pneumonias
Infections following surgery on gastrointestinal tract or septic
  processes such as pyometra
Granulomas
Actinomycotic sulfur granules in pus
Infections near or on mucous membranes
Nonresponse to gentamicin or other aminoglycosides

From Berg, J. N., and Fales, W. H.: Canine and feline anaerobic bacterial infections. Vet. Scope, *21*:2, 1977.

urine for bacterial infection. Microstix* has proved 92 per cent accurate in detecting bacteriuria greater than 10^5 organisms per ml. If urine is collected by cystocentesis, significant bacteriuria may not be observed. Samples positive by Microstix should be recultured using calibrated loop or pour plate techniques.

Tray systems combining multiple bacteriologic media can be used for culturing urine.† Five compartments are available: MacConkey's agar, "streptocol" agar, mannitol salt agar, infusion agar, and a larger Mueller-Hinton area for antimicrobial sensitivity. In urine cultures, the smaller culture areas should be inoculated with a calibrated loop, 0.001 ml of urine.

Catheterization using aseptic technique or antepubic cystocentesis (see pp. 549–552) should be used to collect urine for culture. Specimens of urine should be refrigerated within a few minutes after collection if culture is not immediately performed. Bacterial culture of the specimen should be carried out within 2 hours of collection. Becton-Dickinson supplies a Vacutainer urine transport kit for urine culture. The Vacutainer tube can hold 5 ml of urine, which can be added from a midstream catch or cystocentesis. The collection tube has a bacteriostatic fluid, which preserves unrefrigerated urine specimens for up to 24 hours for culture.

Prostatic Cultures

Inflammation of the prostate or bacterial infection of the prostate may result in a nidus of infection that can cause recurrent urinary tract infection in male dogs. An effective way to evaluate the prostate for bacterial infection is to examine the prostatic fraction of the male ejaculate or, if separation proves to be too difficult, the whole ejaculate specimen can be cultured. To better interpret the results of the prostatic culture, urethral cultures should be obtained prior to the ejaculate sample.

To Culture the Urethra of the Male Dog

Wipe the end of the penis with 1:1000 Zephiran swab. Use a Calgi‡ urethral swab, and insert the swab 5 cm into the urethra. Place the swab in enrichment broth (brain-heart infusion or thioglycollate) by cutting the end of the swab off with sterile scissors. Refrigerate the broth and send it to the laboratory. Subculture using 0.1 ml loops of broth onto blood agar, MacConkey's agar, and mycoplasma media.

To Culture Prostatic Ejaculate

Collect ejaculate fraction into a sterile side mouth container (such as a 12-ml sterile plastic syringe container). Subculture 0.1 ml of ejaculate onto differential media as for urethral swabs.

To determine the significance of prostatic ejaculate culture for bacterial

---

*Microstix, Ames Co., Elkhart, Indiana.
†Bactassay Tray, Pitman-Moore, Washington Crossing, New Jersey.
‡Calgi swabs, Spectrum Diagnostics, 3 Science Road, Glenwood, Illinois 60425.

infection, the number of bacteria in the prostatic culture should be greater than 2 logs of growth compared with the bacteria cultured from the urethra.

Laboratory Diagnosis of Bacterial Diarrhea

Acute infectious diarrhea can be caused by bacteria, viruses (see pp. 252–254), and protozoa (see p. 800). The major bacteria in feces are non–spore-forming anaerobic bacilli, but gram-negative facultatively anaerobic bacteria such as *Escherichia coli* and other members of the Enterobacteriaceae family are usually present.

The clinical picture in acute infectious diarrhea is of frequent loose stools containing pus or blood, abdominal pain, and fever. Damage to the intestinal tract may be produced by an enterotoxin as with *Staphylococcus aureus* or *E. coli* or by invasion of the mucosa of the small intestine and colon. The most common bacterial pathogens of the intestinal tract in small animals are *E. coli*, *Salmonella* sp., and *Campylobacter jejuni*.

Stool specimens can be collected in screw cap glass or plastic containers or waxed cardboard containers with leakproof covers. If feces are not available, a rectal swab can be obtained using a Culturette.* A small amount of stool can be prepared on a slide, stained with Löffler's alkaline methylene blue stain for pus cells, and another slide prepared with Gram stain.

Submission Samples for Chlamydia Psittaci

The importance of chlamydia as the cause of a variety of common diseases in animals and birds is now firmly established. *Chlamydia psittaci* is the causative agent of psittacosis, enzootic abortion of ewes, bovine encephalomyelitis, feline pneumonitis, and ovine polyarthritis. The public health risk and the marked economic losses associated with this agent necessitate rapid and sensitive diagnostic procedures.

Laboratory Diagnosis

Direct Smears. Cell scrapings from conjunctiva during the phase of inflammation (first 10–14 days) and stained with Giemsa may show typical intracytoplasmic inclusions of initial and elementary bodies accompanied by a polymorphonuclear inflammatory cellular reaction.

Isolation and Identification. For isolation, columnar epithelial cells (not exudate) should be obtained. Calcium alginate (not wooden) swabs should be used. Swabs should be placed directly into liquid-holding media on wet ice. The most commonly used transport medium is 2-SP, composed of 0.2M sucrose and 0.02M phosphate (pH = 7.2) with added antibiotics. This can be supplied by the laboratory that is doing the isolations.

Cell monolayers using McCoy and HeLa cells are best for isolation of chlamydia. Egg (yolk sac) inoculation of embryonated eggs has been abandoned. Chlamydial inclusions are detected by fluorescent antibody techniques.

---

*Culturette Culture Collection System, Marion Scientific Laboratories, Kansas City, Missouri 64114.

Laboratory Diagnosis of Viral Infections

The following procedures and materials should be used for diagnosing viral infections:

1. Swabs—Specific types of swabs with carrier media are available for viral culture: Culturette* and Calgi swab.†
2. Media—Several types of media have been used for the transport of viral specimens: modified Stuart, modified Hanks, Leibovitz-Emory, all with added serum.
3. For short-term transit (≤5 days), specimens for viral isolation should be held at 4°C rather than frozen.
4. Submit blood serum samples for possible antibody response (especially paired serum samples) with tissues or tissue fluids for viral isolation.
5. Fluorescent antibody technique—Four types of specimens can be used for immunofluorescence diagnosis: frozen sections, impression smears, lesion scrapings, and resuspended cells in centrifuged sediment.
6. Electron microscopy (EM)—EM techniques are applicable in situations in which viral infections produce titers of virus in the specimen of $10^6 + 10^7$ particles per ml. Specimens such as feces, vesicle fluid, brain tissue, urine, or serum can be negatively stained for EM examinations.

Puncture Fluids

Aspirate material using aseptic technique (see p. 525). Centrifuge the aspirated material at high speed and stain a smear of the sediment with Gram stain. Culture the sediment on blood agar, in thioglycollate media, on Sabouraud's agar or on one of the multiple media plates. Also consider anaerobic cultures.

Wounds and Ulcers

In dealing with an abscess (except those of the eye), clip and clean the abscess site. Aspirate material from the abscess into a sterile syringe and culture in blood agar and thioglycollate broth or on one of the multiple media plates. In open wounds, use a sterile cotton swab and obtain fresh exudate from the deeper portion of the lesion. Also consider anaerobic cultures.

Throat Cultures

It is very difficult to obtain a good representative sample from the throat without contamination from the mouth. Pass a sterile cotton swab over the tonsillar area and posterior pharyngeal walls. In some animals, this may have to be done under a short-acting general anesthetic. Place the swab onto blood

---

*Culturette Culture Collection System, Marion Scientific, Kansas City, Missouri 64114.

†Wilson Diagnostic, Glenwood, Illinois.

agar colymycin nalidixic acid (CNA) blood agar for gram-positive bacteria and MacConkey's agar for gram-negative bacteria. Because of the abundant normal flora, multiple bacteria will usually grow and evaluation of pathogenicity will be difficult.

Spinal Fluid

If the spinal fluid is cloudy, make a direct smear and stain with Gram and Giemsa stains. If the fluid is fairly clear, centrifuge for 10 minutes, make a smear, and stain the sediment with Gram stain. Culture the sediment on blood agar, in thioglycollate medium, or on one of the multiple media plates, and on Sabouraud's agar.

Ear Cultures

Collect material on sterile cotton swabs, make a smear, and stain it with Gram stain. Place the swab on blood agar or CNA blood agar and EMB agar. Look for star-shaped colonies (yeasts) after 48 hours on EMB agar.

Eye Cultures

Use a sterile cotton swab moistened with sterile saline or broth and pass it over the conjunctiva of the inferior fornix of each eye. Use one half of a blood agar and one half of a mannitol plate for each eye. Material should also be placed into thioglycollate medium. Alternatively, use one of the commercial multiple media plates. Make two conjunctival scrapings and stain one with Gram stain and the other with Giemsa stain.

Skin Cultures

Cultures made from the surface of the epidermis or open ulcers are of little significance, because they usually grow a mixture of nonpathogenic organisms. A culture made from the deep tissue of a biopsy specimen may be helpful in the diagnosis of a bacterial, atypical mycobacterial, or subcutaneous mycotic infection. Diagnostic isolates may be obtained from cultures of tissue sections from ulcers, fistulas, abscesses, enlarged nodes, or granulomatous lesions. Smears and cultures made from exudates of deep fistulas and node aspirates may be useful in some cases.

Intact pustules are satisfactory lesions for making smears and cultures. After the skin surface has been carefully sterilized, the pustule's fluid content may be gently aspirated with a sterile needle and syringe for inoculation into appropriate media; or alternatively, the pustule roof may be opened and a culture taken (by swab) from the fluid inside. In all these procedures, the utmost care must be taken to prevent contamination from tissues outside the area of primary involvement.

When any fluid material or tissue is cultured, it is always desirable to use a portion of the sample to make stained smears. These often provide immediate

Table 85. COMMON BACTERIAL CULTURE RESULTS

Site	Commensals	Pathogens
External ear canal		
Dog	*Pityrosporum, Clostridium, Staphylococcus* (a few), *Bacillus* (a few). Never *Streptococcus, Pseudomonas,* or *Proteus*	Many *Staphylococcus* and *Pityrosporum* together; *Pseudomonas, Proteus, Streptococcus, E. coli*
Cat	Not documented	*Staphylococcus aureus,* μ-hemolytic *Streptococcus, Pasteurella, Pseudomonas, Proteus, E. coli, Pityrosporum*
Skin		
Dog	*Micrococcus, Clostridium,* diphtheroids, *S. epidermidis, Corynebacterium, Pityrosporum*	*S. aureus* (coag. pos.), *Proteus, Pseudomonas, E. coli*
Cat	*Micrococcus, Streptococcus, s. aureus (?), S. epidermidis*	*S. aureus, Pasteurella multocida, Bacteroides, B. fusiformis,* hemolytic *Streptococcus*
Conjunctiva	*Staphylococcus, Streptococcus, Bacillus, Corynebacterium,* diphtheroids, *Neisseria, Pseudomonas*	*S. aureus, Bacillus, Pseudomonas, E. coli, Aspergillus*
Vagina	*Staphylococcus, Streptococcus, Enterococcus, Corynebacterium, E. coli, Hemophilus, Pseudomonas, Peptostreptococcus, Bacteroides*	*Brucella canis;* pure culture of organism (esp. *E. coli, Staphylococcus, Pseudomonas*) when accompanied by tissue reaction at vaginal cytology
Urine	Less than 1000* organisms/ml, presence of several organisms suggests contamination	More than 100,000* organisms/ml and often pure culture. *E. coli,* enterobacteria, *Klebsiella, Proteus, P. aeruginosa, P. multocida, Staphylococcus, Streptococcus*

*Absolute numbers of bacteria depend on the collector technique (see p. 499).

Table 86. LABORATORY DIAGNOSIS OF CANINE VIRAL DISEASES

Virus	Disease	Diagnostic Tests	Preferred Specimens
Canine distemper virus	Canine distemper	H	Intestine, bladder, lung, brain (conjunctiva)
		FA	As above; also footpad biopsy and conjunctival scrapings
		SN	Serum, CSF
		VI	Intestine, bladder, lung, brain (conjunctiva)
Canine adenovirus 1	Infectious canine hepatitis	VI, VN, FA, CF	Liver, urine
		H	Liver, gallbladder
		SN	Serum
Canine adenovirus 2	Respiratory disease complex	VI, VN, FA	Lung, nasal swabs
Parainfluenza 2 virus (SV-5)	Parainfluenza	VI, VN, HI	Nasal swabs
Canine parvovirus	Viral gastroenteritis	H, FA	Small intestine, heart
		EM, VI, HA	Feces, rectal swab
		IFA, SN, HI	Serum
Canine coronavirus	Viral gastroenteritis	EM	Feces
		H	Small intestine
		VI	Small intestine, feces, rectal swab
Canine herpesvirus	Neonatal mortality, reproductive disease	H	Lung, kidney, liver
		VI, VN, FA	Same as above
		SN	Serum
Canine reovirus 1 (2)	Upper respiratory infection (pneumonia); enteritis	VI	Nasal swab, lung, feces
Canine rotavirus	Viral gastroenteritis	EM	Feces
		VI	Feces, small intestine
Rabies virus	Rabies		

H = histopathology	CF = complement fixation	
FA = direct fluorescent antibody test	HI = hemagglutination inhibition	
SN = serum neutralization	EM = electron microscopy	
VI = virus isolation	HA = hemagglutination test	
VN = virus neutralization	IFA = indirect immunofluorescent test	

From Kirk, R. W. (ed.): Current Veterinary Therapy 8: Small Animal Practice. Philadelphia, W. B. Saunders Company, 1983, p. 1147.

Table 87. LABORATORY DIAGNOSIS OF FELINE VIRAL DISEASES

Virus	Disease	Diagnostic Tests	Preferred Specimens
Panleukopenia	Feline distemper	VI	Ileum, spleen, lymph nodes, rectal swab
		EM	Feces
		FA	Ileum, thymus, lymph nodes
		H	Ileum, thymus, liver
		SN	Serum
Herpesvirus 1	Feline viral rhinotracheitis	VI	Nasal, oral, ocular swabs; lung, trachea
		H	Nasal turbinates, lung, trachea
		FA	Nasal scrapings
		SN, PRT	Serum
Calicivirus	Feline caliciviral disease	VI, VN, CF	Nasal, oral, ocular swabs; lung, trachea
		FA, H	Lung, trachea; oral ulcers
		SN, PRT	Serum
Feline leukemia	Lymphoma; FeLV-related diseases	IFA	Blood smears
		ELISA	Blood, serum, plasma
		H	Tumor, lymph nodes, bone marrow
		Cyt	Blood, fluid, bone marrow
		VI	Tumor, blood, bone marrow
Feline coronavirus	Feline infectious peritonitis; enteric disease; kitten mortality (?)	H, (FA)	Kidney, liver, lymph nodes, lung, peritoneum, CNS
		AI	Tissue homogenates (lesions), fluids, blood
		IFA	Serum, fluids
		EM	Feces
Rabies virus	Rabies	H, FA, AI	Brain, salivary glands
		VN	Serum
Reovirus	Conjunctivitis	VI	Ocular swab

VI	= virus isolation	EM	= electron microscopy
FA	= direct fluorescent antibody test	H	= histopathology
SN	= serum neutralization	PRT	= plaque reduction test
VN	= virus neutralization	CF	= complement fixation
IFA	= indirect immunofluorescent test	ELISA	= enzyme-linked immunosorbent assay
Cyt	= cytology	( )	= not very commonly applied
AI	= animal inoculation		

From Kirk, R. W. (ed.): Current Veterinary Therapy 8: Small Animal Practice. Philadelphia, W. B. Saunders Company, 1983, p. 1146.

clues to the diagnosis (organisms present [yeast, bacteria, or fungi] and indications as to the host response [cell types, phagocytosis, or eosinophiles]; see p. 525). Examine the slides for the presence of bacteria and cell morphology.

Culture Results

See Table 85.

Viral Isolations

For basic information about tests used for viral isolations, see Tables 86 and 87.

References and Additional Readings

Carter, G. A.: Diagnostic Procedures in Veterinary Bacteriology and Mycology, 3rd ed. Springfield, Charles C Thomas, 1979.
Comitech Series—Published by American Society for Microbiology, 19131 St., N.W., Wash., D.C. 20006: Comitech 9: Collection and Processing Bacterial Specimens; Comitech 12: Laboratory Diagnosis Bacterial Diarrhea; Comitech 13: Laboratory Diagnosis Ocular Infections; Comitch 15: Laboratory Diagnosis Viral Infections.
Cottral, G. E.: Manual of Standardized Methods for Veterinary Microbiology. Ithaca, N.Y., Comstock Publishing, 1978.
Greene, C. E.: Clinical Microbiology and Infectious Diseases of the Dog and Cat. Philadelphia, W. B. Saunders, 1984.
Hirsh, D. C., Jang, S. S., and Bubetstein, E. L.: Blood culture of the canine patient. J. Am.Vet. Med. Assoc. 184:175–178, 1984.
Lennette, E. H., Ballows, A., Hausler, W. J., et al. (eds.): Manual of Clinical Microbiology, 3rd ed. Washington, D.C., American Society for Microbiology, 1980.

FUNGAL CULTURES

Principles of Collection

Positive cultures depend on proper selection of the culture site, proper collection of specimens, and appropriate use of selective media. Cultures are made from hair, skin, nails, and biopsy tissues.

Hair. If the hair is grossly dirty, it should be cleaned with soap and water; if not, wash it carefully with alcohol. Allow it to dry thoroughly. Select a site at the edge of an active lesion, and look for broken or stubby hairs. Use a forceps (curved Kelly or mosquito hemostats), and epilate hair from these areas by pulling parallel to the direction of the hair growth. It is important to get the hair root and not break off the hair shaft. Pluck many hairs and implant (push) the roots of the hair into the selected agar. The hair shaft should then be gently laid down to contact the surface of the medium. Hairs for inoculation can often be selected by choosing those that fluoresce with a Wood's light.

It is desirable to examine some of the plucked hairs with a potassium hydroxide (KOH) or wet mount preparation for spores, hyphae, and so on. Specimens should never be taken from areas that have been treated within 1 week.

If samples are to be sent to a laboratory, the dry hair can be placed in a clean, tightly sealed envelope and mailed.

Skin. Dermatophyte or yeast infections may affect glabrous skin. If necessary, cleanse culture sites with *alcohol gauze swabs* (cotton will leave excess fibers) and allow to dry. Using a fine scalpel blade, collect superficial scrapings of scales, crusts, and epidermal debris at the periphera of typical lesions. Dermatophytes live in a dry state for several weeks, but yeast infections should be cultured immediately or placed in transport medium to prevent drying.

Nails. Although hard keratin fungal infections are rare in animals, diseased nails should be avulsed, scraped, or ground into fine pieces for collection in a sterile Petri dish. Pieces can be examined directly for arthrospores or hyphae and placed on appropriate media for culture.

Tissue Biopsy. Tissue core or excision samples can be sliced and the newly exposed surface used for impression smears or inoculation of media. They also may be chopped or ground and placed in media. Small amounts should be placed in sterile saline or broth for referral to an appropriate laboratory for further processing.

Dermatophyte Media. Sabouraud's dextrose agar has been used traditionally in veterinary mycology for isolation of fungi; however, other media are available with bacterial and fungal inhibitors, such as dermatophyte test medium (DTM), potato dextrose agar, and rice grain medium. Mycosel and mycobiotic agar are formulations of Sabouraud's dextrose agar with cycloheximide and chloramphenicol added to inhibit fungal and bacterial contaminants. If a medium with cycloheximide is used, fungi sensitive to it will not be isolated. Some organisms sensitive to cycloheximide include *Cryptococcus neoformans*, many members of the Zygomycota, some *Candida* species, *Aspergillus* species, *Pseudoallescheria boydii*, and many agents of phaeohyphomycosis. DTM is essentially a Sabouraud's dextrose agar containing cycloheximide, gentamicin, and chlortetracycline as antifungal and antibacterial agents. The pH indicator phenol red has been added. Dermatophytes use protein in the medium first, with alkaline metabolites turning the medium red in color. When the protein is exhausted, the dermatophytes use carbohydrates, giving off acid metabolites. The medium's red color returns to yellow. Most other fungi use carbohydrate first, and only later, protein; so they too may produce a red change in DTM, but only after a prolonged incubation (10–14 days or more). Consequently, DTM cultures should be examined daily for the first 10 days. Fungi such as *Blastomyces dermatitidis, Sporothrix schenckii, Histoplasma capsulatum, Coccidioides immitis, Pseudoallescheria boydii*, some *Aspergillus* species, and others may cause a red change in DTM, so microscopic examination is essential to avoid an erroneous presumptive diagnosis. Because DTM may depress development of conidia, may mask colony pigmentation, and may inhibit some pathogens, fungi recovered on DTM should be transferred to plain Sabouraud's dextrose agar for identification.

Text continued on page 517

Table 88. MICROSCOPIC APPEARANCE OF FUNGI IN THE TISSUE

Disease	Microscopic Examination	Appearance in Tissue
Aspergillosis	Wet mount	Septate hyphae; sometimes mature fruiting heads may be seen
Candidiasis and other yeast infections	Wet mount	Budding and nonbudding yeasts; pseudohyphae may be present
Dermatophytosis (ringworm)	Hematologic stain	Best for smears of yeasts from dog's ears Hair: arthrospores, hyphae, or sheath of spores around hair; skin and nails: arthropores, hyphae
Mycetoma (eumycotic)	Wet mount	Crush granules, observe for dark brown chlamydospores and clear (hyaline) hyphae
Phaeohyphomycosis	Wet mount	Dark hyphae
Rhinosporidiosis	Fluorescent antibody	Spherules (some very large) with and without endospores
Sporotrichosis	Gram or hematologic stain	Yeasts
		These stains may demonstrate yeasts occasionally
Zygomycosis (phycomycosis)	Wet mount	Broad, relatively nonseptate hyphae
	Fungi Causing Systemic Infection	
Blastomycosis	Wet mount	Thick-walled budding yeast; bud has broad base at attachment to mother cell
Coccidioidomycosis	Wet mount	Spherules with and without endospores
Cryptococcosis	India ink and water	Encapsulated yeast
Histoplasmosis	Hematologic stain	Small yeast with narrow neck where bud attaches; found in macrophages and other RE cells
	Actinomycetes Causing Infection	
Actinomycosis	Grain stain (view under oil)	Gram-positive, branching filaments; some show beading; clubs may be seen
	Water mount of flakes or granules (40×)	Clubs
Nocardiosis	Gram stain (view under oil)	Same as Actinomycosis
	Hank's or cold Kinyoun acid-fast stain with 1% Aq H_2SO_4 as decolorizer (oil)	Some nocardiae are totally to partially acid fast; lack of acid fastness does not rule out *Nocardia*
Dermatophilosis	Hematologic stain (view under oil)	Branched tapered filaments that divide transversely and longitudinally to form packets of coccoid cells; sometimes only packets of cells or sparsely scattered cells are found

From Kirk, R. W. (ed.): Current Veterinary Therapy 8: Small Animal Practice. Philadelphia, W. B. Saunders Company, 1983. p. 1159.

Table 89. SEROLOGIC TESTS IN SYSTEMIC FUNGAL DISEASE

	Immunodiffusion (ID)	Complement Fixation (CF)	Counter Immunoelectrophoresis (CIE)	Latex Agglutination (LA)	ELISA	Passive Hemagglutination (PHA)	Tube Precipitation (TP)
Aspergillosis	Used for noninvasive, most widely used test, A. *fumigatus*, A. *flavus*, A. *niger*						
No good test for invasive Aspergillosis except histology							
B. dermatitidis							
Serology testing unreliable, confirm by demonstrating organisms in tissues	Test being done at CDC; commercial kit not proved useful	Titer 1:8 or greater positive (only 50% accurate) cross reactions ocur with *Coccidioides immitis*					
Coccidioidomycosis							
Reaction to coccidioidin which is mycelial-arthrospore antigen; confirm by demonstrating organisms in tissues	Available (IDTP test); detects IgM precipitins	Available; four-fold rise in CF titer is confirmatory; CF titer 1:16 or more suggestive of disseminated infection					Detects positive circulating IgM antibody during 2–3 of illness; *never* performed on CSF

Table continued on following page

Table 89. SEROLOGIC TESTS IN SYSTEMIC FUNGAL DISEASE *(Continued)*

	Immunodiffusion (ID)	Complement Fixation (CF)	Counter Immunoelectrophoresis (CIE)	Latex Agglutination (LA)	ELISA	Passive Hemagglutination (PHA)	Tube Precipitation (TP)
Cryptococcosis Testing for cryptococcal polysaccharide capsular antigen		Available	Available	Highest sensitivity LA test; can be used on CSF; titers 1:8 or greater are diagnostic		Available	
Histoplasmosis Elevated titers may not be evident in fulminant disseminated disease; RIA test also becoming available; titers greater than 1:16 are significant	Available; simpler than CF	Most available; serologic test to antibodies to yeast phase; serum reaction 1:32 or greater or four-fold increase in titer diagnosis	Available Simpler than CF	False positives in LA test; 50%			

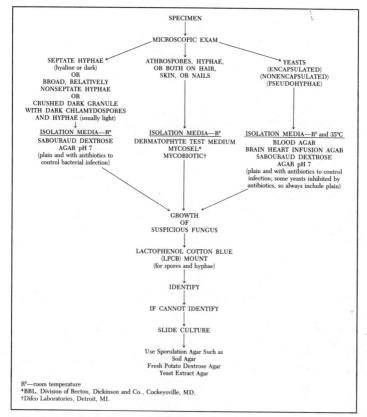

Figure 63. Processing clinical specimens for yeasts, ringworm, and opportunistic fungus infections in veterinary medicine. (From Kirk, R. W.: Current Veterinary Therapy VIII: Small Animal Practice. Philadelphia, W. B. Saunders Company, 1983, p. 1160.)

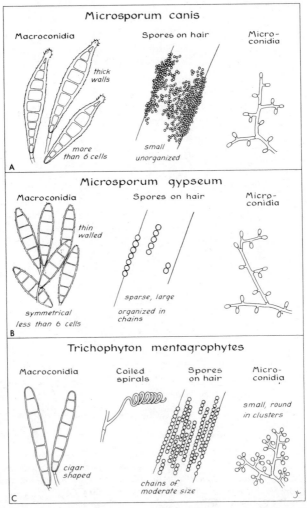

Figure 64. Characteristic microscopic morphologies A, *Microsporum canis*; B, *M. gypseum*; C, *Trichophyton mentagrophytes*. The conidia and spirals are microscopic structures. The hair shafts are much larger. (From Muller, G. H., Kirk, R. M., and Scott, D. W.: Small Animal Dermatology, 3rd ed. Philadelphia, W. B. Saunders Company, 1983, p. 256.)

Potato dextrose agar is useful for promoting sporulation and observing pigmentation. On potato dextrose agar, *Microsporum canis* has a lemon-yellow pigment, whereas *Microsporum audouinii* has a salmon- or peach-colored pigment. Rice agar medium promotes conidia formation in some dermatophytes, especially *Microsporum canis* strains, which produce no conidia on Sabouraud's dextrose agar.

Skin scrapings, nails, and hair should be inoculated onto Sabouraud's dextrose agar, DTM, mycosel, or mycobiotic agar. Cultures should be incubated at 30°C with 30 per cent humidity. A pan of water in the incubator will usually provide enough humidity. Cultures should be checked every 2 to 3 days for fungal growth. DTM may be incubated for 10 to 14 days, but cultures on Sabouraud's dextrose agar should be allowed 30 days to develop.

Practitioners can usually successfully culture and identify dermatophytes in their hospital laboratories.

Diagnosis should depend on characteristic gross culture identification and careful inspection of elements from those cultures using slide preparations and slide cultures for microscopic examination. Tables 88 and 89 and Figures 63 and 64 may be helpful guides. References by Attleberger, McGinnis, McGinnis, et al., and Muller, et al. will provide more detail, if needed.

Fungi other than dermatophytes should probably be cultured by commercial or institutional laboratories with appropriate equipment and special expertise.

References and Additional Readings

Attleberger, M. H.: Practical diagnostic procedures for mycotic diseases. *In* Kirk, R. W. (ed.): Current Veterinary Therapy 8: Small Animal Practice. Philadelphia, W. B. Saunders Company, 1983, p. 1157.

Carter, G. R.: Diagnostic Procedures in Veterinary Bacteriology and Mycology, 3rd ed. Springfield, Illinois, Charles C Thomas, Publisher, 1979.

Jawetz, E., Melnick, J. L., and Adelberg, E. A.: Review of Medical Microbiology, 10th ed. Palo Alto, California, Lange Medical Publications, 1972.

McGinnis, M. R.: Laboratory Handbook of Medical Mycology. New York, Academic Press, Inc., 1980.

McGinnis, M. R., D'Amato, R. F., and Land, G. A.: Pictorial Handbook of Medically Important Fungi and Aerobic Actinomycetes. New York, Praeger Press, 1982.

Muller, G. H., Kirk, R. W., and Scott, D. W.: Small Animal Dermatology, 3rd ed. Philadelphia, W. B. Saunders Company, 1983.

Penn, R. L., Lambert, R. S., and George, R. B.: Invasive fungal infections. Arch. Int. Med., *143*:1215, 1983.

DERMATOLOGIC DIAGNOSTIC PROCEDURES

Skin Scrapings

This is a frequently used diagnostic procedure performed to find and identify microscopic parasites or fungal elements in the skin. Material required is mineral oil in a small dropper bottle, a dull scalpel blade, glass slides, cover slips, and a microscope.

Select undisturbed, untreated skin for a scraping site. It is best to scrape the periphery of skin lesions and avoid the excoriated or traumatized center areas. In scraping for demodectic mange, a small fold of affected skin should be gently pinched and the surface material collected for examinations. This procedure forces the mites out of the hair follicles and onto or near the skin surface. In scraping for sarcoptic mange, large areas should be scraped. Select sites on the elbows, hocks, and ear margins when searching for sarcoptic mange. Many or frequent scrapings may be necessary to demonstrate sarcoptic mange mites or their fecal pellets or eggs.

The accumulated material is placed on a microscope slide and mixed with a small drop of mineral oil. Examine the entire area with a 10X objective thoroughly and carefully. Dry keratin and dead hairs.may also be accumulated by scraping for inoculation of fungal cultures.

Wood's Light Evaluation

Ultraviolet light filtered through nickel oxide produces a beam called *Wood's light*. If an animal is taken into a dark room and its hair and skin are exposed to a Wood's light, fluorescence may show for several reasons. Hair shafts affected by some species of *Microsporum* fungi fluoresce a bright yellow-green (such as the color of a fluorescing watch face). However, iodide medications, petroleum, soap, dyes, and even keratin may produce purple-, blue-, or yellow-colored fluorescence. The positive fungal fluorescence is a valuable aid in selecting affected hairs for culture inoculation. Remember, a negative fluorescence does not eliminate a possible diagnosis of fungal infection. There are both false negatives and false positives.

Acetate (Scotch) Tape Preparation

This is one of the simplest diagnostic procedures. Bend clear (not frosted) acetate tape into a loop around the fingers with the sticky side facing out. Part the animal's hair coat, and press the tape firmly onto the skin and hair. The sticky tape picks up all loose particles it contacts. Cut the loop of tape and place the strip of tape, sticky side down, on a clean microscope slide. Use a low-power microscope to look through the tape at the collected particles. This is an excellent technique for trapping and identifying biting and sucking lice, *Otodectes* and *Cheyletiella* mites, flea dirt and larvae, fly larvae, or dandruff scales.

Acetate (Scotch) tape also is useful in studying hair abnormalities. Use a strong hemostat to securely clamp and quickly avulse a group of 10 to 20 hair shafts. The pointed distal ends can be pressed onto sticky acetate tape (lined up like pickets in a fence), and the hair shafts can be cut off in the middle with a scissors. The butt ends with the hair roots are likewise pressed onto another piece of tape. The tape holding the hair is then pressed onto a microscope slide to allow low-power examination of the hairs through the clear tape. The hairs will be well oriented and controlled; thus, it is easy to evaluate whether they are split, broken, or bitten off and whether the roots are in the anogen or telogen growth stages.

Bacterial Culture (See pages 499–503)

Fungal Culture (See pages 510–517)

Direct and Impression Smears

This simple, direct, and inexpensive technique may reveal significant information within a short period of time. Cytologic examination can be made of material obtained from pustules, vesicles, or the raw, ulcerated, or cut surfaces of a lesion. To make the smear, press a clean microscope slide firmly against a raw or ulcerated lesion to transfer cellular material to the slide. Exudates may be collected by sterile swab or aspirated into a sterile syringe. Roll the swab gently across the slide, or place a drop of fluid from the syringe onto the slide and carefully spread the fluid in a uniform film. Material from a block of tissue can be transferred to the slide by gently pressing the tissue onto the slide in several locations. Use various stains for different conditions.

Rapid stains such as new methylene blue or Diff-Quick are useful and convenient for office procedures, but even Wright's or Gram's stains used for evaluation of bacterial infections are easy to use. Presence of many bacteria, especially mixed types, may mean only surface contamination, whereas single types of bacteria, abundant polymorphonuclear leukocytes, and especially phagocytosis support the diagnosis of infection and the host's response to it. A *few* acantholytic cells (loose epidermal cells) in the smear may be compatible with infectious processes, but large numbers, or "rafts," of acantholytic cells are highly suggestive of autoimmune disorders and imply the need for more complex tests for positive diagnosis.

Large numbers of eosinophils are sometimes found in stained smears. Contrary to popular opinion, they usually do not mean allergy or parasites. They may be associated with the eosinophilic granuloma complex, superficial eosinophilic pustulosis, pemphigus complex, bacterial folliculitis (if ruptured follicle causes a tissue reaction to keratin), and sometimes dermatophytosis. Lactophenol cotton blue and periodic acid–Schiff (PAS) stains enhance the recognition of spores and mycelia, although even new methylene blue or Diff-Quick may be useful in examining hairs, skin, scrapings, and ear smears. Candida and Malassezia *(Pityrosporon)* yeasts are commonly found as budding cells in masses of wax and debris from ear smears.

Tumor cells may be recognized in some impression or aspiration samples where Giemsa is a preferred stain. Although special expertise is needed, cases of mastocytoma, histiocytoma, lymphoma, and "round cell tumors" are most easily recognized. Formalin-fixed tissues for histologic diagnosis should always be prepared in tumor evaluations.

Skin Biopsy

Histologic examination of diseased skin can serve as a means for diagnosis of cutaneous lesions. The etiologic agent is often found in both acute and chronic skin infections.

Core biopsy of the skin is a quick and accurate way to remove a small sample of diseased skin for histopathologic examination. Select a site that is well developed but not traumatized or excoriated. The sample should include both normal and diseased tissue (i.e., biopsy the periphery of the lesion). If the lesion (pustule, vesicle) can be identified early in its development and if only the lesion is biopsied, one may obtain a superior specimen. It is best not to take too large a sample that contains much normal skin. By mistake, the technician might take a section that misses the lesion. Proper selection of the biopsy site is crucial to accurate diagnosis. The hair should be carefully clipped from the lesion. The skin should be lightly blotted with 70 per cent alcohol. Avoid superficial trauma while cleaning the skin. A small subcutaneous bleb should be made with 0.5 per cent lidocaine to deaden the area. Special equipment needed for the biopsy is a 9-mm Keyes punch and 10 per cent formalin solution. After the area has been anesthetized with lidocaine, press and rotate the Keyes punch through the skin until the subcutaneous tissue is penetrated. Remove the biopsy specimen by "spearing" it with a fine needle. Do not grasp it with a forceps. Blot it gently between two pieces of paper towel. Spread the tissue out gently (like a pancake), place the specimen epidermal side up on a piece of cardboard, press it gently to cause adhesion, and drop the specimen into the formalin fixative. The skin defect may be closed with one or two simple interrupted sutures. If deep tissue biopsies are needed, a core biopsy is inadequate. Use a small (No. 15) scalpel blade to obtain an appropriate sample. In all cases in which skin biopsies are made, *multiple* samples should be taken to increase the odds that at least one will have diagnostic lesions. Specimens submitted to laboratories should be accompanied by extensive, detailed clinical information, including a differential diagnosis. Skin biopsies are routinely stained with hematoxylin-eosin (H&E); however, PAS, Gridley's, Gomori's methenamine silver (GMS), and Verhoeff's stains are used for special problems.

Skin Allergy Tests

The intradermal skin test can be used as a means of identifying specific allergens capable of inducing immediate hypersensitivities in dogs. The test will not routinely give positive reactions for delayed hypersensitivities such as those from allergic contact dermatitis. Also, the test has not proved accurate for food-induced allergic dermatitis. Other diagnostic methods such as provocative exposure or patch testing must be used to identify the allergen causing food allergy or contact dermatitis.

Test antigens are purchased in concentrations of 1000 or 1500 PNU per ml. Aqueous antigens are ordered from the manufacturer of human test antigens. The following antigen groups are suggested for routine testing:

Seasonal Allergens (contents of list will vary according to locale; for helpful suggestions contact a local physician allergist).

1. Trees
   a. #1 Tree mix (maple, oak, sycamore, willow)
   b. #2 Tree mix (oak, cottonseed, elm)
   c. #3 Tree mix (hickory, pecan, walnut, beech, birch)

2. Flowers (individual allergens)
   Rose, asters, chrysanthemum, sunflower
3. Grasses
   a. 7 Grass mix (orchard grass, timothy, Kentucky bluegrass, sweet vernal, perennial rye, red top, mixed fescues)
   b. Alfalfa
4. Weeds (individual allergens)
   Sorrel, dock, English plantain, lamb's-quarters, cocklebur, marsh elder, pigweed, spiny pigweed, Kochia, goldenrod, dandelion, mixed ragweed.
5. Fleas

Nonseasonal Allergens

1. Molds (individual allergens)
   Alternaria, Stemphyllium, *Aspergillus*, Mucor, *Penicillium*, Hormodendrum, *Helminthosporium*, Rhizopus, Phoma beta, Epicoccum, Pullaria, Cephalosporium, Botrytis, Fusarium
2. Miscellaneous (individual allergens)
   a. House dust*, barn dust, mixed epidermals, cat dander, human dander, mixed feathers* (chicken, duck, goose), tobacco, cottonseed, newsprint, wool, kapok
   b. Staphylococcus toxoid AB
3. Control Agents
   a. Negative control—diluent or buffered saline
   b. Positive control—histamine phosphate

A negative diluent control and a positive histamine phosphate control are used. Two weeks prior to testing, the animal should be taken off all corticosteroids, antihistamines, and tranquilizers. One to 2 months or longer may be necessary if a long-acting steroid has been given. If there is doubt, a test with histamine can be made to demonstrate the animal's reactivity. The animal should not be tranquilized for the procedure, but it can be given Rompun or can be anesthetized with short-acting barbiturates, if necessary. If the animal is firmly restrained on its side on a comfortable pad and its head is covered with a towel to obscure its vision, it will usually lie quietly after a few moments. Gently clip the hair from the lateral thorax, and do not prep the skin. Make intradermal injections of 0.1 ml of each antigen and each control. Use a 25-gauge 3/8-inch needle attached to a 1-ml disposable syringe. Space the injections about 4 cm apart, and mark each one with a felt pen. The reactions are recorded in terms of cm and are read immediately and again at intervals of 15 minutes and 1 hour after the injection. Flea and staphylococcal injections are also read at 24 hours. A reaction 1 cm larger than the negative control indicates a positive reaction. The histamine control should be diluted 1:10 with saline (1:100,000 histamine phosphate) before injection. This dilution will give a good 4+ reaction (2 cm larger than negative control) in most dogs and is necessary to show that the patient is capable of responding to histamine.

---

*House dust and feathers produce significant reactions in many normal dogs, so they might be omitted from regular tests.

A positive reaction indicates that the patient is hypersensitive to the test antigen or to a similar antigen. A negative reaction could mean any of the following: (1) the patient was not sensitive to the antigens used; (2) the antigen used was not present in sufficient quantity to give a positive reaction (combination antigens); (3) the patient is allergic but does not possess sufficient reagin antibody to give a positive skin test reaction; (4) an improper technique was used; or (5) inhibitory effects of other medications interfered.

One should always remember that a negative skin test does not mean that the patient is not allergic. Positive reactions can be false, too (e.g., feathers, fleas); therefore, the test reactions should correlate with the history if one expects to achieve good results from hyposensitization.

The National Pollen Calendar is helpful in correlating history and reactions with allergens. It is available in the third edition of this text or from manufacturers' of allergy test kits.

Allergy skin testing is expensive and requires dedication, interest, and the experience of many cases to make it a useful diagnostic method. If the clinician is not interested in allergic states and does not see a lot of allergy cases he or she should refer the cases to someone who is more familiar with such cases.

References and Additional Readings

Anderson, W.: Canine Allergic Inhalent Dermatitis. St. Louis, Ralston Purina Co., 1975.

Baker, K. P.: Intradermal tests as an aid to the diagnosis of skin disease in dogs. J. Small Anim. Pract., *12*:445, 1971.

Chamberlain, K. W. (ed.): Allergy in small animal practice. Vet. Clin. North. Am., 4:1974.

Lever, W. F., and Schaumburg-Lever, G.: Histopathology of the Skin, 5th ed. Philadelphia, J. B. Lippincott Co., 1975.

Muller, G. H., Kirk, R. W., and Scott, D. W.: Small Animal Dermatology, 3rd ed., Philadelphia, W. B. Saunders Company, 1983.

Scott, D. W.: Observations on canine atopy. J.A.A.H.A., *17*:91, 1981.

Willemse, A., and vander Brom, W. E.: Evaluation of the intradermal allergy test in normal dogs. Res. Vet. Sci., *32*:57, 1982.

ABDOMINAL PARACENTESIS

Abdominal paracentesis refers to the surgical puncture of the abdominal cavity in order to remove fluids. When removing abdominal fluid, always weigh the animal before and after the procedure. Any subsequent gain in weight indicates a reaccumulation of abdominal fluid. Place the animal in left lateral recumbency and restrain it in this position (Fig. 65). Clip and surgically prepare a 1- to 3-inch square between the bladder and the umbilicus just lateral to the midline. If the bladder is distended, empty it before paracentesis is performed. Infiltrate the paracentesis site with Xylocaine, 0.5 per cent, using a 22- to 24-gauge needle. Abdominal puncture can be made with a 14- to 20-gauge needle. When the abdominal puncture has been made, the animal should be allowed

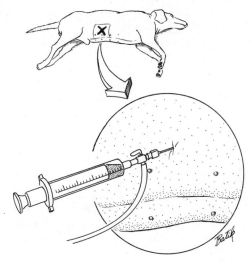

Figure 65. A 3-inch square to the right of the midline between the bladder and umbilicus had been clipped and surgically prepared. Paracentesis is performed using a needle and a three-way valve to facilitate fluid collection.

to stand; this will facilitate drainage of the fluid. Aspiration may be easier if a specially adapted needle with multiple holes drilled in the shaft is used, because it is less likely to become plugged with omentum. An excellent commercial needle is Kormed's Mini Lazarus-Nelson Peritoneal Lavage Kit-MLNK 9001.* Measure the amount of fluid obtained, and examine the fluid to determine whether it is an exudate or transudate. Cytologic examination and culture may also be performed.

THORACENTESIS AND PERICARDICENTESIS

Thoracentesis refers to the aspiration of fluid or air from the thoracic cavity. The procedure may be performed for diagnostic or therapeutic purposes. When fluid or air is present, it may be impossible to remove all of it; however, either of the two should be removed as much as possible. If repeated withdrawal of air or fluid from the chest is contemplated, a chest tube is safer. Clip and surgically prepare the thoracic wall from the fifth to the eighth intercostal spaces. If fluid or air is present on only one side of the thoracic cavity (a rarity in dogs and cats), only that side should be aspirated. If fluid is to be aspirated,

*Kormed Inc., 2510 Northland Dr., St. Paul, Minnesota 55120.

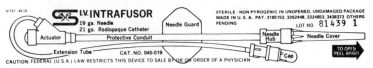

Figure 66. IV Intrafusor: Catalogue #045–014, Sorenson Research Company, Salt Lake City, Utah.

infiltrate Xylocaine, 0.5 per cent into a spot low in the seventh intercostal space using a 1-inch, 22- to 24-gauge needle. Then fit an 18- to 20-gauge needle in a two-way stopcock, which in turn is fitted to a 20-ml sterile syringe. Insert the needle into the thoracic cavity until the tip is just through the pleura but does not lacerate the lung. Any fluid aspirated should be saved and analyzed to determine whether it is a transudate or an exudate. A safer and better way of removing quantities of fluid from the thoracic or pericardial cavity is the use of the IV intrafusor system (Fig. 66).* Needles in this system are available in 14 and 15 gauge, with a radiopaque, through-the-needle catheter attached. The catheter can be passed through the needle in the appropriate cavity, the needle removed, and a three-way valve used to remove fluid or air.

In dogs requiring repeated aspirations of air or fluid from the chest, the suprapubic Cystocath† drainage system works well. Prepare the chest wall over the sixth to eighth intercostal spaces by clipping and surgical preparation. Starting at the sixth rib, make a small incision in the skin and slide the special trocar/cannula to the middle of the dorsal eighth intercostal space. Push the trocar into the chest cavity, leave the cannula in place, and clamp the cannula after removing the trocar. Place the silicone catheter into the chest cavity, attach a three-way valve and a syringe, and aspirate air. Tape the cannula and catheter to the chest wall.

Cytologic examination may be performed and cultures taken of this fluid. Thoracentesis in pneumothorax is carried out in the same manner as the aspiration of fluid; however, because air rises in the thoracic cavity, the thoracentesis puncture should be made high up in the seventh intercostal space.

Pericardicentesis involves the surgical puncture of the pericardium in order to aspirate effusions. Sedate the animal with morphine or a neuroleptanalgesic agent. Surgically prepare both sides of the thorax. Place the animal in lateral recumbency with the right side down. Infiltrate the muscles of the fourth intercostal space at a level with the junction of the ventral and middle thirds of the thorax with Xylocaine, 1 per cent, using a 22-gauge needle. Use a Venocath (16-gauge needle) or an Intrafusor system; place a three-way stopcock on the syringe adapter end of the Venocath. Have an assistant place

*IV Intrafusor, Sorenson Research Company, Salt Lake City, Utah.
†Silastic Cystocath Suprapubic Drainage System, Dow Corning Corp., Midland, Michigan 48640. This system can be reused after cleaning and gas autoclaving.

a 30-ml syringe on the three-way stopcock, and maintain negative pressure on the syringe as the chest is entered. Carefully advance the 16-gauge Intracath needle into the fourth intercostal space, advancing toward the heart, while maintaining negative pressure in the syringe. When fluid enters the syringe, the pericardial sac has been entered. Thread the Intracath polyethylene tubing through the 16-gauge needle so that the end of the tubing lies securely within the pericardial sac, and remove the needle from the intrathoracic space. Continue aspirating fluid. This technique should prevent trauma to the myocardium. Electrocardiographic (ECG) monitoring during pericardicentesis will also warn of trauma to the myocardium. The Intracath tube can be heparinized and the stopcock closed and taped to the body wall, and repeated aspirations can be performed over several days, if necessary. All aspirated fluid should be examined as described on p. 807.

BIOPSY TECHNIQUES

Numerous types of biopsy techniques are available, and the selection of the appropriate technique is based on the tissue to be biopsied, the condition of the patient, and the skill of the examiner.

Excisional Biopsy. This technique refers to the surgical removal of the entire lesion and histologic examination. Excisional biopsy is most frequently used on skin lesions (see Skin Biopsies, p. 519) and in cases in which an entire organ may have to be removed (such as an eye or an internal organ that has developed a tumor).

Incisional Biopsy. This technique refers to the surgical removal of a *portion* of a lesion. A representative area of the lesion should be chosen for biopsy. Include lesion margins, if possible.

Needle Aspiration Biopsy. In this form of biopsy, a variety of needles and a syringe are used to remove a small amount of tissue from the body.

Various types of needles are available for biopsy. The selection of type, gauge, and length of the needle should be based on the site of the biopsy and the characteristics of the tissues to be biopsied. Thick-walled needles with stylet are needed for collecting material from bone and sclerotic tissue. On the other hand, fine-needle aspiration can be used in soft tissues. A 25-gauge needle and 12-ml syringe can be used. The length of the needle is dependent on the location of the tissue biopsied. The Menghini needle is a coring and aspirating biopsy needle. It has an extremely thin wall and a 45-degree convex cutting edge. The needle is available in diameters of 1.0, 1.2, and 1.4 mm and lengths of 3.5 and 7.0 cm. Although only a small number of cells can be obtained, the danger of trauma to tissues with resultant postbiopsy complications is greatly reduced. Needles are available that will remove a small core of tissue by a cutting action. When the overall architecture of a tissue is important in making a diagnosis, a punch (core) biopsy is preferable to a needle biopsy.

Touch imprints is the term referred to when an incised tissue mass has been cut revealing a fresh surface and the mass is gently blotted onto glass slides imprinting cells. *Scrapings* are the result of a scalpel blade or "spatula"-type blade that has scraped the surface of a lesion, thus obtaining exfoliated cells for examination.

Characteristics of Cellular Malignancy

1. Enlargement of nucleus—nuclei larger than 10 microns.
2. Increase in nuclear cytoplasmic ratio.
3. Multinucleation because of abnormal mitosis.
4. Abnormal or frequent mitosis.
5. Variations in size and shape of nuclei.
6. Increase in size and number of nucleoli.
7. Increased basophilia of cellular cytoplasm—increased RNA content.

Needle Punch Biopsy

In this technique, a core or plug of tissue is removed by the cutting action of the biopsy instrument. Both cells and the supporting architecture of the tissue are removed. Examples of needles available for punch biopsies are (1) Franklin-modified Vim-Silverman needle—This needle has an outside 14-gauge cannula and an inner stylet and cutting prongs. (2) Tru-Cut Disposable Biopsy Needle.

Lymph Node Biopsy

Lymph node biopsy is used (1) in generalized lymphadenopathy, (2) in focal lymphadenopathy of unknown etiology, and (3) in suspected instances of tumor metastases. Surgically prepare the skin over the node to be biopsied. With one hand, localize and immobilize the lymph node; with the opposite hand, guide the aspiration biopsy needle into the affected node. Affix a syringe onto the needle and advance the needle into the lymph node. When the needle is in position in the node, gradually draw negative pressure on the syringe. Cellular material within the needle is ejected onto clean glass slides. Lymph node aspirates must be handled gently. To make slides, place two slides together ("squash" sample) and pull the slides apart to avoid shearing the cells.

Lymph node biopsy can be made by excisional or punch (core) techniques, if desired.

Lung Biopsy

Percutaneous aspiration needle biopsy and punch (core) biopsy can be helpful in establishing a diagnosis in many conditions such as (1) chronic inflammatory disease of the lung—for example, granulomatous lung disease caused by mycotic organisms; (2) chronic inflammatory disease; (3) metastatic lung disease; and (4) primary lung tumors. Biopsy may provide enough diagnostic information to preclude performing an exploratory thoracotomy. Lung biopsy is contraindicated in animals with hemorrhagic disease or thoracic disease that produces forceful breathing and coughing.

The biopsy site is clipped and surgically prepared. The skin, subcutaneous tissue, muscle, and parietal pleura are infiltrated with 1 to 2 per cent lidocaine.

In diffuse parenchymal lung disease, it is recommended that the diaphragmatic lobes be biopsied. The dorsal portions of the seventh to ninth intercostal spaces are preferred for percutaneous biopsies. In diffuse lesions, the right lung should be biopsied.

Fewer complications occur with a percutaneous aspiration biopsy than with a punch biopsy; however, a lung aspirate will yield only cells, fluid, and small pieces of tissue. A 20-gauge, 1½-inch disposable needle (such as a Yale spinal needle) with stylet can be used for thoracic aspiration biopsy.

The stylet is left in the needle until the lung substance has been entered. The stylet is then quickly removed, a gloved finger placed over the needle opening to prevent air from entering the thoracic cavity, and a 10- to 20-ml syringe placed on the needle. Using suction and a back-and-forth movement of the needle, the lung material is aspirated.

Contraindications for fine-needle aspiration are bleeding diathesis and coagulopathy, uncontrolled coughing, pulmonary hypertension, pulmonary cysts, and bullous emphysema.

TRANSTRACHEAL ASPIRATION BIOPSY

Transtracheal aspiration provides a safe and clinically useful method for obtaining material for cytologic and bacteriologic examination from the lower respiratory tract of medium to large dogs without invading the oral cavity. The technique can be performed on the unanesthetized animal, although some sedation may be necessary in fractious animals. In small dogs and cats, tracheal aspirates are collected by passing the catheter through sterile tracheal tubes. Light levels of anesthesia are used to accommodate coughing as well as tracheal intubation.

Place the animal in sternal recumbency and elevate and extend the head. Clip the area around the larynx and surgically prepare the skin. The cricothyroid membrane is located by moving the finger cranially along the trachea until the large ventral ridge of the cricoid cartilage is felt. Cranial to this ridge is a triangular depression, the cricothyroid membrane. Use a 16-gauge, 12-inch intravenous (IV) catheter to collect material through the trachea (Fig. 67). Puncture the cricothyroid membrane with the 16-gauge needle, and pass the catheter into the trachea until it reaches the distal trachea or mainstem bronchus. (Alternatively, in large dogs, the catheter can be inserted between the tracheal rings at the junction of the middle third and distal third of the cervical trachea.) Withdraw the needle and leave the catheter in place. Attach a 12-ml syringe containing sterile saline solution to the catheter. Expel 1 to 2

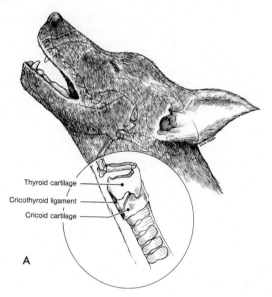

Thyroid cartilage

Cricothyroid ligament

Cricoid cartilage

A

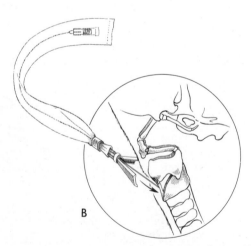

B

Figure 67. A, Diagrammatic representation of anatomic structures involved with transtracheal aspiration technique. The best landmark for percutaneous puncture is the cricothyroid ligament of the larynx, although the tracheal lumen can also be entered between cervical tracheal rings. B, The needle is advanced and directed slightly caudal until the trachea is entered. Once the needle is positioned within the tracheal lumen, the catheter is advanced through the needle and down the trachea. (From Kirk, R. W.: Current Veterinary Therapy VIII: Small Animal Practice, Philadelphia, W. B. Saunders Company, 1983, p. 223.)

ml of saline from the syringe. When the animal coughs, aspirate the syringe to collect cells and mucus for bacteriologic and cytologic examination. When material has been collected, remove the catheter and bandage the animal's neck. Material present in the syringe is cultured in blood agar and in thioglycollate medium. Prepare material from aspiration for cytologic examination. Large plugs of mucus are pressed between two clean glass slides, and thin smears are stained with either Wright's or Giemsa stain.

Complications of transtracheal aspiration biopsy include catheter trauma to the lower airway or needle trauma to the larynx, resulting in bleeding, subcutaneous emphysema, pneumomediastinum, pneumothorax, or airway obstruction.

References and Additional Readings

Bauer, T., and Thomas, W. P.: Pulmonary diagnostic techniques. Vet. Clin. North Am., *13*(2):273, 1983.
Roudebush, P., Green, R., and Digilio, K. M.: Percutaneous fine-needle aspiration of the lung in disseminated pulmonary disease. J.A.A.H.A., *17*(1):109, 1981.

BIOPSY OF THE LIVER

The diagnosis of liver disease can be made based on clinical signs coupled with clinical pathologic findings found when performing a "liver profile." The development of a more specific diagnosis and prognosis in liver disease may be greatly aided by information obtained in a liver biopsy. Liver biopsies are of much greater value in generalized liver disease such as cirrhosis, generalized acute hepatic necrosis, or amyloidosis than in focal hepatic disease. The major indications for performing a liver biopsy are (1) to explain abnormal liver profile, (2) to define reasons for abnormal liver size, (3) to identify possible liver tumor, (4) to obtain a prognosis and rational approach for management, and (5) to identify the cause of ascites.

There are numerous procedures for obtaining liver tissue; however, needle biopsy of the liver, when performed properly, can be very helpful. Careful physical and clinical pathologic examination should precede a liver biopsy. Abnormalities in normal hemostatic mechanisms should be detected and corrected prior to needle biopsy of the liver. Contraindications for hepatic biopsy are (1) possible hemorrhage associated with coagulation abnormality, (2) suspicion of hepatic abscess or cyst, and (3) extrahepatic biliary obstruction.

Equipment

Equipment necessary for liver biopsy includes the following:
1. Local anesthetic.
2. Franklin-modified Vim-Silverman or similar biopsy needle.
3. Cutdown tray (sterile).
4. Suitable fixative for tissue specimen.

Technique

Percutaneous needle biopsy of the liver can be performed under effective sedation and local anesthesia, but general anesthesia is recommended in most cases. Biopsy sites in the liver can best be selected when needle biopsy techniques are done in conjunction with laparoscopy. Blind percutaneous needle biopsies of the liver are easily performed when the liver is enlarged and easily palpated. If the liver is not palpable, blind percutaneous transabdominal and transthoracic liver biopsies should be performed only by experienced clinicians.

A modified percutaneous liver biopsy can be performed by the following method. Prior to biopsy, the animal should be fasted and any ascitic fluid should be removed. The animal is placed in dorsal recumbency and a local block is placed in the midline of the skin and abdomen at the caudoventral aspect of the left hepatic lobe. The incision into the peritoneal cavity should be large enough to accommodate the gloved index finger. Make a separate skin puncture site in the abdominal wall to accommodate the biopsy needle. Use the index finger to manually fix the left hepatic lobe (or other desired hepatic lobe) against the diaphragm or other adjacent structures, and insert the outer cannula and stylet through the abdominal wall into the isolated hepatic lobe. Remove the stylet and rapidly insert the cutting prongs. If properly placed, the cutting prongs should not go through the entire hepatic lobe. Advance the outer cannula over the blades of the cutting prongs, thus entrapping the hepatic tissue material within the cutting prongs. Remove the biopsy needle. Using a wooden applicator stick, very carefully place the biopsy specimen into fixative. Biopsy samples can be used to prepare slides for cytologic examination and the biopsy needle may be cultured. Close the abdominal incision in the routine manner.

References and Additional Readings

Feldman, E. C., and Ettinger, S. J.: Percutaneous transthoracic liver biopsy in the dog. J.A.V.M.A., *169*:805, 1976.

Kasper, J. B., and Chiapella, A. M.: Gastrointestinal biopsy techniques. *In* Kirk, R. W. (ed.): Current Veterinary Therapy VII. Philadelphia, W. B. Saunders Company, 1980.

Strombeck, D. J.: Small Animal Gastroenterology. Davis, Calif., Stonegate Publishing, 1979.

PERCUTANEOUS RENAL BIOPSY

Renal biopsies can be valuable in confirming or eliminating a diagnosis of renal disease that is based on history, physical examination, and radiographic and laboratory data. Additionally, biopsy may be a way of arriving at a prognosis in generalized renal disease and a better means of evaluating what type of treatment should be instituted. The technique we have used for percutaneous renal biopsy in the dog is that outlined by Osborne.

Equipment

Equipment necessary for percutaneous renal biopsy includes the following:
1. A Franklin-modified Vim-Silverman biopsy needle (small size).
2. Sharp, pointed tissue scissors and scalpel.
3. Thumb forceps.
4. Hemostats.
5. Needle holder, skin suture, sponges.
6. Local anesthetic; surgical prep tray; small drape; formalin, 10 per cent, for fixation of specimen.

Technique

Many patients with generalized renal disease are critically ill and debilitated, and general anesthesia is contraindicated. In these cases, a neuroleptan-algesic agent may be used for sedation. If the animal is a good anesthetic risk and renal function will permit it, a general anesthetic can be used.

Surgically prepare the area over the kidney that will be biopsied. Infiltrate the skin and paralumbar muscles caudal to the last rib just below the ventral border of the lumbar muscles with a local anesthetic. Make a paralumbar incision large enough for the index finger in this site over the caudal pole of the kidney. Dissect muscle and fascia until the peritoneum is reached, and enter the peritoneal cavity. With the sterile, gloved index finger, examine the posterior pole and remaining portions of the kidney. Make a small stab incision in the skin just anterior to paralumbar entry into the peritoneal cavity, and insert the biopsy needle into the peritoneal cavity (Fig. 68). Guide the needle toward the posterior pole of the kidney with the index finger. Hold the kidney so that it is immobilized against the body wall, and placing the long axis of the biopsy needle away from the renal pelvis, place the needle just through the renal capsule. Replace the stylet in the needle with the cutting prongs, and rapidly thrust the cutting prongs into the renal cortical tissue. Keeping the cutting prongs in their same position, move the outer cannula down over the blades, rotating the cannula. Remove the cutting prongs and outer cannula, and place the biopsy specimen in fixative. Close the surgical wound, ensuring that excessive hemorrhage is not present.

Alternatively, a Tru-cut biopsy needle* can be used to perform the kidney biopsy. Figure 69 illustrates the use of this biopsy needle.

Fixation and Preparation of Biopsy Material

The choice and concentration of the fixative to be used depends on the type of tissue specimen. In general, when a piece of tissue has been removed for biopsy by excision, the specimen should be no more than 0.5 to 1 cm thick, and a 10:1 volume of fixative to tissue volume should be used.

---

*Travenol Laboratories, Deerfield, Illinois.

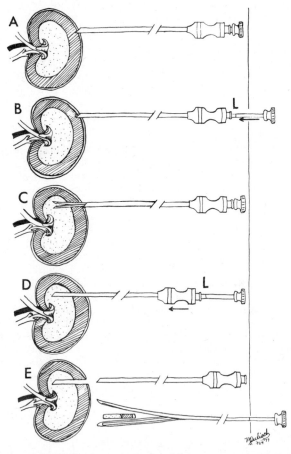

Figure 68. Mechanism of action of Franklin Modified Vim Silverman biopsy needle. *A*, Outer cannula with stylet in place should just penetrate the capsule. *B*, Outer cannula is held in place and stylet is removed. Cutting prongs are introduced until prongs just contact organ or up to line marked on shaft of cutting prongs (L). *C*, Outer cannula is fixed in place while cutting prongs are thrust rapidly into tissue. *D*, The cutting prongs are now held fixed while the outer cannula is gently rotated back and forth over the prongs until the line on the shaft of the prongs can be seen. *E*, Both cannula and prongs are removed together. The prongs are then removed from the cannula and the biopsy is gently removed. (From Withrow, S. J., and Lowes, N.: Biopsy techniques in small animal oncology. J.A.A.H.A., *14*(6):899–902, 1981.)

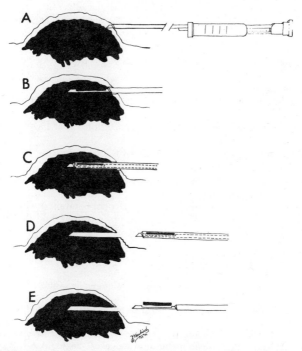

Figure 69. Mechanism of action of Tru-Cut biopsy needle for typical nodular biopsy. A small skin incision is made with a No. 11 blade to allow insertion of the instrument. *A,* With the instrument closed, the outer capsule is penetrated. *B,* The outer cannula is fixed in place, and the inner cannula with specimen notch is thrust into the tumor. Tissue then protrudes into the notch. *C,* The inner cannula is now fixed while the outer cannula is moved forward to cut off the biopsy specimen. *D,* The entire instrument is removed closed with tissue contained within. *E,* The inner cannula is pushed ahead to expose tissue in the specimen notch. (From Withrow, S. J., and Lowes, N.: Biopsy techniques in small animal oncology. J.A.A.H.A., *14*(6):899–902, 1981.)

Various types of fixatives are available for processing tissue biopsies:

1. *Neutral buffered 10 per cent formalin solution*—for routine examination of tissues by light microscopy. The amount of formalin used should be 10 times that of the tissue present. Fix for at least 18 hours.

2. *Bouin's solution*—for fixation of testicular, endocrine, and intestinal mucosal tissue. Fix in Bouin's solution for not more than 24 hours. Bouin's solution is a combination of picric acid, formalin, and glacial acetic acid.

3. *Zenker's–acetic acid solution*—tends to preserve nuclear structures very well. This solution, which is very good for fixation of eyes, is a combination of mercuric chloride and potassium dichromate. Zenker's solution does not remain stable in acetic acid, and 5 ml of acetic acid must be added to 95 ml of Zenker's solution just prior to use.

4. *Freezing*—for frozen sections.

5. *Glutaraldehyde*—used for tissues that are going to be prepared for electron microscopy.

Special techniques are required to prepare fluids that have a low cellular count:

1. Centrifugation of the specimen at 1500 to 2000 rpm's for 10 minutes can allow concentration of cellular material.

2. Special filters such as the Millipore filter 5-pore size or the nucleopore filter can be used to isolate cells.

3. Fluids can be fixed in 40 per cent ethyl alcohol combined with 18 per cent neutral buffered formalin if special stains are required, and the cells can be isolated on filters.

References and Additional Readings

Osborne, C. A. (ed.): Symposium on biopsy techniques. Vet. Clin. North Am., *4*:211, 1974.

Perman, V., Alsaker, R. D., and Riis, R. C.: Cytology of the Dog and Cat. A.A.H.A., South Bend, Ind., 1979.

Rebar, A. H.: Handbook of Veterinary Cytology. St. Louis, Ralston Purina Co., 1978.

Withrow, S.: Biopsy techniques for use in small animal oncology. J.A.A.H.A., *17*(6): 889, 1981.

PROSTATIC BIOPSY (See also p. 503)

A transperineal approach can be used for prostatic biopsy. General anesthesia or neuroleptanalgesia is required to perform this technique. The perineal area is surgically prepared, and an 0.5-cm skin incision is made 2 to 4 cm lateral to the anus on the side of the prostate from which the biopsy is to be obtained. A Tru-cut disposable biopsy needle* is used. The prostate gland should be manually pushed toward the pelvic brim by placing pressure on the abdominal viscera. This can best be done with the dog in lateral recumbency.

---

*Travenol Laboratories, Deerfield, Illinois.

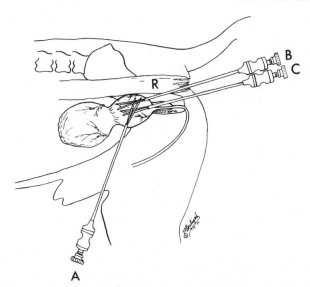

A

Figure 70. Various means of closed prostatic biopsy with needle punch. All penetrations of the prostate should be lateralized to avoid the urethra. Rectum is labeled R. (A) Percutaneous punch lateral to prepuce. (B) Transrectal route uses punch enclosed in glove on index finger while palpating the prostate rectally. (C) Perineal approach enters skin ventral to rectum and travels in pelvic canal up to prostate. (From Withrow, S. J., and Lowes, N.: Biopsy techniques in small animal oncology. J.A.A.H.A., 14(6):899–902, 1981.)

The clinician should wear sterile gloves. Palpate the prostate per rectum with one hand. Hold the biopsy needle with the other hand and insert the needle through the tissue lateral to the anus and medial to the tuber ischii. Direct the needle anteriorly, parallel to the rectum until the prostate is reached (Fig. 70).

The prostate gland may also be biopsied transabdominally or via exploratory laparotomy.

PHARYNGOSTOMY

This technique allows placement of a gastroesophageal tube for repeated oral alimentation required in a wide variety of disease conditions. It obviates the necessity of repeated passage of a stomach tube and is well tolerated by most animals.

Equipment

1. Standard surgical pack and suture material.
2. Plastic or rubber feeding tube. Length from canine teeth to anterior or

midthoracic esophagus. The tube should be of the end-hole type as opposed to the side-hole type.

Technique

A short-acting anesthetic can be used in those animals that are good surgical risks. A neuroleptanalgesic agent with local anesthesia or local anesthesia alone can be used in debilitated patients. Prepare the ventrolateral portion of the neck from the thyroid cartilage to the cranial border of the mandibular ramus. The tube can be placed in the right or left pharynx (Fig. 71). Feel the epihyoid bone and put the gloved finger above the epiglottis (Fig. 72). Use blunt dissection through the skin and a hemostat to place the pharyngostomy tube into the esophagus. For cats, a No. 14–16 French tube should be used, and for dogs, a No. 20 French tube. By going into the esophagus in the posterior pharynx *above* the epiglottis, respiratory difficulties and gagging are avoided. The end of the tube should terminate in the anterior or midthoracic esophagus to prevent reflux esophagitis and ulceration. Occlusion of the jugular vein permits visualization of the external maxillary and linguofacial veins. Palpate the ventral border of the diagrasticus muscle. The hypoglossal nerve and lingual artery are caudal to the pharyngostomy site. The incision is caudal to the diagrasticus muscle and parallel to the facial branch of the linguofacial vein. A safety pin may be placed through the lumen of the

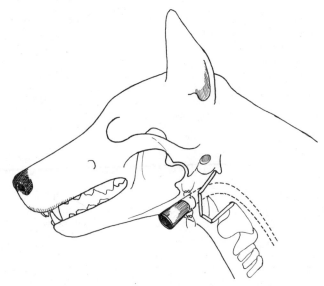

Figure 71. Tube in position within the pharynx and esophagus. (From Bojarab, M. J. (ed.): Current Techniques in Small Animal Surgery, 2nd ed. Philadelphia, Lea & Febiger, 1983, p. 103.)

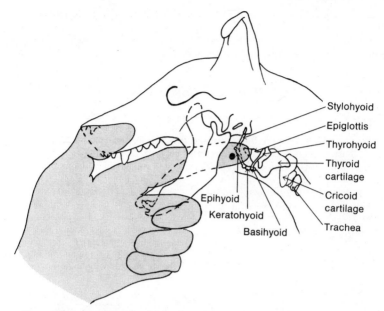

Figure 72. Proper placement of index finger *lateral* to hyoid apparatus. (From Bojarab, M. J. (ed.): Current Techniques in Small Animal Surgery, 2nd ed. Philadelphia, Lea & Febiger, 1983, p. 102.)

tube to maintain its position, or the tube may be taped to the neck. The tube should be capped when not in use.

The incision in the skin and entrance site of the tube should be cleansed daily with soap and water. The wound is allowed to heal by second intention when the tube is removed.

A pharyngostomy incision has also been used to place an endotracheal tube when surgery may be necessary to treat oral or pharyngeal lesions and mandibular or maxillary fractures. See p. 582 for nutrients that can be supplied via pharyngostomy tube. When the pharyngostomy tube is removed, the wound is allowed to heal by second intention.

References and Additional Readings

Bohning, R. H., Jr., et al.: Pharyngostomy for maintenance of the anorectic animal. J.A.V.M.A., *156*:611, 1970.

Crowe, D.: Parenteral hyperalimentation. Veterinary Critical Care Society, 1983.

Hartsfield, S. M., et al.: Endotracheal intubation by pharyngotomy. J.A.A.H.A., *13*:71, 1977.

Lantz, G. C.: Pharyngostomy tube instillation. Compendium on Continuing Education, 3(2):135, 1981.

COLLECTION AND EVALUATION OF CANINE SEMEN

Canine semen should be collected for evaluation of a potential breeder, for investigating infertility, and for artificial insemination.

Method of Collection

Equipment

> ***Sterile and Warmed to Body Temperature*** (use of an incubator is beneficial)
> At least 3 small nonwaxed paper drinking cups.
> A 3-inch glass or Teflon laboratory funnel or a sterile rubber cone connected to a test tube.
> Glass, Teflon or plastic test tubes.
> Saline solution, 0.9 per cent.
> ***Nonsterile***
> Microscope slides and cover slips (warmed).
> India ink (Pelikan), William's stain, Diff Quick Stain, buffered formalin.
> Hemocytometer (counting chamber and 1/100 white blood cell (WBC) dilutor pipette or Unopette).
> Microscope and light.

Collecting Semen

The following procedures should be carried out when collecting semen:

1. Take the male and a female (in heat if possible) to a quiet room where there will be no distractions and good traction (rubber mats or rug) for mounting.
2. Hold the female and allow the male to "flirt" for several minutes. If the female is in heat, a brief period of "foreplay" with both dogs unrestricted is beneficial.
3. Assistants may be needed to hold the muzzled female and to control the male by a collar and leash.
4. If mounting occurs, allow the male to grasp the bitch and start to thrust his pelvis in an attempt to copulate. Gently, from behind the dog, grasp the penis in the prepuce and move the prepuce back over the engorged bulbus glandis and apply pressure with the thumb and forefinger proximal to the exposed bulbus. This can usually be done with one motion as the male is thrusting. If the male is shy and not interested, slight massage of the penis in the prepuce in an attempt to cause erection and masturbation should be attempted. When erection of the bulbus is felt, the prepuce should be reflected posteriorly to free the bulbus. Pressure is applied with the thumb and forefinger behind the bulbus and circling the shaft of the penis. When the erection develops, the penis should be twisted 180 degrees backwards, between the hind legs, so the penis remains in the same plane as in the forward position with the thumb and forefinger still applying pressure proximal to the bulbus. The penis should not be diverted ventrally 180

degrees, because this causes pain. The penis cannot be twisted unless the prepuce is reflected posterior or proximal to the bulbus glandis. Twisting the penis in this position results in a better erection, simulates a natural "tie," and allows the person collecting the semen to better visualize the collection. It is preferable to use a paper cup to collect the semen. It will not conduct heat from the semen collected, is disposable, and is less traumatic if the penis contacts the cup during pelvic thrusting. It is also easier to hold than a funnel and test tube. The cup is preferred to covering the penis with a sterile rubbercone and an attached test tube. This usually contaminates the sample with epithelial cells, inflammatory cells and microflora from the surface of the penis. The first drops of ejaculate may be discarded, especially if any urine is present. The sperm rich fraction should be collected separately. When the ejaculate becomes clear, this is prostatic fluid and should be collected separately for examination.

Following collection, the penis is placed in the forward position, the prepuce is straightened out to avoid paraphimosis, and the female is removed from the room. Allow the stud to lick the erect penis and lose the erection. The stud should be checked for evidence of paraphimosis before he is released or caged.

5. The ejaculate consists of three fractions: (a) urethral secretion (usually clear fluid)—0.1 to 2 ml within 50 seconds, a pH of 0.3. If evidence of urine is present, discard and do not add to the sperm-rich fraction. (b) sperm-containing secretion (milky opaque fluid)—0.5 to 3 ml within 1 to 2 minutes, a pH of 6.1. (c) prostatic secretion (usually clear fluid)—2 to 20 ml within 30 minutes, a pH of 6.5. The total specimen is 0.3 to 20 ml, a pH of 6.4.

6. Because the first and third fractions are clear, water-like material and the second fraction is milky opaque, the clinician can separate them by changing paper cups or collecting tubes as each fraction is ejaculated. It is best to collect only enough prostatic fluid to rinse the sperm fraction into the test tube. Too much is detrimental to sperm longevity in storage. Settergren uses a total collection time of 5 minutes from the beginning of ejaculation when evaluating a stud for fertility. This period allows for some additional fluid collection and will also add a few more sperm to the sample. Collecting individual fractions may be important in determining the site of an inflammatory reaction, but when collecting for artificial insemination, only the sperm-rich, low-volume ejaculate is needed for insemination, dilution, or freezing.

7. The male is returned to his cage. The female is retained until the semen is examined, if actual insemination is to be performed.

Evaluation of Semen

The evaluation of semen should include the following:
1. Immediately after collection, slowly invert the tube several times to mix the semen gently.

2. Determine motility. Place 1 drop of semen on a warmed microscope slide. Cover with a cover slip and observe under low power for general motility. There will be no "waves," but general vigorous forward motion should be evident. If the sample is too concentrated to find individual sperm, mix 1 drop of semen with 1 drop of body temperature saline on a warmed microscope slide. Under high power, count 10 different groups of 10 sperm, observing the number of motile and nonmotile sperm. Total motility for a suitable sample should be 80 per cent or greater. Motility less than 60 per cent is not satisfactory.

3. Determine the number of sperm. Although the number of sperm is determined in a hemocytometer on the basis of sperm per cu mm, this figure varies widely, depending on the dilution by variable amounts of prostatic fluid. More important is the total number of sperm per ejaculate; it should exceed 500 million in a normal male. A minimum number of 200 million sperm per insemination is needed if average conception is to be expected.

4. Determine morphology. Place 1 drop of semen on a slide, add 1 drop of Pelikan India ink, and mix carefully. The mixture is spread carefully like a blood smear and allowed to dry. The carbon particles surround the sperm and outline them so that their structure and form can be observed under high power. One hundred sperm are counted, noting normals and abnormals.

If there is any question about abnormality, it would be best to evaluate 500 sperm cells. It would also be desirable to use a more complex staining technique (William's stain) to make more detailed examinations of the sperm heads. It is prepared as follows: Make fuchsin stock of 10 gm of fuchsin and 100 ml of 96 per cent alcohol. Make phenol solution with 10 ml of liquid phenol (90 per cent) and 170 ml of distilled water. Prepare bluish eosin stock with 1 gm of blue eosin and 100 ml of 96 per cent alcohol. After filtering the fuchsin stock, take 10 ml of it and mix with 100 ml of phenol solution. Take 100 ml of this mixture and add 50 ml of bluish eosin solution. Leave it for 14 days, and filter before using. This solution can be stored for months but is best stored under refrigeration to prevent mold and fungal growth.

William's Staining Method

Spread a film of fresh semen. Air dry it and fix it in a flame. Immerse it in absolute alcohol for 3 or 4 minutes. Allow it to drain and dry. Immerse it in one-half per cent chloramine solution until mucus is removed and the smear appears clear. Wash it in distilled water and then in 96 per cent alcohol. Stain in William's stain for 8 minutes. Wash in water and allow it to dry.

The midpiece and tail of the sperm cell can best be examined by the following technique: Dilute a drop of semen and mix it with buffered formalin. Place a cover slip on the mixture, and examine it with a phase contrast microscope. This type of preparation is ideal for fixing and preserving semen for shipment or for later laboratory examination. To examine other cells, inflammatory epithelial or primordial germ cells, a drop of semen or prostatic fluid is placed on a slide, smeared similar to a blood smear, and allowed to air dry. Stain with a drop of New Methylene Blue on a cover slip or with Diff-Quick Stain.

Normal canine sperm are 68 mμ long; the heads are 7 mμ long. The average percentage of abnormal sperm totals 15. Excellent samples should not exceed 20 per cent of total abnormals. The differential abnormality is important, however, and the following regional abnormals should not be exceeded in any sperm count; abnormality of the head, 10 to 12 per cent; midpiece abnormalities, 3 to 4 per cent; tail abnormalities, 3 to 4 per cent; and protoplasmic droplets, 3 to 4 per cent. Abnormalities that should be counted and recorded are shown in Figure 73. It is important to note the presence and location of distal or proximal protoplasmic droplets, which may indicate cell immaturity.

Damage to the cells within the testis in general is of more serious consequence and may be an indication to consider testicular biopsy for further evaluation. Damage produced after the sperm have left the testis may indicate epididymal disease or may be the result of cold, trauma, or osmotic or urinary contamination. When abnormalities are found, it is always wise to obtain two or three semen samples within a few days for baseline evaluation and then repeat the studies in 4 to 6 weeks to obtain an idea of a healing or regressing trend. There are usually 64 days from date of sperm formation until date of ejaculation—54 days in the testis and 10 days in transport and maturation in the epididymis.

Semen Production

Normal males can be used as studs according to the following schedule without reducing their sperm reserves.
1. Once every other day indefinitely.
2. Once daily for 3 days if 2 days' rest is then allowed.
3. Twice daily for 1 day if 2 days' rest is then allowed.

Inseminating the Bitch

Equipment

Equipment needed for inseminating the bitch includes dry, warm, sterile 5- or 10-ml syringes; rubber adapter tubing, ¾ inch long; a 6- to 9-inch, plastic inseminating pipette; alcohol; and cotton. Do not use lubricating materials.

Procedure

The procedure for bitch insemination includes the following steps:
1. Determine the correct time to inseminate by test teasing with a male, by cytologic examination of vaginal smears, or by vaginoscopic examination when vaginal folds change from round to angular. Breed the day after the

SPERM

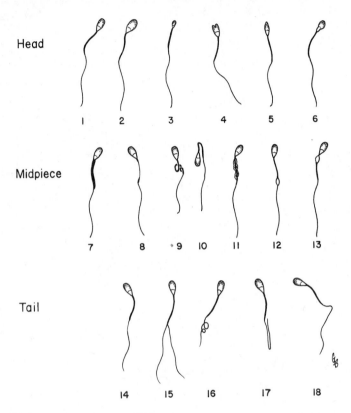

Head

Midpiece

Tail

1	2	3	4	5	6

7　8　· 9　10　11　12　13

14　15　16　17　18

Head
1. Normal
2. Giant
3. Small
4. Indented
5. Pointed
6. Pear-shaped

Midpiece
7. Thickened
8. Thinned
9. Coiled
10. Bent
11. Extraneous
12. Distal cytoplasmic droplet
13. Proximal cytoplasmic droplet

Tail
14. Thinned
15. Double
16. Coiled
17. Folded
18. Kinked

Figure 73. Chart of abnormal sperm.

bitch first stands staunchly to accept service and "flags" her tail or during cytologic indications of estrus, but before leukocytes reappear in the smear. Breed at least twice at 48-hour intervals. Repeat at this interval for up to four inseminations if the vaginal smear still shows signs of estrus.

2. If soiled, clean the vulva thoroughly with alcohol swabs.

3. Gently aspirate semen through the inseminating pipette into the warm syringe.

4. Use no lubricants and insert the pipette through the vulva and dorsally into the vagina and forward to the cervix. With gentle manipulation, in some cases the pipette may be advanced into the uterus. Elevate the bitch's rear quarters by having an assistant pick up the bitch at the hock region so as no pressure is applied to the ventral abdomen and uterus and elevate to a 45-degree angle. The semen is gently and slowly ejected. A bubble of air should be ejected to push all the semen through the pipette. Deposit the semen in the anterior vagina if cervical passage is impossible. The dorsal median vaginal fold may obstruct view of and access to the canine cervix.

5. The pipette is removed, and the bitch, in an elevated position, is held for 4 minutes. During this time, a finger encased in a sterile glove should be inserted into the vagina and the vaginal roof "feathered" to stimulate constrictor activity. This may be important to simulate a "tie" and transport of semen into the uterus.

6. The bitch is lowered to normal position and immediately walked for 5 minutes so that she does not sit down or jump up on a person and allow semen to run back out of the vagina.

7. Undiluted fresh semen should be immediately inseminated for best conception.

8. Refrigerated extended semen should be used within 24 to 48 hours, if possible. However, it has been kept viable for up to 9 days with proper care.

Skim milk has been used as an economical and adequate extender. It is heated to 92° to 94°C for 10 minutes, cooled, and skimmed at room temperature. Each ml should receive 1000 U of crystalline penicillin and 1 mg of streptomycin. Polymyxin B may be added, if *Pseudomonas* sp affect the semen, at 200 U per ml of extender. Semen is diluted with extender at 1:1 to 1:4. Seager extends canine semen for freezing with a diluent containing 11 per cent lactose, 4 per cent glycerine, and 20 per cent egg yolk. The 1:4 diluted semen is refrigerated; then 0.05 ml aliquots are pipetted into depressions in a block of dry ice and held for 8 minutes to freeze. The frozen pellets are then stored in liquid nitrogen. Frozen semen can be thawed in buffered saline at 30° to 37°C. Good semen may be kept satisfactorily for several years and retains 50 per cent of its original motility at thawing. Conception is best when large numbers of thawed motile sperm are deposited in the cervix or uterine cavity. Conception is poor when thawed semen is placed in the anterior vagina, similar to artificial breeding with raw semen.

Feline Semen Collection and Artificial Insemination

Semen can be collected by means of electroejaculation while the tom is anesthetized. In semen collection with an artificial vagina, the tom must be trained over a 2- to 3-week period with teaser queens; thus, this method does not lend itself to breeding problems except in a large cattery. Teaser queens can be produced by injecting spayed females with 0.25 mg of estradiol cyclopentylpropionate (ECP) or by using normal queens in heat. An artificial vagina can be made by cutting off the bulb end of a 2-ml rubber bulb pipette and inserting a 3- × 44-mm test tube into the cut end. The apparatus is placed into a 60-ml plastic bottle filled with warm water (52°C). The rolled end of the rubber pipette is stretched over the rim of the bottle. The opening of the pipette (vagina) is sparingly lubricated with K-Y jelly. A teaser queen is placed in a quiet cage with the tom. As the male mounts and develops an erection, the artificial vagina is placed over the penis. The ejaculation takes 1 to 4 minutes, and the semen volume is 0.05 ml (0.03–0.3) with 50 to 100 million sperm. Motility is normally 80 to 90 per cent, and pH is 7.4. There should be less than 10 per cent abnormal sperm. The semen can be diluted for insemination to contain 10 million sperm in 0.1 ml of saline; then each 0.1 ml is an adequate insemination volume. With such small samples, microequipment is essential to avoid losing semen by surface absorption. Toms can undergo this collection procedure three times weekly and maintain excellent semen quality and libido.

Queens can be detected in estrus by daily stroking their backs and necks and noting the arching of the back and the extended and treading action of the rear feet when they are in receptive heat. Verification of estrus is made by vaginal smears, which show epithelial cell cornification with pyknotic nuclei. Insemination is carried out with a one–fourth-ml syringe and a bulb–tipped 9-cm spinal needle. Ovulation is induced by mechanical vaginal stimulation with a fire-polished glass stirring rod or by an intramuscular injection of 25 to 50 IU of human chorionic gonadotropin. If repeat insemination is made 24 hours later, the conception rate improves from 60 to 75 per cent.

References and Additional Readings

Bartlett, D. J.: Studies on dog semen, I. Morphologic characteristics. II. Biochemical characteristics. J. Reprod. Fertil., 3:174, 1962.

Johnston, S. D.: Diagnostic and therapeutic approach to infertility in the bitch. J. Am. Vet. Med. Assoc., 176:1335–1338, 1980.

Johnston, S. D., Larsen, R. E., and Olson, P. N. S.: Canine Theriogenology. American Society for Theriogenology, 1982.

Larsen, R. E.: Breeding soundness examination of the male dog. In Kirk, R. W. (ed.): Current Veterinary Therapy 8: Small Animal Practice. Philadelphia, W. B. Saunders Company, 1983, pp 956–959.

Seager, S. W. J.: Successful pregnancies utilizing frozen dog semen. Artif. Insem. Dig., 17:6, 1969.

Seager, S. W. J.: Semen collection and artificial insemination in dogs. St. Louis, Ralston Purina Co., 1977.

Settergren, I.: Personal communication, 1974.

Sojka, N. J.: Technique for collecting semen for artificial insemination of cats. Norden News, Fall : 1970.

Sojka, N. J., et al.: Artificial insemination in the cat. Lab. Anim. Care, *20*:198, 1970.

COLLECTION OF URINE

Urine can be removed from the bladder by one of four methods: (1) natural micturition, (2) manual compression of the urinary bladder, (3) catheterization, or (4) cystocentesis.

For routine urinalysis, the collection of urine by natural micturition is often very satisfactory. The major disadvantage is the contamination of the sample with cells, bacteria, and other debris located in the genital tract. The first portion of the stream should be discarded, because it contains the most contamination and debris.

Manual compression of the bladder may be used in collecting urine samples from dogs and cats. Excessive digital pressure should not be used; if moderate digital pressure does not induce micturition, the technique should be discontinued. The technique can be difficult to use in male dogs and male cats.

Urinary catheters are hollow tubes made of rubber, plastic, nylon, latex, or metal and are designed to serve four purposes:

1. To relieve urinary retention.
2. To test for residual urine.
3. To obtain urine directly from the bladder for diagnostic purposes.
4. To perform bladder lavage and instillations.

The size of catheters (diameter) is usually calibrated in French scale with each French unit equivalent to 0.33 mm. The openings adjacent to the catheter tips are called "eyes." Human urethral catheters are routinely used in male and female dogs. No. 4–10 French catheters are satisfactory for most dogs. Catheters should be individually packaged and sterilized by autoclaving or ethylene oxide gas.

Catheterization of the Male Dog

Equipment needed to catheterize a male dog includes a sterile catheter (No. 4–10 French and 18 inches long, with one end adapted to fit a syringe); sterile lubricating jelly; Betadine soap or benzalkonium chloride; sterile rubber gloves or a sterile hemostat; a 20-ml sterile syringe; an appropriate receptacle for the collection of urine; and Furacin or Betadine 1 per cent solution in a 5-ml syringe.

Proper catheterization of the male dog requires two people. Place the dog in lateral recumbency on either side. Pull the rear leg that is on top forward and then flex it (Fig. 74). Alternatively, long-legged dogs can be catheterized easily in a standing position.

Next, retract the sheath of the penis and cleanse the glans penis with a solution of Betadine 1 per cent, Septisol, benzalkonium chloride, or bichloride of mercury solution, diluted 1:1000. The distal 2 to 3 cm of the appropriate size catheter is lubricated with sterile lubricating jelly.* The catheter is never entirely removed from its container while it is being passed, because the container enables one to hold the catheter without contaminating it. The catheter may be passed with sterile gloved hands or by using a sterile hemostat to grasp the catheter and pass it into the urethra.

If the catheter cannot be passed into the bladder, the tip of the catheter may be caught in a mucosal fold of the urethra or there may be a stricture or block in the urethra. In small breeds of dogs, the size of the groove in the os penis bone may limit the size of the catheter that can be passed. Difficulty

---

*K-Y Jelly, Johnson & Johnson, New Brunswick, New Jersey.

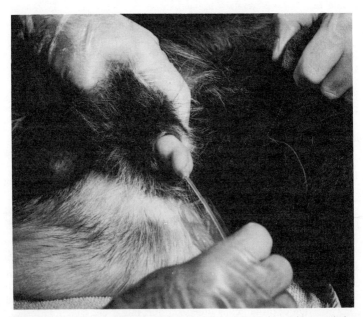

Figure 74. Male canine urethral catheter. The subject is in lateral recumbency with the upper hindleg pulled forward (to the right) and held by an assistant. The penile sheath is retracted, and the glans penis is cleaned. A sterile catheter is protected in its covering until it enters the urethra.

may also be experienced in passing the catheter through the urethra where the urethra curves around the ischial arch. Occasionally, a catheter of small diameter may kink and bend upon being passed into the urethra. When the catheter cannot be passed on the first try, the size of the catheter should be re-evaluated and the catheter gently rotated while being passed a second time. The catheter should never be forced through the urethral orifice.

Effective catheterization is indicated by the flow of urine at the end of the catheter, and a sterile 20-ml syringe is used to aspirate the urine from the bladder. Following catheterization, insert 2 to 5 ml of 1 per cent Betadine solution into the bladder and remove the catheter. Walk the dog immediately following catheterization to encourage urination. An alternative to instilling 1 per cent Betadine solution into the bladder is the oral administration of antiseptics or antimicrobial agents for 3 to 5 days following catheterization.

Catheterization of the Female Dog

Equipment needed to catheterize a female dog includes flexible human ureteral or urethral catheters identical to those used in the male dog. Sterile

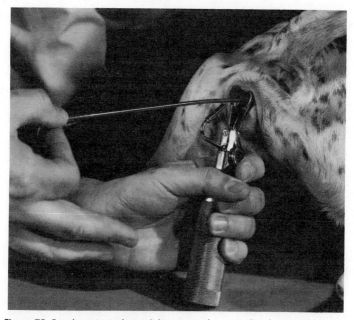

Figure 75. Female canine catheter. Subject is standing or is placed in sternal recumbency. A sterile, lighted, nasal speculum is used to visualize the urethral opening and a catheter is passed. An otoscope cone may also be used effectively.

metal or plastic female catheters can also be used; however, they tend to traumatize the urethra. The following materials should also be on hand: a Brinkerhoff speculum or small nasal speculum; a 20-ml sterile syringe; Xylocaine, 0.5 per cent; sterile K-Y jelly* a focal source of light; appropriate receptacles for urine collection; and 5 ml of Betadine solution.

Strict asepsis should be used. Cleanse the vulva with a solution of Betadine, Septisol, benzalkonium chloride, or bichloride of mercury, diluted 1:1000. The instillation of Xylocaine, 0.5 per cent, into the vaginal vault helps to relieve the discomfort of catheterization. The external urethral orifice is 3 to 5 cm cranial to the ventral commissure of the vulva. In many instances, the female dog may be catheterized in the standing position by passing the female catheter into the vaginal vault, despite the fact that the urethral tubercle is not directly visualized.

In the spayed female in whom "blind catheterization" may be difficult, the use of a Brinkerhoff speculum or nasal speculum with a light source will help to visualize the urethral tubercle on the floor of the vagina (Figs. 75 and 76). In difficult catheterizations, it may be helpful to place the animal in dorsal recumbency and pull the hind legs forward. Insertion of a speculum into the vagina almost always permits visualization of the urethral tubercle and facilitates

---

*K-Y Jelly, Johnson & Johnson, New Brunswick, New Jersey.

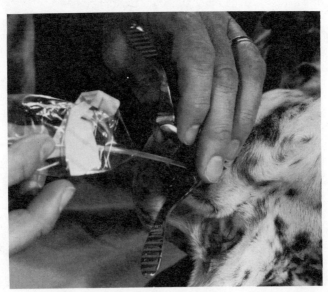

Figure 76. Female canine catheterization. The subject is in dorsal recumbency with the hindlegs pulled forward and held by an assistant. A Brinkerhoff speculum is helpful in visualizing the urethral opening. A sterile plastic catheter is being passed.

passage of the catheter. One should be careful not to pass the catheter into the fossa of the clitoris, because this is a blind passage. Following catheterization, 2 to 5 ml of aqueous Betadine solution diluted to 1 per cent is injected into the bladder.

References and Additional Readings

Lees, G. E., and Osborne, C. A.: Urinary tract infections associated with the use and misuse of urinary catheters. Vet. Clin. North Am., 9:713, 1979.
Lees, G. E., and Osborne, C. A.: Use and misuse of urinary catheters. In Kirk, R. W. (ed.): Current Veterinary Therapy 8: Small Animal Practice. Philadelphia, W. B. Saunders Company, 1983.

Catheterization of Cats

Catheterization of the male cat may require sedation or the use of dissociative anesthesia. Very ill cats or uremic cats can usually be catheterized with systemic sedation, although the use of topical anesthetic such as proparacaine HC1 flushed into the urethral orifice may minimize discomfort. When anesthetized, place the cat on its back and pull the hind legs forward. Draw the penis from the sheath and gently pull it backward. Pass a sterile, flexible plastic or polyethylene (PE 60 to 90) catheter or 3- to 5-inch, No. 3.5 French urethral catheter* into the urethral orifice and gently enter the bladder, keeping the catheter parallel to the vertebral column of the cat. The catheter should never be forced through the urethra. The presence of concretions within the urethral lumen may require the injection of 3 to 5 ml of sterile water, saline, or dilute acetic acid or Walpole's solution† to flush out the concretions so that the catheter can be passed (Fig. 77). (See also p. 127.)

Catheterization of female cats can be accomplished by the use of a plastic, blunt-ended tomcat catheter. The vaginal vault is first anesthetized by instilling Xylocaine, 0.5 per cent. Cleanse the lips of the vulva with an appropriate antiseptic, then grasp and pull them caudally. Insert the tomcat catheter along the floor of the vagina, and gently guide the tip into the urethral orifice. The procedure is usually accomplished without difficulty, even though the urethral orifice is not visualized.

Cystocentesis

Diagnostic cystocentesis involves inserting a needle through the abdominal wall and bladder wall to obtain urine samples for urinalysis or bacterial culture. The technique prevents contamination of urine by urethra, genital tract, or

---

*Monojet, Sherwood Manufacturing Co., St. Louis, Missouri.

†Acetic acid, 0.2 molar—57 ml; sodium acetate, 0.2 molar—43 ml; use millipore filtration and sterilization; otherwise it will grow molds.

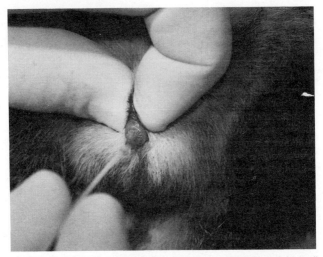

Figure 77. Catheterization of a male cat. With the cat on his back and the hindlegs pulled forward, the penis is withdrawn from its sheath and held. A sterile catheter is passed into the urethra, keeping the catheter parallel to the vertebral column of the cat.

skin and reduces the risk of iatrogenic production of a urinary tract infection. Cystocentesis may also be needed to temporarily decompress a severely overdistended bladder in an animal with urethral obstruction. In these cases, it should only be performed if urethral catheterization is impossible.

Equipment

Equipment required for cystocentesis includes a 22-gauge, 1½- to 3-inch needle (spinal needle); 10- to 30-ml syringe (depending on size of animal); and a three-way stopcock.

Procedure

Clip and surgically prepare the skin over the cystocentesis site on the ventral abdomen. Cystocentesis is performed by placing the needle in the ventral abdominal wall slightly (3–5 cm) cranial to the junction of the bladder with the urethra. Insert the needle at a 45-degree angle (see Figs. 78 and 79). The bladder must contain a sufficient volume of urine so as to permit palpation through the abdominal wall prior to cystocentesis. One hand is used to hold the bladder steady within the peritoneal cavity while the other guides the needle.

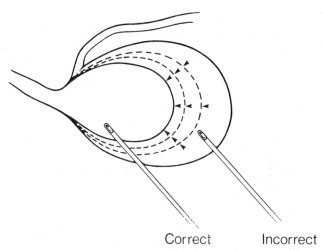

Correct   Incorrect

Figure 78. Schematic drawing illustrating correct and incorrect sites of insertion of a needle into the bladder for the purpose of evacuating urine. The needle should be inserted a short distance cranial to the junction of the bladder with the urethra rather than at the vertex of the bladder. This will permit removal of urine and decompression of the bladder without need for reinsertion of the needle into the bladder lumen. From Osborne, C. A., Johnston, G. R., and Shenk, M. P.: Cystocentesis: indications, contraindications, technique, and complications. Minn. Vet., 17, 1977.

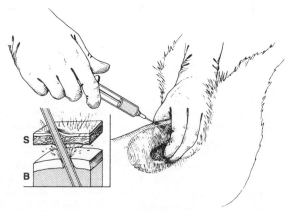

Figure 79. Schematic drawing illustrating escape of urine through the bladder wall adjacent to the needle tract as a result of excessive digital pressure used to localize and immobilize the bladder. S = skin of abdominal wall; B = wall of urinary bladder. (From Osborne, C. A., Lees, G. E., and Johnston, G. R.: Cystocentesis. In Kirk, R. W. (ed.): Current Veterinary Therapy VII: Small Animal Practice. Philadelphia, W. B. Saunders Company, 1980, p. 1153.)

Precautions

Although this procedure is relatively safe, the bladder must have a reasonable volume of urine, the tap should not be made without identifying and immobilizing the bladder, and there must be adequate patient cooperation or sedation. The bladder should be drained completely, if possible.

References and Additional Readings

Osborne, C. A., Lees, G. A., and Johnston, G. R.: Cystocentesis. *In* Kirk, R. W. (ed.): Current Veterinary Therapy VII. Philadelphia, W. B. Saunders Company, 1980.

EXAMINATION OF THE CANINE VAGINA

Vaginal examination involves these procedures: collection of material from the mucosal wall for culture and exfoliative cytology and vaginoscopic examination of vaginal and cervical mucosa. The uterine contents and endometrium can be examined at parturition or in the early post partum period.

Equipment

The following equipment is necessary for examination of the canine vagina: sterile vaginal speculum (adjustable spreading, stainless steel, or disposable plastic; cylindrical; glass, plastic, stainless steel, nylon, etc.); sterile variable size otoscope heads for small dogs; sterile protected culture swabs (Tiegland-type or other); sterile culture swabs (Culturettes); Amies Transport Media with charcoal; viral transport media; glass slides and coverslips; sterile proctoscope (Welch Allyn—human pediatric–type) or other fiberoptoscope, flexible or rigid; and sterile offset biopsy punch.

Technique

Examination of the vagina for culture and cytology or vaginoscopic examination can be done with the aid of an assistant restraining the bitch on an examination table (or on the floor for large breeds). Bitches that can be restrained for other minor examinations (ears, teeth, toe nails, anal sacs, and blood samples) will easily tolerate vaginal examinations. Those that need further restraint may require tranquilization or a short-acting barbiturate anesthetic.

If the bitch has a clean appearing vulva, no preparation prior to examination is needed. If the vulva is soiled or vulvar hair is matted or soiled, trimming of the hair and washing the area with germicidal or surgical scrub such as Betadine or Nolvasan scrub or a general grooming and bath should be done 24 hours prior to examination. If prior preparation is not possible and culturing must be done, any matted hair should be removed and cotton, wet with rubbing alcohol, can be used to remove visible soiling. Water and germicidal soap will usually not control surface contamination of *Pseudomonas* and *Proteus* sp, which frequently contaminate culture swabs. Bitches with long hair should have leg hair pinned to one side with large beautician hair clips and the tail bandaged before examination.

A deep vaginal culture should be obtained before other vaginal examination causes contamination. A sterile, warm vaginal speculum without lubricating jel is passed into the posterior vagina by first having an assistant spread the lips of the vulva open. The sterile, warm speculum is guided into the vagina by placing the speculum into the vulva just at the dorsal commissure of the vulvar lips and applying pressure up and out against the commissure. The speculum is directed dorsally toward the rectum until resistance is met, then redirected horizontally into the cranial vagina. This procedure bypasses the clitoral fossa, urethral opening, and pelvic arch and causes minimal pain. Lubricating jelly is not used, because it contaminates the swabs for culture and cytology.

A guarded culture swab (swab covered by protective plastic pipette) is taken from its individual sterile bag and passed inside the vaginal speculum to the anterior vagina or cervical area or into the cervix and uterus of a bitch during estrus or in the early post partum period. The swab is then exposed from the protective plastic tubing and rotated against the mucosa. It is retracted into the protective plastic tubing and carefully removed from the vagina. The protected swab may then be placed back into the sterile individual plastic bag that it was originally in until it is either processed for culture (½ hour) or placed in Amies Transport Media with charcoal. Amies Transport Media with refrigerator packs and a styrofoam insulated mailing box will retain fastidious organisms for 72 to 96 hours. Bacteria, mycoplasma, and ureaplasma cultures should be processed for potential infectious agents. Viral transport medias can be used for a separate sterile swab if viral agents such as the genital form of canine herpes virus are suspected.

Immediately following the swabbing for culture, while the vaginal speculum is still in place, a moistened (sterile physiologic saline solution) clean or sterile swab should be carefully advanced into the anterior vagina to make a smear for cytology. Protect the swab from the cells of the vulva or caudal vagina by passing it along the inner speculum to the anterior vagina. This is important, because this was the area sampled for culture and is the area of the vagina containing cells that are most representative of ovarian sex steroid hormone changes. Gently rub the swab on the vaginal mucosa. Remove the swab and roll it smoothly onto two or three clean glass slides. The smears may be fixed immediately in 95 per cent alcohol or sprayed with a commercial fixative or hair spray or left to air dry.

A drop of New Methylene Blue stain placed on a coverslip and inverted on the smear can be used as a quick procedure to examine a wet mount preparation immediately. This stain is not permanent, precipitates when it dries, and cannot be used for later comparison with other smears made in the cycle. A better quick permanent method is the use of the Diff Quick stain. Stains such as Giemsa, toluidine blue, Wright's or Shorr's or phase contrast microscopy can also be used. The smear should be examined for stage of estrus cycle and evidence of active inflammation. These findings should be compared with culture results and vaginoscopic findings to interpret evidence of an active genital tract infection, a carrier state of a potential infectious agent, or a possible contaminant at culture. A diagnostic laboratory with the ability to isolate specific infectious agents should indicate the number of organisms (few, moderate, many, or heavy) and report whether the isolates are pure or mixed and their significance.

Examination

The vagina of the bitch is long, and the mucosa forms longitudinal folds. The clitoris is in a well-developed fossa in the floor of the vestibule. We have found that the vagina can be completely visualized with a small sterile proctoscope or fiberoptoscope. Lubricate the warmed, sterile instrument, and pass it to the region of the cervix. Examine first without insufflation for true color and vaginal fluids or discharge. When insufflation is performed while the vulva is compressed around the sterile proctoscope, the vagina balloons and its entire wall can be viewed completely as the instrument is withdrawn.

The normal canine vagina has a uniform light pink color with longitudinal folds. During proestrus and estrus, the folds become more prominent, with cross-striations that give the surface a cobblestone appearance. This cobblestone appearance will remain smooth during high estrogen levels but quickly becomes angular (worn cobblestone appearance) when estrogen drops during the luteinizing hormone (LH) peak (ovulation) and progressive progesterone increases. This change can be used to indicate ovulation time and the ideal time to breed. The hyperemia causes the vagina to appear reddish and congested. The pressure of air insufflation blanches the mucosa. The canine vagina has a large cranial dorsal median fold that may obscure the true cervix. In fact, ridges near the dorsal fold may give a false impression that this fold is the cervix. During estrogen stimulation, the cervix may be open and uterine blood may be escaping. In the management of dystocia, the vaginoscope can be used to diagnose malpositions and aid in the correction of these conditions.

During the endoscopic examination, small tumors or polyps can be removed or large masses sampled with the biopsy punch. Ulcers or erosions can be cauterized, and foreign bodies can be removed.

A complete vaginal examination must include careful palpation of the vaginal wall and pelvic canal. This is accomplished by digital examination through the vulva (using a sterile glove) and is assisted by palpation through the posterior abdominal wall. Evidence of incomplete hymen rings, vaginal fibrous stenotic rings, or pelvic malformation can be diagnosed. A rectal digital examination may be needed for vaginal masses or pelvic deformities.

Characteristics of the Canine Vagina During the Estrus Cycle (See Fig. 80)

The canine reproductive cycle begins at the age of 6 to 12 months and repeats at intervals of 4 to 12 months. Ovulation occurs spontaneously 1 to 3

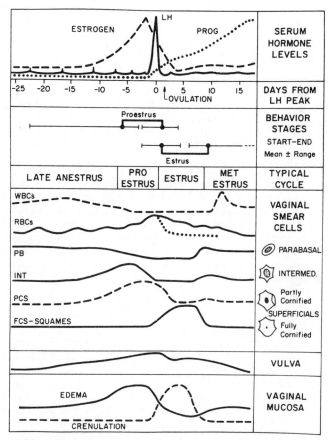

Figure 80. A schematic summary of temporal relationships among periovulatory endocrine events, behavioral and vulval changes, and changes in vaginal exfoliate cytology associated with proestrus and estrus periods in the bitch. (From Kirk, R. W. (ed.): Current Veterinary Therapy VIII: Small Animal Practice. Philadelphia, W. B. Saunders Company, 1983, p. 889.)

days after true estrus. Sperm live in the uterus 4 to 11 days, and the ovum lives 4 days. The fertilized ovum takes 4 to 10 days to reach the uterus, and implantation takes place 18 to 20 days postovulation. The gestation period from the first breeding varies from 57 to 72 days and from the LH peak, 64 to 66 days.

Anestrus

Anestrus is characterized by dryness of the mucosa and a thin vaginal wall with stratified squamous epithelial cells, a few cells to several layers thick but without cornification. There are noncornified epithelial cells and leukocytes in a ratio of 1:5 in the vaginal smear. The leukocytes are polymorphonuclear leukocytes. The noncornified epithelial cells are 25 to 51 mμ in diameter and have round free edges, granular cytoplasm, and large nuclei with distinct chromatin granules (2 to 3 months or longer in some breeds).

Proestrus

In the proestrus cycle, the vaginal wall is thicker and the mucosa shows prominent cornified squamous epithelium (20–30 cells thick) with rete pegging. The longitudinal and transverse vaginal folds are thick, smooth, and round. It becomes impervious to leukocytes, but there is extravasation of red blood cells (RBC) to the surface epithelium. These are discharged. Vaginal smears show predominantly erythrocytes and noncornified epithelial cells, which become cornified as proestrus progresses. Leukocytes are present but decrease as estrus approaches. Debris and bacteria are abundant for 7 to 10 days.

Estrus

The vagina is thick with longitudinal and transverse folds that become angular with decreased estrogen and increased progesterone. There is abundant fluid, often blood tinged. There is an absence of noncornified epithelial cells and leukocytes. There is a dominance of cornified epithelial cells, which are polyhedral and contain pyknotic nuclei or no nucleus; this seems to be related to the appearance of flirting by the bitch and acceptance of the stud. Leukocytes reappear at about 36 to 96 hours after ovulation. Bacteria and debris are absent during estrus, but they return to the smears after ovulation when leukocytes reappear 7 to 10 days later.

Metestrus

Leukocytes rapidly increase in numbers; there is a decrease in cornified and an increase in noncornified epithelial cells. After 5 to 7 days, the number of leukocytes may decrease to 10 to 30 per field.

Following parturition, much cellular debris, leukocytes, erythrocytes, and a few epithelial cells will be present for several days, until placental sloughing is complete. The presence of masses of degenerate leukocytes (and bacteria) indicates metritis or endometritis. Continued blood-tinged fluids containing abundant erythrocytes, a few noncornified epithelial cells, and occasional leukocytes (nontoxic) plus necrotic cells for months post partum are evidence of subinvolution of placental sites.

References and Additional Readings

Lein, D. H.: Examination of the bitch for breeding soundness. *In* Kirk, R. W. (ed.): Current Veterinary Therapy 8: Small Animal Practice. Philadelphia, W. B. Saunders Company, 1983, pp. 909–911.

Lindsay, F. E. F.: Endoscopy of the reproductive tract in the bitch. *In* Kirk, R. W. (ed.): Current Veterinary Therapy 8: Small Animal Practice. Philadelphia, W. B. Saunders Company, 1983, pp. 912–921.

Concannon, P. W.: Reproductive physiology and endocrine patterns of the bitch. *In* Kirk, R. W. (ed.): Current Veterinary Therapy 8: Small Animal Practice. Philadelphia, W. B. Saunders Company, 1983, pp. 886–900.

Examination and Characteristics of the Feline Vagina

Most of the principles just discussed that apply to bitches also pertain to queens. However, the small size of the feline vagina precludes palpation. Use of a sterile warm veterinary small animal otoscope speculum enables fairly good visualization of the vaginal mucosa and provides a sterile speculum for culture procedures using a small 4 mm in diameter sterile swab.* This is easiest following parturition or during estrus.

Vaginal cells for cytologic examination can be obtained with a moistened 3-mm cotton swab (Calgiswab) inserted 2 cm into the vagina. In some cases, flushing the vagina with sterile saline injected and aspirated with a clean glass eye dropper is more successful. This may trigger ovulation as it simulates coitus.

Unlike that occurring in the bitch, there is no diapedesis of erythrocytes in the queen during proestrus or throughout the estrous cycle.

Cytologic examination of feline vaginal smears reveals:
1. *Anestrus or prepuberty:* Scarce debris; numerous small round epithelial cells with high nuclear-cytoplasmic ratios, frequently in groups (seasonal—from September to January in the northern hemisphere).
2. *Proestrus:* Increased debris; fewer but larger nucleated epithelial cells with a low nuclear-cytoplasmic ratio (1 to 2 days).
3. *Estrus:* Markedly less debris; numerous large polyhedral cornified cells with curled edges and small dark pyknotic nuclei or loss of nuclei (3 to 6 days) following coitus or induced ovulation.
4. *Early metestrus:* Hazy, ragged-edged cornified cells; zero to numerous leukocytes with numerous bacteria and increased debris.

---

*Calgiswab Type IV, Inolex Division, American Can Co., Glenwood, IL 60425.

5. *Late metestrus:* Increasing numbers of small basophilic cells with leukocytes still present (total metestrus time—7–21 days). If ovulation does not occur, the smear will return to an anestrous stage with few to no leukocytes.

The feline estrus cycle is continuous every 14 to 36 days if 12 to 14 hours of daily light is present. Ovulation is induced 24 to 30 hours postcoitus. Sperm require 2 to 24 hours for capacitation in the uterus. Implantation occurs 13 to 14 days postcoitus.

References and Additional Readings

Concannon, P. W., and Lein, D. H.: Feline reproduction. *In* Kirk, R. W. (ed.): Current Veterinary Therapy 8: Small Animal Practice. Philadelphia, W. B. Saunders Company, 1983, pp. 932–935.
Concannon, P. W., and Lein, D. H.: Infertility and fertility treatment and management in the queen and tom cat. *In* Kirk, R. W. (ed.): Current Veterinary Therapy 8: Small Animal Practice. Philadelphia, W. B. Saunders Company, 1983, pp. 936–941.

LARYNGOSCOPY AND BRONCHOSCOPY

These techniques may be of value in the diagnosis of upper airway obstructions such as eversion of the lateral ventricles, collapsed arytenoid cartilages, hyperplasia of the vocal cords, the presence of nodules on the vocal cords, overly long soft-palate and traumatic injuries to the neck. Lesions of the trachea and mainstem bronchi, such as collapsed trachea, mediastinal tumors, hilar lymph node enlargement, and parasitic nodules *(Filaroides osleri)*, may also be diagnosed. In addition, bronchoscopy is a valuable technique that permits culturing and cytologic examination of material from bronchi involved in chronic respiratory disease. Upper airway obstruction that is not responsive to conservative therapy is an indication for more extensive diagnostic procedures, such as bronchoscopy.

Equipment

Equipment for laryngoscopy and bronchoscopy includes preanesthetic agents of choice (promazine, Innovar, Numorphan-Thorazine combination, injectable atropine, lidocaine 2 per cent, Surital sodium); syringes; a 3- or 4-inch, 12- to 14-gauge blunt cannula; intubating laryngoscope; mouth speculum; tongue forceps; distal illuminated fiberoptic bronchoscope;* portable power pack; flexible tip aspirating tube 50 cm long; specimen collection bottles (Lukens or Morrison type, 2 ml and 10 ml, sterilized); and a suction source.

Bronchoscopes are available in the following sizes:
3.0 mm by 25 cm; suitable for a 2- to 3-kg animal
3.5 mm by 30 cm; suitable for a 3- to 6-kg animal

---

*American Cytoscope Makers, Inc., Pelham Manor, New York; Olympus Corp., New Hyde Park, New York.

5 mm by 35 cm; suitable for a 6- to 10-kg animal
7 mm by 35 cm; suitable for a 10- to 15-kg animal
8 mm by 45 cm; suitable for a 15- to 22-kg animal
10 mm by 63 cm; suitable for an animal over 22 kg
In addition, a direct vision telescope and biopsying forceps are necessary.

Preparation of the Animal

The animal should be fasted for 18 to 24 hours prior to a bronchoscopic examination. Administer a suitable preanesthetic in combination with atropine one half hour prior to performing bronchoscopy. If the patient is a risk for general anesthesia, local topical anesthesia of the pharynx, vocal cords, and bronchi can be instituted using lidocaine, 2 per cent, administered through a 4-inch blunt cannula; use a neuroleptanalgesic agent for general sedation. In many instances, bronchoscopy can be performed under a short-acting general anesthetic such as thiamylal sodium administered via intravenous (IV) infusion. If bronchoscopy is to be prolonged, the gas delivery tube is attached to the side arm of the bronchoscope, and 4 to 6 liters per minute (LPM) of oxygen containing 1.0 to 1.5 per cent halothane is administered.

Bronchial secretions collected by aspiration of saline lavage should be divided into two parts. One part is submitted for bacteriologic culture. The second part of the sample is transferred from the collecting tube to a centrifuge tube containing 50 per cent ethyl alcohol. The specimen is centrifuged for 30 minutes at 1500 RPM, and the sediment is placed onto clear slides, fixed and stained for cytologic examination. Staining can be accomplished by numerous procedures, including Sano, Giemsa, or Papanicolaou stains.

References and Additional Readings

Roszel, J. F., and O'Brien, J. A.: Bronchoscopy and bronchial cytology in lung disease. Proc. Am. Anim. Hosp. Assoc., 35th Annual Meeting, 1968, pp. 200–203.
Roudebush, P.: Diagnostics for respiratory diseases. In Kirk, R. W.(ed.): Current Veterinary Therapy 8: Small Animal Practice. Philadelphia, W B. Saunders Company, 1983.

GASTROINTESTINAL FIBEROPTIC ENDOSCOPY

Flexible fiberoptic endoscopy is a noninvasive, atraumatic means of visualizing the mucosal surfaces of the esophagus, stomach, and colon. Flexible endoscopes are available from several companies at a wide range of prices. Three affordable endoscopes designed for veterinary use are available from AO Reichert Scientific Instruments (122 Charlton Street, Southbridge, Massachusetts 01550). The characteristics and uses of these endoscopes are summarized in Table 90.

Table 90. SPECIFICATIONS AND APPLICATIONS OF VETERINARY
ENDOSCOPES AVAILABLE FROM AO REICHERT
SCIENTIFIC INSTRUMENTS

	VFS 2	VFS 80	VFS 3
Functional length	80 cm	80 cm	115 cm
Diameter (maximum)	6.3 mm	13.8 mm	13.4 cm
Tip control	2 way	2 way	4 way
Tip deflection			
Up-down	120 degrees	150 degrees	170 degrees
Right-left	—	—	140 degrees
Diameter of channel	2.0 mm	2.5 mm	2.6 mm
Air insufflation	Manual	Automatic	Automatic
Suction control	Petcock	Push button	Push button
Lens cleaning	Manual	Automatic	Automatic
Air/water system	Through biopsy channel	Separate channel	Separate channel
Optical			
Field of view	70 degrees	60 degrees	90 degrees
Depth of field	5 mm–∞	12–7 mm	10–70 mm
Procedures			
Esophagoscopy	X	X	X
Gastroscopy	X	X	X
		(medium-sized and lager dogs)	
Colonoscopy	X	X	X
		(medium-sized and larger dogs)	

X = Instrument satisfactory for indicated procedure.
Courtesy of J. F. Zimmer.

To minimize the risk of injury to the animal and to reduce the possibility
of damage to the endoscope, animals undergoing endoscopic examination are
placed under general anesthesia after routine preanesthetic preparation. A fast
of 12 to 24 hours is recommended for most patients undergoing upper
gastrointestinal endoscopy. However, for those cases with indications of delayed
gastric emptying, a longer fast (24–48 hours) may be needed to empty the
stomach completely. In preparation for colonoscopy, a 24- to 48-hour fast is
recommended. A high warm-water enema is given the evening before and
again 2 to 4 hours before the procedure. Such enemas should be given until
the return is clear.

ESOPHAGOSCOPY

The clinical signs indicating esophageal disease and a potential benefit of
esophagoscopy include repeated regurgitation, excessive drooling, a ballooning
of the esophagus, anorexia or dysphagia, and recurrent pneumonia. Esophagoscopy allows visualization of the mucosal lining of the esophagus, making it

possible to detect inflammation, ulcerations, dilations, diverticula, strictures, foreign bodies, tumors, and parasite infestations.

GASTROSCOPY

Endoscopic examination of the mucosal aspect of the stomach is indicated when the clinical signs or physical findings suggest the presence of gastric disease and/or when there is a need for confirmation or clarification of radiographic findings. In most cases, persistent vomiting is the chief complaint. Other clinical signs suggestive of serious gastric disease include hematemesis, melena, weight loss, anemia, and abdominal pain. Gastroscopy allows visualization of the mucosal lining of the stomach, enabling detection of inflammation, ulceration, foreign bodies, and tumors.

COLONOSCOPY

The primary indication for colonoscopy is the presence of signs of large bowel disease, which typically include tenesmus and the passage of small, frequent stools containing fresh blood and/or excess mucus. (See Table 41 in the section entitled Diarrhea, page 247). Endoscopic examination of the colon allows direct visualization of the effects of mucosal inflammation, ulceration, mucosal polyps, malignant neoplasia, and strictures. Histologic examination of mucosal biopsies will confirm the diagnosis of colonic disease.

References and Additional Readings

Johnson, G. F.: Gastrointestinal Fiberoptic Endoscopy in Small Animal Medicine, White Plains, New York, Gaines Veterinary Symposium, 1979.

Jones, B.: Fiberoptic endoscopy. Proc. Am. Anim. Hosp. Assoc., 1981, pp. 101–103.

Zimmer, J. F.: Gastrointestinal fiberoptic endoscopy. *In* Kirk, R. W. (ed.): Current Veterinary Therapy VII, Philadelphia, W. B. Saunders Company, 1980.

PROCTOSCOPY

Proctoscopy, the technique of examining the descending colon, rectum, and anus, is a valuable procedure. It is helpful in the definitive diagnosis of lower bowel lesions, such as granulomatous colitis, foreign bodies, tumors, lacerations, and other mucosal abnormalities.

Equipment

Equipment needed for protoscopic examination includes a short-acting anesthetic (thiamylal sodium) and lubricating jelly.

A suitable proctoscope such as the Welch Allyn sigmoidoscope with distal illumination is also necessary. The speculum comes in three sizes: one with a

21 mm diameter and that is 25 cm long, one with a 15 mm diameter and that is 25 cm long, and a pediatric size, with a 15 mm diameter and that is 14 cm long. The complete kit usually includes all three sizes of proctoscopes, together with an inflation bulb, biopsy forceps, and portable power pack. This type of set can be completely sterilized.

Technique

In order to visualize the colonic mucosa, the large bowel must be empty. This can be accomplished by withholding food for 24 hours and performing a colonic irrigation the evening before and again 2 hours before the examination. The material used for the enema must be nonirritating and nonoily. Mildly hypertonic saline solutions such as Fleet enemas work well if given 2 hours before examination so that gas and fluid can be passed completely. However, Fleet enemas should not be used in cats or small dogs.

If the general physical condition of the animal is poor and withholding food is not possible, feeding a low-residue diet for 12 to 18 hours preceding proctoscopy can be helpful. This diet could consist of cooked eggs, small amounts of cooked beef or chicken, and small amounts of carbohydrate, such as slice of toast or one-fourth to one-half cup of moist kibble. Maintain good hydration. If all food is contraindicated, oral electrolyte solutions such as Gatorade or Resorb (Bristol) can be used to maintain hydration without moving solids through the intestinal tract.

Give the animal a short-acting anesthetic and place him on a tilted table in lateral recumbency, with the hindquarters elevated. Perform a digital examination of the rectum and pelvic cavity to ensure that there are no strictures, polyps, or other obstructions. Lubricate the proctoscope thoroughly with water-soluble jelly, and pass it gently through the anal sphincter. Press it forward slowly and carefully with a spiral motion. If any resistance is encountered, stop the motion, remove the obturator, and inspect the bowel to determine the cause of resistance. If possible, the obturator should be replaced and forward motion continued until the instrument is passed its full length. Withdraw the obturator, and observe the mucosa.

The major portion of the examination is conducted as the instrument is withdrawn. To view the colonic and rectal walls completely, it is necessary to move the anterior end of the proctoscope around the circumference of a small circle as it is withdrawn. Occasional insufflation with the inflating bulb is helpful in smoothing out folds of tissue. Repeated instrumentation may produce petechiae and minor hemorrhages that are not pathologic.

For examination of the terminal rectum and anus, the Hirshman anoscope provides adequate, convenient visualization.

Newer techniques for visualizing the upper and lower gastrointestinal tract are rapidly being developed and are being used in dogs. The flexible fiberoptic endoscope enables one to visualize and photograph the esophagus, colon, and stomach. One is able not only to directly visualize lesions of the gastrointestinal tract but also to assess motility and biopsy lesions and to remove foreign bodies.

The development of the flexible fiberoptic sigmoidoscope permits examination and biopsy of regions of the colon that cannot be reached by the rigid sigmoidoscope. The flexible fiberoptic sigmoidoscope allows for injection of air and warm water into the colon. Biopsy specimens can be taken while visualizing a lesion. (See Zimmer reference for additional details about such procedures.)

References and Additional Readings

Sherding, R. G.: Canine large bowel diarrhea. Compendium on Continuing Education, 2:279, 1980.

Zimmer, J. F.: Gastrointestinal fiberoptic endoscopy. *In* Kirk, R. W. (ed.): Current Veterinary Therapy VII. Philadelphia, W. B. Saunders Company, 1980.

LAPAROSCOPY

Laparoscopy is a procedure for the visual examination of the peritoneal cavity and its contents after the establishment of pneumoperitoneum. The Needlescope* is a small fiberoptic laparoscope, 1.7 or 2.2 mm in diameter. It requires a bright light source but, because of its small size, can be readily inserted into the abdomen. Some clinicians have successfully used the operating laparoscope (3 mm), manufactured by Richard Wolf Manufacturing Co., Rosemont, Illinois 60018.

Abdominal insufflation and laparoscopy require either general anesthesia, neuroleptanalgesia with local anesthesia, or rarely, (in the critically ill animal) regional local anesthesia alone. The depth and type of anesthesia or analgesia depends on the condition of the patient and the skill and experience of the examiner.

Prior to laparoscopy, a cleansing enema should be performed. The laparoscopy site is surgically prepared.

To insufflate the abdomen, use a Verees pneumoperitoneum needle. Placement of the needle is 3 to 4 cm below the umbilicus, along the linea alba. Saline (10 ml) is injected through the needle, and aspiration is attempted to ensure that a blood vessel or hollow viscus has not been penetrated. If ascitic fluid is present, it must be removed and examined (see p. 807).

Air is injected into the peritoneal cavity through an inline filter using the Verees needle. Insufflation should be slow, and vital signs should be monitored. Following effective insufflation, the needle is removed, a small skin incision is made over the needle entry point, and the larger trocar and cannula are inserted at a 30-degree angle to the animal's longitudinal plane. Extreme care should be taken when placing the trocar into the abdomen. The endoscope (Needlescope) is moved cephalad along the abdominal wall while good insufflation is maintained. Rotate the animal into different positions to enable visualization of various internal organs. Biopsy specimens can be obtained through

---

*Needlescope, Dyonics, Inc., Andover, MA.

the Needlescope or through a separate incision while observing through the Needlescope. When endoscopic inspection has been completed, the Needlescope is removed, the insufflated air is allowed to escape, and skin sutures are placed.

Indications for laparoscopy include biopsy, visual diagnosis, follow-up examinations, and research needs.

Contraindications for laparoscopy include peritonitis, hernias, coagulation defects, obesity, abdominal adhesions, and inexperience of the clinician.

References and Additional Readings

Harrison, R. M., and Wildt, D. E. (eds.): Animal Laparoscopy. Baltimore, Williams & Wilkins, 1980.

Jones, B. D.: The use of fiberoptic endoscopy in veterinary medicine. A.A.H.A. Sci. Proc., Salt Lake City, 1978, p. 241.

Patterson, J. M.: Laparoscopy in small animal medicine. In Kirk, R. W. (ed.): Current Veterinary Therapy VII. Philadelphia, W. B. Saunders Company, 1980.

Zaslow, I. M.: Clinical Endoscopy. In Zaslow, I. M. (ed.): Veterinary Trauma and Critical Care. Philadelphia, Lea & Febiger, 1984.

MEASUREMENT OF CENTRAL VENOUS PRESSURE (DOG)

Measurement of the central venous pressure (CVP) in the dog is an excellent index for determining circulation efficiency. CVP is controlled by interaction of the circulating blood volume, cardiac pumping action, and alterations in the vascular bed. CVP is not a measure of blood volume but an indication of the ability of the heart to accept and pump blood brought to it. CVP reflects the interaction of the heart, vascular tone, and circulatory blood volume. When the heart action and vascular tone remain constant, CVP reflects blood volume. When blood volume and vascular tone are constant, CVP reflects heart action. When blood volume and heart action are constant, CVP can be used to measure vascular tone.

In addition, the placement of a jugular catheter can be helpful in long-term fluid management and in parenteral alimentation of critically ill animals (see p. 610).

Indications

Indications for CVP measurement include (1) acute circulatory failure that has not responded to initial treatment, (2) administration of large volumes of blood or fluids, as may occur in acute shock, (3) as part of the monitoring procedure in poor–risk surgical patients, and (4) abnormal urine production for which fluids are being administered.

Equipment

The following equipment is necessary for CVP measurement:

One Intracath needle, 17 or 18 gauge

One metric rule, 80 cm long

One three-way stopcock

One bottle of isotonic sodium chloride, 500 ml, and intravenous (IV) tubing

One extra piece of tubing, 3 ft long, or a Becton-Dickinson or Batten disposable CVP set

Procedure

In order to measure CVP, a catheter must be placed in the external jugular vein so that it is in direct fluid continuity with the right atrium. Adequate measurement of CVP in the noncomatose animal requires sedation or the use of a short-acting general anesthetic.

Place the animal in lateral recumbency, and clip the hair over the jugular vein. Surgically prepare the skin in the clipped area.

Make a percutaneous puncture of the jugular vein with the Intracath catheter needle, and advance the tip to approximately the third intercostal space (tip of catheter at right atrium). The catheter should be securely fastened to the neck of the patient by passing adhesive tape around the neck incorporating the hub of the catheter needle, so that it comes to lie at the base of the ear. Connect a three-way stopcock to the catheter. Connect an IV setup of isotonic sodium chloride to one end of the stopcock, and to the other end of the stopcock, attach a piece of IV tubing, which should be taped vertically to a pole or a piece of doweling (Fig. 81). The metric rule is placed so that the 0 level is aligned with the midpoint of the trachea at the thoracic inlet, and the rule is taped to the vertical pole.

To fill the CVP manometer, the three-way stopcock is turned so that fluid will flow from the bottle of saline into the manometer and will exceed the 15 cm mark. Next, the stopcock is turned so that a column of fluid exists from the superior vena cava to the manometer. The fluid in the manometer will fall until it reflects the level of the CVP.

It is desirable to allow fluid to flow frequently through the catheter so that the catheter tip will not become plugged with a blood clot. Periodic flushing with heparinized saline will help maintain the patency of the catheter. This setup allows easy administration of fluids and medication IV to the patient and collection of blood, if necessary.

There is no absolute value for a normal CVP. The CVP for the normal dog is -1 to $+5$ cm water. Elevations of $+5$ to $+10$ are borderline; however, values above 10 cm of water may indicate an abnormally expanded blood volume and those above 15 cm of water, possible congestive heart failure. It is the trend of the CVP that should be monitored and correlated with the regimen of treatment. One must be constantly aware of the interrelationship between blood volume, cardiovascular function, and vascular tone.

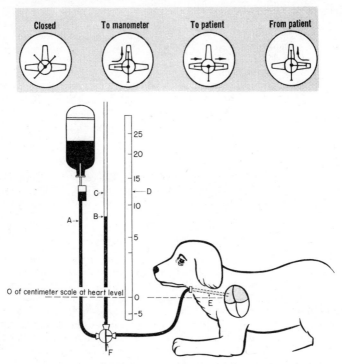

Figure 81. Central venous manometer. *A,* Standard IV infusion tube. *B,* Central venous pressure level. *C,* 30-inch IV extension tube. *D,* Centimeter scale. *E,* Plastic tube in great veins in thorax or right atrium via jugular vein. *F,* Three-way stopcock set in measuring position (open from manometer to catheter). Note: This procedure should be performed with the dog in right lateral recumbency. From Sattler, F. P.: Shock. *In* Kirk, R. W. (ed.): Current Veterinary Therapy III. Philadelphia, W. B. Saunders Company, 1968.

References and Additional Readings

Sattler, F. P., Knowles, R. P., and Whittick, W. G.: Veterinary Critical Care. Philadelphia, Lea & Febiger, 1981.

Zaslow, I. M. (ed.): Veterinary Trauma and Critical Care. Philadelphia, Lea & Febiger, 1984.

SPECIAL TECHNIQUES OF RADIOGRAPHIC EXAMINATION

Gastrointestinal or Small Bowel Studies

Contrast agents available for gastrointestinal studies include barium suspension preparations (Redi-opaque,* which is 30 per cent weight per volume [w/v] of barium sulphate) or Micropaque† and water-soluble agents (Gastrografin,‡ which is 60 per cent meglumine and 10 per cent sodium diatrizoate). Water-soluble agents are used if bowel perforation is suspected. Undiluted water-soluble agents are very hypertonic and should be diluted at a ratio of one part Gastrografin to two parts water.

Procedures

Barium swallows and esophagrams require that the animal be fasted for 12 hours prior to radiography. Remove all leashes from around the animal's neck, and obtain survey radiographs of the thorax. In esophageal contrast studies, 2 to 5 ml of barium suspension contrast medium per kg of body weight should be administered. Barium is contraindicated if a perforation of the esophagus is suspected. When the esophagus has been coated with radiopaque material, lateral, ventrodorsal (V-D), and right V-D oblique thoracic radiographs should be taken to visualize the esophagus.

For barium swallows, the barium should be thick and pasty (like marshmallow fluff). Position the patient and cassette, and have the x-ray technique set up. Give a tablespoonful of barium orally. Make the exposure when the animal makes its second swallow after the barium has been given.

To achieve the maximum information from a gastrointestinal study, the following preliminary steps are necessary:
1. Ensure that the hair of the animal is free from exogenous dirt, paint, and foreign material. Bathe the animal, if necessary.
2. Withhold food for 18 to 24 hours.
3. If the colon is filled with feces, administer a bisacodyl suppository (Dylcolox,§ 5 mg) one-half hour prior to the radiographic procedure or administer a Fleet enema, which leaves no abnormal residual gas patterns in the bowel. A Fleet enema should be given 3 hours prior to the start of the gastrointestinal series. Fleet enemas should not be given to cats; they should receive only a mild soap and warm water enema.

At the start of an upper gastrointestinal series, obtain survey radiographs of the abdomen and establish a technique. A barium sulfate (micropulverized) preparation can be administered by stomach tube, or the animal can be induced to swallow the fluids. Flavored prepared barium suspensions are available.

---

*Redi-opaque, Burns Biotic Laboratories, Oakland, California.
†Micropaque, Picker Corporation, Cleveland, Ohio.
‡Gastrografin, E. R. Squibb & Sons, Lawrenceville, New Jersey.
§Dylcolox, Boehringer Ltd., Burlington, Ontario, Canada.

Dosage levels vary, but approximately 10 ml per kg for barium suspensions is usually given. When using organic iodide liquid preparations, administer 0.5 ml per kg by stomach tube. Obtain lateral and dorsoventral (D-V) radiographs of the abdomen immediately following administration of the barium and at 30-minute, 1-hour, and 2-hour intervals. Water-soluble contrast material passes through the gastrointestinal tract in approximately 30 to 90 minutes. Barium suspensions take 60 to 180 minutes to traverse the intestine. The colon is usually filled with barium 6 hours after oral administration and may contain barium for 2 to 3 days following administration.

Contrast studies of the upper gastrointestinal tract are frequently used in cases of nonresponsive vomiting, refractory diarrhea, hematemesis, suspected enteric foreign bodies, suspected neoplasms and obstructions, and confirmation of misplaced intestinal organs such as may be seen in diaphragmatic hernias.

Barium contrast radiography is contraindicated in suspected cases of perforation of the stomach or upper gastrointestinal tract. In these cases, water-soluble contrast media such as the oral diatrizoates are used, because leakage into the abdomen will produce no foreign body granuloma. In addition, barium sulfate should not be administered when an obstruction of the lower bowel may be present. In these cases, barium may only contribute to the obstipation.

If chemical restraint is needed for gastrointestinal studies, the following tranquilizers can be used: acetylpromazine maleate (Acepromazine,*), triflu-promazine hydrochloride (Vetame,†), and ketamine hydrochloride (Vetalar;‡ for cats only).

The following radiographic views are recommended following the administration of radiographic contrast material:

Survey radiographs of abdomen
    Views: D-V and right lateral (R-L) recumbency.
    Objectives: Evaluate for preparation of patient, interpretation for disease, and reference point for contrast study.

Immediately following administration of contrast material—5 minutes
    Views: D-V, R-L recumbency, and left lateral (L-L) recumbency. The R-L view shows the pylorus of the stomach filled with barium, and the L-L view shows the cardia and fundic portion filled with barium.
    Objective: Evaluate the distended stomach and initial gastric emptying.

Twenty to 30 minutes following administration of contrast material
    Views: D-V and R-L recumbency.
    Objective: Evaluate the stomach, pyloric function, and duodenum.

Sixty minutes following administration of contrast material
    Views: D-V and R-L recumbency.
    Objective: Evaluate the small intestine.

Two hours following administration of contrast material
    Views: D-V and R-L recumbency.

---

*Acepromazine, Ayerst Laboratories, New York, New York.
†Vetame, E. R. Squibb & Sons, Lawrenceville, New Jersey.
‡Vetalar, Parke-Davis, Detroit, Michigan.

Objective: Evaluate the passage of contrast material into the colon and complete emptying of the stomach*—contrast material should be in the terminal portion of the small intestine.

The passage of contrast material through the normal gastrointestinal tract is variable; however, the following guidelines have been suggested:

1. Contrast material in the duodenum within 15 minutes in most patients. Excitement can delay this time to 20 to 25 minutes.
2. Contrast material reaches the jejunum within 30 minutes and is within the jejunum and ileum at 60 minutes.
3. Contrast material reaches the ileocecal junction in approximately 90 to 120 minutes.
4. At 3 to 5 hours postadministration, contrast material has cleared the upper gastrointestinal tract and is within the ileum and the large intestine.

Diatrizoate compounds are hypertonic and irritating to the bowel wall.

In evaluation of gastrointestinal contrast studies, the following criteria may be considered: (1) size of intestinal mass, (2) contour of the mucosal surface, (3) thickness of the bowel wall, (4) flexibility and motility of the bowel wall, (5) position of the small intestine, (6) continuity of the opaque column, and (7) transit time.

Further examination of the upper gastrointestinal tract uses the technique of gastrography and upper gastrointestinal contrast radiography.

In gastrography, the stomach is distended with either negative contrast material (air) or positive contrast material and is radiographically visualized. The animal should be fasted for 12 to 24 hours, and a technique of abdominal radiography should be established. To perform negative contrast gastrography, administer 5 to 10 ml of air per kg of body weight via a stomach tube or 30 to 90 ml of a highly carbonated beverage by stomach tube.

Double contrast gastrography refers to first coating the stomach with barium sulfate suspension and then liberating negative contrast material (air) into the stomach. Radiographs are taken in the V-D, D-V, R-L, and L-L positions.

Barium Enemas

Suspected clinical conditions for which barium enemas are indicated in the dog include ileocolic intussusception and cecal inversion, mechanical and functional large bowel obstruction, invasive lesions of the large bowel, mass outside of the large bowel compressing the bowel, and inflammation of the lower intestinal tract. Barium sulfate enemas are contraindicated in suspected obstruction of the colon and rupture or perforation of the colon.

The following procedures should be followed for giving barium enemas:

1. For the 24 hours preceding radiographs, maintain the animal on a liquid diet only, preferably water or broth.

---

*Modified from O'Brien, T. R.: Radiographic Diagnosis of Abdominal Disorders in the Dog and Cat. Philadelphia, W. B. Saunders Company, 1978.

2. During the 18 to 24 hours before the radiographs, administer a mild high colonic enema or give a saline laxative by mouth.
3. Do not give any irritating enemas within 12 hours of the scheduled radiographic examination; however, isotonic saline solution or plain water enemas should be administered prior to the examination to ensure that the bowel is clear.
4. Obtain survey radiographs of the abdomen, and examine the colon to ensure that this portion of the bowel is clear.
5. Do not force barium into the colon under pressure. Do not elevate the enema bag more than 18 inches above the animal.
6. Do not perform a proctoscopic examination on the same day that the barium enema is given.

Cuffed rectal catheters (Bardex Cuffed Rectal Catheters Nos. 24 to 38 French and Bardex Cuffed Pediatric Rectal Catheter No. 18 French*) can be used in dogs. For very small dogs and cats, smaller catheters are used. A plastic catheter adapter and a three-way stopcock are needed.

Various barium sulfate preparations can be used; however, the final concentration should be 15 to 20 per cent (w/v). A commercially available barium enema kit is helpful.†

In order to effectively perform a barium enema, sedate or anesthetize the animal. Place the cuffed rectal catheter so that the inflated bulb is cranial to the anal sphincter. Place the animal in R-L recumbency and fill the colon with contrast material at a dose of 20 to 30 ml per kg of body weight. Take the radiographs after infusion of a two-thirds dose of barium. If the colon is not filled, infuse more contrast agent. Obtain radiographs in the V-D and lateral positions, and determine whether the colon is adequately distended. Remove as much of the contrast material as possible from the colon, and repeat the radiographs. Then insert 2 ml per kg of air into the colon, and repeat the radiographs. Deflate the cuff on the catheter, and remove it from the rectum. Throughout the procedure of filling the colon with contrast material or air, care should be taken not to overdistend the colon, which may lead to rupture.

In carrying out a barium enema, look for the following radiographic lesions: (1) irregularity of the barium-mucosal interface; (2) spasm, stricture, or occlusion of the bowel lumen; (3) filling defects; (4) outpouching of the bowel wall due to diverticulum or perforation; and (5) displacement of the bowel.

Excretory Urography

Intravenous (IV) administration of organic iodinated compounds in high concentrations permits visualization of the renal pelvis and ureters as the kidneys excrete the substance. Excretory urography does not reveal any quantitative information about renal function and is not a substitute for renal

---

*Bard Hospital Division, C. R. Bard, Inc., Murray Hill, New Jersey.
†Barium enema, E-Z-EM Corporation, Inc., Westbury, New York.

function tests. The degree of visualization of contrast material within the renal excretory system depends on the type of contrast material used—in regard to the concentration of iodine in the contrast medium, the technique of excretory urography to be performed, the state of hydration of the patient, renal blood flow, and functional capacity of the kidneys.

The following routinely used contrast materials contain iodine concentrations of:

Product	mg/ml
Hypaque, 50% (Winthrop Laboratories)	300
Hypaque-M, 75% (Winthrop Laboratories)	385
Renovist II (Squibb & Sons)	310
Renografin-60 (Squibb & Sons)	288
Renografin-76 (Squibb & Sons)	370

Modified from Ticer, J. W.: Radiographic Technique in Small Animal Practice, 2nd ed. Philadelphia, W. B. Saunders Company, 1984, p. 376.

Technique

The following steps should be used in carrying out excretory urography:
1. Fast the animal for 12 to 18 hours.
2. Twelve to 18 hours prior to radiography, administer a high colonic enema or give saline laxative orally.
3. Ensure that the animal's hair is free of dirt and debris.
4. Try to limit the animal's fluid intake for the 12 hours preceding radiography.
5. Empty the animal's bladder immediately before taking radiographs.
6. Take survey radiographs before administering contrast media.

Low-Volume, Rapid Infusion Technique with Abdominal Compression. Rapidly administer 425 mgI per kg of the desired mixture of sodium and meglumine diatrizoates via an indwelling IV catheter. Apply compression to the abdomen in front of the pubis, and obtain lateral and V-D radiographs immediately and 1, 3, and 5 minutes after injection. Remove the compression band, and reradiograph at 10 and 15 minutes.

Low-Volume, Rapid Infusion without Compression. Rapidly administer 850 mgI per kg of iodine compound IV. Obtain a V-D radiograph at 10 seconds postinjection, and repeat V-D and lateral radiographs 1, 3, 5, and 15 minutes following injection.

High-Volume Urography. Mix 1200 mgI per kg of body weight (not to exceed 35 gm) of one of the sodium and meglumine diatrizoates with an equal volume of 5 per cent dextrose and water (D5W). By drip infusion, administer the mixture over a 10-minute period. Obtain abdominal radiographs, and apply compression bandage, repeating radiographs at 10 and 20 minutes. Repeat radiographs at 30 minutes without compression bandage.

Lesions that can be detected using IV urography are renal mass lesions—neoplasia; renal cysts; renal and ureteral traumatic lesions; pyelonephritis; hydroureter, hydronephrosis; renal agenesis, hypoplasia; pelvic and ureteral obstructions—calculi, blood clots; renal parasites; ectopic ureter; and duplication of the collecting system.

Retrograde Contrast Urethrography in the Dog and Cat

Retrograde urethrography is a diagnostic tool that can be used to localize diseases of the lower urinary tract of dogs and cats. Conditions such as urethral neoplasms, strictures, trauma, calculi, or other anomalies can be revealed by this method.

The technique involves the injection of an aqueous iodine contrast medium (such as Hypaque-M, 75 per cent; Renografin-76; or Hypaque Meglumine, 60 per cent) into the urethra using a ureteral or balloon-tipped catheter. The radiopaque contrast material is mixed to a three- to fivefold dilution with sterile petroleum jelly (K-Y jelly) to increase the viscosity of the media. A dilution of 1:3 contrast medium with sterile distilled water or saline can also be used. Prior to performing retrograde contrast urethrography, a cleansing enema should be given. Sedation or anesthesia may be necessary. Five to 10 ml of contrast medium should be injected. Near the end of the injection, while the urethra is still under pressure, a lateral radiograph is obtained.

If the urinary bladder is to be distended with contrast material or air, remove urine from the bladder. In the male dog, position the catheter so that the tip of the catheter is distal to the os penis. Inject 1 to 2 ml of lidocaine into the urethral lumen to anesthetize the urethra adjacent to the balloon-tipped catheter. Extreme care should be taken in the amount of fluid placed in the bladder if the urethra is occluded by a balloon catheter. Overdistention of the bladder results in hematuria, pyuria, urinary bladder rupture, and mild to severe bladder inflammation. Careful palpation of the bladder during distention and noting the back pressure on the syringe used in filling the bladder should be observed.

Retrograde contrast urethrography is a definite aid in defining the extent of urethral damage (stricture) or in demonstrating urethral calculi in male cats. In male cats, a No. 4 French balloon catheter or a No. 3.5 French tom cat open-ended urethral catheter* should be used. The catheter should be inserted 1.5 cm into the penile urethra. If the urethra is patent, 2 to 3 ml of contrast material will enable visualization of the urethra, but increased amounts of contrast material (2–3 ml/lb) injected into the bladder are needed for maximum distention of the preprostatic urethra. A voiding positive contrast urethrogram is necessary to visualize the distal (penile) urethra. Apply external pressure to the bladder (using a wooden spoon or other external compression device), and radiograph the distal urethra.

---

*Monoject, Sherwood Medical Co., St. Louis, Missouri 63103.

Pneumocystography

The following steps should be followed in pneumocystographic examination:

1. Fast the animal for 18 to 24 hours preceding radiography.
2. Administer a high colonic enema, or give saline laxative orally 12 to 18 hours prior to taking radiographs. Administer a mild, warm water enema 2 to 3 hours before the radiographs are to be taken.
3. Ensure that the animal's hair is clean.
4. Take survey radiographs of the bladder, and then empty the bladder of urine. The entire urinary tract—kidneys through urethra—should be included in the radiographs. Avoid the use of metal female catheters, because they may cause traumatic injury to the bladder wall.
5. Using a syringe and a three-way valve, inject 5 to 10 ml of air per kg of body weight into the bladder. Palpate the bladder while filling it with air to avoid overdistention or rupture. Inject air until there is pressure on the syringe barrel or leakage of air around the catheter. If air escapes during the procedure, it should be replaced.
6. Take lateral and V-D views of the abdomen.

Pneumocystography is not an innocuous procedure; fatal venous air emboli have been seen in dogs and cats. Inject air slowly. If possible, use a gas that is readily soluble in blood (such as CO_2 or N_2O) for bladder insufflation. Place the animal in L-L recumbency.

Contrast Cystography

This technique involves injecting radiographic contrast material into the bladder and may be used for the following indications:

Clinical

1. Frequent urination.
2. Intermittent or chronic hematuria and/or small volumes of voided urine.
3. Hematuria that is seen throughout or in the later stages of voiding.
4. Dysuria.
5. Persistent post-traumatic hematuria.

Radiographic

1. Areas of increased or decreased density associated with the urinary bladder.
2. Nonvisualization of the urinary bladder after trauma.
3. Evaluation of abnormal caudal abdominal masses and structures adjacent to the urinary bladder.
4. Evaluation of abnormal bladder shape or location.

The same principles or preparation of the animal apply as when performing a pneumocystogram. Use a urethral catheter with a three-way valve or a small Foley catheter with an inflatable cuff. Organic iodides are the contrast material of choice and should be used in 5 to 10 per cent concentrations.

Table 91. RADIOPACITY OF CYSTIC CALCULI ON PLAIN
ABDOMINAL RADIOGRAPHS

Calculus Composition	Density
Calcium oxalate	Radiopaque
Calcium carbonate	Radiopaque
Triple phosphate	Radiopaque—small calculi may be nonradiopaque
Cystine	Variable density—may have radiopaque stippling
Uric acid and urates	Nonradiopaque
Xanthine	Nonradiopaque
Matrix concretions	Nonradiopaque

From Park, R. D.: Radiology of the urinary bladder and urethra. *In* O'Brien, T. R.: Radiographic Diagnosis of Abdominal Disorders in the Dog and Cat. Philadelphia, W. B. Saunders Company, 1978.

Double contrast cystography can also be performed. Catheterize the urinary bladder and remove all urine. Inject a small volume (2–5 ml) of an aqueous organic iodine contrast medium into the bladder. Roll the animal over in an attempt to coat the bladder with contrast material. Then distend the bladder with air in the same manner as for pneumocystography.

Some of the routine lesions diagnosed with the aid of cystography are: calculi (Table 91); neoplasia; cystitis, if proliferative changes are present; muscle hypertrophy; diverticuli; duplications; adhesions, especially uterine stump; persistent urachus; ruptures; and atonic bladder.

Myelography

Myelography is the study of the spinal cord and vertebral canal made possible by the use of contrast media in the subarachnoid space. Ideally, the contrast material should be relatively nontoxic and absorbable, should provide good contrast, and should be evenly distributed throughout the subarachnoid space. Three contrast agents are used; sodium methiodal (Skiodan,*) isophendylate (Pantopaque,†) and metrizamide‡ (Amipaque§). Water-soluble contrast media such as 40 per cent sodium methiodal provide good radiographic detail; however, they are irritating and can be toxic. Water-soluble contrast media are rapidly absorbed from the cerebrospinal fluid (CSF). The oily preparations such as isophendylate can be used with good diagnostic results, although they may produce a chronic arachnoiditis.

---

*Skiodan, Winthrop Laboratories, New York, New York.

†Pantopaque, Lafayette Pharmacal, Inc., Lafayette, Indiana.

‡Metrizamide, Investigational Drugs, Neygaard & Co., Oslo, Norway, distributed by Gallard-Schlesinger, 584 Mineola Ave., Carole Place, New York.

§Amipaque, Winthrop Laboratories, New York, New York.

The nonionic water-soluble contrast agent, metrizamide, is used almost exclusively for myelographic examinations. This agent has low toxicity and low epileptogenic activity, is inert to nervous tissue, has no long-term side effects, and is resorbed and excreted rapidly from the CSF. Metrizamide can be injected into the subarachnoid space at the cerebellomedullary cistern or at the caudal lumbar spine at a dose level of 0.22 ml per kg. Five minutes after cisternal injection with metrizamide if there is no obstruction, the cervical and thoracic cord segments are outlined, and after 10 to 15 minutes, the entire cord is outlined. Metrizamide can be purchased as an analytical grade substance from chemical supply houses. If the analytical grade is used, it can be dissolved in sterile water and passed through a Millipore filter (0.22 μm) to achieve a final concentration of 350 mg of metrizamide per ml (126–195 mgI/ml). Any unused material should be stored in a lightproof container or refrigerated and used within 5 days. Metrizamide is available commercially as an expensive single dose vial of 10 ml (Amipaque). Preservatives are not added to this reconstituted material. Approximately 15 to 45 per cent of dogs that undergo metrizamide myelography may develop side effects characterized by seizure activity. Several factors influence the rate of seizure development:

1. *Duration of anesthesia of the animal*—the longer the duration of anesthesia following myelography, the lower the risk of convulsive activity.
2. *Weight of the dog and amount of metrizamide administered.* Larger dogs receive more metrizamide and have a greater risk of convulsive activity than small dogs.
3. *Site and rate of contrast injection.* When metrizamide is injected into the cerebellomedullary cisternal space, the head should be tilted up, preventing the material from entering the ventricles. Less seizure activity is noted when the subarachnoid space of the lumbar spine is the area injected.

Animals to be examined with metrizamide should not be given phenothiazine derivatives and should not be anesthetized with neuroleptanalgesic agents, because these lower the epileptogenic threshold.

Technique

Myelographic examination involves the following procedures:

1. Fast the animal for 18 to 24 hours preceding myelography.
2. Anesthetize the animal with a short-acting agent such as thiamylal sodium, and maintain the animal on gas anesthetic of choice.
3. Clip and surgically prepare the skin over the cisterna magna or in the lumbosacral area, depending on where one wishes to enter the spinal canal. For cisterna magna puncture, see p. 496. Lumbar puncture can be made between the fifth and sixth or between the fourth and fifth lumbar vertebrae. A short bevel spinal needle should be used.

To use 40 per cent Skiodan w/v concentration, the material is diluted with 5 per cent dextrose and 5 per cent Xylocaine HCl. The dilution is 4.5 ml of 40 per cent Skiodan, 4.5 ml of 5 per cent dextrose, and 0.2 ml of 5 per cent Xylocaine. The contrast agent is injected into the subarachnoid space between L_{4-5} or L_{5-6} at a dose of 0.3 to 0.5 ml per kg.

Sialography

Sialography is the radiographic examination of the salivary glands and ducts. The glands are visualized by injection of a radiopaque dye into the salivary duct. The technique can be used to outline (via retrograde perfusion) the parotid, zygomatic, mandibular, and sublingual salivary glands. The most common indicator for sialography is the salivary mucocele. The technique is used to help locate the salivary duct tear causing the mucocele and to aid in determining which gland should be removed. General anesthesia is necessary to perform sialography.

Equipment

The equipment needed for sialography includes blunt 22-, 25-, and 26-gauge hypodermic needles; fine tissue forceps; syringes; a mouth gag; and 60 per cent diatrizoate sodium meglumine (Renografin-60).

Technique

The parotid duct opens into the mouth on a papilla on the labial or oral mucosa opposite the upper fourth premolar tooth. The oral mucosa just caudal to the papilla should be grasped with a fine tissue forceps and retracted rostromedially, which will facilitate passage of a blunt 22-gauge needle. Inject 1 to 5 ml of Renografin-60, depending on the size of the animal, and take radiographs immediately.

The major zygomatic salivary duct opens into the mouth approximately 1 cm caudal and slightly dorsal to the parotid duct papilla. A 25- or 26-gauge blunt needle is inserted into the duct while the mucosa around the duct opening is held with a small forceps.

The mandibular ducts open into the mouth on the lateral surface of the lingual caruncles (sublingual folds). The sublingual duct enters the mouth 1 to 2 mm caudal to the mandibular duct. The sublingual opening is smaller than the mandibular opening. It has been estimated that in one dog out of three, the two ducts (mandibular and sublingual) join before entering the mouth. In large dogs, a 22-gauge blunt needle is used to cannulate the mandibular duct, and in small dogs, a 25-gauge needle is used. A 26-gauge blunt needle is used to cannulate the sublingual duct.

Bronchography

The following procedures should be used in bronchographic examination:
1. The animal should be fasted for 24 hours prior to beonchography.
2. The animal should be preanesthetized with promazine, Innovar, or a Numorphan-Thorazine combination and atropine. Following this, a short-acting general anesthetic (thiamylal sodium) may be given. If general

anesthesia is contraindicated, lidocaine, 2 per cent, may be applied topically to the pharynx, vocal cords, and bronchi.

3. Only one half of the chest is examined at a time, with a 24- to 48-hour wait before the other side is examined. Aqueous Dionosil can be used, 5 to 10 ml per side, as the contrast medium. A 50 to 60 per cent w/v suspension of barium sulfate in carboxymethylcellulose base (Redi-Flow, 100 per cent w/v) can also be used. It is best to position the contrast material in the appropriate bronchi using a nontraumatic polyethylene catheter and radiographic visualization. Excessive bronchial secretions must be removed by suction through a bronchoscope before the radiographic contrast material is administered.

4. Contraindications for bronchography are pneumonia and congestive heart failure.

Nonselective Angiocardiography (See p. 374)

Cholecystography

Use of this technique depends on the ability of selected radiopaque compounds to be removed from the blood and excreted via active transport by hepatocytes. Contrast agents for cholecystography can be administered either orally or IV. Oral cholecystographic examination requires that the contrast agent (1) enter the small bowel, (2) be absorbed and enter the portal circulation, and (3) be excreted into the bile and concentrated in the gallbladder. IV cholecystography eliminates some of the variables within the digestive tract and may be a more reliable technique in dogs and cats.

Following the administration of a selected contrast agent to produce cholecystography, (D-V) and standing lateral projections for radiography are indicated at time intervals appropriate for the contrast material used.

References and Additional Readings

Barsanti, J. A., Crowell, W., Losonsky, J., et al.: Complications of bladder distention during retrograde urethrography. Am. J. Vet. Res., 42:819, 1981.

Davis, E. M., Glickman, L., Rendano, V. T., and Short, C. M.: Seizures in dogs following metrizamide myelography. J.A.A.H.A. 17(4): 642, 1981.

Fox, P. R., and Bond, B. R.: Nonselective and selective angiocardiography. Vet. Clin. North Am., 13(2): 259, 1983.

Johnston, G. R., Osborne, C. A., and Jessen, C. R.: Retrograde contrast urethrography in the dog and cat. Sci. Proc. Am. Anim. Hosp. Assoc., 44th Annual Meeting, 1977, p. 423.

Kleine, L. J.: Radiography in the diagnosis of intestinal obstruction in dogs and cats. Compendium on Continuing Education, Small Anim. Pract., 1:44, 1979.

Kleine, L. J.: Radiology of acute abdominal disorders in the dog and cat. Compendium on Continuing Education, Small Anim. Pract., 1:520, 1979.

Lord, P. F., and Olsson, S. E.: Myelography with metrizamide in the dog: a clinical study in its use for the demonstration of spinal cord lesions other than those caused by intervetebral disk protrusions. J. Am. Vet. Radiol. Soc., 17:42, 1976.

O'Brien, T. R.: Radiographic Diagnosis of Abdominal Disorders in the Dog and Cat. Philadelphia, W. B. Saunders Company, 1978.

Owens, J. M.: Radiographic Interpretation for the Small Animal Clinician. St. Louis, Ralston Purina Co., 1982.

Rendano, V. T.: Radiology of the gastrointestinal tract of small animals. Can. Vet. J., 22:331, 1981.

Root, C. R.: Contrast radiology of urinary system. In Ticer, J. W.: Radiographic Technique in Small Animal Practice. Philadelphia, W. B. Saunders Company, 1975.

Ticer, J. W.: Radiographic Technique in Small Animal Practice, 2nd ed. Philadelphia, W. B. Saunders Company, 1984.

Therapeutic Procedures ━━━━━━━━━━━━

ADMINISTRATION OF MEDICATIONS

Oral Administration of Capsules and Tablets

Dogs

Solid medications should be given to dogs quickly and decisively so that the "pilling" is accomplished before the animal realizes what has happened. With fairly large, placid dogs, hold the tablet between the tips of the second and third fingers of the right hand. Slip the thumb of the left hand through the interdental space, and press up on the hard palate. Use the thumb of the right hand to press down on the space behind the mandibular incisors (Fig. 82). Push the pill deep into the pharynx, withdraw the hands quickly, and close the animal's mouth. Often a brusque tap under the chin startles the dog and facilitates its swallowing. When the animal licks its nose, you can be confident that it has swallowed.

Dogs who offer more resistance can be induced to open their mouths by compressing the upper lips against the teeth. As they open their mouths, the lips are rolled medially so that if they attempt to close, they will pinch their own lips.

Dogs that struggle and slash with their teeth are most difficult, especially if they are aggressive toward the medicator. They can often be medicated by placing the tablet over the base of the tongue with a 6-inch, curved Kelly hemostat or special pill forceps.

Cubes of canned food or dried meat can often be "pushed down" a placid but anorexic patient by using the thumb as a lever. The fingers are kept out of the mouth but the thumb is inserted behind the last molar of the open mouth and pushes the bolus down. Alternatively, pills can often be "tossed" to a dog hidden in a cube of meat or cheese and swallowed in a single gulp.

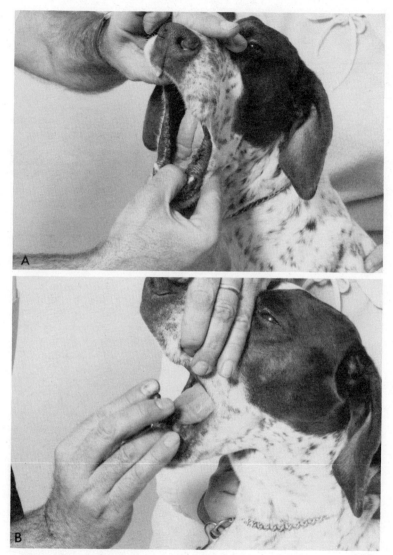

Figure 82. *A,* Placement of thumbs for opening dog's mouth. *B,* Administering capsule to dog. It should be placed deeply into the pharynx.

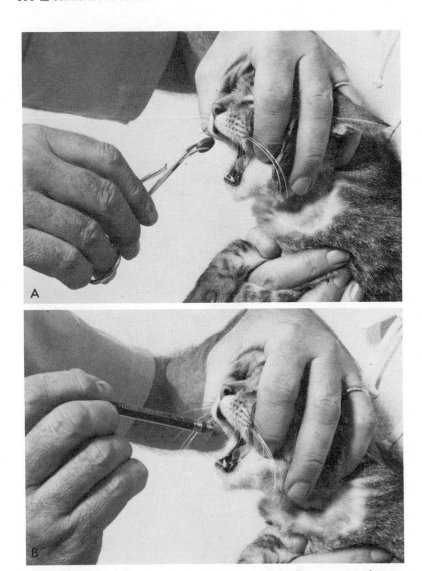

Figure 83. A, Administering capsule to cat using a curved Kelly or a mosquito forceps to place the capsule deep in the pharynx. B, Using the eraser end of a pencil to touch the posterior pharynx and/or the capsule to stimulate swallowing.

Cats

Two methods of pilling are useful in cats. In both methods, the cat's head is elevated and tipped back. Use the left hand to hold the head from behind with the index finger at one commissure of the mouth and the thumb at the other. Use the index finger of the right hand to open the mouth by pressing down on the incisor teeth. Hold the mouth open by compressing inward with the fingers at the angle of the jaw. A tablet can be placed deep in the pharynx with the curved Kelly hemostat, the forceps removed and the mouth closed quickly, and the cat tapped under the jaw or on the tip of the nose to facilitate swallowing (Fig. 83). Licking of the nose signals success. The alternate method is similar except that the tablet is dropped deep into the mouth and the eraser-end of a pencil is used to tap the pill (or even the posterior pharynx) and stimulate the swallowing reflex.

Oral Administration of Liquids

Without the Stomach Tube

Small amounts of liquid medicine can be given successfully to dogs and cats by pulling the commissure of the lip out to form a pocket (Fig. 84). The patient's head should be held level so that the medication will not ooze into the larynx. Spoons are ineffective. They measure fluids inaccurately and materials spill easily. A small prescription bottle or an old hypodermic syringe

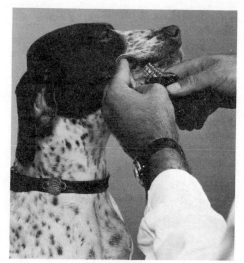

Figure 84. Administering liquid medication to a dog. The flap of the lip should be used as a funnel to direct liquids into the mouth.

with a metal tip makes a convenient, easy-to-use measuring device. Often the medicine is deposited in the "cheek pouch," and it can be encouraged to flow between the teeth by using a hemostat or the metal syringe tip to push gently between the teeth. Patience and gentleness are needed for success.

With the Stomach Tube

Stomach tubes can be passed through the nostrils (nasogastric), but the small lumen limits the types of solutions that can be administered. Nasogastric intubation can be done using a variety of tube sizes (Tables 92 and 93). Newer polyurethane tubes* when coated with a Xylocaine lubricating jelly are nonirritating and may be left in place with the tip at the level of midthoracic esophagus. When placing the nasogastric tube, instill 4 to 5 drops of 0.5 per cent proparacaine HCl in the nostril of the cat or 0.5 to 1.0 ml of 2 per cent lidocaine HCl in the nostril of the dog. Elevate the head and direct the tube dorsomedial to the alar fold. After the tip has been inserted 1 to 2 cm into the nostril, direct the tube ventrally down the esophagus. If the turbinates block the passage of the tube, reinsert the tube. The position of the tube can be checked by injecting 1 ml of sterile saline. If the animal coughs, reinsert the tube because the trachea has been intubated. Nasogastric tubes can be left in place by securing them with a butterfly bandage that is taped and sutured to

---

*Dobbhoff Enteral Feeding Tube or Entriflex Feeding Tubes, Bioresearch Medical Products, 35 Industrial Parkway, Somerville, New Jersey.

Table 92. TUBES FOR NASOGASTRIC AND NASOENTERAL FEEDING

Composition	Sizes (French × cm length)	Tip Weight	Name	Manufacturer
Polyvinylchloride†	5×16	no	Infant	
	5×42	no	feeding	National Catheter Co
	8×42	no	tube	
	3½×12	no		
	5×16, 5×36	no		Argyle, division of
	8×16, 8×42	no		Sherwood Medical
	10×42	no		
Polyurethane	5×20, 5×36	no	Indwell	
	8×42			
	6×31	no	Entron	Biosearch Medical Pdts.
	8×36, 8×43	yes	Entriflex	
Silicone	5×15, 8×15	no	Nutrifeed	American Pharmaseal
	6×42, 8×42	yes		
	6×36	yes	Keofeed	Ivac Corporation
	7.3×36, 7.3×42			

†Will harden if left in stomach for more than 2 weeks. From Lewis, L. D., and Morris, M. L.: Small Animal Clinical Nutrition. 1984.

Table 93. SIZE OF NASOGASTRIC TUBES TO USE

Animal Weight (kg)	Tube Size (French)
< 5	3.5–5*
5–15	5–8
> 15	8–10

*A 19- to 21-gauge butterfly catheter (Abbott Laboratories) may also be used. From Lewis, L. D., and Morris, M. L.: Small Animal Clinical Nutrition. 1984.

external nares and using a collar or bucket to prevent the animal from removing the tube. Always flush the tube with sterile saline after having infused fluids or food. Orogastric tubes are simpler and more practical. Little restraint is needed to pass a stomach tube in a placid or depressed dog or cat.

Gavage in puppies and kittens can be effected by passing a soft rubber urethral catheter as an orogastric tube. A No. 12 French catheter is of an adequate diameter to pass freely, but it is too large to enter the larynx of infant animals up to 14 days of age. Mark the tube with tape or a ballpoint pen at a point equal to the distance from the tip of the nose to the eighth rib. It is merely pushed into the pharynx and down the esophagus to the midthoracic level. A syringe can be attached to the flared end and medication is injected slowly.

Larger puppies and adult dogs tolerate intubation with little fuss, although they may have to be placed on a table and restrained. In some animals, the finger can be used to hold the jaws slightly apart. In most, a wooden spacer-block or a partially used roll of adhesive tape should be inserted behind the canine teeth to keep the mouth open. Pass the tube through a central hole in the tape or block (Fig. 85). A No. 22 French urinary catheter, 30 inches long, is an ideal tube. It is attached to a funnel, bulb, or syringe that delivers the medication. In most cases, the tip of the tube should be wet or lubricated with catheter jelly and then gently pushed into the pharynx.

When the dog swallows, advance the catheter down the esophagus to the level of the eighth or ninth rib. It is advisable to measure this distance on the tube first and mark it with a ballpoint pen or with a piece of tape. It is almost impossible to pass the tube into the trachea in a conscious dog with his head held in a normal position. Always palpate the neck, however, to be certain that the tube can be located in the esophagus.

Cats usually offer more resistance to oral intubation than do dogs. They can be restrained in a bag or cat stocks, but taping the legs together seems to be more practical. With taping, the cat can be held in a vertical position by an assistant. The operator then grasps the cat's head, as for pilling, and quickly passes the prelubricated tube 6 to 10 inches down the esophagus. A No. 12 to 16 French soft rubber catheter, 16 inches long, makes a suitable tube, and the plastic adapter on the end for attaching a syringe makes medication easy to administer (Table 94).

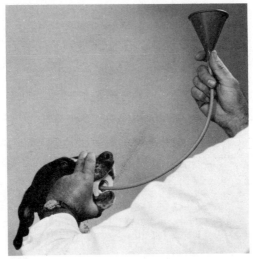

Figure 85. Administering liquid medication to a dog via a stomach tube. Note the roll of adhesive tape used as a gag.

Table 94. MAXIMUM STOMACH CAPACITY OF CATS*

Body Weight (kg)	Stomach Volume* (ml/kg)
0.5–1	100
1–15	70
1.5–4	60
4–6	45

*Amount of water that will produce vomiting or distress. From Lewis, L. D., and Morris, M. L.: Small Animal Clinical Nutrition. 1984.

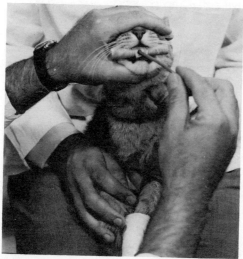

Figure 86. Administering liquid medication to a cat via a stomach tube. Note the wooden gag with a hole in the center for passage of the tube. There are vertical holes at the ends to accommodate the canine teeth.

For most cats, a block of soft wood should be used for a speculum to prevent severe damage or severance of the stomach tube. Drill a vertical hole in each end of the block (wooden dowel) so that the upper and lower canine teeth can pass through. A horizontal hole in the center allows the tube to pass through. Force the cat to bite down on the block and close the jaws while intubation proceeds (Fig. 86).

Types of solutions given for oral alimentation are listed in Tables 95 to 98.

Topical Medications

Ocular

There are numerous ways of applying medication to the eyes, including drops, ointments, subconjunctival injections, and subpalpebral lavage. The route and frequency of medication depend on the disease being treated.

If more than 2 drops of aqueous material are administered, the fluid will wash out of the conjunctival sac and be wasted. Most drops should be applied every 2 hours (or less) to maintain effect. Ointments should be applied sparingly, and their effect may last a maximum of 4 to 6 hours.

Drops should be placed on the inner canthus without touching the eye with the dropper. Ointment (⅛ inch long strip) should be placed on the cornea or lower palpebral border.

Table 95. LIQUID DIET FOR DOGS OR CATS

¼ cup vegetable oil
½ can Prescription Diet i/d (Hill's)
2½ cups water

Blend to liquid consistency in a blender. Yield 885 ml. Feed 30 ml per lb body weight daily divided into 2–4 feedings. This provies 30 kcal, 0.75 gm of protein, and 25 ml of water/lb body wt.

ANALYSIS

Moisture 84.6%
Protein. 2.4%
Fat 7.8%
Carbohydrate 5.2%
Kcal/ml 1.0%

From Lewis, L. D., and Morris, M. L.: Small Animal Clinical Nutrition. 1984.

Table 96. LIQUID DIETS FOR CATS*

Use	Formula	kcal/oz	Protein (%)	Fat (%)	Carbo-hydrate (%)
Anorexia other than the following	Equal parts egg yolk† and water, or 2 parts c/d‡ blended with 1 part water	34 / 32	5.3 / 8.6	8.9 / 5.0	0.3 / 4.4
Renal failure, hepatoses, or enteritis	1 part egg yolk,† 1 part corn syrup, and 2 parts water, or 2 parts k/d‡ blended with 1 part water and 1 part 50% glucose solution	45 / 43	2.6 / 4.4	4.4 / 5.4	14.0 / 18.1
Fever or cachexia without uremia, enteritis, or hepatosis	3 oz egg yolk,† 3 oz water, 1 tsp cooking oil, 1 T corn syrup, or 1 oz p/d‡; 0.5 oz water, 1 tsp cooking oil	46 / 50	5.0 / 7.8	13.0 / 13.2	6.0 / 3.0

*Feed 1 oz/lb body wt/day divided into 2–4 feedings.
†Strained baby food.
‡Canned Feline Prescription Diets (Hill's).
From Lewis, L. D., and Morris, M. L.: Small Animal Clinical Nutrition. 1984.

Table 97. COMMERCIALLY PREPARED LIQUID DIETS

Product (Company)	Caloric Density (kcal/ml)	Osmolality (mOsm/l)	Nutrients (% of total kcal)			Electrolytes (mEq/l)		
			Protein	Fat	Carbohy-drate	Sodium	Potas-sium	Chlo-ride
Osmolite HN (Ross)	1.06	310	Casein (16.7)	Corn oil and MCT (30)	Hydrolysed cornstarch (53.3)	39.5	38.6	40
Isocal HCN (Mead-Johnson)	2.0	690	Casein (15)	Soy oil and MCT (40)	Corn syrup (45)	35	36	34
Ensure Plus HN (Ross)	1.5	650	Casein (16.7)	Corn oil (30)	Hydrolysed cornstarch and sucrose (53.3)	50.2	45	44.8
Vital HN (Ross)	1.0	460	Hydrolysate of whey, meat, and soy, and essential amino acids (16.7)	Safflower and MCT oil (9.3)	Hydrolysed cornstarch and sucrose (74)	16.7	29.9	18.8
Criticare HN (Mead-Johnson)	1.54	650	Hydrolysed casein (30%) and amino acids (70%) (14)	Safflower oil (3)	Malto-dextrins and modified cornstarch (83)	27.5	33.8	29.6
Vivonex HN (Nor-wich-Eaton)	1.0	810	Crystalline amino acids (17)	Safflower oil (0.8)	Glucose and oligosacch-arides (82.2)	33.5	17.9	52.3

From Lewis, L. D., and Morris, M. L.: Small Animal Clinical Nutrition. 1984.

Table 98. NUTRIENT PRODUCTS FOR ADDING TO LIQUID DIETS

| Product (Company) | kcal | Osmo-lality | Nutrient Source | | | Electrolytes (mEq/l) | |
			Protein	Fat	Carbohy-drate	Sodium	Potas-sium
Protein:							
Pro-mix (Navaco)	4/gm	—	Whey			7	410
Casec (Mead-Johnson)	4/gm	—	Casein			7	30
Propac (Organon)	4/gm	—	Whey			10	13
Fat:							
Microlipid (Organon)	4.5/gm	80		Safflower oil			
MCT Oil (Mead-Johnson)	7.7/gm	—		Fractionated coconut			
Vegetable Oil	9.4/gm	—		Corn, saf-flower, soy, etc.			
Carbohydrate:							
Polycose (Ross)	4/gm 2/ml	850			Hydro-lysed cornstarch	25	5
Moducal (Mead-Johnson)	4/gm 2/ml	725			Maltodex-trin	15	6
Sumacal (Organon)	4/gm	—			Maltodex-trin	4	<1
Corn Syrup	2.9/ml	—			Primarily maltose	30	1
50% Glucose	2/ml	2800			Glucose	0	0

From Lewis, L. D., and Morris, M. L.: Small Animal Clinical Nutrition. 1984.

Otic

Powders and aqueous solutions are generally contraindicated in the external ear canal. Thin films of ointments or propylene glycol solutions may be effective vehicles. A few drops generally suffice, and the ear should be massaged gently after instillation to spread the medication over the lining of the ear canal.

Nasal

Isotonic aqueous drops are used and should be applied without touching the dropper to the nose. Oily drops are not advised, because they may damage the nasal mucosa or may be inhaled and produce a lipid pneumonia.

Dermatologic

There can be several objectives that have to be met when treating dermatologic disorders: (1) eradication of causative agents; (2) alleviation of symptoms, such as reduction of inflammation; (3) cleansing and débridement; (4) protection; (5) restoration of hydration; and (6) reduction of scaling and callus. Many different forms of skin medications are available, but the vehicle in which they are applied is an extremely critical factor. In all cases, topical medications should be applied to a clean skin surface in a very thin film, because only the medication in contact with the skin is effective. In most cases, clipping hair from an affected area enhances the effect of medication.

Vehicles

The following is a list of vehicles in which skin medications are made available:
1. *Lotions* are suspensions of powder in water or alcohol. They are used for acute, eczematous lesions. Because they are less easily absorbed than creams and ointments, they need to be applied 2 to 6 times a day.
2. *Pastes* are mixtures of 20 to 50 per cent powder in ointment. In general, they are thick, heavy, and difficult to use.
3. *Creams* are oil droplets dispersed in a continuous phase of water. Creams permit excellent percutaneous absorption of ingredients.
4. *Ointments* are water droplets dispersed in a continuous phase of oil. They are very good for dry, scaly eruptions.
5. *Propylene glycol* is a stable vehicle and spreads well. It allows good percutaneous absorption of added agents.
6. *Adherent dressings* are bases that dry quickly and stick to the lesion.

Making Injections

Preparing the Skin

Before medications are aspirated from multiple dose vials, carefully wipe the rubber diaphragm stopper with the same antiseptic used on the skin. This basic rule should be observed with all medication vials, even with modified live virus vaccines.

It would be admirable to prepare the skin surgically before making all needle punctures to administer medications. Because this is not practical, we should carefully part the hair and apply a good skin antiseptic such as Zephiran in 70 per cent alcohol. Place the needle directly on the prepared area, and thrust it through the skin.

Subcutaneous Injections

The dog and cat have loose alveolar tissue and can easily accommodate large volumes of material in this subcutaneous space. Infection may be introduced inadvertently or vessels may rupture, causing hematomas. Because these accidents are more difficult to handle in this location and because the skin of the dorsal neck is very thick, this region should not be used for injections. The dorsal back from the shoulders to the rump makes an ideal site for subcutaneous injection. Pick up a fold of skin in this region, prepare it with antiseptic, and pinch. Pinch the area a second time while making the injection. The patient rarely feels the injection. Gentle massage of the area after the injection is completed facilitates spreading and absorption of the medication. Only isotonic, buffered, or nonirritating materials should be given subcutaneously.

Intramuscular Injections

Because the tightly packed muscular tissue cannot expand and accommodate large volumes of injectables without trauma, medications given by this route should be small in volume. They are often depot materials that are poorly soluble and some may be mildly irritating. Intramuscular injections should never be given in the neck because of the fibrous sheaths there and the complications that may occur. We also feel that injections in the hamstring muscles may cause severe pain, lameness, and occasionally peroneal paralysis due to local nerve involvement. Unless the animal is extremely thin, we advise giving injections into the lumbodorsal muscles on either side of the dorsal processes of the vertebral column. Manufacturers' and legal requirements (as for rabies vaccination) may dictate use of the hamstring muscles, however.

After proper preparation of the skin, insert the needle through the skin at a slight angle (if the animal is thin) or at a perpendicular angle (if the animal is obese). When any medication is injected by a route other than the intravenous one, it is *imperative* to retract the plunger of the syringe before injecting to be certain that a vein was not entered by mistake. This is especially crucial in oil suspension, microcrystalline suspension, or potent dose medications.

Intravenous Injections (see p. 610.)

SIMPLIFIED FLUID THERAPY

Proper administration of fluids can be a difficult and challenging experience for the veterinarian. Proper management of fluid therapy depends on understanding the abnormal physiology present as well as the advantages and disadvantages of the various forms of fluid therapy. Assessment of each animal's needs—lacks and excesses—and of its renal and cardiovascular function must be made.

In this section, the basic principles of fluid therapy are discussed.

General Principles

1. Although administration of salt, dextrose, and water may ameliorate temporary emergencies, the addition of other electrolytes in balanced or especially tailored formulas is better definitive therapy.
2. Fluids and electrolytes, and especially calories, can be given more cheaply and effectively by mouth than by injection (unless contraindicated).
3. If renal function is adequate, the body can adjust itself by selectively retaining or excreting water and electrolytes. However, enough fluids and electrolytes must be given to allow the kidneys to function.
4. If renal function is inadequate, the animal is in a critical condition and should be referred to a center with adequate laboratory and therapy facilities for intensive treatment.
5. Water and some electrolytes are in a state of constant flux between the body fluid compartments.
6. Use fluids in proper relation to the total medical problem.
7. Select laboratory tests that when repeated frequently will indicate *trends* in the patient's condition (see p. 737).

Normal Values in Fluid Therapy

The percentage of body weight as water in the total body for the average animal is 60 per cent; for the fat animal, 50 per cent; and for the thin animal, 70 per cent.

Fluid Compartments

Total water, 60 per cent:
  Intracellular water, 40 per cent.
  Extracellular water, 20 per cent.
   Interstitial water, 15 per cent.
   Intravascular water, 5 per cent.

Rules Pertaining to Blood

1. Canine total blood volume is approximately 88 ml per kg.
2. Most dogs can donate 20 ml of blood per kg every 3 weeks.

Table 99. NORMAL WATER TURNOVER DATA

	Dog (ml/lb)	Cat (ml/lb)
Total water turnover/24 hours	30	42
Input		
Oral (food and drink)	23	36
Metabolic (released from carbohydrates and fat)	7	6
Output		
Urine	10	20
Other (sweat, feces, insensible, incorporated into new protoplasm)	20	22

3. Most cats can donate 40 ml of blood every 3 weeks.
4. Total blood volume is 7 per cent of body weight.
5. Plasma volume is 4 per cent of body weight (dogs, 50 ml/kg; cats, 45 ml/kg).
6. Erythrocyte volume is 3 per cent of body weight.

Normal Blood Plasma Electrolytes

Cations and anions always balance, and the total approximates 155 mEq per L (Tables 99 and 100).

Major extracellular ions are Na, Cl, and HCO_3. Major intracellular ions are K, PO_4, and proteins (see p. 737).

Types of Fluid and Electrolyte Imbalance

Water and electrolytes are lost in various proportions. There are four major types of imbalance; the first two are more commonly encountered than the last two.

Water Loss (Type One Imbalance)

In water loss or desiccation, more water than sodium is lost. It is caused by decreased water intake or increased loss by transpiration in fevers or heatstroke. Thirst is evident. Urine contains large amounts of sodium and chloride ions and has a high specific gravity.

Table 100. BLOOD PLASMA ELECTROLYTES*

Cations (mEq/L)		Anions (mEq/L)	
Na l	145.0	HCO_3	24
K	5.0	Cl	110
Ca + Mg	5.0	Inorganic anions	5
		Anion gap	16

*Approximately 155 mEq/L.

Sodium Loss (Type Two Imbalance)

In sodium loss, more sodium than water is lost. It is caused by osmotic loss through vomiting, diarrhea, wound drainage, polyuria, sequestration of fluid in tissues, and diabetes. There is little thirst. Urine specific gravity is normal but sodium and chloride content is low. In vomiting animals, the gastric secretions contain high concentrations of hydrogen and chloride and moderate amounts of sodium (30–90 mEq/L) and potassium (5–25 mEq/L.). When vomitus comes exclusively from the stomach, the animal is alkalotic. Vomiting associated with disease of the pylorus and duodenum results in higher concentrations of sodium (80–120 mEq/L) and bicarbonate (30–50 mEq/L) loss. The presence of yellowish-green or green fluid in the vomitus indicates bile. Animals with these factors are acidotic rather than alkalotic.

Water Excess (Type Three Imbalance)

Water excess is usually caused by treatment error, such as giving plain water for sodium loss problems. This problem rarely occurs.

Sodium Excess (Type Four Imbalance)

Sodium excess is associated with various states of edema. Usually it is a chronic problem. It is not usually considered a problem of fluid therapy.

Basics of Acid-Base Physiology

Blood pH represents the balance between those processes in the body that produce acidosis and those that produce alkalosis. The normal pH ranges between 7.35 and 7.45. Blood pH is maintained by three major mechanisms: (1) blood buffer systems, (2) respiratory mechanisms that alter pCO_2, and (3) metabolic mechanisms (mainly renal) that alter HCO_3^- and H^+ (Fig. 87).

Hyperventilation decreases blood pCO_2 and decreases the H^+ ion concentration, producing alkalosis of respiratory origin. Hypoventilation increases the pCO_2, producing acidosis of respiratory origin. The normal canine pCO_2 in arterial blood is 36 to 42 mm Hg. In cats, it is 28 to 34 mm Hg. Changes in the pCO_2 values directly influence the level of hydrogen ion concentration, and, in dogs, values below 35 mm Hg or above 45 mm Hg indicate respiratory alkalosis or acidosis.

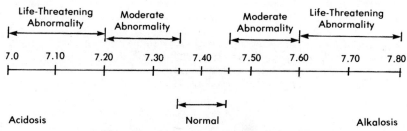

Figure 87. Indications of severity of changes in PTT.

The metabolic influence on pH can be examined by looking at whole blood buffer base and base deficit/excess. Base deficit/excess is the titratable acid or base when the blood is titrated to a pH of 7.4 and pCO_2 of 40 mm Hg with complete hemoglobin saturation. Base deficit/excess can be used to calibrate qualitative determinations of surplus acid or base. To help in arriving at a level of base deficit/excess, the Sigaard-Andersen blood acid–base alignment nomogram can be used (see Fig. 88). The normal base excess or deficit is 0 ± 4 mEq/L. Base deficit values less than −4 indicate metabolic acidosis, whereas base excess values greater than +4 indicate alkalosis. The hemoglobin concentration should be interpreted with regard to the "effective" hemoglobin concentration in extracellular fluid, which is 20 per cent of the actual hemoglobin concentration. Thus, when reading and using the nomogram, take 20 per cent of the actual hemoglobin value as the "effective" value to be read on the chart.

To interpret the acid base status of an animal:
1. First examine the blood pH—below 7.35 = acidosis; above 7.45 = alkalosis.
2. Next examine the pCO_2 (respiratory component).
3. Then examine the base excess/deficit (metabolic component)—<22 mEq HCO_3^-/L = metabolic acidosis; >25 mEq HCO_3^-/L = metabolic alkalosis.

Frequently, there are combinations of respiratory and metabolic alkalosis. Note which component is deviated furthest from normal; this is often the primary cause, whereas the other component is often a secondary cause.

In evaluating the acid-base status, the following two points are important: (1) when the site of an acid-base lesion is respiratory, the physiologic compensation is renal; and (2) when the site of the lesion is metabolic, the physiologic compensation is respiratory. Therapeutic treatment of acid-base abnormalities should be undertaken in the same mode as the pathophysiology of the underlying lesion—namely, respiratory abnormalities are treated with respiratory intervention.

The most sophisticated and desirable method of measuring the acid-base status of an animal is with blood gas and pH electrodes. Arterial samples are preferred over venous samples, and heparin is used as an anticoagulant. Arterial samples are sometimes difficult to obtain, so venous samples are often used. Capillary blood can be collected from the ear and is satisfactory provided that there are no capillary circulation alterations and capillary blood is free flowing. Obtain blood samples in plastic syringes and seal the needles. Blood samples can be stored for up to 30 minutes at room temperature without significant change in acid-base values. Storage in an ice-water bath allows extending the time in which analysis will be accurate to 3.5 hours for pH and 6 hours for pCO_2.

The acid-base status of an animal can also be evaluated by using a commercial kit* to measure total carbon dioxide and an expanded pH meter to measure blood pH. This type of testing has the advantage of being a more economical and practical office procedure. The CO_2 test measures the amount

---

*Harleco CO_2 Apparatus Set, Harleco Division, American Hospital Supply Corp., Philadelphia, Pennsylvania.

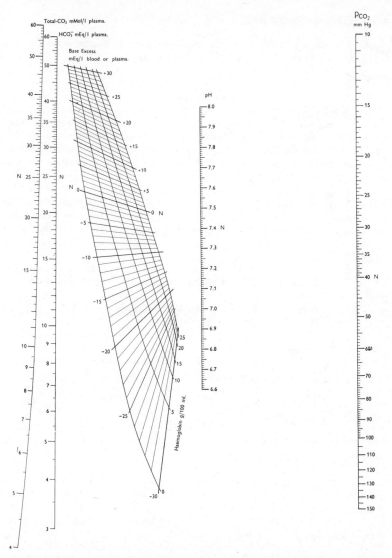

Figure 88. Blood acid–base alignment nomogram according to Sigaard-Andersen. Measure blood PCO_2 and pH with appropriate electrodes. Connect values and read bicarbonate concentration in milliequivalents per liter left. Determine hemoglobin and read base-excess where PCO_2–ph–bicarbonate line crosses the base-excess nomogram, the appropriate hemoglobin concentration. N: normal. This nomogram is designed for use with blood 38° C. (From Sigaard-Andersen: Scand. J. Clin. Lab. Invest., 15:211, 1963; also see Severinghaus, J.: Chapter 61 in Handbook of Physiology, Vol. II, Sec. 3, Respiration. American Physiology Society, 1965.) Modified from Schwartz, G. R.: Principles and Practice of Emergency Medicine. Vol. 1. Philadelphia, W. B. Saunders Company, 1979, p. 304.

of CO_2 released when HCO_3^- in the serum is mixed with lactic acid. This test is a useful indication of plasma HCO_3^- concentration.

Metabolic Acidosis

Metabolic acidosis exists when the pH is less than 7.35, and the HCO_3^- is less than 24. The condition may be acute, as with diabetic ketoacidosis, or chronic, as seen in chronic renal failure. Metabolic acidemia is diagnosed when arterial pH is depressed and the base deficit is elevated. Additional parameters that may be helpful in establishing an etiology are blood sugar, ketones, creatinine, BUN, and electrolytes. Some common causes of metabolic acidosis are diabetic ketoacidosis, renal failure (both acute and chronic), poisonings with aspirin and ethylene glycol, severe diarrhea, and renal tubular acidosis. The major physiologic response to metabolic acidosis is via hyperventilation. The major physiologic response to metabolic acidemia is respiratory compensation, resulting in increased alveolar ventilation and decreased $PaCO_2$. If the $PaCO_2$ remains elevated and fails to compensate for metabolic acidosis, a combined metabolic and respiratory acidosis may result.

Metabolic acidosis can produce hyperventilation, depressed myocardial activity, ventricular fibrillation, vomiting, depression, and hyperkalemia (see p. 35).

The treatment of metabolic acidosis should include:
1. Correcting the underlying problem, if possible.
2. Ensuring that the animal is well ventilated, and correcting any underlying respiratory disease.
3. Giving alkali therapy with sodium bicarbonate, even while correcting underlying problems, if the pH is below 7.2 (life threatening).

The mEq of bicarbonate required to bring the base excess to zero equals the base deficit (in mEq/L) $\times$ ⅓ of the body weight (in kg). It can be determined by the formula:

mEq HCO_3^- required $= 0.3 \times$ BW (kg) $+$ (desired HCO_3^- $-$ observed HCO_3^-), where the desired HCO_3^- is usually 25 mEq per L.

In administering sodium bicarbonate, infusions should be slow to minimize red blood cell damage and hyperosmolality, and hypokalemia should be corrected if present before administering a bicarbonate load. The electrocardiogram should be monitored for evidence of electrolyte-induced change, and potassium should be administered if needed.

When the amount of bicarbonate needed has been determined: (1) give up to ¼ of this calculated dose by IV bolus—place the remaining HCO_3^- in IV fluids. (2) Monitor if possible with blood gas or HCO_3^- determinations (see p. 608).

Metabolic Alkalosis

Metabolic alkalosis exists when the pH > 7.45, and $HCO_3^- > 28$. This condition is not as common as metabolic acidosis. It may be associated with profuse vomiting and loss of fixed acid, administration of diuretics and excessive alkali administration. Measurement of blood electrolytes indicates a lowered potassium and chloride level. Correction of the electrolyte imbalance necessitates the administration of KCl and normal saline IV (see p. 607). The same formula used to determine bicarbonate depletion can be used to calculate bicarbonate excess. The bicarbonate excess in mEq is roughly equal to the chloride depletion in mEq. Thus, NaCl and KCl can be used to replace the HCO_3^- deficit (see p. 602).

Respiratory Acidosis

Respiratory acidosis exists when the pH < 7.35 and $PaCO_2$ > 40. The condition is associated with hypoventilation. When the condition is acute, there may be little compensation; however, chronic cases are usually compensated for by metabolic means. Etiology can involve severe pulmonary disease, hypoventilation caused by central nervous system disease, drug intoxications, anesthetic accidents, or respiratory failure associated with muscular or nervous disease. The treatment of choice is the correction of the underlying respiratory problem.

Respiratory Alkalosis

By definition, this condition exists if the pH is greater than 7.45, and the $PaCO_2$ is less than 40. Primary respiratory alkalosis is rarely seen in animals, and in those situations in which respiratory alkalosis is present, it is generally iatrogenic or compensatory.

References and Additional Readings

Haskins, S. C.: Sampling and storage of blood for pH and blood gas analysis. J.A.V.M.A., 170:429, 1977.

Haskins, S. C.: Fluid and electrolyte therapy. Compendium on Continuing Education, 6(3): 244, 1984.

Muir, W. W., and Diabartola, S. P.: Fluid therapy. In Kirk, R. W. (ed.): Current Veterinary Therapy 8: Small Animal Practice. Philadelphia, W. B. Saunders Company, 1983.

Schwartz, F. R., Safar, P., Stone, J. H., et al.: Principles and Practice of Emergency Medicine. Philadelphia, W. B. Saunders Company, 1978, pp. 301–309.

van Slvijs, F. J., deVries, H. W., DeBroijne, J. J., and van den Brom, W. E.: Capillary and venous blood compared with arterial blood in the measurement of acid-base blood gas states of dogs. Am. J. Vet. Res., 44(3): 459, 1983.

Planning Fluid Therapy

General Considerations

1. Keep the animal in water and electrolyte balance, and modify treatment as the clinical course varies (Table 101).
2. Recognition of trends and patterns of shifts is more important than observation of one abnormal laboratory test.

Table 101. DAILY REQUIREMENTS OF DOGS FOR CALORIES, WATER, AND SODIUM

Body wt (kg)	Total kcal/day or water ml/day	ml per kg	ml/hr	Sodium mEq/L	Total (mEq)	Potassium mEq/L	Total (mEq)
1	140	140	6	Final	4.2	Final	2.8
2	232	116	10	solution	7.0	solution	4.6
3	312	104	13	should	9.4	should	6.2
4	385	96	16	contain	11.6	contain	7.7
5	453	91	19	30–40	13.6	20 mEq/L	9.1
6	518	86	22	mEq/L	15.5		10.4
7	580	83	24		17.4		11.6
8	639	80	27		19.2		12.8
9	696	77	29		20.9		13.9
10	752	75	31		22.6		15.0
11	806	73	34		24.2		16.1
12	859	71	36		25.8		17.2
13	911	70	38		27.3		18.2
14	961	68	40		28.8		19.2
15	1011	67	42		30.3		20.2
16	1060	66	44		31.8		21.2
17	1108	65	46		33.2		22.2
18	1155	64	48		34.7		23.1
19	1201	63	50		36.0		24.0
20	1247	62	52		37.4		24.9
25	1468	59	61		44.0		29.4
30	1677	56	70		50.3		33.5
35	1876	54	78		56.3		37.5
40	2068	52	86		62.0		41.4
45	2254	50	94		67.6		45.1
50	2434	49	101		73.0		48.7
60	2781	46	116		83.4		55.6
70	3112	44	130		93.4		62.2
80	3431	43	143		102.9		68.6
90	3739	41	156		112.2		74.8
100	4038	40	168		121.1		80.8
150	5428	36	226		162.8		108.6

Daily calorie requirements are increased during certain physiologic states and the maintenance allowance should be increased proportionately: early growth (0–6 months of age)—2× maintenance; preadult (6–12 months)—1.5×; pregnancy—1.5×; lactation or heavy exercise—2–3×; trauma, surgery, etc.—2×.

From Haskins, S.: Fluid and electrolyte therapy. Compendium on Continuing Education, 6(3): 244, 1984.

Table 102. NORMAL VALUES FOR LABORATORY TESTS COMMONLY USED TO EVALUATE DEHYDRATED DOGS

Test	Normal Value
Packed cell volume (PCV) or hemoglobin*	37–55 per cent
	12–18 gm/100 ml
Plasma protein*	5.3–7.5 gm/100 ml
Blood urea nitrogen	10–20 mg/100 ml
Plasma or serum osmolality	280–305 mOsm/L
Plasma or serum sodium	140–155 mEq/L
Plasma or serum potassium	3.7–5.8 mEq/L
Plasma or serum chloride	100–155 mEq/L
Plasma HCO_3	16–25 mEq/L
Blood pH	7.30–7.45
Blood pCO_2	29–42 mm Hg

*Most important in objectively evaluating fluid problems. The PCV and plasma protein values are usually considered together so that anemia (if present) will be evident as fluids are replaced.

3. With rare exceptions, potassium is of much less importance in fluid problems of dogs than of humans.
4. Caloric balance is difficult to obtain by any route other than oral and is of small importance during short, acute illness, because it can be corrected during convalescence.
5. Determine whether a fluid imbalance exists by history of losses, body weight loss, plasma protein, and packed cell volume (Tables 102 and 103).

Specific Considerations

Determine the Volume Deficit (4–6–8 Rule)

1. The loss of 4 per cent of the body weight in fluid is indicated only by a history of fluid loss. Thus, a 10-kg (22-lb) dog with 4 per cent loss would have a volume deficit of 0.04 times 10, or 0.4 kg, or 400 ml.
2. The loss of 5 per cent of body weight is the level at which clinical signs of dehydration are first observed. The skin lacks pliability; the mouth is dry.
3. The loss of 6 per cent represents moderate and obvious fluid deficits. It is indicated by "tacky" skin, dry red mucosa, concentrated urine or decreased volume, etc.
4. The loss of 8 per cent represents severe fluid losses. The pulse may be weak, there is oliguria, and the animal is depressed.
5. Loss of 10 to 12 per cent or even higher is extremely serious and may be life threatening. The general signs are those of shock.

Table 103. TESTS TO ASSESS SEVERITY OF DEHYDRATION

Test	Result	Interpretation
Urine		
Volume	Lower than normal	Intake low or extrarenal loss of water is increased
Chloride	Present	Water depletion with little salt depletion
	Absent or very low	Salt depletion
Albumin	Present with oliguria	Dehydration
	Present after fluid replacement	Renal disease
Blood		
Hemoglobin content and hematocrit	Raised	Dehydration; degree helps assessment of case
Plasma protein	Low after treatment	1. Sodium retention and over-expansion of extracellular fluid phase
		2. True anemia as complicating feature
Blood urea nitrogen (BUN)	Raised slightly	Dehydration
	High and persistent	Renal disease
Total carbon dioxide; chloride	Low CO_2, with normal or raised chloride	Acidosis
	High CO_2, with normal or low chloride	Alkalosis
	Low chloride level	Suggests chloride or sodium chloride depletion
Plasma sodium	Low	Sodium deficit
	High	1. Loss of water in excess of base
		2. After relief of dehydration: suggests excessive sodium administration
Plasma potassium	Low	Potassium deficit: may be due to giving sodium without potassium in replacement
	High	Severe dehydration despite absolute potassium deficit
		May follow too rapid administration of potassium by infusion
Plasma calcium	Low	Hypocalcemia may occur after relief of acidosis, especially if animal is undernourished

Determine the Osmolar Deficit

The object is to determine whether the animal has lost more water than electrolytes (type one imbalance) or more electrolytes than water (type two). The clinical signs and history will give helpful clues, but determining the plasma sodium level can be useful. If the sodium is *less* than approximately 143 mEq/L, the plasma is hypotonic and the fluid losses were hypertonic (contained much electrolyte in proportion to water). If the sodium is more than approximately 143 mEq/L, the plasma is hypertonic and losses have been hypotonic. Replacement is made accordingly.

Osmolal Gap

Serum osmolality must be kept within a relatively narrow range in healthy animals (see p. 815). Normal serum osmolality is 285 to 310 mOsm per kg. See p. 815 for the formulas used to estimate serum osmolality. These formulas estimate serum osmolality when azotemia or hyperglycemia does not exist. If these conditions are present, the formula for serum osmolality is

$$1.86 \ (Na \ + \ K) \ + \ \frac{Glucose}{18} \ + \ \frac{BUN}{2.8} \ + \ 9$$

In normal dogs, changes in serum osmolality parallel changes in serum sodium concentration.

The difference between the measured osmolality and the calculated serum osmolality is called the *osmole gap*. The normal osmole gap is 0 to 10 mOsm/ kg.

Increased Osmole Gap Indicates Increased Solute

1. Ethylene glycol poisoning (see p. 194).
2. Ethanol, salicylate poisoning.
3. Shock, lactic acidosis.
4. Increased serum protein—monoclonal gammopathy or polyclonal gammopathy (see p. 724).
5. Septicemias.
6. Infusion of hyperosmotic fluids (mannitol, sorbitol, glucose).

The measurement of serum osmolality can be used to estimate existing fluid deficits.

In those cases in which an animal is azotemic (see p. 122) and osmolality is used to calculate fluid deficits, the calculated osmolality should be corrected for the elevated BUN by dividing the existing BUN by 2.8 and subtracting the answer (which is the mOsm contributed by the urea) from the calculated osmolality.

Estimate Sodium Level

If the animal is not acidotic, the sodium level can be estimated by adding the factor of 11 to HCO_3^- and chloride levels. For example, 11 + 24 + 110 = 145 (normal). Estimate ongoing loss requirements, and determine the maintenance requirements of the animal for sodium and chloride.

Hyponatremia develops with serum sodium levels of less than 137 mEq/L. Hyponatremia produces weakness and a reduction in extracellular fluid volume. There can be hyperosmolar hyponatremia as seen in hyperglycemia of diabetes mellitus. Hyposmolar hyponatremia produces a decreased extracellular fluid (ECF) volume and is seen with vomiting, diarrhea, salt-wasting renal disease, Addison's disease, and extensive burns and following diuretic administration.

To correct hyponatremia (1) correct the underlying cause, (2) stop giving sodium-free solutions, and (3) administer NaCl, 0.9 per cent, or lactated Ringer's solution (percentage of dehydration × 0.3 × weight (kg) = volume replacement (ml).

The following equation can be used to calculate sodium replacement needed:

existing Na level mEq/L × wt of dog (kg) × 0.3 = mEq of sodium required

Hypernatremia exists when serum sodium is greater than 155 mEq/L. Hypernatremia produces hyperosmolality, resulting in neurologic signs of weakness, depression, seizures, and coma. Causes can be diabetes insipidus, nephrogenic diabetes insipidus, hyperventilation-heat prostration, salt water ingestion, sodium bicarbonate administration, hypertonic saline enemas, and primary aldosteronism.

To correct hypernatremia:
1. Stop administering sodium-containing solutions.
2. If pure water loss is occurring, administer 5 per cent dextrose in water (D5W).

$$\left(0.3 \times \text{body wt (kg)} \times \left(1 - \frac{140}{\text{serum Na}} \right) = \text{L of water} \right)$$

3. If pulmonary edema is associated because of extensive ECF expansion, begin furosemide therapy (see p. 209).
   Determine Special Ion Involvement (Potassium, Calcium, Phosphorus).
   When the ionic composition of the ECF is measured, all cations should equal anions according to the law of electroneutrality, that is,

$$\text{Na}^+ + \text{K}^+ + \left(\begin{array}{c} \text{undetermined cations} \\ \text{Ca}^{++} \text{ and } \text{Mg}^{+++} \end{array} \right) = \text{Cl}^- + \text{HCO}_3^- +$$

(undetermined anions such as PO_4^{---}, SO_4^{--}, proteinate, or organic acids)

In reality, an anionic gap (AG) of 16 (15–25) normally exists for dogs. Abnormal changes in the AG may be helpful in determining the causes of acid-base imbalances.

The total CO_2 concentration is often substituted for HCO_3^- concentration.

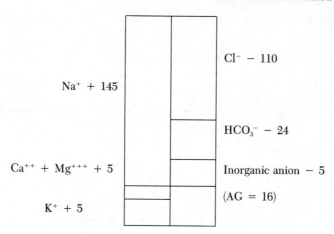

Cations Anions

Causes of Increased AG:
1) Decreased unmeasured cations
   a) Hypokalemia, hypocalcemia, hypomagnesemia
2) Increased unmeasured anions
   a) Organic anions: lactate, ketoacids
   b) Inorganic anions: phosphate, sulfate
   c) Protein: hyperalbuminemia (short-lived)
   d) Exogenous anions: salicylates
   e) Medications: penicillin
   f) Toxic agents: paraldehyde, ethylene glycol
   g) Endogenous anions: uremia, hyperosmolar hyperglycemic nonketotic coma

Causes of Decreased AG:
1) Increased unmeasured cations
   a) Hyperkalemia, hypercalcemia, hypermagnesemia
2) Retention of abnormal cations
   a) Myeloma globulins
3) Decreased unmeasured anions
   a) Hypoalbuminemia

Metabolic Acidosis and Anion Gaps
Metabolic acidosis associated with a normal or decreased anion gap:
1) Renal loss of bicarbonate
   a) Renal tubular acidosis
2) Gastrointestinal loss of bicarbonate
   a) Diarrhea

3) Other causes of normal anion gap
    a) (Hyperchloremic) metabolic acidosis
    b) Dilutional acidosis
Metabolic acidosis associated with an increased anion gap:
1) Increased acid production—uremic acidosis
    a) Increased ketone production
    b) Increased lactic acid production
    c) Unknown organic acid (ethylene glycol ingestion, paraldehyde poisoning, methanol poisoning, salicylate poisoning)
2) Decreased acid secretion
    a) Acute renal failure
    b) Chronic renal failure
3) Hyperchloremic acidosis
    a) Diarrhea
    b) Renal causes (early renal failure, renal tubular acidosis)
    c) Drugs (carbonic anhydrase inhibitors, acidifying agents—NH_4Cl, $CaCl_2$, methionine)
    d) Ketoacidosis with renal ketone loss

The ability of the kidneys to excrete the anions of the accumulated acid determines whether a high AG acidosis or hyperchloremic acidosis will develop.

When the increase in the AG is greater than the decrease in plasma HCO_3^- concentration, combined high AG metabolic acidosis and metabolic alkalosis should be suspected.

Mixed acid base disturbances can occur such as metabolic alkalosis and high AG metabolic acidosis in uremic animals that have been vomiting; the HCO_3^- values in these cases may be variable.

Mixed high AG levels and hyperchloremic metabolic acidosis can develop in dogs with uremia and diarrhea.

The normal serum potassium level in the dog ranges from 3.9 to 5.6 mEq per L, and, in the cat, it ranges from 4.0 to 4.5 mEq per L. More than 90 per cent of the total ingested potassium is excreted by the kidneys. Acid-base balance affects potassium excretion, acidosis decreases potassium, and alkalosis increases potassium excretion. Diuretics increase sodium loss as well as increasing potassium loss.

Hypokalemia refers to serum potassium levels below 3.5 mEq per L. The most frequently associated causes are metabolic and respiratory alkalosis associated with vomiting, excessive administration of sodium bicarbonate, excessive use of diuretics; dilutional hypokalemia when inadequate levels of potassium are present in fluids being administered; vomiting; diarrhea; ketoacidotic diabetes; and postobstructive diuresis.

Signs of hypokalemia may be metabolic. resulting in altered tolerance to carbohydrate and elevated fasting blood glucose determination, neuromuscular weakness, depression, lethargy, confusion, coma, decreased muscle tone, gastrointestinal atony, vomiting, constipation, and cardiovascular changes (see p. 36). Renal function may also be impaired as a result of reduced glomerular filtration rate (GFR).

Treatment of Hypokalemia
1) Correct underlying disease process, replace potassium.
2) Use oral route when possible in mild deficits—bananas, meat, vegetables, or potassium elixirs such as Kaon elixir mixed with food.
3) Moderate or severe hypokalemia with less than 3.0 mEq per L—use parenteral administration of potassium chloride. Rate of administration should not exceed 0.5 mEq per kg per hr or the total should not exceed 3 to 5 mEq per kg per 24 hours. Potassium supplementation is contraindicated in oliguric states. Guidelines for estimating the dose of KCl to be given are contained in the following table:

ESTIMATED DOSE OF POTASSIUM CHLORIDE*

Serum K$^+$ mEq/L	mEq K$^+$ Supplementation/250 ml Fluid*
Normal	5
3.0–3.5	7
2.5–3.0	10
2.0–2.5	15
2.0	20

*Calculated dose based on total daily fluid requirements, knowledge of actual serum potassium, and adequate urine output.

Hyperkalemia exists when serum potassium is 7.0 to 7.5 mEq per L or greater (see also p. 748). Most common causes of hyperkalemia are acute renal failure, obstructive urinary disease, adrenocortical hypofunction, too much potassium administered to the animal, and severe metabolic and respiratory acidosis. (See p. 147 for hyperkalemia and cardiac function; see p. 148 for medical treatment hyperkalemia.)
Serum calcium levels (see also p. 744).

Mean values of calcium for mature dogs are approximately 10.0 mg per dl and for cats, 9.0 mg per dl. Young dogs have higher serum calcium levels; however, this is not true for cats. Changes in serum proteins (albumin) can alter plasma calcium levels (see p. 744 for formula to correct). See page 659 for disorders resulting in hypercalcemia. See Metabolic Emergencies (p. 146) for the treatment protocol for severe hypercalcemia.

The most common cause of hypocalcemia is hypoalbuminemia. See page 744 for formula to adjust calcium levels obtained. Hypoalbuminemia-producing calcium levels in the range of 7 to 9.5 mg per dl usually are not associated with any clinical deficit. For further causes of hypocalcemia, see page 744, and for emergency treatment of hypocalcemia, page 146.

Serum phosphorus mainly measures inorganic phosphorus and is expressed in mg per dl. The most common cause of hyperphosphatemia associated with disease is renal failure (see p. 122). See page 125 for management of hyperphosphatemia associated with renal disease.

Table 104. ACID-BASE PARAMETERS IN ACUTE UNCOMPENSATED DISTURBANCES

Disturbance	pH	pCO_2	CO_2 Combining Power	HCO_3^-	$\dfrac{HCO_3}{H_2CO_3}$
Metabolic acidosis	↓	—	↓	↓	< 20
Respiratory acidosis	↓	↑	—	—	< 20
Metabolic alkalosis	↑	—	↑	↑	> 20
Respiratory alkalosis	↑	↓	↓	↓	> 20

Determine the Acid-Base Status.

The preservation of normal hydrogen ion concentration is of vital importance to normal enzyme activity, cardiac and skeletal muscle contraction, and nerve conduction. Conclusions regarding clinical acid-base status are not precise but are probably best drawn from measurements of ECFs, especially arterial blood. History, clinical signs, and even measurement of urine pH may be helpful.

The four states of altered acid-base physiology are metabolic acidosis, respiratory acidosis, metabolic alkalosis, and respiratory alkalosis. Each of these changes induces a compensatory response in the body to minimize the changes in pH (Table 104).

Implementing the Plan

1. *Supply fluids to replace deficits from previous losses* and to improve renal function. (Hydrate the patient!) See Table 105.
   Use the 4–6–8 per cent rule times body weight to give volume needed.
   Use the history and sodium data to estimate osmolar needs. For hypotonic needs, use water orally or D5W or dextrose 2.5 per cent in half-strength lactated Ringer's solution; these agents provide "free water." For isotonic needs, use lactated Ringer's solution or 0.9 per cent saline in ⅙ molar (M) sodium lactate at a ratio of 3:1. For hypertonic needs, use dextrose 5 or 10 per cent in saline or in lactated Ringer's solution or use 3 per cent sodium chloride solution, which is very hypertonic. Hypertonic solutions should be administered slowly to prevent circulatory overload.
2. *Supply fluids to meet daily normal maintenance needs* (for urine, feces, insensible losses). The volume should be 55 ml per kg per day, supplied as water orally or as dextrose or invert sugar in water for injection. Normal urine has a sodium concentration of 60 to 80 mEq per L and a potassium concentration of 30 to 50 mEq per L, although concentrations may vary widely. One half of the daily losses are from urine, and the other half are due to insensible water loss. It is important to record urine volume and the weight of the animal (see also p. 236).

Table 105. COMPOSITION OF SOLUTIONS

	Glucose (gm/L)	NaCl	Na Lactate	KCl	CaCl$_2$	MgCl$_2$	NH$_4$Cl
				(mEq/L)			
5% D/W	50						
10% D/W	100						
20% D/W	200						
5% D/S	50	145					
2.5% dextrose in half-isotonic saline	25	73					
0.85% saline (isotonic saline; N/S)		145					
0.9% saline		154					
3% saline		513					
5% saline		856					
1/6 molar sodium lactate (1.9%)			167				
1/6 molar ammonium chloride (0.9%)							167
2% ammonium chloride							374
Ringer's solution		147		4	5		
Hypotonic Ringer's solution (modified)		103		5	5	3	
Lactate Ringer's solution		103	27	4	4		

From Freitag, J., and Miller, L. W. (eds.): Manual of Medical Therapeutics. 23rd ed. Boston, Little, Brown & Co., 1980.

Other daily requirements to be met include sodium, 1.0 mEq per kg; potassium, 2 mEq per kg; protein, 4 to 8 gm per kg; and calories, 40 to 100 per kg. Protein will be used for energy unless adequate calories are provided from other sources. Replacing calories by injection is difficult (see p. 617). Probably it is best accomplished orally by gavage unless the need is likely to be short-term. Fat emulsions by injection may be impractical for dogs and dangerous for cats. Invert sugar and fructose are retained better than dextrose, which is readily lost in the urine. Administration of 20 per cent or higher concentrations of dextrose intravenously results in a net water loss unless the rate is *very* slow. About 20 calories per kg of body weight must be given daily as dextrose to provide for obligatory central nervous system (CNS) requirements.

3. *Supply fluids to meet the special losses* that occur during the course of treatment (vomiting, diarrhea, wound drainage). Replace these losses by selecting fluids that match the volume and composition of those lost. Replace blood loss with fresh blood and wound drainage with plasma or lactated Ringer's solution. Give plain water for insensible losses of fevers.

Table 106. ESTIMATION OF BICARBONATE DEFICIT IN PATIENTS
WITH METABOLIC ACIDOSIS*

Severity of Signs	Estimated HCO_3^- Deficit (mEq/L)	HCO_3^- Needed to Correct (mEq/kg)
Mild	5	1.5
Moderate	10	3.0
Severe	15	4.5

*Four grains of sodium bicarbonate = 0.25 gm = 3.0 mEq HCO_3^-.

In diarrhea, large amounts of Na^+, K^+, Mg^{++}, and Ca^{++} and water are needed. A vomiting dog requires replacement of large amounts of Cl^-, Na^+, and K^+ and water. Potassium is lost in regurgitated gastric fluid and in the urine.

4. *Supply fluids to assist in the therapy of acid-base disorders.* Because most acid-base disturbances are secondary to pathologic processes, the initial therapy should be aimed at proper diagnosis and management of the primary disease.

Many of the standard injectable solutions (0.9 per cent NaCl, lactated Ringer's solution, Ringer's solution) have a pH below 7.0, and the addition of 5 to 10 mEq of bicarbonate to each liter of these solutions makes an excellent buffer that can be used routinely. When moderate to severe acidosis is present, larger amounts are indicated. Table 106 provides useful guidelines. In all cases and regardless of the route used, bicarbonate deficit should be corrected over a period of 24 hours. Add B complex vitamins to all fluids administered 1 ml per L.

ROUTES AND RATES OF ADMINISTRATION

Intravenous

Any solution for injection can be given by the intravenous (IV) route, and it is the *only* route for hypotonic or hypertonic solutions.

The rate of administration depends on the animal, but usual routines call for 4 to 5 ml per minute. Rates up to 30 to 40 ml per minute may be indicated in some animals for short periods of time.

Use special care in determining the rate and volume administered to old animals with cardiopulmonary disease, because rapid and extensive expansion of the vascular volume may cause severe overloading problems.

Intravenous Infusions

Establishing Rates of Flow
Differences among IV infusion sets:
Cutter   —20 gtt* per ml

---

*gtt = drops.

Abbott   —15 gtt per ml
McGaw   —15 gtt per ml
Travenol—10 gtt per ml
Calculate the drops per minute and, thus, the proper rate of infusion.

$$\frac{\text{total amount solution in ml } \frac{(\text{gtt})}{(\text{ml})}}{\text{number of hours to infuse } \frac{(60 \text{ min})}{(1 \text{ hr})}} = \times \text{ gtt/min}$$

Drops per ml for the various IV manufacturers can be established as constants: Cutter, 1/3; Abbott or McGaw, 1/4; and Travenol, 1/6. For example, if one wishes to infuse 500 ml in 4 hours, what will be the rate of flow in drops per minute? First, whose set is being used, and what is the fluid rate per hour?

$$\frac{500 \text{ ml}}{4 \text{ hr}} = \frac{\text{x ml}}{1 \text{ hr}} \qquad \text{answer: 125 ml/hr}$$

(125 ml/hour) × (manufacturer's constant fraction) = gtt/min.

To calculate the IV rate in microdrips, use the following equation:

$$\text{microdrip tubing} = 60 \text{ gtt} = 1 \text{ ml}$$

Readjusting Intravenous Rates
When the rate of an already infusing IV must be changed, it is better to recalculate it than to arbitrarily change it. For example, suppose there are 800 ml left in an infusing bottle of 1000 ml D5W. What is the rate of fluid to be infused over the next 5 hours if the Abbott equipment is used?

$$\frac{(800 \text{ ml}) \frac{(15 \text{ gtt})}{(\text{ml})}}{(5 \text{ hr}) \frac{(60 \text{ min})}{(1 \text{ hr})}} = \times \text{ gtt/min}$$

$$\times = 40 \text{ gtt/min}$$

To calculate the macrodrip rate: For 10 drops/ml

$$\frac{\text{ml}}{\text{hr}} \times \frac{1 \text{ hr}}{60 \text{ min}} \times \frac{60 \text{ gtt}}{\text{min}} = \text{gtt/min}$$

The IV fluid bottle should be marked with tape to indicate how much fluid should be expended in a given period of time.

Subcutaneous and Intraperitoneal

These are "pool" routes in which a depot of fluid is accumulated for absorption later. Fluids used should approach isotonicity and should contain at least half (80 mEq/L) the normal sodium level of plasma.

Large volumes can be given rapidly (100 to 200 ml subcutaneously over a local area; 100 to several thousand ml intraperitoneally).

Frequency

Continuous infusion IV is necessary initially or if peripheral circulation is poor. It may also be given intermittently.

Intermittent infusions into a "pool" should be repeated as the "pool" is absorbed. Usually every 12 hours is adequate.

TECHNIQUE OF ADMINISTRATION

Assembling Equipment

1. Use unopened, pyrogen-free sterile equipment.
2. Provide an air vent and attach the recipient set with bubble trap and drip chamber.
3. Set up the bottle and fill the tubing to the needle adapter. Be sure that the bubble trap is half full of fluid.

Venipuncture for Intravenous Route

For short-term infusions of drugs or fluids, a simple needle inserted into a vein is the least expensive method of establishing an IV infusion. The difficulty with this technique is the tendency of the needle to go through the vessel wall, resulting in fluids or medication being administered extravascularly. A better method is the use of a scalp vein needle or a butterfly needle. The needle is attached to a medium length of small-gauge polyethylene tubing. The plastic butterfly can be taped to the leg to maintain the needle in position.

Use of Intravenous Catheters in Animals

The percutaneous placement of catheters into large veins such as the jugular has made the IV administration of fluids to animals a more feasible procedure. Additionally, the use of catheters in the jugular vein allows easy recording of central venous pressure (CVP). The success of long-term maintenance of an IV catheter involves proper insertion of the catheter under sterile conditions, a secure bandaging technique, and careful maintenance (Fig. 91).

Types of Intravenous Catheters

Needles and catheters are sized according to their outside diameter or gauge. The larger the gauge, the smaller the outside diameter (see p. 833).

The lumen or inside diameter of the catheter controls the rate of fluid delivery, and the flow rate varies according to a fourth power of the diameter. Doubling the lumen diameter increases the fluid flow rate 16 times.

There are three basic types of catheters: (1) those that introduce the catheter through a needle (Fig. 89); (2) those that introduce the catheter over a needle (Fig. 90A and B); and (3) a combination of types (1) and (2).

Careful preparation of the skin site is mandatory to avoid contamination, and, if possible, a percutaneous placement is made. A cutdown procedure is used only when a vein of adequate size cannot be located. Catheter contamination is reduced by using a closed system. Care should be taken to avoid excess traumatic injury to vessel walls; this may predispose to phlebitis and thromboembolism. A soft, pliable catheter reduces these risks.

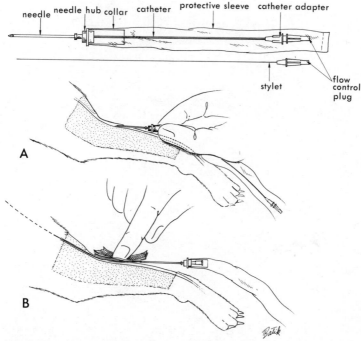

Figure 89. A, Percutaneous needle puncture of cephalic vein. It should be inserted close to the carpus. The catheter is advanced through the needle into the vein. B, After placing the catheter in the vein, the needle is withdrawn, pressure applied over the venipuncture site, the catheter taped in place, and the needle guard placed around the needle.

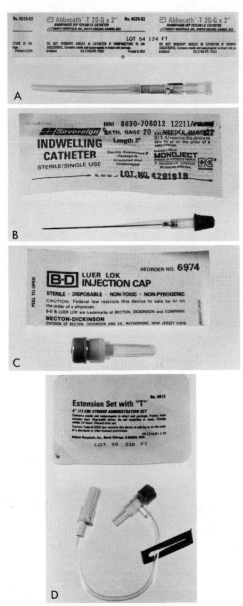

Figure 90. *A,* Abbocath T (Teflon catheter outside the needle). *B,* Sovereign indwelling catheter (catheter outside the needle). *C,* B-D Luer Lok injection cap (can be used to plug catheter yet allow intermittent injections). *D,* Abbott extension set with "T" (allows open flow line with cap for intermittent injections).

612

Selection of types of catheters and gauges depends on: (1) species and size and fragility of veins to be used, (2) length of time that the catheter will be in place, and (3) type of fluid to be delivered—viscosity, rapidity of flow desired.

	Cephalic or Tarsal Vein (catheter gauge)	Jugular (catheter gauge)
Cat or small dog	20–24	18–22
Medium-sized dog	19–23	18–20
Large dog	17–20	14–18

Equipment

Bardic Inside Needle Catheter* with stylet (available in various sizes [see Fig. 89]. Both 18-gauge and 14-gauge are used commonly; larger sizes are best).

Argyle Medicut Intravenous Cannula†

Sovereign Indwelling Catheter† (available in 14-, 18-, and 20-gauge catheter size—that is, an over-the-needle catheter fitting over 16-, 20,- or 22-gauge, 2-inch needles [see Fig. 90*B*]. These catheters are a good size for placing in the cephalic vein).

Another catheter that works well in both dogs and cats is the Abbocath T Catheter (see Fig. 90*A*).‡

Abbott also makes a useful extension set with a T (Fig. 90*D*).

The Vasculon TM§ Catheter System is an effective cephalic vein catheter in small animals.

The B-D injection cap is useful for intermittent closure of catheters, which also allows injections (see Fig. 90*C*).

Technique (Catheter Inside Needle)

The catheter can be placed into the jugular, cephalic, or recurrent tarsal vein. Prepare the skin site by clipping the hair, scrubbing the skin over the vein or artery with a povidone-iodine scrub, and wiping with iodine and alcohol. Open the sterile package and remove the needle guard, which should be retained for later use. Distend the vein by appropriately positioning the animal, and make a percutaneous needle puncture into the vein. Most problems arise at this point, because the needle and catheter tip are not in the lumen of the vessel. When the catheter tip is felt to enter the vessel lumen, blood should enter the catheter. At this time, *elevate the tip* of the catheter to remain in the vessel lumen, and holding the stylet with one hand, gently push the

---

*Bard Hospital Division of C. R. Bard, Inc., Murray Hill, New Jersey.
†Sherwood Medical Industries, 1831 Olive Street, St. Louis, Missouri 63103.
‡Abbott Laboratories, North Chicago, Illinois 60064.
§Pioneer Viggo, Inc., 4650 Southwest Pacific Avenue, Beaverton, Oregon 97005.

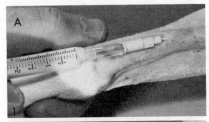

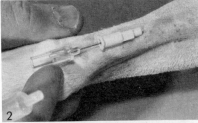

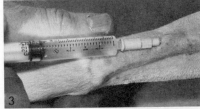

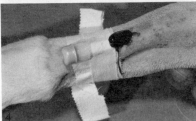

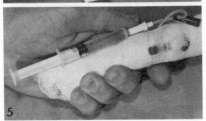

Figure 91. Placement and fixation of catheters.

A, Cephalic vein placement.

1. Syringe with catheter *and* needle inserted into cephalic vein.
2. Needle being removed from inside catheter.
3. Heparin and saline solution injected to flush catheter and check proper placement.
4. Catheter/skin insertion site has been coated with Betadine ointment. Catheter hub has B-D cap occluding entrance, and tape is wrapped around hub and leg for fixation. Note tape folded back on tag ends for easy removal.
5. Extension set with "T" is attached to catheter.

Illustration continued on opposite page

Figure 91. *Continued.*

B, Jugular vein placement.

1. Syringe with catheter *and* needle inserted into jugular vein.
2. Catheter slightly withdrawn and secured with two pieces of tape. Needle punctures tape and skin and back out tape so suture can be used to secure catheter to skin (suture needle could also be used for this technique).
3. Suture tied and Betadine ointment applied at catheter/skin junction.
4. Knit bandage wrap used to secure and protect catheter. Note extension set with "T" attached for versatility of injections.

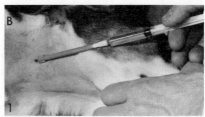
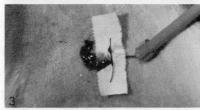
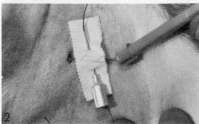
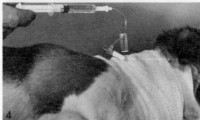

catheter gently into the vein. Place the thumb in back of the flow control plug, and push the catheter gently into the vein. Do not attempt to pull the catheter back out through the needle; the sharp edge may cut the catheter. If venipuncture is unsuccessful, remove the needle and catheter together.

When the catheter has been placed into the vein, remove the needle from the vein. Apply pressure over the venipuncture site for 30 seconds with a gauze sponge. Cover the venipuncture site with Neomycin polymixin B ointment or Betadine ointment and a sterile gauze sponge, and tape it in place. Discard the collar and protective sleeve from the needle hub and seat the IV fluid adapter into the needle hub. Remove the stylet from the catheter.

Place the needle within the needle guard. Tape the needle guard to the skin and connect the IV infusion set to the adapter. Check for leakage or infiltration, and ensure that the IV solution is running freely.

It is necessary to completely cover the catheter apparatus and needle holder with bandage and tape.

The following should be kept in mind to avoid problems with long-term continuous fluid administration.

1. Use T-connectors in the female attachments of the IV catheter. This enables coupling the male end of the IV set and allows IV injections without disengaging the IV set from the catheter hub (see Fig. 90C).

2. If an animal is hyperactive and is in a large cage, the 80-inch Venosets* may allow the animal to move without undue tension of the catheter.

3. If fluids are to be discontinued for a period of time, it is desirable to leave the catheter in place. The catheter can be closed with an injection cap, secured in place, and flushed with heparinized saline (1000 units of heparin, 250 ml of saline) (see Fig. 90B). If the catheter is not used for more than 12 hours, the catheter should be flushed through the injection cap with heparinized solution once or twice a day. If an injection cap is not available, 2 or 3 ml of heparinized solution in a small syringe can be taped to the catheter.

Percutaneous catheterization of the femoral or dorsal metatarsal artery can be accomplished using the same technique as just described; however, a 4- to 6-inch catheter should be used. Care must be taken on removal of these catheters; pressure over the artery should be maintained for enough time to prevent hematoma formation (5–10 min).

Ways to Prevent Phlebitis

1. Use aseptic technique.
2. Use appropriate needles and catheters.
3. Dilute irritating medications.
4. Be cautious about administering hypertonic solutions, even dextrose.
5. Replace sterile IV catheters every 48 to 72 hours.

Technique (Catheter Outside Needle)

IV catheters that are assembled *outside* the needle and used for insertion can be used as just described except for some slight differences in emphasis.

It is important for over-the-needle catheters to be inserted well into the vessel before advancing the catheter independent of the needle. There is a

---

*Venoset, Abbott Laboratories, North Chicago, Illinois 60064.

small amount of needle exposed distal to the catheter. If insertion into the vessel only involves the exposed needle, there may not be a large enough opening in the vessel to accommodate the insertion of the catheter as it slides over the needle.

When the catheter has been inserted fully into the vessel, remove the needle and attach an injection cap. Flush the catheter with heparinized saline. The catheter is then secured as previously described.

Intravenous Cutdowns

In cases in which it is not possible to place an IV cannula percutaneously—for example, because of collapsed or damaged veins or because of extensive subcutaneous fat—a venous cutdown is indicated. The cephalic or external jugular vein can be used.

Equipment

A scalpel, several hemostats, small blunt straight-tipped scissors, small fine-pointed scissors, suture material, No. 15 Bard Parker blade, sponges, and local anesthetic are necessary.

Technique

1. Clip the hair over the vein and cleanse the skin with an antiseptic solution. Apply sterile drapes around the area to prevent contamination. The operator wears gloves, a cap, and a mask.
2. Infiltrate the regions of the incision with local anesthetic.
3. Make a longitudinal incision through the dermis and subcutaneous tissue over the vein. If the vein cannot be easily located by palpation, make a transverse incision across the vein to locate the vein.
4. Spread the subcutaneous tissue with a hemostat in the direction of the vein. Pass a curved hemostat under the vein, and pull two ligatures around the vein. Tie the distal ligature, and leave the proximal ligature *untied.*
5. Using the ends of the distal-tied ligature for control, hold the vein and, using a No. 15 blade, incise the vein halfway across.
6. Insert a cannula into the venotomy incision. Small forceps on the lips of the venotomy wound or a small silk stay suture may help in placement of the cannula. Tie the proximal suture around the catheter securely enough to prevent bleeding but not so tight as to prevent eventual removal of the cannula.
7. Suture the skin around the cannula. Place an antibiotic or Betadine dressing on the skin, and bandage the dressing and cannula in place. When connecting the IV, ensure that the cannula is not pulled out of the vein.

Subcutaneous Injection

1. Use a 3-inch, 15- or 16-gauge needle attached to tubing.
2. Clean the skin, and push the needle to the entire depth under the skin in the region of the shoulder, back, or loin.

3. Pull the folds of the skin up to the needle hub to allow the needle to penetrate fully.
4. As fluid fills the subcutaneous space, allow the skin folds to retract and gradually withdraw the needle.
5. *Do not* "fan" the needle under the skin to spread the fluid; however, the needle may be redirected in a straight line in another direction.
6. Use multiple sites as needed to give additional volumes.

Intraperitoneal Injection

1. Thoroughly clip and cleanse the skin over the abdominal injection site (just lateral to the linea alba and midway between the umbilicus and pelvic brim).
2. Insert a 2- or 3-inch, 16- or 18-gauge needle into the peritoneal cavity.
3. Fill the cavity until the abdomen is distended or until lesser dosage is given.

General Considerations

Solution bottles can be changed easily or Y-tube infusion sets can be used with impunity except in IV infusions. In the latter case, extreme care must be used to avoid air embolism during bottle changes. Do not permit an unattended bottle to become empty.

With hypertonic or hypotonic solutions, care must be exercised to avoid subcutaneous infiltration. Constant supervision is needed during IV infusions.

SOLUTIONS NEEDED

Use commercial solutions. These solutions should be simple unless you have a good laboratory and the interest to follow cases closely. Give solutions IV only when warmed to body temperature.

Necessary Basic Solutions

1. Dextran (plasma substitute), 500 ml; dextran, 6 per cent, in D5W; or dextran, 6 per cent, in sodium chloride, 0.9 per cent.
2. CPD blood collection and administration packs or ACD solution in blood collecting vacuum bottle (see p. 624).
3. Electrolyte solutions (500 and 1000 ml)
   D5W
   Sodium chloride, 0.9 per cent
   Sodium lactate, 1/6 molar
   Lactated Ringer's solution

Optional Helpful Solutions

1. Invert sugar, 10 per cent (5 per cent dextrose, 5 per cent fructose), in water
2. Dextrose, 50 per cent in water

3. Sodium chloride, 3 per cent
4. Gastric replacement solution
5. Duodenal replacement solution
6. Calcium gluconate, 10 per cent in water
7. Dextrose, 5 per cent, in sodium chloride, 0.9 per cent
8. Amino acid solution, 5 per cent
9. Intestinal replacement and general electrolyte solution

Parenteral Nutrition

Parenteral nutrition is the process of supplying nutrients—namely, proteins, carbohydrates, fats, electrolytes, vitamins, and fluids by an IV route. Total parenteral nutrition indicates that the animal is receiving all its nutritional maintenance needs IV. This form of therapy may be indicated for short periods of time in the animal who cannot or will not take in adequate nutrients orally; that is, animals with acute renal failure, inflammatory bowel disease, protracted vomiting, or severe oral or esophageal disease or during postoperative days following enteric surgery.

General Considerations

1. Total energy requirement for a dog is approximately 70 kcal per kg per day (more in small or pyrexic animals, less in large breeds).
2. Protein requirement for a dog is approximately 2.5 gm per kg per day.
3. Glucose or dextrose yields 4 kcal per gm.
4. Protein yields 4 kcal per gm.
5. Dextrose solutions greater than 10 per cent should not be given via a peripheral vein.

The first goal of parenteral nutrition is to supply energy to the patient. Providing 25 kcal per kg per day IV will help inhibit the anorectic patient from using body protein as an energy source. It is usually possible to meet this need for several days using 10 per cent dextrose. Longer term or total energy requirements are difficult to meet using dextrose solutions because of the high osmotic pressure of the required concentrated solutions. Commercially available isotonic lipid emulsions (such as Intralipid* 10 per cent, 1.1 kcal/ml) may be used to supply energy without giving a high volume of hyperosmolar solution. However, these preparations are expensive, have short shelf lives, and have been reported to cause occasional adverse reactions (e.g., dyspnea, cyanosis, hives, and pyrexia). If used to supply energy, injectable fat emulsions should provide only 60 per cent of the caloric requirement of the patient. To spare body protein, some carbohydrate (usually dextrose) must be supplied, too. When calculating caloric requirements, remember to include any parenteral protein supplement being given in the total available calories, because protein will provide approximately 4 kcal per gm.

---

*Cutter Medical, Berkeley, California 94710.

FORMULAS

For Central Veins		For Peripheral Veins	
Dextrose	25%	Dextrose	5% or 10%
Amino acids	4.25%	Amino acids	4.25%
Na^+	35 mEq	Na^+	35 mEq
K^+	33mEq	K^+	33 mEq
Mg^{2+}	5 mEq	Mg^{2+}	5 mEq
Ca^{2+}	—mEq	Ca^{2+}	—mEq
Phosphates	15 mM	Phosphates	15 mM
Acetate	71 mEq	Acetate	71 mEq
Chloride	49 mEq	Chloride	49 mEq
Total kcal	1020/L	Total kcal	349 or 510/L
Osmolarity	1848	Osmolarity	833 or 1085
Approximate volume	1000 ml	Approximate volume	1000 ml

Although-it is usually unnecessary to administer protein IV to patients on parenteral nutrition for only a few days, if therapy is prolonged it may be wise to give either protein hydrolysates or amino acid solutions such as Vein Amine* or Aminosyn†.

A total parenteral nutrition formula for small animals can be made using crystalline amino acid preparations available in 3 to 10 per cent concentrations. Abbott Laboratories Aminosyn, 8.5 per cent, in 500 ml bottles is mixed under sterile conditions with 500 ml of 50 per cent dextrose solution. The shelf life of the finished solution is 21 days if refrigerated at 4° C. Because the resultant mixture is hyperosmotic, it must be administered via a large-bore indwelling venous catheter in the jugular vein. A peripheral vein solution that is not as hyperosmotic can be made using 5 to 10 per cent dextrose solution.

The administration of total parenteral nutrition should be initiated slowly and tapered off gradually. During the initiation of parenteral nutrition, it is important to evaluate serum electrolytes daily. If parenteral nutrition continues for several weeks, electrolyte levels should be measured biweekly.

Complications

The major complications associated with total parenteral nutrition in small animals are
1. The time consumed and expense of administration.
2. Thrombophlebitis and embolic phenomena from long-term catheterization.
3. Metabolic complications such as acidosis and azotemia.

References and Additional Readings

Chew, D., and Meuten, D. J.: Disorders of calcium and phosphorus metabolism. Vet. Clin. North Am., 12(3):411, 1982.

*Cutter Medical, Berkeley, California 94710.
†Abbott Laboratories, North Chicago, Illinois 60064.

Cornelius, L. M.: Fluid therapy in small animal practice. J.A.V.M.A., *176*:110, 1980.
Gleed, R.: Personal communication, 1984.
Haskins, S.: Maintenance fluid therapy. Proc. A.A.H.A., p. 489, 1982.
Polzin, D. J., Stevens, J. B., and Osborne, C. A.: Clinical application of anion gap in evaluation of acid-base disorders in dogs. Compendium on Continuing Education, 4(12):1021, 1982.
Schaer, M. (ed.): Symposium on fluid and electrolyte balance and disorders of potassium metabolism. Vet. Clin. North Am., *12*(3):399–409, 1982.
Scott, R. C.: Disorders of sodium metabolism. Vet. Clin. North Am., *12*(3):375, 1982.
Southwick, L.: Catheterization. *In* Zaslow, I. M.: Veterinary Trauma and Critical Care. Philadelphia, Lea & Febiger, 1984.
Spencer, K. R.: Intravenous catheters. Vet. Clin. North Am., *12*(3):533, 1982.

Peritoneal Dialysis

The peritoneum serves as a passive, semipermeable barrier to the diffusion of plasma water and peritoneal fluid. The movement of solutes from plasma water to dialysis solution is thought to result from diffusion and/or solvent drag effects of bulk flow.

Factors that alter peritoneal clearance are blood flow to the peritoneum and changes in peritoneal membrane permeability. Peritoneal clearance can be increased by (1) increasing dialysate exchange volume, (2) decreasing the time dialysate fluid stays in the peritoneal cavity, (3) increasing the temperature of the dialysate fluid to body temperature, or (4) adding glucose in hypertonic concentration to the dialysis fluid. Commercial dialysis solutions made for human patients can be used in dogs but are lower in both sodium and chloride ions. Additional sodium and chloride ions should be added to commercially available solutions. Commercially available dialysate solutions may contain 1.5 per cent or 4.25 per cent glucose. The 1.5 gm per 100 ml dextrose solution is moderately hypertonic to normal plasma (350 mOsm/L), whereas the 4.25 gm per 100 ml solution (490 mOsm/L) can be used to produce negative fluid balance in overhydrated animals.

The major use of peritoneal dialysis in dogs is to treat and maintain patients with acute oliguric renal failure until they compensate for renal damage.

Technique

The ability to perform peritoneal dialysis in the dog has been greatly improved by a special column disc catheter developed by Thornhill.

In performing peritoneal dialysis, place the animal in left lateral recumbency. Clip and surgically prepare a site midway between the umbilicus and pelvis.

Empty the bladder if it is filled. Using local anesthetic (such as 2 per cent Xylocaine), infiltrate the skin and abdominal musculature just lateral to the midline and a few centimeters posterior to the umbilicus. Commercial peritoneal dialysis sets* are available, or ⅛-inch ID Silastic tubing† with multiple fenestrations can be used. When the catheter is placed, suture it to the skin and bandage the abdomen and catheter. Inject enough warm (38° to 39° C) dialysate fluid to mildly distend the abdomen (200–2000 ml). Lactated Ringer's solution with added glucose (to 2 per cent) is a satisfactory lavage fluid, but Peridial, 1.5 per cent, and Inpersol, 1.5 per cent, are balanced more correctly. After 1 hour, drain the abdomen of solution. Remove the dialysate by siphoning it back into the original sterile container. During the first dialyzing period, some fluid will be absorbed; thus, the entire volume that was placed in the peritoneal cavity will not be collected. In severe renal failure cases, peritoneal dialysis may have to be repeated three to five times a day.

A major complication to peritoneal dialysis in the dog has been the inability to keep the indwelling catheter from becoming blocked. Commercial human peritoneal dialysis sets may function for a short period of time in the dog but then become blocked with tissue and fibrin. The Column Disc Peritoneal Dialysis Catheter‡ developed in the dog by Dr. J. Thornhill of Purdue University has permitted continuous ambulatory peritoneal dialysis in dogs without catheter obstruction. Using a surgical incision, insert the catheter within the abdomen. Place it paramedially alongside the bladder in the lower medial quadrant of the abdomen. Pull the disc firmly against the parietal peritoneum, and close the peritoneum over the base of the catheter. The abdominal muscle layers should be sutured tightly around the first dacron velour cuff to prevent fluid leakage and ascending infection. Take the free end of the catheter and tunnel it subcutaneously to exit in the skin through a stab incision at a point beyond the second dacron velour cuff. Suture the body wall closed, secure the catheter to the ventral abdominal wall, and flush the catheter with heparinized saline. In this type of dialysis technique, called *CAPD* (Continuous Ambulatory Peritoneal Dialysis), Dianeal 137 with 1.5 per cent dextrose§ is used. The dialysis solution is available in 250-ml, 500-ml, 1-L, and 2-L bags. For each 2 L of dialysate, add 2 ml of heparin to prevent fibrin from plugging the catheter. (Instill a sufficient volume of warmed dialysate solution to mildly distend the abdomen. An infusion adapter is available for the catheter‖; a clamp to seal the catheter is also available from the same company. Peritoneal dialysis must be done under aseptic conditions. A mask and gloves must be worn. As the fluid rapidly flows from the silastic bag into the peritoneum, roll up the bag; when the bag is empty, tape it to the body wall. Dialysate solution is allowed to remain in the peritoneal cavity for 45 to 50 minutes. Document the volume of solution instilled and removed from the abdomen during each

---

*Stylocath and Inpersol Peritoneal Catheter (with stylet), Abbott Laboratories, N. Chicago, Illinois 60064; Diacath, Travenol Laboratories, Inc., Deerfield, Illinois, 60015.

†Silastic brand medical grade tubing, Dow Corning Corp., Midland, Michigan.

‡Vetcath-Physio-Control, 11811 Willows Road, Redmond, Washington 98052.

§Dianeal-Viaflex-Transfer Set Tubing, Travenol Laboratories, Inc., Deerfield, Illinois 60015.

‖Beta-Cap Adapter, Quinton Instruments Co., Seattle, Washington 98121.

exchange. When dialysis fluid is to be collected, unroll the bag; gravity permits collection of dialysate. As the patient improves, dialysis may be reduced to three or four times per day, and the dwell time for the fluid in the abdomen may be increased to 4 to 6 or even 8 to 12 hours.

There is always a danger of peritonitis resulting from peritoneal dialysis. Daily peritoneal infusion of a very dilute iodine solution prevents bacterial contamination of the dialysis catheter and peritoneal cavity. The technique should be performed as follows: once each day following removal of dialysate, instill physiologic saline (same quantity as used for dialysate exchanges) and immediately remove it. Next, instill physiologic saline to which has been added 0.2 ml of 2 per cent solution of iodine USP per L. Allow the solution to remain in the abdominal cavity for 4 minutes. Remove the iodine-saline solution. Repeat the routine dialysis procedure as necessary. Peritoneal infection is indicated by the presence of turbid drainage fluid with white blood cell (WBC) counts exceeding 100 to 200 cells per mm^3. Gram stain as well as culture and sensitivity should be done on the fluid. Blood culture media should be inoculated with dialysate fluid and culture plates should be inoculated to identify gram-positive and coliform organisms.

If peritonitis is suspected, Thornhill suggests that antimicrobial therapy should be begun by adding 16 mg of tobramycin per 2 L of dialysate and 250 mg of cephathin sodium per 2 L of dialysate per each exchange. Systemic cephalexin should be used at 20 mg per kg BID. Other antibiotics that may be added to dialysate fluid depending on bacterial sensitivity results are penicillin G (50,000 units/L), ampicillin (50 mg/L), cloxacillin (100 mg/L), ticarcillin (100 mg/L), vancomycin (30 mg/L), amikacin (50 mg/L), clindamycin (50 mg/L), and sulfadiazine:trimethoprim (25:5 mg/L).

Additional complications that can occur are intra-abdominal trauma or perforation during catheter placement, electrolyte imbalances and excessive protein loss, and cardiovascular and respiratory complications resulting from too rapid fluid injections.

References and Additional Readings

Gourley, I. M., and Parker, H. R.: Peritoneal dialysis. *In* Kirk, R. W. (ed.): Current Veterinary Therapy VI. Philadelphia, W. B. Saunders Company, 1977, pp. 1144–1149.

Thornhill, J. A.: Peritoneal dialysis in the dog and cat. Compendium on Continuing Education, 3(1):20, 1981.

Thornhill, J. A.: Peritonitis associated with peritoneal dialysis. J.A.V.M.A., *182*(7):721, 1983.

Vaamonde, C. A.: Peritoneal dialysis. Postgrad. Med., *62*:148, 1977.

BLOOD TRANSFUSIONS

Cats

Blood transfusions for cats are usually administered for medical reasons, and repeated small doses of fresh whole blood are desirable. Cats have an AB blood group system. Studies indicate that approximately 73 per cent of cats are type A, 26 per cent are type B, and 1 per cent are type AB. Cats with type B usually have anti-A in their serum and will hemolyze red blood cells (RBCs) of type A when their anti-A titers are as low as 1:64. Cats with type A blood have a low incidence of anti-B antibody, with titers rarely exceeding 1:2.

The chance of an incompatible transfusion (A→B) or (B→A) in random population of cats is estimated to be 36 per cent. If cats are to be kept as in hospital blood donors, their blood can be typed*; type A donors are preferred.

Equipment

The following equipment is necessary for blood transfusions: thiamylal sodium; two 20-ml siliconized syringes; one 2-inch, 18-gauge siliconized needle; one scalp vein infusion set; adhesive tape, 1 inch wide; blanket; a clear plastic bag; an oxygen tank; a flow meter; and rubber tubing. If desired, an acid citrate dextrose (ACD) blood collection bottle or a 150-ml or citrate phosphate dextrose (CPD) plastic bag (Fenwal Blood Pak) can be used.

Technique

Donor cats can be anesthetized by barbiturates and euthanized by complete exsanguination by a left ventricular puncture with a 2-inch, 18-gauge needle. In such cases, about 150 ml of blood can be harvested and stored in ACD or CPD solution. In many instances, a donor cat is kept in the hospital for repeated collections. These animals are lightly anesthetized with barbiturate or ketamine, the left thorax is prepared as for surgery, and ventricular puncture is accomplished by inserting a 2-inch, 18- to 20-gauge needle through the left third or fourth intercostal space. The needle is attached to a 20-ml siliconized glass syringe, and blood is aspirated to fill the syringe. Two syringes are filled in this manner. It is advisable to use ACD solution or heparin as an anticoagulant in the syringe to prevent clotting while readministering the blood. A safer procedure than cardiac puncture is jugular vein aspiration, although it takes more time. Use a scalp vein set for venipuncture and collection of blood.

Donor cats should be healthy, vigorous, and free of blood disorders. In these animals, a 40-ml donation can be repeated safely every 3 weeks. All donor cats should be checked for feline leukemia virus. Cat blood should not be stored. Obtaining fresh blood is preferable.

---

*Blood can be typed by Stormont Laboratories, 1237 E. Beamer St., Suite D, Woodland, California 95695.

Administering Blood

Cats needing blood are usually extremely depressed, toxic, or anoxic and require blood to correct anemias or for other medical reasons. Struggling or violent exertion may cause these patients to collapse and die. Therefore, extreme gentleness and care are mandatory in handling and restraint. Critically anemic cats should be cradled gently on a towel or blanket and the head placed in a clear plastic bag into which oxygen is being infused at 4 to 6 L per minute.

Blood can be administered intravenously (IV) by way of the jugular, cephalic, or femoral vein, using a 22- to 24-gauge scalp vein infusion set. Intramedullary infusion is possible through the femur by way of the intratrochanteric fossa. However, this may be impractical and present dangers of intramedullary infection. Intraperitoneal infusion can be used safely with good utilization of erythrocytes. About 45 per cent of the infused red blood cells are in the circulation within 24 hours, and 65 per cent within 48 hours.

The average 2- to 3-kg cat can accept 30 to 40 ml of blood injected IV over a period of 30 minutes. Small, repeated injections are safer and more desirable than a large, single injection. Single intraperitoneal injections (40 ml) are safe (Table 107).

Table 107. VOLUME OF BLOOD IN ML NEEDED FOR TRANSFUSION PER POUND OF RECIPIENT CAT*

		PCV of Donated Blood (including anticoagulant)									
		30%	32%	34%	36%	38%	40%	42%	44%	46%	48%	50%
PCV of Recipient	4%	16.3	15.3	14.4	13.6	12.9	12.3	11.7	11.1	10.6	10.2	9.8
	6%	14.0	13.1	12.4	11.7	11.1	10.5	10.0	9.5	9.1	8.8	8.4
	8%	11.7	10.9	10.3	9.7	9.2	8.8	8.3	8.0	7.6	7.3	7.0
	10%	9.3	8.8	8.2	7.8	7.4	7.0	6.7	6.4	6.1	5.8	5.6
	12%	7.0	6.6	6.2	5.8	5.5	5.3	5.0	4.8	4.6	4.4	4.2
	14%	4.7	4.3	4.1	3.9	3.7	3.5	3.3	3.2	3.0	2.9	2.8

Example: PCV of recipient   6%
PCV of donated blood   46%
Weight of recipient   7 lbs

Volume of blood needed per pound   9.1 ml *(See above table)*
Multiplied by weight of recipient   ×7 lbs

Total volume of blood needed   = 63.7 ml

*Based on a post-transfusion PCV of 18%.
From Norsworthy, G. D.: Blood transfusion in the cat. Feline Pract., 7:29, 1977.

Dogs

The blood group system of the dog has been worked out and the nomenclature is as follows:

CANINE BLOOD GROUPS

New Nomenclature*	Common Name	Incidence†
DEA–1.1	A_1	40
DEA–1.2	A_2	20
DEA–3	B	5
DEA–4	C	98
DEA–5	D	25
DEA–6	F	98
DEA–7	Tr	45
DEA–8	He	40

*Dog erythrocyte antigen system.
†In random dog population.

The ideal blood donor should be (DEA – 1) A and (DEA – 7) Tr negative, healthy, and 1 to 6 years of age and should weigh 20 kg (44 lb) or more and should not have been transfused. Donor dogs can be bled at a rate of 10 to 20 ml per kg every 3 weeks. In clinical practice, few transfusion reactions are observed because about 40 per cent of the random dog population is A-negative and multiple transfusions are usually not required. When dogs are to be kept as blood donors, their blood can be typed by a commercial laboratory.*

Equipment

The following equipment is necessary for blood transfusions:
Thiamylal sodium
Blood donor kit, preferably a CPD containing blood pak (Fenwal) or an SMB anticoagulant.
Blood recipient kit containing a 5-ml syringe with saline and an IV catheter.
Sterile IV cutdown kit containing a scalpel; thumb forceps; a needle holder; sharp, pointed scissors; two pairs of mosquito forceps; a curved needle; plain catgut; fine silk; and sponges.

Collecting Blood

Blood may be drawn from a donor dog aseptically via the jugular vein or femoral artery or by left ventricular puncture. When repeated withdrawals of blood are to be made from a donor dog, the femoral artery or jugular vein

---

*Stormont Laboratories, 1237 E. Beamer St., Suite D., Woodland, California 95695.

should be used. Femoral artery puncture has a distinct advantage in that blood under pressure can be obtained. This is helpful if bags are being used in collection. Left ventricular puncture can be used; however, it is dangerous. Dogs are given a short-acting IV anesthetic prior to bleeding.

The way in which blood is removed, preserved, and stored determines its viability. Blood is routinely collected in plastic bags containing CPD solution and allowed to flow through the solution while the bag is gently agitated. When the bag is filled, the tubing should be clamped without allowing air to enter.

Recent experiments have demonstrated the advantage of collecting canine blood in a solution consisting of ascorbate phosphate, citric acid, sodium citrate, sodium phosphate, and dextrose. With this solution, viability remained above 70 per cent for 6 weeks when blood was kept at 4° C. Oxygenated blood so collected can be stored under refrigeration at 4° C. In general, do not use stored whole blood more than 3 weeks old. Plasma can be harvested from blood and frozen for later use. The donor dog should be healthy, parasite-free, vaccinated for the usual diseases, and legally owned by the veterinarian. A mature, thin, 22-kg (48-lb) animal makes an ideal donor.

Component storage of blood is the most efficient way to use whole blood or blood products for treatment of bleeding patients. This involves separating and freezing the plasma from fresh units of whole blood. The remainder can be stored as packed cells at 4° C for up to 6 weeks for blood collected in CPD or SMB and 3 to 4 weeks in ACD. The clotting factors in plasma are preserved by freezing, and the packed red cells are available for immediate use.

A blood bank centrifuge is required to effectively separate cellular components. If a centrifuge is not available, the red cells can be allowed to settle by gravity overnight at 4° C and the supernatant plasma is removed. Plasma stored at $-40°$ to $-70°$ C will last for up to 1 year. At household freezer temperatures of $-20°$ C, plasma will last for 2 to 4 months.

Administering Blood

In dogs, blood is invariably given IV. The cephalic vein is commonly used, but the jugular vein is routinely used when an IV catheter is placed in the animal. The recipient set should be filled, so that blood in the drip chamber covers the filter. Blood can be administered at variable rates, but the routine figure of 4 to 5 ml per minute is often used. Volume is given as needed. To calculate the approximate volume of blood needed to raise hemoglobin levels, the following formula can be used:

$$\frac{\text{volume of blood}}{\text{required (ml)}} = \frac{\text{recipients wt (kg)} \times \text{Hb rise wanted (gm/dl)} \times 70}{\text{donors Hb concentration (gm/dl)}}$$

(See Table 108.) Surgical emergencies and shock may require several times this volume within a short period (see p. 59).

Table 108. EXAMPLE OF ESTIMATING VOLUMES IN BLOOD THERAPY

30-kg dog with PCV = 10%; desired PCV = 18%; anticoagulated donor blood with PCV = 50%
Total blood volume = (90 ml/kg)(30 kg) = 2700 ml
Existing red cell mass = (2700 ml)(10%) = 270 ml
Desired red cell mass = (2700 ml)(18%) = 490 ml
Required red cell mass = 490 ml − 270 ml = 220 ml
Required blood volume = (220 ml)(50%) = 440 ml

From Kirk, R. W. (ed.): Current Veterinary Therapy 8: Small Animal Practice. Philadelphia, W. B. Saunders Company, 1983.

If the blood type of the patient is unknown and CEA-1 or CEA-2 (type A negative blood) is not available, any dog blood can be given to patients in acute need if they have not had previous transfusions. If mismatched blood is given, however, the patient will become sensitized; and, after 9 days, destruction of the donated erythrocytes will begin. In addition, any subsequent mismatched transfusions may cause an immediate reaction (usually mild) and rapid destruction of the donated cells.

The clinical signs of blood transfusion reaction are seen only when type A blood is given to a non–type A recipient that has been previously sensitized. Incompatible blood transfusions to breeding females can result in isoimmunization, resulting in hemolytic disease in puppies. The A negative bitch transfused with A positive blood who produced a litter from an A positive stud can have neonatal isoerythrolysis of puppies. The signs of a transfusion reaction are usually seen within 1 hour of the time of the beginning of the transfusion. Hemoglobinemia and hemoglobinuria result. Fever, emesis, incontinence of urine, tremors, hives, and transient prostration may be observed.

If a transfusion reaction is observed: (1) discontinue the transfusion if it is still in progress; (2) give soluble corticosteroids IV; (3) ensure complete rest; (4) give oxygen, if necessary; and (5) if blood is necessary, cross-match blood of donor with that of recipient. Crossmatching blood is important when repeated transfusions are to be performed (see p. 686).

References and Additional Readings

Aver, L., and Bell, K.: The AB blood group system in the domestic cat. Anim. Blood Groups Biochem. Genet., 11:63, 1980.

Breznock, E. M., and Strack, D.: Blood volume of nonsplenectomized and splenectomized cats before and after acute hemorrhage. Am. J. Vet. Res., 43(10):1811, 1982.

Dodds, W. J.: Management and treatment of hemostatic defects. In Bojrab, J. (ed.): Pathophysiology in Small Animal Surgery. Philadelphia, Lea & Febiger, 1982.

Eisenbrandt, D. L., and Smith, J. E.: Evaluation of preservatives and containers for storage of canine blood. J.A.V.M.A., 163:988, 1973.

Ou, D., Mahaffey, E., and Smith, J. E.: Effect of storage on oxygen dissociation of canine blood. J.A.V.M.A., 167:56, 1975.

Smith, J. E., Mahaffey, E., and Board, P.: A new storage medium for canine blood. J.A.V.M.A., 172:701, 1978.

Stormont, C. J.: Blood groups in animals. J.A.V.M.A., 181(10):1120, 1982.

TRACHEOTOMY

Indications

Tracheotomy is indicated in the following situations:

To relieve upper respiratory tract obstructions.

To facilitate removal of respiratory secretions.

To decrease the dead air space.

To provide a route for inhalant anesthesia when oral or facial surgery is complex.

To reduce resistance to respiration.

To reduce the risk of closed glottis pressure (cough) following pulmonary or cranial surgery.

To facilitate artificial respiration.

Technique

In an emergency situation with asphyxiation imminent, any cutting instrument will suffice in making a tracheotomy. Moistening the hair over the ventral neck facilitates midline incision over the trachea. The first few tracheal rings (2–3, 3–4) are incised to allow placement of any firm tube (ballpoint pen barrel), or the knife blade may be rotated 90 degrees to maintain the tracheal opening.

A specialized instrument has been developed for emergency tracheostomy/cricothyroidotomy. This is a percutaneous special–slotted 13-gauge needle that is passed into the trachea through the cricothyroid ligament. A special tracheostomy tube* is guided through the split needle into the tracheal lumen.

In less demanding circumstances, aseptic surgical technique should be followed. Make a midline skin incision just caudal to the larynx to permit incision and retraction of the paired sternohyoid muscles, exposing the trachea. Then elevate and immobilize the trachea by passing ¼-inch umbilical tapes around it as traction sutures. A transverse incision is made through the annular ligament between the third and fourth tracheal rings. Two or three tracheal rings may be incised or partially resected to allow placement of the tracheotomy tube. Following tube placement, the soft tissues are loosely approximated with absorbable sutures and the skin is closed with nonabsorbable sutures.

Tracheotomy Tubes

Many of the shortcomings of the old curved metal tracheotomy tubes are overcome by the utilization of the newer plastic tubes. These are often better tolerated by the patient, because they are lighter in weight, more flexible, less irritating, and contoured better for the canine or feline trachea. Crusting of secretions has been less of a problem with the PVC tubes.

The uncuffed Morrant-Baker and cuffed Bassett tubes are available in a wide variety of sizes for the dog (2–21 FG), with and without adapters for

---

*Available from Pertrach, Inc., 1760 Termino Avenue, Suite 301, Long Beach, California 90804.

connection to respirators or anesthesia machines. The infant tracheotomy tubes (Great Ormond St. Hospital pattern) have proved ideal for small dogs and cats. We also use the Portex* cuffed tracheostomy tubes that have an obturator permitting cleaning of the tube.

Postoperative Care

Postoperative care is as important as the surgery itself. The following procedures should be used:
1. Humidify the inspired air. This can be accomplished by nebulizing water into the cage or by instilling 1 to 3 ml of sterile saline into the trachea.
2. Use systemic antibiotics prophylactically.
3. Cleanse the wound and the tracheal tube frequently. By using the traction sutures, the tube can be easily removed and replaced.
4. Frequent aspiration of respiratory secretions should be performed. A soft urethral catheter (12-French) is attached to a T-tube and to a vacuum pump so that suction can be applied or released at will. This tube is passed through the wound to the large bronchi. Instillation of 3 to 5 ml of saline into the trachea helps to loosen mucous debris. Then suction out the debris.
5. Tracheotomy wounds heal within 7 to 10 days following removal of the tube. They should be allowed to heal by second intention, because primary closure may predispose to subcutaneous emphysema.

The major complications resulting from tracheotomy are tubes becoming plugged with mucus, blood, or debris; the tube falling out or being pulled out; coughing because of intubation; gagging when the tracheotomy tube is aspirated; respiratory distress with the tracheotomy tube in place; and tracheal wall necrosis.

Reference

Harvey, C. E., and O'Brien, J. A.: Tracheotomy in the dog and cat. J.A.A.H.A., *18*(4):563, 1982.

---

*Portex Blue Line Tracheostomy Unit, Industrial Way, Wilmington, Massachusetts 01887.

ENDOTRACHEAL INTUBATION

General Considerations

The two types of endotracheal tubes most commonly used in the dog are the Magill and the Murphy. The tubes are usually constructed of rubber or plastic, and their appropriate size can be classified by several different scales of measurement. In selecting an appropriate-sized endotracheal tube, consider the size of the animal and select the tube with the largest diameter that can be introduced without force (Table 109).

Table 109. RECOMMENDED SIZES FOR ENDOTRACHEAL TUBES

	Body Weight (kg)	Magill Size	French Size	Internal Diameter (mm.)
Dogs	2	2	22	6.0
	4	4–5	26–28	8.0
	6	6–7	28–30	9.0
	9	8	32	10.0
	12	9–10	34–36	11.0–12.0
	14	9–10	34–36	11.0–12.0
	16	10–11	36–38	11.0–12.0
	18–20	11–12	38–44	12.0
Cats	1	00	13	4.0
	2	0	16	5.0
	4	1	20	5.0

Equipment

Materials needed for endotracheal intubation include an appropriate-sized endotracheal tube, a laryngoscope, a mouth gag, a water-soluble lubricating material such as K-Y jelly, lidocaine spray, gauze pads, and 1-inch gauze.

Tubes should be cleansed with soap and water, both inside and outside, scrubbed, and thoroughly rinsed. The dry tubes may be sterilized by steam heat, liquid chemicals, or ethylene oxide gas. We prefer gas sterilization. Tubes are stored in a dry clean area.

It is better to use high-volume, low-pressure cuffs on endotracheal tubes. Overinflation of tracheal cuffs can lead to tracheal ulceration, tracheitis, hemorrhage, tracheomalacia, fibrosis, and stenosis. Occlusion of high-volume, low-pressure cuffs can be achieved at 25 mm Hg or less.

Always check the cuff of a cuffed tube to ensure that there are no leaks and that it is working properly. Prior to intubation, the selected endotracheal tube should be lubricated with material such as K-Y jelly. Intubation is carried out under a short-acting anesthetic or while the animal is under the influence of an analgesic-tranquilizer combination. Intubation in the dog and cat may cause an increase in sympathetic activity or vagal stimulation, resulting in cardiac arrhythmias. Atropine or glycopyrrolate may be given to canine and feline patients to avoid certain arrhythmias that are often associated with induction of anesthesia and intubation. They should always be given when narcotic analgesics or xylazine are used or when ocular surgery is being performed.

Caution in the use of atropine is warranted, and animals should have cardiovascular function monitored during surgery. Atropine will (1) increase anatomic dead space in the pulmonary compartment by 50 to 100 per cent; (2) remove vagal control over myocardium and increase cardiac rate, thus increasing oxygen demand and irritability of damaged myocardial tissue; and (3) change the nature of bronchial secretions to become more tenacious.

Atropine *should not* be given to animals with heart rates over 140 beats per minute, or with insulinomas, or to dogs receiving xylazine for cystometry. Glycopyrrolate may have some distinct advantages over atropine.

Technique

Direct visualization of the larynx is the best method for intubating dogs and cats. A laryngoscope should be used for intubation. The blades are detachable from rechargeable handles. MacIntosh, Miller, or Bizarri-Guiffrida blades work well in animals. Small blades (pediatric) are needed in cats and small dogs. Place the animal in lateral, sternal or dorsal recumbency, according to preference. Hold the laryngoscope in the left hand, and open the mouth with the right hand. In large dogs or animals under light anesthesia, the use of a mouth gag may be helpful. Pull the tongue forward with the right hand, being careful not to lacerate the ventral aspect of the tongue on the lower incisor teeth. In large dogs, it may be helpful to hold the tongue between the small and ring fingers to prevent it from moving excessively. Place the tip of the laryngoscope blade at the base of the tongue at the glossoepiglottic fold. Press the tip of the blade ventrally. This will move the epiglottis and expose the glottis. In some dogs, especially those that are brachycephalic, it may be necessary to put the laryngoscope tip directly on the epiglottis. Holding the endotracheal tube in the right hand, insert the endotracheal tube. A piece of aluminum wire temporarily placed inside a very flexible plastic tube will provide enough rigidity to make intubation simpler. Place the tube between the vocal folds, using a slight rotating motion rather than trying to push the tube through. Never try to force too large a tube into position. If partial closure of the glottis or laryngeal spasm occurs during attempted intubation, deepen the level of anesthesia, administer a muscle relaxant such as succinylcholine, or apply a local anesthetic spray such as 2 per cent lidocaine to the larynx using a spray or soaked Q-tip.

The cuff of a cuffed endotracheal tube should be at a level just beyond the larynx. Overinflation of the cuff may lead to a pressure necrosis of tracheal epithelium.

In cats induced with thiamylal sodium, intubation may be difficult because of laryngospasm. It is easier to intubate cats if ketamine is administered as a preanesthetic at a dosage of 6 to 8 mg per kg. A Warne neonatal endotracheal tube has proved to be very easy to use in the cat. The tube is noncuffed. It should be coated with 4 per cent lidocaine jelly prior to being placed in the trachea.

Reference

Sawyer, D.: Canine and feline endotracheal intubation and laryngoscopy. Compendium on Continuing Education. 6:973, 1984.

OXYGEN THERAPY

TISSUE OXYGENATION

The basic indication for oxygen therapy is inadequate tissue oxygenation (hypoxia).

The partial pressure of oxygen (pO_2) is a convenient figure to use in following oxygen utilization. Inspired air has a pO_2 of 150 mm Hg. As it is mixed with air in the alveolus, the pO_2 drops to 100 mm Hg. Arterial blood saturated with oxygen has a pO_2 of 95 mm Hg, and when tissues have been supplied, the pO_2 of venous blood is about 40 mm Hg. Oxygen tissue levels normally approximate 35 mm Hg.

Oxygen is transported in the blood in combination with hemoglobin and in physical solution in the plasma. If an adequate amount of hemoglobin is normally saturated with oxygen while breathing room air, breathing high concentrations of oxygen will only slightly increase that carried by hemoglobin. However, significant increases in dissolved plasma oxygen will be obtained. On the other hand, if inadequate hemoglobin saturation is obtained by breathing normal air, breathing high concentrations of oxygen may markedly raise hemoglobin saturation and improve tissue-oxygen tensions. The additional oxygen in physical solution would be helpful, too.

MONITORING PULMONARY FUNCTION

1. Observe the physical signs of the animal; rate (8–25 breaths/min); rhythm.
   a. Hypoventilation—lower than normal alveolar minute volume.
   b. Cheyne-Stokes breathing—cyclic hyperventilation and hypoventilation associated with acidosis and alterations in medullary center response.
   c. Biot's breathing—hypoventilation with periods of apnea, indicating severe medullary disease.
   d. Tachypnea—rapid rate of breathing without any comment on the volume of air moved.
2. Auscultate the thorax (see p. 452).
3. Evaluate mucous membranes—capillary perfusion.
4. Radiograph the chest if the procedure will not decompensate (overly stress) the animal.
5. Obtain some idea of ventilation volume—normals are 10 to 20 ml per kg for tidal volume; 150 to 250 ml per kg for minute volume, and 8 to 20 breaths per minute. Ventilometers are valuable when placed on the expiratory end of the breathing circuit.
6. Measure arterial blood gases, if possible (see p. 593).

SIGNS OF HYPOXIA

Measurement of arterial blood gases and pH is the only reliable means of measuring hypoxia.

The clinical signs of hyperpnea, dyspnea, tachycardia, and cyanosis may be dominant features in some patients, but they are nonspecific and unreliable.

TYPES OF HYPOXIA

Hypoxic Hypoxia

Alterations of respiratory function may lead to a lowered pO_2 of arterial blood, which in turn may be caused by:

1. *Alveolar hypoventilation,* which is the result of depressed respirations of increased resistance to chest movements. Hypercapnia is present. With a normal lung, adequate ventilation with air should help to correct the problem. In acute pneumothorax caused by leakage of air into the pleural cavity from ruptured lung or bronchi (see p. 212), additional administration of air or oxygen under positive airway pressure will further increase the tension pneumothorax and kill the animal. In this case, air must be effectively removed from the pleural space.

2. *An arteriovenous shunt* within the heart or lungs due to congenital defect or to perfusion of a section of lung that is not ventilated (consolidated or atelectatic segment). If the rest of the lung is hyperventilated, hypercapnia will not develop. Correction of the shunt is necessary, and oxygen inhalation is only partially helpful.

3. A *diffusion defect* in which the alveolar membrane is altered by fibrosis, emphysema, or thromboembolic disease. Hypercapnia usually is not present, because carbon dioxide can diffuse 20 times as fast as oxygen. Inhalation of oxygen may be helpful.

4. *Uneven blood flow and ventilation* throughout the lung may be caused by many pulmonary diseases and is probably the most common cause of hypoxia. Hypercapnia may or may not be present. Hyperventilation with air and oxygen inhalation are helpful.

Reduced oxygen-carrying capacity of the blood may be due to low or abnormal hemoglobin. Therapy must increase the amount of active hemoglobin.

Circulatory Hypoxia

Inadequate perfusion of tissues may be due to shock, low cardiac output, or vascular obstruction. Tissues do not live on oxygen alone, so improved circulation is imperative.

Histotoxic Hypoxia

Toxic tissue cells may be unable to use oxygen. Inhalation of oxygen is of no value.

Indications for Oxygen Therapy

In the following situations, oxygen therapy is necessary:

1. In veterinary medicine, oxygen is indicated in acute cases of respiratory insufficiency (hypoxic hypoxia) leading to a low arterial oxygen tension. It is rarely indicated for any chronic condition because of economic and practical considerations.
2. Altered ventilation-perfusion relationships are often indications for oxygen therapy. However, measures designed to treat infection, reduce airway obstruction, or improve the mechanics of breathing may reduce the need for oxygen.
3. Circulatory failures such as shock and reduced cardiac output cause hypoxia because of poor perfusion. Giving oxygen is an ancillary treatment, subordinate to the measures directed at the primary cause. However, oxygen therapy may be the critical factor in raising oxygen tissue levels above hypoxic levels.
4. In anemic hypoxia, blood transfusions are needed, and oxygen therapy is helpful only if the hemoglobin is abnormal (carboxyhemoglobin).
5. Histotoxic hypoxia is unlikely to be benefited by oxygen therapy, but it should be administered.
6. When possible, arterial blood gas analysis should be used to assess the need for oxygen therapy. Analysis should include oxygen tension, carbon dioxide tension, and blood pH.

Normal Values

1. pO_2: 85 to 95 mm Hg (arterial); 40 to 60 mm Hg (venous).
2. pCO_2: 29 to 36 mm Hg (arterial); 29 to 42 mm Hg (venous).
3. Blood base excess: ±2.5 mEq/L.
4. Plasma bicarbonate: 17 to 24 mEq/L.
5. Blood pH: 7.31 to 7.42.

ADMINISTERING OXYGEN

The goal of oxygen therapy is to increase the oxygen carried in the blood by raising the arterial oxygen tension to normal in hypoxic hypoxia, and by increasing the arterial oxygen tension above normal in circulatory and anemic hypoxia.

The requirements of an oxygen tent environment include the following:

1. Usually 30 to 40 per cent oxygen is more than adequate to treat cases of hypoxia correctable by oxygen therapy. (Higher concentrations may be needed for severe circulatory failure.) Initially, high flow rates of 10 L per minute are required to wash out residual nitrogen in the cage. A maintenance flow of 5 L per minute is usually sufficient.
2. Adequate humidification (often 40–60 per cent) is absolutely essential.

3. Maintenance of carbon dioxide at less than 1.5 per cent is necessary. Oxygen tents equipped with CO_2 absorbers can maintain CO_2 levels at 0.7 per cent.
4. Control of environmental temperature at 65° to 70° F is necessary in almost all cases.

Methods of oxygen administration include face mask, tracheal catheter, nasal catheter, oxygen tent, endotracheal tube, and intermittent positive pressure breathing (IPPB) respirator. Obviously, endotracheal intubation and IPPB can be used only in the anesthetized or comatose animal. Tight-fitting masks are usually resented by the animal, and its struggles cause further hypoxia.

Supplemental oxygen may be administered via a catheter placed either through the cricothyroid ligament or between the tracheal rings. Either of these techniques overcomes the total lack of patient cooperation that is common with nasal catheters. It has proved especially useful for the administration of supplemental oxygen to dogs too large for the oxygen cages. A large, sterile, pliable male urinary catheter is utilized. Humidified oxygen at a flow rate of 5 to 8 L per minute should achieve an oxygen concentration of 30 to 50 per cent.

For controlled positive pressure ventilation, either orotracheal intubation or a tracheostomy is indicated. Awake animals will not tolerate orotracheal intubation. The technique is used in comatose, anesthetized, or heavily sedated (with neuroleptanalgesic) animals. Neuromuscular blocking agents are *not* recommended for any but the most minimal of time duration positive pressure procedures.

In orotracheal intubation (see p. 631), high-volume, low-pressure endotracheal cuffs are used and the time limit for maintaining intubation depends on the condition of the patient and the degree of chemical restraint required. Prolonged tracheal intubation necessitates a tracheostomy (see p. 629).

For a discussion of tracheostomy, see page 629, and for positive controlled pressure ventilation, see page 82.

Another excellent way to administer oxygen is to pass a soft, flexible catheter through the cricothyroid membrane into the trachea. The catheter tip should be multiple fenestrated. Oxygen is bubbled through a heated water nebulizer and allowed to flow through the catheter at 2 to 4 L per minute and is adjusted as needed. The catheter is taped to the neck.

Oxygen tent equipment to provide these conditions is rarely found in veterinary hospitals. The best equipment includes a mechanical, thermostatically controlled compressor cooling unit, a circulatory fan, nebulizers or humidifiers to moisten the air, and a CO_2 absorber. The OTC-2 intensive care oxygen therapy unit manufactured by Kirschner Scientific fulfills these requirements; other professionally designed tents meet some of the requirements. The ice-chest oxygen diffusion tents are *very poor* for long-term maintenance therapy in hypoxemic animals. Small incubator isolettes have been used with good success in cats and puppies.

The animal should be continuously maintained in the tent, not on an intermittent basis. Animals with chronic respiratory disease or hypoxemia from other causes such as depressant drugs or cerebral trauma have become adjusted to a high CO_2 level and rely on the chemoreceptor reflex to maintain respiration.

Administration of high levels of oxygen may depress the "hypoxic drive," resulting in a lowered respiratory rate, apnea, and increased hypoxia. Therefore, animals with chronic hypoxia should be observed closely for respiratory depression when oxygen therapy is administered.

OXYGEN TOXICITY

Toxicity problems are not encountered with short-term, low concentration therapy. Convulsions and atelectasis from nitrogen washout of obstructed areas of lung may be found as special complications of prolonged high concentration therapy. Avoid concentrations above 50 per cent. Pulmonary irritation (pulmonary congestion, exudation, and edema) occurs after continuous exposure to 80 to 100 per cent concentrations of oxygen. It will also produce retrolental fibroplasia in young animals, but 40 per cent oxygen appears to be safe. Elevated levels of CO_2 may also be toxic and should be avoided, especially in oxygen tent use.

NEBULIZATION THERAPY

Inhalation therapy is most useful to humidify air in the respiratory tract and to moisten the mucous membranes. Drying causes irritation—which in turn causes swelling, bronchial gland hypertrophy, goblet cell proliferation, and loss of ciliary epithelium. Respiratory secretions become thick and tenacious, and efficient bronchial drainage is impaired.

The aims of aerosol therapy are:
1. Humidification of bronchial mucous membranes.
2. Deposition of minuscule amounts of potent drugs in smaller airways to obtain optimal topical therapeutic effects with minimal systemic side effects (e.g., bronchodilators).
3. Deposition of moderate amounts of potent agents, or agents that are only effective topically (e.g., antibiotics and mucolytics).
4. Deposition of relatively large quantities of bland substances that promote bronchial drainage with minimal irritation (e.g., saline, propylene glycol, glycerine, detergents).

The indications for nebulization therapy are: (1) in combination with oxygen therapy; (2) in tracheostomy care; (3) in acute respiratory diseases: tracheobronchitis, bronchiolitis, upper respiratory disease of cats, pneumonia, and postoperative atelectasis and pneumonia; and (4) in chronic respiratory diseases: chronic bronchitis, bronchopneumonia, collapsed trachea with secondary tracheobronchitis, emphysema, and bronchiectasis.

Principles of Action

Large water particles (10–60μ) in the high velocity air flow of the nose and throat settle on the mucosa of the larynx, nose, and throat. Particles smaller than 10μ (2–10μ) are deposited in the bronchi, but only the smallest reach the bronchioles. Ultrasonic aerosol generators are the most effective machines for nebulization. Their mists can be directed into a cage or a face mask. If nebulization is used with an endotracheal or tracheostomy tube, inspired gases should be warmed to body temperature.

Dense mist from an unheated jet-nebulizer contains only slightly more water than is needed to humidify air with temperature increasing from 22° to 37° C. The evaporation of the aerosol solution can be prevented by stabilization, that is, by heating it to 53° C or by reducing the vapor pressure by adding 10 per cent propylene glycol. Because distilled water and hypertonic solutions are irritating to the mucosa, only isotonic or half-strength isotonic saline should be used.

Although continuous, low-level humidification of the oxygen tent atmosphere is necessary, periodic medication by aerosol spray is permissible. High levels of water can be introduced several times daily for 10 to 15 minutes per treatment, or drugs can be added to the solution during these times. Many drugs have been used; isoproterenol, epinephrine, and phenylephrine are some of the drugs that may cause bronchodilatation and decreased airway resistance.

It is important to differentiate obstruction of the bronchi due to pulmonary edema from that due to bronchial secretions. In both cases, the patient cannot ventilate because of fluids or semifluid liquids in the bronchi. In pulmonary edema, the fluid turns to a frothy, bubbly material that produces a "rattling" in the throat. Patients suffering from pulmonary edema should be treated with antifoaming substances such as 12 per cent alcohol in water, given by nebulization. If used to treat tenacious exudates, these agents increase viscosity and, thus, the obstruction.

Thick, inflammatory exudates, on the other hand, need to be thinned by detergent materials that liquefy bronchial secretions. However, these agents increase frothing and, indirectly, anoxia if used in pulmonary edema.

In pulmonary edema, antifoaming agents (12 per cent alcohol) should be used. In bronchial exudates (thick), detergents (liquefying agents such as acetylcysteine) should be used.

Heated aerosol units (vaporizers) produce water droplets of large particle size, which do not penetrate small bronchioles and may overheat the patient. They should not be used for intensive therapy.

Drugs that can be applied by nebulizer include:
1. Bronchodilators—always use when administering drugs that may be irritating and constricting.
   a. Bronkosol (Isoetharine HCl 1 per cent, and phenylephrine 0.25 per cent)— 0.5 to 1.0 ml in 2 to 3 ml of saline TID.
2. Antibiotics—poorly absorbed from the respiratory mucosa.
   a. Kanamycin—250 mg in 5 ml saline BID.
   b. Gentamicin—50 mg in 5 ml saline BID.
   c. Polymixin B—333,000 IU in 5 ml saline BID.
3. Bland solutions—use in large volume for prolonged mist effect.
   a. Saline—5 to 200 ml as needed.
   b. Glycerine—5 per cent in saline.

c. Detergents (see below).

d. Propylene glycol—10 to 20 per cent solution in saline.

4. Detergents and mucolytics.

a. Acetylcysteine (Mucomyst)—5 to 10 per cent solution in saline, 2 to 10 ml TID; in cage use 100 to 200 ml as needed.

5. Antifoaming agents.

a. Ethyl alcohol—70 per cent solution, 5 to 10 ml BID.

References and Additional Readings

Bolton, G. R.: Aerosol therapy. *In* Kirk, R. W. (ed.): Current Veterinary Therapy VI. Philadelphia, W. B. Saunders Company, 1977, pp. 12–15.

Haskins, S. C.: Management of pulmonary disease in the critical patient. *In* Zaslow, I. M. (ed.): Veterinary Trauma and Critical Care. Philadelphia, Lea & Febiger, 1984, pp. 339–384.

Shoemaker, W. C., Thompson, W. L., and Holbrook, P. R.: The Society of Critical Care Medicine: Textbook of Critical Care. Philadelphia, W. B. Saunders Company, 1984.

PHYSICAL THERAPY

Most physiotherapeutic modalities have a stimulating effect and their action is directed toward the musculoskeletal system or the skin.

Hydrotherapy

Water baths or soaks are one of the easiest and most versatile ways of using physical therapy in small animal practice. Wet packs, water soaks, or whirlpool baths can be helpful in adding moisture (hydrating) or removing moisture (dehydrating) from the skin. Cyclical repetitions of moisture and drying applied to the skin many times a day serve to dehydrate (this is similar to the chapped lip and hand syndrome seen in people). Constant moisture hydrates and even macerates the skin.

Whirlpool baths are the most efficient and popular way to apply the benefits of hydrotherapy and, often, antiseptic medication to the skin. They combine moist heat, gentle massage, and the solvency properties of water with or without the mechanical impact of water from a whirlpool, to remove dirt, pus, and necrotic debris. Dry or scaly skin will be softened and moisturized. Whirlpools may increase edema and are contraindicated in acute traumatic and inflammatory conditions or in cases of impaired sensation or circulation (unless treated with extreme caution). Whirlpools are particularly beneficial for skin infections, chronic dryness, open or infected wounds, skin grafts, adhesions, arthritis, postsurgical fractures, amputations, muscle spasms, and stiff joints. This modality is especially useful to clean and stimulate the skin of patients who are predisposed to decubital ulcers.

The patient should be placed in an appropriate water bath at a temperature of 39° to 42° C (102° to 108° F). A low-sudsing detergent or antiseptic solution (Betadine, chlorine, chlorhexidine) can be added for cleansing and germicidal effects. Allow the water turbine to circulate the water around and against the affected parts for 10 to 15 minutes once or twice daily. Support and reassure the animal during treatment, and never leave an animal unattended. Following therapy, ensure that the tub and turbine are thoroughly cleaned and sanitized.

Commercial whirlpool baths or Jaccuzi type agitators are a good investment for a busy practice. A less expensive alternative is a variable temperature bath with agitation provided by a pressure hose.

Heat

Effects

The effects of heat in physical therapy include the following:
1. Hyperemia and dilation of cutaneous vessels.
2. Increase in pulse, blood pressure, and pulmonary ventilation.
3. Increased metabolite transfer across capillary membranes.
4. General muscle relaxation.
5. Sedative and analgesic effect.
6. Improved extensibility of connective tissue.

In the presence of trauma, swelling, and edema, circulation may be impeded and the application of heat may cause necrosis. Cold is more beneficial in the early acute stages of inflammation and edema.

SUPERFICIAL HEAT

Infrared radiation is produced by long-wave generators that glow red and produce heat that penetrates only 1 to 2 mm. Short-wave generators produce visible light, and heat penetrates 10 to 12 mm, so it reaches blood-carrying layers of tissue, where the heat is dispersed by the circulation. Because of this, short waves do not produce a burning sensation; however, one should meticulously check the skin during therapy to ensure that it is not overheated. Warm sensation is normal. If the skin feels hot to the touch, the heat is too intense. This therapy is contraindicated for acute trauma and inflammation. It is beneficial for subacute and chronic problems, skin infections, and abscesses. Treat for 15 to 20 minutes once or twice daily.

Hot packs or wet towels can be used to apply mild, gentle heat. They have the same indications as infrared heat, but there should be additional precautions. Hot packs may spread contagious skin disease, and the weight of the packs, in an insensitive area, is more likely to cause burns or tissue damage. This modality has the advantage of providing moist heat, which is particularly beneficial for chronic soft-tissue problems such as arthritis, myositis, and contractures. Hot packs should be applied for 10 to 15 minutes several times each day. Check the skin under the packs frequently during therapy.

Whirlpool baths combine moist heat, gentle massage, and the solvency properties of water to remove dirt, pus, and necrotic debris. The moist heat aspects are especially indicated for extensive involvement of musculoskeletal disorders. Warm water baths can be repeated two to three times daily for 10 to 15 minutes. They can often be followed with a gentle massage and passive flexion and extension exercises to improve range-of-motion and soft-tissue flexibility.

DEEP HEAT

Shortwave diathermy transmits physical energy deep into tissues, and because the body tissues resist the flow of high frequency current (27 million cps), heat is produced. In dissipating heat, there is marked vascular dilation, sedation, analgesia, and relief of muscle spasm. However, edema may increase. Absolute contraindications are use in the presence of metal, ischemia, malignancy, or pregnancy. No water can be in the field, and splints and bandages must be removed. This therapy has potential shock danger to both the patient and the technician, so all cables, electrodes, and other equipment must be in excellent condition. Safety cannot be overemphasized. Each unit should be calibrated and adjusted individually to produce only a sensation of warmth. Daily treatment is applied for 15 to 20 minutes.

Microwave techniques produce about the same effects as diathermy except that more localized heating occurs (so only one side of a joint may be treated at a time). Microwaves are more readily absorbed by water, so great care must be used around the eye or in the presence of edema to ensure that the effects are not excessive.

Ultrasound produces the deepest heat. It produces mechanical vibrations (one million/sec.) in the elastic media of the body. Ultrasonic waves are reflected from boundaries between different types of tissues. The vibrations produce a micromassage that accelerates fluid absorption by increasing permeability. Ultrasonic therapy can be dangerous if the intensity or application is concentrated too long in a small area. Burn or tissue destruction may result. It is contraindicated over neoplasms, the eye, heart, spine, and brain; near growing bony epiphyses; and in acute infections. Otherwise, its beneficial effects are similar to other forms of deep heat. It is particularly indicated in softening scar tissue and in reducing the pain of neuromas and degenerative joint disease. It can be used over and around metal implants.

Ultrasound therapy is applied via a transducer using coupling media such as water or contact gels. The transducer is moved constantly over a small area (usually 6 to 8 inches square, depending on the size of the transducer). It is best to shave the skin before therapy to enhance contact (or use a water bath).

Dosage varies with each patient. Most ultrasonic generators have an output of 700,000 to 1,000,000 cps at intensities of 0.1 to 1.0 watt per sq cm. It is best to use the lowest intensity possible. The maximum dosage should be 1.0 watt per sq cm for 5 minutes of application to the affected tissues. This can be repeated once daily for 5 days, then every other day for 5 treatments. Then, it should not be repeated for at least 1 month. Do not use in acute injuries, inflammations, or infections.

For cervical intervertebral disease, use 0.3 watts per sq cm for 3 minutes daily for 5 days; then every other day for 5 treatments.

For arthritis, bursitis, and myositis, use 0.2 watts per sq cm for 3 minutes for joints of the extremities. Repeat two times weekly.

Cold

Cold can be applied by blowing cold air on the skin, by evaporation of volatile liquids from the skin, or by direct contact of the cooling substance with the skin surface.

Effects

The effects of cold in physical therapy include:
1. Decreased tissue temperature.
2. Decreased blood flow, vasoconstriction.
3. Decreased tendency to edema.
4. Decreased delivery of nutrients, phagocytes.
5. Decreased phagocytic action.
6. Brief cold applications produce transient vasoconstriction followed by vasodilation and increased blood flow.

Cold reduces extravasation of blood and fluid into tissues after trauma. It reduces pain and spasticity and is indicated in acute traumatic and inflammatory conditions.

Overtreatment with cold may produce maceration and frostbite. Prolonged cold produces a vascular response with stasis of blood, occlusion of vessels, and tissue anoxia and necrosis.

Cold packs over a damp towel applied to the affected area and covered with a folded dry towel to prevent rapid warming can be used for 15 to 20 minutes. Treatment is repeated several times daily. It is important to keep the rest of the patient's body warm, dry, and comfortable during treatment. Cold treatments are often more effective when alternated with heat treatments (immersion bath or moist warm packs). This is most effective when heat is applied for 3 to 4 minutes, alternated with 1 to 2 minutes of cold. This can be repeated for 15 to 20 minutes and should always end with the hot phase.

Cold immersion baths for one or several extremities may be useful. The temperature should be 15.5° to 21° C (60° to 70° F) and can be decreased by adding ice or cold water. Continue treatment until the muscles are relaxed or the animal cannot tolerate the cold, usually 2 to 5 minutes. Modification of this technique can be used for heat stroke, but one must be careful not to overchill such patients.

Electricity

Medical galvanism is the physiologic use of direct current. It will produce the same effects as heat except that it has no tendency to produce edema. It is beneficial for acute, subacute, or chronic traumatic and inflammatory problems, that is, arthritis, decubiti, neuralgia, tenosynovitis, or postfracture repair. It should not be used near the brain, heart, or neoplasms.

Low intensity therapy (0.5–1.0 milliampere of intensity/sq in. of electrode) is desirable. Electrodes should be wet and held in firm contact with the skin. No metal should be in or near the area being treated. Halfway through the treatment, the intensity of current should be reduced to zero, the polarity reversed, and the intensity returned to starting levels.

Electrical stimulation of partially or wholly innervated muscle is possible with alternating current. Intact *or* denervated muscle will contract when stimulated with interrupted pulses of direct current. These kinds of stimulation improve circulation and nutrition of the muscle, help venous return, remove lymph, relax spasm, reduce edema, and assist in muscle re-education. Muscle atrophy and weakness can be retarded or controlled. Each muscle or group can be stimulated 10 to 20 times for one procedure, depending on the condition. Avoid overtreatment. See Downer (1978) for specific details of therapy.

Massage

Massage is the use of the hands and fingers to manipulate soft tissues. It is usually used in combination with heat, cold, or whirlpool treatments. Massage improves circulation, reduces edema, loosens and stretches fibrotic or contracted tissue, and has a soothing or sedative effect.

Massage should not be used in acute, inflammatory, traumatic, and painful lesions or with tumors, hemorrhages, and possibly contagious conditions. It is indicated for tight or contracted tendons, ligaments, or muscles, chronic traumatic or inflammatory problems, and subacute or chronic edema.

In performing massage, keep the strokes in the direction of venous flow. Firm, rapid pressure tends to be stimulating, whereas slow, light strokes are soothing. Some type of lubricating powder or oil can be used to reduce friction. The massage can be stroking, kneading, or applied with friction. Stroking and kneading assist circulation, whereas friction and kneading tend to loosen adhesions and scars and to stretch tissues. Massage should last 15 to 20 minutes and can be repeated several times daily if desired.

Exercise

Therapeutic exercise should strengthen musculoskeletal function, improve range-of-motion flexibility, improve endurance or coordination, and increase cardiovascular and respiratory capabilities. It should never be forced, but kept within safe tolerance of the patient's cardiac and respiratory capacity. Active exercise (such as walking, running, or swimming) is most desirable, because endurance and strength increase with repetition. Passive exercise is useful when paralysis or traumatic injuries preclude active exercise. Movements should never be forced, but stabilization of parts and controlled pressure should be used to activate only those structures of concern. When attempting to increase range of motion, use smooth, controlled pressure to move the joint slightly beyond its limited range; hold the stretch for a count of 5; and slowly release the traction. Several repetitions can be performed 2 or 3 times daily. Gradual improvement can be expected within several weeks.

References and Additional Readings

Downer, A. H.: Physical Therapy for Animals. Springfield, Illinois, Charles C Thomas, Publisher, 1978.

Krusen, F. H.: Handbook of Physical Medicine and Rehabilitation. Philadelphia, W. B. Saunders Company, 1971.

Purdy, S. R.: Senior Seminar, Cornell University, 1981.

Schirmer, R. G.: Ultrasound therapy. In Kirk, R. W. (ed.): Current Veterinary Therapy III. Philadelphia, W. B. Saunders Company, 1968.

SECTION 5

Interpretation of Laboratory Tests

In this section, the interpretation of results of laboratory tests that vary from normal are discussed. This section provides information about the possible causes of these variations and touches on points of differential diagnosis. However, the discussion is *not* a complete evaluation of the differential merit of each test.

The information discussed here is not intended to give specific directions for performing laboratory tests. For this, the reader should consult standard texts on clinical pathology.

CEREBROSPINAL FLUID

Analysis of cerebrospinal fluid (CSF) is a valuable aid in establishing a diagnosis in neurologic disease. Changes in CSF mainly depend on the location and extent of the lesion.

CSF in the dog and cat is collected by puncture of the cerebellomedullary cistern (see p. 496). After the needle has entered the subarachnoid space, a pressure recording manometer should be attached immediately, and the opening and closing pressures should be recorded. When the pressure has been recorded, slowly remove 2 ml of CSF for further examination. Record the closing CSF manometric pressure. Normal cerebellomedullary fluid pressure does not usually exceed 170 mm. Closing CSF pressure is not usually less than one half of opening pressure. If closing pressure is markedly reduced, this may indicate a decreased CSF volume from subarachnoid space and a possible space-occupying lesion. Elevated CSF pressure may be associated with space-occupying central nervous system (CNS) lesions such as tumor formation, hemorrhage, abscess, cerebral edema, communicating hydrocephalus, and meningitis.

GROSS APPEARANCE

Color

Normal CSF is clear and colorless. A pinkish or reddish color usually indicates hemorrhage, which may be caused by the spinal tap itself or may be due to CNS disease. The supernatant will be clear following centrifugation if the hemorrhage was caused by the tapping procedure. A yellow, or xanthochromic, color of the spinal fluid indicates previous hemorrhage from injury or cerebrovascular accident or progressive brain disease (such as inflammation or neoplasia). Mild CSF contamination with blood will not alter white blood cell (WBC) or protein determinations. Leukocytosis of 10,000 per cm in the CSF indicates gross blood contamination, and the tap should be repeated. In some cases of previous hemorrhage, centrifuging the CSF will reveal the supernatant to be yellow and the sediment to be red or brown. In other cases, a clot forms, resulting in few loose cells. A gray or green color may indicate suppuration.

Turbidity

A cloudy CSF usually indicates the presence of a high cell count (pleocytosis). Neutrophils are found in bacterial meningitis, bacterial encephalitis, abscess, and hemorrhage. Increased numbers of mononuclear cells are found in the CSF in viral encephalitis, fungal infections, postvaccinal reactions, uremia, and chronic and toxic conditions.

Cytologic examination should be done within 30 minutes after obtaining the sample; otherwise, cell disintegration will take place. The normal cell count is under 5 per µl.

Coagulation

Normal CSF does not coagulate. Increased fibrinogen, found in inflammation such as acute suppurative meningitis, produces coagulation.

PROTEIN

The main protein in normal CSF is albumin. Increases in the total protein in disease usually reflect increases in the globulin levels. If blood is present within the CSF, the globulin levels will also be high. Protein examination may be qualitative or quantitative. The Pandy test used for qualitative determination of proteins measures only globulins. Quantitative protein determinations are more critical, measuring lower levels of protein, including both albumins and globulins.

BACTERIOLOGIC EXAMINATION

If the CSF is turbid, it should be cultured and a Gram or new methylene blue (NMB) stain should be made. Gram and NMB will also show cryptococci. NMB will also show the capsule. Culture the CSF on blood agar, in thioglycollate medium, or in Sabouraud's medium, depending on the findings in the direct smear. If the fluid is not turbid, centrifuge it before staining and culturing the sediment. India ink can be used to see the capsule of the cryptococcal organisms in a smear. Small amounts of proteins, mainly albumins, are present in the CSF fluid (up to 15–25 mg/100 ml). CSF protein levels above 25 to 30 mg per 100 ml are considered abnormal.

CREATININE KINASE

Creatinine kinase (CK) elevations in serum (see p. 743) usually indicate muscle disease, and when elevated in the CSF, CK is usually independent of its serum concentration. Elevated CK in CSF is of little value in differential diagnosis; however, it may indicate a guarded to poor prognosis.

References and Additional Readings

de Lahunta, A.: Veterinary Neuroanatomy and Clinical Neurology, 2nd ed. Philadelphia, W. B. Saunders Company, 1983.
Oliver, J. E., and Lorenz, M. D.: Handbook of Veterinary Neurologic Diagnosis. Philadelphia, W. B. Saunders Company, 1983, Chap. 8, pp. 106–110.

ENDOCRINE FUNCTION

Disturbances in the secretion of some hormones may be recognized clinically if careful attention is given to the history and physical examination. Particular attention should be paid to the rate of growth and physical development; subsequent changes in body weight and conformation and distribution of body fat; sexual development and reproductive performance; changes in physical activity and stamina; the condition of the skin and hair; and the occurrence of polyphagia, polydipsia, or polyuria.

Adrenal Cortex

Cortisol, corticosterone, and aldosterone—the principal hormones secreted by the adrenal cortex—regulate carbohydrate and electrolyte metabolism. Cortisol is the main glucocorticosteroid produced by the adrenal cortex, and its rate of secretion is controlled primarily by adrenocorticotropin (ACTH) from the adenohypophysis. Aldosterone is the main mineralocorticoid, and corticosterone has both mineralo- and glucocorticosteroid functions. The prime regulator in controlling aldosterone release is the renin-angiotensin system, which is dependent on variations in fluid volume. Aldosterone stimulates sodium and chloride reabsorption, increases the excretion of potassium, and increases the retention of water, thus expanding the vascular compartments.

The Effect of Mineralocorticoids

The mineralocorticoids increase resorption of sodium and chloride, increase the excretion of potassium, and allow an exchange of intracellular potassium with extracellular sodium.

The Effect of Glucocorticosteroids (Cortisol)

Glucocorticosteroids increase protein catabolism, resulting in an increased breakdown of muscle protein, interference with the normal production of bone matrix, and increased gluconeogenesis from amino acids. Antibody formation initially increases, but later decreases because of the lysis of lymphocytes and lymph nodes. Glucocorticosteroids tend to conserve energy derived from circulating glucose by (1) inhibiting glucose utilization in peripheral tissues, (2) mobilizing fatty acids for energy production, and (3) increasing the flow of amino acids to liver for new glucose production. Glomerular filtration is increased, and an "anti-ADH" effect results in diuresis. Electrolyte effects are evidenced by retention of small amounts of sodium and excretion of potassium. Arteriolar tone and blood pressure are maintained. Inflammatory reactions are reduced because of a decrease in fibroplasia as well as a decrease in the production of histamine and histamine-like substances (serotonin).

EVALUATION OF ADRENOCORTICAL FUNCTION

Clinical Syndromes

Canine hyperadrenocorticism can occur spontaneously from excessive administration of glucocorticoids or from two forms of spontaneous hyperadrenocorticism: pituitary-dependent and cortisol-producing adrenocortical tumor.

Clinical signs of hypercorticism (Cushing's disease) are associated with the long-term effects of excessive glucocorticosteroids; polydypsia and polyuria; polyphagia; pendulous abdomen associated with loss of abdominal muscle tone and hepatomegaly; muscle weakness; alopecia due to atrophy of the hair follicles, skin, and sebaceous glands; accumulation of keratin plugs within hair follicles, resulting in comedones; thin skin and hyperpigmentation; ectopic calcification, which may accumulate in the skin (calcinosis cutis); testicular atrophy in the male or clitoral hypertrophy and anestrus in the female; poor wound healing; and decreased exercise tolerance. Muscle atrophy and gait abnormalities can also be associated with long-term elevated glucocorticosteroid levels. Additional systemic problems that can be associated with hyperadrenocorticism are urinary tract infection, corneal ulceration, acute pancreatitis, pulmonary calcification, diabetes mellitus, and salmonellosis.

Approximately 80 per cent of hyperadrenocorticism cases are associated with adrenocortical hyperplasia. Adrenocortical hyperplasia secondary to a functional ACTH-producing pituitary tumor occurs in many animals. These tumors are usually chromophobe adenomas and appear small, not producing neurologic signs. Adrenocortical neoplasms may constitute about 5 per cent of hyperadrenocorticism cases.

Laboratory Tests

The total leukocyte, differential, hematocrit, and total eosinophil counts should be evaluated. Serum sodium, potassium, chloride, urea, and protein determinations may also be valuable.

The following laboratory tests are helpful in confirming the diagnosis of hyperadrenocorticism: a complete blood count (CBC) that exhibits a stress pattern, including leukocytosis, neutrophilia, lymphopenia, eosinopenia, and monocytosis; slight elevation of SGPT value; elevated alkaline phosphatase, associated with an induction of the steroid liver isoenzyme of alkaline phosphatase by glucocorticosteroid excess; mild to moderate elevations in serum cholesterol; and a slight to moderate elevation in fasting blood glucose, associated with increased hepatic gluconeogenesis. Urine specific gravity is low in polyuria-polydypsia cases; resting thyroid hormone levels are low; and systolic and diastolic blood pressures are elevated. Urinalysis often reveals proteinuria and evidence of cystitis.

Analysis of Hypothalamic–Pituitary–Adrenocortical Axis
(Fig. 92)

Dexamethasone Suppression Test

The dexamethasone-ACTH test is indicated in cases in which there is need to distinguish between adrenal hyperplasia, pituitary-dependent adrenal hyperplasia, and adrenal neoplasia.

In normal dogs, dexamethasone acts to suppress plasma cortisol concentration essentially to 0 and to maintain suppression for several hours. In dogs with pituitary-dependent Cushing's disease, there is decreased sensitivity to the suppression; thus, a larger dose of dexamethasone is required.

The low-dose dexamethasone screening test should be run first. The high-dose dexamethasone suppression test can be begun 48 hours later. For the screening test, inject dexamethasone (Oradexon; Organon Laboratories) intravenously (IV) 0.01 mg per kg at start and collect baseline, 3-hour, and 8-hour samples. Collect blood in heparin; centrifuge; remove plasma, and freeze.

In normal dogs, plasma cortisol is reduced below 1.5 μg per 100 ml within 3 hours and remains suppressed for 8 hours or more. In most dogs with pituitary-dependent Cushing's disease, there is a slight decrease at the 3-hour point, but by 8 hours there is no suppression. No cortisol suppression occurs in the majority of dogs with adrenal tumors and in 25 per cent of those with pituitary-dependent hyperadrenocorticism (Peterson). An intramuscular (IM) low-dose dexamethasone test can also be run using 15 μg per kg of dexamethasone and collecting plasma at 2, 4, 6, and 8 hours postinjection. *The low-dose dexamethasone test can confirm Cushing's disease but cannot reliably differentiate between pituitary-dependent and adrenal tumors.*

A high-dose dexamethasone suppression test can be used in some cases to differentiate between the presence of pituitary-dependent Cushing's disease and autonomous adrenal tumor. Inject dexamethasone IV, 1.0 mg per kg, and collect a prior baseline and a later response sample at 8 hours postinjection.

In using 1.0 mg of dexamethasone per kg of body weight, complete suppression is defined as plasma cortisol values (1) less than 50 per cent of the baseline or (2) less than 1.5 μg per dl, according to Peterson (using his RIA technique). Dogs with pituitary-dependent hyperadrenocorticism (90 per cent) often will fulfill this suppression criteria, whereas dogs with adrenocortical tumors may not suppress.

New radioimmunoassay tests for endogenous ACTH production can be used to screen dogs for Cushing's disease and to distinguish pituitary-dependent from adrenocortical tumor hyperadrenocorticism. In normal dogs, the resting ACTH levels on early morning samples have been determined at 46.0 ± 16.85 pg per ml with a range of 20 to 100 pg per ml. In dogs with pituitary-dependent

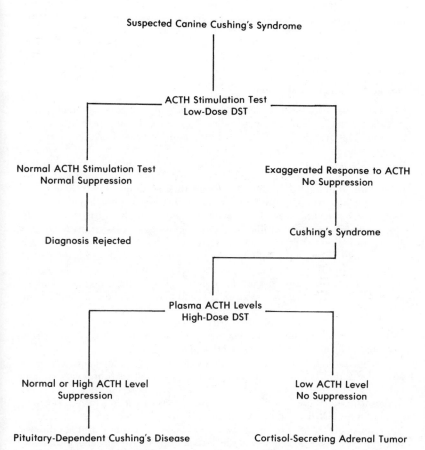

Figure 92. Flowchart for evaluation of suspected canine Cushing's synrome (DST = Dexamethasone suppression test). From Peterson, Mark. Hyperadrenocorticism; *In* Symposium on Endocrinology, Vet. Clinics North America, Vol. 14, No. 4, July 1984, p. 742.

functional hyperplasia, ACTH levels are usually greater than 40 pg per ml, with means reported as 98 ± 48.6 pg per ml and 132 pg per ml ± 68, with ranges from 29 to 340 pg per ml. In dogs with adrenocortical tumors, ACTH concentrations were usually less than 20 pg per ml, with averages being 16 pg per ml ± 2.0 (range 16–36). This form of testing coupled with dexamethasone suppression testing is extremely helpful in evaluating the pituitary-adrenal axis in hyperadrenocorticism. Blood for ACTH assay should be drawn in cold, heparinized, plastic syringes; iced; and spun immediately in plastic tubes in a refrigerated centrifuge. Plasma should then be separated into plastic tubes and kept frozen until assayed.

Plasma Cortisol Determinations

Plasma cortisol levels can be valuable diagnostic aids in hyperadrenocorticism. Plasma cortisol levels can be determined by competitive protein-binding, fluorometric techniques, and radioimmunoassay. Cortisol values may differ significantly from laboratory to laboratory. The radioimmunoassay test is the most sensitive test. In the evaluation of plasma cortisol levels, blood is taken pre- and postadministration of synthetic ACTH (Cortrosyn). This test can be performed immediately after the dexamethasone suppression test. An early morning venous sample, 3 to 5 ml, is obtained in heparin; the blood sample is centrifuged; and the plasma is removed. Plasma should be separated from the blood cellular elements within 15 to 30 minutes. The plasma must be kept frozen until the test is run; otherwise, cortisol levels will decrease greatly. Cortrosyn (0.25 mg in 1 ml of saline solution) is administered IM. At 60 minutes post-ACTH injection, the second venous sample is removed.

ACTH gel can also be used to evaluate adrenocortical function, and 2.2 IU of ACTH gel per kg can be given IM, and plasma can be collected 2 hours later.

The normal levels of plasma cortisol measured by radioimmunoassay are variable, depending on which laboratory performs the test. It is recommended that normal levels be established for the laboratory used.

Single plasma cortisol determinations cannot be used to adequately access adrenal function because of normal variation in blood cortisol levels. Testing cortisol levels and response with ACTH is much more effective. In hyperadrenocorticism, there is a hyper-response of plasma cortisol to ACTH stimulation. In normal dogs, post-ACTH cortisol concentrations are at least two to three times higher than basal levels. In pituitary-dependent Cushing's disease, post-ACTH cortisol is higher than the normal response (usually above 15 μg/dl). In dogs with adrenocortical tumors, there is a variability in response to ACTH, with some dogs having normal (two to three times cortisol increases) and other dogs having exaggerated increases. Dogs with carcinoma of the adrenal gland may show an especially elevated cortisol response. Dogs with adrenocortical tumors (approximately 25 per cent of these cases) may show a below normal response to ACTH stimulation; however, 75 to 80 per cent of dogs with adrenocortical tumors *do not* show at least 50 per cent suppression of baseline cortisol levels when evaluated with dexamethasone, 0.1 mg per kg.

A subnormal response to ACTH and a greater than 50 per cent suppression of plasma cortisol by high-dose dexamethasone indicate a diagnosis of iatrogenic hyperadrenocorticism.

The ACTH test is valuable as a screening test for Cushing's disease. However, if the test is normal, Cushing's disease cannot be ruled out, because dogs with adrenal tumors can respond normally to ACTH. The test alone cannot reliably distinguish between pituitary-dependent and adrenal tumor causes of Cushing's disease.

Normal Cortisol Levels for Cats

Controls—cortisols, 4.2 to 19 μg per dl

Normals—ACTH response, 8.5 to 20 μg per dl

Megestrol acetate administered to cats causes significant depression of cortisol, and ACTH-stimulated cortisol response is still abnormal for at least 1 or 2 weeks after discontinuance of megestrol.

Hypoadrenocorticism (Addison's disease) is the result of primary adrenocortical failure. The disease is more common in female than male dogs. Lack of aldosterone leads to inability to conserve sodium and excrete potassium. Loss of sodium leads to a decrease in extracellular fluid volume, weight loss, decreased blood pressure, decreased cardiac output, azotemia, generalized weakness, and depression. Hyperkalemia and mild acidosis also develop. Hyperkalemia causes decreased excitability of cardiac muscle, increase in the refractory period of the myocardium, and slowing of conduction. Anorexia, vomiting, abdominal pain, lethargy, and decreased tolerance to stress are seen. Major presenting clinical signs are depression, weakness, slow pulse, dehydration, and occasionally shocklike signs (p. 147).

The following laboratory tests are helpful in confirming the diagnosis of hypoadrenocorticism: elevated BUN associated with prerenal azotemia from reduced renal perfusion and decreased glomerular filtration rate, and electrolyte changes consisting of hyponatremia, hypochloremia, and hyperkalemia. Normal sodium:potassium ratio is 27:1 to 32:1. Hypoadrenocorticism results in alterations to 20:1 or below. Hypoadrenocorticism is associated with hyperkalemia, hyponatremia, hypochloremia, and hypercalcemia in 25 to 30 per cent of the cases.

Normal serum sodium and potassium levels cannot rule out the possibility of hypoadrenocorticism in all cases. Diagnosis of hypoadrenocorticism should be based on lack of response to ACTH. Clinical signs include lethargy, weakness, anorexia, vomiting, weight loss, *pre-renal azotemia* (urine specific gravity of 1.042), *eosinophilia, microcardia, hypoglycemia, and anemia.*

The Electrocardiogram

In hyperadrenocorticism with hypokalemia, the Q-T interval is prolonged and U waves may be seen. Sinus bradycardia and sinus arrest may be seen.

In hypoadrenocorticism with hyperkalemia (serum potassium between 6 and 7 mEq/L), the T waves may become increased in amplitude, spiked, and narrow based. Serum potassium levels of 7 and 8 mEq per L produce a depression of the P wave. Serum potassium levels above 8 mEq per L produce bradycardia (50–70 beats/min), absence of P waves, and a widened QRS wave. Concentrations of potassium in the range of 11 to 14 mEq per L lead to ventricular asystole or ventricular fibrillation.

Growth Hormone (Somatotropin)

Growth hormone (GH) is a polypeptide hormone secreted by the anterior pituitary gland. It stimulates cell growth and mitosis and results in increased cell size and increased numbers of cells. The ability to reach normal body size is dependent on GH. Absence of effective levels of GH results in retarded growth called *dwarfism*. Overproduction of GH can result in acromegaly.

GH is affected by many physiologic factors believed to be mediated by factors produced by the hypothalamus. The release of GH from the anterior pituitary is mediated by a hypothalamic growth hormone releasing factor (GHRF). A GH inhibiting factor, somatostatin, has been located in the median eminence of the hypothalamus and can block GH release.

Growth Hormone Excess in Dogs (Acromegaly)

Eigenmann has described acromegaly in dogs associated with elevated levels of GH resulting from the treatment of dogs with progestational compounds or, in older dogs, occurring spontaneously during the corpus luteum phase (progestational phase) of the ovarian cycle.

Using radioimmunoassay of GH, Eigenmann has established normal GH levels for the dog to be 10 ng per ml or less.

Evidence of excessive GH production is characterized by: (1) inspiratory stridor caused by increased soft tissue around the neck and increased soft-tissue density around the abdomen; (2) reduced exercise tolerance; (3) poly-uria–polydypsia (PU–PD); and (4) enlargement of interdental space.

The condition is controlled by ovariohysterectomy, thus reducing the GH levels into the normal range. (See p. 667 for the influence of GH on diabetes.)

Growth Hormone Deficiency (Dwarfism)

Endocrine dwarfism occurs most frequently in the German shepherd breed of dogs, where it is believed to be inherited as an autosomal recessive trait. The condition in German shepherds is associated with abnormal development of Rathke's pouch and produces partial or total pituitary insufficiency. See the review article by Eigenmann for the clonidine stimulation test to release GH and for the treatment regimen.

The Posterior Pituitary

Antidiuretic hormone (ADH), or vasopressin, and the oxytocic hormone involved in parturition are both produced in the hypothalamus and released from the pars nervosa of the pituitary.

THE EFFECT OF ANTIDIURETIC HORMONE

Arginine vasopressin is formed in the supraoptic and paraventricular nuclei of the hypothalamus and stored in the posterior lobe of the pituitary. Under normal conditions, the major physiologic controls governing vasopressin release are plasma osmolarity and changes in blood volume. The major physiologic effect of ADH is to increase the permeability of the distal tubules to the kidneys to water.

DIABETES INSIPIDUS (See Polydypsia-Polyuria, p. 236)

Diabetes insipidus is a syndrome of excessive excretion of water due to insufficient production or release of ADH. In affected animals, urine volume is increased from 3 to 10 times the normal amount per day; urine specific gravity ranges in value from 1.001 to 1.005; and urine osmolarity ranges from 50 to 200 mOsm per kg.

There are two prerequisites to a diagnosis of diabetes insipidus: (1) persistent diuresis in the presence of stimuli that normally provoke the secretion of ADH, and (2) antidiuresis in response to administered ADH.

The release of ADH and its effect on the urine should be measured by urine and plasma osmolality rather than by specific gravity. (Osmolality is a measurement of the number of particles in a given weight of fluid and is proportional to the osmotic pressure of that fluid. Osmolality is measured by freezing point depression in an osmometer. See p. 815.)

Tests for Diabetes Insipidus (See also Differential Diagnosis Polyuria-Polydypsia, p. 236)

Vasopressin Response Tests

Aqueous ADH Test

1. Place the indwelling catheter in the vein; flush with heparinized saline.
2. Empty the bladder of residual urine.
3. Make a fresh solution of aqueous ADH (pitressin) in 5 per cent dextrose and water (DSW).
4. Administer ADH IV, 5mU per lb over a 60-minute period. (An addition of 5 units of aqueous vasopressin in 1 L of D5W produces a vasopressin concentration of 5mU per ml; thus, 1 ml per lb administered over a 60-minute period.)
5. Collect urine at 30, 60, and 90 minutes following vasopressin infusion.
6. Response in dogs with diabetes insipidus may not be as great as in normal dogs, and specific gravity may reach only 1.012 or higher, but this is diagnostic for insipidus.

Repositol ADH Response Test

1. Inject (after warming and shaking) 5 units of pitressin tannate in oil subcutaneously. The effects can last 2 to 3 days.
2. Withhold fluids and food during the test period.
3. Empty the bladder immediately, and collect all urine at 9 and 12 hours following ADH administration.

Although precise responses of dogs to this test have not been established, a urine specific gravity value of 1.020 to 1.025 or higher represents a normal response.

DDAVP intranasal drops (Minirin) can be used by administering one drop in the nose (20 μ [0.1 ml]) every 12 hours. Urine specific gravity and osmolality can then be checked.

Infusion of Hypertonic Saline

Infusion of hypertonic saline may also be used to determine whether ADH can be released, but it is rarely required and should be used with caution.

1. Withhold food for 12 hours (however, water may be given free choice).
2. Administer 30 ml of water per kg by stomach tube.
3. One hour later, urine and plasma samples are collected and the osmolality is checked. An indwelling catheter is left in the bladder.
4. Ten ml per kg of 5 per cent saline is administered IV over a period of 30 minutes *under close observation.* (This infusion occasionally produces mild to moderately severe seizures and should be discontinued immediately if they occur.)
5. At the 15 and 30 minute marks after the infusion, urine and plasma samples are collected and their osmolality is checked. The hypertonic saline will cause a rise in plasma osmolality, and urine osmolality must be increased to above that of the corresponding plasma sample to demonstrate ADH secretion.

The Thyroid Gland

Thyroid hormone affects the rate of metabolism, growth, and development. Thyroxine and triiodothyronine are iodinated amino acids, and their synthesis and secretion are principally under the control of the thyroid-stimulating hormone (TSH). In the formation of thyroid hormones, iodine is absorbed from the gastrointestinal tract, is transported to the follicular cells of the thyroid gland, and becomes part of the follicular colloid. When iodine is bound to tyrosine, this monoiodotyrosine is again iodinated to form diiodotyrosine, and the oxidative condensation of two diiodotyrosine molecules forms thyroxine (T_4), or one monoiodo and one diiodotyrosine form triiodothyronine (T_3). Thyroxine is transported in the blood of the dog by at least four serum proteins. Only "free" T_3 and T_4 are physiologically active and maintain the euthyroid state of the animal. Metabolism of thyroid hormones occurs primarily in the liver by both diiodination and conjugation.

Maintenance of normal thyroid secretion is established through the anterior pituitary via TSH and the "free" T_3/T_4 feedback system. The control of TSH production is also regulated by the hypothalamus through the production of thyrotropin-releasing hormone (TRH).

Normal blood level of thyroxine in the dog is approximately 1 to 4 μg per dl and, for triiodothyronine, between 60 and 200 ng per dl. Protein-bound iodine (PBI) levels would then be at about 2.00 μg per 100 ml for the dog and approximately 1.60 μg per 100 ml for the cat. In the cat, T_4 levels as measured by radioimmunoassay range from 1.18 to 2.95 μg per dl and T_3 levels, 39 to 112 ng per dl, although these estimates vary with different laboratories.

EVALUATING THYROID FUNCTION

Disorders in thyroid function can result in either a hyperfunctional or hypofunctional state. Hyperthyroidism is rare and is mainly associated with animals having functional tumors of the thyroid gland. Signs seen in the dog are nervousness, weight loss, polydypsia, and polyuria. Hyperthyroidism in cats 10 to 15 years of age is associated with functional thyroid tumors. The major presenting clinical signs are weight loss, polyphagia, hyperactivity, PU–PD, hyperdefecation with marked steatorrhea, heat intolerance, panting, and muscle tremors. Mild to moderate cardiomegaly may develop, and there is tachycardia (heart rate greater than 240 beats/min), ventricular hypertrophy, and increased voltage of R waves. Cardiovascular disease may produce a hypertrophic congestive heart failure with pleural effusion. Electrocardiographic changes are recorded in 80 per cent of the cats with this condition with tachycardias greater than 240 beats per minute. Increased R-wave amplitudes in lead II (greater than 0.9 mv), ventricular tachyarrythmias, and intraventricular conduction disturbances developed.

T_4 radioimmunoassay tests in hyperthyroid cats averaged 8.0 to 24.0 μg per dl (1.4–4.0 μg/dl is normal), and T_3 levels were 277 ± 49 μg per dl (25–100 μg/dl is normal). Clinical pathology indicates an increased packed cell volume (PCV) in 45 per cent of the cases, eosinopenia in 40 per cent of the cases, and erythrocytosis in 20 per cent of the cases.

Treatment of feline hyperthyroidism involves the surgical removal of one or both tumorous thyroid glands (with sparing of the parathyroids, if possible). Another form of treatment is the administration of radioactive iodine [131]I (1–5 mc), which will take 7 to 14 days to be effective and must be administered in a facility with licensing for administration of radioactive drugs as well as an isolation facility for the treated animal.

Prior to surgical removal of the thyroid tumor, affected cats should be made euthyroid by the oral administration of propylthiouracil, 50 mg TID for 2 weeks, or Tapazole (methimazole), 5 mg TID for 2 weeks. Propylthiouracil has produced side effects, including vomiting, lethargy, hemolytic anemia, thrombocytopenia, and granulocytopenia; thus, its use is discouraged. With administration of antithyroid drugs, blood samples for CBC should be obtained at least weekly. T_4 levels usually normalize within 2 weeks of treatment with antithyroid medication. In very severe thyrotoxicosis, stable iodine given IV, 50 to 100 mg per day for 1 week, may be given to lower the T_4.

Cardiac arrythmias may be controlled with the daily administration of propranolol (see p. 36).

Following surgical removal of thyroid tumors, T_4, T_3, and serum calcium should be evaluated. Thyroid supplementation in the form of triiodiothyronine, 0.1 mg per day, is administered.

In the dog, most hypothyroidism cases are of primary origin, resulting from idiopathic follicular atrophy or an entity that is being more commonly recognized: immunologically mediated lymphocytic thyroiditis. Hypothyroidism is seen most commonly in middle age, in mid- to large-sized breeds of dogs.

Hypothyroidism is characterized by lethargy and easy fatigability, intolerance to cold, changes in skin and hair coat, abnormal estrous cycle, infertility, decreased libido, constipation or mild diarrhea, bradycardia, weight gain, and, occasionally, normocytic-normochromic anemia. In the skin, there is atrophy of the hair follicles, myxedema, and bilaterally symmetrical alopecia. Inability to tolerate cold is associated with decreased metabolic rate. A myopathy can be produced that is characterized by type II fiber atrophy and decrease in muscle function. Approximately 20 per cent of the cases develop seborrhea. Another manifestation of hypothyroidism in dogs may be laryngeal paralysis. This condition and case summaries have been reported by Harvey.

Laboratory Tests

There are numerous tests for the evaluation of thyroid gland function in dogs; however, the measurement of serum T_4 levels by T_4 radioimmunoassay is the most accurate method available, especially when combined with TSH response.

T_4 Test

This test determines the total circulating serum thyroxine level. The two most commonly used methods for T_4 analysis are competitive protein–binding (CPB) assay and radioimmunoassay. T_4 determination by radioimmunoassay has largely supplanted competitive protein-binding and is the preferred thyroid test. Normal values for T_4 radioimmunoassay in the dog are 2.3 ± 0.8 µg per dl. There is variability in normal T_4 levels in the dog, depending on the laboratory used. Also, there is an overlap in dogs that may be hypothyroid and those that are euthyroid. The TSH response test is helpful in these situations.

The use of a test response dose of TSH is a much more accurate method of measuring thyroid function and is the test of choice. The IV TSH response test is faster and less expensive. Obtain baseline T_4 levels and inject 2 units of TSH (Dermathycin) IV. Collect a second blood sample 3 to 6 hours after administration for T_4 determination. Another method is the IM administration of TSH. Obtain baseline values of T_4 radioimmunoassay, and administer 0.4 U per kg of aqueous TSH IM. Obtain a second sample for T_4 radioimmunoassay 16 hours later. The minimal normal thyroid response is a doubling of the zero time thyroid response at 16 hours post-TSH injection.

The major action of thyroid hormones is primarily mediated by T_3 at the cellular level. T_4 serves as a prohormone for T_3 (T_4 is converted to T_3). There can be clinical cases in which T_4 levels are normal; however, T_4 is inadequately converted to T_3 and the animal exhibits clinical hypothyroidism. Therefore, T_3 testing can also be done using radioimmunoassay. In interpreting T_4 values, it is important to realize that certain extrathyroidal factors can influence the levels:

1. Excess endogenous (Cushing's disease) or exogenous corticosteroids can cause lowered T_3 and T_4 test results. Lowered T_4 results from a decrease in thyroid-binding globulin levels and suppression of TSH release.
2. Other diseases resulting in lowered T_4 and T_3 levels are acute infections, diabetes mellitus, malignant disease, and renal disease.
3. Drug-induced interference such as propranolol salicylate therapy, phenylbutazone, phenytoin, phenobarbitol, or o,p'DDD (Mitotane).

The efficacy of thyroidal replacement hormones can be checked using T_4 and T_3 testing (following replacement with L-thyroxine). The animal should be evaluated 4 to 6 weeks after beginning medication. T_4 should be measured 4 to 8 hours following administration, and T_3 should be measured 2 to 3 hours following administration. These tests are called post-pill tests.

The thyroid gland's ability to trap iodide can be evaluated by its ability to take up [131]I. This procedure is limited to institutions that are equipped to perform this work. Decreased thyroid uptake indicates hypothyroidism. Serum cholesterol determinations should be coupled with thyroid function tests.

Thyroid Gland Biopsy

This procedure is very helpful in confirming the diagnosis of hypothyroidism and in distinguishing primary from secondary hypothyroidism. Because most cases of hypothyroidism in dogs are due to primary atrophy of the thyroid gland or destructive thyroiditis, biopsy of the thyroid is almost equal in diagnostic value to measurement of ^{131}I uptake. Furthermore, it often provides confirmatory evidence in cases in which the results of other tests are equivocal or invalidated by iodine contamination.

Calcium Metabolism and Disorders of the Parathyroid Glands

Calcium is involved in many biologic processes of the body, including neuromuscular excitability, membrane permeability, muscle contraction, enzyme activity, hormone release, and blood coagulation. Normal serum calcium ranges from 8.8 to 10.8 mg per dl and is available in the serum in two forms: The nondiffusable form is protein bound (mainly to albumin) and constitutes about 45 per cent of the measurable calcium. This form is biologically inactive. The ionized forms of calcium are biologically active. The serum calcium level of immature dogs is approximately 10 to 12 mg per dl.

Primary control of blood calcium is dependent on: (1) parathyroid hormone (PTH) secretion, (2) calcitonin hormone secretion, and (3) the presence of cholecalciferol (vitamin D). Major control of calcium is dependent on PTH production. Parathyroids are composed of chief cells whose secretory activity is related to circulating levels of ionized blood calcium. The biologic effects of parathyroid hormone are numerous (see Table 110): (1) elevates blood calcium concentration; (2) decreases the blood phosphate concentration; (3) increases the urinary excretion of phosphate and decreases calcium loss in urine; (4) increases the rate of skeletal or modeling and bone resorption; (5) increases the urinary excretion of hydroxy–proline-containing peptides; (7) activates adenyl cyclase in target cells; and (8) accelerates the formation of active vitamin D metabolites by the kidney.

Levels of calcium within the body are also controlled by the hormone calcitonin. Calcitonin is secreted by the parafollicular cell population within the mammalian thyroid gland. Calcitonin-secreting cells are derived embryologically from cells of the neural crest. Calcitonin produces a hypocalcemic effect by decreasing the entry of calcium from the skeleton into plasma due to a temporary inhibition of PTH-stimulated bone resorption. Additionally, calcitonin increases the rate of movement of phosphate out of plasma into soft tissue and bone, and PTH and calcitonin are synergistic in decreasing the renal tubular reabsorption of phosphorus. The hypocalcemic effects of calcitonin are primarily the result of decreased entry of calcium from the skeleton into plasma due to a temporary inhibition of PTH-stimulated bone resorption. Regulation of calcitonin secretion is governed by the ionized calcium level.

The final major hormone involved in the regulation of calcium metabolism is 1,25-dihydroxyvitamin D_3 (1,25-DHCC). The target tissue for this metabolite is the small intestine, where it stimulates calcium and phosphate absorption and increases calcium and phosphate utilization from bone. Ultraviolet irradiation of ergosterol produces vitamin D_2. Vitamin D_2 or D_3 is transformed by the

Table 110. ACTIONS OF HORMONES INFLUENCING
CALCIUM METABOLISM

Vitamin D
  Increased intestinal absorption of calcium and phosphorus through increased
    synthesis of calcium-binding protein.

Calcitonin
  Decreased bone resorption causing diminished entry of calcium and phosphorus into
    the blood.
  Decreased phosphorus level from enhanced movement of phosphorus from the blood
    into soft tissues.
  Decreased renal resorption of phosphorus.

Parathormone
  Increased intestinal absorption of calcium.
  Increased bone lysis causing increased release of calcium and phosphorus into the
    blood.
  Decrease resorption of phosphorus by the kidney.
  Increased resorption of calcium by the kidney.
  Increased activation of vitamin D_3.

From Blank, R. E.: Differential diagnosis of hypercalcemia in dogs. Compendium on Continuing Education, *1*:220, 1979.

liver to 25-hydroxyvitamin D and is then actively metabolized in the kidney to 1,25-hydroxyvitamin D. In the skin, ultraviolet light converts 7-dehydrocholesterol to vitamin D_3 (cholecalciferol).

DISORDERS OF PARATHYROID GLANDS

Primary hypoparathyroidism signifies subnormal amounts of PTH, or it may indicate that the hormone secreted cannot react normally with the target cells. Decreased secretion of PTH results in hyperphosphatemia and hypocalcemia and impairs 1,25-dihydroxyvitamin D production. The two most common causes of primary hypoparathyroidism are idiopathic atrophy or destruction of parathyroid tissue, probably immune mediated, and the removal of and injury to parathyroid glands during thyroid surgery. Idiopathic hypoparathyroidism has been found in mature, female, small breed dogs. The clinical manifestations of hypoparathyroidism develop because of reduced bone resorption and progressively diminishing calcium levels (4–6 mg/100 ml). Lowered calcium levels result in nervousness, ataxia, weakness, muscle cramps, hypophosphatemia (without azotemia), prolongation of the Q-T interval on electrocardiogram, tremors with possible generalized tetany, convulsions, PD–PU, vomiting, and disorientation. Increased renal tubular resorption of phosphorus results in elevated blood phosphorus levels.

PTH levels can be measured by radioimmunoassay tests. One study reports serum PTH levels in the dog as $128 \pm 85 \mu$ mEq per ml with variations from 65 to 213. Results depend on what laboratory performs the test and what test kit is used.

Treatment of hypoparathyroidism involves the use of calcium and vitamin D. The following points may be helpful:
1. Hypocalcemia resulting in tetany and convulsions requires immediate IV calcium (see p. 146), 1.0 to 1.5 ml per kg of 10 per cent calcium gluconate administered slowly over 20 minutes, with cardiac monitoring. When bradycardia and shortening of the Q-T interval appear, discontinue treatment. Slow IV 10 per cent calcium gluconate can be used over 6 to 8 hours (2 ml/kg). Animals require 50 to 75 mg of elemental calcium per kg per day, which is 500 to 750 mg per kg per day of calcium gluconate or 400 to 600 mg per day of calcium lactate in 3 to 4 divided doses.
2. Oral calcium can be supplemented as calcium gluconate or calcium lactate tablets. Calcium gluconate contains 9 per cent elemental calcium and calcium lactate contains 13 per cent calcium.
3. Vitamin D products should be administered (Table 111). If D_2 is used, there is a long onset of establishment of effective levels—2 to 4 weeks—an initial dosage of 4,000 to 6,000 units per kg per day, then reduced after blood calcium is normalized to 1,000 to 2,000 units per kg per day. Dihydrotachysterol is more potent than D_2, raising the serum calcium more rapidly—0.03 mg per kg per day for 2 days, then 0.02 mg per kg per day for 2 days, then 0.01 mg per kg per day, observing serum calcium and adjusting the dosage as needed. 1,25-dihydroxyvitamin D has a very short half-life (less than 1 day) and a very rapid onset of action, not needing intermediary metabolic

Table 111. VITAMIN D PREPARATIONS

Product	Dosage Form*	Commercial Name	Dosage† (kg body wt/day)	Time for Response After Giving	Time for Response After Discontinuing
Vitamin D₂	Capsules (50,000 units)	Calciferol (K-U) Drisdol (Winthrop) Deltalin (Lilly)	Until response 4,000–6,000 units, then 1,000–2,000	2 weeks	1 week
	Oral solution (8,000 units/ml)	Drisdol (Winthrop)			
	IM injectable (50,000 units/ml)	Calciferol (K-U) Vitadee (Gotham)			
Dihydrotachysterol	Tablets (0.12–0.4 mg)	Dihydrotachysterol (P-R)	0.03 mg for 2 days 0.02 mg next 2 days, then 0.01 mg	1 week	Several days
	Capsules or Oral solution 0.125 mg/ml and capsule)	Hytakeral (Winthrop)			
1,25-dihydroxyvitamin D₃	Capsules (0.25 and 0.5 mg)	Rocaltrol (Roche)	0.06 μg	1–4 days	1 day

*40,000 units has an activity of 1.0 mg.

†Dosage must be adjusted to each individual patient to maintain a plasma calcium concentration of 9 to 11 mg/dl. If it does not increase by at least 0.5 mg/dl within 4 weeks, double the dosage. Do not give vitamin D if the plasma calcium concentration exceeds 10 mg/dl or if the plasma calcium times phosphorus concentration exceeds 55.

From Lewis, L. D., and Morris, M. L.: Small Animal Clinical Nutrition. Topeka, Kansas, Mark Morris Associates, 1984.

action. The dosage is approximately 0.06 μg per kg per day. The major problem is the expense of the drug.

4. When the animals have been stabilized on a vitamin D supplement regimen, calcium supplementation can usually be withdrawn. Periodic checks in serum calcium are very important, and vitamin D therapy may be markedly reduced or even stopped.

Secondary hyperparathyroidism may be nutritional or renal in origin. Both conditions result in altered calcium:phosphorus ratios. In nutritional secondary hyperparathyroidism, there is an increased secretion of PTH to compensate for altered mineral levels associated with dietary abnormalities. Dietary abnormalities that may lead to nutritional secondary hyperparathyroidism are: (1) low level of calcium in diet, (2) excessive phosphorus with normal or low calcium, and (3) inadequate amounts of vitamin D₃. Hypocalcemia results in parathyroid stimulation. Nutritional secondary hyperparathyroidism has been reported in a wide variety of species, including the dog, cat, and primate (Table 112).

Table 112. DIFFERENTIAL DIAGNOSIS OF PRIMARY HYPERPARATHYROIDISM, RENAL SECONDARY HYPERPARATHYROIDISM, PSEUDOHYPERPARATHYROIDISM, AND HYPERCALCEMIA DUE TO NEOPLASTIC OSTEOLYSIS

Factors	Primary Hyperparathyroidism	Renal Secondary Hyperparathyroidism	Pseudohyper-parathyroidism	Neoplastic Osteolysis*
Serum calcium	Elevated	Normal to decreased	Elevated	Elevated
Serum phosphorus	Decreased unless uremic; then normal to increased	Increased	Decreased unless uremic; then normal to increased	Frequently increased
Serum alkaline phosphatase	Normal to increased	Normal to increased	Normal to increased	Normal to increased
Blood urea nitrogen; creatinine	Normal unless uremic; then increased	Increased	Normal unless uremic; then increased	Normal unless uremic; then increased
Bone radiographs	Varying degrees of demineralization	Varying degrees of demineralization	Varying degrees of demineralization	Disseminated osteolytic lesions

*Findings reported in human beings.
From Osborne, C. A., and Stevens, J. B.: Hypercalcemic nephropathy. *In* Kirk, R. W.: Current Veterinary Therapy VI. Philadelphia, W. B. Saunders Company, 1977, p. 1083.

Secondary hyperparathyroidism of renal origin is a complication of chronic renal failure, with progressive loss of glomerular function and retained phosphorus, resulting in progressive hyperphosphatemia. Hyperphosphatemia results in lowering of blood calcium levels and secondary stimulation of PTH release. Additionally, chronic renal disease is involved in altered vitamin D metabolism, leading to hypocalcemia. Chronic renal disease impairs the production of 1,25-dihydroxyvitamin D_3 by the kidney.

The clinical signs associated with hypercalcemia are variable and are associated with changes in cell membrane excitability. Decreased neuromuscular excitability can result in weakness, vomiting, constipation, and bradycardia. Bone changes associated with increased resorption of calcium may be evidenced radiographically.

The most severe systemic manifestation of hypercalcemia is associated with renal disease. In early or mild cases, there is calcification, degeneration, and necrosis of the epithelium of ascending Henle's loop, distal tubules, and collecting ducts. Severe states of hypercalcemia are associated with calcification of tubular epithelium and basement membranes. Severe hypercalcemia results in the distribution of calcium throughout the renal parenchyma. The clinical signs associated with renal disease are polyuria, polydypsia, dehydration, and uremia of variable degree. A marked inability to concentrate urine (isothenuria and hyposthenuria) associated with glomerulotubular imbalance usually develops.

Consistently elevated blood calcium levels above 11.5 to 12.0 mg per 100 ml can be associated with any of a series of lesions: (1) primary hyperparathyroidism, (2) vitamin D intoxication, (3) malignant neoplasms with osseous metastases, and (4) other malignant neoplasms (pseudohyperparathyroidism) of which lymphosarcoma is the most common.

In primary hyperparathyroidism, hormone secretion is autonomous and is usually associated with an adenoma composed of active chief cells. Hypercalcemia results in the clinical signs of anorexia, vomiting, constipation, generalized muscular weakness, demineralization or fracture of long bones, bradycardia, depression, polyuria, and polydypsia.

Pseudohyperparathyroidism is a metabolic abnormality in which parathyroid-like hormone is produced by some malignant tumors of nonparathyroid origin. Pseudohyperparathyroidism has been reported in dogs and cats with malignant lymphoma, mammary adenocarcinoma, and apocrine gland adenocarcinoma of the anal sac.

Dogs with lymphosarcoma and hypercalcemia have increased osteoclastic bone resorption, which appears to be dependent on infiltration of bone marrow by neoplastic cells and the production of a bone resorption–stimulating factor.

Glucose Metabolism—Diabetes Mellitus

The islets of Langerhans secrete two hormones that have important functions in intermediary metabolism: glucagon and insulin. Glucagon is a polypeptide hormone that elevates blood glucose by stimulating hepatic glycogenolysis. Secretion of glucagon is stimulated by lowered blood glucose and sympathetic nerve stimulation. It may help maintain blood glucose levels during starvation. The principal actions of insulin are: (1) to promote glucose oxidation and triglyceride formation in adipose tissue; (2) to promote protein and glycogen synthesis in muscle; and (3) to promote glycogen and triglyceride synthesis in the liver. Changes in blood glucose levels produce reciprocal changes in the levels of these two hormones. Many other hormones are important in regulating carbohydrate metabolism. The catecholamines epinephrine and norepinephrine enhance glucose production by enhancing hepatic glycogenolysis, gluconeogenesis, lipolysis, and proteolysis. Growth hormone has a catabolic effect on carbohydrate metabolism. Cortisol raises blood sugar by increasing gluconeogenesis. Excessive thyroid hormone production can cause increased glucose oxidation.

The major disease associated with an abnormality in the metabolism of glucose is diabetes mellitus. Persistent hyperglycemia caused by diabetes mellitus may result from subnormal levels of circulating insulin or reduced responsiveness of the organs upon which insulin has its effect. Hyperglycemia does not mean a lack of insulin in all cases. It is possible to classify spontaneous diabetes mellitus of dogs into types I, II, and III, according to fasting plasma insulin concentration, insulin peak response following IV glucose tolerance test, insulinogenic index ($\Delta I/\Delta G$), and total insulin secreted (Table 113).

Type I, insulin dependent diabetes, is characterized clinically by sudden onset of symptoms, absence of immunoreactive insulin, need for insulin to sustain life, and tendency to develop ketotic diabetes. Most cases of type I are found in mature and older dogs.

Type II, noninsulin dependent diabetes mellitus, is characterized by glucose intolerance and typical signs of diabetes. Plasma insulin concentrations are usually within acceptable limits in dogs that are not obese but are higher in obese dogs. In both obese and non-obese dogs, there is no insulin response to a glucose load. Breed predilection indicates that dachshunds and poodles are at increased risk.

In type III diabetes in dogs, fasting plasma glucose concentrations are nondiagnostic, but there is glucose intolerance and subnormal insulin response to a glucose load. In obese dogs, glucose intolerance may be improved after weight loss. The major clinical signs with diabetes mellitus are increased water consumption, excessive frequency and amount of urination, increased appetite, and weight loss. Affected animals may be dehydrated and ketotic (see p. 138). Gastrointestinal upset may be manifested by vomiting and anorexia. Severe gastrointestinal signs can be associated with acute pancreatitis and secondary diabetes mellitus (see p. 119). Diabetic neuropathy may produce leg weakness associated with a distal axonopathy. A large percentage (90 per cent) of dogs with diabetes develop cataracts.

Because classification of diabetes mellitus based on insulin levels usually does not help with diagnosis, a classification based on other possibly associated diseases is more significant.

In older female dogs that have a higher incidence of diabetes, disease factors may develop that alter their peripheral resistance to insulin. Two factors

Table 113. SUMMARY: CLINICAL GLUCOSE, AND INSULIN MEASUREMENTS IN CANINE DIABETES MELLITUS*

Diabetes type	Clinical signs	Glucose, glucose tolerance, and insulin values						
		G_o	GTT	K	I_o	IPR	$\Delta I/\Delta G$	TIS
Type I	Marked	Incr	Intol	Decr	None	None	None	None
Type II nonobese	Marked	Incr	Intol	Decr	Normal	None	None	None
Type II obese	Marked	Incr	Intol	Decr	Incr	None	None	None
Type III nonobese	None	Incr	Intol	Decr	Normal	Decr	Decr	Decr
Type III obese	None	Incr	Intol	Decr	Incr	Incr	Incr	Incr

*G_o = plasma glucose; GTT = glucose tolerance test; K = glucose disappearance coefficient; I_o = initial plasma insulin; IPR = insulin peak response; TIS = total insulin secretion; Incr = increase; Intol = intolerant; Decr = decrease.

From Mattheeuws, D., et al.: Diabetes mellitus in dogs: relationship of obesity to glucose tolerance and insulin response. Am. J. Vet. Res., 45(1):102, 1984.

that can produce this are increased levels of GH or excesses of glucocorticoids, as seen in hyperadrenocorticoidism. Elevated GH levels greater than 10 ng per ml (radioimmunoassay measurement) have been found in female dogs treated with medroxyprogesterone acetate or have been seen naturally during diestrus. These dogs have altered IV glucose tolerance test results associated with insulin insensitivity and glucose intolerance. In this group of dogs, withdrawal of artificial progestational compounds is indicated or an ovariohysterectomy should be performed.

Another factor that can play an important role in diabetes is hyperadrenocorticoidism. Abnormal glucocorticoid levels lead to insulin resistance and glucose intolerance. Dogs with diabetes and concurrent hyperadrenocorticism may prove very difficult to manage and may also have to be treated with o,p'-DDD (Mitotane) therapy.

Diabetes mellitus occurs predominantly in cats over 5 years of age, and male cats are at increased risk for developing the disease. The following signs are most often present in cats with diabetes mellitus: depression, anorexia, weight loss, weakness, polydypsia, polyuria, vomiting, and diarrhea. Cats may show a polyneuropathy characterized by "dropped hocks" in the hind legs, with absent patella reflexes. Approximately 30 per cent of diabetic cats are icteric. Predisposing factors in the cat leading to the development of diabetes are the use of progestational compounds such as Ovaban, acute pancreatitis, pancreatic amyloidosis, prolonged use of systemic glucocorticoids, and hepatic lipoidosis.

Early onset diabetes mellitus is uncommon in dogs but has been described in one form as a primary atrophy of beta cells of the pancreas in genetically related keeshonds. Early onset diabetes in keeshonds develops at 2 to 6 months of age. Affected animals are hypercholesterolemic, ketotic, insulinopenic, and eugluconemic. Early onset diabetes mellitus is inherited as an autosomal recessive trait with incomplete penetrance. Diabetic phenotype has been found to be expressed in 80 per cent of the dogs with diabetes mellitus genotype. Diabetes has also been found in a variety of breeds and mixed dog populations as a delayed finding related to systemic disease and secondary pancreatic damage.

GLUCOSE TOLERANCE TEST EVALUATING GLUCOSE METABOLISM

The glucose tolerance test is used to help confirm a diagnosis of diabetes mellitus when other tests are equivocal. Either oral or IV tests may be used. The oral glucose tolerance test in the dog is started by obtaining a baseline fasting blood sugar. Next, 2.0 gm of glucose per kg of body weight is administered in a solution through a stomach tube. The concentration of glucose should not be greater than 25 per cent. Blood samples are taken at 30, 60, 120, 170, and 240 minutes. In nondiabetic animals who have been on a high carbohydrate intake for 3 days prior to testing, the fasting blood sugar is less than 110 mg per 100 ml. It does not rise above 160 mg per 100 ml at the end of the first hour and returns to normal by the end of the second hour. In diabetic animals, the baseline fasting blood sugar is usually over 150 mg per

100 ml, rises markedly during the test, and does not return to pretest levels within 2 hours.

The standard IV glucose tolerance test is performed by administering 0.5 gm of glucose per kg of body weight following a 15-hour fast. A 50 per cent glucose solution is used. A baseline blood sample is obtained prior to testing and again at 5, 15, 30, 45, and 60 minutes.

Lorenz and Cornelius developed a procedure using a high-dose IV glucose tolerance test for the dog. Following a baseline fasting blood sugar sample, 1 gm of glucose (given as 50 per cent glucose) per kg of body weight is administered IV and blood samples are taken at 5, 15, 30, 45, and 60 minutes. To shorten the procedure, blood samples can be taken at 5 and 60 minutes. The glucose disappearance coefficient (K) is calculated from the formula: $K = \dfrac{698}{T_2 - T_1}$. Values for K that are 2.0 or less can be considered evidence for latent diabetes mellitus.

PROVOCATIVE TESTS FOR INSULIN RELEASE

Several diagnostic tests have been used to document the diagnosis of hypoglycemia secondary to functional beta cell tumors in dogs. Pancreatic adenocarcinomas are functional tumors of the beta cells of the islets of Langerhans. The tumors occur in older dogs, with German shepherds, collies, and setters having the highest incidence, with median age being 9 years; most of the tumors are malignant. The major clinical signs are associated with hypoglycemia: (1) weakness; (2) incoordination, especially of the rear legs; (3) generalized muscle twitching; (4) neurologic abnormalities characterized by convulsions, changes in behavioral patterns (such as increased barking), crying, and increased irritability; and (5) relief of neurologic disturbances by feeding or administering glucose (Whipples Triad, see p. 144).

Most dogs with clinical signs referable to insulinomas have clinical and biochemical evidence of Whipples Triad. Blood glucose levels are usually below 70 mg per dl and are often in the 40 to 50 mg per dl range. Some dogs have normal blood glucose levels until they are fasted, then they develop low glucose levels. Fasting should not be carried out for more than 8 hours, which is usually sufficient to see altered blood glucose levels. The clinical signs in insulinomas appear to be episodic rather than constant.

Plasma insulin levels can be measured by immunoreactive insulin (IRI) concentrations. Estimates of IRI concentrations in normal dogs average 20μU per ml; values above 54μU are considered abnormal (Table 114).

Insulin concentrations closely parallel plasma glucose concentrations. Another test that has used this principle, the "amended insulin–glucose ratio" (AIGR), is obtained by using the formula:

$$\frac{\text{serum insulin } (\mu U/ml) \times 100}{\text{plasma glucose } (mg/100ml) - 30}$$

Normal ratios are less than 30. Because dogs with functional islet cell adenomas may have normal serum insulin levels, the AIGR may be helpful in

Table 114. CONCENTRATIONS OF INSULIN IN SERUM OF CLINICALLY NORMAL DOGS*

Condition	No. of Animals	μIU/ml (X ± SE)	Range (μIU/ml)
Males	8	14.70 ± 6.70	4.20–60.52
Lactating bitches	10	26.12 ± 4.76	3.72–47.82
Estrous bitches	9	22.79 ± 8.56	4.32–87.40
Pregnant bitches	6	22.94 ± 4.13	8.96–31.79
Metestrous bitches	3	24.46 ± 5.38	18.20–35.18
Proestrous bitches	5	26.57 ± 5.90	16.99–49.31

*Radioimmunoassay of insulin can be determined using the IV glucose tolerance test (see p. 667). Values of 50 μU per dl or greater, 1 minute after injection, are abnormal and suggest the presence of a beta cell tumor.

From Reimers, T. J., Cowan, R. G., McCann, J. P., and Ross, M. W.: Validation of a rapid solid-phse radioimmunoassay for canine, bovine, and equine insulin. Am. J. Vet. Res., *43*(7):1274, 1982.

making a tentative diagnosis of pancreatic tumor when coupled with clinical signs.

Another evaluation of serum insulin levels is the simple glucose:insulin ratio, with normal being greater than 5.0 and abnormal being less than 2.5

$$\frac{\text{plasma glucose mg/100 ml}}{\text{serum insulin } \mu\text{U/ml}}$$

Glucagon Tolerance Test

The hormone glucagon raises the blood sugar by stimulating glycogenolysis of liver glycogen. The elevation of blood glucose thus stimulates the release of insulin from pancreatic beta cells. Glucagon also has a secondary effect—to directly stimulate the release of insulin from pancreatic beta cells. These two effects of glucagon are used in the glucagon tolerance test for functional beta cell tumors in dogs. Take a fasting blood sample. The length of the fast must be critically observed, because in animals with insulin-secreting tumors, coma can be produced. The fast should be from 2 to 4 hours. Give 0.03 mg per kg of glucagon IV. Take blood samples for glucose and insulin (critical periods are 1, 3, and 5 minutes) at 5, 15, 30, 45, 60, 90, 120, and 180 minutes. In the normal dog, a rise in blood glucose occurs initially and returns to the control level in 2 to 3 hours.

The following findings in a glucagon tolerance test are indicative of excessive production of insulin: (1) a decrease in blood glucose concentration 1 or 2 minutes after injection; (2) peak blood glucose concentrations less than 135 mg per 100 ml; (3) hypoglycemia with blood sugar levels less than 50 mg per ml at 60 to 120 minutes postinjection; (4) one minute after injection, immunoreactive insulin concentrations of values greater than 50 μU per ml or an average increase (from fasting to 1 minute postinjection) of greater than 18 μU per ml.

References and Additional Readings

Atkins, C. E., Hill, J. R., and Johnson, R. K.: Diabetes mellitus in the juvenile dog: A report of four cases. J.A.V.M.A., *175*:362, 1979.

Becker, M. J., Holland, D., and Becker, D. N.: Serum cortisol (hydrocortisone) values in normal dogs as determined by radioimmunoassay. Am. J. Vet. Res., *37*:1102, 1976.

Belshaw, B. E., and Rijnberk, A.: Radioimmunoassay of plasma T4 and T3 in the diagnosis of primary hypothyroidism in dogs. J.A.A.H.A., *15*:17, 1979.

Blank, R.: Differential diagnosis of hypercalcemia in dogs. Compendium on Continuing Education, *1*:220, 1979.

Capen, C. C., and Martin, S. L.: Calcium metabolism and disorders of the parathyroid glands. Vet. Clin. North Am., *7*:513, 1977.

Capen, C. C., Belshaw, B. E., and Smith, S. L.: Endocrine disorders. *In* Ettinger, S. J. (ed.): Veterinary Internal Medicine, Vol. 2. Philadelphia, W. B. Saunders Company, 1975.

Caywood, D. D., Wilson, J. W., Hardy, R. M., and Shull, R. M.: Pancreatic islet cell adenocarcinoma: Clinical and diagnostic features in six cases. J.A.V.M.A., *174*:714, 1979.

Feldman, E. C., and Tyrell, J. B.: Hypoadrenocorticism. Vet. Clin. North Am., *7*:549, 1977.

Harvey, H. J., Irby, N. L., and Watrous, B. J.: Laryngeal paralysis in hypothyroid dogs. *In* Kirk, R. W. (ed.): Current Veterinary Therapy VIII. Philadelphia, W. B. Saunders Co., 1983.

Kallfeltz, F. A.: Thyroid function in the dog. Vet. Clin. North Am., *7*:497, 1977.

Kaneko, J. J., Comer, K., and Ling, G. V.: Thyroxine levels by radioimmunoassay (T4-RIA) and thyroid stimulating hormone response in normal dogs. Calif. Vet., *32*:9, 1978.

Kaneko, J. J., et al.: Renal clearance, insulin secretion and glucose tolerance in spontaneous diabetes mellitus of dogs. Cornell Vet., *69*:375, 1979.

Ling, G. V., Lowenstine, L. J., Pulley, L. T., et al.: Diabetes mellitus in dogs: a review of initial evaluation, immediate and long-term management and outcome. J.A.V.M.A., *170*:521, 1978.

Lorenz, M. D., and Cornelius, L. M.: Laboratory diagnosis of endocrinological disease. Vet. Clin. North Am., *6*:687, 1976.

Meijer, J. C., deBruijne, J. J., Rijnberk, A., and Croughs, R. J. M.: Biochemical characterization of pituitary-dependent hyperadrenocorticism in the dog. J. Endocrinol., *77*:111, 1978.

Owens, J. M., and Drucker, W. D.: Hyperadrenocorticism in the dog: Canine Cushing's syndrome. Vet. Clin. North Am., *7*:583, 1977.

Peterson, M. E.: Symposium on endocrinology. Vet. Clin. North Am. *14*:721–946, 1984.

Scott, D. W.: Hyperadrenocorticism. Vet. Clin. North Am., *9*:3, 1979.

HEMATOLOGY: INTERPRETATION OF LABORATORY FINDINGS

Hematology is the branch of medicine that deals with the relationship of changes in the hemogram to underlying primary or secondary disease states and includes the study of morphology of the blood and blood-forming tissues.

Hematologic studies in veterinary medicine have five major functions:
1. To confirm the diagnosis of the presence or absence of a blood abnormality.
2. To determine the extent of the disease process.
3. To find out why there is a blood abnormality.
4. To serve as a guide in the prognosis of clinical cases.
5. To serve as a guide during therapy in the treatment of clinical disorders.

This section on hematology covers the interpretation of results obtained from hematologic examination. It includes evaluation of the erythron, the leukogram, leukemias, the sedimentation rate, coagulation disorders, blood parasites, and blood chemistry.

Evaluation of the Erythron

The erythron refers to the circulating erythrocytes in the blood, their precursors, and all the elements of the body concerned with their production. Abnormalities in the erythron may manifest themselves as anemia, polycythemia, hemodilution, or hemoconcentration (Fig. 93).

TESTS

There are several basic tests that enable one to evaluate the state of the erythron.

The Hematocrit (Packed Cell Volume)

This test measures the relative red blood cell (RBC) mass. It is an accurate test (error of 1 to 2 per cent). The use of the microhematocrit enables one to use a small amount of blood and conduct the test rapidly.

Following high-speed centrifugation, the blood in the hematocrit tube will be divided into three layers: the bottom or packed erythrocyte layer; the middle or buffy coat, containing leukocytes and thrombocytes; and the upper plasma layer.

The hemoglobin concentration can be predicted from the packed cell volume (PCV) in all conditions except iron deficiency anemia and during the remission phase of acute blood loss and hemolytic anemia. The value of the hemoglobin is approximately equal to one third the PCV. The approximate total erythrocyte count (normocytic, normochromic erythrocytes) can be estimated by dividing the PCV by one sixth. In the dog, the following PCV values are estimated according to the animal's age: 2 to 4 months, 32 to 45 per cent; 4 to 6 months, 35 to 52 per cent: 6 to 8 months, 41 to 55 per cent.

Approximate leukocyte counts can be made by measuring the buffy coat (useful only in the Wintrobe hematocrit tube). The first mm of the buffy coat is equal to approximately 10,000 leukocytes, and each additional 0.1 mm equals 2000 leukocytes per cu mm. (This is only a means of obtaining a rough estimation of the total leukocyte count.)

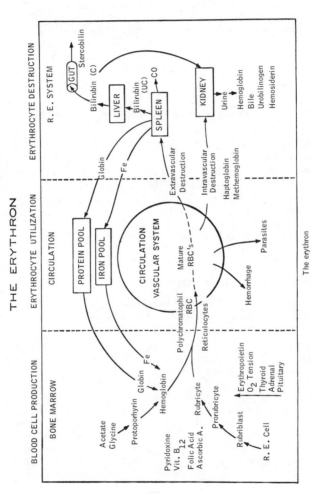

Figure 93. The erythron. (Used by permission of Dr. John Switzer.)

Always examine the color of the plasma layer in the hematocrit tube: a yellow plasma may indicate icterus, a pale to colorless plasma may indicate bone marrow depression, a cloudy plasma may indicate lipemia, and a red-tinged plasma is indicative of hemolysis. The PCV varies with the age, breed, state of nutrition, environment, degree of activity, and state of hydration of the animal. Care should be taken to avoid anticoagulant excess (EDTA), because this can result in a reduction of the PCV by as much as 25 per cent.

Hemoglobin

Hemoglobin tests measure the oxygen carrying ability of the erythrocytes. The hemoglobin (Hb) should be approximately one third of the hematocrit (Hct) if the red cells are of normal size.

Erythrocyte Counts

This determination is the most inaccurate of the tests used to evaluate the erythron (the error may be as high as 20 to 40 per cent). RBC numbers vary with the age of the animal and, in general, total RBC count is used only in obtaining RBC indices.

Red Blood Cell Indices

These values are based on knowing the PCV, total RBC count, and Hb. Because both the total RBC and Hb suffer from inaccuracies, the blood cell indices may also reflect these inaccuracies. Basically, these indices determine whether the erythrocyte population is made up of small cells, large cells, or cells with adequate or inadequate amounts of Hb. The average volume of erythrocytes is called the *mean corpuscular volume* (MCV). The average weight of Hb in the average cell is called the *mean corpuscular hemoglobin* (MCHb). The mean corpuscular hemoglobin concentration (MCHC) is the percentage concentration of Hb in the RBC mass. The same basic information obtained in the RBC indices may also be obtained subjectively by careful examination of the blood smear.

The MCV expresses the average volume of the individual erythrocyte, as summarized in Table 115. Normal MCV is seen in normocytic anemias as may

Table 115. MORPHOLOGIC CLASSIFICATION OF ANEMIA

Classification	MCHC Normal	MCHC Decreased
MCV normal	Normocytic Normochromic	Normocytic Hypochromic
MCV increased	Macrocytic Normochromic	Macrocytic Hypochromic
MCV decreased	Microcytic Normochromic	Microcytic Hypochromic

From Benjamin, M. M.: Outlines of Veterinary Clinical Pathology, Vol. 3 (3rd ed.), Iowa State University Press, 1978, p. 129.

be present with acute hemorrhage and hemolysis, whereas increased MCV (macrocytic cells) are associated with increased activity of the bone marrow or deficiencies in hematopoietic factors. Decreased MCV or microcytic cells are associated with iron deficiency or deficiency in hematopoietic factors.

$$\frac{\text{MCV}}{\text{Expressed in femtoliters}} = \frac{\text{PCV in ml/10 ml}}{\text{RBC count, millions/}\mu\text{L}}$$

$$\frac{\text{MCHb}}{\text{Expressed in pg}} = \frac{\text{Hb in gm/dl} \times 10}{\text{RBC count, millions/}\mu\text{L}}$$

$$\frac{\text{MCHC}}{\text{Expressed in gm/dl}} = \frac{\text{Hb in gm/dl} \times 100}{\text{PCV}}$$

The normal range for MCHC is 30 to 36 gm per dl for all mammals (with few exceptions). Normal MCV (femtoliters) for dogs is 60 to 77, and for cats, 39 to 55. Normal MCH (pg) for dogs is 19.5 to 24.5, and for cats, 12.5 to 17.5.

Blood Smears and Erythrocyte Morphology

The stem cells for mature RBCs located in the bone marrow generate a continuous supply of nucleated erythyroid precursors. Precursor cells undergo a series of divisions in which nuclear and cytoplasmic maturation take place. As the RBC matures, the number of polyribosomes and mitochondria decrease, the cells become smaller in size, and the cytoplasm loses its basophilic staining properties. During maturation, Hb is synthesized.

Thin blood smears using a good staining technique are needed to evaluate the morphology of RBCs. Examine the smear; evaluate the size, shape, and color of the erythrocytes; and determine the presence of any intra- or extracellular parasites.

Anisocytosis refers to an abnormal variation in the size of the RBCs due to the presence of both mature and immature RBCs in the circulation. It may be slight, moderate, or marked. Mild anisocytosis is normal in cats.

Macrocytosis refers to an increase in the MCV of the RBC, and it is most frequently seen in responsive anemias and, rarely, with B_{12} and folic acid deficiency. Macrocytosis has been seen in miniature poodles and chondroplastic malamutes, where the etiology is unknown.

Poikilocytosis refers to any unusual shape of the RBCs. This usually occurs in chronic anemia in which the RBCs are not stable and undergo fragmentation and indicates premature destruction of erythrocytes or defective erythrocyte formation. Poikilocytosis is seen in disseminated intravascular coagulation (DIC) (see p. 63) and the fragmentation anemia that rapidly develops presents an acute hemolytic anemia. Other disease entities that have been associated with poikilocytosis are massive heartworm disease, hemangiosarcomas, disseminated neoplasia, and chemotherapy with Cytoxan.

Polychromatophilia refers to the bluish tinge of young RBCs.

Howell-Jolly bodies are remnants of nuclear material found in young RBCs.

Normoblasts are immature RBCs, both orthochromophilic and polychromatophilic, that contain Hb, are nucleated, and are capable of carrying oxygen. They indicate that immature RBCs are in demand. Because nucleated RBCs are ordinarily counted as leukocytes in the process of counting white blood cells (WBCs), the WBC count should be corrected for circulating normoblasts.

Nucleated RBCs may be released during periods of accelerated erythropoiesis (if the response is appropriate for the need, it is called *appropriate;* when nucleated RBCs are released and the numbers are not related to the degree of stimulation, the response is called *inappropriate*). Nucleated RBC release is associated with the following:

Congestive heart failure
Chronic pulmonary disease
Endotoxemia
Bone marrow neoplasia
Myelofibrosis
Myelosclerosis
Bone marrow necrosis
Spinal cord disease

Lead poisoning
Extra medullary hematopoiesis
Some healthy schnauzers
Anemias of increased red cell production
Anemia of decreased red cell production
Others

There are three diseases in which nucleated RBCs are frequently seen: canine hemangiosarcoma (HSA), autoimmune hemolytic anemia (AIHA), and lead toxicity (Table 116).

Leptocytes are thin erythrocytes that have an increased surface area without an increase in cell volume; this gives the cell distinctive morphologic characteristics. The cells are usually seen in chronic disease leading to anemia. "Target cells" are a form of leptocyte seen most frequently in the dog.

Acanthocytes are RBCs with numerous projections. These cells have been "fractured" or damaged, and this damage is associated with hepatic disease and

Table 116. DIFFERENTIAL DIAGNOSIS OF NUCLEATED RBCs

Hemogram	HSA	AIHA	Lead Poisoning
Anemia	Mild to moderate	Severe	Mild
Reticulocytes	Many	Many	Many
Nucleated RBCs	Moderate (80 per cent in anemia cases)	Moderate	Moderate to many
Basophilic stippling	Few	Few	Frequent
Spherocytosis	Rare	Yes	No
Icterus	Mild	Usually	No

Adapted from Fees, D., and Withrow, S. J.: Canine hemangiosarcoma. Compendium on Continuing Education. 3(12):1049, 1981.

lipid abnormalities. Keratocytes are RBCs with variable numbers of elongated, irregularly spaced projections and are associated with damage from intravascular fibrin as occurs in DIC.

Hereditary stomatocytosis is a rare hereditary disorder in chondrodysplastic Alaskan malamutes. The RBCs are abnormal, possibly associated with abnormalities in the red cell cation pump. The RBCs have a short life span and appear as stomatocytes.

Hypochromasia refers to a decrease of Hb in erythrocytes. In Wright's- or Giemsa-stained smears, the cells appear abnormally pale.

Punctate basophilia or stippling of the erythrocytes may be due to degenerative changes in the cytoplasm involving ribonucleic acid (RNA) in the young cells. Stippling may also occur in lead poisoning.

Spherocytes are RBCs of decreased diameter in relation to their volume. They appear hyperchromatic and lack central pallor. They are readily detected in the dog and are observed in autoimmune and isoimmune hemolytic anemias and following transfusions. These cells are removed from the circulation by the spleen. They are seen in AIHA. When the percentage of cells that are spherocytes is less than 25, the mechanism may be fragmentation or immune mediated. When the spherocytes number 25 to 50 per cent, the mechanism is most likely immune mediated. When spherocytes comprise more than 50 per cent of the RBCs, the mechanism is immune mediated. Usually those cases with 50 to 75 per cent of spherocytes have good reticulocyte responses and respond readily to treatment. When the spherocytes range from 75 to 100 per cent, the reticulocyte response is lower or nonexistent.

Reticulocytes are immature, nonnucleated erythrocytes that still retain basophilic staining material (RNA). Although reticulocytes do not contain a nucleus, the cell still possesses polyribosomes and mitochondria and can therefore synthesize hemoglobin and utilize oxygen. The number of reticulocytes in the peripheral blood is the most commonly used clinical index of erythropoietic activity. Another way of expressing reticulocyte response is:

Reticulocyte Response	Normal	Slight	Moderate	Marked
Dogs, % reticulocytes	1	1–4	5–20	21–50
Cats, % reticulocytes	0–0.4	0.5–2	3–4	5–10

These cells can only be identified by supravital staining methods, such as with new methylene blue (NMB) stain. The degree of reticulocyte count indicates increased erythrogenesis. The cat has a delayed maturation time for reticulocytes. Peak levels of reticulocytes are reached after 11 days (following blood loss of 50 per cent). The normal reticulocyte count in the cat ranges from 1.4 to 10.8 per cent, with a mean of 4.6 per cent. The reticulocyte count should be corrected for PCV:

$$\text{Reticulocyte count} \times \frac{\text{measured Hct}}{\text{normal Hct}} = \text{corrected reticulocyte count.}$$

The reticulocyte index can be computed in the dog and may be helpful in defining nonregenerative vs other forms of anemia:

$$\text{corrected reticulocyte count} \times \dfrac{1}{\text{maturation factor}} = \dfrac{\text{reticulocyte}}{\text{index}}$$

HCT	Maturation Factor
45	1.0
35	1.5
25	2.0
15	2.5

A reticulocyte index of less than 1.0 is found in nonregenerative anemias, 1.0 to 3.0 is found in hemorrhagic anemia, and greater than 3.0 is found in hemolytic anemia.

Erythrocyte refractile bodies (ERB) are round or angular refractile bodies consisting of denatured Hb particles that are best seen with NMB and are commonly called *Heinz bodies*. Healthy cats can have variable numbers of erythrocytes with Heinz bodies, and there is no indication of a shortened erythrocyte survival time (normal cat, 69–79 days). The refractile bodies are 1 to 3 μ in diameter and are located at the periphery of the cell.

Heinz Body Anemia. Heinz bodies result from denatured Hb during periods of excessive oxidative stress. These anemias are acquired and, in the dog, are often associated with the ingestion of onions (the toxic principle of which is N-propyl nitrite). The degree of severity of the hemolytic anemia is variable, and the changes in erythrocytes can best be demonstrated with NMB staining. Heinz body anemia has also been associated with a variety of toxic drugs, including phenothiazines, urinary antiseptics containing methylene blue and phenazopyridine (in the cat), sodium nitrate, and naphthalene. Acetaminophen in the cat can cause severe Heinz body hemolytic anemia (see p. 191).

The life span of RBCs in the dog is approximately 110 to 122 days; in the cat, approximately 69 to 79 days. The stimulus for increased RBC production is persistent anoxia at the level of the renal cortex, resulting in the elaboration of the hormone erythropoietin by the kidney.

Anemias

Anemia is a condition in which there is a diminution in the numbers of erythrocytes or a deficiency in Hb or both. It is a clinical sign of disease, not a diagnosis. The significant clinical signs associated with anemia are pallor, weakness, collapse and shortness of breath, tachycardia, systolic bruits, and malaise. Anemia, a sign of disease, should not be treated without first trying to understand and eliminate the cause.

Anemias may be classified in two basic ways, by either morphology or etiology (Tables 117 and 118).

Table 117. MORPHOLOGIC CLASSIFICATION OF THE ANEMIAS

Macrocytic Normochromic
  Pernicious anemia
  Vitamin B_{12} and folate deficiencies
  Erythemic myelosis in cats
  Macrocytosis of poodles
Macrocytic Hypochromic (occurs during recovery from massive blood loss)
  Hemorrhage
    Injury
    Neoplasms
    Thrombocytopenia
    Blood-clotting disorders
  Hemolytic destruction erythrocytes
    Hemoparasites
    Autoimmune hemolytic anemia (AIHA)
    Heinz body anemia associated with drug toxicity
    Erythrocyte pyruvate kinase deficiency in Basenji dogs
Normocytic Normochromic (a chronic disease producing depression of erythrogenesis)
  Chronic infections
  Nephritis with uremia
  Malignancies
  Hormone deficiencies (i.e., hypothyroidism)
Microcytic Hypochromic
  Iron deficiency
  Vitamin B_6 (pyridoxine) deficiency
  Chronic blood loss (internal parasites)

Adapted from Schalm, O. W.: Morphological classification of the anemias. J. Vet. Clin. Pathol., 7:6, 1978. No. 1, March/April 1978.

Table 118. ETIOLOGIC CLASSIFICATION OF ANEMIA

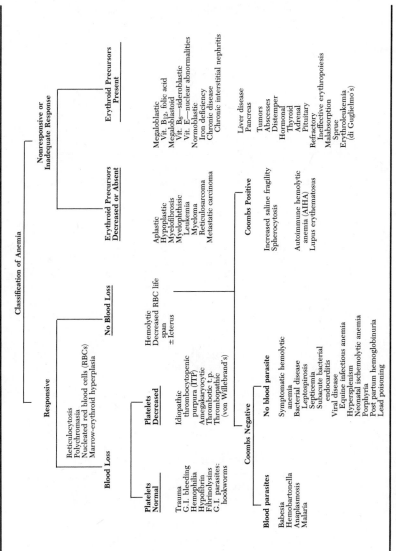

Classification of Anemia

Responsive

Reticulocytosis
Polychromasia
Nucleated red blood cells (RBCs)
Marrow-erythroid hyperplasia

Blood Loss

Platelets Normal

Trauma
G.I. bleeding
Hemophilia
Hypofibrin
Fibrinolysins
G.I. parasites: hookworms

Platelets Decreased

Idiopathic thrombocytopenic purpura (ITP)
Amegakaryocytic
Thrombotic t.p.
Thrombopathic (von Willebrand's)

No Blood Loss

Hemolytic
Decreased RBC life span
± Icterus

Coombs Negative

Blood parasites

Babesia
Hemobartonella
Anaplasmosis
Malaria

No blood parasite

Symptomatic hemolytic anemia
Bacterial disease
Leptospirosis
Septicemia
Subacute bacterial endocarditis
Viral disease
Equine infectious anemia
Hypersplenism
Neonatal ischemolytic anemia
Porphyria
Post partum hemoglobinuria
Lead poisoning

Coombs Positive

Increased saline fragility
Spherocytosis

Autoimmune hemolytic anemia (AIHA)
Lupus erythematosus

Nonresponsive or Inadequate Response

Erythroid Precursors Decreased or Absent

Aplastic
Hypoplastic
Myelofibrosis
Myelophthisic
Leukemia
Myeloma
Reticulosarcoma
Metastatic carcinoma

Erythroid Precursors Present

Megaloblastic
Vit. B₁₂, folic acid
Megaloblastoid
Vit. B₆—sideroblastic
Vit. E—nuclear abnormalities
Normoblastic
Iron deficiency
Chronic disease
Chronic interstitial nephritis

Liver disease
Pancreas

Tumors
Abscesses
Distemper
Hormonal
Thyroid
Adrenal
Pituitary
Refractory
Ineffective erythropoiesis
Malabsorption
Sprue
Erythroleukemia (di Guglielmo's)

Used by permission of Dr. John Switzer.

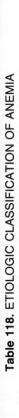

ETIOLOGIC CLASSIFICATION

Anemias can be subdivided into two categories on the basis of excessive loss of erythrocytes owing to hemorrhage or hemolysis and inadequate production of erythrocytes.

Blood Loss Anemias

The anemia of acute blood loss occurs when 25 to 40 per cent of the circulating blood volume is lost over a relatively short period of time. Blood loss anemia may result from overt hemorrhage following trauma or surgery, clotting defects, or rupture of highly vascular malignant tumors such as hemangioendotheliomas. Chronic loss of blood from parasitism may also result in blood loss anemia. Acute uncomplicated blood loss anemia exhibits a marked regenerative response, and the anemia is characteristically normochromic-normocytic. Chronic blood loss anemia associated with parasitisms, gastrointestinal bleeding, or genitourinary tract bleeding may result in a hypochromic microcytic anemia.

Hemangiosarcomas in dogs can present as acute collapse with shock associated with tumor rupture in the peritoneal cavity, thoracic cavity, pericardium, or brain. Dogs with hemangiosarcoma may also present with a history of weakness, intermittent or progressive lethargy, very pale mucous membranes, panting, and exercise intolerance.

The response of the dog to acute external blood loss is predictable. By the third day following blood loss, reticulocytes in increased numbers are present in the peripheral blood. Peak reticulocyte response occurs between the fifth and sixth day. Normoblasts, Howell-Jolly bodies, and anisocytosis are also markedly evident at the time of peak reticulocyte response. Packed cell volume increases from the fourth day to the twenty-first day, after which it is normal. Cats do not respond as rapidly to blood loss, and the peripheral blood smears do not reflect marked polychromasia and anisocytosis.

Internal blood loss into body cavities results in marked absorption by lymphatics, so that two thirds of the lost blood may be absorbed in 24 hours and the balance completely absorbed after 48 to 72 hours.

Hemolysis

A hemolytic state exists when the life span of the red cell is decreased. If destruction is balanced with erythropoiesis, no anemia exists.

Accelerated red cell destruction can be associated with two basic causes: (1) intracorpuscular defects (inherited red cell defects), and (2) extracorpuscular defects (acquired).

Hemolytic anemias are characterized by: (1) signs of regenerative anemia (such as reticulocytosis, polychromasia, and Howell-Jolly bodies); (2) decreased red cell life span; (3) increased osmotic fragility; (4) hyperbilirubinemia and hyperbilirubinuria; (5) elevated fecal urobilinogen; (6) hemoglobinemia and hemoglobinuria; (7) splenomegaly; (8) spherocytes in peripheral smear; and (9) Heinz bodies. (Table 119.)

Table 119. HEMOLYTIC ANEMIA

Type	Red Blood Cell Parasites	Bacterial and Viral Diseases	Autoimmune Hemolytic Anemia	Abnormal Red Blood Cell Metabolism	Symptomatic Idiopathic Hemolytic
Marrow	Erythroid hyperplasia	Erythroid hyperplasia	Erythroid hyperplasia There may be depression	Erythroid hyperplasia	Erythroid hyperplasia
Peripheral blood Reticulocytosis Nucleated red blood cells Polychromasia	Demonstration of parasites Animal inoculation	Morphology: normal siderocytes (EIA)	Spherocytes Poikilocytes Red blood cell fragments	Normochromic Normocytic	Normocytic Normochromic
White blood count	Moderate neutrophilia Atypical lymphocytes	Neutrophilia with left shift Viral—leukopenia, lymphocytosis	Moderate neutrophilia	Normal	Normal to elevated
Platelets	Normal	Normal	Normal to decreased with ITP	Normal	Normal
Saline fragility	Normal to slight increase	Normal to extreme fragility Autohemolysis marked	Increased fragility with characteristic curve	Normal Autohemolysis corrected with glucose or ATP	Usually normal
Coombs' test	Negative	Negative	Positive	Negative	Negative

Used by permission of Dr. John Switzer.

Hemolytic anemias can be peracute, acute, or chronic. In the peracute cases, all signs of regeneration are absent and jaundice and hemoglobinuria may rapidly develop. The spleen may be congested and markedly enlarged.

Acute hemolytic anemia may develop over a period of 1 week. Regenerative signs are usually prominent; jaundice is usually present.

In determining the cause of a hemolytic anemia, the location of the site of RBC destruction is important.

Intravascular Hemolysis. This type of hemolysis usually causes a peracute or acute hemolytic syndrome resulting in hemoglobinemia, hemoglobinuria, increased MCHC, and red discoloration of plasma. If hemolysis is extensive enough and of sufficient duration for bilirubin to be formed and to exceed the liver's capability of conjugating bilirubin, hyperbilirubinemia will be evident. Intravascular hemolysis can be associated with: (1) bacterial infection (e.g., *Leptospira* sp); (2) RBC parasites (e.g., *Babesia* sp); (3) chemicals, that is, those that can produce a Heinz body anemia (e.g., phenothiazines, onion, methylene blue, acetaminophen, phenazopyridine, copper, castor bean, severe hypophosphatemia, and the venae cavae syndrome of dirofilariasis); and (4) immune-mediated etiology (e.g., neonatal isoerythrolysis, incompatible transfusion).

Extravascular Hemolysis. This type of hemolysis usually follows a chronic clinical course. Hb is not evident in plasma or urine. In chronic cases, bone marrow hyperplasia may compensate for RBC destruction, and PCV may be within the normal range. Extravascular hemolysis can be associated with: (1) RBC parasites (e.g., Hemobartonella); (2) immune-mediated etiology (e.g., AIHA, lupus erythematosus); (3) intrinsic erythrocytic defects (e.g., pyruvate kinase deficiency in basenjis and beagles); and (4) increased fragmentation of erythrocytes, as seen in DIC.

Depression Anemia

Bone marrow depression anemias are those anemias in which erythrocytes are produced at a decreased rate or are improperly formed within the bone marrow (hypoproliferative or hyperproliferative with abnormal maturation). The anemia may be hypoplastic if there is partial or incomplete production of erythrocytes or aplastic if there is no development of new erythrocytes.

Bone marrow depression anemias can be caused by:
1. Adverse physical agents such as excessive irradiation.
2. Chemical agents, such as arsenicals, estrogens, and hydrocarbons, and antibiotics, such as chloramphenicol and streptomycin.
3. Metabolic inhibition of bone marrow such as occurs with any chronic infection, chronic interstitial nephritis, chronic liver disease, and endocrine diseases (hypothyroidism and hypopituitarism).
4. Myelophthisic tumors such as lymphosarcoma.

Anemia can also be associated with a variety of other systemic abnormalities. Anemia is seen in chronic inflammatory disease and is characterized by a shortened erythrocyte life span, disordered iron metabolism, depressed bone marrow response, and disordered iron storage. Abnormalities exist in the release of iron storage from the reticuloendothelial system. The anemia is usually normocytic-normochromic. In anemia of inflammatory disorders, there is hypoferremia, a decrease in transferrin, reduced saturation of transferrin, and decreased bone marrow sideroblasts.

The normal serum iron content in the dog is 84 to 233, with a mean of 149 μg per dl; the total iron binding capacity is 284 to 572, with a mean of 391 μg per dl; and the total iron binding capacity saturation is 33 to 37 per cent.

Chronic iron deficiency anemia is found in dogs in whom there is chronic blood loss associated with internal parasitism such as hookworm disease, fleas, chronic bleeding from tumors, hemorrhagic colitis, or gastrointestinal bleeding of unknown etiology. Characteristically, animals with iron deficiency anemia have an Hct below 37 per cent, an Hb below 12 gm per dl, microcytosis with a mean cell volume of less than 60 fl, and lowered serum iron, below 84 μg per dl. Total iron binding capacity is generally normal, and absolute reticulocyte counts may be elevated.

The condition of low serum iron concentration and anemia must be differentiated from the anemia of inflammatory disease (AID; see p. 678). In AID, there is normal to increased storage of iron in the body, but it is inadequately released into the plasma to be transported to and metabolized in developing erythroid cells in the bone marrow.

When stained for iron, bone marrow aspirates show minimal to no iron in iron deficiency anemia, whereas stainable iron is present in normal or increased amounts in AID.

In iron deficiency anemia, ferrous salts can be administered orally at a dosage of 100 to 300 mg of ferrous sulfate (33–100 mg of elemental iron) per day. For systemic administration, iron dextran is the most commonly administered drug. Iron dextran can be administered at 10 mg of elemental iron per kg, divided BID, until the total required dose of iron is attained. The total dose of iron needed can be estimated by using the formula:

$$TD \ (mg) \ = \ BW \ (kg) \ + \ (4.5 \ [15-Hb] \ + \ 30)$$

where TD = total dosage and BW = body weight.

Leukoerythroblastic anemia exists where there is a pronounced elevation in nucleated circulating erythrocytes and immature WBCs. This type of anemia is characteristic of myelophthisis, which is caused by metastatic carcinoma of leukemic infiltration of the bone marrow.

Histiocytic medullary reticulosis is characterized by phagocytosis of RBCs by malignant histiocytes leading to anemia.

Anemias are often associated with feline leukemia virus infection. There may be associated bone marrow hypoplasia. Aplastic anemia may be associated with pancytopenia or may be only RBC aplasia. In some cases, there may be abnormal maturation of RBCs, although there still is adequate bone marrow cellular elements.

Pure red cell aplasia exists when the patient's bone marrow fails to produce RBCs, but normal numbers of WBCs and platelets are produced. Reticulocytes are extremely depressed or absent from peripheral blood, as are RBC precursors from the bone marrow. Although a distinct etiology for this condition is not known, factors to be considered include immune-mediated agents, thymoma, infections, chemicals, and systemic lupus. Treatment involves use of immuno-suppressive agents such as prednisolone and androgens to attempt to stimulate the marrow.

DIAGNOSIS OF ANEMIAS

There are several major questions that should be answered in order to begin to classify anemia as to etiology:

Does a true anemia exist? This can be determined by evaluating the Hb and PCV together with the presenting clinical signs.

Is the anemia hemolytic or nonhemolytic? This question can be answered by examining the urine for excessive bilirubin or hemoglobinuria, presence of free Hb in the plasma, the presence of icterus, increased urobilinogen in the urine and feces, and signs of increased bone marrow activity.

Is the anemia responsive (are the bone marrow and other hematopoietic centers responding to the stress) or unresponsive? A response to an anemia is indicated by increased leukocytes and a shift to the left, increased reticulocytes, nucleated erythrocytes present in the peripheral circulation, polychromatophi-lia, Howell-Jolly bodies, and increased platelet count.

The signs of a nonresponsive anemia are a pale or colorless plasma, decreased leukocytes, absence of reticulocytes, no nucleated erythrocytes, and normal erythrocyte indices.

Exceptions to normal erythropoietic indices would be iron and vitamin B_6 (microcytic hypochromic), or folic acid and vitamin B_{12} (macrocytic hypochromic) deficiencies.

Of primary importance in evaluating nonresponsive anemias is the bone marrow examination. The myeloid-erythroid ratio determines whether eryth-rocytic precursors are present. Examination for abnormally shaped erythroid precursors or for the presence of leukemic or tumor cells has diagnostic importance in refractory anemias.

Examination of the bone marrow can be very helpful in differentiating whether only erythroid precursors are involved in the clinical problem or whether there is also a granulopoietic abnormality.

A. Erythroid hypoplasia and normal granulopoietic response.
   1. Lack of erythropoietin production.
   2. Anemia of chronic inflammatory or neoplastic disease associated with low serum, low iron binding capacity.
   3. As part of the feline leukemia virus (FeLV) complex.
B. Erythroid hypoplasia and granulopoietic hypoplasia. This entity suggests a problem at the stem cell level.
   1. Aplastic anemia that may be associated with radiation.
   2. Myelophthisic anemia—replacement of bone marrow by abnormal ac-cumulation of neoplastic cells.

   3. Infections—feline panleukopenia virus, FeLV complex, ehrlichiosis.
   4. Chemical toxins—chloramphenicol, primidone, phenylbutazone, sulfas.
   5. Chronic renal failure—impaired erythropoietin.
   6. Endocrine disorders—hypothyroidism, lack of androgens; hypoadreno-corticism.
   7. Impairment of DNA synthesis (macrocytic anemia) can involve vitamin B_{12} and folic acid deficiency, with resultant cell arrest in the prorubricyte and rubricyte stages.

C. Defective erythropoiesis with hyperproliferative erythroid bone marrow and defective maturation. In this situation, erythropoietic precursors are numerous in the bone marrow, but abnormal maturation of cells leads to defective RBC function and anemia.
   1. Abnormal nucleic acid synthesis associated with B_{12} and folic acid deficiency.
   2. Impaired hemosynthesis—iron deficiency, pyridoxine deficiency, copper deficiency, lead poisoning.
   3. Erythemic myelosis and erythroleukemia.

Polycythemia

    Polycythemia refers to an increase in the erythrocyte count, Hb concentration, or PCV. *Absolute polycythemia* is an excess of erythrocytes in the circulation accompanied with an increase in total blood volume. Absolute polycythemia can further be divided into secondary polycythemia and primary polycythemia. *Relative polycythemia* refers to an increase in RBC, associated with a decrease in the volume of plasma and signs such as water deprivation, vomiting, diarrhea, fever, general malnutrition, and acute shock. Shifting of body fluids from plasma to interstitial tissue such as occurs with shock, especially abdominal problems that induce shock and burns, can result in polycythemia. The distinction between absolute polycythemia and relative polycythemia can be made by examining the hemogram (or "blood picture"*).

    In absolute secondary polycythemia, there is an increase in the total RBC mass (erythron) as a response to hypoxia (Table 120).

    Abnormalities with erythropoietin production may be associated with renal tumors, renal vascular impairment, renal cysts, hydronephrosis, release of erythropoietin-like substance from hepatomas, uterine myoma, or cerebellar hemangiomas. In the dog, secondary polycythemia has been associated with renal carcinomas.

    Most cases of secondary polycythemia are associated with generalized hypoxia that can be caused by: (1) low ambient oxygen tension, (2) respiratory hypoventilation, (3) obstructive pulmonary disease, (4) AV shunting, or (5) abnormal Hb. Renal ischemia can result in increased RBC production.

---

   *From Dorland's Illustrated Medical Dictionary, 25th ed. Philadelphia, W. B. Saunders Company, 1974.

Table 120. DIFFERENTIAL FEATURES OF POLYCYTHEMIA

Feature	Relative	Polycythemia Vera	Secondary Hypoxia	Secondary Renal Disease
Red cell volume	Normal	Increased	Increased	Increased
Plasma volume	Decreased	Usually normal	Normal to decreased	Variable
Leukocyte count	Increased	Man—increased Animals—variable	Normal	Usually normal
Arterial oxygen saturation	Normal	Normal	Decreased	Normal
Erythropoietin level	Normal	Decreased to normal	Increased	Increased

From Benjamin, M.: Outline of Veterinary Clinical Pathology, 3rd ed. Ames, Iowa, Iowa State University Press, 1979.

Primary polycythemia (polycythemia vera) is considered to be a myeloproliferative disease, with the development of myeloid metaplasia and acute leukemia as a possible outcome. No excessive erythropoietin is required for this abnormal cloning of erythocytic precursors. In primary polycythemia, increased RBC mass results in increased RBC viscosity and hypoxia, thromboembolism, and rupture of damaged vessels. This is a disease in middle-aged dogs and has no gender predilection.

The use of radioactive chromium (^{51}Cr) labeling of RBC mass can be used to document abnormal RBC masses.

A variety of techniques have been used to treat polycythemia vera, including bleeding and various immunosuppressive and chemotherapeutic agents, such as hydroxyurea. Hydroxyurea is initially given in a loading dose of 30 mg per kg per day for 7 to 10 days, followed by 15 mg per kg per day in single or divided doses. The PCV is initially reduced to less than 60 per cent, with repeated phlebotomies withdrawing 20 ml per kg of blood and replacing fluid volume.

Blood Groups and Crossmatching (See also p. 622)

There are at least 15 different blood factors known in the dog. Only CEA-1* and CEA-2, and possibly CEA-7, are antigenic enough to pose a threat in transfusion reactions. Factors CEA-1 and CEA-2 (old blood Type A) appear to be dominant. Thirty-seven per cent of dogs are CEA-1 and CEA-2 negative, and 63 per cent are CEA-1 and CEA-2 positive. Transfusion of CEA-1 and CEA-2 positive blood into CEA-1 and CEA-2 negative dogs may lead to the development of anti–CEA-1,2 antibodies, which are potential hemolysins in

---

*CEA = canine erythrocyte antigens

both in vivo and in vitro conditions. On the first random transfusion, approximately 25 per cent of these transfusions have the potentiality for the production of anti–CEA-1,2 antibodies. If a CEA-1,2 negative dog that has been previously immunized receives CEA-1,2 positive blood, a transfusion reaction occurs within 1 hour, which is characterized by hemoglobinemia, hemoglobinuria, thrombocytopenia, leukopenia, fever, emesis, incontinence, urticaria, and weakness. With a second transfusion, the probability of receiving incompatible blood from randomly selected donors is about 15 per cent. The major danger is in administering CEA-1,2 positive blood for a second and third time to a CEA-1,2 negative recipient. A CEA-1,2 negative bitch sensitized to CEA-1,2 positive blood through transfusions and mated to a CEA-1,2 positive sire may also produce puppies with neonatal isoerythrolysis after suckling.

All blood donors should be CEA-1,2 negative to prevent transfusion reactions due to the CEA-1,2 factor. The A positive dog is a universal recipient. Blood typing is commercially available through Stormont Laboratories, 1237 E. Beamer St., Suite D, Woodland, California 95695.

BLOOD CROSSMATCHING

The test of the recipient's serum with the donor's RBCs is known as a *major crossmatch;* when the donor's plasma and recipient's RBCs are used, it is called *minor crossmatch.* Under most circumstances, a major crossmatch is performed.

BLOOD CROSSMATCHING

	Donor (vol ml)		Recipient (vol ml)	
	Red Cells	Serum	Red Cells	Serum
Major crossmatch	0.1	—	—	0.1
Minor crossmatch	—	0.1	0.1	—
Donor control	0.1	0.1	—	—
Recipient control	—	—	0.1	0.1

*Performed at 37°C, room temperature, and 4°C (see text)

Note: Blood for replacement to treat bleeding disorders should be collected in ACD, CPD, or similar anticoagulant and *not* in heparin.

Fresh blood of the donor and recipient should be used in crossmatching. Two drops of a 4 per cent suspension of the donor's RBCs suspended in donor's serum are mixed with 2 drops of recipient's serum in a 7 × 60 mm test tube. The tube is incubated at room temperature for 15 minutes. After centrifuging the tube for 1 minute at 1000 rpm, examine the contents for hemolysis and agglutination. Using a similar procedure, set up a control with the donor's serum and RBCs in the same tube. The presence of significant hemolysis or agglutination in the crossmatched tube indicates incompatibility of blood donor and recipient.

Interpretation of Bone Marrow

Bone marrow is a site of production of erythrocytes, granulocytes, and thrombocytes. For methods by which bone marrow can be obtained from the dog and cat, see p. 494. When the bone marrow material has been obtained, a differential count of 500 nucleated cells should be made. The myeloid to erythroid (M:E) ratio should be determined by dividing the number of nucleated RBCs into the sum of all cells belonging to the granulocytic series. When the total leukocyte count is within the normal range for the species, the M:E ratio can be used to indicate depression or acceleration of erythrogenesis. Different areas of the bone marrow smear should be included in the cell count. Normal values for M:E ratio range from 0.75 to 2.5, with a mean of 1.20:1.0. The normal M:E ratio in the cat is 0.60 to 3.90, with a mean of 1.6:1.0 (Schalm et al., 1975). An elevated M:E ratio indicates myeloid hyperplasia, and/or erythroid hypoplasia; a low M:E ratio indicates the opposite situation. The M:E ratio may appear normal in bone marrow hypoplasia if both erythroid and myeloid elements are depressed. Evaluation of the M:E ratio is not as important as are the cellularity and the types of cells found in the bone marrow.

Examples of conditions in which an increased M:E ratio may occur are leukocytosis, leukemoid reaction, granulocytic leukemia, lymphosarcoma, and erythemic hypoplasia. A decreased M:E ratio may be associated with a reduction in the number of myeloid cells, hyperplasia of erythropoietic tissue, metarubricytic (normoblastic) response associated with hemorrhage, hemolysis, iron deficiency, lead poisoning, cirrhosis of the liver, polycythemia vera, and rubriblastic (megaloblastic) response associated with a deficiency of vitamin B_{12} and/or folic acid. Tumors of RBC-producing tissues (as in erythemic myelosis) can also alter the M:E ratio.

The Thrombon

The thrombon consists of circulating blood platelets and megakaryocytes and megakaryoblasts in the bone marrow. Megakaryocytes do not divide, but platelets are formed when invaginations of the megakaryocyte membrane coalesce and platelets are released as ribbons which fragment into individual platelets. Approximately 150 to 200 platelets are formed from a single megakaryocyte by fragmentation of a ribbon. Thrombopoietin is a plasma factor that stimulates this fragmentation. Maturation time for the development of a mature platelet is 3 days, and normal platelet life span is 7 to 10 days.

Blood platelets are involved in both the intrinsic and extrinsic pathways of coagulation and are essential for the formation of the prothrombin-converting enzyme complex in the intrinsic coagulation pathway. The platelet component is called *platelet factor 3* (PF-3). Other platelet factors have been found that are involved in the intrinsic blood-clotting pathway.

The normal range of blood platelets is from 200,000 to 500,000 per μL of blood.

Abnormalities of the thrombon can be either quantitative or qualitative.

Effective management of thrombocytopenia involves the correction of the underlying problem where possible. Infectious agents such as *Ehrlichia* or *Rickettsia rickettsii* should be eliminated and DIC should be treated. Avoid the administration of drugs with antiplatelet activity.

When platelet numbers fall to the level that petechiation and bleeding develop, transfusions of fresh platelets are necessary (see p. 709). Whole fresh blood taken in plastic bags should be used. Enough fresh whole blood should be given to increase the patient's platelet count to 100,000/mm³. If platelet-rich plasma can be prepared, it has distinct advantages when administered at a rate of 6 to 10 ml per kg.

Immune-mediated thrombocytopenia is treated with corticosteroids. If corticosteroids are not helpful, the use of vincristine in low doses can be added and has resulted in increased levels of circulating platelets. The dose of vincristine is 0.01 to 0.025 mg per kg. Corticosteroids reduce the titre of antiplatelet antibody, platelet sequestration, and splenic and hepatic destruction of platelets. Prednisolone may be administered in dosages of 0.5 to 1.5 mg per kg every 12 hours during the acute phase of thrombocytopenia. Therapy should continue until the platelet count is greater than 100,000 per mm³; then corticosteroids should be tapered off very slowly.

Evaluation of the Leukocyte Response

Leukocytes serve the function of protecting the body against foreign substances. The two basic mechanisms involved are phagocytosis and antibody production.

Phagocytes consist of the granulocytes—neutrophils, eosinophils, and basophils—and monocytes.

The immunocyte system is concerned with the production of antibody and with cell-mediated immunity. Cells of the immunocyte system are the thymic-derived lymphocytes (also known as T-l, T-lymphocytes, and T cells)— concerned with direct cell-mediated immunity—and the "bursa-equivalent" lymphocytes (also known as B-1, B-lymphocytes, and B cells)—concerned with antibody production.

Leukocytic changes in the peripheral blood can be associated with (1) diseases that affect the blood-forming organs (such as the bone marrow, lymphoid tissue, spleen, and reticuloendothelial system) and (2) diseases that affect other body tissues in such a way as to mobilize leukocytes to the area of injury or disease. In order to obtain the maximum information from leukocyte examinations, the total leukocyte count must be correlated with the differential count.

Clinical Interpretation of the Leukogram

The *leukogram* consists of the total and differential leukocyte count and the morphologic assessment of blood leukocytes. Included in the interpretation of the leukocyte response is the total leukocyte count and differential cell patterns, along with any distinctive morphologic changes.

General Leukocyte Responses

Leukopenia

Leukopenia refers to a decrease in the total number of circulating leukocytes. Leukopenia can be associated with infections of viral etiology, destroying young myeloid cells. In the early stages of an infectious disease that is bacterial in origin, there can be a depletion of peripheral blood leukocytes until the bone marrow produces more leukocytes. In cases of shock, leukocytes can become sequestered in capillaries of the lung, liver, and spleen. Bone marrow abnormalities can lead to abnormal production of leukocytes or to an abnormal life span of leukocytes. Bone marrow can be affected by some of the following abnormalities: (1) hypoplasia associated with metabolic abnormalities, ionizing radiation, or chemical agents; (2) bone marrow dysplasia, with normal marrow becoming replaced with tumor cells (myelophthisic); (3) abnormalities of maturation of cells associated with vitamin B_{12} deficiency; and (4) the action of chemical agents on the bone marrow.

Leukocytosis

Leukocytosis refers to an increased number of leukocytes beyond the normally accepted range per μL. In most instances, only one predominant cell type is elevated in numbers; however, simultaneous increases of several types may occur. Increases in total number of neutrophils exceed any other cell type; thus, leukocytosis usually implies neutrophilia unless another specific cell type is designated.

The degree of leukocytosis may be related to numerous factors, including cause, severity of the infection, resistance of the animal, location of the inflammatory response, and species variation. Estimations of the neutrophil-leukocyte ratio can be used to predict an animal's ability to handle leukocytic response (see table below).

	N/LE Ratio	Leukopenia	Leukocytosis *Moderate*	*Marked*	*Extreme*
Dog	3.5	6000/μL	18–30	30–50	50–100
Cat	1.8	8000/μL	20–30	30–50	50–76

Neutrophil Responses

The interpretation of neutrophil responses depends on the total number of neutrophils present per μL of blood and the presence or absence of morphologic changes within the cells. The following information is pertinent when interpreting neutrophil responses:

1. The primary functions of neutrophils are phagocytosis and bactericidal action.
2. Neutrophil maturation proceeds through morphologic stages in the bone marrow.
3. Regulation of neutrophil production is by granulopoietin (or a colony-stimulating factor), which is produced by stimulation of bacterial products.
4. Neutrophil release from the bone marrow is promoted by a leukocytosis-inducing factor.

Neutrophilia Without a Left Shift

Physiologic events such as increased blood flow associated with muscular activity, increased heart rate, increased blood pressure, and increased production of epinephrine can mobilize neutrophils normally located in the margins of small vessels.

Corticosteroids of either endogenous or exogenous origin cause neutrophilia without a left shift, as well as lymphopenia, eosinopenia, and occasional monocytes.

Neutrophilia can accompany inflammatory disorders in cases in which the tissue reaction does not stimulate large numbers of immature neutrophils to be present.

Neutrophilia With a Left Shift

Neutrophilia with a left shift is an increase in the peripheral blood of immature cells of the granulocytic series. It indicates the presence of inflammation with a tissue demand for neutrophils. Neutrophil release from the bone marrow is age related, with the most mature cells being released the earliest. The increase in neutrophils is usually orderly, with increased numbers of band neutrophils usually exceeding neutrophilic metamyelocytes. If immature neutrophile production is not orderly, granulocytic leukemia could be present.

Normal Neutrophil Count With a Left Shift

The presence of a low, normal, or slightly elevated total leukocyte count with an increase of immature cells in the peripheral blood is called *a degenerative shift to the left*.

If this response exists, it is important to interpret subsequent leukocytic responses to determine whether immature neutrophils are accompanied by an increased WBC count. If continued stress for production of neutrophils is placed on the bone marrow, if total neutrophil numbers fail to increase, and if immature neutrophils persist, this may signify severe purulent inflammatory disease and the release of toxic products as occurs in septicemia or bacterial sepsis.

Neutropenia With or Without a Left Shift

Neutropenia indicates a lower than normal WBC count and is associated with a deficiency of functional neutrophils in the peripheral blood.

Neutropenia can result from (1) a sudden demand for increased numbers of neutrophilic leukocytes, (2) sequestration of circulating neutrophils, and (3) decreased bone marrow production of neutrophils.

Neutropenia may indicate severe bacterial infection and toxemia such as occurs in acute metritis, aspiration pneumonia, acute peritonitis, and bacterial pneumonia. Bone marrow depression can be associated with myelophthisic tumors as a manifestation of systemic disease (such as feline leukemia). Neutropenia can also be associated with a reduction of granulopoiesis in the bone marrow that may be drug-induced or associated with chronic infection or malignancies replacing bone marrow elements. Deficiencies in vitamin B_{12} and folic acid can impair the development of mature neutrophils. Congenital defects of neutrophil development are also known, such as cyclic neutropenia in gray collies.

Immune-Mediated Neutropenia

Immune-mediated neutropenia is a disease in which there is a persistent neutropenia with monocytosis while other blood cells remain normal. The bone marrow may be hypocellular but has greatly reduced numbers of more mature neutrophils. Progranulocytes and myelocytes predominate, and the M:E ratio is usually high. The absence of more mature, postmitotic granulocytes is described as a "maturation arrest"; however, this term should be used only when direct evidence of inhibition of mitosis or intramarrow granulocyte destruction can be shown. A definitive diagnosis of immune-mediated neutropenia depends on whether an antineutrophil antibody is evident.

A wide variety of causes for immunoneutropenia have been demonstrated, including idiopathic, viral, or bacterial infections; drug therapy; neoplasia; isoimmune neonatal neutropenia; and transfusion-induced isoimmune neutropenia. These causes have most frequently been described in man.

Antineutrophil antibody in the circulation changes the neutrophil membrane, making the neutrophil more susceptible to damage and resultant phagocytosis by marrow macrophages. These neutrophils have a shortened intravascular survival time. The circulating antineutrophil antibody is predominantly of the IgG type.

Lymphocyte Responses

Lymphocytes are part of the immunocyte system of the body that responds to foreign antigens by producing antibody and mounting a direct cellular response. Subpopulations of lymphocytes are functionally different: the thymic-derived T cells are concerned with direct cell-mediated immunity, whereas the gut-derived B cells are concerned with antibody production.

Lymphocytes can be produced in several areas of the body. Lymphocyte production occurs chiefly in the thymus and bone marrow. The circulating small lymphocytes represent two populations of cells—namely, B- and T-lymphocytes. Lymph nodes are not sites of intense lymphocyte production but, rather, are sites of phagocytic activity, with antigen draining into regional lymph nodes and stimulating B-lymphocytes. Lymph nodes, spleen, and gut-associated lymphatic tissue are seeded by lymphocytes formed elsewhere; with antigenic stimulation, local lymphopoiesis occurs.

Lymphopenia

Lymphopenia denotes reduced numbers of circulating lymphocytes. In the dog, this would be less than 1000 cells per μL and, in the cat, less than 1500 cells per μL. Lymphopenia is associated with (1) lymphocyte destruction or cell redistribution associated with increased endogenous or exogenous corticosteroid levels; (2) loss of lymphatic fluid as in chylothorax or chronic enteric disease; and (3) lysis of lymphocytes, which is associated with systemic infections such as canine distemper, canine hepatitis, radiation injury, and use of immunosuppressive drugs.

Lymphocytosis

Lymphocytosis is an increase in the total lymphocyte count above normal and can be associated with (1) physiologic lymphocytosis accompanying fear, excitement, and handling (this is especially prevalent in the cat; also, young animals have higher lymphocyte counts than older animals); (2) prolonged or abnormal antigenic stimulation; (3) hypoadrenocorticism; and (4) lymphocytic leukemia.

Eosinophil Responses

Eosinophils originate in the bone marrow where a high percentage of cells are mature (75 per cent) and serve as a reservoir of cell release. Eosinophils are found in various tissues that are portals of entry of antigenic agents and potential histamine release. These tissues are gut, respiratory, and urinary tracts. Eosinophilia in the dog refers to the presence of more than 750 cells per μL.

Two characteristics distinguish the eosinophil from the neutrophil and other leukocytes: (1) eosinophils can inactivate mediators released from mast cells and reduce the reaction associated with IgE-mediated degranulation of mast cells; and (2) eosinophils can damage the larval stage of helminth parasites, such as Shistosoma mansoni. Eosinophils can also react chemotactically to mediators released in other immunologic reactions, including split products of complement and products of activated lymphocytes (eosinophil-stimulation promoter and eosinophil chemotactic factor).

The eosinophil cell contains specific enzymes that reduce IgE-mediated inflammation: (1) Ten to 20 times as much arylsulfatase-B as found in neutrophils; (2) phospholipase D; (3) lysophospholipase activity; and (4) histaminase.

Evidence indicates that degranulation of the eosinophil cell releases major basic protein, which, when it comes into contact with antibody-coated parasites, may destroy them.

Diseases and organ function problems that involve the release of histamine, serotonin, and bradykinin can produce elevated levels of eosinophils. Some of the causes are (1) parasitisms; (2) allergies involving the skin, gastrointestinal tract, and upper respiratory tract; (3) adrenocortical insufficiency; (4) eosinophillic myositis and panosteitis; (5) eosinophilic leukemia; and (6) degeneration of body tissue and proteins.

Lower than normal levels of eosinophils result in eosinopenia, which can be induced by (1) hyperadrenocorticism; (2) administration of corticosteroids or ACTH; and (3) prolonged systemic stress associated with inflammation, trauma, or intoxications.

Basophil Responses

Basophils are produced in the bone marrow and may be present in cellular immune reactions. Basophilic granules contain heparin in a bound form with histamine, serotonin, and hyaluronic acid. Tissues that contain mast cells (basophil cells within tissues) are skin and subcutaneous tissue, lung, gastrointestinal tract, uterus, scrotum, and serosal linings.

Monocyte Responses

Monocytes are produced in the reticuloendothelial system and are transformed into macrophages when present in tissues. Monocytes are phagocytic cells that persist for longer periods of time in tissues than do neutrophils and, when present in increased numbers in the leukogram, may indicate chronic suppurative inflammation or acute stress.

Erythrocyte Sedimentation Rate (ESR)

If blood containing anticoagulant is allowed to stand in an upright tube, the erythrocytes will gradually settle to the bottom. The rate at which the settling takes place is an index of the reaction of the body to disease or injury. To interpret the sedimentation rate, one must compare the obtained value with the value expected for the PCV of the animal. The corrected value is expressed as "minus" when the sedimentation rate is less than expected and "plus" when it is more than expected.

The following are the anticipated ESR values for the dog:

PCV (per cent)	ESR at 60 min
10	79
15	64
20	49
25	36
30	26
35	16
40	10
45	5
50	0

The following factors can influence the sedimentation rate:

1. Alterations in the composition of the plasma may occur in inflammatory, neoplastic, and metabolic diseases. Increased levels of globulin and fibrinogen may produce clumping or aggregation of erythrocytes, followed by rapid settling of these cells.
2. Alterations in the numbers of erythrocytes present in the circulation can affect the sedimentation rate. Negative sedimentation values are often related to the presence of young erythrocytes in large numbers in anemia in remission. These young blood cells do not form rouleaux, and they stay dispersed in the plasma. Young cells also have a lower specific gravity than mature RBCs, which does not permit them to settle as rapidly. A reddish tinge in the lower portion of the plasma fraction of the sedimentation tube indicates the presence of young erythrocytes (diphasic reaction).
3. The size of the erythrocytes can influence the sedimentation reaction. The presence of macrocytes and spherocytes increases the sedimentation rate whereas microcytes, leptocytes, and poikilocytes retard the sedimentation rate.
4. The type of anticoagulant used, the age of the blood sample (samples more than 2 hours old have decreased sedimentation rates), the diameter of the sedimentation tube, and the position of the tube influence the sedimentation rate.

The sedimentation rate is a nonspecific test. It is a valuable procedure in determining the presence of some diseases and in following the course of a disease. A normal sedimentation rate, however, does not rule out the presence of disease. The sedimentation rate can be used as a guide to prognosis.

Increased sedimentation rates can be found in:

1. Infectious diseases such as leptospirosis and canine distemper.
2. Some neoplastic diseases.
3. Systemic infections, such as bacterial endocarditis, and in localized infections, such as pneumonia, myocarditis, and pleuritis.
4. Parasitism such as infestation with heart worms.
5. Secondary skin disorders in which there is alteration in plasma proteins.
6. Pregnancy.
7. Radiation injury.
8. Metabolic abnormalities such as hypercholesterolemia.

References and Additional Readings

Benjamin, M. M.: Outlines of Veterinary Clinical Pathology, 3rd ed. Ames, Iowa, Iowa State University Press, 1978.

Butterworth, A. E., and David, J. R.: Eosinophil function. N. Engl. J. Med., 304(3):154, 1981.

Chickering, W. R., and Prasse, K. W.: Immune-mediated neutropenia in man and animals. Vet. Clin. Pathol., 10(1):6, 1981.

Cotter, S. M.: Anemia associated with feline leukemia virus infection. J.A.V.M.A., 175:1191, 1979.

Cramer, D. V., and Lewis, R. M.: Reticulocyte response in the cat. J.A.V.M.A., 160:61, 1972.

Davenport, D. J., and Breitschwerdt, E. B.: Platelet disorders in the dog and cat. Compendium on Continuing Education, 4(10):788, 1982.

Duncan, J. R., and Prasse, K. W.: Veterinary Laboratory Medicine. Ames, Iowa, Iowa State University Press, 1977.

Fees, D. L., and Withrow, S. J.: Canine hemangiosarcoma. Compendium on Continuing Education, 3(12):1047, 1981.

Feldman, B. F., Kaneko, J. J., and Farver, T. B.: Anemia of inflammatory disease in the dog. Clinical characterization. Am. J. Vet. Res., 42(7):1109, 1981.

Greene, C. E., et al.: Vincristine in the treatment of thrombocytopenia in five dogs. J.A.V.M.A., 180(2):140, 1982.

Harvey, J. W.: Canine hemolytic anemias. J.A.V.M.A., 176:970, 1980.

Harvey, J. W., French, T. W., and Meyer, D. J.: Chronic iron deficiency anemia in dogs. J.A.A.H.A., 18(6):946, 1982.

Lewis, H. B., and Rebar, A. H.: Bone Marrow Evaluation in Veterinary Practice. St. Louis, Missouri, Ralston Purina Company, 1979.

Payne, B. J., Lewis, H. B., Murchison, T. E., et al.: Hematology of laboratory animals. In Melby, E. C., and Altman, N. H. (eds.): Handbook of Laboratory Animal Science, Vol. III. Cleveland, Ohio, CRC Press, 1976, pp. 383–461.

Peterson, M. E., and Randolph, J. F.: Diagnosis of canine primary polycythemia and management with hydroxyurea. J.A.V.M.A., 180(4):415, 1982.

Schalm, O. W., Jain, N. C., and Carroll, E. J.: Veterinary Hematology, 3rd ed. Philadelphia, Lea & Febiger, 1975.

Tasker, J. B.: Symposium on clinical laboratory medicine. Vet. Clin. North Am., 6:1976.

Hematopoietic Neoplasms

This group of blood disorders is characterized by malignant neoplasia of the hematopoietic tissues, which may include bone marrow, lymphoid tissue, the reticuloendothelial system, and the plasma cell system. The disease can be classified according to the predominant cell type; however, the parent neoplastic tissues may all be of one stem cell type. (Table 121.)

Leukemia is the generalized, neoplastic malignant growth of one of the leukocytic tissues and refers to the presence of neoplastic cells in the circulating blood.

Lymphosarcoma refers to a neoplastic proliferation of abnormal lymphocytes or their precursors in lymph nodes or other lymphatic tissue, resulting in enlarged lymphatic tissue and infiltration of various tissues by neoplastic cells.

Reticulum cell sarcoma is a neoplastic proliferation of reticulum cells of lymph nodes or other reticuloendothelial areas, resulting in tumor formation and infiltration of various tissues.

Myeloproliferative disorders are a complex of cellular abnormalities arising in the bone marrow. The stages of myeloproliferative disorders can be categorized into reticuloendotheliosis, erythemic myelosis, erythroleukemia, granulocytic leukemia, monocytic leukemia, and myelomonocytic leukemia.

Myelogenous tumor refers to the presence of primary neoplastic cells within the bone marrow.

Erythemic myelosis, erythroleukemia, and reticuloendotheliosis refer to hematopoietic tumors of erythroid precursors.

Table 121. CLASSIFICATION OF HEMOPOIETIC NEOPLASMS

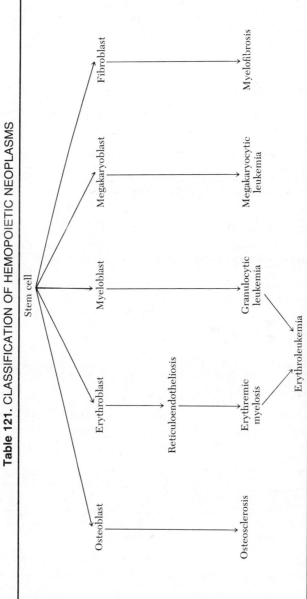

From Benjamin, M.: Veterinary Clinical Pathology, 3rd ed. Ames, Iowa, Iowa State University Press, 1979, p. 155.

Erythroleukemia is characterized by abnormal proliferation of both erythroid and myeloid cell lines. Myeloproliferative disorders may begin as erythemic myelosis, progress to erythroleukemia, and terminate as granulocyticleukemia.

Reticuloendotheliosis refers to a myeloproliferative disorder of the cat with immature, undifferentiated reticuloendothelial cells in the blood and bone marrow.

Feline Leukemia Virus (Feline Leukemia Complex)

Leukemia complex is a term used to describe all the neoplastic diseases of hematopoietic or blood-forming cells originating in bone marrow or lymphoid tissue. Approximately one third of all cat tumors are hematopoietic tumors, and 90 per cent are lymphoid tumors. The cause of the feline leukemia complex is an RNA virus termed *C-type virus* and classified in the Oncorna virus genus and Retrovirus family. The virus contains an enzyme, reverse transcriptase, which allows the virus to produce DNA copy and more viral RNA, thus being able to form new complete viral units. Cells infected with C-type viruses can begin to neoplastically proliferate. Virus-infected tissue can be identified by: (1) demonstration using electron microscopy; (2) demonstration of feline leukemia virus (FeLV) structural proteins and glycoproteins in the cytoplasm and on the surface of infected cells as indicated by positive immunofluorescent techniques; and (3) cytotoxicity test.

FeLV can cause a variety of hematopoietic neoplasms and anemias, as well as some immune-deficiency conditions.

Most tumors caused by FeLV are classified as lymphosarcomas and consist of solid masses of proliferating lymphocytes. Lymphosarcomas are seen in thymic, alimentary, renal, generalized, or miscellaneous forms.

FeLV is very widespread in nature. It has been estimated that 1.8 to 3.5 per cent of cats in the general free-roaming cat population are chronic virus carriers. Cats in urban areas and catteries show a much higher incidence of exposure to the virus. FeLV is shed in the saliva, urine, and feces of infected cats and is present in the blood cells and platelets. The virus can also be transmitted from mother to offspring, either in utero or following birth.

The period of disease development in healthy cats infected with FeLV is variable; however, studies indicate that 83 per cent of FeLV-infected cats die within 3 years.

Diagnosis of lymphosarcoma in the cat depends on what primary tissues are affected. In the gastrointestinal form, vomiting, diarrhea, constipation, and anorexia are the signs most often seen. In the multicentric form, icterus and uremia are often present when there is extensive infiltration of the liver and kidneys. The anterior mediastinal form may be characterized by difficulty in swallowing, dyspnea, coughing, and vomiting after eating. Often, there are nonspecific signs such as lethargy, anemia, loss of weight, anorexia, and dehydration.

Enlargement of peripheral lymph nodes is not commonly found in lymphosarcoma of the cat; nevertheless, all lymph nodes should be carefully examined. In addition, the liver, spleen, mesenteric lymph nodes, and kidneys should be examined for any indication of enlargement. Aspiration of fluid (thoracentesis or paracentesis) may be helpful when exfoliative cytology is performed.

Examination of peripheral blood smears in cats with lymphosarcoma reveals that a pronounced normocytic-normochromic anemia is present in 65 to 70 per cent of the cases. A high percentage of these cases involves a nonresponsive anemia. There is an absolute leukocytosis in 30 per cent of the cases, an absolute leukocytopenia in 10 per cent of the cases, and an absolute lymphocytopenia in 40 per cent of the cases. Leukemia is present in 10 to 30 per cent of the cases, depending on the stage of the disease at examination.

Most feline lymphosarcomas are of T-cell origin; however, B-cell lymphosarcoma is observed in the alimentary form. Seventy per cent of cats with lymphosarcoma are FeLV positive, and 30 per cent have no detectable FeLV antigens. Both FeLV positive and FeLV negative lymphosarcoma cells have tumor-specific feline oncornavirus–associated cell membrane antigen (FOCMA).

Ancillary examinations that may be helpful include radiographs of the thorax and abdomen, thoracentesis and paracentesis coupled with exfoliative cytology, intravenous pyelogram (IVP) examination, pneumoperitoneogram, and biopsy of any suspicious tissue.

FeLV is infectious for cats and is transmitted primarily via the saliva and urine. The prevalence of FeLV among cats depends on their environment. It has been estimated that 33 per cent of cats in a multicat household may be infected, less than 1 per cent of cats living alone are infected, and only 0.9 per cent of stray cats with an unknown history of FeLV exposure are infected. In hospital blood donor cats, 12 per cent have been found to be infected with FeLV.

The extent of disease in FeLV–exposed cats is dependent on the immunologic response to FeLV envelope antigens and to the FeLV– and FeSV–induced tumor-specific antigen. Forty per cent of cats exposed to FeLV envelope antigen produce high neutralizing antibody titers and become immune to infection; 30 per cent of FeLV–exposed cats do not produce an effective immune response and become persistently infected; 30 per cent of exposed cats neither become infected nor become immune to FeLV and are susceptible to FeLV infection.

Immunity to FeLV antigen can be developed, and two kinds of antibodies have been described: (1) a virus neutralizing antibody, and (2) FOCMA antibodies, which are antibodies against feline oncornavirus–associated cell membrane antigens. The standard tests that are used to demonstrate the presence of FeLV in a host are the FeLV immunofluorescent antibody (IFA) test and the FeLV enzyme–linked immunoabsorbent assay (ELISA) test. A positive IFA test is indicative of the presence of infectious FeLV in the cat. About 97 per cent of IFA–positive cats remain infected for life, and 3 per cent of those cats reject the virus and develop immunity to FeLV and become IFA negative.

The ELISA test detects soluble $FeLV_{p27}$ antigens in the plasma or serum of FeLV–infected cats. Controversy exists concerning whether the ELISA test should be the final conclusive test in determining whether a cat is infected with FeLV. The ELISA test has been positive in cases in which the FeLV IFA test is negative, and the virus could be isolated from 68 per cent of the cats with ELISA–positive tests and from 98.5 per cent of the cats with IFA-positive tests. The FeLV IFA test can be used to confirm ELISA–screening findings.

Cats that have protective titers of FOCMA antibody will not develop lymphosarcoma; however, they can develop the other diseases associated with FeLV.

Most unexposed cats in the general pet cat population and the majority of FeLV–exposed cats, do not have protective titers (>1:10) of FeLV–neutralizing antibody. FeLV–infected cats do not have FeLV–neutralizing antibody.

Hardy has used information obtained from data on FeLV–neutralizing antibody and FOCMA–antibody status to classify healthy cats into one of six categories, as described in Tables 122 through 124.

FeLV is capable of growing in canine or human tissue culture cells. However, FeLV antigen has never been found in any human tumors thus far examined. The cat, a known harborer of an oncogenic virus, is always in very close contact with man. For this reason, the public health significance of FeLV is being carefully investigated. At this time, there is no definitive proof that vertical transmission of FeLV may occur between the cat and man; however, it is strongly recommended that cats afflicted with lymphosarcoma be euthanized and not held for treatment.

Cats exposed to FeLV can respond in several different ways:
1. Not become infected at all.
2. Become temporarily infected, develop immunity, and overcome the infection.

Table 122. IMMUNE CLASSES OF HEALTHY CATS: CLASSES OF HEALTHY CATS BASED ON THEIR FeLV STATUS AND THEIR ANTIBODY RESPONSE TO FeLV AND FOCMA

Class of Healthy Cat	Exposure History	FeLV Status	Protective FeLV Neutralizing Antibody ($\geq$1:10)	Protective FOCMA Antibody ($\geq$1:32)	Susceptibility or Resistance	
					to FeLV Infection	to LSA Development
1	not exposed	−	−	−	susceptible	susceptible
2	exposed	−	−	+	susceptible	resistant
3	exposed	−	+	−	resistant	susceptible
4	exposed	−	+	+	resistant	resistant
5	exposed	+	−	−	infected	very susceptible
6	exposed	+	−	+	infected	resistant

From Hardy, W. D.: Current status of FeLV diseases. Friskies Res. Digest, 5:1, 1979.

Table 123. FeLV DISEASES

Cell Type	Proliferative Diseases (Neoplastic)	Degenerative Diseases (Blastopenic)
Diseases known to be caused by FeLV		
Lymphoid cells	Lymphosarcoma	Thymic atrophy (kittens)
	Reticulum cell sarcoma	Immunosuppressive diseases (adults)
Bone marrow cells		
Primitive mesenchymal cell	Reticuloendotheliosis	—
Erythroblast	Erythremic myelosis	Erythroblastosis (regenerative anemia)
	Erythroleukemia	Erythroblastopenia (nonregenerative anemia)
		Pancytopenia
Myeloblast	Granulocytic leukemias (neutrophilic) (basophilic)	Myeloblastopenia (panleukopenia-like syndrome)
Megakaryocyte	Megakaryocytic leukemia	Thrombocytopenia
Fibroblast	Myelofibrosis	—
Osteoblast	Medullary osteoclerosis	—
	Osteochrondromatosis	
Kidney	—	FeLV immune complex glomerulonephritis
Diseases thought to be caused by FeLV		
Placenta and uterus	—	Abortions and resorptions
Neural cells	—	Neurologic syndrome
FeSV disease*		
Skin fibroblast	Multicentric fibrosarcoma	—

*FeSV is derived from recombination of FeLV with cat cellular genes.
From Hardy, W. D.: Hematopoietic tumors of cats. J.A.A.H.A., *17*(6):921, 1981.

Table 124. FeLV IMMUNOFLUORESCENT ANTIBODY TEST AND REMOVAL PROGRAM

1. Remove all FeLV–infected sick cats from the household.
2. If there are no other cats at home, wait 10 days before bringing another cat into the household.
3. Immediately test all remaining cats for FeLV.
4. Remove all FeLV–infected healthy cats from the household.
5. Clean dishes, litter pans, and bedding with detergents.
6. Quarantine all remaining FeLV–uninfected cats in the household.
7. Retest all FeLV–uninfected cats 3 months after the first test. The incubation period for FeLV infection can be as long as 3 months.
8. The household can be considered free of FeLV–infected cats only when all cats have tested FeLV negative in 2 tests done 3 months apart.
9. Test all new cats for FeLV before they are introduced into the household.

From Hardy, W. D.: Hematopoietic tumors of cats. J.A.A.H.A., *17*(6):921, 1981.

3. Become infected and continue to shed virus indefinitely without becoming ill.
4. Become infected and develop leukemia or another of the FeLV–related diseases. Cats infected with FeLV show a generalized syndrome of immunosuppression and numerous systemic diseases. The basic information that a veterinarian needs is whether a cat is infected with FeLV virus. Basically, FeLV–negative cats (even if they have neutralizing antibody or FOCMA titers) should not be housed on the same premises with a FeLV–infected cat (as proved by at least 2 positive IFA tests done 3 months apart).

Other forms of diseases associated with infection by FeLV may include:

1. Myeloproliferative diseases, which refer to neoplastic proliferation of cells formed in the bone marrow. There are four stages of feline myeloproliferative disease: (1) erythemic myelosis; (2) erythroleukemia with mixed populations of erythemic and granulocytic cellular proliferation; (3) myeloblastic leukemia; and (4) proliferation of erythroid and myeloid cells in the bone marrow and spleen and proliferation of fibrous tissue and cancellous bone, producing medullary osteosclerosis or myelofibrosis.
2. Anemia. Various types of anemia have been associated with FeLV: nonregenerative anemia unassociated with hematopoietic neoplasia, nonregenerative anemia associated with a panleukopenia-like syndrome, hypoplastic anemia with no bone marrow involvement, myelophthisic-type anemia, and regenerative and nonregenerative anemia associated with *Hemobartonella felis*.
3. Immune suppression associated in young cats with thymic involution.
   a. Feline infectious peritonitis
   b. Poor healing wounds and abscesses
   c. Chronic general infections
   d. Glomerulonephritis
   e. Panleukopenia-like syndrome
   f. Abortions
   g. Stomatitis
   h. Respiratory diseases

References and Additional Readings

Barlough, J. E.: Diagnosis and management of feline leukemia virus infections. *In* Kirk, R. W. (ed.): Current Veterinary Therapy VIII: Small Animal Practice. Philadelphia, W. B. Saunders Company, 1983.

Hardy, W. D., Jr.: Hematopoietic tumors of cats. J.A.A.H.A., *17*(6):951–980, 1981.

Hardy, W. D., Jr., Essex, M., and McClelland, A. J. (eds.): Feline Leukemia Virus. New York, Elsevier Science Publishing Co., Inc., 1980.

Hardy, W. D., Jr.: Feline leukemia virus. J.A.A.H.A., *17*(6):951, 1981.

Jarrett, O.: Recent advances in epidemiology of feline leukemia virus. Vet. Ann., *23*:287–293, 1983.

Canine Lymphosarcoma

The most common type of lymphosarcoma in the dog appears to be lymphoblastic and prolymphocytic lymphosarcoma of the disseminated variety. The affected animal is usually between 5 and 10 years of age. Dog breeds reported to have epidemiologically confirmed higher incidences of lymphosarcoma are the boxer, basset hound, St. Bernard, Scottish terrier, airedale, bulldog, and Labrador retriever. Most dogs with lymphosarcoma develop bilateral lymphadenopathy and visceral organ involvement (e.g., spleen, liver, kidneys, or intestines; see Table 125).

The signs associated with lymphosarcoma are often related to sites of involvement. In suspected cases of canine lymphosarcoma, examine all peripheral lymph nodes, carefully palpate the spleen and liver, and visually examine the tonsils. The eyes, respiratory, and nervous systems may also be involved. Other more rarely observed sites of lymphosarcoma are the skin and mediastinum.

A true leukemic blood picture with greater than 100,000 cells per μL rarely develops, although examination of peripheral smears may reveal primitive or atypical cells in more than 60 per cent of the cases. Approximately 50 per cent of dogs may have protein values lower than normal age-matched dogs. Anemia is present in about one third of the cases.

Most canine lymphosarcomas appear to be of B-cell origin, based on lymphocyte surface markers. The major cell types associated with canine lymphosarcoma are lymphocytic, lymphoblastic, or histiocytic. Lymphoblastic is the most common cell type in the dog. Histiocytic lymphosarcoma is the most poorly differentiated of the cell types. The survival time of dogs treated for lymphoblastic lymphosarcoma ranges from 6 to 18 months, averaging 9 months. In histiocytic lymphosarcoma, survival times range from 1 to 6 months.

Canine lymphosarcoma is the most common cause of hypercalcemia in the

Table 125. CLINICAL CLASSIFICATION OF CANINE LYMPHOSARCOMA

Classification*	Description of Clinical Stage
I	Involvement limited to one lymph node or group in one anatomic region
II	Involvement of multiple nodes but limited to one side of the diaphragm
III	Generalized involvement of lymphoid tissue (i.e., lymph nodes, spleen, tonsils, and thymus gland)
IV	Involvement of any nonlymphoid tissues, including viscera, blood, bone marrow, CNS, and eyes

*Each classification was subclassified into (a) none to slight systemic signs, mild fever, anorexia, lethargy, and normal blood chemical values; or (b) severe systemic signs, weight loss, anemia, leukopenia, vomiting, diarrhea, and abnormal clinical-chemical analysis.

Table 126. PROCEDURE FOR TREATING CANINE LYMPHOSARCOMA

Drug	Dosage
Vincristine sulfate	0.5 mg/m², IV, once a week
Cytosine arabinoside	100 mg/m², IV, 1 dose a day for first 4 days of first week; repeat the 4 doses if animal relapses
Cyclophosphamide	50 mg/m², per os, 1 dose a day, 4 days a week for 8 weeks
Prednisone	20 mg/m², per os, twice a day for first 7 days, then 10 mg/m², twice a day on alternate days
L-asparaginase*	20,000 IU/m², IP, once on weeks 9 and 10
Vaccine†	0.25 ml, deep IM, once on weeks 10, 11, 12, 14, and 16; discontinue if relapse occurs before week 16

*Supplied by National Cancer Institute, National Institutes of Health, Bethesda, Maryland.
†Autogenous vaccine or Freund's complete adjuvant.
m² = square meters of body surface.

dog (see pp. 744). Additional examinations that may be helpful are exfoliative cytology in lymph nodes or fluid aspirates, lymph node biopsy, bone marrow examination, radiology, and exploratory surgery.

Altered serum calciums are frequently associated with bone marrow involvement (see p. 494). Dogs with hypercalcemia associated with lymphosarcoma are very ill, and serum calcium levels may be in the 15 to 20 mg per dl (emergency) range. Hypercalcemia in lymphosarcoma is associated with production of an osteoclast-activating substance stimulating bone resorbing activity.

Unlike feline lymphosarcoma, no evidence of viral etiology has been obtained in dogs, and there are no reports of case clusters. Canine lymphosarcoma and lymphocytic leukemia are transplantable to neonatal pups or to canine fetuses in utero. Dogs with lymphosarcoma have an immune deficiency in the cellular (T-cell) component, as measured by lymphocyte blastogenesis.

The treatment for lymphosarcoma in the dog should be individualized, depending on the staging of the disease, the location of tumor tissue, and possibly the cell type (Table 126). For further information about treatment protocols, see the suggested readings.

References and Additional Readings

Barton, C.: Canine lymphosarcoma. Proc. A.A.H.A., p. 345, 1983.

Cline, M. J., and Haskell, C. M.: Cancer Chemotherapy, 3rd ed. Philadelphia, W. B. Saunders Company, 1980.

DeVita, V. T., and Hellman, S.: Cancer Principles and Practices of Oncology. Philadelphia, J. B. Lippincott Co., 1982.

Holmberg, C. A., and Wilson, F. D.: Lymphoid neoplasia in the canine. In Shifrine, M., and Wilson, F. D. (eds.): The Canine as a Biomedical Research Model. Immunological, Hematological, and Oncological Aspects. Springfield, Virginia, National Technical Information Service, 1980.

Jeglum, A. K.: Treatment of lymphosarcoma. *In* Kirk, R. W. (ed.): Current Veterinary Therapy VIII: Small Animal Practice. Philadelphia, W. B. Saunders Company, 1983.

MacEwen, E. G., et al.: Diagnosis and treatment of canine hematopoietic neoplasms. Vet. Clin. North Am., 7:105, 1977.

Theilen, G. H., Worley, M., and Benjamini, E.: Chemoimmunotherapy for canine lymphosarcoma. J.A.V.M.A., 70:607, 1977.

Weller, R. E., Holmberg, C. A., Theilen, G. H., and Madewell, B. R.: Histologic classification as a prognostic criterion for canine lymphosarcoma. Am. J. Vet. Res., 41(8):1310, 1980.

Feline Infectious Peritonitis

Feline infectious peritonitis (FIP) is a chronic, progressive viral disease of domestic and wild Felidae. When first characterized, the disease was recognized as a chronic fibrinous peritonitis with abdominal effusion. Both effusive and noneffusive forms of the disease can exist. Effusive FIP can be seen as pleuritis and/or peritonitis. Noneffusive FIP is characterized by pyogranulomatous inflammation and necrosis of a variety of organs, including kidney, eye, brain, lung, and liver (Table 127).

FIP is caused by a small RNA virus of the coronavirus variety. The virus is shed by sick, subclinically ill, and asymptomatic carrier cats. The natural route of infection is unknown, although there have been reports that the virus can be transmitted orally. The disease is readily reproduced by parenteral inoculation of infected fluids or tissues and is present in the blood of infected cats. Maternal transmission, either in utero or neonatal, may also occur.

Morbidity (Infection Rate) Versus Mortality

The FIP virus is widespread in nature. In problem catteries, the overall morbidity approaches 90 per cent or more. In the general population, the

Table 127. CLINICAL SITUATIONS IN WHICH A DIAGOSIS OF FIP SHOULD BE CONSIDERED

Abdominal distension due to peritoneal effusion
Dyspnea due to pleural effusion
Enlarged, lumpy kidneys
Mesenteric lymphadenopathy
Unexplained neurologic signs
Ocular lesions of anterior uveitis or chorioretinitis
Granulomatous lung disease
Icterus
Chronic, fluctuating nonresponsive fever
Chronic, unexplained malaise (e.g., anorexia, depression, and weight loss)
Lymphopenia with neutrophilic leukocytosis or leukopenia
Elevated total plasma protein (hypergammaglobulinemia)
Unexplained nonregenerative anemia

From Sherding, R. G.: Feline infectious peritonitis. Compendium on Continuing Education, 1:95, 1979.

morbidity is about 20 per cent. When the virus is introduced into a susceptible population of cats for the first time, the overall mortality during the first 6 months to 1 year may approach 25 per cent or more in some instances.

There is no apparent breed or sex predilection to the clinical disease. The peak incidence of clinical disease is in cats that are approximately 1 to 2 years of age.

The incubation period of FIP is variable. In the experimental case, the incubation period may be days, whereas in the naturally occurring case, the incubation period may be weeks or months. The average duration of clinical illness is 2 to 5 weeks; however, the condition may become protracted with a course of 6 months.

There appears to be a wide degree of variability in the presenting signs of this disease. It has been stated that only 1 in 15 cats will show classical signs of FIP.

FIP produces a generalized vasculitis associated with phlebitis, thrombophlebitis, and thrombosis in numerous organs. Microscopic disseminated fibrinonecrotic or pyogranulomatous inflammation and necrosis are found in almost every body organ. The form of periphlebitis and the generalized inflammation suggest that the inflammatory reaction is immune mediated.

Cats infected with FIP may also develop DIC characterized by thrombocytopenia, prolonged one-stage prothrombin time, partial thromboplastin time, and increased fibrin split products, along with decreased factors VII, VIII, IX, X, XI, and XII activity.

Clinical Forms

Effusive Form (Wet Form, Nonparenchymatous FIP, Peritoneal Form). The classical wet or effusive form of FIP is characterized by chronic weight loss, fever, depression, and ascites. The peritoneal form of dry FIP presents mainly as chronic weight loss, fever, and lethargy, and signs referable to specific organ involvement.

Noneffusive or Dry Form. The noneffusive form of FIP is characterized by the development of multifocal granulomatous lesions in several different organs.

The ocular lesions of FIP can range from a slight clouding of the aqueous humor to an exudative retinitis and choroiditis with retinal detachment. Central nervous system (CNS) involvement is common in the noneffusive or dry form of FIP. A kitten mortality disease complex also is associated with FIP virus.

Among the clinical pathologic abnormalities found in FIP is a mild to moderate normochromic-normocytic nonregenerative anemia. The absolute WBC is elevated, associated with an increase in the absolute numbers of neutrophils. Lymphocyte numbers are reduced. Elevation in total plasma protein as determined by means of a refractometer is a characteristic feature of FIP. The hyperproteinemia is due to elevations in the concentrations of α-2, β-2, and gamma globulins on protein electrophoresis. (Serum fibrinogen levels of 400 mg/dl or greater can be seen.)

Approximately 40 to 50 per cent of all field cases of FIP have concurrent

FeLV infections. FIP is also a more significant clinical problem in catteries where concurrent FeLV infections exist.

References and Additional Readings

Barlough, J., and Weiss, R. C.: Feline infectious peritonitis. *In* Kirk, R. W. (ed.): Current Veterinary Therapy VIII: Small Animal Practice. Philadelphia, W. B. Saunders Company, 1983, pp. 1186–1193.

Horzinek, M. C., and Osterhaus, A. D. M. E.: The virology and pathogenesis of feline infectious peritonitis. Arch. Virol., 59:1, 1979.

Nielsen, S. B., et al.: Feline infectious peritonitis and viral respiratory diseases in feline leukemia–infected cats. J.A.A.H.A., 17(5):759, 1981.

Pedersen, N. C.: Feline infectious diseases. Corona viral infections of cats. Proc. A.A.H.A., 40th Annual Meeting, 1981, p. 83.

Weiss, R. C., and Scott, F. W.: Pathogenesis of feline infectious peritonitis. Nature and development of viremia. Am. J. Vet. Res., 42:382, 1981.

Weiss, R. C., Dodds, J. W., and Scott, F. W.: Disseminated intravascular coagulation in experimentally induced feline infectious peritonitis. Am. J. Vet. Res., 41:663, 1980.

FELINE INFECTIOUS PERITONITIS TEST

A number of tests are available for the interpretation of coronaviral antibody (FIP) test in cats, including an indirect fluorescent antibody test and computer-assisted, kinetics-based ELISA called *KELA*.*

The IFA test measures antibody to the FIP virus in the serum of cats. The test uses frozen (liver) tissue of cats that have been infected with FIP.

Cross-reacting coronaviridae such as TGE virus are also frequently used. Serologic surveys indicate that previous exposure of cats to other coronaviridae (other than FIP) is widespread and that 10 to 40 per cent of cats will be sero positive for coronaviral antibodies. Serial fourfold dilutions (1:25–1:25,600) of test serum are made with phosphate-buffered saline solution. In rapid screening tests, serum dilutions of 1:25, 1:100, and 1:400 are used. Rabbit anticat IgG, conjugated with fluorescein isothiocyanate, is used to detect liver cells that have reacted with feline immunoglobulins in the serum samples.

In the KELA test, the KELA titer represents the absolute amount of antibody present in the sample (i.e., the true antibody end-point); thus, titers will be reported as, for example, 1:27, 1:381, and 1:3252 and are not limited to a rigid dilution scheme.

In addition, the KELA has been calibrated to report results using the same scale of measurement as the IFA. Thus, KELA results may be considered as "IFA-equivalent" titers. For example, a KELA titer of 1:1300 would have been reported as 1:1600 by IFA, whereas a KELA titer of 1:250 might have been reported as either 1:100 or 1:400 by IFA. In both cases, the discontinuous

---

*KELA—Available through Diagnostic Laboratory, New York State College of Veterinary Medicine, Ithaca, New York 14853.

Table 128. GENERAL RECOMMENDATIONS FOR CONTROL OF FIPV
INFECTION IN CATTERIES

Coronaviral Antibody–Positive Catteries

Maintain cats in as good health as possible. Provide adequate air circulation, but keep temperature conditions warm. Avoid stress by providing good nutrition, vaccinating against other viruses, eliminating feline "psychosomatic" conditions, etc.

Isolate or remove any FeLV–positive cats.

Remove breeding queens with repeat problems of bloody vaginal discharge, reproductive failure, and neonatal deaths.

Wean all kittens as early as possible, and hand rear them away from other cats.

Keep premises thoroughly cleaned with an effective virucidal disinfectant, such as standard bleach diluted 1:32 in water.

Coronaviral Antibody–Negative Catteries

Keep premises clean and sanitary.

New cats should come from catteries with no past history of FIP diagnosis and should have tested negative for coronaviral antibodies within the past 30 days. All new cats should be kept in quarantine for 2 to 3 weeks before entering the cattery and then should be retested for coronaviral antibodies. Cats testing negative both times can be allowed to enter the cattery.

Cattery cats should not be sent to coronaviral antibody–positive catteries for breeding and should not be allowed to contact coronaviral antibody–positive cats in any way.

All cats returning from shows should be kept in quarantine for at least 2 weeks. If signs of upper respiratory infection are noted, quarantine should be continued and a coronaviral antibody titer should be determined after 3 to 4 weeks.

From Scott, F. W., et al.: Feline Info. Bull. No. 4, 1978; Scott, F. W., et al.: Proc. A.A.H.A. 46th Annual Meeting, 1979; Scott, F. W.: J.A.V.M.A. *175*:1164, 1979.

nature of the IFA dilution scheme would have made it difficult to accurately determine the true antibody end-point of the sample.

The presence of FIP antibodies in the serum indicates that the cat has had previous contact with the virus; however. the diagnostic significance of this is not known. A very high percentage of normal, healthy cats (in FIP virus–free catteries, 83 per cent of the cats had positive FIP titers) have antibody to FIP virus. Antibodies to other coronaviruses, particularly corona enteritis virus of young cats, TGE virus of swine and canine coronavirus may cross-react in both the IFA and KELA tests. Antibody titers (IFA) of cats that have been exposed to coronavirus but are asymptomatic generally range from 1:25 to 1:400. Clinically normal animals have KELA titers below 1:250. Animals with clinical signs of FIP correlated with laboratory supportive data may have IFA titers of 1:1600 or greater or KELA titers of 1:250 or greater. Rising high titers over a period of several weeks with either test is also supportive evidence for active infection (Table 128).

References and Additional Readings

Barlough, J. E.: Evaluation of a computer-assisted, kinetics-based enzyme linked immunosorbent assay for detection of coronavirus antibodies in cats. J. Clin. Microbiol. 17(2):202, 1983.

Jacobson, R. H., Downing, D. R., and Lynch, T. J.: Computer-assisted enzyme immunoassays and simplified immunofluorescence assays: applications for the diagnostic laboratory and veterinarians office. J.A.V.M.A., *181*:1166, 1982.

Pederson, N. C., Boyle, J. F., Floyd, K., et al.: An enteric coronavirus infection of cats and its relationship to feline infectious peritonitis. Am. J. Vet. Res., *42*:368, 1981.

Bleeding and Blood Coagulation

A good medical history can be helpful in evaluating animals with a bleeding problem. Basically, the causes of abnormal bleeding can be divided into five major categories: (1) vascular trauma, (2) defective production of hemostatic factors, (3) dilution of hemostatic factors, (4) use of systemic anticoagulants, and (5) DIC.

Most bleeding is the result of local injuries from a variety of causes. The following types of bleeding should cause the clinician to suspect possible abnormalities in blood coagulation:

1. Bleeding at multiple sites throughout the body involving several body systems.
2. Development of spontaneous deep hematomas.
3. Unusually prolonged bleeding after injury.
4. Delayed onset of extensive hemorrhage after bleeding.
5. Inability to find an organic cause for bleeding.

In obtaining a history of the bleeding patient, the following information is important:

1. How old was the animal when the bleeding first occurred? Hereditary defects usually develop in very young dogs.
2. Do immediate relatives have similar bleeding problems? Are both genders affected?
3. Is the animal in question allowed to roam freely having exposure to rodenticides? Has the animal recently received any drugs known to interfere with hemostasis or depress the production of platelets?

Bleeding and altered mechanisms of blood coagulation may have varied manifestations, including petechial hemorrhages, epistaxis, melena, hematuria, and bleeding into body cavities, joints, and the spinal cord. The clinician must determine whether the bleeding has a local cause or is the manifestation of a disease producing alteration in bleeding or clotting mechanisms. It is important to establish the site and duration of the bleeding, its history (including any previous episodes of bleeding), and the presence of another disease.

(For further discussion on blood-clotting factors, see Figure 94 and Table 129.)

Collection and Handling of Blood Samples To Be Used in Evaluation of Coagulation Abnormalities

1. All blood samples should be taken with plastic- or silicone-coated glass syringes by *careful* venipuncture.
2. Trisodium citrate or sodium oxalate is the anticoagulant of choice for

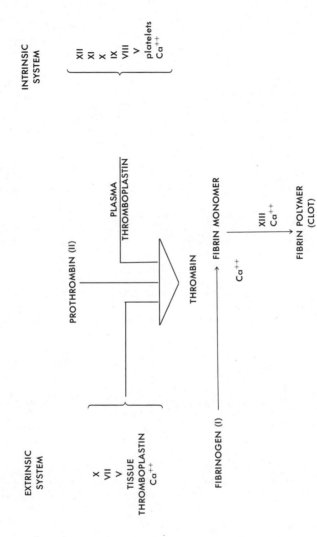

Figure 94. Factors involved in blood coagulation. From Dodds, W. J., and Kaneko, J. J.: Hemostasis and blood coagulation. In Kaneko, J. J., and Cornelius, C. E. (eds.): Clinical Biochemistry of Domesitc Animals, 2nd ed. Vol. II. New York, Academic Press, 1971.

Table 129. BLOOD CLOTTING FACTORS AND SYNONYMS

International Classification*	Synonyms
Factor I	Fibrinogen
Factor II	Prothrombin
Factor III	Tissue thromboplastin
Factor IV	Calcium
Factor V	Proaccelerin
	Labile factor, accelerator globulin (AcG)
Factor VII	Proconvertin
	Serum prothrombin conversion accelerator (SPCA), stable factor, autoprothrombin I
Factor VIII	Antihemophilic factor (AHF)
	Antihemophilic globulin (AHG), platelet cofactor I, plasma thromboplastic factor A
Factor IX	Christmas factor
	Plasma thromboplastin component (PTC), platelet cofactor II, autoprothrombin II, plasma thromboplastic factor B
Factor X	Stuart factor
	Stuart-Prower factor
Factor XI	Plasma thromboplastin antecedent (PTA)
Factor XII	Hageman factor
Factor XIII	Fibrin stabilizing factor (FSF)
	Fibrinase, Laki-Lorand factor

*As recommended by the International Committee for the Nomenclature of Blood Clotting Factors (1962). The most commonly used synonym for each factor is listed first.

From Dodds, W. J., and Kaneko, J. J.: Hemostasis and blood coagulation. *In* Kaneko, J. J., and Cornelius, C. E. (eds.): Clinical Biochemistry of Domestic Animals, 2nd ed., Vol. II. New York, Academic Press, 1971.

coagulation and platelet work (e.g., 1 part 3.8 per cent trisodium citrate plus 9 parts whole blood). The anticoagulant should be added to the syringe first and the blood drawn directly into the syringe in the required volume.

3. All samples must be kept in plastic- or silicone-coated glass test tubes.
4. Plasma samples should be prepared for fresh blood and tested immediately or frozen for testing later. Plasma frozen at −20°C can be stored for a few days while samples frozen at −40° to −80° C can be stored for several months to a year. Samples to be shipped for specialized coagulation assays should be sent in dry ice. Samples should be assayed in duplicate and kept at refrigerator temperature when tested.
5. Platelet tests must be done on fresh samples within 2 hours of collection. Polycarbonate is an ideal plastic surface for platelet preparation. Samples should be kept at room temperature, because platelet shape is altered by heat or cold.

Practical Screening Diagnostic Tests in Bleeding Disorders
(See Table 130)

The following tests can be helpful in differentiating the course of bleeding

Table 130. DIFFERENTIAL DIAGNOSIS OF ACQUIRED
BLEEDING DISORDERS

	Vitamin K Deficiency and/or Liver Disease	Primary Fibrinolysis
Coagulation Factors decreased	II, VII, IX, X (I, V—liver only)	I, V, VII (mild)
Clotting time PTT PT	prolonged	prolonged
Platelets (Activity and number)	normal	normal
RBC distortion Leptocytosis Poikilocytosis Burred cells	none	none
Increased Fibrinolytic Activity by FDPs Euglobin lysis or Plasminogen assay	none*	present
Paracoagulation Tests Ethanol gelation Protamine Precipitation	negative	negative

*May be present with fibrinolysis complicating liver disease.
From Greene, C. E.: Disseminated intravascular coagulation in the dog. J.A.A.H.A., 11:674, 1975.

disorders in animals. It should be stressed that evaluation of paired samples using a normal control dog can be very helpful in evaluating abnormalities.

Activated Coagulation Time (ACT) of Whole Blood. Measurements of whole blood clotting time can be performed by the Lee-White whole blood clotting time and the capillary tube clotting time. The activated coagulation time is technically more dependable, because it obviates variations of blood temperature during the test, aids in eliminating some of the variables produced by tissue thromboplastin, and provides a more reliable vehicle for contact activation of the blood sample. Qualitative or quantitative abnormalities of platelet function may result in prolongation of the ACT test. Platelet numbers may have to be reduced to below 10,000 per mm³ before an effect of the ACT test is produced. Low fibrinogen levels can also influence the ACT test.

To perform the ACT test, make a cephalic or jugular venipuncture using a disposable 20-gauge, 1-inch needle screwed into a plastic tube holder. Insert

Table 130. DIFFERENTIAL DIAGNOSIS OF ACQUIRED BLEEDING DISORDERS *(Continued)*

Acute DIC	Chronic DIC	Primary Platelet Consumption	Circulating Anticoagulants
I, II, V, VIII, X, XIII	mild decrease, as in acute, or normal (may be increased)	normal	normal
prolonged	slightly prolonged or normal normal but most likely	normal decreased	prolonged normal
decreased	decreased		
present	variable	none	none
present	none or present	none	none
positive	positive or negative	negative	negative

a 5-ml Vacutainer Tube,* partially evacuated, into the needle holder; withdraw 2 ml of blood to eliminate any tissue thromboplastin that is present when the needle entered the vein. Remove the first tube, and replace it with a second tube containing 12 mg of diatomite (siliceous earth), partially evacuated to withdraw 2 ml of blood. Prewarm the diatomite tube to 38°C in a calibrated heating block.† When blood first appears in the diatomite tube, begin timing with a stop watch. When 2 ml of blood are present in the tube, return the tube to the heating block. After 1 minute and at each 5-second interval thereafter, remove the tube from the block; tilt and observe for evidence of clotting. Normal values are median 75.0 seconds; mean, 77.5; standard deviation (SD), 14.7 seconds.

Platelet Count. Make a direct platelet count using a hemocytometer. For

---

*Vacutainer Tube, No. 3206 or 3865, Becton-Dickinson Co., Rutherford, New Jersey.

†Dow Diagnostest Heating Block, Model 12/1A, Dow Chemical Co., Midland, Michigan.

most animal species, the range is 175,000 to 500,000 per mm^3. The tendency for bleeding problems to develop in association with thrombocytopenia will depend on the number and function of the available platelets.

Platelet Function. This can be estimated by clot retraction.

Activated Partial Thromboplastin Time (APTT). This measures the cumulative effects of clotting factors in the intrinsic or intravascular system. The normal range for the APTT of healthy dogs is 14 to 25 seconds.

Prothrombin Time (PT). PT measures the effects of the extrinsic or tissue fluid system of clotting. Most of these factors are synthesized in the liver, and PT is one of the screening tests used in liver function. The prothrombin-complex clotting factors are II, VII, and X; these interact with factor V and fibrinogen in the presence of tissue thromboplastin and $CaCl_2$.

Thrombin Time. This measures the amount of functional fibrinogens in plasma. The test is used in DIC when fibrinogen levels may be low. Fibrinogen levels may be normal in DIC; however, the thrombin time may be altered because fibrinogen function is changed by in vivo fibrinolysis.

Fibrin Degradation Products (FDP). Elevated levels occur in DIC (see p. 63). This test uses a latex-agglutination method for measuring FDP. Because the human test cross-reacts with the dog, this test can be used in canine DIC.

Important Bleeding Disorders in Small Animals (See Table 131)

Deficiency of Factor VIII, Hemophilia A. This disease is an X-chromosome-linked, recessive trait, carried by females and manifested in males. Female hemophiliacs can be produced by breeding hemophiliac males to carrier females. The disease has been reported in a wide variety of dog breeds and cats. The clinical disease can manifest itself in mild, moderate, or severe forms, producing both internal and external bleeding. Signs may be observed shortly after weaning and may include umbilical cord bleeding, gingival bleeding, gastrointestinal hemorrhage, hemarthrosis, and hematoma development. Laboratory tests reveal a prolonged APTT and normal PT, bleeding time, and thrombin times. Affected animals have very low factor VIII coagulant activity but normal or elevated levels of factor VIII–related antigen. Carrier female animals can be detected by low factor VIII activity (30–60 per cent of normal), and a normal or elevated factor VIII antigen.

Another type of hereditary defect in which there is a factor VIII deficiency is known as *von Willebrand's disease* (VWD). The disease is caused by an insufficient concentration or a functional abnormality of von Willebrand factor (VWF), a plasma protein necessary for normal platelet plug formation. Factor VIII coagulation activity, factor VIII–related antigen, and VWF are usually low in animals with VWD. This defect can be inherited as an autosomal recessive disease in which clinically affected animals are homozygous for the VWD gene or as an autosomal, incomplete dominant with variable expression. Homozygosity is often lethal. The disease has been found in numerous breeds of dogs: German shepherds, Golden retrievers, miniature schnauzers, Doberman

Table 131. TRANSFUSION THERAPY OF BLEEDING DISORDERS

I All Types (transfusion not to exceed 4–6 ml/min)*	II Inherited disorders	
	Disease	Treatment
PCV less than 20 per cent with platelet defects: Fresh, preferably typed and/or cross-matched, *homologous* whole blood—12–20 ml/kg body weight repeated as necessary once or twice during first 24 hours	Factor VII deficiency	Mild condition; treatment not required
	Factor VIII deficiency (Hemophilia A)	Fresh or fresh-frozen plasma, plasma cryoprecipitates,† or special FVIII concentrates
	Von Willebrand's disease	
Plasma defects with PCV at or above 20 per cent: Fresh or fresh-frozen *homologous* plasma	Factor IX deficiency (Hemophilia B; Christmas disease)	Fresh or fresh-frozen plasma, supernatant from plasma cryoprecipitates,† or special FIX concentrates
6–10 ml/kg body weight every 6–8 hours until bleeding stops		
6–10 ml/kg body weight once or twice daily for next 3–5 days, if required	Factor X deficiency	Fresh or fresh-frozen plasma
	Factor XI deficiency	
	Fibrogen deficiencies	Fresh or fresh-frozen plasma, plasma cryoprecipitates, or fibrinogen concentrates
Platelet defects with PCV at or above 20 per cent: Fresh, *homologous*, platelet-rich plasma	Prothrombin deficiencies	Fresh or fresh-frozen plasma or prothrombin concentrates
6–10 ml/kg body weight 1–3 times daily until bleeding stops	Platelet function defects	Fresh platelet-rich plasma

*PVC = packed cell volume. If PCV is less than 20 per cent, treat with fresh, matched whole blood *or* with packed RBCs and plasma and/or platelet compounds. If PCV is at or above 20 per cent, treat with plasma and/or platelet components.
†The treatment of choice for severe hemostatic defects is concentrate therapy.
Note: Blood should be collected in ACD or CPD anticoagulants and *not* in heparin.
Modified from Dodds, J.: Inherited coagulation disorders in the dog. In Practice 5(2):54–58, 1983.

pinschers, standard Manchester terriers, Pembroke Welsh corgis, and Scottish terriers. The recessive disease has been recognized in Scottish terriers and Chesapeake Bay retrievers. The incomplete dominant has been recognized in 25 breeds of dogs.

Routine screening tests of coagulation defects are nondiagnostic in this disease. Diagnosis is based on finding reduced or undectable levels of factor VIII; antigen and/or platelet-related activities of VWF. Animals with the recessive form of the disease are homozygotes and have zero FVIII:Ag/VWF; heterozygotes have reduced levels, 15 to 60 per cent of normal. In the incompletely dominant form, reduced VWF antigen is present (less than 7–60 per cent). Signs vary from mild to severe and are usually associated with surgery. Other forms of bleeding that may be associated with VWD are hematuria; diarrhea with melena; penile bleeding; lameness; hematoma formation; excessive bleeding when nails are cut, tails are docked, ears are cropped, and so on; prolonged estrual or post partum bleeding; nose bleeds; and neonatal deaths. Definitive diagnosis is established by assays for factor VIII activity and an immunologic assay for factor VIII VWF and factor VIII antigen.

Deficiency of Factor IX (Christmas Factor or Hemophilia B). This disease has occurred in the dog and has been reported in black and tan coonhounds, Cairn terriers, Scottish terriers, Shetland sheepdogs, St. Bernards, cocker spaniels, French bulldogs, Old English sheepdogs, and Alaskan malamutes. It is inherited as a sex-linked, recessive trait. The clinical signs are more severe than those seen with hemophilia A. Carrier females have low (40–60 per cent of normal) factor IX activity.

Deficiency of Factor VII. This disease has also occurred in the dog. Congenital deficiencies of factor VII have been reported in beagles, although bleeding tendencies are very mild. It appears to be inherited as an autosomal, incompletely dominant characteristic with heterozygotes having 50 per cent factor VII deficiency. There is a prolonged prothrombin time and prolonged serum prothrombin consumption time.

Factor X Deficiency. This has been found in cocker spaniels. The disease very closely resembles the fading puppy syndrome in newborn dogs. Bleeding may be internal or through the umbilicus, and affected dogs frequently die. In adult dogs, bleeding may be mild. In severe cases, factor X levels are reduced to 20 per cent of normal; levels are 20 to 70 per cent in mild cases.

Factor XII deficiency, or Hageman trait deficiency, has been found as an inherited autosomal recessive trait in domestic cats. Heterozygotes can be detected because of a partial deficiency of factor XII, averaging 50 per cent of normal activity levels. Homozygote cats with factor XII deficiency have less than 2 per cent activity. Deficiency of Hageman factor usually does not result in bleeding or other major disorders.

Factor XI deficiency is an autosomal disease in English springer spaniels, Great Pyrenees, and Kerry blue terriers. Protracted bleeding may be observed following surgery, and hemozygotes have low factor XI activity (less than 20 per cent); heterozygotes have 40 to 60 per cent factor XI activity.

PLATELET FACTORS (See also p. 688)

Platelets are essential for normal blood coagulation. When vasoconstriction occurs in an injured vessel, the blood flow is retarded, and platelets attach to the injured endothelium. Following adhesion, platelets undergo primary aggregation, a release of chemical mediators for the coagulation mechanism, secondary aggregation and contraction. Certain plasma proteins, including calcium, fibrinogen, VWF, and a part of factor VIII are required for normal platelet adhesion. The release factors produced by degranulating platelets include vasoactive substances, ADP, prostaglandins, serotonin, epinephrine, and thromboxane A_2. The formation of secondary aggregation is accompanied by the production of platelet factor 3 (thromboplastin).

Qualitative Disorders of Platelets

Alterations in platelet function can affect platelet adhesion, aggregation or release of vasoactive substances. In VWD, there is a deficiency of VWF (a subunit of factor VIII), resulting in altered platelet adhesion (see p. 711). Vascular purpuras are reported and are seen in collagen abnormalities such as Ehlers-Danlos syndrome, which, in dogs such as the German shepherd, dachshund, and St. Bernard, may be inherited as an autosomal dominant with complete penetrance.

Thrombasthenic thrombopathia is a hereditary abnormality of platelet aggregation described in otter hounds, foxhounds, and Scottish terriers. This is inherited as an autosomal dominant trait. Platelets do not aggregate normally in response to ADP and thrombin stimulation.

Evaluation of blood platelets is based on a total thrombocyte count, a clot retraction test, and a bleeding time.

Platelet function defects (thrombopenia, thrombopathia) are autosomally inherited and affect both genders. This familial disorder has been reported in otter hounds and basset hounds.

The clinical signs may resemble VWD. Laboratory tests indicate a prolonged bleeding time but normal platelet count and clotting tests.

Causes of Thrombocytopenia

A decrease in the number of circulating platelets (thrombocytopenia) can result in increased bleeding time and prolonged clot retraction time. Causes of thrombocytopenia can be divided into two categories: (1) increased platelet destruction, utilization, or sequestration; and (2) decreased platelet production by the bone marrow. Primary thrombocytopenia of unknown cause has been called *idiopathic thrombocytopenic purpura (ITP)*. Recent information indicates that 80 per cent of the thrombocytopenia cases are secondary to other diseases such as immune-mediated disorders, including AIHA, systemic lupus erythematosus, rheumatoid arthritis, DIC, and other diseases that can affect the bone marrow. Platelet production in the bone marrow can be reduced primarily or secondarily. The bone marrow hypoplasia can involve either only platelets or all cell lines. Antibody to an animal's own platelets is usually of the IgG type. A specialized test—namely, the platelet factor 3 release test—can be used to demonstrate antiplatelet antibody. Thrombocytopenia is usually associated with bleeding of the purpuric or capillary type and is characterized by petechiation and ecchymoses of the skin, mucous membranes, and conjunctiva; and gingival bleeding, epistaxis, melena, and hematuria.

A summary of the etiology of thrombocytopenia follows:

1. Primary (etiology unknown)—idiopathic thrombocytopenia purpura, AIHA, amegakaryocytic thrombocytopenia.
2. Secondary
   a. Aplastic anemia.
   b. Destruction of thrombocytes in peripheral blood caused by incompatible blood transfusions, hypersplenism, sensitivity or allergy to various drugs and chemicals, extensive burns, massive transfusions of citrated stored blood, excessive platelet consumption in pulmonary thrombosis, chronic infection, irradiation, infectious disease, or live virus vaccination.
   c. Platelet sequestration and increased utilization: hypersplenism, hepatomegaly, endotoxemia, DIC, hypothermia, or prolonged hemorrhage.
   d. Myelophthisic—leukemia and bone marrow tumors.
   e. Abnormal platelet function—that is, thrombocytopathic thrombocytopenia resembling VWD in man. This is a familial disorder in Samoyed dogs.

Abnormal function of blood platelets is referred to as *thrombopathia*. Abnormal function of platelets does not usually affect the platelet count. Functional abnormalities can be produced by uremia, drug therapy (aspirin, phenyl, butazone, promazine, tranquilizers, estrogens, nitrofurans, sulfonamides, penicillins), liver disease, and injection of modified live viruses.

Immunologically Mediated Thrombocytopenia in the Dog

Idiopathic and secondary thrombocytopenia are characterized by petechiae and ecchymoses of the skin and mucous membranes, gingival bleeding, epistaxis, melena, and hematuria. The disease occurs as a primary disease entity associated with an immunologic mechanism and secondary to the effects of certain drugs or toxic agents or to a variety of disease states. Some of the disease states that have been cited are septicemia, lymphoproliferative disorders, incompatible blood transfusions, malignancy, and autoimmune diseases (for example, AIHA, systemic lupus erythematosus, and rheumatoid arthritis). In systemic lupus, 20 to 30 per cent of ANA positive dogs may have thrombocytopenia that is immune mediated. Coombs' positive anemias are often associated with thrombocytopenia (see p. 728). *Ehrlichia canis* infection often produces extensive thrombocytopenia. Other infectious organisms that can cause thrombocytopenia are *Ehrlichia equi* and *Rickettsia rickettsii*, which causes Rocky Mountain spotted fever (see p. 723).

Primary immune–mediated thrombocytopenia has an unknown etiology and is most frequently seen in middle-aged female dogs. Antibody-positive thrombocytopenias are chronic and recurrent. A 7S immunoglobulin has been found to cause the release of platelet factor 3 from fresh homologous platelets. The spleen is the major site of production of this non–complement-fixing antibody. Platelet factor 3 can be demonstrated in the blood of numerous cases (up to as high as 70 per cent). Not only are peripheral platelets affected by platelet factor 3; megakaryocytes in the bone marrow are also affected.

Other Causes of Bleeding Disorders

Monoclonal gammopathies. Bleeding tendencies, including epistaxis, gingival bleeding, and retinal hemorrhages, may be associated with a wide variety of gammopathies. Abnormal proteins may coat platelets, combine with clotting factors, or damage capillaries—all leading to bleeding tendencies.

Vitamin K deficiency. Vitamin K–dependent clotting factors—namely, factors II, VII, IX, and X—can be significantly lowered in several situations, including warfarin poisoning, pindone and diphacinone poisoning, administration of the coccidiostat sulfaquinoxaline, and possible malabsorption syndromes. Vitamin K is required for the postribosomal carboxylation of glutamyl residues in the vitamin K—dependent coagulation factors. The coumarin compounds inhibit the expoxidase reaction and deplete active vitamin K, producing coagulopathies.

References and Additional Readings

Byars, T. D., Ling, D. V., Ferris, N. A., et al.: Activated coagulation time (ACT) of whole blood in normal dogs. Am. J. Vet. Res., 37:1359, 1976.

Davenport, D. J., Breitschwerdt, E. B., and Carakostas, M. C.: Platelet disorders in the dog and cat. Compendium on Continuing Education, 4(9):762, 1982.

Dodds, W. J.: Physiology of hemostasis. *In* Slatter, D. H. (ed.): Textbook of Small Animal Surgery. Philadelphia, W. B. Saunders Co., 1985.

Dodds, W. J.: Hemostasis and blood coagulation. *In* Kaneko, J. J. (ed.): Clinical Biochemistry of Domestic Animals, 3rd ed. New York, Academic Press, 1980.

Dodds, W. J.: Immune mediated diseases of the blood. Vet. Sci. Comp. Med., 27:150–196, 1983.

Green, R. A.: Hemostasis and disorders of coagulation. Vet. Clin. North Am., 11:289, 1981.

Kier, A. B., Bresnahan, J. F., White, F. J., and Wagner, J. E.: The inheritance pattern of factor XII (Hageman) deficiency in domestic cats. Can. J. Comp. Med., 44:309, 1980.

Mount, M. E., Feldman, B. F., and Buffington, T.: Vitamin K and its therapeutic importance. J.A.V.M.A., 180(11):1354, 1982.

Blood Parasites

HEMOBARTONELLA FELIS (FELINE INFECTIOUS ANEMIA)

H. felis is the rickettsial agent that causes a disease in cats that may be characterized by fever, anorexia, lethargy, emaciation, splenomegaly, macrocytic normochromic anemia *without* hemaglobinuria, and occasionally icterus.

Cats may carry *H. felis* and be perfectly normal; however, during periods of stress, overt clinical infection may develop. The parasite is seen as coccoid, rodlike, or ringlike bodies on the RBCs in smears stained with Wright's, Giemsa, NMB, or acridine orange. Parasitemic episodes are variable but may last up to a month. Fever is present during parasitemic episodes. Cats become anemic following a parasitemic episode. *Hemobartonella* parasites alter the erythrocyte membrane and produce immune-mediated damage leading to increased red cell fragility and destruction. The direct Coombs' test can become positive in cats infected with *H. felis*. Parasitized cells become spherical and have a markedly shortened life span. Response to the anemia produced is characteristic of a markedly regenerative anemia.

Hemobartonella can be disseminated by blood-sucking arthropods such as fleas, and hemobartonella organisms can be transmitted from female cats to their offspring. Infections can also be transmitted iatrogenically through blood transfusions. The numbers of parasites present in the peripheral blood at any one time can vary greatly; therefore, repeated smears may be needed (3 to 5 consecutive days). In cases of severe infection with *H. felis* and a resultant very low PCV (below 20), a whole blood transfusion can be administered (see p. 622).

Treatment of *H. felis* is controversial. Oral tetracycline (20 mg/kg administered three times daily for 3 weeks) and IV thiacetarsamide sodium (1 mg/kg administered in two injections 48 hours apart) have been recommended as effective chemotherapeutic agents. Neither drug totally eliminates the parasite from infected cats, and animals remain chronically infected. Cats should be treated for 3 weeks with oxytetracycline orally and with prednisolone 1 to 2 mg per kg because of the associated immunologic disorder characterized by the direct positive Coombs' test.

HEMOBARTONELLA CANIS

H. canis is the rickettsial agent that causes a disease in dogs that may be characterized by fever, anorexia, weakness, splenomegaly, macrocytic normochromic anemia, and (rarely) icterus. The infection is usually latent and may be activated by stress or splenectomy. The parasite is seen as coccoid or chainlike forms on the RBCs in smears stained with Wright's, Giemsa, NMB, or acridine orange. The numbers of parasites present in the peripheral blood at any one time can vary greatly; therefore, repeated smears may be needed (3 to 5 consecutive days). Treatment consists of tetracycline hydrochloride orally, 20 mg per kg three times a day for 21 days, or oxyphenarsine hydrochloride (Mapharsen) IV, 4 mg per kg in a 0.4 per cent solution.

BABESIA CANIS

B. canis is the hematozoan agent that causes a disease in dogs that may be characterized by recurrent fever, anorexia, lethargy, splenomegaly, macrocytic normochromic anemia, hemoglobinuria, and variable icterus. Acute babesiosis may produce a shock syndrome. Blood transfusions and other mechanisms of treating hypoxic shock should be instituted (see p. 59). Laboratory findings include hemolytic anemia, thrombocytopenia, bilirubinemia, bilirubinuria, hemoglobinuria, azotemia, and possible development of DIC. An IFA test is available to detect dogs with patent or subpatent parasitemia. The parasite is seen as multiple, basophilic, pear-shaped bodies within the RBCs in smears stained with Wright's, Giemsa, or NMB. The numbers of parasites present in the peripheral blood at any one time can vary greatly; therefore, repeated smears *may be needed (3 to 5 consecutive days). Ehrlichiosis and babesiosis may occur simultaneously, and leukocytes should be examined for *Ehrlichia canis* morulas. The brown dog tick, *Rhipicephalus sanguineus*, is the principal vector in the United States. Treatment consists of quinuronium sulfate (Acaprin) subcutaneously, 0.25 mg per kg; phenamidine subcutaneously, 0.50 ml per 10 kg in a 3 per cent solution (may be repeated in 24 hours); trypan blue IV, 2 ml per 10 kg in a 1 per cent solution; or diminazene aceturate (Berenil) IM, 11 mg per kg in a 1 per cent solution (two doses, 5 days apart). Animals that recover from babesiosis remain carriers.

BABESIA GIBSONI

B. gibsoni is the protozoan agent that causes a disease in dogs that may be characterized by recurrent fever, anorexia, lethargy, splenomegaly, macrocytic normochromic anemia, hemoglobinuria, and (very rarely) icterus. The parasite is seen as multiple, basophilic, annular or oval bodies within the RBCs in smears stained with Wright's, Giemsa, or NMB. The numbers of parasites present in the peripheral blood at any one time can vary greatly; therefore, repeated smears may be needed (3 to 5 consecutive days). Treatment consists of diminazene aceturate (Berenil) IM, 11 mg per kg in a 1 per cent solution (two doses, 5 days apart) or metronidazole (Flagyl) orally, 250 mg per day for 10 days.

BABESIA FELIS (BILIARY FEVER OR MALIGNANT JAUNDICE)

B. felis is the protozoan agent that causes a disease in cats that may be characterized by fever, anorexia, lethargy, macrocytic normochromic anemia, and icterus. The parasite is seen as multiple, basophilic, oval or round bodies within the RBCs in smears stained with Wright's, Giemsa, or NMB. The numbers of parasites present in the peripheral blood at any one time can vary greatly; therefore, repeated smears may be needed (3 to 5 consecutive days). Treatment consists of tetracycline hydrochloride orally, 20 mg per kg three times a day, along with trypan blue IV, 2 ml per 10 kg in a 1 per cent solution for 2 days, or quinuronium sulfate (Acaprin) subcutaneously, 0.25 mg per kg.

EHRLICHIA CANIS (CANINE EHRLICHIOSIS)

Canine ehrlichiosis appears to be distributed widely throughout the world. The greatest incidence is reported from tropical and subtropical areas, including

Vietnam, Thailand, Singapore, and Tunisia. The disease is also prevalent in the southern and southwestern regions of the United States. Any dog exposed to the infestation of infected ticks—namely, *Rhipicephalus sanguineus* can become infected—however, the German shepherd breed appears to be the most at risk. This disease is characterized by the following signs: blood-tinged oculonasal discharge, neurologic signs, normocytic-normochromic anemia, epistaxis, edema of the limbs and scrotum, peripheral lymphadenopathy, and pancytopenia. The clinical and hematologic findings in ehrlichiosis are varied depending on the stage of illness of the animal. In the acute stage, there is fever, anorexia, weight loss, lymphadenopathy, and pancytopenia. In the subsequent subclinical stage, there are hemorrhagic episodes, thrombocytopenia, epistaxis, melena, weakness, weight loss, anorexia, dyspnea, ascites, limb edema, and hypergammaglobulinemia. Concurrent infection with *Babesia canis* can lead to marked icterus. The parasite is seen as basophilic, raspberry-shaped obligate rickettsial parasites. When grouped together in the cytoplasm of WBCs, they are called *morulae*. A strain of Ehrlichia that parasitizes neutrophils has also been found, and this strain may be similar to *Ehrlichia equii* in the horse. *E. canis* persists in infected dogs for at least 29 months and probably for life unless appropriate antibiotic therapy is administered. The vector of *E. Canis* is *Rhipicephalus sanguineus*. In the tick, trans-stadial (larva to nymph to adult) transmission occurs, and the tick transmits the disease only if engorgement develops during the acute phase of the disease. The brown dog tick is the natural reservoir of the organism and can transmit infection and disease to susceptible dogs for at least 155 days after engorgement. Stained blood smears will reveal the morulae of *E. canis* in monocytes. An indirect fluorescent antibody test is available for serologic diagnosis. Serum antibodies to *E. canis* can be detected as early as 7 days past exposure, but some dogs may not become positive for detectable antibodies until 28 days. Antibody to *E. canis* does not guarantee immunity to it. Treatment of ehrlichiosis is with oral tetracycline hydrochloride 10 mg per lb of body weight TID for 14 days. With tetracycline treatment, numerous cases recur following 1 to 2 months of treatment. Another form of treatment that has been used is imidocarb dipropionate (Imizol, Wellcome, England). Two doses of 5 to 7 mg per kg are administered IM at 14-day intervals. There is pain on IM injections, and side effects may include salivation, serous ocular discharge, diarrhea, and depression. Delayed reactions may include high fevers in response to the drug. Additional supportive care, including blood transfusions and fluids, may be needed.

HEPATOZOON CANIS

H. canis is the protozoan agent that causes a disease in cats and dogs that may be characterized by cyclic fever, emaciation, anemia, and hepatosplenomegaly. The parasite is seen as basophilic, elongate, rectangular bodies with dark, red-purple nuclei and pink cytoplasmic granules within the leukocytes in smears stained with Wright's. There is no effective treatment.

INFECTIOUS CYCLIC THROMBOCYTOPENIA IN THE DOG

This disease is caused by a platelet-specific rickettsial organism ultrastructurally similar to *E. canis,* but it does not cross-react with *E. canis* serologically. The organism has been tentatively classified as *E. platys.* The disease can be transferred from infected to noninfected dogs via blood inoculation, and, presumably, this is also a tick-transmitted disease. The geographic distribution of this disease is similar to *E. canis.* An IFA test has been developed for detection of serum antibodies to the platelet-specific rickettsial organism that causes this disease.

ROCKY MOUNTAIN SPOTTED FEVER (RICKETTSIA RICKETTSII)

Rocky Mountain spotted fever is a tickborne rickettsial disease, with dogs being a readily susceptible host. Clinical signs exhibited by infected dogs are high fever, anorexia, depression, abdominal pain, myalgia, hemorrhages, uveitis and retinal hemorrhages, lymphadenopathy, epistaxis, and DIC. Neurologic signs may develop and include ataxia, nystagmus, and seizures.

Hematologic changes include anemia, thrombocytopenia, and leukopenia proceeding to leukocytosis. Serum chemistries may reveal elevation of SGPT and serum alkaline phosphatase.

Determination of serum Rickettsia titer on paired acute and convalescent samples is confirmatory for the diagnosis of Rocky Mountain spotted fever. A fourfold rise in titer is considered diagnostic.

Many dogs infected with *Dermacentor andersoni* or *D. variabilis* develop subclinical rickettsial infections. Epizootiologic studies indicate titers to Rocky Mountain spotted fever in dog populations ranging from 4 to 64 per cent, with the highest incidence found in working breeds.

Treatment consists of eliminating ticks and using appropriate antibiotic therapy—tetracyclines or chloramphenicol. Supportive therapy with fluids and treatment for shock may be indicated.

References and Additional Readings

Breitschwerdt, E. B., et al.: Babesiosis in the greyhound. J.A.V.M.A., *182*(9):978, 1983.

French, T. W., and Harvey, J. W.: Serologic diagnosis of infectious cyclic thrombocytopenia in dogs using an indirect fluorescent antibody test. Am. J. Vet. Res., *44*(12): 2407, 1983.

Harvey, J. W., and Gaskin, J. M.: Experimental feline haemobartonellosis. J.A.A.H.A., *13*:28, 1977.

Hribarnik, T.: Canine ehrlichiosis. Compendium on Continuing Education. *3*(11):997, 1981.

Kelly, D. J., Osterman, J. V., and Stephenson, E. H.: Rocky Mountain spotted fever in areas of high and low prevalence: survey of canine antibodies. Am. J. Vet. Res., *43*(8):1429, 1982.

Price, J.: Canine ehrlichiosis. Proc. Satellite Symposium on Diseases of Small Animals. Tel Aviv, Israel, 1980.

Troy, G. C., Vulgamett, J. C., and Turnwald, G. H.: Canine ehrlichiosis: a retrospective study of 30 naturally occurring cases. J.A.A.H.A., *16*:181, 1980.

LABORATORY DIAGNOSIS OF IMMUNOLOGIC DISORDERS IN THE DOG AND CAT

Four distinct classes of immunoglobulins have been identified in normal canine serum and are designated immunoglobulin G (IgG), immunoglobulin A (IgA), immunoglobulin M (IgM), and immunoglobulin E (IgE). IgG, IgA, and IgM have also been described in normal feline serum. IgG is the most abundant of the immunoglobulins and is involved as a systemic mediator of numerous systemic infections. IgM is the major immunoglobulin produced in a primary immune response. IgA is the major immunoglobulin found in external secretions of the body and plays an important role in protecting the intestinal, respiratory, and urogenital tracts.

Gammopathies

Abnormalities in serum immunoglobulins characterized by increased levels are termed *gammopathies.* Basically, categories of gammopathies can be defined as polyclonal increases and monoclonal increases.

The monoclonal gammopathies are a group of disorders characterized by proliferation of a single clone of plasma cells, which produce a homogeneous, monoclonal (M) protein. Monoclonal gammopathies are designated by capital letters that correspond to the classes of their heavy chains that are designated by the Greek letters: γ for IgG, α for IgA, μ for IgM, δ for IgD, and ϵ for IgE. Subclasses are IgG, IgG_2, IgG_3, and IgA_1 and IgA_2. Myeloma proteins in the dog are usually IgG or IgA. Lymphosarcoma produces proteins of the IgM class.

Initial evaluation of serum for monoclonal gammopathies should be done with electrophoresis on cellulose acetate membrane. Specific identification of an abnormal protein level can be accomplished with immunoelectrophoresis.

Monoclonal gammopathies are characterized by a narrow peak in any of the electrophoretic zones. The abnormal, dense, sharply defined electrophoretic band is composed of a homogeneous monoclonal protein, or M-component of paraprotein. Examples of monoclonal gammopathies are: multiple myeloma, macroglobulinemia, lymphoproliferative disorders, and essential benign hypergammaglobulinemia (rare in animals; see Fig. 95).

Plasma cell dyscrasias are a group of diseases resulting from the uncontrolled proliferation of B-lymphocytes, which synthesize abnormal amounts of monoclonal immunoglobulins. Multiple myeloma is the most common form of monoclonal gammopathy seen in veterinary medicine. Multiple myelomas result in monoclonal antibody proliferation other than IgM, plasmacytic cellular infiltration into the bone marrow, Bence Jones proteinuria, and osteolytic lesions seen on radiographic evaluation of skeletal system (which are often difficult to locate). Bence Jones proteins refer to light chain proteins (22,000 daltons) that pass through the renal glomerulus and are passed in the urine. These proteins are toxic for renal tubular cells and may be associated with

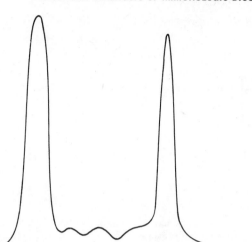

Figure 95. Monoclonal pattern of serum protein as traced by densitometer after electrophoresis on cellulose: tall, narrow-based peak of mobility. Modified from Kyle, R. A., and Greipp, P. R.: Laboratory investigation of monoclonal gammopathies. Mayo Clin. Proc., 53:719, 1978.

renal failure. These proteins precipitate when heated to 60°C but redissolve as the temperature is raised to 80°C.

Polyclonal gammopathies are characterized by the increased production of several immunoglobulin types. This condition usually arises in association with persistent stimulation of the immune system. In the dog, elevation usually occurs in the β region; and in the cat, in the γ region. Abnormalities that can result in polyclonal gammopathies are protracted infections; chronic parasitisms; cirrhosis of the liver; and immunologically mediated diseases such as systemic lupus erythematosus, rheumatoid arthritis, thyroiditis, idiopathic hypergammaglobulinemia, Aleutian disease of mink, myasthenia gravis, and feline infectious peritonitis (see Fig. 96).

In addition to routinely evaluating the serum for abnormal levels of blood proteins, other tests should be performed, including:

1. Evaluation for cryoglobulins. Serum samples should be evaluated at 0°C and incubated at this temperature for 24 hours to detect the presence of a precipitate gel. Dissolution of this precipitate gel at 37°C for 30 minutes indicates the presence of a cryoglobulin.

2. The urine should be evaluated for abnormal proteins. It is recommended that electrophoresis of the urine be performed. A 24-hour urine sample will have to be collected for this test.

Major clinical signs associated with monoclonal gammopathies include:

1. Bleeding diathesis, which can often be recognized on retinal examination by hemorrhages and exudative retinal detachments.

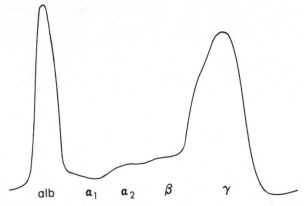

Figure 96. Polyclonal pattern from densitometer tracing after paper electrophoresis: broad-based peak of mobility. Modified from Kyle, R. A., and Greipp, P. R.: Laboratory investigation of monoclonal gammopathies. Mayo Clin. Proc., 53:719, 1978.

2. Hyperviscosity syndrome. Serum viscosity is related to the type, size, shape, and concentration of the abnormal immunoglobulin in the blood. Hyperviscosity is particularly severe in animals suffering from IgM myeloma.
3. Nephrotoxicity caused by proteins in renal tubules.
4. Cryoglobulinemia, which can cause animals to develop gangrenous sloughs of the ear tips, eyelids, digits, and tip of the tail.
5. Hypercalcemia.
6. Skeletal lesions.
7. Infections.
8. Anemia.

Clinical treatment of dogs with hyperviscosity syndrome associated with an IgA monoclonal gammopathy resulting from multiple myeloma is available. It involves continuous plasmapheresis (at least once) to remove abnormal protein constituents, followed by a program of chemotherapy with alkylating agents such as melphalan and cyclophosphamide coupled with systemic prednisolone administration.

Autoimmune Hemolytic Anemia

Autoimmune hemolytic anemia (AIHA) is a disease in which the body attempts to destroy its own red blood cells (RBCs). The clinical signs of AIHA are referable to a responsive anemia that may be acute or chronic. The disease can be seen in dogs of all ages but is more common in females. Antibody may be directed against unaltered RBC's (primary AIHA) or against RBCs that have been antigenically altered by reaction with chemicals or microorganisms (secondary AIHA).

Autoantibodies in AIHA may be of the IgG or IgM class. Most cases of AIHA in dogs and cats are caused by IgG antibodies in combination with complement and react with RBCs at 37°C. IgG does not fix complement efficiently, and acute, intravascular hemolysis is not commonly seen. AIHA may coincide with other autoimmune diseases, including systemic lupus erythematosus and immune-mediated thrombocytopenia. Other diseases that have been associated with Coombs' positive anemia in dogs and cats are lymphosarcoma, hemangiosarcoma, feline leukemia virus (FeLV), hemobarto-nellosis, ehrlichiosis, dirofilariasis, piroplasmosis, leishmaniasis, and glomeru-lonephritis.

Dodds, in reviewing immune-mediated diseases of the blood, states that an increasing number of cases of these types of disorders are being recognized. There are predominating incidences in Old English sheepdogs. Additionally, certain families of dogs have been found to have increased incidences of these problems (American cocker spaniels, long-haired dachshunds, German shepherds, Irish setters, miniature and toy poodles, Shetland sheepdogs, Scottish terriers, vizslas).

Dodds has reported on 223 dogs tested for immune-mediated hemolytic disease between 1980 and 1982. Of 214 dogs tested by direct Coombs' test, 72 per cent were positive, 51 per cent had IgG and complement on RBCs, and 38 per cent were complement mediated alone; 50 per cent were also thrombocytopenic, of which 62 per cent of those were positive for platelet factor 3.

AIHA is seen in cats, and affected animals often have an underlying systemic disease such as FeLV, myeloproliferative disease, and *Haemobarto-nella felis* infection. Cats frequently show autoagglutination of blood, hepato-splenomegaly, and icterus. Cats do not exhibit good spherocytosis, because the RBCs are normally small and dense.

There are several forms of AIHA:

1. *In-vivo hemolysins.* Animals in this condition are very ill. There is massive destruction of RBCs in the circulation, and both hemoglobulinuria and hemoglobinemia can result. In these cases, IgM in combination with complement is the mediating antibody.
2. *In–saline-acting agglutinins.* Animals in this condition are ill and the prognosis is poor. The blood agglutinates as soon as it is drawn and placed upon a slide, regardless of the precautions taken to prevent a drop in temperature.
3. *Incomplete or nonagglutinating antibodies.* This is the most common form of AIHA. The blood cells themselves are not actually destroyed by the allergic reaction, but RBCs coated with antibody tend to be removed by the reticuloendothelial system, particularly the spleen; thus, there is an accelerated destruction of RBCs. The onset of the disease is usually gradual.
4. *Cold agglutinins.* This form of AIHA is usually mediated by IgM antibodies. In this condition, there is often hemoglobulinuria; the blood agglutinates when placed on a slide and allowed to cool. If the slide is heated to 37°C,

the agglutination disappears. Skin manifestations involving the extremities arise because of ischemia associated with intravascular agglutination in small blood vessels. Coombs' test results are negative at 37°C, but positive at 4°C.

The most important mechanism of RBC destruction is removal by the reticuloendothelial system—namely the spleen.

Development of clinical signs in AIHA depends on whether the onset is acute or gradual and whether thrombocytopenia is also involved. Acute clinical signs are depression, anorexia, pale mucous membranes, splenomegaly, peripheral lymphadenopathy, hemoglobinemia, and icterus. Thrombocytopenia presents with clinical signs of petechiation of the skin, mucous membranes, and sclera.

COOMBS' TEST (ANTIGLOBULIN TEST)

Confirmatory diagnosis of AIHA is based on demonstration of a positive Coombs' antiglobulin test for the presence of autoantibody on the surface of erythrocytes or in the serum. Antibodies directed against RBCs can be classified by serologic characteristics into warm autoantibodies, which have maximal activity at 37°C and which are usually IgG, and cold autoantibodies, which usually have maximal activity at 2° to 4°C and are of the IgM class.

In immune-mediated hemolytic anemia, the RBCs may be coated with immunoglobulins, immunoglobulins and complement, or complement alone.

In the Coombs' test, a suspension of washed RBCs of the animal (direct test) or of normal homologous RBCs exposed to the animal's serum (indirect test) is allowed to react with species-specific antiglobulin to effect visible agglutination. The direct antiglobulin test demonstrates the presence of autoantibodies on the surface of the erythrocytes. The indirect test reveals the presence of antibodies in the serum. The indirect Coombs' test is not reliable because of the variability of isoagglutinins present. The direct Coombs' test is usually performed with pooled antisera; however, additional information can be obtained by evaluating agglutination with anti-IgG and anti-C_3 (anti-C_3 is the most frequent agglutinating agent in dogs).

For the direct Coomb's test, the blood sample is collected in EDTA, which prevents in-vitro binding of C_3 to RBCs.

ERYTHROCYTE OSMOTIC SALINE FRAGILITY TEST

Spherocytes are less resistant than normal cells, because their spherical shape does not allow for an increase in volume, which occurs when water enters the cell.

The increased susceptibility of erythrocytes to lysis in hypotonic saline is associated with spherocytosis. The presence of spherocytes associated with AIHA is of sufficient magnitude to produce gross changes in the saline fragility curve.

Autoimmune Thyroiditis
(Lymphocytic Thyroiditis)

Immune-mediated thyroiditis appears to be a common cause of thyroid disease in dogs, resulting in clinical hypothyroidism. Biopsies of thyroid tissue from dogs with hypothyroidism reveal infiltration of the gland with plasma cells and small lymphocytes.

Experimentally, the disease has been found most frequently in beagles, where its occurrence may be genetically determined. Antibodies to thyroglobulin, against follicular microsomes, and against unidentified colloid antigen are usually present. Focal lymphocytic thyroiditis in laboratory beagles is not usually associated with the severe clinical signs and alterations in thyroid function tests observed in pet dogs (see p. 656). Beagles have lower maximal thyroid uptake of ^{131}I and more rapid loss of ^{131}I compared with dogs with mild or no thyroiditis.

Myasthenia Gravis

Myasthenia gravis is a disease of neuromuscular transmission associated with a deficiency of acetylcholine receptors in the neuromuscular postsynaptic membrane. The disease is autoimmune, and autoantibodies to acetylcholine receptors are detected in the sera of affected patients.

Myasthenia gravis occurs both as a congenital and developmental disease in the dog and cat.

In congenital myasthenia gravis, there is a deficiency of acetylcholine receptors; however, this is not associated with autoantibodies against acetylcholine receptor sites. Congenital myasthenia gravis is usually recognized at 8 weeks of age and has been described in Springer spaniels, Jack Russell terriers, smooth fox terriers, and Siamese cats.

Acquired myasthenia gravis has no breed or sex predilection and is usually a disease of middle-aged dogs 7 to 11 years of age. The signs of myasthenia gravis are weakness following muscle activity; this weakness responds to rest. The eyelids and ears droop, although marked ptosis is not evident. The animal may not be able to hold up the head, close the jaw, or adequately chew and swallow food. Often, a megaesophagus is present. A change in the character of the bark may develop. All neurologic reflexes are depressed. Routine screening of complete blood-count (CBC) and blood chemistry results in animals with myasthenia are usually normal. Ninety per cent of dogs with acquired myasthenia gravis have antiacetylcholine receptor autoantibodies in their sera.

Electromyographic findings in myasthenic patients reveal a decrease in amplitude of action potentials recorded from skeletal muscles during stimulation of motor nerves.

The diagnosis of myasthenia gravis is based on clinical history, signs, physical and radiographic examination, and response to anticholinesterase agents. The short-acting anticholinesterase agent edrophonium chloride (Tensilon) is given intravenously (IV) at a dosage of 1 to 2 mg. Within 10 to 30 seconds following injection, there should be obvious clinical improvement. Caution should be used with this test, and atropine and positive pressure ventilation equipment should be available in case of emergency.

Animals with acquired myasthenia gravis have a fair to guarded prognosis. They are usually treated with corticosteroids and anticholinesterase agents such as neostigmine (Prostigmin) or pyridostigmine/bromide (Mestinon):

	Peak Effect	Duration	Dose
Pyridostigmine	2 hr	4–6 hr	60 mg 3–4 times/day
Neostigmine	1.5 hr	2–4 hr	15 mg

Muscarinic side effects may be controlled with atropine.

Systemic Lupus Erythematosus

Systemic lupus erythematosus (SLE) is a generalized immunologic disorder resulting from a generalized loss of overall control of the specificity of the B cell, possibly associated with abnormal suppressor cell function. Affected animals, namely dogs (rarely reported in cats), produce autoantibodies against a wide range of normal organs and tissues, including nucleic acids, namely DNA.

SLE may be mild or severe in dogs and is associated with the following signs, either individually or in combination:
1. Hemolytic anemia (Coombs' positive) and/or thrombocytopenia (platelet factor 3 positive), nonregenerative anemias.
2. Severe polyarthritis characterized by a shifting leg lameness; the arthritis is nonerosive.
3. Glomerulonephritis and proteinuria. DNA-immune complexes become deposited in glomeruli, resulting in a membranous glomerulonephritis. Immune complexes may also be deposited in arterial walls, producing an immune-mediated vasculitis, fibrinoid necrosis, and fibrosis.
4. Skin lesions, usually involving the face and ears (and sometimes mucotaneous junctions), that are frequently symmetrical. The cutaneous manifestations of SLE are variable and may include discoid LE, macular-papular rashes, vesiculobullous eruptions, mucocutaneous ulceration, alopecia, seborrhea-erythema, panniculitis, vasculitis, secondary pyodermas, lymphedema, and nasal dermatitis.
5. Antimuscle antibodies can lead to myositis; antimyocardial antibodies can lead to myocarditis.
6. Leukopenia.
7. Fever of unknown origin, myocarditis, oral ulcers, and polymyositis.

LE AND ANA TESTS

SLE is a multisystem autoimmune disease involving blood vessels, kidneys, skin, joints, the hematopoietic system, and the gastrointestinal tract. Immune complexes bind with a complement, producing multisystemic inflammatory reaction.

Diagnosis of SLE is based on serologic evidence, using the LE test and antinuclear antibody (ANA) test. The LE test is less reliable than the ANA test. Positive LE tests have been found in AIHA, rheumatoid arthritis, lymphosarcoma, leukemia, pulmonary granulomatosis, and warfarin poisoning. In the LE test, nuclear material from fragmenting cells is incubated with leukocytes and serum from patients with SLE. In this case, antinuclear factors shown to be IgG antibody to native DNA nuclear protein coat the nuclear material, opsonizing it for phagocytosis by polymorphs. The LE cell is a polymorph that has ingested nuclear material. Approximately 60 per cent of animals with SLE have a positive LE test on initial examination; therefore, the absence of LE-positive cells does not rule out SLE.

The ANA test refers to the demonstration of ANA by immunofluorescence or by radioimmunoassay procedures for detecting antibody activity against native (double-stranded) DNA. The ANA test is not specific for any single immunologic disease and is positive in a variety of chronic inflammatory disorders. The mean titer of ANA values has been shown to be much higher in proven cases of SLE, and there is a greater predisposition to the peripheral staining pattern in dogs with SLE, whereas in other autoimmune diseases, the diffuse staining pattern is more evident.

Low titer ANA is found in many normal dog sera. Because of this, indirect immunofluorescence using mouse liver or tissue culture cells gives more accurate results for ANA titers, with a titer of 1:20 regarded as significant.

The ANA test is not specific for LE, and positive ANA tests may be found in pemphigus erythematosus, pemphigus vulgaris, lymphocytic thyroiditis, rheumatoid arthritis, idiopathic polymyositis, AIHA, thrombocytopenia, demodicosis, heartworm disease, and endocarditis.

DISCOID LUPUS ERYTHEMATOSUS (See Dermatologic
Examination, p. 456)

Rheumatoid Arthritis

(For discussion of clinical signs of illness, see p. 301.)

ROSE-WAALER TEST FOR RHEUMATOID FACTOR

Because canine or feline rheumatoid latex reagent is not commercially available, the Rose-Waaler test has been used. This test is performed using rabbit antibody against sheep RBCs. Inactivate the antibody against complement by heating. Ascertain the agglutinating titer of the antibody by using washed sheep RBCs. Prepare the indicator cells for use in the test by incubating washed sheep RBCs with the lowest dilution of antiserum not resulting in agglutination. Agglutinating titer of 16 or higher is regarded as positive, 8 as questionable, and 2 to 4 as not significant.

Many dogs with rheumatoid arthritis are negative for rheumatoid factor. The Rose-Waaler test best detects IgM rheumatoid factor. Rheumatoid factor may be present in very low levels in the serum and may be sequestered in circulating immune complexes.

LATEX PARTICLE TEST

This test is used to determine the presence of rheumatoid factor. It is predicated on the fact that IgG can be absorbed onto latex particles to form a substrate for the rheumatoid factor test. A latex reagent specific for the dog (*not for man*) must be used; the suspected serum and latex reagent are tested by mixing dilutions on a microscope slide. Commercially available rabbit anti-dog IgG serves as a reproducible standard. The test detects an agglutinin that most closely exhibits the properties of IgM rheumatoid factor.

Glomerulonephritis

Immunologic factors contribute to the production of many forms of glomerulonephritis. Two pathogenetic mechanisms appear to be operative in the mediation of immunologic glomerular injury, as indicated on the accompanying table. The first is the nephrotoxic or antiglomerular basement mem-

	Nephrotoxic	**Immune Complex Disease**
Antibodies	Directed against the glomerular basement membrane	Directed against circulating antigens (immune complexes are deposited in glomeruli secondarily)
Fluorescence	Linear (γG, complement)	Granular (antigen, γG, complement)
Histology	Neutrophil accumulation	Membranous or mesangiocapillary

brane type, which produces antibodies capable of reacting with glomerular basement membrane antigens. The second is the immune complex type, which passively traps circulating complexes in the glomerular capillary walls. The antibody involved in this reaction is not directed against glomerular antigens. The antigen may be either endogenous or exogenous in origin. This form of glomerulonephritis has been described in the dog in association with neoplastic, inflammatory, infectious, and autoimmune diseases. Renal lesions associated with dirofilariasis have been described (see p. 789).

Table 132. CONDITIONS IN DOMESTIC ANIMALS WITH PROVEN AUTOALLERGIC COMPONENTS

Condition	Antibodies Directed Against
Autoimmune hemolytic anemia	RBCs
Systemic lupus erythematosus	RBCs, WBCs, platelets, nuclear material
Idiopathic thrombocytopenia	Platelets
Autoallergic thyroiditis	Thyroglobulin
Rheumatoid arthritis	Altered immunoglobulin, heart muscle
Glomerulonephritis	Glomerular basement membrane
Myasthenia gravis	Muscle, thymus
Pemphigus	Intercellular cement substance
Phacoanaphylaxis	Lens tissue
Keratitis sicca	Lacrimal gland

Adapted from notes of Dr. Arthur Hurvitz.

In order to detect immune complexes in renal tissue, a needle or wedge biopsy of kidney tissue is required. For the immunofluorescence test, an anti-canine IgG and anti-canine C_3 labeled with FITC are used to detect immune complexes in the mesangium and/or on the glomerular basement membrane. Glomerular damage associated with humoral immunologic disease results in a discontinuous granular fluorescent pattern along the glomerular basement membrane when examined with fluorescent microscopy.

Skin Diseases

Immunologically mediated skin diseases in the dog involve the bullous autoimmune abnormalities, including pemphigus vulgaris, pemphigus vegetans,

Table 133. CONDITIONS IN DOMESTIC ANIMALS WITH POSSIBLE AUTOALLERGIC COMPONENTS

Condition	Antibodies Directed Against
Canine distemper	Myelin
Old dog encephalitis	Brain tissue
Diabetes mellitus	Beta cells (insulin)
Addison's disease	Adrenal cortex
Biliary cirrhosis	Liver parenchyma
Pancreatitis	Pancreatic epithelium
Ulcerative colitis	Mucosal glands
Endocardiosis	Heart tissue
Chronic interstitial nephritis	Renal tissue
Renal disease—secondary to *E. coli* enteritis or pyometra	Renal tissue

Adapted from notes of Dr. Arthur Hurvitz.

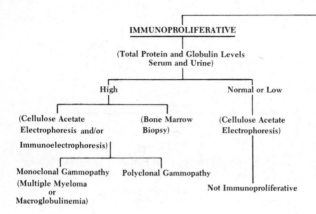

IMMUNOPROLIFERATIVE

(Total Protein and Globulin Levels
Serum and Urine)

High   Normal or Low

(Cellulose Acetate
Electrophoresis and/or

Immunoelectrophoresis)   (Bone Marrow Biopsy)   (Cellulose Acetate Electrophoresis)

Monoclonal Gammopathy   Polyclonal Gammopathy
(Multiple Myeloma
or
Macroglobulinemia)   Not Immunoproliferative

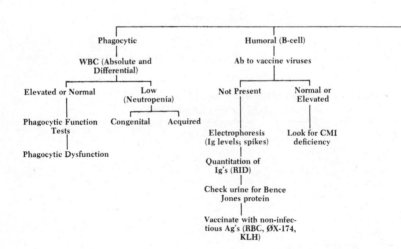

Phagocytic   Humoral (B-cell)

WBC (Absolute and
Differential)   Ab to vaccine viruses

Elevated or Normal   Low (Neutropenia)   Not Present   Normal or Elevated

Phagocytic Function Tests   Congenital   Acquired

Phagocytic Dysfunction

Electrophoresis
(Ig levels; spikes)   Look for CMI deficiency

Quantitation of
Ig's (RID)

Check urine for Bence
Jones protein

Vaccinate with non-infec-
tious Ag's (RBC, ØX-174,
KLH)

1. History (Age of onset, site of infection, type of organism, family history and medications).
2. Physical Examination (Lymphadenopathy, splenomegaly, etc.).
3. Laboratory Tests.

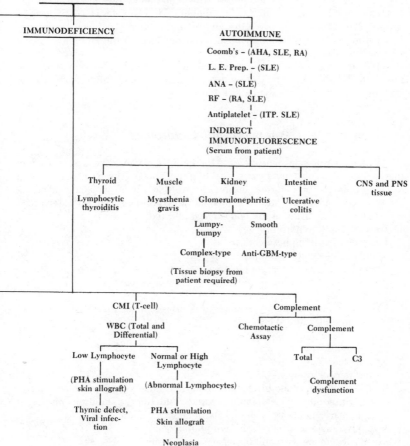

Figure 97. Approach to the clinical and laboratory evaluation of an animal with immunologically based problems. From Schultz, R. D.: Laboratory diagnosis of immunologic disorders. *In* Kirk, R. W. (ed.): Current Veterinary Therapy 6. Philadelphia, W. B. Saunders Company, 1977, p. 455.

pemphigus foliaceus, pemphigus erythematosus, bullous pemphigoid, and discoid LE and SLE. Antibodies may be directed against intercellular cement substance and epithelial cell wall or basement membrane zone. Bullous eruption, ulceration, crusting, and scarring characterize these diseases.

Diagnosis is based on skin biopsies that are frozen or stored in Michel's medium and sectioned and examined with immunofluorescence for abnormal location of antibody in the diseased epithelium. However, for all these diseases definitive diagnosis must correlate clinical signs, clinical pathology tests, and histopathology with the immunologic tests. Reliance on the latter tests alone may lead to diagnostic errors.

Further discussion of conditions having autoallergic components can be found in Tables 132 and 133, and a summary of laboratory diagnosis for immunologic disorders is shown in Figure 97.

Paraneoplastic Syndromes

Paraneoplastic syndromes refer to the indirect, noninvasive, systemic effect that certain types of tumors can produce in their hosts. The effects are related to the production of abnormal hormones or other protein molecules affecting the metabolism of the host. Paraneoplastic syndromes can be categorized according to the portion of the body that is affected:

1. Hematopoietic syndromes
   Leukocytosis—lymphosarcoma
   Leukopenia—lymphosarcoma
   Thrombocytopenia—lymphosarcoma
   Anemias—FeLV; reduced RBC maturation (see p. 698)
   Erythrocytosis—renal tumors
2. Excessive production of serum proteins—gammopathies (see also p. 724)—hyperviscosity syndromes
   Multiple myeloma tumors (see also   )
   Lymphoproliferative diseases
3. Ectopic hormone production
   a. Pituitary adenomas—ACTH
   b. PTH–like hormone-producing hypercalcemia—lymphosarcoma, leukemia, thyroid adenocarcinoma, parathyroid tumors, multiple myeloma, mammary adenocarcinoma, perianal adenocarcinoma
4. Hypoglycemia—associated with lymphosarcoma
5. Mast cell tumors—histamine, heparin, serotonin
6. Non–beta cell tumors of pancreas
   a. Production of gastrin leading to Zollinger–Ellison syndrome
7. Metastatic and primary lung tumors, spirocercosis, rhabdomyosarcoma of the bladder, and carcinoma of the liver
   a. Can produce hypertrophic pulmonary osteoarthropathy
8. Hyperestrogenism—Sertoli cell tumors

References and Additional Reading

Aronsohn, M. G., Schunk, K. L., Carpenter, J. L. and King, N. W.: Clinical pathologic features of thymoma in 15 dogs. J.A.V.M.A. *184*:1355–1362, 1983.

Barlough, J. E., Jacobson, R. H. and Scott, F. W.: Immunoglobulins of the cat. Cornell Vet. *71*:397–407, 1981.

Brown, N. O.: Paraneoplastic syndromes of humans, dogs and cats. J.A.A.H.A. *17*:911–918, 1981.

Dodds, W. J.: Immune mediated disease of the blood. Ad. Vet. Sci. Comp. Med. 27:163–196, 1983.

Haines, D. M., Lording, P. M., Penhale, W. J.: Survey of thyroglobulin autoantibodies in dogs. Am. J. Vet. Res. *45*:1493–1497, 1984.

Halliwell, R. E. W.: Autoimmune disease in the dog. Adv. Vet. Sci. Comp. Med. *22*:222–233, 1978.

Hurvitz, A. I.: Gammopathies. *In* Ettinger, S. J. (ed.): Textbook of Veterinary Internal Medicine. Philadelphia, W. B. Saunders Co. 1975, pp. 1704–1708.

Kelly, M. J.: Myasthenia gravis—a receptor disease. Comp. Cont. Ed. *3*:544, 1981.

Matus, R. E., Leifer, C. E., Gordon, B. R., MacEwen, G. E., and Hurvitz, A. I.: Plasmapheresis and chemotherapy of hyperviscosity syndrome associated with monoclonal gammopathy in the dog. J.A.V.M.A. *183*:215–218, 1983.

Meuten, D. J.: Hypercalcemia, Vet. Clin. North Am. *14*:891–910, 1984.

Quimby, F. W., Jensen, C., Nawrocki, D. and Scollin, P.: Selected autoimmune diseases of the dog. Vet. Clin. North Am. 8:665–682, 1978.

Quimby, F. W., Smith, C., Brushwein, M., and Lewis, R. W.: Efficacy of immunodiagnostic procedures in the recognition of canine immunologic disease. Am. J. Vet. Res. *41*:1662–1666, 1980.

Scott, R. C.: Immune mediated renal disease. *In* Kirk, R. W. (ed.): Current Veterinary Therapy VIII. Philadelphia, W. B. Saunders Co., 1983., pp. 966–971.

Tizard, I.: An Introduction to Veterinary Immunology. 2nd ed., Philadelphia, W. B. Saunders. Co., 1982.

Werner, L. L. and Gorman, N. T.: Immune mediated disorders of cats. Vet. Clin. North Am. *14*:1039–1064, 1984.

Werner, L. L.: Coombs' positive anemias in the dog and cat. Comp. Cont. Ed. *11*:96–102, 1980.

Williams, D. A.: Gammopathies. Comp. Cont. Ed. *3*:815–822, 1981.

CLINICAL CHEMISTRY

The measurement of various constituents of the blood can be an invaluable aid in confirming a diagnosis and in determining the prognosis and course of a clinical disease. Several facts should be remembered when the use of blood chemistry tests is contemplated.

1. Blood chemistry tests are important only when combined with an adequate history and physical examination.
2. Blood chemistry tests should not be used indiscriminately. Selected tests should be used to evaluate a differential diagnosis or confirm a diagnosis. See table at end of this list.

3. The clinician must realize the limitations of the test being used and must be able to interpret the results of the test.
4. The clinician must be familiar with reference laboratory values used at a given commercial laboratory. In general, reference values include 95 per cent of all values obtained from normal animals. The other 5 per cent of normal animals will have values falling outside the reference interval in the third standard deviation above or below the mean. The larger the number of tests run on a serum sample, the greater the chance that a normal animal will have at least one test being abnormal. *Do not base clinical diagnoses on one aberrant test result!*

Tests That Reflect Liver Disease

Glucose	Urea N	Uric acid
Cholesterol	Total protein	Albumin
Alkaline phosphatase	Lactic dehydrogenase	GOTransaminase

Tests That Reflect Pancreatic Disease

Glucose	Cholesterol	Calcium
Lipase	Amylase	

Tests That Reflect Kidney Disease

Urea N	Phosphorus	Total protein
Albumin	Na, K, Cl, CO	Creatinine

Tests That Reflect Hyperadrenocorticism

Glucose	Cholesterol	Alkaline phosphatase

Tests That Reflect Muscle Disease

SGOT	CPK

Tests That Reflect Thyroid Disease

Cholesterol

Tests That Reflect Parathyroid or Bone Disease

Calcium	Phosphorus	Alkaline phosphatase

Tests That Reflect Autoimmune Disease

Direct Coombs'	Antinuclear antibodies	LE cell
Rheumatoid factor	Antiplatelet factor	

Coagulation Screening Tests

Prothrombin time	Activated partial thromboplastin time
Platelet count	Fibrin split products

Lipid Screening Tests

Triglycerides	Total lipids

PREPARATION OF BLOOD SAMPLES FOR MULTICHANNEL BIOCHEMICAL ANALYZERS

Automated multiphasic blood chemistry analyzers such as the Technicon SMA 12/60* are available to veterinarians for laboratory screening procedures. In the preparation of blood samples for multichannel biochemical analyzers, several factors are important in obtaining accurate results:
1. Hemolysis should be avoided.
2. Serum or plasma should be separated from cells within 45 minutes of obtaining the blood sample.
3. Plasma should be stored at 4°C if delay is experienced in having samples run. No significant change in parameters is noted in samples held at 4°C for up to 24 hours.
4. For automated clinical chemistry profiles on the SMA 12/60, it is necessary to have a minimum of 2.5 ml of serum.

When commercial laboratory services are being used for evaluating other clinical pathology profiles, the following table may be of value:

BASIC 12- to 16-UNIT CHEMSCREEN USUALLY AVAILABLE VIA AUTOMATED CHEMISTRY

Calcium	Bilirubin, total	Alkaline phosphatase
Phosphorus	SGPT	SGOT
Glucose	Albumin	LDH
Blood urea nitrogen	Total protein	Creatinine

Although laboratories may differ somewhat in the type of collection vials used for submitting specimens, most laboratories accept or use Vacutainer collection vials (see p. 888).

For those tests requiring serum, the serum must be separated from the cells within 45 minutes of the venipuncture. Blood should be allowed to clot for 30 to 60 minutes, then centrifuged at 3000 RPM to separate the serum fraction.

For submittal of specimens for clotting function, see page 709.

SERUM PROTEINS

The liver produces all the albumin and most of the globulins; a small amount of gamma globulin is produced by reticuloendothelial tissue.

Fibrinogen, albumin, and globulins constitute the major proteins of the blood plasma. In determining serum proteins, serum or plasma must be free

---

*Technicon SMA 12/60, Technicon Corporation, Tarrytown, New York.

Table 134. NORMAL VALUES FOR SERUM PROTEIN

Serum Protein	Dog	Cat
Total protein (serum) (gm/dl)	5.40–7.10	5.40–7.30
Albumin (gm/dl)	2.30–3.20	2.10–3.30
Globulin (gm/dl)	2.70–4.40	2.60–5.10
Alpha-1	0.20–0.50	0.20–1.10
Alpha-2	0.30–1.10	0.40–0.90
Beta-1	0.60–1.20	0.30–0.90
Beta-2	—	0.60–1.00
Gamma-1	0.50–1.30	0.30–2.50
Gamma-2	0.40–0.90	1.40–1.90
Albumin:globulin ratio	0.59–1.11	0.45–1.19

Source: Kaneko, J. J.: Standard values in domestic animals. University of California, Davis. From Benjamin, M.: Outline of Clinical Veterinary Pathology, 3rd ed. Ames, Iowa, Iowa State University Press, 1978.

of hemolysis. Fibrinogen is removed in coagulation; therefore, fibrinogen determinations cannot be done on serum.

In general, plasma proteins are low in young animals (usually less than 5.0 gm/100 ml of plasma). Older animals may have total plasma proteins in the range of 7.0 to 8.0 gm per dl (see Table 134).

Gamma globulins are formed by the reticuloendothelial cells of the body, whereas albumin, fibrinogen, prothrombin, and alpha and beta globulins are formed in the liver. (See p. 755 for information about globulins and A/G ratio.)

Determination of plasma protein levels may be important when:
1. The nutritive state of the animal is being assessed.
2. Kidney and liver functions are being evaluated.
3. The role of the reticuloendothelial system in a clinical situation is being assessed.
4. Fluid balance in states of shock, dehydration, and hemorrhage is being determined.

The albumin fraction exerts the greatest effect on the total volume of plasma protein. Decreases in albumin levels usually result in lowered total plasma volume. A decrease in total serum albumin may be the result of a lowered protein intake resulting from malnutrition that may be diet related or associated with malabsorption, deficient synthesis of albumin by the liver associated with chronic hepatic disease (see p. 762), excessive protein breakdown that may occur with prolonged fever, diabetes mellitus, postsurgical conditions and trauma, or excessive loss of protein that may occur with acute nephritis, nephrosis, burns, parasitism, ascites, and hemorrhage associated with damaged vessels and tissue.

The concentration of proteins in the blood determines the colloidal osmotic pressure of the plasma. Lipemic plasma, cloudy plasma, or hemolysis will affect the total serum protein determinations. The concentration of protein in the plasma can be influenced by the nutritional state of the animal, hepatic function (see p. 762), renal function, blood loss, dehydration, various diseases, and metabolic abnormalities. Various individual fractions of the plasma proteins may be helpful in diagnosing certain diseases. These plasma protein fractions may be separated by plasma electrophoresis.

Disorders that cause hypoproteinemia can be associated with diminished production of proteins or increased loss of proteins. Diminished production of proteins, specifically hypoalbuminemia, can be associated with primary or secondary intestinal malabsorption, exocrine pancreatic insufficiency, malnutrition, parasitism, and liver disease. Increased loss of proteins resulting in hypoalbuminemia could be associated with renal disease (specifically glomerular disease), protein-losing enteropathies, severe exudative skin diseases, and chronic blood loss.

Hyperproteinemia can occur in dehydration, shock, administration of quantities of concentrated amino acids, certain neoplasms, and infections.

Plasma fibrinogen levels have been used in the interpretation of the response and severity of certain diseases in small animals. The normal range of fibrinogen is 200 to 400 mg per 100 ml of plasma. The total plasma protein (PP):fibrinogen (F) ratio is variable, depending on the age of the animal. In general, a PP:F ratio of less than 15.0:1.0 would indicate an increase in fibrinogen over plasma protein. A ratio below 10.0:1.0 indicates a marked increase in fibrinogen. Fibrinogen is a soluble plasma protein produced in the microsomes of hepatic parenchymal cells and stored in the liver. The half-life of canine fibrinogen is 2.3 to 2.7 days. Normal ranges of fibrinogen level are 200 to 400 mg per dl in the dog and cat.

Increased fibrinogen levels are associated with inflammation (both acute and chronic) and tissue destruction. Decreased fibrinogen levels can be associated with clotted blood samples, liver disease, disseminated intravascular coagulation (DIC), fibrinous exudation into serous cavities, shock, and nutritional disorders.

BLOOD AMMONIA

Ammonium is normally absorbed from the lower intestinal tract, removed via the portal circulation, transported to the liver, and converted to urea. Ammonia is normally converted to urea in the liver by the urea cycle. Abnormalities in blood ammonia levels can be seen in the hepatoencephalopathy conditions in veterinary medicine. The most common of these conditions is congenital portacaval shunts; however, acquired diseases such as cirrhosis, toxic hepatopathy, and hepatic neoplasia can also lead to this condition.

In animals with congenital portal vein anomalies, ammonium biurate crystals may be found in the urine of approximately one third of the cases, and fasting venous blood ammonia levels are usually greater than 120 μg per dl. An ammonia tolerance test can be run in the dog. The animal must be fasted for 6 hours. Blood samples should be collected in ammonium-free heparin and placed in ice when held for analysis. Separate the plasma within 30 minutes after sampling by centrifugation after chilling the sample. Administer 0.1 gm of NH_4 Cl per kg of body weight orally following a fast. A maximum of 3 gm is administered in 20 to 50 ml of warm water. Samples are collected at 30 minutes, and results are compared with control values. Values are dependent on the testing procedure being used; thus, paired samples should be run with a normal dog. (Normals are usually 19 to 120. Levels above 300 are abnormal.)

Blood ammonia levels for the cat following the oral administration of 100 mg per kg of ammonium chloride have been reported to be 0.26 to 0.53 mg per dl, with normal fasting blood ammonia levels being 0.1 to 0.35 mg per dl.

SERUM AMYLASE

In normal animals, a small amount of serum amylase from the pancreas and salivary glands is present in the blood. Inflammation of the pancreas may release abnormal amounts of this enzyme into the blood. Conditions such as renal insufficiency, corticosteroid elevations, and factors that increase the production of pituitary and adrenal glands could also elevate serum amylase levels. Hyperamylasemia associated with renal failure is associated in part with the impaired clearance of amylase by glomerular filtration. Primary renal failure is usually associated with an azotemia, impaired ability to concentrate or dilute urine (specific gravity = 1.007–1.024), and moderate to severe hyperamylasemia (two to three times normal). In dogs, acute pancreatitis is associated with marked hyperamylasemia, which may be up to seven times normal, occasional prerenal azotemia, and ability of the kidneys to concentrate urine to a specific gravity greater than 1.025.

Normal values for serum amylase levels in dogs are modified Caraway units (amyloclastic)—under 1000, Harding units (amyloclastic)—under 3200, Gomori (amyloclastic)—0 to 800, DyAmyl (saccharogenic)—under 3200, IU per L—185 to 700, and Somogyi units—100 to 400.

PLASMA BICARBONATE (See p. 608)

The bicarbonate–carbonic acid buffer is one of the most important buffer systems in maintaining the normal pH of the body fluid. Normally, these constituents are present in a ratio of 1 part of carbonic acid to 20 parts of bicarbonate.

Serum bicarbonate is elevated in metabolic alkalosis such as occurs with prolonged vomiting or in respiratory acidosis due to hypoventilation. Serum bicarbonate is reduced in metabolic acidosis in conditions such as diabetic ketosis, persistent diarrhea, renal insufficiency, shock, or respiratory alkalosis due to hyperventilation.

CARBON DIOXIDE (See p. 593)

Serum contains HCO_3^-, physically dissolved CO_2 (proportional to the pCO_2), and H_2CO_3. At normal blood pH, the ratio of HCO_3^- to dissolved CO_2 and H_2CO_3 is 20:1. In reliably assessing acid-base status, measurement of arterial blood pH or pCO_2 and total CO_2 is desirable. When the value of any two of these three parameters is known, a nomogram can be used to calculate the other.

Practical office evaluation of acid-base abnormalities often depends on the availability of CO_2 determinations interpreted along with clinical findings. When one measures the CO_2 content of blood allowed to be exposed to the air, the total CO_2 that is measured is almost exclusively bicarbonate. The development of rapid, inexpensive office screening procedures for CO_2 determination makes this a practical test. A low CO_2 level may indicate either metabolic acidosis or respiratory alkalosis, and a high CO_2 level may indicate metabolic alkalosis or respiratory acidosis.

SERUM BILIRUBIN (See p. 755)

BLOOD UREA NITROGEN (BUN)–SERUM UREA NITROGEN (SUN)

Ammonium oxalate or "double oxalate" cannot be used as an anticoagulant if this test is to be performed, because the ammonia will be measured as urea.

Urea, an end product of protein metabolism, is excreted by the kidneys. Some 40 per cent or more of this urea is reabsorbed by the kidney tubules. Thus, blood urea levels are one indication of kidney function and can serve as a rough index of glomerular filtration rate. The BUN varies directly with protein intake and inversely with the rate of excretion of urea. Nonrenal variables may cause variable increases in urea nitrogen levels: (1) ingestion and absorption of large quantities of protein; (2) absorption of protein from gastrointestinal hemorrhage; (3) catabolic states in fever, infection, or trauma; and (4) administration of catabolic drugs such as glucocorticoids or thyroid hormones.

BUN may be elevated in renal insufficiency (acute or chronic); increased nitrogen metabolism associated with diminished renal blood flow or impaired renal function, as may occur in dehydration and shock; adrenal insufficiency and congestive heart failure; and postrenal obstruction preventing normal urination, as may occur with urethral calculi.

Repeated BUN tests are usually indicated to follow the progress of the animal. An elevation of BUN will not become evident until 70 to 75 per cent or more of the nephrons of both kidneys become nonfunctional.

Azotemia is the presence of abnormally high concentrations of urea, creatinine, and other nonprotein nitrogenous substances in the blood.

CREATININE

Creatinine is derived from creatine and phosphocreatine during muscle metabolism and is excreted by way of the glomerulus of the kidney, with a small amount secreted by the proximal tubules. Blood creatinine levels are not affected by dietary protein, protein catabolism, age, gender, or exercise. Excretion is almost entirely dependent on the process of glomerular filtration. Creatinine clearance can be used as a reasonable measurement of the glomerular filtration rate (GFR). Estimation of the degree of reduction of glomerular filtration from the concentration of creatinine in plasma has a basis because of a steady state relationship between the GFR and the concentration of creatinine in the plasma. For every 50 per cent reduction in GFR, the creatinine concentration should double. The normal plasma creatinine concentration is 0.5 to 1.0 mg per 100 ml. Twenty-four–hour endogenous urine creatinine assays are more reliable in evaluating GFR but are more difficult to run. Serial determinations of creatinine should be used when determining the prognosis in renal disease. The significance of an elevated creatinine can be determined only after analyzing other renal function tests. A high creatinine level that persists despite appropriate therapy justifies a guarded prognosis.

URIC ACID (See also p. 764)

BLOOD CALCIUM

Calcium is necessary for the normal function of muscle contraction, transmission of nerve impulses, blood coagulation, neuromuscular excitability, and cell membrane permeability. The main store of body calcium is in the bones. Serum calcium exists in two forms: (1) an inactive form that is combined with a serum protein fraction (mainly albumin), and (2) an active form that is not combined with a protein. When total serum calcium is measured in the laboratory, the measurement includes ionized calcium, chelated calcium, and protein-bound calcium.

Approximately 50 per cent of the measured total plasma calcium is bound to serum proteins. Hyperproteinemia can increase the measured calcium, and hypoproteinemia can decrease the measured calcium.

Changes in serum calcium relative to blood albumin levels can be estimated using the following formula:

corrected calcium (mg/dl) = Ca (mg/dl) − albumin (gm/dl) + 3.5

There are several clinical situations in which serum calcium levels should be determined, including bone disorders, convulsions, parathyroid abnormalities, renal insufficiency, malabsorption syndromes, pseudohyperparathyroidism, and vitamin D intoxication. Various forms of neoplasia in the dog have been associated with hypercalcemia, including lymphosarcoma, multiple myeloma, mammary gland adenocarcinoma, fibrosarcoma, perianal gland adenoma, perirectal adenocarcinoma, and abdominal adenocarcinoma. Of these, lymphosarcoma is the most common tumor associated with calcium abnormalities (see p. 696). The incidence of hypercalcemia in dogs with lymphosarcoma ranges from 10 to 40 per cent. The anterior mediastinal form of lymphosarcoma is commonly associated with high calcium levels. Cats with lymphosarcoma rarely demonstrate hypercalcemia.

Several factors can alter the ionized (active) serum calcium levels:
1. Alkalosis lowers ionized calcium levels, whereas acidosis may increase ionized calcium levels.
2. Vitamin D levels influence serum calcium levels. Deficiencies of vitamin D may lead to low blood-calcium levels. Large excesses of vitamin D cause high levels of serum calcium and may result in dystrophic calcification. The

ingestion of the house plant, day blooming jasmine (*cestrum diurnum*) can produce vitamin D intoxication.

3. The parathyroid glands, by producing parathormone, can greatly influence the serum calcium levels. Parathormone controls calcium mobilization from the bones and the renal excretion of phosphorus, thus controlling the calcium:phosphorus ratio.

4. The calcium:phorphorus ratio in the diet can also affect the serum calcium levels.

Increased serum calcium levels are seen in primary hyperparathyroidism. Primary hyperparathyroidism is very rare and is usually caused by a functioning adenoma of the parathyroid gland. It has been reported in dogs (see also p. 659).

Secondary hyperparathyroidism may result from an improper calcium or phosphorus ratio in the diet or from renal insufficiency. The normal calcium:phosphorus ratio in the diet is 1.2:1. Excessively high phosphorus ratios, as seen in cats on all red meat diets, lead to hyperparathyroidism and mobilization of calcium from the bones. Secondary hyperparathyroidism in renal insufficiency is associated with a retention of phosphorus, leading to hyperphosphatemia and hypocalcemia, which stimulates the production of parathormone. It is important to remember that in secondary hyperparathyroidism, the serum calcium levels may be normal, decreased, or elevated, depending on the stage of the disease.

Thus, repeated serum calcium, phosphorus, and alkaline phosphatase determinations are needed to assess the condition of an animal with secondary hyperparathyroidism.

Other causes of high serum calcium may be primary hyperparathyroidism (tumor, hyperplasia); pseudohyperparathyroidism; tertiary hyperparathyroidism; overzealous oral or parenteral calcium supplementation; recovery phase of acute renal failure; drug induced (thiazides, spironolactone); adrenocortical insufficiency; hyperthyroidism and hypothyroidism; hypophosphatasia; generalized periostitis; immobilization; use of calcium ion–exchange resins in hemodialysis; and sarcoidosis.

Decreased levels of blood calcium can be seen in hypoparathyroidism, azotemia, hypoalbuminemia, starvation, eclampsia, rickets, vitamin D deficiency, and malabsorption syndromes. Excessive dietary calcium produces hypercalcitonism, either by increasing plasma calcium with direct stimulation of the thyroid C cells, or indirectly, via stimulation of gastrin produced by the G cells, mainly in the distal pylorus of the stomach. The ultimate results of excessive dietary calcium in balanced proportion to phosphorus are hypocalcemia, hypophosphatemia, and hypophosphatasemia. Hypoalbuminemia is the most common condition associated with hypocalcemia. It involves a reduction in protein bound calcium, although ionized calcium may remain normal.

Other causes for lowered serum calcium include hypoparathyroidism (surgical, idiopathic); eclampsia; intoxications (ethylene glycol), reduction in serum albumin (malabsorption, short-bowel syndrome, chronic liver disease, nephrotic syndrome, malnutrition); pancreatitis; renal disease (acute and chronic renal tubular dysfunction, renal tubular acidosis); adrenal corticosteroid excess; commercial phosphate–containing enemas when used in small dogs and cats can produce hypocalcemia, because phosphate is absorbed through the colonic wall; increased skeletal avidity due to osteoblastic metastases; infusion of chelating agents; hyperphosphatemia (renal failure, phosphate infusions); rickets and osteomalacia; magnesium deficiency; glucagon administration; mithramycin administration; pseudohypoparathyroidism; medullary carcinoma of the thyroid; and calcitonin-secreting tumors.

CREATINE PHOSPHOKINASE

The enzyme creatine phosphokinase (CPK) splits creatine phosphate in the presence of ADP to yield creatine and ATP. CPK is most abundant in mammalian skeletal muscle, heart muscle, and nervous tissue. Variations in CPK values can be related to gender, age, and physical activity. They are elevated in the presence of muscle damage that could result from trauma, infarction, muscular dystrophies, or inflammation. Elevated CPK values can also be observed following intramuscular injections of irritating substances, and this factor should be considered in measurement of this enzyme. Elevated CPK values do not reveal what the underlying muscle pathology is. Muscle diseases may be associated with abnormalities of the muscle fiber itself or with neurogenic diseases resulting in secondary damage to muscle fibers. High increased CPK values are usually associated with myogenic disease.

DELTA–AMINO LEVULINIC ACID

Delta–amino levulinic acid (DALA) is one of the precursors of heme; and from two moles of DALA, one mole of porphobilinogen is formed. This conversion requires an enzyme, amino levulinic acid (ALA) dehydrase, which is partially inhibited by lead. The influence of lead in blocking the normal metabolism of ALA results in the appearance of an abnormally large amount of DALA in the plasma and urine. This abnormal level of DALA can be used as a diagnostic test for lead poisoning. Normal background urinary DALA levels in the dog have ranged from 120 to 190 µg per 100 ml.

Increased levels of DALA are usually attributed to the inhibitor of ALA dehydrase activity in the conversion of DALA to porphobilinogen (PGT) in heme synthesis.

References and Additional Readings

Barnes, J. R., Smith, P. E., and Drummond, C. M.: Urine osmolality and Δ-amino levulinic acid excretion. Arch. Environ. Health, 25:450, 1972.

SERUM PHOSPHORUS (INORGANIC PHOSPHORUS)

Normal phosphorus values are measured in mg per dl and may be variable in the dog depending on age and diet. Young, rapidly growing large breed dogs will have phosphorus levels of 8.0 to 9.0 mg per dl. Mature dogs have phosphorus values ranging from 2.5 to to 6.1 mg per dl; cats vary from 3.5 to 7.1 mg per dl.

The level of inorganic phosphorus in the plasma can be influenced by the parathyroid glands, intestinal absorption, renal function, bone metabolism, nutrition, and ionized serum calcium levels.

Hyperphosphatemia can occur in renal failure with phosphorus retention; hypoparathyroidism with an excessive tubular reabsorption of phosphorus in the absence of adequate levels of parathormone; and excessive vitamin D intake, associated with phosphate enemas and hemolysis. The most common reason for abnormally elevated phosphate levels is renal failure (see p. 123).

Hypophosphatemia can occur in inadequate intake of phosphorus, primary hyperparathyroidism due to the elimination of larger amounts of phosphorus in the urine, and after insulin administration.

Diabetes mellitus may be associated with hypophosphatemia because of osmotic diuresis and abnormal tubular reabsorption of phosphorus.

SERUM SODIUM AND CHLORIDE

Chloride is the principal inorganic anion of the extracellular fluid. It is important in the maintenance of acid-base balance. When chloride in the form of hydrochloric acid or ammonium chloride is lost, alkalosis follows; when chloride is retained or ingested, acidosis follows. Abnormalities in serum chloride are uncommon but, when found, may be associated with metabolic acidosis as seen in diarrhea, chronic draining fistulas, renal tubular acidosis, and administration of ammonium chloride.

Sodium and chloride ions provide the greatest part of the osmotically active solute in the plasma and can greatly influence the distribution of the water. The shift of sodium ions into cells or a loss of sodium from the body produces a decrease of extracellular fluid that greatly affects circulation, renal function, and the nervous system.

Increases in sodium may occur in dehydration or a primary water deficit, hyperadrenocorticoidism, and central nervous system (CNS) trauma or disease.

Decreased serum sodium levels can be seen in adrenal insufficiency, inadequate sodium intake, renal insufficiency, physiologic response to burns or trauma, losses from the gastrointestinal tract (as in diarrhea or intestinal obstruction), water intoxication, and uncontrolled diabetes mellitus.

Metabolic acidosis with evidence of increased anion gap is usually associated with hyperchloremia. Hyperchloremia can be associated with hemoconcentration, hyperchloremic metabolic acidosis, or chronic respiratory alkalosis.

Hemoconcentration can be evaluated by comparing serum chloride and sodium. Careful evaluation of the respiratory system and any evidence of hepatic coma can eliminate respiratory alkalosis.

Most cases of hyperchloremic metabolic acidosis are associated with dehydration, loss of sodium bicarbonate or conjugate base from the extracellular space, and increased renal tubular resorption of chloride.

One unusual and interesting disease observed in dogs with hyperchloremia is renal tubular acidosis. Two forms have been described. In proximal renal tubular acidosis (type II), there is abnormal tubular resorption of bicarbonate and loss of HCO_3 in the urine, with retention of chloride. Additionally, glycosuria, aminoaciduria, and phosphaturia may be present. The combination of these syndromes in the dog has been described as a "Fanconi-like" syndrome in man and is seen in the Basenji breed.

Distal renal tubular acidosis is associated with the inability of the distal renal tubules and collecting ducts to secrete hydrogen ions against a pH gradient. Metabolic acidosis develops with retention of chloride and sodium. The urine pH becomes elevated in relationship to blood pH. Confirmation of this problem is based on the ability of the kidneys to excrete an acid load such as ammonium chloride.

Elevated serum chloride levels can be seen in renal insufficiency following administration of ammonium chloride; chronic pyelonephritis; dehydration; overtreatment with saline solutions; congestion and edema associated with cirrhosis of the liver; and carbon dioxide deficit (as occurs in hyperventilation). Clinical manifestations are polydipsia-polyuria (PD-PU), anorexia, weight loss, weakness associated with loss of potassium, acidosis, and progressive renal failure.

Decreased serum chloride levels can be seen in gastrointestinal disease (producing vomiting and diarrhea), renal insufficiency with salt deprivation, overtreatment with certain diuretics, diabetic acidosis, adrenal insufficiency, and hypoventilation (as occurs in pneumonia, emphysema, and pulmonary edema), resulting in respiratory acidosis.

SERUM POTASSIUM (See p. 602)

Potassium represents the major cation of intracellular fluid. The concentration of potassium in the extracellular fluid normally varies over a narrow range from 3.9 to 5.6 mEq per L in the dog and from 4.0 to 4.5 mEq per L in the cat. Cells are highly permeable to K^+ ions, and they move passively and freely in and out. Numerous mechanisms are responsible for the regulation of potassium levels: (1) ingestion in the diet, (2) sodium pump (renal), (3) arterial pH, (4) insulin levels, and (5) cell breakdown.

Abnormalities associated with abnormal decreases in potassium can produce metabolic, neuromuscular, cardiovascular, and renal changes:

1. Hypokalemia produces glucose intolerance—release of insulin is impaired.
2. Neuromuscular—skeletal muscle weakness; impaired smooth muscle function.
3. Inability to concentrate urine, resulting in nocturia, PD-PU.
4. Abnormal repolarization of cardiac cell membranes—depression of S-T segment, prolongation of Q-T interval, slow heart rate.

Clinically significant hyperkalemia occurs when serum potassium exceeds 7.0 to 7.5 mEq per L.

Hyperkalemia is often associated with impaired renal excretion of potassium. Potassium excretion is largely accomplished by tubular secretion, not by glomerular filtration; therefore, hyperkalemia does not occur until late in the course of renal disease, with marked alteration in glomerular filtration and existing uremia. Urethral obstruction, especially in cats, is often associated with elevated serum potassium levels (see p. 49). The major cardiovascular effects of hyperkalemia are reviewed on p. 49. Hypokalemia is not usually of clinical importance until serum potassium levels fall below 3.5 mEq per L. Metabolic acidosis contributes to the development of severe hyperkalemia, as does adrenal insufficiency.

Hypokalemia can result from excessive loss of potassium associated with protracted vomiting or diarrhea. Alkalosis results in the migration of potassium ions from the extracellular to intracellular fluid and increased urinary loss of potassium. Urinary loss of potassium occurs by secretion in the distal tubules. Excessive potassium is lost in hyperadrenocorticism and renal tubular acidosis. Hypokalemia may be evident following the administration of K^+-depleting diuretics. Hypokalemia can also be seen in ketoacidotic diabetes following the administration of insulin, which causes K^+ ions to enter the cell (see p. 607). Fluid administration of fluids low in potassium can result in hypokalemia; lactated Ringer's solution contains only 4 mEq of K per L (see p. 607).

A summary of electrolyte changes in certain clinical disorders is shown in Table 135.

BLOOD GLUCOSE (See p. 664)

Blood glucose levels are usually determined after a 12-hour fast. Serum is the sample of choice; however, plasma is acceptable. Sodium fluoride is the anticoagulant to use.

The glucose level in the blood is maintained within a relatively narrow physiologic limit. Several factors control blood glucose levels, including hepatic gluconeogenesis and glycogenolysis, renal excretion and reabsorption, removal of glucose by the tissues, effects of hormonal processes on tissue metabolism, and intestinal absorption of glucose.

Elevated blood glucose levels (hyperglycemia) can occur in diabetes mellitus, hyperthyroidism, hyperadrenocorticoidism, hyperpituitarism, anoxia (because of the instability of liver glycogen in oxygen deficiency), production of epinephrine, certain physiologic conditions (digestion, exposure to cold, following general anesthesia), administration of glucose-containing fluids, and acute pancreatic necrosis.

Decreased blood glucose levels (hypoglycemia) may occur in hyperinsulinism due to a tumor of the pancreas (islet cell adenoma) or from an overdose of exogenous insulin, following severe excretion, starvation, adrenal insufficiency, hypopituitarism, and hepatic insufficiency, as well as in a functional hypoglycemic von Gierke–like syndrome.

SERUM TRANSAMINASE (See Table 136.)

Aspartate aminotransferase (AST; formerly SGOT) is found in high levels in the liver, myocardium, and skeletal muscles. Alanine aminotransferase (SGPT) is found in large concentrations in the liver of the dog and cat.

Table 135. CHANGES IN ELECTROLYTES AND URINE VOLUME IN CLINICAL DISORDERS*

| Disorder | Blood Sodium | Electrolytes | | | Urine Volume |
		Potassium	Bicarbonate	Chloride	
Congestive heart failure	N or D	N	I	D	D
Diarrhea	D	D	D	D	D
Pyloric obstruction	D	D	I	D	D
Dehydration	I	N	N or D	I	D
Adrenal cortical insufficiency	D	I	N or D	D	N or d
Diabetes insipidus	N or I	N	N	I	I
Diabetic acidosis	D	N or I	D	D	I
Chronic renal failure	D	N or D	D	D or N	V
Acute renal failure	D	I	D	I	D
Renal tubular acidosis	D	D	D	I	I
Diamox administration	D	D	D	I	I

*N = normal; D = decreased; I = increased; V = variable.

Table 136. LIVER FUNCTION TESTS

Condition	SGOT	SGPT	AP	BSP
Passive congestion	±	+	+	+
Fatty degeneration	+	+	+	+
Necrosis	+ +	+ + +	+ +	+ + +
Biliary obstruction	+	+ +	+ + +	+ + +

From Benjamin, M.: Outline of Veterinary Clinical Pathology, 3rd ed. Ames, Iowa, Iowa State University Press, 1978, p. 249.

Destruction of liver cells can release these enzymes, resulting in an increase in their concentration in the plasma. Half-lives of SGPT in normal dogs average 2.5 hours. If persistently high levels of SGPT are present, it suggests the presence of a hepatocellular necrosis.

Increased SGPT in the dog and cat is usually specific for hepatic necrosis. SGPT values of 10 to 50 Sigma-Frankel units are considered normal; values of 50 to 400 units indicate moderate liver necrosis; and severe necrosis is indicated by values of more than 400 units.

The simultaneous use of Bromsulphalein BSP and SGPT is of value in differentiating between advanced fibrosis and liver necrosis. In fibrosis, the BSP excretion is decreased and the SGPT is normal, whereas in necrosis, the reverse situation usually occurs.

SGOT is not specific for liver necrosis. Pathologic conditions involving the cardiac or skeletal muscles that produce necrosis will also elevate the SGOT.

Cats with cholestatic liver disease may show signs of lethargy, weakness, vomiting, anorexia, diarrhea, weight loss, jaundice, pyrexia, bleeding disorders, and ascites. Elevation of ALP in the cat is not an accurate indication of cholestatic disease (see p. 764). A much better indication is the SGPT test, and elevations in serum bile acids and total cholesterol and a marked elevation in liver copper content are present in long-present cholestasis.

ALKALINE PHOSPHATASE (See p. 764)

Serum alkaline phosphatase activity is a summation of different isoenzymes derived from different body tissues.

Alkaline phosphatase is present in high concentrations in bone, intestinal mucosa, renal cortex, placenta, and bile. The alkaline phosphatase in serum consists of a mixture of isoenzymes that can be separated by electrophoresis. Significant increases in alkaline phosphatase can be observed in both intrahepatic cholestasis and extrahepatic bile duct obstruction. High levels of serum alkaline phosphatase are not usually observed in the cat, even with hepatobiliary obstruction. The half-life for hepatic-derived alkaline phosphatase in the cat is 5.8 hours. This enzyme is rapidly cleared from the blood.

Increased serum alkaline phosphatase activity in clinical cases is associated with liver or bone abnormalities; the serum half-life for these isoenzymes is 3 days.

Serum alkaline phosphatase may be increased in bone diseases, in increased osteoblastic and osteoclastic changes such as secondary hyperparathyroidism, in obstruction of bile ducts, in certain bone tumors such as osteogenic sarcomas, and in hyperadrenocorticism. Phenobarbital is a potent activator of alkaline phosphatase.

Biliary obstruction results in the most dramatic increases of serum alkaline phosphatase. The obstruction is not usually a complete extrahepatic obstruction, but intrahepatic, associated with swelling of hepatocytes and bile stasis. Alkaline phosphatase is membrane bound and produced by epithelial cells forming bile canaliculi. In biliary obstruction, these cells proliferate to increase enzyme activity. Serum alkaline phosphatase activity is also increased with steroid-induced hepatopathy, either iatrogenic or associated with Cushing's disease.

A more sensitive test than serum alkaline phosphatase elevations for biliary obstruction is the gamma glutamyl transpeptidase (GGT) test. GGT is absent from skeletal tissues and may more clearly reflect obstructive problems in the biliary system.

SERUM LIPIDS

Serum lipids in the dog are composed of cholesterol, both free and esterified; triglycerides; phospholipids; and unesterified (free) fatty acids.

The normal lipid profile in the dog includes (1) serum character—either clear, turbid, or lactescent; (2) cholesterol; (3) triglyceride; and (4) lipoprotein electrophoresis.

Triglycerides are the main form in which lipids are stored. Triglycerides are the predominant class of dietary lipids. Variabilities in triglyceride level depend on the diet of the animal in question. Animals should be fasted for 12 hours prior to taking blood samples for lipid analysis. Normal triglyceride levels have been found to range from 30 to 150 mg per dl, with mean triglyceride levels around 60 mg per dl.

Cholesterol is a precursor of bile salts and endogenous steroids as a part of cell wall membranes. Total cholesterol levels in the dog have been estimated to range from 80 to 280 mg per dl.

Chylomicrons in the blood following the ingestion of a meal are absorbed by the liver within 4 hours. Remaining plasma lipids, including triglycerides, cholesterol, and phospholipids, are bound to proteins, forming lipoproteins. Lipoproteins can be separated by ultracentrifugation and classified according to density or separated by electrophoresis and scanned by a densitometer. Four major classes of endogenous lipoproteins have been characterized in the dog: (1) very low-density lipoproteins (VLDL); (2) low-density lipoproteins (LDL); (3) high-density lipoprotein-1 (HDL_1); and (4) high-density lipoprotein-2 (HDL_2). Electrophoretic examination has revealed the following lipoproteins: beta (LDL), pre-beta (possibly VLDL), alpha-2 (HDL_1), and alpha-1 (HDL_2).

Hyperlipidemia refers to an abnormally high concentration of lipid or lipoprotein in the blood. Hyperlipidemia is not always characterized by a lactescent serum, and the character of the blood depends on the type of lipid present within the blood. The hyperlipidemic state can be categorized into primary hyperlipidemias and secondary hyperlipidemias. The primary hyper-lipidemias in man are an inherited disorder of lipid metabolism and have not been characterized in dogs.

Secondary hyperlipidemias are commonly found in dogs and are associated with pancreatitis, diabetes mellitus, hypothyroidism, and various liver abnormalities. When an animal presents with hyperlipidemia, it is important to evaluate the dietary status. A complete physical examination, including clinical pathology, should be performed to evaluate the possible role of systemic diseases.

SERUM LIPASE

Lipase determinations are made on serum samples. Lipase is excreted by the kidneys, and the presence of oliguria or anuria can result in increased levels of serum lipase. Normal values of serum lipase in the dog are Sigma-Tietz units, 0–1; Ree-Byler units, 0.8 to 12; and International, 13 to 200.

Normally, a low concentration of this fat-splitting enzyme is present in the blood. In acute pancreatitis, pancreatic lipase is released into the circulation in elevated amounts. A new serum lipase–turbidimetric test is available through Boehringer-Mannheim Diagnostics.* The basic principles of the test are that pancreatic lipase catalyzes the two-step hydrolysis of triglycerides with rapid formation of diglycerides, followed by the somewhat slower formation of monoglycerides:

$$\text{Triolein} + H_2O \xrightarrow{\text{lipase}} \text{diglyceride} + \text{fatty acid}$$

$$\text{Diglyceride} + H_2O \xrightarrow{\text{lipase}} \text{monoglyceride} + \text{fatty acid}$$

The decrease in turbidity of a triolein suspension undergoing lipase-catalyzed hydrolysis is measured in the ultraviolet range. The rate of turbidity decrease is a measure of serum lipase activity. The advantage of this test is that the results can be obtained in 15 minutes at reasonable costs.

SGPT AND AST (SGOT) (See p. 764)

SERUM LDH (LACTIC DEHYDROGENASE)

LDH catalyzes the reaction:

$$\text{Lactate} + NAD\dagger \rightleftarrows \text{pyruvate} + NADH + H^+$$

LDH is found in body tissues that use glucose for energy.

---

*Boehringer Mannheim Diagnostics, 7800 Westpark Drive, Houston, Texas 77063.
†NAD = nicotinamide adenine dinucleotide.

Assay of total serum LDH, because of its ubiquitous origins and consequent difficulties encountered in interpretation of altered levels,.has not been widely used as a diagnostic aid in veterinary medicine. Analysis of LDH isoenzymes, however, provides more specific diagnostic information. In normal canine serum, 5 isoenzymes of LDH are demonstrable, with $LDH_1 > LDH_3 > LDH_4 > LDH_2 > LDH_5$. This distribution may be altered following damage to tissues. The nature of the alteration provides a more accurate indication of the organs involved than does assay of total serum LDH. Sources of LDH isoenzyme fractions are LDH_1 and LDH_2—heart, erythrocytes, kidney, and brain; LDH_3—lung, pancreas, adrenal, spleen, thymus, and thyroid; LDH_4 and LDH_5—skeletal muscle and liver.

LDH isoenzyme analysis provides a reliable and fairly specific aid to the diagnosis of active myocardial damage in the dog. There is a rapid rise and fall in the activity of LDH_1 and LDH_2 following experimentally induced myocardial damage in the dog. The presence of increased activity of these isoenzymes in serum provides good supportive evidence of recent or continuing myocardial damage. Conversely, the absence of elevated activity of these isoenzymes suggests that myocardial damage is not the cause of the problem or is no longer active or is proceeding at such a low level as not to be reflected in the serum.

Because of the abundance of LDH (LDH_1 and LDH_2) in erythrocytes, samples for analysis should be free of hemolysis; otherwise, pronounced alterations in LDH activity are observed.

Increases in both total LDH and LDH isoenzymes have also been observed in dogs with neoplasia. The isoenzyme patterns observed in these cases vary, but the major increases have been observed in the isoenzymes of intermediate and slow electrophoretic mobility.

With liver disease and skeletal damage, assay of LDH isoenzymes does not appear to offer any advantage over the more commonly assayed enzymes.

References and Additional Readings

Bass, D. V., Haffman, W. E., and Dorner, J. L.: Normal canine lipid profiles and effects of experimentally induced pancreatitis and hepatic necrosis on lipids. Am. J. Vet. Res., 37:1355, 1976.

Benjamin, M. M.: Outline of Veterinary Clinical Pathology, 3rd ed. Ames, Iowa, Iowa State University Press, 1979.

Bovée, K. C., and Joyce, T.: Clinical evaluation of glomerular function: 24-hour creatinine clearance in dogs. J.A.V.M.A., 174:488, 1979.

Bovée, K. C., et al.: Characterization of renal defects in dogs with a syndrome similar to the Fanconi syndrome in man. J.A.V.M.A., 174:1094, 1979.

Coles, E. H.: Veterinary Clinical Pathology, 3rd ed. Philadelphia, W. B. Saunders Company, 1980.

DiBartola, S. P., and Tasker, J. B.: Elevated serum creatinine phosphokinase: a study of 53 cases and a review of its diagnostic usefulness in clinical veterinary medicine. J.A.A.H.A., 13:744, 1977.

Duncan, R. J., and Prasse, K. W.: Veterinary Laboratory Medicine and Clinical Pathology. Ames, Iowa, Iowa State University Press, 1978.

Epstein, M. E., Barsanti, J. A., Finco, R., and Cowgill, L. M.: Postprandial changes in plasma urea nitrogen and plasma creatinine concentrations in dogs fed commercial diets. J.A.A.H.A. *20*:779–782, 1984.

Everett, R. M., Duncan, J. R., and Prasse, K. W.: Alkaline phosphatase, leucine aminopeptidase, and alanine aminotransferase activities with obstructive and toxic hepatic disease in cats. Am. J. Vet. Res., *38*:963, 1977.

Everett, R. M., Duncan, J. R., and Prasse, K. W.: Alkaline phosphatases in tissues and sera of cats. Am. J. Vet. Res., *38*:1533, 1977.

Ford, R. B.: Clinical application of serum lipid profiles in the dog. Proceedings of 27th Gaines Veterinary Symposium, College Station, Tex., 1977, pp. 12–16.

Haffman, W. E., Renegar, W. E., and Dorner, J. L.: Serum half-life of intravenously injected intestinal and hepatic alkaline phosphatase isoenzymes in the cat. Am. J. Vet. Res., *38*:1637, 1977.

Meyer, D. J.: The recognition and diagnosis of canine hepatic encephalopathy. Fla. Vet. J., *7*:20, 1978.

Meyer, J., Strombeck, D. R., Stone, E. A., et al.: Ammonia tolerance test in clinically normal dogs and in dogs with portosystemic shunts. J.A.V.M.A., *173*:377, 1978.

Rogers, W. A., Donovan, E. F., and Kociba, G. J.: Lipids and lipoproteins in normal dogs and dogs with secondary hyperlipoproteinemia. J.A.V.M.A., *166*:1092, 1975.

Strombeck, D. R., and Rogers, Q.: Plasma amino acid concentrations in dogs with hepatic disease. J.A.V.M.A., *173*:93, 1978.

Strombeck, D. R., Weiser, M. G., and Kaneko, J. J.: Hyperammonia and hepatic encephalopathy in the dog. J.A.V.M.A., *167*:1105, 1975.

Wilkins, R. J., Hurvitz, A. I.: Profiling in Veterinary Clinical Pathology—Dog and Cat, Vol. 1. Tarrytown, N.Y., Technicon Corporation, 1978.

LIVER FUNCTION TESTS

The liver has many varied functions, and no one laboratory test can be used as an indication of normal or abnormal liver function. Because of its tremendous size and regeneration capability, a large portion of the liver (80 per cent) may be injured before alterations in liver function are noticed. Repeated liver function tests are frequently needed to follow the course of liver diseases. The use of a limited battery of tests is indicated to obtain a liver profile to help determine what anatomic units of the liver are diseased.

Liver function tests are used to determine the presence of liver disease, the type of disease, the extent of damage, and the disease prognosis. Liver function tests should not be used alone but should be correlated with clinical signs and liver biopsy (see p. 755) to develop an overall picture.

LIVER EXCRETION TESTS

Bile Pigment Formation

The liver is composed of four anatomic systems–namely, hepatocytes, biliary network, vascular system, and Kupffer's cells (reticuloendothelial system). The main anatomic unit of the liver is the lobule. There is a central efferent vein surrounded by hepatocytes and portal circulation at the periphery of the lobule. The biliary flow is opposite to that of the blood flow, with bile flowing toward the portal tracts.

The major part of bilirubin excreted by the liver into the bile is derived from the turnover of erythrocytic hemoglobin. Fifteen per cent of the bilirubin, however, is derived from the catabolism of various hepatic hemoproteins such as cytochrome P-450, peroxidase, and catalase, as well as from the overproduction of heme by bone marrow. Hemoglobin released by the red cells is normally transported in the plasma by haptoglobin and alpha-2 mucoprotein to the reticuloendothelial cells, where heme is enzymatically degraded, first, to biliverdin by heme oxygenase and, subsequently, to bilirubin by biliverdin reductase. The bilirubin is then transported in the plasma firmly bound to albumin. It next enters the hepatic cell and is bound to ligandin (an intracellular protein) prior to its conjugation to various sugars. Bilirubin must be conjugated to become water soluble, a process necessary for its excretion into the bile. Any obstruction preventing the excretion of bile pigment results in elevations in conjugated bilirubin in the blood and urine.

Bile pigment formation can be summarized as follows:
1. Bile pigments result from the breakdown of hemoglobin, produced when erythrocytes are destroyed.
2. Heme is converted to biliverdin and then to free bilirubin (unconjugated by the reticuloendothelial system).
3. The free bilirubin is conjugated in the smooth endoplasmic reticulum of the liver to bilirubin glucuronide (direct-reacting bilirubin).
4. Conjugated bilirubin is secreted by the bile ducts, stored in the gallbladder, and excreted in the small intestine. In the intestine, the bacterial flora reduces bilirubin to compounds collectively called *urobilinogen*.

Increased Bile Pigment Formation

Increases in bile pigment can result in the production of clinical jaundice. Excess bile pigment may be produced by the following:
1. Increased destruction of erythrocytes, producing elevated amounts of hemoglobin.
2. Decreased excretion or retention of conjugated bilirubin diglucuronide as a result of cellular disease of the liver or blockage of the excretory ducts of the liver or both.

Bile that is delivered to the common duct is composed of three fractions: (1) a bile salt–dependent fraction from liver cells; (2) a fraction from liver cells resulting from active sodium transport; and (3) a fraction secreted by the bile ducts, which is controlled by secretin.

Normal plasma bilirubin is less than 0.6 mg per dl. With hepatocellular disease, the hyperbilirubinemia is usually half conjugated bilirubin and half unconjugated. Total plasma bilirubin levels exceeding 5 mg per dl are usually associated with hepatic disease involving both biliary obstruction and hepatocellular damage. The greatest increments in serum bilirubin are associated with hepatic problems involving the periportal area.

Cholestasis refers to the stagnation of bile and may be associated with: (1) abnormal bile salt concentrations, which alter hepatic membranes by detergent action; (2) interference of drugs and abnormal bile acids with micelle formation;

(3) interference with sodium transport from hepatic cells to bile; (4) changes in bile canalicular membranes; and (5) increased intraluminal biliary pressure resulting from intrahepatic or extrahepatic obstruction of ducts.

Measurement of Increased Bilirubin Levels

The icterus index is based on a comparison of the color of the patient's serum or plasma to potassium dichromate solutions of different concentrations. This test gives only a rough index of the amount of elevation of plasma bilirubin.

van den Bergh Reaction

In the plasma, bilirubin exists in both a conjugated water-soluble form that reacts quickly (directly) with a diazo reagent and a nonconjugated form that is not water-soluble and that reacts slowly (indirectly) with diazo reagents. Elevated levels of indirectly acting bilirubin indicate increased erythrocyte breakdown, resulting in high levels of unconjugated or free bilirubin. Elevated levels of bilirubin that react directly indicate hepatocellular damage or obstructive disease of the liver. The low renal threshold for bilirubin conjugates in the dog produces low serum levels of bilirubin in intrahepatic and obstructive disease.

Urine Bilirubin

The greatest portion of detectable bilirubin found in the urine is in the conjugated form. In the dog, bilirubin can also be formed in the renal tubules following reabsorption of filtered hemoglobin, and renal tubular epithelial cells have the ability to conjugate bilirubin. Male dogs have a statistically higher level of bilirubin in their urine than female dogs.

The renal threshold for urine bilirubin is low in the dog, so that levels of a trace to 1+ may normally be present in the urine of specific gravity of 1.040 or greater. A small amount of glucuronyl transferase is located in the renal tubular epithelial cells of the canine kidney and has the ability to excrete free bilirubin in limited quantities. A 2+ to 3+ bilirubin reaction in the urine of a dog with a normal urine volume and a specific gravity between 1.020 and 1.035 usually indicates hyperbilirubinemia owing to hepatocellular or obstructive disease.

Bilirubinuria is not a normal finding in cats, even when the urine is concentrated. Therefore, the presence of bilirubin in the urine of cats is quite significant and is most frequently associated with altered biliary metabolism in the liver.

Urine Urobilinogen

Urobilinogen is normally formed from bilirubin by the reaction of bacteria on bilirubin in the bowel. Most urobilinogen is excreted in the feces, but a small portion is taken up by the portal circulation, returned to the liver, or finally excreted by the kidneys into the urine (Fig. 98).

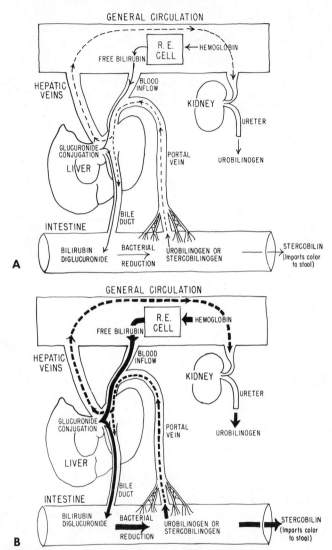

Figure 98. A, The normal enterohepatic circulation of bile pigments.

B, Hemolytic crisis. Observe the increase in the quantity of free bilirubin in the serum (unable to pass the renal filter), stercobilin in the stool (imparts a darker color to the stool), and urinary urobilinogen. Increased urinary urobilinogen may be due partly to the increased quantity of bile pigments metabolized owing to erythrocyte hemolysis. If secondary liver damage is extensive from hemosiderosis or bile pigment overload, some bilirubin glucuronide may be regurgitated and lost to urine (not in diagram).

Illustration continued on following page

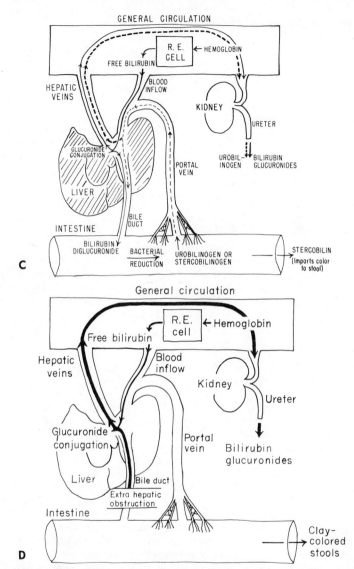

Figure 98. *Continued. C,* Hepatocellular pathology. Observe the presence of bilirubin glucuronide and increased amounts of urobilinogen in the urine. Increased urinary urobilinogen is due to the inability of the altered hepatic cells to quantitatively reexcrete this pigment into the bile. Free bilirubin may also be elevated in the serum owing to a decreased hepatic uptake of the pigment.

D, Extrahepatic obstruction. Observe regurgitation to the serum and subsequently the increased urinary excretion of bilirubin diglucuronide conjugated in the liver. Urinary urobilinogen and fecal stercobilin are absent. From Kaneko, J. J., and Cornelius, C. E. (eds.): Clinical Biochemistry of Domestic Animals, 2nd ed. New York, Academic Press, 1971, pp. 172–175.

Increased urine urobilinogen can result from impaired liver function or from "overloading" of the liver because of increased bilirubin production in hemolytic jaundice. In hemolytic anemias, greater amounts of urinary urobilinogen are associated with both an increased amount of circulating bile pigments and a secondary hepatic insufficiency.

Decreased or absent urobilinogen production can result from a delay in running the test, a complete obstruction of the biliary passages, decreased destruction of erythrocytes, changes in the intestinal flora due to intestinal disease or excessive treatment with antibiotics, or a dilution of the urine such as may occur with polydypsia and polyuria (e.g., chronic interstitial nephritis).

Increased levels of bilirubin producing icterus with an absence of urobilinogen in the urine is indicative of obstructive jaundice (Table 137).

Fecal Urobilinogen (Stercobilinogen)

Stercobilinogen contributes to the normal brown color of the feces. Increased amounts of stercobilinogen produce a dark orange stool, whereas decreased amounts produce a light gray or clay-colored stool. Increased amounts of stercobilinogen occur when blood destruction is increased. Decreased amounts or the absence of stercobilinogen occurs in obstruction of the biliary passages or alterations in the intestinal flora by disease or antibiotics.

Bromsulphalein Excretion (BSP Test)

BSP retention should be determined on animals in a fasting state. The process of uptake, conjugation, and excretion by the liver of foreign dyes measures both the biochemical integrity of hepatic cells and hepatic blood flow. The disappearance of intravenously (IV) injected BSP is dependent on: (1) hepatic circulation; (2) plasma protein binding—hypoproteinemia can markedly reduce BSP retention time, with the liver removing the dye more rapidly; (3) BSP uptake and conjugation in hepatocytes; and (4) rate of secretion of BSP into the biliary system. BSP is given as an IV dose, 5 mg per kg. Extravascular injection will cause marked tissue edema and inflammation.

BSP dye is removed from the vascular system by the reticuloendothelial and parenchymal cells of the liver. It is a satisfactory means of testing the excretory capabilities of the liver when no jaundice is present. Competition for hepatic uptake between foreign dyes such as BSP and bilirubin exists; thus, interpretation of this testing procedure is difficult in cases of hyperbilirubinemia. In the dog, less than 5 per cent retention at 30 minutes is considered within normal limits. In the cat, less than 3 per cent retention at 30 minutes is considered within normal limits.

Reduced hepatic circulation may markedly affect BSP retention: (1) extrahepatic vascular shunting (portasystemic shunt), (2) intrahepatic shunting (cirrhosis), (3) cardiac failure, (4) hypovolemia, and (5) hypoproteinemia. BSP retention time becomes abnormal when two thirds of the liver is lost. This can be associated with: (1) impairment of BSP secretion into the bile along with

Table 137. DIFFERENTIAL DIAGNOSIS OF JAUNDICE

Icterus	Anemia	Blood van den Bergh	Urine Bilirubin	Urine Urobilinogen	Feces Color
Increased production or deficient conjugation (hemolytic disease)	Present	Indirect elevated	+	4+	Dark
Impaired secretion into biliary passage (hepatocellular damage)	Absent usually	Direct elevated	2+–4+	2+–4+	Normal
Impaired excretion (extrahepatic obstruction)	Absent	Direct elevated	4+	0–1+	Clay-colored

biliary obstruction; (2) abnormal BSP metabolism in uptake, storage, or conjugation; and (3) deficiency in intracellular-binding proteins.

Indocyanine green (ICG) is another dye that has been used to estimate clearance by the liver.

In the cat, ICG is administered IV at 1.5 mg per kg. The 30-minute retention (per cent) is 7.3 ± 2.9. Because BSP results in very minimal retention values following 30 minutes (0.6 ± 0.8 per cent) and greater than 3.0 per cent retention at 30 minutes abnormal, the ICG test is a valuable test in the cat.

In the dog, the 30-minute retention (per cent) for ICG at a dose of 1.0 mg per kg is 14.7 ± 5.0, and at a dose of 1.5 mg per kg, 11.4 ± 3.0.

ICG is 90 per cent protein bound and is entirely dependent on hepato-biliary excretion, with 97 per cent recovery in the bile.

EVALUATION OF SYNTHESIS IN THE LIVER

Protein Metabolism

Albumin, prothrombin, fibrinogen, and small amounts of globulin—α (alpha) and β (beta)—are all formed in the liver. The rate of albumin synthesis is determined by hepatic function and the animal's nutritional status. Albumin represents 25 per cent of the proteins synthesized by the liver. The α-1 globulin fraction contains high- and very high-density lipoproteins, haptoglobulin, glycoprotein, and mucoprotein. The α-2 component consists of ceruloplasmin that carries copper, plasminogen, prothrombin, glycoprotein, and macroglobulin. The β globulins consist of low- and very low-density lipoproteins and transferrin.

The liver is also involved in the synthesis of blood clotting factors. The liver synthesizes factors I, II, V, VII, VIII, IX, and X. The production of activated prothrombin complex factors II, VII, IX, and X is dependent on vitamin K. The half-lives of clotting factors in the prothrombin complex are about 2.5 days for prothrombin, 0.2 days for factor VII, 1.2 days for factor IX, and 1.7 days for factor X. Factors V, VII, and XIII are available in fresh-frozen plasma only.

Hyperglobulinemia in liver disease is generally polyclonal. The α-2 globulins and β globulins will be increased.

Serum proteins can be affected both quantitatively and qualitatively in liver disease; however, changes in serum proteins are not specific for liver disease. In some diseases of the liver, especially chronic diseases, the level of serum albumin is decreased; this lowers the total serum protein and may reverse the albumin/globulin (A/G) ratio. In many liver diseases, however, there is a compensatory rise in serum globulin in an attempt to maintain the serum protein level. In obstructive jaundice, the level of serum albumin is lowered late in the course of the disease after secondary liver damage has taken place. In cirrhosis or fibrosis of the liver, serum albumin is lowered, but the level of serum albumin is dependent on the extent of damage to the liver (see Serum Proteins, p. 739).

Prothrombin Concentration—Coagulopathies in Liver Disease

Coagulation defects seen in severe liver disease can be associated with the following: deficiency of one or more clotting factors, increased fibrinolysis, circulating anticoagulants, an increased level of circulating thromboplastin, and abnormalities in or reduced numbers of thrombocytes. Disseminated intravascular coagulation (DIC) can be precipitated by thromboplastic substances released from the liver during acute hepatic disease (see p. 63).

In a study of coagulation defects occurring in spontaneous forms of hepatic disease, the following was found: decreased factor XI in dogs with hepatic degeneration; increased factor VIIIR antigen in dogs with hepatic inflammation; shortened prothrombin time, decreased factors IX, X, and XI, and increased factor VIIIR antigen in dogs with hepatic cirrhosis; and shortened prothrombin time, decreased factor VIII complement, and increased factor VIIIR antigen in dogs with hepatic neoplasia.

The synthesis of prothrombin is a function of the liver. A low prothrombin concentration may result from inadequate absorption of vitamin K in the intestinal tract because of an absence of bile, inability of a damaged liver to convert vitamin K to prothrombin, and ingestion of poisons such as warfarin.

In low prothrombin levels with evidence of clinical jaundice, give 5 to 10 mg of vitamin K_1 intramuscularly (IM) and recheck the prothrombin time in 12 to 24 hours. If the prothrombin time has returned to between 85 and 90 per cent of normal, the liver cells still retain their capacity to synthesize prothrombin. If a poor response to vitamin K administration is seen, severe hepatocellular disease probably exists. Plasma concentrations of prothrombin are not usually altered to the extent to produce overt clinical signs unless almost all the liver's function is lost. Prothrombin time should be evaluated, however, before performing a hepatic biopsy (see p. 709).

Cholesterol and Cholesterol Esters

The liver is involved in lipid metabolism, including the esterification and excretion of cholesterol. The liver esterifies cholesterol with linoleic acid and converts cholesterol to cholic acid. Cholesterol is secreted with the bile, and it is also metabolized in the liver to cholic acid. Increased cholesterol levels can be observed in intrahepatic and posthepatic cholestasis, with lowered chylomicron formation and cholesterol absorption and increased hepatic synthesis of cholesterol. In obstructive liver disease, cholesterol esters can reflux into the blood from the liver. Other systemic diseases can produce elevated cholesterol levels. High total serum cholesterol levels have been reported in diabetes mellitus, fatty degeneration of the liver, hypothyroidism (highly variable), and hyperadrenocorticism.

Because normal blood cholesterol levels are so highly variable, they cannot be relied on to reflect hepatic disease. The ratio of esterified to total cholesterol is more reliable. Normal ratios range from 0.64 to 0.80. Values less than 0.64

have been reported in 90 per cent of dogs with hepatic disease (Strombeck, 1979).

Abnormally low levels of cholesterol and triglycerides can be seen in dogs with portacaval shunts.

DETOXIFICATION IN THE LIVER

Uric Acid

Uric acid is converted to allantoin in the liver by uricase except in man, monkeys, and the Dalmatian dog. In liver disease, the amount of uric acid in the blood may be elevated. This test is extremely variable in the results produced in the dog and cat with liver disease.

EVALUATION OF ENZYME ACTIVITY

Increases in the concentration of enzymes in the blood occurring with liver disease may be associated with the escape of enzymes from damaged hepatic parenchymal cells with necrosis or altered membrane permeability or altered biliary secretion, as occurs with obstructive jaundice. (See also Alkaline Phosphatase, p. 751, and Serum Transaminase, p. 749.)

The aminotransferases, specifically serum alanine amino transferase (SALT; SGPT), are elevated in hepatocellular damage. These enzymes are located in hepatocyte cytoplasm. Altered cellular metabolism and elevated SALT levels are also seen in some congenital portal vascular anomalies, idiopathic feline hepatic lipidosis and steroid-induced hepatopathy, and the prolonged administration of anticonvulsant drugs, especially primidone, phenobarbital, and diphenylhydantoin.

Serum alkaline phosphatase (SAP) is a membrane-bound enzyme; after extrahepatic bile duct obstruction in dogs, the amount of SAP increases over days to weeks. Increases of SAP in cats with cholestasis is less prominent than in dogs because of faster clearance of SAP in cats. The enzyme that is of greater significance in cholestasis in the cat is SALT.

Gamma-glutamyl transpeptidase (GGTP) and arginase are new enzyme tests for liver function, which can be measured in conjunction with SALT. In acute hepatocellular injury, arginase levels may rapidly increase and then quickly return to normal if hepatocellular injury is corrected (Table 138).

Another test that may be useful in evaluation of liver disease is measurement of bile acids.

Bile acids are synthesized from cholesterol by the liver. Bile acids are secreted into the intestinal tract and undergo enterohepatic recirculation. Normal hepatic uptake, deconjugation, secretion, and liver synthesis are necessary to maintain normal levels of bile acids. Liver disease and impaired enterohepatic circulation can cause increase in bile acids. Normal bile acid levels are 0 to 8 μ moles per L, with a level of 8 to 12 being slightly elevated. Greater than 250 μ moles per L indicates severe liver disease.

Table 138. PLASMA ENZYME VALUES IN CLINICALLY NORMAL DOGS

No. of Dogs	Test	Enzyme Value*
4	Plasma aspartate aminotransferase (Sigma-Frankel units/ml)	14.1 (10–21)
9	Plasma alanine aminotransferase (Sigma-Frankel units/ml)	20.0 (14–40)
9	Plasma sorbitol dehydrogenase (milli-International units/ml)	9.6 (5.5–18.0)
9	Plasma alkaline phosphatase (Sigma units/ml)	0.85 (0.71–1.5)
9	Plasma arginase (International units/L)	1.9 (0–6.0)
9	Total plasma bilirubin (mg/dl)	0.13 (0–0.37)
9	Plasma γ-glutamyl transpeptidase (Sigma units/ml)	0.92 (0–2.26)

*Data expressed as mean (minimum-maximum values).
From Noonan, N. E., and Meyer, D. J.: Use of plasma arginase and gamma glutamyl transpeptidase as specific indicators of hepatocellular or hepatobiliary disease in dogs. Am. J. Vet. Res., *40*:942, 1979.

COPPER TOXICOSIS OF THE LIVER IN DOGS

A genetically linked liver disease affecting Bedlington terriers and Doberman pinschers has been associated with abnormal concentrations of copper (5–50 times normal) in the liver. The disorder may remain latent or may result in an acute hepatic crisis. In affected dogs, the copper accumulation is progressive, resulting in chronic hepatitis and eventual cirrhosis.

Tissue biopsy specimens from the liver can be assayed for copper by atomic absorption spectrophotometry and stained differentially for copper with rubeanic acid.

LIVER BIOPSY (See p. 529)

References and Additional Readings

Benjamin, M.: Veterinary Clinical Pathology, 3rd ed. Ames, Iowa, Iowa State University Press, 1979.
Center, S. A., Bunch, S. E., Baldwin, B. H., Hornbuckle, W. E. and Tennant, B. C.: Comparison of sulfobromophthalein and indocyanine green clearances in the cat. Am. J. Vet. Res. *44*:727–730, 1983.
Center, S. A., Bunch, S. E., Baldwin, B. H., Hornbuckle, W. E. and Tennant, B. C.: Comparison of sulfobromophthalein and indocyanine green clearances in the dog. Am. J. Vet. Res. *44*:722–726, 1983.
Cornelius, C. E.: Biochemical evaluation of hepatic function in dogs. J.A.A.H.A., *15*:259, 1979.
Hardy, R. M.: Diseases of the liver. *In* Ettinger, S. (ed.): Textbook of Veterinary Internal Medicine, Vol. 2. Philadelphia, W. B. Saunders Company, 1975, pp. 1219–1246.

Lees, G. E., Hard, R. M., Stevens, J. B. and Osborne, C. A.: Clinical implications of feline bilirubinuria. J.A.A.H.A. 20:765–771, 1984.

Noonan, N. E., and Meyer, D. J.: Use of plasma arginase and gamma glutamyl transpeptidase as specific indicators of hepatocellular or hepatobiliary disease in dogs. Am. J. Vet. Res., 40:942, 1979.

Strombeck, D. R.: Small Animal Gastroenterology. Davis, California, Stonegate Publishing Company, 1979.

Strombeck, D. R., and Rogers, Q.: Plasma amino acid concentrations in dogs with hepatic disease. J.A.V.M.A., 173:93, 1978.

Strombeck, D. R., Rogers, W., and Gribble, D.: Chronic active hepatic disease in a dog. J.A.A.H.A., 169:802, 1976.

Zawie, D. A. and Garvey, M. S.: Feline hepatic disease. Vet. Clin. North Am. 14:1201–1230, 1984.

ANTIMICROBIAL SENSITIVITY TESTING

Susceptibility of microorganisms to antibiotics can be measured in commercial laboratories by dilution techniques, which report minimal inhibitory concentrations (MIC). Smaller laboratories use the agar diffusion technique, in which the zone of inhibition of microbial growth around a disc containing a fixed amount of antibiotic is directly related to the MIC of the organism being tested.

This in vitro test is classically performed using a pure culture growth of the infecting agent obtained by culture isolation from the primary specimen (see p. 499). The test serves to indicate organism susceptibility or resistance to specific antimicrobial agents. A response showing resistance should eliminate that agent from therapeutic consideration; however, a test showing susceptibility may not always guarantee similar results in vivo. In general, the following holds true: If the test shows resistance, the organism is not likely to respond to therapy with the antibiotic. If the test response is intermediate, the organism is susceptible if dosage is high or if the antibiotic is concentrated, as in the urine. If the test shows susceptibility, the organism is susceptible to ordinary dosage. The tests, properly performed, do serve as a useful guide.

The test *is not* indicated in the following circumstances:

1. When organisms are of unvarying susceptibility. Beta-hemolytic *Streptococcus, Pasteurella, Actinobacillus, Actinomyces,* and anaerobes (except for *B. fragilis*) are susceptible to penicillin or ampicillin.

2. When the number of organisms as determined by culture is deemed to be insignificant for infection.

3. When the primary specimen yields a mixture of infecting organisms so that uncertainty is created as to which, if any, is the etiologic agent. Interpretation of tests run on such samples is difficult and unreliable.

The test *is* indicated in the following circumstances:

1. When body defenses may be defective and the utmost antimicrobial efficacy is necessary.

2. When the antibiotic such as streptomycin allows the organisms to develop resistance easily.

3. When infections are caused by bacterial species that commonly have many strains of differing antibiotic susceptibility. Among bacteria that commonly show variable strains are *Staphylococcus aureus* and members of the Enterobacteriaceae family (such as *E. coli, Proteus, Enterobacter, Klebsiella,* and *Salmonella*).

The antimicrobial paper disc method is practical for small office laboratories. In carefully performed tests, the following points should be emphasized:

1. Use Mueller-Hinton medium for the tests. (Sulfonamides often will not give satisfactory zones on media that contain blood.)

2. Transfer 4 or 5 similar colonies from the primary isolation medium to 5 ml of β lacto-tryptic soy broth. This can be done with a sterile wire loop or by using the Prompt* veterinary sensitivity standardizing system to streak the Mueller-Hinton plates.

A direct colony pickup system (Prompt) allows more rapid standardization of bacterial colonies and thus more rapid results of antibiotic sensitivity. Using this system, antibiotic sensitivity readings using the disc system can be made with 90 per cent accuracy 8 hours following the inoculation of Mueller-Hinton plates, with the exception of ampicillin and penicillin discs.

The bacterial inoculum should be between 5×10^7 and 5×10^8 colony forming units (CFU) per ml. Streak the entire agar plate surface in three different directions by rotating the plate to 60-degree angles after each streaking. Place the antibiotic discs 20 to 25 mm apart on the plate. A 150-mm plate can hold 12 or 13 disks.

3. When a package of sensitivity discs has been opened, it should be stored in the refrigerator and the discs should be either used or discarded within 1 month.

4. Select discs pertinent to the type of infection usually encountered in the organ system involved. For example, urinary tract infections are rarely caused by gram-positive organisms *(Staphylococcus* or *Streptococcus),* and respiratory infections are rarely caused by gram-negative organisms. Use only high-level discs for urinary infections because the kidney hyperconcentrates the antibiotic. Urine levels, not serum levels, are crucial.

5. Veterinary clinicians usually select drugs from the following list for sensitivity tests: penicillin, erythromycin, chloramphenicol, tetracycline, streptomycin, neomycin, polymyxin, nitrofurantoin, sulfonamide, ampicillin, oxacillin, lincomycin, kanamycin, gentamicin, and cephaloridine.

6. Drug sensitivity extrapolation must be done carefully. Results from methicillin may apply to any of the penicillinase-resistant penicillins; similarly, tetracycline and sulfonamide tests may hold for others of their groups. Polymyxin and colistin too are similar, and neomycin and kanamycin often cross-react. Cephalothin discs may be used to determine susceptibility to the major cephalosporins.

---

*3M Manufacturing Co., St. Paul, Minnesota.

Table 139. INTERPRETATION OF INHIBITION ZONES OF TEST CULTURES

Antibiotic	Disk Content	Resistant mm or less	Intermediate mm Range	Sensitive mm or more
Amikacin	10 mcg	11	12–13	14
Ampicillin[1] when testing gram-negative microorganisms and enterococci	10 mcg	11	12–13	14
Ampicillin[1] when testing staphylococci and penicillin G–susceptible microorganisms	10 mcg	20	21–28	29
Ampicillin[1] when testing *Hemophilus* species	10 mcg	19		20
Bacitracin	10 units	8	9–12	13
Carbenicillin when testing *Proteus* species and *Escherichia coli*	50 mcg or 100 mcg	17	18–22	23
Carbenicillin when testing *Pseudomonas aeruginosa*	50 mcg	12	13–14	15
	100 mcg	13	14–16	17
Cephalothin[2] when reporting susceptibility to cephalothin, cephaloridine, and cephalexin	30 mcg	14	15–17	18
Cephalothin[2] when reporting susceptibility to cephaloglycin	30 mcg	14		15
Chloramphenicol	30 mcg	12	13–17	18
Clindamycin[3] when reporting susceptibility to clindamycin	2 mcg	14	15–16	17
Clindamycin[3] when reporting susceptibility to lincomycin	2 mcg	16	17–20	21
Colistin[4]	10 mcg	8	9–10	11
Erythromycin	15 mcg	13	14–17	18
Gentamicin	10 mcg	12		13
Kanamycin	30 mcg	13	14–17	18
Methicillin[5]	5 mcg	9	10–13	14
Neomycin	30 mcg	12	13–16	17
Novobiocin[6]	30 mcg	17	18–21	22
Oleandomycin[7]	15 mcg	11	12–16	17
Penicillin G, when testing staphylococci[8]	10 units	20	21–28	29
Penicillin G, when testing other microorganisms[8, 9]	10 units	11	12–21	22
Polymyxin B[4]	300 units	8	9–11	12

	5 mcg	24	25
Rifampin when testing *Neisseria meningitidis* susceptibility only			
Streptomycin	10 mcg	11	15	12–14
Tetracycline[10]	30 mcg	14	19	15–18
Tobramycin	10 mcg	11	14	12–13
Vancomycin	30 mcg	9	12	10–11
Chemotherapeutic Agents				
Furadantin (nitrofurantoin)[11]	300 mcg	14	17	15–16
Nalidixic acid[11]	30 mcg	13	19	14–18
Oxolinic acid[6]	2 mcg	10	11	
Trimethoprim/sulfamethoxazole[6]	1.25/23.75 mcg	10	16	11–15
Triple sulfa[12]	300 mcg	12	17	13–16

[1]The ampicillin disk is used for testing susceptibility of both ampicillin and hetacillin.

[2]Staphylococci exhibiting resistance to the penicillinase-resistant penicillin class disks should be reported as resistant to cephalosporin class antibiotics. The 30 mcg cephalothin disk cannot be relied upon to detect resistance of methicillin-resistant staphylococci to cephalosporin class antibiotics.

[3]The clindamycin disk is used for testing susceptibility to both clindamycin and lincomycin.

[4]Colistin and polymyxin B diffuse poorly in agar, and the accuracy of the diffusion method is thus less than with other antibiotics. Resistance is always significant, but when treatment of systemic infections due to susceptible strains is considered, it is wise to confirm the results of a diffusion test with a dilution method.

[5]The methicillin disk is used for testing susceptibility of all penicillinase-resistant penicillins, that is, methicillin, cloxacillin, dicloxacillin, oxacillin, and nafcillin.

[6]Not applicable to medium that contains blood.

[7]The oleandomycin disk is used for testing susceptibility to oleandomycin and trioleandomycin.

[8]The penicillin G disk is used for testing susceptibility to all penicillinase-susceptible penicillins except ampicillin and carbenicillin, that is, penicillin G, phenoxymethyl penicillin, and phenethicillin.

[9]This category includes some organisms such as enterococci and gram-negative bacilli that may cause systemic infections treatable with high doses of penicillin G. Such organisms should be reported only susceptible to penicillin G and not to phenoxymethyl penicillin or phenethicillin.

[10]The tetracycline disk is used for testing susceptibility to all tetracyclines, that is chlorotetracycline, demeclocycline, doxycycline, methacycline, oxytetracycline, rolitetracycline, minocycline, and tetracycline.

[11]For urinary tract infections only.

[12]All 300-mcg sulfonamide disks may be similarly interpreted.

Adapted from Manual of Clinical Microbiology, 3rd ed. Washington, D.C. American Society of Microbiology, 1980.

7. After placement of the discs, the plate is turned upside down and incubated at 35 to 37°C for 18 hours. (It may be read with magnification after 5 to 6 hours.)

8. The zones of inhibition should be measured as diameters from zone edge to zone edge. Sulfonamides may give a soft inner zone of partial growth. Use the outer definite zone for measuring the diameter of inhibition.

9. *Do not compare the inhibition zone size of various antibiotics for determination of relative therapeutic merit.* For example, a polymyxin zone of 12 mm may be just as effective as chloramphenicol at 18 mm (Table 139).

10. Report the organism as resistant if there is no inhibition of growth around the disc. Do not expect good therapeutic results with such an antibiotic.

11. Report the organism as susceptible if a clear zone of inhibition of *significant size* is evident around the disc. In vivo results do not always conform to in vitro tests, however. Consult Table 139 for evaluation of inhibition sizes.

12. Disc potency, diffusion of the agent, and other factors mentioned modify the size of the zone inhibition.

One of the difficulties of interpretation is caused by the inability to balance antibacterial concentration in the disc with that which can be obtained in the tissue at the infection site. For estimation of the effect of individual agents, see p. 190.

The appendix contains two tables that may be helpful.

1. Use of Antimicrobial Agents for Treatment of Infection (Table 190, p. 921).
2. Most Effective pH for Optimal Antibacterial Activity (Table 191, p. 924).

References and Additional Readings

Carter, G. R.: Diagnostic Procedures in Veterinary Bacteriology and Mycology, 3rd ed. Springfield, Illinois, Charles C Thomas, Publisher, 1979.

Cottral, G. E.: Manual and standardized methods for veterinary microbiology. Ithaca, New York, Cornell University Press, 1978.

Ward, G. E., and Bates, F.: Improved antimicrobial susceptibility testing. Mod. Vet. Pract., *64*:795, 1983.

MYCOLOGY

Dermatophytes

Wood's light fluorescence of affected hair and skin may be observed in many infections due to *Microsporum canis,* a common dermatophyte of small animals. A similar response often is observed with *M. audouini* and *M. distortum,* rare animal dermatophytes. Not all specimens of these fungi fluoresce. When they do, the typical fluorescence is a yellow-green color. Other colors of fluorescence (purple, blue) may be due to medications, mineral oil, scales, or mineral particles. Fluorescing hair and skin make excellent samples for culture, and the distribution of these areas may indicate foci of infection not otherwise apparent.

Potassium hydroxide, 20 per cent, for digestion of hair and scale preparations may clear the sample of debris so that fungal mycelia can be observed more easily. Unless the fungous growth is abundant, the test may be negative, and even if mycelia are observed, one cannot make valid conclusions about the pathogenicity of the organism. A positive test does help confirm suspicions and is a mandate for cultures and further identification.

Fungous cultures (see p. 510) afford the only accurate way to identify pathogenic organisms, and positive laboratory reports provide a definitive diagnosis.

1. The great majority of dermatomycoses of small animals are caused by *Microsporum canis,* or *gypseum,* or *Trichophyton mentagrophytes.* Other pathogenic dermatophytes are listed in Table 140.

2. *Candida albicans,* a yeast, causes a mycosis of intermediate depth (moniliasis) that may affect skin and mucous membranes. It often is an opportunist associated with moist or macerated skin or mucous membrane, and the clinician should search carefully for another etiologic agent. *Candida albicans* and *Malassezia pachydermatis* are yeasts commonly found in otitis externa, but they may be present as secondary invaders.

Wet mount or acetate tape preparations can be made from fungal cultures for precise identification of fungal species. To visualize the morphologic aspects, collect small masses of cultured growth with a sterile loop, suspend in saline and place them under a coverslip. Another method is to press clear acetate (Scotch) tape onto the surface growth of a fungal culture. Place a drop of lacto cotton phenol blue stain onto a microscope slide. Then place the tape, sticky side down, on top of the stain, cover with a coverslip, and examine for morphologic identification.

Deep Mycoses

Subcutaneous mycoses develop in the host at the site of inoculation and are usually soil saprophytes that do not spread to other animals. Debilitating diseases, immune deficiencies, and long-term antibiotic or corticosteroid therapy are common findings in affected animals.

Systemic mycoses are usually chronic, low-grade, debilitating, nonpainful infections that are not usually transmitted naturally between animal hosts. Young animals that may have a depressed immune system show enlarged nodes, abscesses, draining fistulas, or granulomatous lesions. The rare acute infections are usually diagnosed at necropsy.

Direct smears from exudates or node aspirates and scrapings from granulomas or affected skin are suitable specimens (Table 141). Centrifuge transtracheal washings, cerebrospinal fluid (CSF), or urine, and collect the sediment. Suspend the material in 10 to 20 per cent potassium hydroxide (KOH) and Parker Ink (1 part ink, 2 parts KOH) to help outline the fungi. India ink and water can also be used to help outline cryptococcosis budding yeast forms. The ink outlines the clear capsule so that it appears as a halo.

Text continued on page 777

Table 140. TENTATIVE DIAGNOSIS OF RINGWORM IN
SMALL ANIMALS FROM CLINICAL MATERIALS

Fungus Species	Animals Affected	Location and Appearance of Lesions
		MICROSPORUM INFECTIONS
Microsporum canis	COMMON: Cats Dogs OCCASIONAL: Horses Monkeys RARE: Rabbits Rodents Chinchillas	Scattered lesions, but especially on head. Adult cats and dogs: infections may be clinically inapparent or may be represented by loss of hair only. Young animals: lesions usually more clearly defined. Discrete circular areas of hair loss with scaling and occasionally inflamed borders are common. Heavy crusts may develop in these areas. Severe clinical cases may appear in both young and adult animals, with heavy crusted areas or widespread loss of hair, scaling, and erythema. Horses: lesions particularly in harness areas ("girth itch").
Microsporum gypseum	COMMON: Dogs OCCASIONAL: Cats Horses Wild rodents	Infection may be clinically inapparent. Often a single lesion on head or leg or scattered discrete lesions over body. Circular areas with loss of hair and some scaliness, or heavy yellowish brown crusts which later fall off leaving a "moth-eaten" appearance to animal. Hairs loose at edges of crusts. Some hairs embedded in crusts.
Microsporum audouinii	RARE: Dogs Monkeys Guinea pigs	Single or scattered lesions, circular with loss of hair, scaling, and some erythema. Eczematous lesions reported.
Microsporum distortum	OCCASIONAL: Monkeys RARE: Dogs	Single or scattered lesions, circular with loss of hair and scaling.

Table continued on opposite page

Table 140. TENTATIVE DIAGNOSIS OF RINGWORM IN
SMALL ANIMALS FROM CLINICAL MATERIALS (*Continued*)

Wood's Light Examination	Direct Examination in KOH Mounts	
	Skin Scrapings	**Hair**
Bright yellow-green fluorescence of infected hairs.	Mycelium and chains of arthrospores.	Sheath of small spores (2–3 μ) in mosaic, completely surrounds hair at base. Easily dislodged from hair in preparation. Mycelium within hair running parallel to its length.
No fluorescence.	Mycelium and masses of very large arthro-spores, some in chains.	Large spores (5–8 μ) in chains or in irregular masses on surface of hairs. Mycelium within hair, running parallel to its length.
Bright yellow green fluorescence of infected hairs.	Mycelium and chains of arthrospores.	Sheath of small spores (2–3 μ) in mosaic, completely surrounds hair at base. Easily dislodged from hair in preparation. Mycelium within hair running parallel to its length.
Bright yellow green fluorescence of infected hairs.	Mycelium and chains of arthrospores.	Same as above.

Table continued on following page

Fungus Species	Animals Affected	Location and Appearance of Lesions
		TRICHOPHYTON INFECTIONS
Trichophyton mentagrophytes	COMMON: Dogs Cats Rabbits Chinchillas Guinea pigs Mice Rats	Most common on head near mouth and eyes or at base of tail, but may be anywhere on body. Infection may be clincally inapparent. Usually irregularly defined areas of hair loss with considerable scaling are found. Heavy crusts may form. Occasionally, pustules form at edges of lesion and suppuration beneath crusts.
	OCCASIONAL: Horses Cows Muskrats Opposums Squirrels Foxes RARE: Swine	Horse: lesions particularly in harness areas ("girth itch"). Wild rodents: infections often clinically inapparent. In rodent epizootics, lesions may be heavy raised crusts of "favic type."
Trichophyton gallinae	COMMON: Chickens Turkeys RARE: Wild birds Dogs	White powdery scaliness, which tends to form concentric rings on comb and wattles. Later, heavy white crusts form in these areas ("white comb" or "favus of chickens"). In rare cases, infection may spread over body showing scaliness of the skin. Does not involve the feathers.
Trichophyton equinum	COMMON: Horses RARE: Dogs	Scattered lesions especially in saddle area ("girth itch"). Circular lesions with matting of hair followed by hair loss and development of crusts. As lesions heal, crusts fall off leaving bald areas and giving the animal a "moth-eaten" appearance.
Trichophyton schoenleinii	OCCASIONAL: Dogs Cats Mice Monkeys	Commonly on the head, and occasionally on the back. Heavy yellowish crusts depressed at their centers to form "cups" or "scutula." Crusts may be agglomerated to form large masses. These are tightly adherent to the skin, which bleeds when they are removed.
Trichophyton rubrum	RARE: Dogs Cows	Single or scattered lesions, showing loss of hair, scaling, and erythema.

Table continued on opposite page

Wood's Light Examination	Direct Examination in KOH Mounts	
	Skin Scrapings	**Hair**
No fluorescence.	Mycelium and chains of arthrospores.	Sheath or isolated chains of spores (3–5 μ) on surface of hair. Mycelium within hair.
No fluorescence.	Mycelium and chains of arthrospores.	Feathers not affected.
No fluorescence.	Mycelium and chains of arthrospores.	Sheath or isolated chains of spores (3.5–8 μ) on surface hair. Mycelium within hair.
Not reported in animals. (In human infections, none or dull whitish fluorescence has been reported.)	Masses of very irregular mycelium and arthrospores, some in chains.	Hair invasion not reported in animals. In human infections, hairs are invaded throughout their length by branching mycelium that contain vacuoles and fat droplets.
No fluorescence.	Branching mycelium.	Hair invasion rare. In experimental animal infections, chains of spores have been observed on outside of hair, and mycelium within hair.

Adapted from George, L. K.: Animal Ringworm in Public Health. Washington, D.C., U.S. Dept. of Health, Education and Welfare, 1959, and Jungerman, P. F., and Schwartzman, R. M.: Veterinary Medical Mycology. Philadelphia, Lea & Febiger, 1972.

Table 141. HELPFUL FEATURES FOR IDENTIFICATION
OF SOFT-TISSUE MYCOSES

Agent	Important Features
Systemic Mycoses	
Blastomycosis	Direct smear with Parker ink and KOH. Large, thick-walled budding yeast.
Coccidioidomycosis	Direct smear with Parker ink and KOH. Thick-walled spherules with endospores and smaller spherules devoid of spores.
Cryptococcosis	Direct smear in India ink and water. Small, round budding yeast surrounded by a capsule (halo). Culture at both 20° and 37°C without cyclohexamide, which inhibits growth.
Histoplasmosis	Usually need culture. Direct smear with blood stain may show small oval bodies, yeast cells within macrophages.
Subcutaneous Mycoses	
Aspergillosis	Nasal washings, biopsies, and scrapings in KOH for hyphae and aspergillus heads. Culture on Sabouraud's agar.
Mycetoma	*Actinomycotic*—crush granules and use Gram stain to observe Gram + filaments. Culture granules after washing in sterile saline, and place on Sabouraud's agar without antibiotics and on blood agar. Incubate one set at 37°C, and one at 25°C. *Eumycotic*—crush granules, mix with KOH, and examine for hyphae and chlamydospores.
Phaeohyphomycosis	Exudate or tissue mixed with KOH to see black septate hyphae with unusual dilations. Culture on Sabouraud's dextrose agar at 25°C.
Phycomycosis	Exudates and tissue mixed with KOH and examined for wide, non-septate hyphae. Culture on Sabouraud's agar at 25°C.
Prototwhecosis	Exudates mixed with KOH and examined for oval to globose structures containing 2 or more autospores. Easily cultured on blood or Sabouraud's agar. Yeast colonies in 24 hours.
Rhinosporidiosis	Crush a polyp, mix with KOH, and examine for sporangia with endospores. Culture not needed.
Sporotrichosis	Direct smears of little value. Dimorphic. Culture on Sabouraud's agar; use special fungal stains on tissues.

Cultures require up to 6 weeks of growth and an extensive isolation procedure. Attleberger's description* is helpful in planning the identification; however, a commercial or institutional laboratory evaluation is a mandatory aid.

Histopathology is often helpful in diagnosis. Soft-tissue specimens of affected organs should be fixed in 10 per cent buffered formalin. Stains of special value for preparation of these specimens are hematoxylin-eosin, Gridley, Gomori-Methenamine silver, and periodic acid–Schiff (PAS).

References and Additional Readings

Attleberger, M. H.: The deep mycoses and the actinomycetes. *In* Kirk, R. W. (ed.): Current Veterinary Therapy VII. Philadelphia, W. B. Saunders Company, 1980.

Muller, G. H., Kirk, R. W., and Scott, D. W.: Small Animal Dermatology, 3rd ed. Philadelphia, W. B. Saunders Company, 1983.

Rebell, G., Toplin, D., and Blank, H.: Dermatophytes. Their Recognition and Identification, 2nd ed. 1020 Northwest 16th St., Miami, Florida 33136, Dermatology Foundation of Miami, 1970.

Rippon, J. W.: Medical Mycology: The Pathogenic Fungi and the Pathogenic Actinomycetes. Philadelphia, W. B. Saunders Company, 1982.

---

*Attleberger, M. H.: Practical diagnostic procedures for mycotic diseases. *In* Kirk, R. W. (ed.): Current Veterinary Therapy VIII. Philadelphia, W. B. Saunders Company, 1983.

INTERNAL PARASITES OF DOGS AND CATS

Ancylostomiasis
(Ancylostoma caninum, Ancylostoma braziliense, Uncinaria stenocephala)

The life cycle of all three species of hookworm are similar. Infection with hookworms can occur in the following ways:

1. Skin penetration—third stage larvae can infect by active skin penetration followed by somatic migration. The minimum prepatent period is 14 to 17 days in puppies.
2. Oral infection—the minimum prepatent period is 14 to 17 days.
3. Transmammary/intrauterine infection—for *Ancylostoma caninum*.

Adult worms live in the small intestine. Growth and maturation after the ingestion of infective ova require between 18 and 21 days. Females lay large quantities of eggs that are passed in the feces and, under the proper conditions, hatch in 48 to 72 hours. The larvae develop to the infective third stage within 5 to 7 days.

Clinical Picture

The clinical picture in hookworm disease is dependent on the virulence of the species of hookworm involved, the degree of exposure to infective larvae, and the degree of resistance of the host (including immunologic resistance). The major signs are associated with blood loss and gastrointestinal irritation. Weakness, unfitness, anemia, diarrhea, bloody or tarry stools, anorexia, depression, and death may occur. Anemia created by blood loss is initially normocytic and normochromic; however, with the development of iron deficiency, the anemia becomes hypochromic microcytic. Larvae may wander through other internal organs, such as the liver and lungs, producing secondary signs of hepatitis and pneumonia. Infection of young puppies with hookworms *in utero* or after birth may produce a peracute syndrome with rapid blood loss, anemia, shock, and death. Prenatal infection does not become patent until the eleventh postnatal day; therefore, fecal examination of puppies with peracute hookworm disease may be negative.

Transmission to Man

Infective larvae can penetrate the skin of man, causing cutaneous larval migrans (creeping eruption).

Diagnosis

A diagnosis can be made by demonstrating eggs or larvae in the feces. In puppies prenatally or neonatally infected with hookworms, severe clinical disease may occur during the prepatent period, and diagnosis must be based on signs of the disease.

Chemotherapy

Drugs preferred for the treatment of hookworm include pyrantel pamoate (Nemex), pyrantel pamoate plus oxantel pamoate (Nemex Plus), mebendazole (Telmin), Dichlorvos (Task), and thenium closylate (Canopar) (Table 142).

The insoluble benzimidazole anthelmintics, mebendazole and fenbendazole, are also efficient against hookworms.

Control

When hookworm disease is prevalent, the following control measures may prove helpful:
1. Feces should be removed regularly from earth runs and should not be left on the ground for more than 24 hours.
2. Soil can be periodically treated with salt, 160/gm per L of boiling water or sodium borate, 14 kg per sq meter. (Borate on the ground in this amount may be toxic to young dogs.)
3. Concrete runs should be hosed and washed well.
4. Bitches should be wormed prior to whelping.

Table 142. ANTHELMINTICS FOR DOGS AND CATS

Drugs	Efficacy*					Dosage	Comments
	Hook-worms	Ascarids	Whip-worms	Tape-worms	Strongy-loides		
Canopar (thenium closylate) (Burroughs Wellcome)	89%	±	—	—	—	1 tablet (500 mg) for dogs over 10 lb (5 kg), regardless of weight; ½ tablet (125 mg) BID (q 12 hr) for 5- and 10-lb (2.5 to 5 kg) dogs	Some emesis. Cannot use in nursing pups or those less than 5 lb (2.5 kg). Occasional deaths (collies and airedales).
Piperazine (many manufacturers)	—	52–100%	—	—	—	45–65 mg base/kg orally, maximum of 250 mg for pups under 2.5 kg and for cats and kittens	No contraindications except long standing renal or liver disease.
Caricide (diethylcarbamazine) (American Cyanamid)	—	80%	—	—	—	6.6 mg/kg/day orally as a preventive	Substantial adult ascarid burden is eliminated when DEC is given as a heart-worm preventive. Contraindicated if micorfilariae are present.
Styrid-Caricide (DEC + styrylpyridinium chloride) (American Cyanamid)	80%	80%	—	—	—	6.6 mg DEC and 5.5 mg Styryl. Cl./kg/day orally	Used as a heartworm preventive and as an aid in control of ascarids and hookworms.
Milibis-V (glycobiarsol) (Winthrop)	—	—	90%	—	—	220 mg/kg daily × 5 days	Developed for treatment of amebiasis. ½ dose × 10 days recommended for debilitated dogs.

Table continued on following page

Table 142. ANTHELMINTICS FOR DOGS AND CATS *(Continued)*

Drugs	Efficacy* Hook-worms	Ascarids	Whip-worms	Tape-worms	Strongy-loides	Dosage	Comments
Thiabendazole (Merck Sharp & Dohme)	±	±	—	—	95%	55 mg/kg daily × 3 days orally	Some emesis. Repeat treatment monthly if needed.
Nemex-2 (pyrantel pamoate) (Pfizer)	95%	95%	±	—	—	18 mg/kg in tablet or suspension (Nemex-2, Strongid-T, Imathal)	Used in dogs of all ages, including nursing pups. No contraindications.
Task (dichlorvos) (Shell)	95%	95%	90%	—	—	Dogs: 27–33 mg/kg. Puppies & cats: 11 mg/kg	Contraindications include heartworm disease and liver or kidney damage. Do not use in conjunction with other cholinesterase inhibitors. Split dosage for debilitated animals.
Styquin (butamisole HCl) (American Cyanimid)	92%	—	99%	—	—	2.4 mg/kg SC	A fourfold overdose is lethal; do not use simultaneously with Scolaban or in heartworm-positive or debilitated dogs.
Telmintic (mebendazole) (Pitman-Moore)	95%	95%	95%	85% T† 0% D	—	22 mg/kg in food daily × 3 days (nematodes) or 5 days (*Taenia*)	Approved for dogs; experimental in cats. Evidence suggests occasional drug-induced acute hepatic necrosis in dogs.

Drug				Tapeworms†	Dose	Remarks
Vermiplex (toluene and dichlorophene) (Pitman-Moore)	82%	90%	—	72% T / 85% D	—	Size capsule as directed by manufacturer	Incoordination, emesis, toxicity in excess.
Scolaban (bunamidine HCl) (Burroughs Wellcome)	—	—	—	100% T / 56–90% D / 86–100% E	—	25–50 mg/kg on empty stomach; feed lightly in 3 hr	Occasional idiosyncratic reaction. Do not use simultaneously with Styquin.
Yomesan (niclosamide) (Chemagro)	—	—	—	80% T / 18–56% D	—	100–157 mg/kg orally	Heavy mucus interferes with elimination of scolex.
Droncit (praziquantel) (Haver Lockhart)	—	—	—	100% T, D, E	—	Dogs: 5 mg/kg, single oral, SC, or IM dose Cats: 11 mg total (1–3 lbs) 22 mg total (3–11 lbs) 33 mg total (>11 lbs)	10 mg/kg required for Echinococcus juveniles. Effective against tapeworm larvae in many intermediate hosts. No effect on nematodes.
Panacur (fenbendazole) (American Hoechst)	98%	99%	100%	88–100% T / 0% D	—	50 mg/kg/day × 3 consecutive days	Suspension or granules (added to moist food). Single dose, even at 150 mg/kg, is not effective in dogs or cats.

*Percentages in "Tapeworms" column refer to % of dogs cleared of infection; all others refer to % of nematodes expelled.

†T = *Taenia* sp.; D = *Dipylidium caninum*; E = *Echinococcus* sp.

Modified from Roberson, E., and Cornelius, L. M.: Gastrointestinal parasitism. *In* Kirk, R. W. (ed.): Current Veterinary Therapy VIII: Small Animal Practice. Philadelphia, W. B. Saunders Company, 1983.

Ascariasis
(Toxocara canis, Toxocara cati, Toxascaris leonina)

The pattern of migration of these three helminths is variable. In the dog, *Toxocara canis* and, in the cat *Toxocara cati* follow a tracheal migration route. Second stage larvae hatch in the stomach after ingestion, penetrate the bowel wall, enter the portal blood stream, wander in the hepatic parenchyma, enter the post cava, and arrive in the lungs—breaking out of the capillaries to the alveoli and migrating up the bronchial tree and trachea to the pharynx where they are swallowed. Following a moult in the stomach wall, the parasite matures in the small intestine. The prepatent period for direct infection in young puppies is 4 to 5 weeks.

If the *Toxocara* larvae hatch in numerous foreign hosts, the pattern of migration is altered, resulting in somatic migration.

T. canis infections in puppies less than 1 month of age are produced by migration of second stage larvae from the bitch to the pups in utero. Infected puppies can have third stage larvae in their lungs when born, and a moult from third stage to fourth stage larvae occurs during the first week of life; fourth stage larvae may be present in the intestinal tract at 3 days after birth. The prepatent period for intrauterine infection of puppies is 19 to 23 days.

T. canis has a life span averaging 4 months. Females can produce up to 200,000 eggs per day within a temperature range of 15°C to 35°C and humidity of 85 per cent. Toxocara eggs can become infective within 2 to 5 weeks, whereas Toxascaris eggs may require only 1 week. Infective larvae are third stage.

Toxascaris leonina follows a mucosal migration in both dogs and cats. The second and third moults occur in the intestinal wall, and the fourth stage larvae enter the lumen of the gut to mature. The prepatent period is normally 10 to 11 weeks.

The life cycle of *T. cati* is similar to *T. canis*; however, there is no placental transfer of larvae. Neonatal infection of kittens can develop via transmammary passage of larvae in the queen's milk.

When the eggs of *T. canis* hatch, they can be ingested by several noncanid species, including man. The invading larvae do not invade the intestinal tract but may reach other tissues, including the skin, liver, and eye. Other species such as earthworms, mice, rats, chickens, pigeons, lambs, and pigs may be infested by *T. canis* larvae, and if dogs eat infected tissues, the encysted larvae may mature within the dog. This is called a *paratenic cycle*.

Signs

Heavy prenatal *Toxocara* infections can produce abdominal cramps and distention in young puppies. Obstruction of the intestinal tract may occur, or the severely affected puppy may be predisposed to intussusception.

The signs associated with ascariasis are related to the migration of the parasite through the liver and lungs, as well as gastrointestinal irritation. Pulmonary edema is seen with migration of second stage larvae; signs are cough, nasal discharge, and increased respiratory rate. Migration of third stage larvae through the stomach produces distention, emesis, and vomiting of immature worms.

Heavy adult *T. canis* infections in the small intestine can lead to gastrointestinal signs such as vomiting, diarrhea, abdominal pain, partial obstruction, a "pot-bellied" appearance, emaciation, a dull harsh hair coat, and restlessness.

Prenatally acquired *T. canis* infections can be difficult to diagnose in puppies younger than 3 weeks of age. History of vomiting, diarrhea, coughing, debility, stunted growth, and painful abdomen suggest ascariasis.

A diagnosis is based on finding parasitic eggs on fecal examination, parasites in the stool, or vomitus.

Chemotherapy

Administer piperazine, dichlorvos, mebendazole, fenbendazole, or pyrantel pamoate (see Table 142).

Control

The complexity of the life cycle of *T. canis* makes both the bitch and pups sources of infection. Intrauterine and postparturient infections in the bitch can cause reinfection of suckling pups, as well as transmammary infection. The following control measures are important:

1. Puppies should be reared in an enclosed environment until weaning. All fecal material should be removed daily and disposed of.
2. Puppies should be screened for *T. canis* at 4 and 8 weeks of age.
3. Bitches should be screened for parasites during the first 4 weeks of pregnancy and wormed if necessary.
4. The feces of the bitch should be collected daily and disposed of during the suckling period.

Transmission to Man

Toxocara larvae have been implicated in an increasing number of cases of visceral larval migrans infestations in the liver and eyes of young children. It is the responsibility of the veterinarian to keep pets as free as possible of *Toxocara* and to inform pet owners that children should avoid contact with parasite-laden feces. An ELISA test has been developed for detecting exposure to ascarids. The public health article by Shantz (see references) should be read by all veterinarians.

Trichuriasis
(Whipworms, Trichuris vulpis)

This parasite inhabits the large bowel and cecum. Eggs are passed in the stool and require a higher temperature for embryonation than do ascarid eggs.

The infective eggs are ingested by the host, hatch in the small intestine where the larvae develop in the jejunal glands, and then migrate posteriorly where they mature. The prepatent period is 70 to 197 days. Adult *Trichuris vulpis* may live in the cecum and colon for 16 months, and eggs may remain viable under proper conditions for 5 years.

Signs

Signs depend on the numbers of parasites present and include intermittent diarrhea, loss of weight, emaciation, anemia, abdominal pain, flatulence, and "flank suckling." Many animals with light infections may show no signs.

Diagnosis

A diagnosis is based on finding eggs in the feces. Repeated fecal examinations may have to be performed, using a flotation fluid with a specific gravity of 1.4 in order to find eggs.

Chemotherapy

Administer mebendazole or fenbendazole for 3 days orally. Because trichuris larvae take 3 months to develop and may be more resistant to treatment than adults, repeated medication may be required, along with good sanitation measures to prevent reinfection (see Table 142).

Strongyloidosis
(Strongyloides stercoralis)

This parasite lives in the mucosae of the anterior half of the small intestine in dogs, cats, foxes, and man. The parasitic worms are all females, and the eggs develop parthenogenetically. The eggs develop rapidly and hatch before evacuation in the feces. Some of the larvae develop into infective larvae, whereas others develop into free-living males and females. Infective larvae may enter by the oral route or may penetrate the skin. Percutaneous infections may cause focal dermatitis. First-stage larvae are usually found in fresh feces. After a fecal culture has been made for at least 18 hours, the diagnosis may be confirmed by finding free-living adult worms and infective third-stage larvae. Larvae migrate by way of the circulation and lungs, going to the intestine as fourth stage larvae. Progeny may be shed in the feces 7 to 20 days after infection.

Signs

Geographical strains of *Strongyloides* differ greatly in their virulence and infectiousness for hosts.

Signs include diarrhea, which usually contains blood, loss of weight, anorexia, listlessness, and bronchopneumonia.

Diagnosis

A diagnosis is based on recovery of the characteristic infective larvae in the feces after incubation in sterile sand for 48 hours. Examination of fresh fecal smears is also helpful.

Transmission in Man

Strongyloidiasis in man is a chronic debilitating disease. Man and dog can readily infect each other; therefore, caution should be used in handling infected dogs. Infected dogs should be isolated, and extreme care should be taken to avoid human contamination.

Chemotherapy

Administer thiabendazole orally for 3 consecutive days. Monthly fecal examinations should be made for 1 year following infection and therapy (see Table 142).

Tapeworms

In the United States, most dogs and cats are domesticated and eat prepared, cooked foods; therefore, cestode parasitism in both man and animals is not a major problem. Exceptions to this general statement can be found with infections in dogs of *Dipylidium caninum* in which the intermediate host is the flea, and *Taenia pisiformis* in which the natural reservoir is the rabbit. Cats frequently harbor *Taenia taeniaeformis*, the larval stage of which is found in rats and mice (Table 143).

Treatment

Recommended drugs for tapeworms include: praziquantel (Droncit), fenbendazole mebendazole (Telmin), bunamidine (Scolaban), and niclosamide (Yomesan). Fenbendazole and mebenazole are highly effective for *Taenia* spp. only. These drugs are reasonably effective (usually at higher than normal dose rates). However, unless re-infection is prevented (by the provision of an adequate diet and attempts to stop scavenging), dogs will rapidly become reinfected and may again be passing large numbers of eggs within 14 days of treatment.

Table 143. CESTODES FOR DOGS AND CATS

Name	Definitive Host	Intermediate Host	Remarks
Dipylidium caninum	Dog, cat, wolf, fox, other animals	Fleas and biting lice	Proglottids are shaped like cucumber seeds; probably the most common tapeworm of dogs
Taenia taeniaeformis	Cat, dog, fox, and other animals	Various rats, mice, and other rodents	A common tapeworm of cats
Taenia pisiformis	Dog, cat, fox, wolf, and other animals	Rabbits and hares, rarely squirrels and rodents	Common in hunting dogs and farm dogs who eat rabbits
Taenia hydatigenia	Dog, wolf, rarely cat	Domestic and wild cloven-hoofed animals, rarely rodents	More frequently found in farm dogs.
Diphyllobothrium species	Man, dog, cat, and other fish-eating animals	Found encysted in organs and free in body cavity of various fish	Found in northern United States and Canada
Echinococcus granulosus	Dog, wolf, fox, and other wild carnivores	Sheep, goats, cattle, swine, horses, deer, moose, and some rodents; occasionally man and other animals	Public health significance is important
Multiceps multiceps	Dog, fox, and coyote	Sheep, goats, and other ruminants	Found rarely in western North America

Lungworms

The metastrongyloid nematodes *Aelurostrongylus abstrusus*, *Paragonimus kellicotti*, and *Capillaria aerophilia* are parasites that reproduce in the air passages and pulmonary vessels or parenchyma of the lungs.

Adult *Aelurostrongylus* worms live in the terminal respiratory bronchioles, alveolar ducts and small branches of the pulmonary arteries. Eggs are forced into the alveolar ducts and alveoli. The first stage larvae escape into the airways and are coughed up and swallowed, thus passing into the feces. The first stage larvae can survive in moist soil for up to 5½ months, in live mollusks for 5 months, and in dead mollusks for 3 weeks. Various transport hosts (amphibians, birds, reptiles and rodents) may eat infected mollusks and serve as a source of infection when eaten by cats and dogs. When ingested, the infective, third stage larvae penetrate the mucosa of the esophagus, stomach, and small intestine, traveling to the blood stream and lymphatics and finally to the lungs. The prepatent period is 34 to 42 days.

The life cycle of *Capillaria aerophilia* may be direct or may involve earthworms as facultative intermediate hosts. *Paragonimus* lung flukes have a natural host, the mink, but also occur in the dog, cat, pig, and other animals. Eggs that are coughed up and/or swallowed by the adult host are passed in the feces or sputum, and the miracidia hatch. The miracidia then enter a snail. Crayfish become infected by eating snails and/or cercariae. The definitive host becomes infected by eating the crayfish. Geographic distribution of this parasite is the Great Lakes and Midwest and southern United States.

Adults live in the trachea and produce eggs, which are coughed up and passed in the feces. The eggs are ingested, and the prepatent period is about 6 weeks.

Clinical Picture

Cats affected with *Aelurostrongylus* exhibit few clinical disturbances. When severe infestations or debilitation occurs, signs of illness may include a chronic cough with gradually increasing dyspnea, anorexia, and fever. Occasionally, sneezing and oculonasal discharge may be present. The most dangerous period is 6 to 13 weeks after infection, when large numbers of eggs and larvae are produced. Thoracic radiographs reveal solid or cavitating parenchymal lesions that may be more prominent in the caudal lung lobes.

Infection of dogs with *Paragonimus* or *Capillaria* can produce severe interstitial and bronchial-alveolar pneumonia characterized by a productive cough. Transtracheal washes (see p. 527), and fine needle biopsies of the lungs may be very helpful in revealing large numbers of eosinophils and parasite eggs. *Paragonimus kellicotti* produces radiographically evident lung cysts in affected animals. These cysts can spontaneously rupture, leading to pneumothorax and hemoptysis.

Diagnosis

Fecal examination is the most practical diagnostic technique. First-stage larvae of *Aelurostrongylus* have a characteristic notched or S-shaped tail and appear in the feces. The Baermann apparatus is the most accurate way of finding larvae in the feces. Fecal examination will not reveal early infections (less than 5 to 6 weeks) of *Aelurostrongylus* when adult parasites are not yet mature or late infections when eggs are no longer produced. In addition to fecal examination, the use of transtracheal washes and lung needle biopsies can be very helpful.

Chemotherapy

Various chemotherapeutic agents have been used to treat *Aelurostrongylus* infections. Although data are limited, it appears that the oral administration of levamisole hydrochloride (Levasole) 25 mg per kg per day per os for 5 days or Fenbendazole 50 mg per kg for 3 days may be effective. The anthelmintic choice for *Paragonimus* infection is albendazole. Dosage is 25 mg per kg orally BID for 10 days.

Control

Prevention of *Aelurostrongylus* infection requires preventing cats from catching mollusks or transport hosts, which is extremely difficult.

In *Capillaria aerophilia* infection, placing animals in wire bottom pens or on sanitized concrete runs will prevent recurrence of infestation.

Experimental evidence indicates that dogs infected with *Paragonimus* can be treated with Fenbendazole, 100 mg per kg each day for 10 to 14 days.

There has been recent experimental and clinical evidence of low-grade infection of the lungs of dogs with *Filaroides hirthi*. These are very small nematodes, 0.5 to 2.0 mm long, found in the alveolar spaces and terminal bronchioles of dogs. These infections are most prevalent in beagle colonies. The first stage larvae of *Filaroides hirthi* are infectious directly from the feces. Zinc sulfate flotation is much more efficient than a Baerman technique in concentrating larvae and demonstrating them in the feces; however, eggs may be difficult to find. Transtracheal washes may be helpful in finding parasites. Albendazole, given at a dosage rate of 25 to 50 mg per kg twice daily for 5 days, has killed all but a small proportion and sterilized the few surviving *Filaroides hirthi* worms in artificially infected beagle pups. Extensive tissue reaction around the dead worms persisted for an undetermined length of time.

Spirocerca lupi

The life cycle of *Spirocerca lupi* requires passage through coprophagous beetles and a range of facultative paratenic hosts, which can include lizards, chickens, and mice. Dogs and cats may ingest infected insects or paratenic hosts that feed on insects or crustaceans. When infected larvae are ingested by a dog, they migrate in the adventitia of the visceral arteries and aorta to the walls of the esophagus and stomach. The degree of clinical signs present in *Spirocerca* infection depends on the degree of trauma and functional obstruction caused by the migrating larvae. *Spirocerca* infection may produce signs of clinical disease characterized by vomiting, anorexia, dysphagia, aortic aneurysm, esophageal neoplasms, and secondary pulmonary osteoarthropathy. Diagnosis may be difficult; however, the demonstration of eggs in feces or vomitus is helpful.

Dirofilariasis
(Heartworm Disease)

Heartworm disease is endemic in the eastern and southern United States, and its distribution is gradually spreading north and west. Any area that has a high mosquito population may be subject to this disease. Furthermore, the transient nature of today's lifestyle and the rapid modes of transportation allow frequent movement of people and their pets. The life cycle of *Dirofilaria immitis* requires a female mosquito as both an intermediate host and a vector. The main mosquitos involved are *Culex pipiens*, *Culex quinquefasciatus*, *Anopheles*, and *Aedes* species.

Mosquito vectors feed on the muzzle, eyes, and perineum of dogs. If a dog carries microfilariae, the microfilariae are ingested by the mosquito, along with the blood. After a 2-week maturation, the larvae are infective (third stage) and dwell in the mouth parts of the mosquito. When the mosquito feeds again, these infective larvae enter the host through the puncture wound. They live there for 2 to 2½ months, going through two additional molts before becoming mature adults; then they invade the venous system. Young adult heartworms can reach the right ventricle in 8 to 10 weeks postinfection. They are not capable of releasing microfilariae into the blood until 6 to 7 months postinfection. Adult heartworms can live 5 years, and microfilariae can live for 2 to 3 years in the bloodstream (Table 144).

Diagnosis

History

A suggestive history of exposure to an endemic heartworm region of the country should prompt a laboratory examination.

Symptoms

The animal may be asymptomatic. The diagnosis is generally made during a routine blood check. However, possible symptoms include loss of stamina, weight loss, poor physical condition, a soft, moist cough (especially on exertion), and ascites. The dog may stand with elbows abducted, and syncope, seizures, and anemia may occur. There may be acute vena caval or liver failure syndrome,

Table 144. DIFFERENTIATION OF MICROFILARIAE OF
D. IMMITIS AND *D. RECONDITUM*

Characteristic	*D. immitis*	*D. reconditum*
Average width (in microns)* (Lindsey, 1961, 1962)	6.8(6.1–7.2)	5.2 (4.7–5.8)
Average length (in microns) (Lindsey, 1961, 1962)	314 (286–340)	270 (258–292)
Mobility (Schalm and Jain, 1966)	Sluggish	Active
Presence of "button hook" on posterior extremity (Newton and Wright, 1956)	Absent	Present
Shape of anterior extremity	Tapered	Blunt
Presence of cephalic hook (Sawyer *et al.*, 1965)	Absent	Present
Degree of straightness	Straight	Crescent-shaped
Dye uptake using Coriphosphine 0 (Rothstein and Brown, 1960)	Stained in 10 minutes	Stained in 30 minutes
Acid phosphatase activity (Chalifoux and Hunt, 1971)	Two distinct zones	Generalized

*Width measured at 50 or 60 microns from tip of anterior extremity.
From Kelly, J.D.: Canine heartworm disease. *In* Kirk, R. W. (ed.): Current Veterinary Therapy VII. Philadelphia, W. B. Saunders Company, 1980.

in which signs develop over a 12- to 24-hour period. The dog displays weakness, collapse, anorexia, and hemoglobinuria. Death occurs in 12 to 72 hours. Usually no ascites is present.

Physical Examination

Heart murmurs are usually absent. A split-second heart sound may be present due to the pulmonary hypertension that develops. Signs of right heart failure such as venous engorgement, jugular pulse, or ascites may be present.

Electrocardiography

The electrocardiogram (ECG) is often normal with heartworm disease. Abnormalities may occur in the form of a moderate right axis deviation. Occasionally, severe changes are seen. The lead CV_6LU has sometimes been helpful. The presence of an S wave deeper than 0.7 mv would establish right ventricular hypertrophy.

Radiography

Radiographs are very helpful, especially when the disease has progressed. Right ventricular enlargement and a bulge in the area of the pulmonary artery may be seen on the dorsoventral view. The pulmonary arteries may be large.

Rather than tapering to a fine point as a normal pulmonary artery, it tends to end abruptly. This plus the presence of diffuse patchy densities in the lung fields are evidence of pulmonary embolization.

Radiographs may be used to make the diagnosis when the ECG and blood tests are negative. Any animal that has right ventricular enlargement on x-ray examination should have its blood checked for microfilariae, and an ECG should be obtained. Additionally, radiographs may show hepatomegaly, splenomegaly, ascites, or pleural effusion.

Clinical Pathology

The diagnosis of heartworm disease is made by finding microfilariae of *D. immitis* in the bloodstream. They must be differentiated from the microfilariae of *Dipetalonema* spp. Several different tests have been advocated for the detection of microfilaria, including the direct wet smear, membrane filtration test, capillary sedimentation test, saponin lysis test, and modified Knott test. The most reliable test is still the modified Knott procedure.

The presence of eosinophilia may be associated with heartworm disease, but it is a nonspecific finding. Any animal with an unexplained eosinophilia should have a blood check, a chest x-ray examination and an ECG.

Occult dirofilariasis refers to *D. immitis* infestation without circulating microfilariae in peripheral blood. The percentage of cases of adult heartworm disease without microfilaremia is variable, being anywhere from 20 to 67 per cent. The importance of occult dirofilaria infection can be clinically important in three major disease situations: (1) in determining that a dog is free of heartworm disease before beginning a preventative program with diethyl carbamazine; (2) in demonstrating the presence of adults and microfilariae in heartworm infected dogs; and (3) in determining heartworm infection in dogs as a cause of cardiopulmonary disease.

There are several demonstrated causes of occult dirofilariasis: (1) prepatent infections in which clinical, pulmonary arterial signs may develop but microfiliaria are not produced, and indirect fluorescent antibody (IFA) testing for antimicrofilarial antibody is negative; (2) unisexual infections with nongravid female worms; (3) drug-induced sterility of adult *D. immitis;* and (4) immune-mediated sterile infection, which is negative on routine microfiliariae check but positive on IFA testing.

Clinical signs include weight loss, extreme fatigue, chronic cough, and dyspnea. Radiographic findings are enlargement of the right ventricle, enlargement of the pulmonary outflow tract, and pulmonary infiltrative disease that is most demonstrable radiographically in the peripheral areas of the diaphragmatic lobes. ECG changes of right ventricular hypertrophy are seen in advanced heartworm disease (see p. 335). The clinical pathology may reveal an eosinophilia, basophilia, and hypergammaglobulinemia. The IFA test for occult dirofilariasis is commercially available from numerous laboratories, including Paradiagnostics Inc., P.O. Box 6, Davis, California. The ELISA heartworm test is used to measure antibody to the parasite and is more sensitive than the IFA method. The ELISA test can detect antibodies to heartworms within 60 to 90 days after the bite of an infected mosquito. The commercial ELISA method (Mallinkrodt chemical ELISA test) cannot be used in cats.

The lung pathology is associated with an immunologically mediated reaction around pulmonary end arterioles. The affected animals should be treated with aspirin prior to treatment for adult *Dirofilaria* infestations.

Cats are also susceptible to heartworm disease; however, antemortem diagnosis, routine screening procedures, and prophylactic therapy are rarely used. Clinical signs in cats include coughing, dyspnea, lethargy, and increased bronchovesicular sounds with systolic murmur (Table 145). The most consistent laboratory signs are hyperglobulinemia and eosinophilia. Enlarged pulmonary caudal lobar arteries and right ventricular enlargement can be seen. Occult dirofilariasis appears to be common. Only 20 per cent of cats with adult *D. immitis* may have circulating microfilariae. Both the serologic IFA-microfilaria slide test and the ELISA test are very useful in detecting prepatent or nonpatent infection.

Treatment

Heartworm disease can be treated medically or surgically. Because of the drawbacks of surgery and the success of medical therapy, most dogs are treated

Table 145. DIFFERENTIAL DIAGNOSIS OF FOUR FELINE DISEASES WITH SIMILAR CLINICAL SIGNS

Abnormality	Heartworm Disease	Asthma	Lungworm Infection	Cardio-myopathy
Coughing	±	+	+	−
Dyspnea	±	±	±	±
Heart murmur	±	−	−	±
Gallop rhythm	±	−	−	±
Hyperglobulinemia	+	−	−	−
Eosinophilia	±	±	±	−
Right ventricular enlargement (electrocardiography)	±	−	−	−
Right ventricular enlargement (radiography)	±	−	−	±
Enlarged pulmonary arteries	+	±	±	±
Tortuosity or blunting of pulmonary arteries	+	−	−	−
Pulmonary edema	−	−	−	±
Pleural effusion	±	−	−	±

+ = abnormality present; − = abnormality absent; ± = abnormality variably present.

From Calvert, C. A., and Mandell, C. D.: Diagnosis and management of feline heartworm disease. J.A.V.M.A., *180*(5):550, 1982.

medically. Occasionally, surgery is done when large numbers of adult *Dirofilaria* are present; however, this is difficult to determine. The number of microfilariae present in the peripheral circulation does not correspond with the number of adult microfilariae that may be present.

Medical Treatment

1. CBC, BUN, urinalysis, and liver profile are obtained prior to treatment for heart worms. Renal function can be markedly altered in dirofilaria infection. This is associated with glomerulonephritis. Urine protein loss should be carefully evaluated. If any of these test results are abnormal, appropriate supportive therapy, such as fluids, B vitamins, vitamin C, lipotrophic agents, antibiotics, and steroids has been advocated. If the dog is in heart failure, it should be digitalized prior to treatment.

2. Sodium caparsolate (1 per cent) is administered 0.22 ml per kg of body weight twice a day for 2 days. The drug is potentially nephrotoxic and hepatotoxic, and therapy should be discontinued if persistent vomiting, anorexia, or icterus occurs. The irritant action of this drug mandates a perfect intravenous (IV) injection. No drug can be administered perivascularly. The animal is hospitalized or kept at cage rest for 10 to 14 days after treatment. The drug kills the adult heartworms over a 1- to 3-week period. Exercise is restricted for 4 to 6 weeks or longer, depending on the severity of the case.

   The use of aspirin systemically at dosage levels of 10 mg per kg daily for 4 weeks following adulticide therapy reduces possible platelet involvement in thromboembolism and in myointimal proliferation of damaged arterial walls.

   Complications of therapy for dirofilariasis are drug toxicity or thromboembolism in the lungs from dead worms. Signs of drug toxicity include bilirubinuria, vomiting, icterus, and dehydration.

3. Dithiazanine (Dizan), 8.8 mg per kg, is administered PO daily for 7 days as a microfilaricide. Microfilariae testing is performed on Day 8 and if positive, the dithiazanine dosage is increased to 13 to 14 mg per kg per day for a maximum of 10 days. Dizan is started 6 to 8 weeks after the caparsolate therapy. Gastrointestinal disturbances with vomiting and diarrhea are often seen with Dizan treatment. Dizan discolors the stool, making it blue-green. Dizan may be nephrotoxic.

   Many dogs have been treated with levamisole as a microfilaricide. Levamisole has proved effective against the microfilariae of *D. immitis*. The oral preparation of levamisole used for sheep is administered daily at a dosage of 11 to 15 mg per kg for 6 days, and the blood is re-examined. Dosage can be repeated for up to 15 days of medication. If microfilariae are not eliminated by this time, a new microfilaricide should be used. Levamisole is potentially toxic and may produce vomiting, nervousness, restlessness, and visual disturbances; it does not have FDA clearance for use in dogs.

   The side effects of levamisole administered to the dog may occasionally be severe and may manifest as generalized neurologic deficits associated with granulomatous encephalomyelitis or encephalitis and perivascular cuffing of nonspecific etiology.

The new class of drugs, the avermectins, are effective against microfilariae. Ivermectin has been used as a microfilaricide at a single dosage of 0.25 mg per kg orally two weeks after adveticide therapy. The agent is also effective against developing stages of *D. immitis* when used once a month. As of December 1984, the drug has not received FDA clearance for use in dogs.

4. Diethylcarbamazine (Caricide) is used as a preventive agent. It is not a microfilaricide. It is effective against the third-stage infective larvae. Caricide should not be used in dogs that test microfilaria-positive because of the high percentage of allergic reactions in those dogs.

Caricide is given at a dosage of 6.6 mg per kg once daily. Treatment should be begun 30 days before entering an endemic heartworm area and the regimen should be continued for at least 60 days after leaving the area. It should be administered year round in heartworm endemic areas.

Ollulanus tricuspis
(Gastric Nematode in Cats)

Persistent vomiting in cats may be associated with parasitisms by the *Ollulanus* parasite. This is a minute nematode whose life cycle is viviparous with the third- and fourth-stage larvae and adults existing in the host's stomach and expelled in vomitus. The parasites cause chronic gastritis. They can be recognized when vomitus is examined with a dissecting microscope. The parasites are 0.8 to 1 mm long. Aleurostrongylus parasite infection may cause similar clinical signs, but the larvae migrate or are coughed up in the trachea, are swallowed, and then passed in the feces. Aleurostrongylus adults are much larger than Ollulanus adults, which are 4 to 9 mm in length.

Platynosum concinnum
(Liver Fluke)

In the southern part of the United States and in similar climates, especially south Florida and Hawaii, the digenetic trematode platynosum may infect the liver of cats. In stray cats and "ranging" feral cats that have access to the intermediate host—namely, land snails or intermediate hosts such as lizards and toads—the incidence may be as high as 50 per cent. The adult flukes are 1.1 mm wide and 2.7 mm long, and their eggs are 30 to 40 microns in size. Infected cats develop fibrotic livers, portal fibrosis, and biliary epithelial hyperplasia and become chronically debilitated and icteric, signs associated with chronic liver disease.

The drug of choice in treatment at this time appears to be albendazole.

References and Additional Readings

Calvert, C. A., and Mandell, C. D.: Diagnosis and management of feline heartworm disease. J.A.V.M.A., *180*(5):550, 1982.

Calvert, C. A., and Rawlings, C. A.: Diagnosis and management of canine heartworm disease. *In* Kirk, R. W. (ed.): Current Veterinary Therapy VIII:Small Animal Practice. Philadelphia, W. B. Saunders Company, 1983.

Carlisle, C. H.: Canine dirofilariasis: its radiographic appearance. J. Am. Coll. Vet. Radiol., *21*(3):123, 1980.

Dillon, R., Sakas, P. S., Buxton, B. A., and Schultz, D.: Indirect immunofluorescence testing for diagnosis of occult *Dirofilaria immitis* infection in three cats. J.A.V.M.A., *180*(1):80, 1982.

Georgi, J. R.: Parasitology for veterinarians, 4th ed. Philadelphia, W. B. Saunders Co., 1984.

Hargis, A. M., Prieur, D. J., and Wescott, R. B.: A gastric nematode (Ollulanus tricuspis) in cats in the Pacific Northwest. J.A.V.M.A., *178*(5):475, 1981.

Hitt, M. E.: Liver flukes in cats—*Platynosum concinnum.* Feline Pract., *11*(3):26, 1981.

Rawlings, C. A., Dawe, D. L., McCall, J. W., et al.: Four types of occult *Dirofilaria immitis* infection in dogs. J.A.V.M.A., *180*(11):1323, 1982.

Rawlings, C. A., Keith, J. C., Lewis, R. E., et al.: Aspirin and prednisolone modification of radiographic changes caused by adveticide treatment in dogs with heartworm infection. J.A.V.M.A., *182*(2):131, 1983.

Shantz, P. M.: Roundworms in dogs and cats: veterinary and public health considerations. Compendium on Continuing Education, 3(9):773, 1981.

Sutton, R. H., and Atwell, R. B.: Nervous disorders in dogs associated with levamisole therapy. J. Small An. Pract., 23:391, 1981.

Vandevolde, M., Boring, J. G., Huff, E. J., and Gingreich, D. A.: Effect of levamisole on canine central nervous system. J. Neuropath. Exp. Neurol., 37:165, 1978.

Wong, M. M., Pedersen, N. C., and Cullen, J.: Dirofilariasis in cats. J.A.A.H.A., *19*:855, 1983.

Coccidiosis

Isospora bigemina, Isopora rivolta, and *Isospora felis* are the three common types of organisms causing coccidiosis in the United States.

Coccidiosis usually affects young dogs and cats, especially those from kennels, pet shops, catteries, or other places where large numbers of animals are kept together. The disease is characterized by anorexia, diarrhea (frequently hemorrhagic), and loss of weight.

Infection of the host results from ingestion of infective oocysts. The coccidia undergo repeated cycles of asexual multiplication (schizogony), which finally terminate in the formation of sexually differentiated gametes that combine to form zygotes. At this stage, a protective covering is formed (oocyst.) Sporulation (sporogony) may occur in the intestinal tract or after the oocyst is eliminated in the feces. In the genus *Isospora,* there are two sporocysts, each containing four sporozoites.

Diagnosis

Diagnosis is based on finding oocysts in the feces coupled with the clinical history. The diarrhea may precede a heavy outpouring of oocysts by a few days and may continue even after oocyst levels become low. It is, therefore, not always possible to confirm a clinical diagnosis of coccidiosis by finding oocysts in the feces. Other intestinal parasites and systemic diseases such as distemper may also complicate the picture.

Treatment

There is no good treatment for coccidiosis in dogs and cats once the signs of disease have appeared. Prophylaxis of clinical coccidiosis depends on good sanitation and controlling the natural intake of sporulated oocysts by young animals. With good hygiene and sanitation, coccidiosis is a self-limiting disease. Treatment of patients with coccidiosis should be aimed at controlling the diarrhea, reducing the population of coccidial organisms, correcting fluid and electrolyte imbalances, and establishing good principles of animal hygiene and sanitation. Intestinal sulfonamides, neomycin, Furacin, tetracycline, and chloramphenicol have all been used to help control secondary infections and to reduce the population of coccidial organisms.

Toxoplasmosis

Toxoplasma is an intestinal coccidian of cats, with a wide range of intermediate hosts. Cats, especially kittens younger than 6 months of age, can become infected and shed *Toxoplasma* oocysts after eating mice, rats, birds, or meat containing *Toxoplasma* cysts. Cats can acquire infection by ingesting any of three infectious stages of *Toxoplasma*—namely, tachyzoites, bradyzoites in the encysted form in muscle tissue, and oocysts or zygote found within the feces of definitive hosts. Less than 50 per cent of cats shed oocysts after ingesting cysts. The prepatent period to the shedding of oocysts is 3 to 5 days after the ingestion of mice or meat containing *Toxoplasma* cysts and 20 to 34 days after the ingestion of oocysts. Oocysts are shed by infected cats for 1 to 5 weeks during primary infection and in reduced numbers or not at all following reinfection. The oocysts are not infectious until sporulation, which requires 1 to 5 days (or longer, depending on environmental temperature and oxygenation). Under favorable circumstances, oocysts remain infectious for several months to a year or longer.

The oocysts of toxoplasma develop two sporocysts and four sporozoites. *Isospora felis* and *Isospora rivolta* are the two common coccidian parasites found in young cats. The oocysts of *Isospora felis* measure 40 by 30 microns and *Isospora rivolta*, 25 by 20 microns. Oocysts of *Toxoplasma* are much smaller, 10 by 12 microns, or about twice the size of a red blood cell.

Standard techniques of fecal flotation at 1.15 specific gravity will concentrate the oocysts in the supernatant. Cats infected with toxoplasma shed oocysts for only a 2-week period; finding oocysts in cat feces during this limited time period is unlikely.

From serologic evidence, it would appear that man and animals can suffer from asymptomatic infections with *Toxoplasma* organisms. *Toxoplasma* antibodies have been found in varying percentages of cats, depending on the types of populations tested. Forty to 60 per cent of cats in the Kansas-Iowa area had *Toxoplasma* antibodies, and reports indicate that 24 to 57 per cent of dogs in the United States have *Toxoplasma* antibodies.

Clinically, symptomatic toxoplasmosis may involve many organs. Following the oral ingestion of oocysts, the gastrointestinal tract is infected; there can then be hematogenous and lymphogenous dissemination of the organism to other organs, including the liver, lungs, lymph nodes, eyes, central nervous system, and muscle.

Confirmation of *Toxoplasma* infection can be based on serologic evidence or isolation of *Toxoplasma* organisms by inoculating tissues into mice. Serologic examination should consist of paired sera examination taken 1 or 2 weeks apart.

The serologic tests include the Sabin-Feldman dye test, fluorescent antibody test, haemagglutination test, complement fixation test, direct agglutination test, latex agglutination slide test, and enzyme linked immunosorbent assay.

Diagnosis of toxoplasmosis can be made based on clinical signs, isolation of the organism, or demonstration of antibody determinations on serum specimens. The antigen-antibody curves of the dye test (seldom run anymore), the complement fixation, direct agglutination, and IgG/IgM fluorescent antibody tests run closely parallel and probably measure the same antibody level. The indirect haemagglutination test appears to be distinct from the other tests, because antibody rises to a maximum later in infection. The curve for IgM also differs in that this titer may go up more rapidly and decline more rapidly in acute infections.

The most specific of the tests is the IgM-ELISA test, although it is not yet widely commercially available. When compared to the IgM-IFA test, this test is positive more frequently and at higher titers. IgM-ELISA titers may persist for as long as 9 months after the clinical onset of disease.

Titers of greater than or equal to 1:64 by the IgM-IFA test suggest recently acquired infection or exposure and the corresponding titers in the IgM-ELISA are greater than or equal to 1:256.

Treatment

Sulfadiazine and pyrimethamine interfere in sequential steps with the biosynthesis of dihydrofolate and act synergistically against *Toxoplasma*. The toxic side effects can be alleviated and prevented with yeast and folinic acid. The shedding of oocysts by kittens can be almost eliminated by treating with sulfadiazine, 120 mg per kg per day, or with 60 mg per kg per day of sulfadiazine together with 0.5 mg per kg per day of pyrimethamine. Cats passing oocysts in the stool should be handled according to the precautions mentioned in the following discussion.

Prevention of Infection by Toxoplasma

Animals may become infected with *Toxoplasma* in the following ways: in the bradyzoite encysted stage—from eating infected uncooked meat; in the oocyst stage—from cats and soil; and from tachyzoites—transplacentally. Feeding dried, cooked, or canned food to a cat that is kept indoors and has no opportunity to hunt mice or birds eliminates the risk of acquiring toxoplasmosis. Meat that has been frozen is less infectious but may still harbor *Toxoplasma* cysts. Litter pans should be cleaned daily with boiling water or dry heat. Cat feces should be burned or flushed down a toilet. A pregnant woman should wear plastic gloves to clean the litter pan. The following points are important in the control of toxoplasmosis:

1. Do not feed cats raw meat products. Heat meat to 66°C (150°F) throughout before eating, or feed canned or dry food to cats.
2. Control flies, cockroaches, and other coprophagous animals that can serve as hosts of *Toxoplasma*.
3. Avoid contact with soil and sand that can be contaminated by cat feces. Change litter boxes daily. Clean litter pans by immersion in boiling water or use disposable litter pans.
4. Wash hands after handling cats or their excrement.
5. Wear gloves while working in the garden, and keep children's sandboxes covered when not in use.
6. The presence of antibody against *Toxoplasma* does not mean that a cat is presently infected or in need of treatment. There is no need to "get rid of" the cat. In fact, immune cats are safer pets than nonimmune cats, because on reinfection, they shed few or no oocysts.

References and Additional Readings

Burridge, M.: Toxoplasmosis. Compendium on Continuing Education, 2:233, 1980.
Dreesen, D. W., and Lubroth, J. S.: Life cycle of *Toxoplasma gondii*. Compendium on Continuing Education, 5(6):456, 1983.
Dubey, J. P.: *Toxoplasma, Hammondia, Besnoitia, Sarcocystis*, and other tissue cyst-forming coccidia of man and animals. *In* Kreier, J. P. (ed.): Parasitic Protozoa, Vol. III. New York, Academic Press, 1977, pp. 101–237.
Sikes, R. K.: Toxoplasmosis. J.A.V.M.A., *180*(8):857, 1982.

FECAL SAMPLE COLLECTION AND EXAMINATION

Collection

Fresh fecal samples are always desirable. Two-to-4-ounce closed containers are best suited for fecal collections. Fecal samples can be picked up with disposable wooden tongue blades after the animal defecates, or they can be taken directly from the rectum. An enema may be administered; however, soapy or oily enemas should not be used, because they interfere with good examinations of the stool. Material left on thermometers is not usually adequate for fecal examinations except in a few heavy parasitic infestations. If samples must be kept for a few hours to several days, refrigeration or chemical fixation should be used. Refrigeration at 4°C preserves eggs and larvae for up to 72 hours. Formalin may be added to fecal specimens, 1 part 10 per cent formalin to 4 parts fecal specimen, to preserve parasite material.

Gross Examination

Examine the stool for adult worms or tapeworm segments. Note the presence of blood, mucus, fat, or other undigested material. Characterize the odor of the stool. Note the amount of stool passed, and observe whether it is formed or unformed. Fecal volume is determined by the content of water and fiber. Normal feces contain 60 to 70 per cent water. Volume of formed feces in a 15-kg dog should be about 40 ml per day (Strombeck). The longer the total gastrointestinal passage time, the firmer the feces. If the stool is formed, note its shape and diameter.

Color

Feces are usually brown in color due to the pigments urobilin and stercobilin derived from the bacterial action of bilirubin. A dark brown to black tarry stool can indicate that the animal is on a high meat diet or that there are blood pigments in the stool from upper gastrointestinal bleeding. Excessive amounts of bilirubin may produce a darker orange-brown stool. Charcoal and bismuth can produce black feces, whereas sulfonbromophthalein causes the feces to be purple. A grayish white, clay-colored stool is associated with biliary obstruction and pancreatic acinar insufficiency. A light brown or tan-colored stool is frequently seen in nursing puppies or dogs on a diet high in milk. A very white or acholic stool can be associated with an absence of bile pigments, overt bacterial infections of the gastrointestinal tract, or diarrhea with rapid passage of material through the intestinal tract. A green stool may be seen in dogs with unchanged bilirubin in the stool. Fresh red blood in the stool indicates recent bleeding into the colon or rectum.

Mucus

Normal stools contain only a small amount of mucus, which may not be easily observed. Excess mucus in the stool is a sign of lower bowel disease and is associated with acute and chronic inflammatory disease of the terminal ileum, cecum, and colon.

Odor

Odor is produced by indole and skatole, which are products of bacterial action in tryptophan. By-products of the breakdown of sulfur-containing amino acids and hydrogen sulfide also contribute to the odor. Alterations in the diet or bacterial flora can markedly change fecal odor.

MICROSCOPIC EXAMINATION OF THE FECES

Smear technique. This technique is used when small quantities of material are available or when the fecal examination must be completed in a short period of time. This procedure involves mixing a small amount of fecal material in a drop or two of saline placed on a slide and examining it microscopically. This method is qualitative and is useful only if positive; a negative result is inconclusive.

Qualitative concentration method. This is the routine method for parasite examination. The concentration of parasite ova or oocysts may be determined in a number of ways. All the methods depend on mixing the fecal sample with a material whose specific gravity is heavier than most of the parasitic ova or oocysts, yet is lighter than the fecal debris. Solutions of sodium chloride, sucrose, glycerine, zinc sulfate, or magnesium sulfate may be used to float the parasitic ova. Sugar flotation, although satisfactory for most parasitic ova, will not float the ova of tapeworms and flukes. Saturated sodium nitrate is routinely used for fecal flotation in the dog. Tapeworms are most easily diagnosed by gross examination of the feces for the typical segments. Fluke eggs can be found using the technique of Dennis, Stone, and Swanson (Benbrook) or the technique of Joy (described by Farrell).

Methods for protozoa examinations. The protozoan parasites, *Trichomonas*, *Giardia*, and *Balantidium*, disappear rapidly from fecal samples. In order to identify these parasites, the stool must be either examined or placed in a fecal fixative immediately after removal from the rectum. Polyvinyl alcohol is a good fecal fixative. Wet smears are satisfactory in some cases of protozoan infections if the feces can be examined immediately and the infection is heavy. The wet smears can be stained with Lugol's iodine to better visualize Giardia cysts. Routine fecal examination using sugar and salt solutions destroy Giardia cysts, and they are microscopically not recognizable. The zinc sulfate centrifugation technique allows Giardia cysts to be recognized. $ZnSO_4$ solution is prepared by mixing 331 g $ZnSO_4$ in 1 L of warm tap water to a specific gravity of 1.18. Fecal smears stained with iron hematoxylin, trichrome, or Giemsa are best for visualizing Giardia organisms. Better results are obtained in isolating Giardia from dogs when duodenal aspirations are used, as compared with fecal examinations (88 per cent recovery in duodenal aspirates vs. 39 per cent recovery in a single fecal flotation).

A second technique involving fixed feces provides the advantages of concentration and delayed examination. Prepare PAF fixative: phenol crystals (white), 20.0 gm; normal saline (0.85 per cent), 825.0 ml; ethanol (95 per cent), 125.0 ml; and formaldehyde solution, 50.0 ml (23 ml of liquified phenol may be substituted for the crystals). Cover the fresh feces with the PAF fixative, and allow them to stand at room temperature for 1 hour or longer. Strain the fixed sample through gauze, and then centrifuge the collective fluid at 1000 rpm for 2 or 3 minutes. Decant the excess fluid, and wash and centrifuge the sediment twice with normal saline. Stain several drops of the sediment with thionin or azure A, to allow for easy identification. If concentration is not desired, directly examine the sediment from the fixed feces.

Methods for Strongyloides examination. The rhabditiform larvae of *Strongyloides stercoralis* can be found in smears prepared from fresh feces. These larvae can be easily confused with other larval parasites and can be definitively identified by incubating the fecal specimen for 24 hours at room temperature or by culturing the feces on sterile sand for 48 hours. The infective filariform larvae will develop and can be identified by the esophageal length (one third of the total body length). A Baermann apparatus may also be used for examination of the larvae.

The feces should also be examined for the presence of undigested muscle (creatorrhea), fat (steatorrhea), or starch (amylorrhea) and for the presence or absence of pancreatic proteolytic enzymes. Fat droplets are demonstrated with a Sudan III stain. Muscle fibers are seen microscopically in direct fecal smears. One drop of Lugol's solution will turn undigested starch blue. Fecal trypsin can be identified by using the film strip digestion test or the more accurate gelatine tube test.

References and Additional Readings

Kirkpatrick, C., and Farrell, J. P.: Giardiasis. Compendium on Continuing Education. 4(5):367, 1982.

Sloss, M. W., and Kemp, R. L.: Veterinary Clinical Pathology, 5th ed. Ames, Iowa, Iowa State University Press, 1978.

Strombeck, D. R.: Small Animal Gastroenterology. Davis, California, Stonegate Publishing Company, 1979.

Theinpont, D., Rochette, F., and Vanparijs, O. F. J.: Diagnosing Helminthiasis through Coprological Examination. Indianapolis, Indiana, Pitman-Moore Co., 1979.

Specific Tests for Evaluation of Gastrointestinal Function

Fecal Weight

Twenty-four hour fecal weight depends on the nature of the diet and the level of fluid content in the feces. Dogs fed dry dog food have bulkier, softer feces that weigh roughly twice as much as dogs fed canned dog food that contains 70 per cent water, most of which is absorbed in the gastrointestinal tract. To attempt to standardize fecal weight against a norm, feed a dog a canned meat-based dog food, 50 gm per kg of body weight, once daily for 2 or 3 days, then make a 24-hour collection, weigh the feces, and divide by the weight of dog in kg. (Fig. 99.)

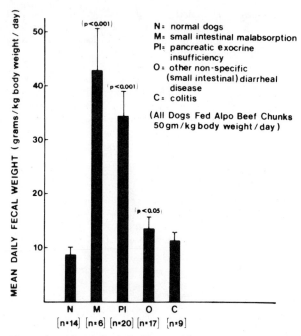

Figure 99. Fecal weight in diarrheal disease. The fecal weight of dogs with diarrhea associated with either small intestinal malabsorption or pancreatic exocrine insufficiency is significantly higher than the fecal weight of normal dogs and dogs with other types of nonsteatorrheic diarrheal disease. (Adapted from Burrows, C. F., et al.: Determination of fecal fat and trypsin output in the evaluation of chronic canine diarrhea. J.A.V.M.A. 174:62, 1979 with permission; reprinted with permission from Burrows, C. F.: The assessment of canine gastrointestinal function: recent advances and future needs. Gaines Vet. Symp. 31:3, 1981.)

Exocrine Pancreatic Function

In the gelatin tube test, two tubes containing 2 ml of 7.5 per cent gelatin are warmed to 37°C to liquify the gelatin. To one tube, 2 ml of a feces mixture is added, and to both tubes, 2 ml of 5 per cent sodium bicarbonate is added. Incubate both tubes at 37°C for 1 hour and refrigerate for 20 minutes. Failure to gel indicates the presence of trypsin, which has digested the gelatin.

Evaluation of feces for proteolytic enzyme activity can be performed using the "film test" to detect digestion of the gelatin in the film emulsion and the tube test of gelatin to detect digestion of the gelatin.

These tests usually identify animals with complete loss of pancreatic exocrine function. False-positive results to the test (identifying animals as having no proteolytic enzymes) may occur because pancreatic enzymes can be destroyed by intestinal bacteria and autodigestion.

Another test for evaluating the secretion of pancreatic enzymes (specifically chymotrypsin) by the pancreas involves the oral administration of n-benzoyl,-1-tyrosyl and para-aminobenzoic acid (BT-PABA). This peptide is specifically cleaved by chymotrypsin to release PABA, which is then reabsorbed into the blood and excreted by the kidneys. PABA can be measured in either blood or urine. In initial investigations, the substrate (PABA) is administered as a solution containing 1 gm of the peptide per 15 ml of water or propylene glycol. Administer at a level of 0.25 ml per kg by stomach tube following an 18-hour fast. Then give an additional 25 to 100 ml of water via stomach tube. Dogs must be confined for 6 hours following oral administration of the PABA, so that urine can be collected and analyzed. At the end of 6 hours, all urine is collected by catheterization. Normal renal function must be present for accurate PABA test results. Mean excretion in clinically normal dogs is 73.6 plus or minus 13.7 per cent, and PABA excretions beyond 2 standard deviations from the mean are abnormal. PABA excretions of less than 46 per cent are abnormal. If blood samples are taken, they are obtained at the beginning of the test and every 30 minutes for 3 hours. If the initial dose of PABA is given at 15 mg per kg and mixed with 10 ml per kg of body weight of tap water, PABA concentrations should reach a peak at 300 mg per dl at 120 to 150 minutes following administration. Dosages given to dogs with pancreatic insufficiency should never exceed 85 mg per dl. Some dogs with chronic diarrhea associated with small intestinal disease will have abnormal PABA test results.

The major value of this test is to determine whether a dog is deficient in pancreatic enzymes and needs replacement therapy. Dogs require enzyme replacement therapy when their PABA excretion is less than 15.8 per cent (see Fig. 99).

FECAL FAT

The presence of excessive amounts of fat in the feces (steatorrhea) can be a prominent sign of a severe gastrointestinal disturbance, such as malabsorption. The normal dog excretes 3 to 5 gm of fat in the stool per day and is not greatly affected by normal dietary intake of fat.

Demonstration of steatorrhea can be done by staining a fresh stool with a lipophilic stain such as Sudan II and examining it under the microscope. Levels of split and unsplit fats in fecal samples can be detected with Sudan III. Mix a 3-mm diameter pellet of fecal material with a drop of 36 per cent acetic acid on a glass slide. Add one drop of Sudan III stain, apply a cover slip, and pass it over a bunson burner or alcohol lamp, bringing the mixture to a boil three times. Under the microscope, split fats will appear as orange globules when cooled. When 10 or more 20-micron or larger globules of fat are seen per high-power field, the test is positive for split fats.

Fat Absorption and Excretion Tests

To perform a gross fat absorption test (plasma turbidity test), draw a heparinized blood sample from a fasted animal and separate the plasma. Feed the animal a meal enriched with corn oil (2 ml/kg) or peanut oil (0.5–2.0 ml/kg). An alternate product is Lipomal,* 3 ml per kg. Take a second blood sample 2 hours after ingestion of the fat meal, and compare plasma turbidity between pre- and post-fat ingestion samples. If the blood sample is not lipemic after 2 hours, wait until 4 hours and take a second blood sample. In the normal situation, the second plasma sample shows increased turbidity because of neutral fat droplets or chylomicrons. If both plasma samples are clear, either pancreatic exocrine function is inadequate or the intestine is not absorbing nutrients properly. Pancreatic exocrine insufficiency can be eliminated by repeating the test, but by predigesting the fat meal with pancreatic extracts. If the second sample of plasma still remains clear, a diagnosis of malabsorption should be considered.

For a 24-hour fecal fat excretion test, the animal should be placed on a constant diet for 72 hours. This diet should be meat based and should contain 8.5 to 9 per cent fat. The animal should be fed at a level of 50 gm per kg of body weight. All stool should be collected for 24 hours and sent to a laboratory for total fecal fat. Values for fecal fat are expressed in gm per kg of body weight per day; normal dogs excrete 0.25 gm per kg of fat per day. Normal values are 4 to 5 gm of fat in the stool per day. Steatorrhea is present when the total fecal fat exceeds 7 gm per day.

D-Xylose Absorption Test

The D-xylose absorption test measures the ability of the proximal jejunum to absorb five-carbon sugar. The rate at which xylose is absorbed in determined by the amount administered, rate of gastric emptying, size of the area of absorption in the small intestine, and intestinal circulation. To adequately evaluate the test, the gastric emptying time should be normal. The major

---

*Upjohn Co., Kalamazoo, Michigan.

FECAL FAT OUTPUT IN NORMAL DOGS AND DOGS WITH DIARRHEAL DISEASE*

	Fat Output (gm/kg body weight/day)†
Normal dogs (N = 14)	0.24 ± 0.01
Pancreatic insufficiency (N = 20)	2.08 ± 0.36
Intestinal malabsorption (N = 6)	1.14 ± 0.11
Colitis (N = 9)	0.19 ± 0.02
Other nonsteatorrheic small intestinal disease (N = 17)	0.18 ± 0.03

*Adapted from Burrows, C. F., et al.: Determination of fecal fat and trypsin output in the evaluation of chronic canine diarrhea. J.A.V.M.A., *174*:62, 1979, with permission.
†Fat output is expressed as mean ± SEM.

defects leading to abnormal xylose absorption are abnormalities in mucosal absorption area and circulation. Lymphangiectasia has no effect on xylose absorption. Fast the patient for 24 hours, and empty the bladder prior to the administration of D-xylose. Administer 500 mg per kg of a 10 to 25 per cent solution of D-xylose in 200 ml of warm water by stomach tube. Collect all urine for the next 5 hours; the bladder must be rinsed on final collection. Eight to 12 gm of D-xylose can indicate a malabsorption problem. Kidney function must be normal for the accurate interpretation of this test. Serum xylose levels can also be measured. Serum may be the preferred method over urine collection. Blood samples are taken every 30 minutes for 3 hours. Peak concentrations at 60 to 90 minutes are 60 to 70 mg per dl of D-xylose. In the normal dog, serum xylose levels peak between 1 and 2 hours after admission (mean concentration 142 mg/100 ml). Values at 30 minutes range from 25 to 160 mg per 100 ml. At 1 hour, serum levels of D-xylose were 63 plus or minus 12 mg per ml. Values of less than 45 mg per dl after 1 hour are considered abnormal. A control dog (normal) should be evaluated with the animal being tested.

The oral glucose tolerance test measures the ability of the proximal jejunum to absorb a six-carbon sugar (see p. 664).

Combined BT-PABA and Oral Xylose Tolerance Test

Xylose and PABA are absorbed independently, and the two tests have been combined in attempting to detect the etiology of chronic diarrheal disease of small bowel origin. The combination of these tests can be used in an attempt to differentiate maldigestion from malabsorption, but this discrimination does not always hold true. PABA uptake can be impaired in dogs with chronic diarrhea, especially in those that show abnormalities in xylose uptake (Fig. 100).

Vitamin A Absorption Test

The oral vitamin A absorption test measures the ability of the intestine to digest and absorb lipids. Administer 300,000 units of vitamin A (White's cod liver oil concentrate drops) to the fasting dog. Collect heparinized blood samples prior to the administration, and after 2, 4, 6, 8, and 24 hours. Mean fasting serum vitamin A concentrations range from 112 to 278 µg per 100 ml. Normal dogs show a two- or threefold increase in vitamin A levels over fasting. A flat curve may indicate a lack of bile, pancreatic enzymes, malabsorption, or disease of the ileum.

Triolein[131] Test

Another test is oral administration of ^{131}I-labeled triolein. On the day before the test, administer 0.3 ml of Lugol's iodine in a capsule orally to block the thyroidal uptake of ^{131}I label. On the day of the test, administer 20 microcuries of ^{131}I triolein. Collect blood samples over 2, 4, 6, 8, and 10 hours. Normal dogs show 8 to 15 per cent absorption after a 10-hour period.

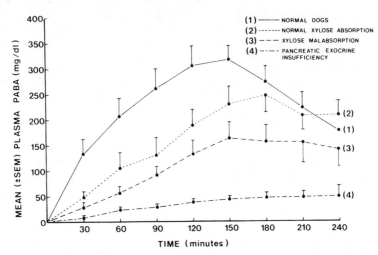

Figure 100. Plasma PABA concentrations after oral administration of BT-PABA (15 mg/kg) in normal dogs and dogs with chronic diarrheal disease. Mean plasma PABA concentration in dogs with pancreatic exocrine insufficiency never rises above 50 mg/dl and is significantly lower than that in both normal dogs and dogs with chronic diarrhea (with or without xylose malabsorption). Dogs with chronic diarrhea also have significantly lower plasma PABA concentrations than normal dogs. (From Burrows, C. F.: The assessment of canine gastrointestinal function: recent advances and future needs. Proceedings 31st Gaines Veterinary Symposium, 1981.)

Oral administration of ^{131}I-labeled oleic acid is similar to the test as described for triolein, substituting ^{131}I oleic acid. Normal values are 10 to 15 per cent absorption in 10 hours.

Performance of the ^{131}I triolein and oleic acid tests in sequence aids in differentiating steatorrhea. In steatorrhea associated with a lack of pancreatic lipase, absorption of oleic acid will be normal; however, absorption of triolein, which requires lipolysis, will be reduced. The absorption of both compounds is reduced in malabsorption syndrome. Absorption of oleic acid may also be reduced in long-standing cases of pancreatic insufficiency.

References and Additional Readings

Burrows, C. F.: The assessment of canine gastrointestinal function: recent advances and future needs. Proceedings of the 31st Gaines Veterinary Symposium, 1981.

Hayden, D. W., and van Kruinigen, H. J.: Control values for evaluating gastrointestinal function in the dog. J.A.A.H.A., *12*:31, 1976.

Lorenz, M. D.: Canine malabsorption syndromes. Compendium on Continuing Education, 2(11):885, 1980.

Strombeck, D. R.: Small Animal Gastroenterology. Davis, California, Stonegate Publishing Co., 1979.

PUNCTURE FLUIDS EXAMINATION

All serous cavities and tissue spaces of the body contain a small amount of fluid. Under normal circumstances, this consists of a low-protein blood filtrate. Abnormal amounts of fluids in body cavities are termed *effusions*. Aspirates of these fluids are studied in an attempt to classify the origin of these fluids as transudative (a noninflammatory accumulation of fluid associated with a physiochemical disturbance) or exudative (an accumulation of fluid associated with an inflammatory response). Not all body fluids can be strictly classified as transudates or exudates. Transudates that are long-standing can be transformed into modified transudates by the accumulation of inflammatory cells, chemotactic substances, and increased protein levels.

PHYSICAL EXAMINATION

1. Measure the volume of fluid removed.
2. Evaluate fluid for color and transparency.
   a. A pinkish to reddish color usually indicates the presence of erythrocytes.
   b. A yellowish color is imparted by excessive bilirubin, a high protein content, or degenerated erythrocytes.
   c. A milky white color may indicate chyle. If the cloudiness of the fluid is caused by the presence of chylomicrons, the fluid will clear upon adding ether and shaking.
   d. A thick, creamy fluid usually indicates the presence of a large number of leukocytes.
3. Note whether the fluid coagulates. The ability to clot is dependent on the amount of fibrin present. Exudates may show rapid coagulation, whereas transudates usually do not coagulate. Lysis of the clot may occur in exudates and may not be demonstrated.
4. Determine the specific gravity of the fluid. In general, the specific gravity is closely correlated with the protein content of the fluid. If a refractometer is used to measure specific gravity, a specific gravity of 1.020 is approximately equivalent to 3 gm per dl of protein with an additional 1 gm per dl of protein, increasing specific gravity 0.0004 units. Attempt to characterize the fluid as being a transudate, modified transudate, septic exudate, nonseptic exudate, chylous effusion, a neoplastic effusion, or hemorrhage.
5. Smell the fluid for odor. Puncture fluids are usually odorless unless contaminated by putrefying bacterial organisms such as *Escherichia coli* from the intestinal tract or urine from a ruptured bladder.

CHEMICAL EXAMINATION

Seromucin Test

This test can be used to help distinguish a transudate from an exudate. Exudates are usually seromucin positive and transudates are usually seromucin negative.

Total Proteins

Exudates usually have a high protein content (more than 3 gm/100 ml), whereas transudates usually have a lower total protein content.

Urea Nitrogen

Urea nitrogen determinations can be used in determining the presence of nitrogenous material within the abdominal cavity in such conditions as rupture of the bladder or in evaluating the efficiency of fluid that has been used in peritoneal dialysis.

A transudate is clear and has a specific gravity less than 1.017, a protein concentration of less than 2.5 gm per dl, and less than 500 cells per unit.

A modified transudate has been altered by protein and cells and often appears serosanguinous. Protein concentration is 2.5 gm per dl, with 1000 to 5000 cells of mixed population. Effusions associated with right heart failure or neoplasia are usually modified transudates.

Exudates may be nonseptic or septic. Septic exudates are usually more cellular and contain degenerating neutrophils, high protein levels, degenerating red blood cells, and infectious organisms.

MICROSCOPIC EXAMINATION

Total Cell Counts

The cell content of fluid, in regard to numbers and cell type, will depend on how the fluid within the body cavity accumulated. Pure transudates are usually acellular with small numbers of macrophages and lymphocytes coming from the blood. The accumulation of fluids in body cavities is usually associated with changes in mesothelial lining cells. Mesothelial cells exfoliate, become cuboidal, enlarge in size, and assume a strong basophilic staining cytoplasm.

The presence of large numbers of inflammatory cells and elevated protein content generally characterize an exudate. The presence of polymorphonuclear leukocytes and elevated protein levels in exudative fluid is not always indicative of a septic inflammation. If neutrophils exhibit degenerative morphologic changes (karyolysis, karyorrhexis, and pyknosis), the presence of microorganisms should be suspected.

The following cell types may also be found in pleural and peritoneal effusions:

1. *Macrophages* can be found in both acute and chronic effusions.
2. *Neutrophils* are nondegenerative in transudates, nonseptic exudates, and in septic exudates where the etiologic agent is of low toxicity. Neutrophils are degenerative in most severe septic infections.
3. Plasma cells indicate chronicity.
4. Giant cells indicate granulomatous inflammation.
5. Neoplastic cells.
6. Eosinophils, basophils, mast cells, and other cells that have exfoliated from body cavities may be present in exudates or modified exudates.

7. Traumatic or neoplastic rupture of major lymphatic ducts can result in the accumulation of chyle in the pleural or peritoneal cavity. Chyle usually has a milky appearance when removed. Microscopically, chyle contains large numbers of lymphocytes, chylomicrons, and red blood cells.

8. Diagnosis in chronic pleuritis, pleural effusion, and pneumonias can be aided by the thoracentesis (see p. 523) and fine needle aspiration biopsy of the lung. The presence of a bloody exudative fluid with yellow flecks or granules may be indicative of Nocardia or actinomycotic infection. The granules should be crushed on a microscope slide and examined, as well as the fluid cultured. In actinomycotic infections, the granules contain gram-positive branching filamentous rods and *Actinomyces viscosus* is the most common organism isolated from the thoracic cavity of dogs. If a modified acid-fast staining technique is used, *Nocardia* will stain acid-fast and *Actinomyces* will not stain.

Differential Smear

Large numbers of neutrophils indicate a purulent exudate, and one should look for a causative organism. Lymphocytes indicate a chronic exudative or viral reaction. Very young, bizarrely shaped lymphocytes may indicate tumor formation. If an allergy or parasitic problem is causing the formation of an exudate, eosinophils may be found. If a tumor is suspected, examination of cells by a competent cytologist may prove very helpful in making a diagnosis. Smears should be fixed while still wet with a commercial fixative such as Spraycyte (Clay Adams Co.). These smears can be stained by the method of Papanicolaou or Sano and then examined. Veterinary schools and hospitals have pathologists trained in the field of exfoliative cytology.

BACTERIOLOGIC EXAMINATION

Bacteriologic examination involves the following procedures:
1. Prepare new methylene blue or Gram stain of aspirated material.
2. Culture (see p. 499).
3. Animal inoculations may be indicated.

References and Additional Readings

Hardie, E. M., and Barsanti, J. A.: Treatment of canine actinomycosis. J.A.V.M.A., *180*(5):537, 1982.

Perman, V., Osborne, C. A., and Stevens, J. B.: Laboratory evaluation of abnormal body fluids. Vet. Clin. North Am., *4*:255, 1974.

Prasse, K. W., and Duncan, J. R.: Laboratory diagnosis and pleural and pericardial effusions. Vet. Clin. North Am., *6*:625, 1976.

Rebar, A. H.: Diagnostic cytology in veterinary practice. *In* Kirk, R. W. (ed.): Current Veterinary Therapy VII. Philadelphia, W. B. Saunders Company, 1980, pp. 16–27.

Stevens, J. B., Perman, V., and Osborne, C. A.: Biopsy sample management, staining, and examination. Vet. Clin. North Am., *4*:233, 1974.

SYNOVIAL FLUID

Synovial fluid is a protein dialysate of plasma that contains mucin produced by the synovial cells.

Synovial fluid can be obtained by arthrocentesis (the aseptic aspiration of a joint cavity).

Examination of Synovial Fluid

1. The physical characteristics should be noted including color, turbidity, viscosity, clot formation, and quantity. Normal synovial fluid does not clot but forms a gel that returns to a liquid following shaking. Clotting of synovial fluid is abnormal and is associated with abnormal vascular permeability or degeneration of synovial membrane.
2. A determination of the total cell count and a differential count should be performed. Collect synovial fluid in a EDTA-containing vial to prevent clotting.
3. A total protein estimation should be made.
4. A mucin clot test can be performed (Duncan and Prasse, 1977). A poor mucin clot may indicate a septic arthritis producing bacterial enzymes or excessive effusions into the joint. (Table 146.)
5. Bacteriologic examination, including culture, should be performed. Cell counts made in dogs with aspirates from the carpal, elbow, shoulder, hip, stifle, and hock joints showed that from 0 to 2900 cells, with a mean of 430 cells per cu mm, could be found. The anticoagulant to be used with synovial fluid is EDTA.

The cell count of normal synovial fluid should contain less than 10 per cent polymorphonuclear leukocytes (polymorphs). The following mean per cent values have been reported for the dog: monocytes, 39.72; lymphocytes, 44.16; clasmatocytes, 4.20; and polymorphs, 1.38.

In traumatic osteoarthritis, clasmatocytes increased in number.

In traumatic or degenerated joint lesions, there may be an increase in the nonmucin protein content of the joint fluid because of the degeneration or change in permeability of blood vessels. Mucin concentration is usually decreased in infectious arthritis but stays normal in traumatic or degenerative joint lesions.

Polyarthritis associated with systemic lupus has been described in the dog and lupus erythematosis (LE) cells have been located in the synovial fluid.

When joint effusions of unknown etiology are present, it can be advantageous to obtain a synovial membrane biopsy.

Normal joint fluid should be sterile when cultured (see p. 499).

References and Additional Readings

Duncan, R. J., and Prasse, K. W.: Veterinary Laboratory Medicine. Ames, Iowa, Iowa State University Press, 1977.

Table 146. SYNOVIAL FLUID ABNORMALITIES ASSOCIATED WITH VARIOUS CAUSES OF ARTHRITIS

Classification	Turbidity	Color	Volume	Factor Mucin Clot	Fibrin Clot	Total WBC	Cytology
Degenerative joint disease	Nonturbid	Clear to pink	Normal; increased in acute disease	Good	Absent	Normal to mild elevation early	Normal to slight increase in mononuclear cells.
Nonseptic arthritis	Often turbid	Pink	Normal to increased	Good to poor	Present	Mild to marked elevation	Neutrophilia; sometimes LE cells or ragocytes
Septic arthritis	Turbid	Pink	Increased	Poor to very poor	Present	Marked elevation	Neutrophilia; sometimes bacteria

From Miller, J. B., Perman, V., Osborne, C. A., et al.: Synovial fluid analysis in canine arthritis. J.A.A.H.A., *10*:392, 1974.

Fernandez, F. R., Grindem, C. B., Lipowitz, A. N., and Perman, V.: Synovial fluid analysis: preparation of smears for cytologic examination of canine synovial fluid. J.A.A.H.A., *19*(5):727, 1983.

Perman, V.: Synovial fluid. *In* Kaneko, J.: Clinical Biochemistry of Domestic Animals, 3rd ed. New York, Academic Press, Inc., 1980, pp. 749–783.

Perman, V., Alsaker, R. D., and Riis, R.: Cytology of the Dog and Cat. South Bend, Indiana, Am. Anim. Hosp. Assoc., 1979.

Rebar, A. H.: Handbook of Veterinary Cytology. St. Louis, Missouri, Ralston Purina Company, 1978.

URINALYSIS

PHYSICAL EXAMINATION

Collection (See also p. 545).

Use a clean, transparent container. Do not collect the first part of the urine stream, but then collect 2 or 3 ounces of an early morning sample. This first part is not likely to be concentrated and/or to contain constituents of diagnostic significance. Samples can be collected by catheterization (see pp. 545–549) or cystocentesis (see p. 549).

A fresh sample is desirable; thus, it should be presented promptly for laboratory evaluation (especially culture) or refrigerated for adequate preservation for several hours.

Short-term preservation of casts and cellular elements can be made effective by acidification of the urine. If urine is alkaline, add 0.1 ml of normal hydrochloric acid a drop at a time until the pH is on the acid side. To prevent microbial growth in a urine sample, add one drop of 40 per cent formalin per 30 ml of urine, or thymol, 5 to 10 ml.

Volume

Normal urine volume is variable and dependent on diet, fluid intake, environmental factors, body size and weight, and exercise. A normal dog will produce 12 to 20 ml of urine per kg per 24 hours (see p. 592).

Color and Appearance

Normal urine is usually yellow to amber in color (due to urochrome pigments) and is clear.

A very pale yellow colorless urine indicates a very dilute urine such as may occur in diabetes insipidus, chronic interstitial nephritis, hyperadrenocorticism, pyometra, or excessive fluid intake.

A dark yellow to orange urine usually indicates a concentrated urine such as occurs in dehydration, fever, or reduced fluid intake.

A cloudy appearing urine usually indicates crystalluria or the presence of a high cell content as may occur with an infection of the urinary tract.

An orange urine may indicate excessive amounts of urobilinogen or the presence of the metabolic end products of agents such as Azo gantrisin.

A red urine may indicate hemorrhage, food pigments, or the presence of dyes such as phenolsulphonphthalein.

Greenish urine may indicate increased levels of bilirubin. Greenish blue urine can be produced by such drugs as dithiazanine iodide and methylene blue.

Transparency

Urine is usually clear upon being voided. Highly concentrated urine or urine with a high crystal or cell count may be cloudy. If the urine is allowed to stand after being collected, precipitates of crystals form and the urine becomes cloudy. The cause of urine turbidity is best evaluated by sediment examination.

Reaction (pH)

The pH of the urine usually depends on the diet and metabolism of the animal. The kidneys can adjust the pH of the urine between 4.5 and 8.5. The urine pH of dogs and cats usually lies between 5.5 and 7.0.

If the urine is retained in the bladder for greater than 24 hours or if urinalysis is obtained within 8 hours after eating, the urinary pH will be greater than 7.0. Urine pH is most significant if the animal is fasted for 8 to 14 hours prior to sampling and the pH is recorded immediately after the sample has been obtained.

Increased acidity of the urine can be produced by an all-meat diet, fever, metabolic and respiratory acidosis, diabetic ketoacidosis, primary renal failure, severe diarrhea, severe vomiting, starvation, prolonged vigorous exercise, or the administration of acidifying drugs such as ammonium chloride, ascorbic acid, or DL-methionine.

An alkaline urine can be produced by urinary retention, cystitis (especially those infections caused by *Proteus* that split urea to form ammonia), metabolic and respiratory alkalosis, vomiting, or renal tubular acidosis (see p. 602) or by treatment with drugs such as sodium bicarbonate, sodium lactate, potassium citrate, acetazolamide, and chlorothiazide.

ODOR

Abnormal urine odors are significant only in freshly voided specimens. An odor of ammonia (NH_3) is the most common abnormal odor of urine; it can occur if urea has been degraded by urea-splitting bacteria, as may occur in cystitis, or in states of metabolic acidosis. NH_4^+ (no smell) is degraded to NH_3 (odor) by heat. A putrid odor to the urine indicates degradation of large quantities of protein. Ketonuria may impart a fruity odor to the urine.

Specific Gravity (See also p. 236)

Urine specific gravity is the ratio of the weight of a volume of urine compared with the weight of an equal volume of water at a specified temperature. The specific gravity of urine will vary depending on the proportion of each respective solute and the type of solute present.

Urine specific gravity may range from 1.001 to 1.065 in normal dogs and from 1.001 to 1.080 in normal cats. The range of 1.015 to 1.045 is more commonly found in dogs and 1.035 to 1.060 is most often seen in cats. A urine specific gravity of 1.008 to 1.012 is often seen in normal animals. The concept that an average normal specific gravity may be 1.025 is misleading, because it may indicate that a specific gravity above or below this level is abnormal. In dogs, a urine specific gravity of greater than or equal to 1.025 is indicative of an adequate population of nephrons to prevent clinical signs of uremia. Renal disease may be present in dogs that are able to concentrate their urine to a specific gravity of 1.025. Cats with less than 25 per cent of functional nephrons can concentrate their urine to a specific gravity of greater than 1.025. Animals with an elevated BUN and a urine concentration of greater than 1.025 have either prerenal uremia or primary glomerular disease. In those with prerenal uremia, normal renal function should be re-established by restoring vascular volume and perfusion pressure. Animals with primary glomerular disease have a persistent proteinuria.

The kidneys have a very large reserve capacity. Impairment of concentrating ability of the kidney is not detectable until at least two thirds of the total population of nephrons are nonfunctional. The loss of the ability to concentrate and dilute urine may develop gradually. If dehydrated azotemic animals have impaired ability to concentrate urine, the animal has generalized renal disease in most situations. The renal dysfunction may be acute or chronic, reversible, partially reversible, or irreversible.

Random sample specific gravities are unreliable. Repeated tests are much more valuable, especially in animals with urine of low specific gravity. A lowered specific gravity may be associated with polyuria. It occurs in chronic interstitial nephritis, diabetes insipidus, pyometra, advanced uremia, adrenocorticohyperplasia, and pyelonephritis. It may be produced by excessive increase in fluid intake (polydipsia) or by the reabsorption of edema fluid.

Animals with a low urine specific gravity require a water deprivation test to determine whether they can concentrate their urine (see p. 236). However, dogs with urine specific gravity of 1.007 to 1.029 and cats with urine specific gravity of 1.007 to 1.034 associated with clinical dehydration or azotemia usually have primary renal disease.

No set time should be established for a water deprivation test. Animals should be examined and weighed several times during the test period. The test should be discontinued if: (1) the urine specific gravity is greater than 1.025; (2) the animal has lost 5 per cent of its body weight; or (3) the specific gravity remains below 1.025 but the concentration of BUN becomes abnormally elevated.

Following a water deprivation test, if a nonazotemic patient still has polyuria and specific gravity below 1.025, further tests are required (see p. 239).

An increased specific gravity can be seen in cystitis, acute nephritis (in the oliguric phase), diabetes mellitus, reduction in fluid intake, fever, and dehydration from any cause.

Osmolality

Osmolality is the measure of osmotic pressure of a fluid dependent on the number of particles of solute per unit volume of solvent. Urinary osmolality is independent of the kind of solute present, and renal concentrating ability is best assessed by osmolality. Osmolality is measured by determining the freezing point depression of a solution. Normal values for serum osmolality in the dog and cat are 280 to 310 mOsm per kg. Blood to be processed for osmolality determination should be collected in heparin, because EDTA, oxalate, and citrate alter osmolality determinations. Total osmolality of the serum can be calculated by determining the partial osmolal contribution of each solute. Sodium and its associated anionic components account for 93 per cent of normal serum osmolality. The following formula has been used in estimating serum osmolality:

$$1.86 \, (Na + K) \, \frac{Glu}{18} + \frac{BUN}{2.8}$$

The osmotic concentration of urine is variable, depending on the fluid and electrolyte balance of the body. In normally hydrated dogs and cats, urine osmolality is usually 500 to 1200 mOsm per kg. If an osmometer is not available, urine osmolality can be estimated by multiplying the last two digits of the specific gravity value by 36. Levels obtained are plus or minus 20 mOsm per kg compared with osmometry. The ratio of urine osmolality to plasma osmolality (U/P Osm) has been used as an index of renal function:

1. A U/P Osm ratio above 1 indicates that the kidneys are capable of concentrating urine above the concentration of plasma. If the animal is deprived of water for 24 hours, the normal canine U/P Osm ratio is 3 or higher.
2. A U/P Osm ratio of 1 indicates that water and solute are being excreted in a state that is iso-osmotic with plasma.
3. A U/P Osm ratio below 1 indicates that the kidneys are capable of absorbing solute in excess of water.

Chemical Examination of the Urine

Protein

Urinary proteins are derived from variable amounts of plasma proteins, proteins from the urinary tract, and proteins from the genital tract. Protein measurements should be made from the supernatant of centrifuged urinary samples. The major mechanisms of protein handling by the kidneys involve selective glomerular permeability, tubular resorption, and disposal of absorbed proteins. The passage of proteins through glomerular capillary walls is primarily related to the molecular size, weight, and shape of the proteins; electrical charge; and renal hemodynamics. Proteins larger than $MW = 68,000$ are not present in the normal glomerular filtrate. In lesions of renal nephrons, the greater the severity of the lesion, the greater the chance of loss of high molecular weight proteins. Filtered proteins are absorbed and degraded by tubular epithelial cells. This happens almost exclusively in the proximal tubules of the kidney, which can be saturated when increasing amounts of proteins cross the glomerulus, thus resulting in proteinuria.

Protein in the urine of normal animals cannot be demonstrated by normal qualitative methods. If the glomerular membrane is damaged or if bleeding occurs anywhere in the urogenital tract, protein may be found in the urine. Albumin is the first protein to leak through a damaged glomerular membrane, followed by fibrogen and alpha, beta, and gamma globulin.

Prerenal proteins should, by definition, arise from nonrenal sources, and may be found in hemoglobinuria, myoglobinuria, or multiple myeloma.

The development of proteinuria in primary renal disease can be explained by three mechanisms: (1) increased glomerular filtration of protein, (2) reduced tubular reabsorption of protein, and (3) addition of protein by renal tubules.

The presence of abnormal levels of protein in the urine can be classified as being prerenal, renal, or postrenal in origin:

1. Prerenal proteinuria
   a. Hemoglobinuria
   b. Myoglobinuria
   c. Bence Jones proteinuria (multiple myeloma)
2. Renal proteinuria
   a. Glomerular disease
   b. Tubular disease—increased secretion, decreased reabsorption, damage to tubules with leakage
   c. Renal parenchymal inflammation
3. Postrenal proteinuria
   a. Diseases of the lower urinary tract, specifically inflammatory disease, tumors, chronic irritation
   b. Genital diseases, specifically inflammatory disorders

Proteins may appear in the urine under certain physiologic conditions, such as excessive muscular activity, convulsions, consumption of a large amount of protein in the diet, or emotional and physical stress.

Trace and 1+ results are commonly observed with colorimetric dipstick tests in concentrated urine samples obtained from normal dogs and cats. Elevation of proteins in the urine generally refers to increased levels of plasma proteins, specifically albumins. Persistent proteinuria in the absence of hematuria and pyuria generally indicates glomerular disease. The specific gravity of the urine is important in determining the significance of protein levels in the urine, with mild proteinuria in a urine specific gravity of 1.005 implying a greater loss of protein than mild proteinuria in a more concentrated sample of 1.040.

The magnitude of proteinuria is correlated more with the nature of the glomerular lesion than with the stage of renal disease. Amyloidosis of the kidneys results in the greatest amount of protein being lost. Twenty-four hour urinary excretion of less than 400 mg per day is considered normal. Normal dogs may excrete 13.9 plus or minus 7.71 mg per kg per day of protein in the urine.

Extraurinary causes of proteinuria include metastatic neoplastic disease, altered circulation associated with embolic phenomena, and increased abdominal pressure with resultant altered blood flow to kidneys. Nonrenal causes of increased urinary proteins can include inflammation of the lower urinary tract, hematuria, or contamination of the urine from genital tract infection; prostatitis in males; and chronic passive congestion of the kidneys associated with cardiac insufficiency, dirofilaria infections, liver disease, neoplasms, and emboli.

Elevated amounts of protein in the urine can be found in kidney diseases such as nephritis, amyloidosis, pyelonephritis, and glomerular disease.

Urinary proteinuria of nonrenal origin is usually associated with hemorrhagic or inflammatory lesions of the ureters, urinary bladder, and/or urethra. Contamination of urine with inflammatory exudate or blood can cause proteinuria.

Bence Jones proteins are light-chain immunoglobulins that are present in the urine. Both kappa and lambda (22,000 MW and 44,000 MW) can pass through glomerular capillary walls. They are commonly associated with multiple myeloma; however, they have been associated with other immunologic disorders such as macroglobulinemia and leukemia complex.

There are numerous clinical methods available for measurement of urinary proteins; however, the "dipstick" tests are used most frequently. In comparing the developed color on the dipstick after placing it in the urine, the following interpretation can be made:

$$
\begin{aligned}
\text{trace protein} &= 20 \text{ mg/dl} \\
1+ \text{ protein} &= 30 \text{ mg/dl} \\
2+ \text{ protein} &= 100 \text{ mg/dl} \\
3+ \text{ protein} &= 300 \text{ mg/dl} \\
4+ \text{ protein} &= \geq 1000 \text{ mg/dl}
\end{aligned}
$$

Proteinuria should always be interpreted in conjunction with specific gravity.

Glucose

Normal urine does not contain glucose; the glucose that has been filtered at the glomerular membrane has been reabsorbed in the proximal convoluted tubules. If the glucose level in the blood exceeds 175 mg per 100 ml of blood, glucose will appear in the urine. A few normal dogs have a low renal threshold for glucose and may produce urine that constantly contains small amounts of glucose.

Elevated levels of glucose in the urine (fasted sample) may be present in the following:

1. Emotional glycosuria induced by fear, excitement, or violent exercise in which the level of epinephrine is increased and glucocorticosteroids are mobilized .

2. General anesthesia, which promotes a rapid release of glucose from storage compartments in the liver.

3. Diabetes mellitus.

4. Hyperthyroidism—because of the rapid uptake of glucose from the gastrointestinal tract.

5. Acute pancreatic necrosis.

6. Hyperpituitarism.

7. Overactivity of the adrenal cortex.

8. Nephritis due to damage of the resorptive capabilities of the proximal convoluted tubules.

9. Primary renal glycosuria caused by a renal tubular enzymatic defect.

10. Animals given drugs such as glucocorticosteroids or glucose solutions, or those ingesting excessive amounts of carbohydrates in the diet.

The administration of certain drugs will produce a false-positive reaction for glycosuria when tested by a method depending on the reduction of copper. Some of these are antibiotics such as streptomycin, Aureomycin, Terramycin, Chloromycetin, penicillin; and chemicals such as lactose, pentose, ascorbic acid, morphine, salicylates, chloral hydrate, and formaldehyde.

There are several methods of measuring sugar in the urine. Most of these tests are based on colorimetric determinations proportional to the amount of glucose in the urine as measured by enzymatic tests. The type of test (enzymatic) should be known, its limitations should be understood, and it should be determined whether refrigerated urine samples should be brought to room temperature before testing. Important points to keep in mind regarding these tests are:

1. Clinitest reagent tablets are used for obtaining a semiquantitative estimation of sugar in the urine. Reducing substances other than glucose may give a positive reaction. This system is based on copper reduction methods and color changes associated with reduction of cupric ions (blue) to cuprous oxide (orange-red). The color change is dependent on the concentration of reducing compounds, including glucose in the urine.

2. Clinistix* reagent strips and Tes-Tape* are colorimetric strip tests for glycosuria. False negatives can be obtained, especially in detecting high and low glucose concentrations. These tests involve the reaction of urine with the enzyme glucose oxidase. It is important that the urine sample be at *room temperature* when performing analysis using a glucose oxidase test.

A negative glucose oxidase test and a negative copper reduction test indicate the absence of significant quantities of glucose in urine.

A positive glucose oxidase test and a negative copper reduction test indicate less than 250 mg per dl of glucose in the urine, or false-positive glucose oxidase reaction.

A positive glucose oxidase test and a positive copper reduction test indicate glucosuria in excess of 250 mg per dl.

A negative glucose oxidase test and a positive copper reduction test indicate nonglucose-reducing substances in the urine (Fig. 101).

*Ames Division, Miles Laboratories, Elkhart, Indiana.

ALGORITHM for GLUCOSURIA

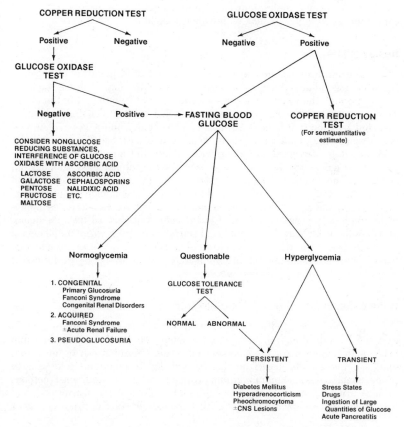

Figure 101. Algorithm for localization of glucosuria. (Reprinted with permission from Osborne, C.A., Stevens, J. B., et al. Clinical significance of glucosuria. Minn. Vet. 20, 1980.)

Ketone Bodies

The ketone bodies are acetone, acetoacetic acid, and betahydroxybutyric acid. Most commercial tests are based on the reaction of acetoacetic acid and acetone with nitroprusside in an alkaline environment and do not measure betahydroxybutyric acid. The intensity of color is proportional to the quantity of ketones present: + = 5 to 40 mg per dl; + + = 40 to 100 mg per dl; and + + + = more than 100 mg per dl. If these substances increase, ketosis is present. Any decrease in carbohydrate utilization results in increased fatty acid oxidation and increased ketone formation. Conditions such as starvation, diabetes mellitus, pyrexia; low-carbohydrate (high-fat) diets, impaired liver function, prolonged vomiting and diarrhea, and hypoglycemic syndromes can produce ketonuria. Young animals tend to develop ketonuria with starvation more rapidly than do older animals. Ketone bodies have a diuretic action and contribute to the polyuria seen with diabetes mellitus.

Hemoglobin

When intravascular hemolysis occurs, the released hemoglobin becomes bound to a globulin and haptoglobin, forming a stable complex that is too large to pass through the renal glomerulus and, therefore, is not found in the urine. This complex is removed by reticuloendothelial cells. When haptoglobin is depleted by excessive hemolysis, uncompleted hemoglobin can circulate and pass through the glomerulus, where some of it is absorbed by renal tubular cells and it is converted to hemosiderin. When the amount of hemoglobin produced exceeds the reabsorptive capacity of the tubular cells, hemoglobin and methemoglobin are found in the urine. In the renal processing of hemoglobin, the excretion of hemosiderin alone (slight hemolysis) can occur, hemosiderin and hemoglobin (chronic marked hemolysis) can occur, or hemoglobin only (acute marked hemolysis) can occur. Commercial tests for hemoglobin in the urine may detect red blood cells (RBCs) and myoglobin. Chemical tests are based on the pseudoperoxidase activity of the heme fraction of hemoglobin. A urinary sediment examination should always be performed if tests for occult urinary blood are positive.

Urine Bilirubin (See also p. 736 in Edition III of this handbook)

Only the conjugated form of bilirubin can be present in the urine. To examine for bilirubin, the urine sample should be fresh, because bilirubin oxidizes to intermediary products and biliverdin. Bilirubin can be measured with icto test tablets, based on the diazotization reaction and color change proportional to the amount of bilirubin present in the urine. Additional methods for measuring bilirubin are the Ames Reagent sticks* and Chemstrips 6, 7, and 8.† Drugs, such as phenazopyridine, that change the color of urine may alter

---

*Ames Division, Miles Laboratories, Elkhart, Indiana.
†Bio-Dynamics, Indianapolis, Indiana.

the reading of these tests by causing an artificial color reaction. The sensitivity of tests for detecting bilirubinuria depend on the test and the manufacturer, but, in general, it ranges from 0.1 to 0.4 mg per dl. The presence of bilirubin in the urine usually precedes the formation of bilirubinemia.

Urobilinogen

Tests for urobilinogen must be performed on fresh urine samples, because the oxidation of urobilinogen produces urobilin, which turns the urine brown. Urobilinogen is formed by the action of bacteria in the intestinal tract on bilirubin. Some of the urobilinogen is excreted in the feces, and some is reabsorbed and returned to the liver by the portal circulation, where it is excreted into the bile. However, some of the reabsorbed urobilinogen is circulated to the kidneys and excreted in the urine. Urobilinogen in dilutions of 1:32 to 1:64 may normally be found in canine and feline urine.

Decreased amounts of urobilinogen are usually found in obstructive jaundice; disease of the intestinal tract, which impairs absorption; overtreatment with oral antibiotics, which change the normal intestinal bacterial flora; or chronic interstitial nephritis, resulting in a polyuria with a low specific gravity and dilution of the urine.

Increased amounts of urobilinogen can be found in hepatitis, cirrhosis of the liver, or hemolytic jaundice. Screening tests for urobilinogen in the urine of dogs and cats is probably unreliable, and results should be interpreted in light of other clinical and clinicopathologic findings.

Substances that interfere with the test for urobilinogen are indole, bile and nitrates, sulfonamides, procaine, and formalin. Phenazopyridine produces a red color in the reagent pad.

The daily excretion of selected electrolytes in the urine is determined by measuring the concentration of pooled electrolytes in 24-hour urine samples and multiplying the concentration by the 24-hour volume. The fractional clearance of an electrolyte in the urine has been reported as its calculated clearance divided by the clearance of creatinine.

Chlorides

Urine chloride content varies greatly with diet, acid-base balance, water balance, endocrine function, and the amounts of other electrolytes present within the body. Only 24-hour urine collections are of value in determining urine chlorides. Urine chloride values are of real significance only in a complete study of acid-base balance.

Decreased urine chloride values can be seen in animals given salt-free diets, in fasting animals, and in those with symptoms of excessive vomiting and diarrhea, congestive heart failure, or ascites.

Increased urine chlorides can be seen in animals with increased salt intake, Addison's disease (where low mineralocorticoid levels lead to an inability to conserve salt), and in some forms of diuretic therapy.

Calcium

Twenty-four hour urine samples are needed for calcium determinations. Repeated urinary calcium determinations are usually needed to interpret the results adequately.

Decreased urinary calcium levels can be seen in animals with canine puerperal tetany or in hypoparathyroidism.

Increased urinary calcium levels may be present in animals with nutritional secondary hyperparathyroidism, hypervitaminosis D, or hyperthyroidism or in those given calcium-containing solutions.

Blood

Hematuria, or the presence of blood in the urine, may be associated with metabolic, infectious, toxic, neoplastic, or traumatic disorders. Free hemoglobin in urine is associated with hemolytic disease. Myoglobin reacts with most tests for hemoglobin and is present because of muscle injury that can be associated with trauma, abnormal metabolism, or toxic or altered circulation.

Hematuria can be found in conditions such as nephritis, urolithiasis, cystitis, cystic calculi, prostatitis, pyelonephritis, neoplasms of the kidney, prostate or bladder, during estrus in females, and in thrombocytopenia.

Hemoglobinuria may be produced in babesiasis, hemolytic disease of the newborn, autoimmune hemolytic anemia (AIHA), incompatible blood transfusions, severe burns, chemical toxins, and numerous plant poisonings.

Confirmation of a positive occult blood test for hematuria depends on sediment examination of the urine. RBCs may be crenated or distorted in concentrated urine samples and may be lysed in dilute urine samples. They appear as faint shadows, called *ghost cells*.

Microscopic Examination of the Urine

Normal urine contains very little sediment. Centrifuge 10 ml of the fresh urine sample (at 1500 RPM for 5 min) to concentrate the sediment. Examine and note the amount, color, and consistency of the sediment. A red sediment indicates the presence of erythrocytes, a white sediment indicates the presence of crystals or cellular debris, and a yellow tinge may indicate bile pigments. Resuspend and stain the urine sediment (new methylene blue or Sternheimer-Malbin stain) for further examination, if necessary. Interpret sediment findings in light of the urine specific gravity. It is also important to note whether catheterization was used to obtain the sample or whether it is a "catch" sample. The number of RBCs and white blood cells (WBCs) are counted in ten microscopic fields and reported as average number per high-power microscopic field. Casts are reported as average number per low-power field. Bacterial, urinary crystals, and sperm are reported as few, frequent, or many.

Organized Sediment

Epithelial Cells

All urine contains a few epithelial cells. Renal tubular epithelial cells are small and round, with granular cytoplasm. The presence of accumulated numbers of these cells in casts is indicative of renal disease. Transitional epithelial cells vary in size and shape, being spindle, caudate, or polygonal. They originate from the renal pelvis, ureters, urinary bladder, and urethra and are increased in cystitis, pyelonephritis, calcium formation, ureteritis, prostatitis, and urethritis. The number may be increased because of catheterization procedures. Large squamous cells come from the urethral or vaginal epithelium. These cells may be increased in vaginitis. Squamous epithelial cells, which are thin with irregular borders and a small dense nucleus, are largest of the cells in normal urine. They may be either single or in sheets. Tumors of the bladder may exfoliate tumor cells into the urine. Cells in urine accumulating from transitional cell carcinomas are usually large, occur in groups, and may have large vacuoles in the cytoplasm. Characteristics of abnormalities of malignant cells are described on p. 526).

Erythrocytes (Hematuria)

Erythrocytes usually appear as pale, light-refractive discs. Crenation of erythrocytes occurs in concentrated urine, and swelling, in dilute urine. Erythrocytes may appear in the urine because of inflammation, necrosis, trauma, shock, infarction, congestion, calculi formation, clotting defects, parasites, and poisons such as mercury, arsenic, or thallium. See gross hematuria (p. 286).

Leukocytes (Pyuria)

The appearance of WBCs in the urine is dependent on specific gravity, pH, the volume of urine in which they are found, and the ability to distinguish the cells from nonsquamous epithelial cells of the kidney, which may be difficult. In fresh urine samples, WBCs are one and a half times larger than RBCs. The nucleus of the cells have often degenerated. Less than 5 WBCs per high-power field is normal.

Increased numbers of leukocytes usually indicate an inflammatory process within the genitourinary tract. Such conditions as cystitis, urethritis, pyelonephritis, nephritis, prostatitis, vaginitis, metritis, or balantitis may produce pyuria. The presence of numbers of bacteria in addition to WBCs is usually significant, indicating primary or secondary bacterial infection. If the origin of leukocytes cannot be determined after examining the sediment from a "catch" sample of urine, a sample should be obtained by catheterization or cystocentesis (see p. 545).

Bacteria

Normal, freshly voided urine should be sterile. Urine that is not fresh or that has been contaminated during collection will contain bacteria. Bacteriuria is significant only if the urine sample was taken aseptically (see p. 549). Infections of the urinary or genital tract may produce large numbers of bacteria together with erythrocytes and leukocytes. Quantitative urine culture is advantageous in determining whether active urinary tract infection is present. A count of greater than 100,000 bacteria per ml of freshly collected and cultured urine is significant. Stain urine sediment containing bacteria by Gram's method and culture the sediment (see p. 501).

Parasites

The eggs of *Diocytophyma renale* (dog and mink) and *Capillaria plica* (dog, cat, and fox) may be found in the urine. The urine sample also may be contaminated by feces containing parasite ova.

Spermatozoa

Spermatozoa may be frequently seen in the urine of male dogs but has no clinical significance.

Casts

Urinary casts are cylindrical-shaped structures similar to renal tubular lumens. The matrix of the casts is primarily composed of Tamm-Horsfall (T-H) mucoproteins that are locally secreted by epithelial cells that line the loops of Henle, the distal tubules, and the collecting ducts. Casts are most frequently seen in concentrated, acidic urine. The detection of significant numbers of casts in urine sediment indicates tubular involvement in an active pathologic process; however, casts should not be interpreted as an index of renal function. Material present within the lumen of renal tubules at the time T-H mucoprotein gels are deposited will become entrapped within the tubules; therefore, casts are commonly classified on the basis of morphologic appearance.

The presence of casts in urinary sediment indicates pathology of the renal tubules; however, the number of casts is not a good index of the severity, duration, or reversibility or irreversibility of the disease process.

When examining urinary sediment, it is important to centrifuge the specimen at no greater than 1500 to 2000 RPMs for 5 minutes.

Different types of casts will have different clinical significance:

1. Hyaline casts are primarily composed of T-H mucoproteins and are commonly seen in association with proteinuria. Hyaline casts are usually colorless, homogeneous, and semitransparent in unstained sediment. A few hyaline casts may be found in normal sediment, but increased numbers are usually indicative of renal irritation.

2. Granular casts are a form of hyaline casts, which contain granules consisting of degenerating tubular epithelial cells. These casts indicate a degeneration of tubular cells and are usually indicative of nephritis.

3. Epithelial, fatty, granular, and waxy casts represent different stages of degeneration of epithelial cells in casts. The degenerating epithelial cells are attached to a hyaline matrix. Epithelial, granular, and waxy casts are usually associated with diseases that cause degeneration and necrosis of tubular epithelial cells.

4. Waxy casts indicate severe kidney damage, usually acute nephritis, renal degeneration, or amyloidosis; the finding of these casts indicates an unfavorable prognosis.
5. Fatty casts will stain orange or red with Sudan III stain. These casts are produced in degenerative diseases of the kidneys, with the deposition of lipid material in the tubules.
6. Blood casts indicate glomerulonephritis or hemorrhage within the nephron of the kidney.
7. Leukocyte casts indicate inflammation within the kidney tubules (as an acute nephritis).

Mucus

Mucus threads within the urine indicate irritation of the genitourinary tract. Mucus is produced by genital secretions and is a normal occurrence.

Unorganized Urinary Sediment

From 0.4 to 2.8 per cent of all dogs develop urolithiasis. The age of greatest incidence is 2 to 10 years. In 95 per cent of the cases, the uroliths occur in the bladder or urethra.

The presence and amount of crystals in the urine are dependent on the concentration and pH of the urine (Table 147). Chemical analysis of the crystals is important, because many of them have a mixed composition.

Acid urine may contain amorphous urates (more so in Dalmatians), uric acid, and calcium oxalate crystals. Triple phosphate crystals may be found in slightly alkaline urine.

Alkaline urine may contain triple and amorphous phosphate crystals. Urate uroliths in dogs are ammonium urate. Most affected male Dalmations have

Table 147. GUESSTIMATION OF UROLITH TYPE

	Struvite	**Oxalate**	**Urate**	**Cystine**[b]
All breeds (%)[a]	70–80	3–15	3–15	1–15
Basset, bulldog, Chihuahua, Irish and Yorkshire terriers (%)	25	10	5	60
Dalmation (%)	25	0	75	0
Nephroliths (%)[c]	78	22	0	0
Radiographic density	+ + +	+ + +	−	+
Urine pH	Alkaline	Varies	Varies	Acid[d]
Urine crystals[e]	Phosphate	Oxalate	Urate	Cysteine

[a]Recurrence is generally the same type. More than 90 per cent are struvite in dogs that are 1 year old or younger.

[b]Occur only in males.

[c]Generally struvite if urine culture is + and oxalate if − in a sample obtained by cystocentesis.

[d]Alkaline if urinary tract infection is present and in urine produced within 12 hours after eating.

[e]Only helpful if uroliths are present.

urate uroliths, although almost one fourth have phosphate uroliths. Dalmatians excrete a high quantity of urate in the urine because of an abnormality in the hepatic enzyme uricase, necessary to convert urate to allantoin. In other breeds, abnormalities (usually cogenital portosystemic shunts) can result in urate accumulation and urate crystaluria.

Cystinuria is a metabolic disorder in male dachshunds, Labrador retrievers, Irish setters, Cairn terriers, cocker spaniels, boxers, poodles, Scottish terriers, corgis, and shelties. Cystine uroliths occur as a result of an inherited defect in renal tubular reabsorption of cystine and lysine. In dogs, it is a gender-linked disease and occurs only in males.

Silicate uroliths are not common and have been reported in several breeds of dogs; they occur most commonly in German shepherds.

Oxalate urolithiasis is prevalent in diseases that alter calcium oxalate excretion, including hypercalciuria and hyperparathyroidism, and when there is excessive vitamin D intake, osteolytic neoplasms, hypercalcitonism, and proximal renal tubular damage.

Crystals that may indicate the presence of a pathologic process include tyrosine (liver disease), ammonium urate (portacaval shunt), calcium oxalate (ethylene glycol toxicity), and cystine (congenital cystinuria) (Fig. 102).

Uroliths are polycrystalline concretions that contain greater than 95 per cent of inorganic crystalloids and less than 5 per cent of organic matrix. Uroliths may be present in the bladder and may be detected on palpation, or they may present in animals with bladder or urethral disease. Nephroliths are located in the renal pelvis, and 75 to 80 per cent are struvite, especially if urine cultures are positive; 20 per cent are oxalate with negative urine cultures.

Examination of uroliths may be very significant in the proper postoperative management of the animal with stone formation. All uroliths that are surgically removed should be washed and stored in a sterile container for analysis. The number, size, and shape of the stones should be recorded. The urolith should be cut in half with a knife, bone saw, or jeweler's saw, and the nucleus and cortex of the stone should be examined separately. Qualitative and quantitative analysis of stone content can be performed by a commercial laboratory; kits* are available for the qualitative identification of phosphates, ammonium, magnesium, calcium, cystine, oxalates, uric acid, and carbonates.

Uroliths that are composed of struvite (magnesium ammonium phosphate) may be dissolved on a dietary regimen of Stone diet (see p. 862). There are several factors responsible for struvite calculi, and the control (not just dietary management) of these factors is important (see p. 872):

1. Control bacterial urinary tract infection. The urine becomes supersaturated with magnesium ammonium phosphate and calcium phosphate when the urine is alkaline, resulting in urease (bacterial origin) breakdown of ammonia. *Staphylococci* and proteus bacterial organism are urease producers.
2. Measure pH of urine.
3. Culture urine and possibly calculi.

---

*Urolithiasis Laboratories, Box 25475, Houston, Texas, 77005.

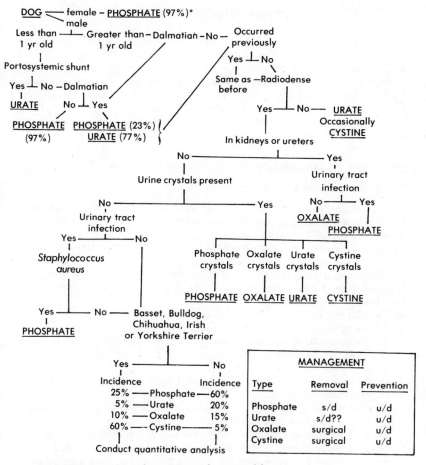

Figure 102. Diagnosis and management of canine uroliths.
*Indicates the percentage of cases due to this type of urolith. (From Lewis, L. D. and Morris, M. L.: *Small Animal Clinical Nutrition.* Mark Morris Assoc., Topeka, Kan., 1984.)

4. Control urinary tract infection with appropriate antibiotic treatment (see p. 920).

5. Administer urinary acidifiers (in phosphate uroliths), 200 mg per kg per day of ammonium chloride in the animal's food.

6. Increase urinary volume. Increase water consumption and frequency of voiding. Supplement the diet with sodium chloride, 0.5 to 1.0 g per day, provided that there is no medical contraindication to this.

7. Initiate treatment with low-protein, low-phosphorus magnesium, or Stone diet (s/d) (see p. 872).

RENAL FUNCTION TESTS

Precise and specific renal function tests are impractical for use in everyday veterinary practice. There are several tests that are useful in estimating renal function and in detecting kidney disease; however, even these do not provide a specific diagnosis—that depends on results of renal biopsy, urography, pyelography, or renal angiography. The tests that can be useful to the clinician for measuring renal function are urinalysis, urine specific gravity, plasma creatinine, creatinine clearance, 15-minute urine phenolsulfonphthalein excretion test, and the 60-minute plasma phenolsulfonphthalein test.

PRACTICAL MEASUREMENTS OF GLOMERULAR FUNCTION

Creatinine Clearance

Creatinine is an important part of the make-up of muscle, brain, and blood, where, in the form of creatinine phosphate, it functions as a high energy substance. Normally, small amounts of creatinine can be found in the urine. In cachectic states, starvation, febrile diseases, and muscular diseases (where there is muscle wasting) the urinary levels of creatinine may be elevated.

Finco and associates have described the following technique for glomerular filtration rate (GFR) measurement in the dog by the administration of a creatinine solution simultaneously:

1. Fast the dog for 8 hours, allowing free access to water.
2. Obtain the accurate weight of the dog to the nearest 0.1 kg.
3. A creatinine solution of 50 mg per ml is injected subcutaneously at a dose of 2.0 ml per kg for dogs weighing up to 20 kg (44 lb), and 1.5 ml per kg for larger dogs.
4. Pass a stomach tube, and give a volume of warm water equal to 3 per cent of body weight of the dog.
5. Catheterize the dog using aseptic technique. At 58 to 60 minutes post creatinine injection, remove all residual urine from the bladder, perform two bladder flushes with sterile saline (50 ml), and discard the flushes.
6. Obtain a blood sample at 60 minutes, and save it for creatinine analysis.
7. Save all urine produced between 60 and 80 minutes after administering creatinine. At 78 to 80 minutes, aspirate all urine, perform one bladder flush with 50 ml of saline, and save it with the saline.
8. Obtain a second blood sample at 80 minutes for creatinine value.
9. Record the volume of fluid collected between 60 and 80 minutes.

$$\frac{\text{creatinine}}{\text{clearance}} = \frac{\text{urine vol (ml)} \times \text{urine creatinine concentration (mg/ml)}}{\text{mean plasma creatinine concentration (mg/ml)}}$$

GFR ml/min/kg = creatinine clearance/20 min/weight of dog in kg

In the normal dog, creatinine is neither reabsorbed nor secreted, and creatinine clearance can be used to measure GFR. Commonly used tests overestimate serum creatinine levels because of measurement of noncreatinine chromagens and because of the falsely lower estimates for GFR.

Method for Performing Endogenous Creatinine Clearance Studies in Dogs

1. Catheterize and empty the urinary bladder. Rinse the bladder with several ml of sterile saline. Discard urine and saline.
2. Collect *all* urine produced during a timed period. If an extended collection period is used, either place the animal in a metabolism cage or frequently collect voluntarily voided urine.
3. At the midpoint of the timed urine collection, obtain a blood sample for determination of serum creatinine concentration (S_c).
4. At the end of the timed urine collection, catheterize and empty the bladder. Rinse the bladder with several ml of sterile saline. Urine *and* saline should be added to the urine that has already been collected. Record the total time elapsed during urine collection (T). The total urine volume produced (including the final saline rinse) should be measured (V). A well-mixed aliquot of urine should be submitted for determination of urine creatinine concentration (U_c).
5. Accurately determine the dog's body weight (BW).
6. Calculate clearance of creatinine (C_{cr}) using the following formula:

$$\text{creatinine clearance} = \frac{U_{cr} \times Y^\circ}{P_{cr} \times BW}$$

where;

U_{cr} = urinary creatinine/24 hr
P_{cr} = plasma creatinine mg/dl
Y° = urine flow in ml/min/24 hr or urine volume in 1440 min
BW = body weight in kg

Mean GFR in the dog is 2.98 ± 0.96 ml/min/kg and 3.7 ± 0.77 ml/min/kg.

PRACTICAL MEASUREMENTS OF TUBULAR FUNCTION

Urine Specific Gravity (See p. 814)
Phenolsulfonphthalein Urine Test (PSP)

Because this dye is about 85 per cent protein-bound, only a small amount is filtered by the glomeruli. The rest is excreted by the tubules and thus is used to estimate effectively tubular function in dogs. It also gives an estimate of renal plasma flow (not as accurately as para-amino hippurate (PAH) clearance, however), because 50 to 60 per cent of PSP is removed normally with the first pass through the kidneys. With a prolonged test period, even a severely damaged kidney may excrete normal amounts of dye. Thus, the amount excreted in the first 15 minutes is used as an indication of renal plasma flow. The total amount excreted over 1 hour may be helpful in evaluating tubular function (normally 50 to 60 per cent). Excretion of less than 25 per cent of the 6 mg test dose in 15 minutes is evidence of severe renal damage.

The method is carried out as follows: The patient must be well hydrated. The bladder is emptied, and the catheter is left in situ. Six mg of PSP is given intravenously (IV). All urine is collected for 15 minutes and measured for PSP (alkalinize with NaOH and use colorimeter). All urine is collected for 60 minutes and measured for PSP.

Sixty–Minute Plasma Phenolsulfonphthalein Concentration Test

PSP dye can also be used to evaluate renal function in this test. It is especially useful in the evaluation of function before evidence of extensive kidney disease is established by other diagnostic criteria, such as the BUN test or serum creatinine determination. This test is not specific for any particular renal function but is used to indicate tubular excretion and glomerular function.

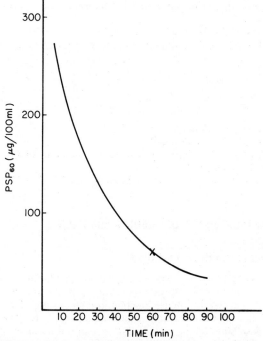

Figure 103. Typical plasma disappearance curve for PSP in the dog after IV injection of 1 mg PSP/kg of body weight. (From Kaufmann, C. F., and Kirk, R. W.: The 60-minute plasma phenolsulfonphthalein concentration as a test of renal function in the dog. J. Am. Anim. Hosp. Assoc., 9:67, 1973.)

A pretest heparinized blood sample of 4 ml is obtained, and then PSP dye, 1 mg per kg of body weight, is injected IV. A 4-ml heparinized blood sample is withdrawn exactly 60 minutes after injection.

The normal range of PSP_{60} is less than 80 μg per 100 ml for all dogs. A value of 120 or greater is indicative of functional problems, and values between 80 and 120 μg per 100 ml can indicate renal disease.

The total amount of PSP excreted by the kidney in a given period of time is dependent on how much PSP is delivered to the kidney by the circulation. The PSP_{60} is elevated in cases of renal tubular dysfunction, glomerular disease, or conditions that affect renal plasma flow (Fig. 103).

References and Additional Readings

Benjamin, M.: Outlines of Veterinary Clinical Pathology, 3rd ed. Ames, Iowa, Iowa State University Press, 1979.

Bovée, K. C., and Joyce, T.: Clinical evaluation of glomerular function: 24-hour creatinine clearance in dogs. J.A.V.M.A., *174*:448, 1979.

DiBartola, S. P., Chew, D. J., and Jacobs, G.: Quantitative urinalysis including 24-hour protein excretion in the dog. J.A.A.H.A., *16*(4):537, 1980.

DiBartola, S. P., and Chew, D. J.: Canine urolithiasis. Compendium on Continuing Education, *3*(3):226, 1981.

Finco, D. R., Coulter, D. B., and Barsanti, J. A.: Procedure for a simple method of measuring glomerular filtration rate in the dog. J.A.A.H.A., *18*(5):804, 1982.

Graver, G. F., and Allen, T. A.: Chronic renal failure in the dog. Compendium on Continuing Education, *3*(11):1009, 1981.

Green, R. A.: Perspectives in clinical osmometry. Vet. Clin. North Am., *8*:287, 1978.

Kaufman, C. F., and Kirk, R. W.: The sixty-minute plasma phenolsulfonphthalein concentration as a test of renal function in the dog. J.A.A.H.A., *9*:66, 1973.

Lewis, L. D., and Morris, M. M., Jr.: Small Animal Clinical Nutrition. Topeka, Kansas. Mark Morris Associates, 1983.

Mulnix, J. A., Rijnberk, A. D., and Hendriks, H. J.: Evaluation of a modified water deprivation test for diagnosis of polyuric disorders in dogs. J.A.V.M.A., *169*:1327, 1976.

Osborne, C. A., et al.: Clinical significance of glucosuria. Minn. Vet., *20*:16, 1980.

Osborne, C. A., and Stevens, J. B.: Handbook of Canine and Feline Urinalysis. St. Louis, Missouri, Ralston Purina Company, 1981.

Osborne, C. A., et al.: Medical dissolution of canine struvite uroliths. Minn. Vet., *22*(2):14, 1982.

Osborne, C. A., and Polzin, D. J.: Azotemia: a review on what's old and what's new. Part 1. Compendium on Continuing Education, *5*(6):497, 1983.

Stevens, J. B., and Osborne, C. A.: Urinalysis: indications, methodology, and interpretation. Proc. A.A.H.A., *10*:359, 1974.

Charts
and
Tables

TABLES OF WEIGHTS AND MEASURES
(See end sheets)

Table 148. CONVERSION TABLE OF WEIGHT TO BODY SURFACE AREA IN METERS FOR DOGS*

Kg	M²	Kg	M²
0.5	0.06	26.0	0.88
1.0	0.10	27.0	0.90
2.0	0.15	28.0	0.92
3.0	0.20	29.0	0.94
4.0	0.25	30.0	0.96
5.0	0.29	31.0	0.99
6.0	0.33	32.0	1.01
7.0	0.36	33.0	1.03
8.0	0.40	34.0	1.05
9.0	0.43	35.0	1.07
10.0	0.46	36.0	1.09
11.0	0.49	37.0	1.11
12.0	0.52	38.0	1.13
13.0	0.55	39.0	1.15
14.0	0.58	40.0	1.17
15.0	0.60	41.0	1.19
16.0	0.63	42.0	1.21
17.0	0.66	43.0	1.23
18.0	0.69	44.0	1.25
19.0	0.71	45.0	1.26
20.0	0.74	46.0	1.28
21.0	0.76	47.0	1.30
22.0	0.78	48.0	1.32
23.0	0.81	49.0	1.34
24.0	0.83	50.0	1.36
25.0	0.85		

*Although the above chart was compiled for dogs, it can be used for cats, too. A formula for more precise values follows:

$$\text{BAS in M}^2 = \frac{K \times W^{2/3}}{10^4} \quad \textit{Given that}$$

BSA = body surface area
M² = sq meters
W = weight in gm
K = 10.1 (dogs), 10.0 (cats)

From Ettinger, S. J.: Textbook of Veterinary Internal Medicine, Vol. I. Philadelphia, W. B. Saunders Company, 1975, p. 146.

Table 149. CANINE–HUMAN AGE EQUIVALENTS (YEARS)

Age of Dog	Age of Man	Age of Dog	Age of Man
1	15	11	60
2	24	12	64
3	28	13	68
4	32	14	72
5	36	15	76
6	40	16	80
7	44	17	84
8	48	18	88
9	52	19	92
10	56	20	96

Table 150. CONVERSION TABLE FOR STANDARD FRENCH (CHARRIÉRE) GAUGE

The standard French, or Charriere, Scale (abbreviated F or Fr) is generally used in the size calibration of catheters and other tubular instruments. It is based on the metric system, with each unit being approximately 0.33 mm, and a difference of 0.33 mm in diameter between consecutive sizes. Example: 27F indicates a diameter of 9 mm; 30F, a diameter of 10 mm.

A convenient conversion table from the French Scale to the English and American Scales that is sometimes used for certain instruments is given below.

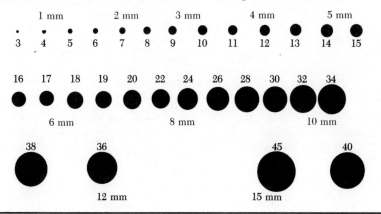

HEREDITARY DEFECTS OF DOGS (Patterson)

Table 151. A CATALOGUE OF CONGENITAL/HEREDITARY DISORDERS
OF DOGS (BY BREED)

Breed	Mode*	Disorders
Aberdeen Terrier		Primary uterine inertia
Afghan Hound	R	Cataract (bilateral)
		Elbow joint malformation
	R	Necrotizing myelopathy
Airedale Terrier		Cerebellar hypoplasia
		Trembling of the hind quarters
		Umbilical hernia
Alaskan Malamute		Anemia with chondrodysplasia
	R	Dwarfism
	R	Factor VII deficiency
	R	Hemeralopia
		Renal cortical hypoplasia
American Foxhound		Deafness
		Microphthalmia
Antarctic Husky	D	Entropion
	SLR	Hemophilia A
Australian Shepherd	R	Microphthalmia/multiple colobomas
Basenji		Coliform enteritis
	R	Hemolytic anemia
		Inguinal hernia
	D	Persistent pupillary membrane
		Pyruvate kinase deficiency
		Umbilical hernia
Basset Hound	D	Achondroplasia
	SLR	Anomaly of third cervical vertebra
		Inguinal hernia
	ID	Platelet disorder
		Primary glaucoma
Beagle		Atopic dermatitis
		Bladder cancer
		Bundle branch block
		Cataract (unilateral)
	D	Cataract with microphthalmia
	P	Cleft lip and palate
		Distemper
	R, P	Epilepsy
	R	Factor VII deficiency
	SLR	Hemophilia A
		Hypercholesterolemia
		Intervertebral disc disease
		Lymphocytic thyroiditis
	R	Mononephrosis
		Multiple epiphyseal dysplasia
		Necrotizing panotitis

Table continued on opposite page

Table 151. A CATALOGUE OF CONGENITAL/HEREDITARY DISORDERS
OF DOGS (BY BREED) (*Continued*)

Breed	Mode*	Disorders
	P	Otocephalic syndrome
	R	Primary glaucoma
	P	Pulmonic stenosis
		Renal hypoplasia
	R	Retinal dysplasia
	R	Short tail
		Thyroiditis
		Unilateral kidney aplasia
Bedlington Terrier		Renal cortical hypoplasia
	R	Retinal dysplasia
Bernese Sennehund	P	Cleft lip and palate
Black and Tan Coonhound	SLR	Hemophilia B
Bloodhound		Distemper
Blue Tick Hound		Globoid cell leukodystrophy
Border Collie		Central progressive retinal atrophy
Border Terrier		Aortic and carotid body tumors
	R	Cataract (bilateral)
		Craniomandibular osteopathy
		Hemivertebra
		Mastocytoma
		Oligodendroglioma
		Patella luxation
		Pituitary tumor
Boxer		Abnormal dentition (extra incisor)
		Aortic and carotid body tumors
		Aortic stenosis
		Atrial septal defects
	SLR	Cystinuria
		Dermoid cysts
		Endocardial fibroelastosis
		Fibrosarcoma
		Gingival hyperplasia
		Histiocytoma
		Intervertebral disc disease
		Mastocytoma
		Melanoma
		Oligodendroglioma
		Persistence of right venous valve
		Pulmonic stenosis
	P	Subaortic stenosis
		Superficial corneal ulcer
Brussels Griffon		Short skull
Bull Mastiff		Abnormal dentition (extra incisor)
Bull Terrier	R	Deafness
		Inguinal hernia
		Umbilical hernia

Table continued on following page

Table 151. A CATALOGUE OF CONGENITAL/HEREDITARY DISORDERS
OF DOGS (BY BREED) (*Continued*)

Breed	Mode*	Disorders
Cairn Terrier		Craniomandibular osteopathy
	SLR	Cystinuria
	R	Globoid cell leukodystrophy
	SLR	Hemophilia A
	SLR	Hemophilia B
		Inguinal hernia
Ceylon		Hairlessness
Chihuahua		Collapsed trachea
		Dislocation of the shoulder
	SLR	Hemophilia A
	R	Hydrocephalus
		Hypoplasia of dens
		Mitral valve defects
		Patella luxation
		Pulmonic stenosis
Cocker Spaniel	P	Behavioral abnormalities
	R	Cataract (bilateral)
		Cataract with microphthalmia
	P	Cleft lip and palate
	R	Cranioschisis
		Distichiasis
	D	Factor X deficiency
		Hip dysplasia
	R	Hydrocephalus
		Inguinal hernia
		Intervertebral disc disease
		Over- and undershot jaw
	P	Patent ductus arteriosus
		Primary glaucoma
		Primary peripheral retinal dystrophy
		Renal cortical hypoplasia
		Skin neoplasms
	R	Tail abnormalities
		Umbilical hernia
	P	Ununited anconeal process
Collie		Bladder cancer
	R	Collie eye anomaly
	R	Cyclic neutropenia
		Deafness
	R, P	Epilepsy
	SLR	Hemophilia A
		Inguinal hernia
	ID	Iris heterochromia
		Microphthalmia
		Nasal solar dermatitis
		Optic nerve hypoplasia
	P	Patent ductus arteriosis
		Umbilical hernia
	D	Achondroplasia
Dachshund	P	Cleft lip and palate
	SLR	Cystinuria

Table continued on opposite page

Table 151. A CATALOGUE OF CONGENITAL/HEREDITARY DISORDERS
OF DOGS (BY BREED) (*Continued*)

Breed	Mode*	Disorders
	ID	Deafness Diabetes mellitus Ectasia syndrome Intervertebral disc disease Iris heterochromia Microphthalmia Osteopetrosis Over- and undershot jaw (longhaired Dachshund) Renal hypoplasia
Dalmatian	R	Atopic dermatitis Deafness Excess uric acid excretion Globoid cell leukodystrophy
Doberman Pinscher		His bundle degeneration Polyostotic fibrous dysplasia Renal cortical hypoplasia Spondylolisthesis Liver copper storage disease Persistent primary hyperplastic vitreons
English Bulldog	P R	Abnormal dentition (extra incisor) Anasarca Arteriovenous fistula Cleft lip and palate Hemivertebra Hydrocephalus Hypoplasia of trachea Mitral valve defects Oligodendroglioma Predisposition to dystocia Pulmonic stenosis Short skull
	R	Short tail Spina bifida
English Cocker Spaniel	SLR R R	Hemophilia A Juvenile amaurotic idiocy Neuronal ceroidlipofuscinosis
English Springer Spaniel	D ID R	Cutaneous asthenia Factor XI deficiency Retinal dysplasia
Foxhound		Deafness Osteochondrosis of the spine
Fox Terrier	R	Ataxia Atopic dermatitis Deafness Dislocation of the shoulder Esophageal achalasia Glaucoma Goiter Lens luxation

Table continued on following page

Table 151. A CATALOGUE OF CONGENITAL/HEREDITARY DISORDERS OF DOGS (BY BREED) (*Continued*)

Breed	Mode*	Disorders
		Oligodontia
		Pulmonic stenosis
French Bulldog		Hemivertebra
German Shepherd		Atopic dermatitis
	P	Behavioral abnormalities
	D	Cataract (bilateral)
	P	Cleft lip and palate
	SLR	Cystinuria
		Dermoid cyst
		Ectasia syndrome
		Enostosis
	R, P	Epilepsy
		Esophageal achalasia
		Eversion of nictitating membrane
	SLR	Hemophilia A
	P	Hip dysplasia
	R	Pancreatic insufficiency
	P	Persistent right aortic arch
		Pituitary dwarfism
		Renal cortical hypoplasia
	P	Subaortic stenosis
	P	Ununited anconeal process
	D	Von Willebrand's disease
German Shorthaired Pointer	R	Amaurotic idiocy
	R	Eversion of nictitating membrane
		Fibrosarcoma
	D	Lymphedema
		Melanoma
		Subaortic stenosis
Golden Retriever	D	Cataract (bilateral)
		Cataract with microphthalmia
Gordon Setter		Generalized progressive retinal atrophy
Great Dane	SLR	Cystinuria
		Deafness
		Eversion of nictitating membrane
	ID	Iris heterochromia
		Mitral valve defects
		Spondylolisthesis
	P	Stockard's paralysis
Great Dane × Bloodhound		Paralysis of the hind limbs
Greyhound		Esophageal achalasia
	SLR	Hemophilia A
		Predisposition to dystocia
	R	Short spine
Griffon		Dislocation of the shoulder
Griffon Bruxellois × Dachshund		Susceptibility to rickets

Table continued on opposite page

Table 151. A CATALOGUE OF CONGENITAL/HEREDITARY DISORDERS
OF DOGS (BY BREED) (*Continued*)

Breed	Mode*	Disorders
Irish Setter	SLR	Carpal subluxation
		Generalized myopathy
	R	Generalized progressive retinal atrophy
	SLR	Hemophilia A
		Persistent right aortic arch
	R	Quadriplegia with amblyopia
Irish Terrier	SLR	Cystinuria
Jack Russell Terrier		Ataxia
		Lens luxation
Keeshond	P	Conus septal defects
	R, P	Epilepsy
		Mitral valve defects
	P	Tetralogy of Fallot
Kerry Blue		Hair follicle tumor
	P	Ununited anconeal process
King Charles Spaniel		Diabetes mellitus
Labrador Retriever		Carpal subluxation
	ID	Cataract (bilateral)
		Craniomandibular osteopathy
	SLR	Cystinuria
	SLR	Hemophilia A
	R	Retinal dysplasia
Labrador × American Foxhound		Diaphragmatic hernia
Labrador × Poodle	D	Lymphedema
Lhaso Apso		Inguinal hernia
		Renal cortical hypoplasia
Mexican, Turkish, and Chinese Breeds	D	Hairlessness
Miniature Pinscher		Dislocation of the shoulder
Miniature Poodle	R	Achondroplasia
		Cerebrospinal demyelination
	SLR	Cystinuria
		Dislocation of the shoulder
		Ectasia syndrome
		Ectodermal defect
	R	Generalized progressive retinal atrophy
		Globoid cell leukodystrophy
		Hypoplasia of dens
		Partial alopecia
		Patella luxation
	P	Patent ductus arteriosus
Miniature Schnauzer	R	Cataract (bilateral)
		Pulmonic stenosis
	D	Von Willebrand's disease

Table continued on following page

Table 151. A CATALOGUE OF CONGENITAL/HEREDITARY DISORDERS OF DOGS (BY BREED) *(Continued)*

Breed	Mode*	Disorders
Mongrel		Black hair follicular dysplasia
	SLR	Cystinuria
		Multiple cartilaginous exostoses
Newfoundland		Eversion of nictitating membrane
	P	Subaortic stenosis
Norwegian Dunkerhound		Deafness
		Microphthalmia
Norwegian Elkhound	R	Generalized progressive retinal atrophy
		Keratoacanthoma
		Renal cortical hypoplasia
Old English Sheepdog	R	Cataract, bilateral
Otterhound	ID	Platelet disorder
Pekingese		Distichiasis
		Hypoplasia of dens
		Inguinal hernia
		Intervertebral disc disease
		Short skull
		Trichiasis
		Umbilical hernia
Pointer		Bithoracic ectomelia
	R	Cataract (bilateral)
	R	Neuromuscular atrophy
	R	Neurotropic osteopathy
		Umbilical hernia
Pomeranian		Dislocation of the shoulder
		Hypoplasia of dens
		Patella luxation
	P	Patent ductus arteriosus
		Tracheal collapse
Poodle (see also Miniature, Standard, and Toy Poodle)	P	Atopic dermatitis
		Behavioral abnormality
	SLR	Cystinuria
		Distichiasis
	R	Epilepsy
	P	Patent ductus arteriosus
Pug		Male pseudohermaphroditism
		Trichiasis
Rhodesian Ridgeback		Dermoid sinus
Rottweiler		Diabetes mellitus
St. Bernard		Aphakia with multiple colobomas
		Dermoid cysts of cornea
		Eversion of nictitating membrane
	SLR	Hemophilia A
	SLR	Hemophilia B
	P	Stockard's paralysis
St. Bernard × Great Dane		Paralysis of the hind limbs

Table continued on opposite page

Table 151. A CATALOGUE OF CONGENITAL/HEREDITARY DISORDERS OF DOGS (BY BREED) (*Continued*)

Breed	Mode*	Disorders
Samoyed		Atrial septal defects
		Diabetes mellitus
	SLR	Hemophilia A
		Pulmonic stenosis
Scottish Terrier		Bladder cancer
		Atopic dermatitis
		Achondroplasia
		Craniomandibular osteopathy
	SLR	Cystinuria
		Deafness
		Melanoma
		Primary uterine inertia
	R	Scottie cramp
	D	Von Willebrand's disease
Sealyham Terrier		Atopic dermatitis
		Lens luxation
	R	Retinal dysplasia
Shetland Sheepdog		Bladder cancer
	R	Collie eye anomaly
	SLR	Hemophilia A
		Hip dysplasia
	ID	Iris heterochromia
		Nasal solar dermatitis
	P	Patent ductus arteriosus
Shiba Ina	R	Short spine
Shih Tzu	P	Cleft lip and palate
		Renal cortical hypoplasia
Siberian Husky	ID	Iris heterochromia
Silver Grey Collie		Cyclic neutropenia
	ID	Iris heterochromia
Skye Terrier	R	Hypoplasia of the larynx
Springer Spaniel	D	Ehlers-Danlos syndrome
	ID	Factor XI deficiency
	R	Retinal dysplasia
Staffordshire Bull Terrier	R	Cataract (bilateral)
	P	Cleft lip and palate
Standard Poodle	R	Cataract (bilateral)
Swedish Lapland	R	Neuronal abiotrophy
Swiss Dogs		Generalized progressive retinal atrophy
Swiss Sheepdog	P	Cleft lip and palate
Tervueren Shepherd	R	Epilepsy
Toy Poodle		Ectasia syndrome
		Fibrosis of the plantaris muscle
	R	Generalized progressive retinal atrophy
		Patella luxation
	P	Patent ductus arteriosus
		Tracheal collapse

Table continued on following page

Table 151. A CATALOGUE OF CONGENITAL/HEREDITARY DISORDERS OF DOGS (BY BREED) *(Continued)*

Breed	Mode*	Disorders
Vizsla	SLR	Hemophilia A
Weimaraner		Eversion of nictitating membrane
		Fibrosarcoma
	SLR	Hemophilia A
		Melanoma
		Spinal dysraphism
		Umbilical hernia
Welsh Corgi	SLR	Cystinuria
		Generalized progressive retinal atrophy
		Predisposition to dystocia
West Highland White Terrier		Atopic dermatitis
		Craniomandibular osteopathy
	R	Globoid cell leukodystrophy
		Inguinal hernia
Whippet		Partial alopecia
Yorkshire Terrier		Hypoplasia of dens
		Patella luxation
	R	Retinal dysplasia
All Breeds	D	Blood group incompatibility
Brachycephalic breeds		Pituitary cysts
		Stenotic nares and elongated soft palate
Giant Breeds		Elbow dysplasia
		Hip dysplasia
		Osteogenic sarcoma
Many Breeds	P	Behavioral abnormalities
	SLR	Cryptorchidism
		Demodectic mange
	D	Dewclaws
		Ectropion
		Elbow dysplasia (especially large and giant breeds)
		Entropion
		Esophageal dilation
		Hip dysplasia (especially large and giant breeds)
Many Miniature Breeds		Collapsed trachea
		Glycogen storage disease
		Legg-Calvé-Perthes syndrome
		Patellar luxation
		Predisposition to dystocia
		Tracheal collapse
Miscellaneous		White breed deafness

*Mode of inheritance: R = recessive; D = dominant; ID = incomplete dominance; SLR = sex-linked recessive; and P = polygenic.

From Kirk, R. W. (ed.): Current Veterinary Therapy. Philadelphia, W. B. Saunders Company, 1983, pp. 1225–1230.

TAIL DOCKING

The data on tail docking and dewclaw removal were based on official standards published by the American Kennel Club or on information obtained directly from judges, veterinarians, dog breeders, and professional handlers (Table 152). However, because of the ambiguous descriptions used in many standards and because of the changes in breed fashions, veterinarians are cautioned *to use these figures as suggestions only!* Always obtain *specific instructions* from the owner as to length of dock or whether to remove dewclaws.

Table 152. TAIL DOCKING*

Breed	Length at Less Than One Week of Age
Sporting Breeds	
Brittany Spaniel	Leave 1 inch‡
Clumber Spaniel	Leave 1/4–1/3
Cocker Spaniel	Leave 1/3 (about 3/4 in.)
English Cocker Spaniel	Leave 1/3
English Springer Spaniel	Leave 1/3
Field Spaniel	Leave 1/3
German Shorthaired Pointer	Leave 2/5†
German Wirehaired Pointer	Leave 2/5†
Sussex Spaniel	Leave 1/3
Vizsla	Leave 2/3†
Weimaraner	Leave 3/5 (about 1 1/2 in.)
Welsh Springer Spaniel	Leave 1/3–1/2
Wirehaired Pointing Griffon	Leave 1/3†
Working Breeds	
Bouvier des Flandres	Leave 1/2–3/4 in.
Boxer	Leave 1/2–3/4 in.
Doberman Pinscher	Leave 3/4 in. (two vertebrae)
Giant Schnauzer	Leave 1 1/4 in. (three vertebrae)
Old English Sheepdog	If necessary—close to body (leave one vertebra)‡
Rottweiler	If necessary—close to body (leave one vertebra)‡
Standard Schnauzer	Leave 1 in. (two vertebrae)
Welsh Corgi (Pembroke)	Close to body (leave one vertebra)‡
Terrier Breeds	
Airedale Terrier	Leave 2/3–3/4§
Australian Terrier	Leave 2/5†
Fox Terrier (Smooth and Wirehaired)	Leave 2/3–3/4§
Irish Terrier	Leave 3/4†
Kerry Blue Terrier	Leave 1/2–2/3
Lakeland Terrier	Leave 2/3§
Miniature Schnauzer	Leave about 3/4 in.—no more than 1 in.

Table continued on following page

Table 152. TAIL DOCKING (*Continued*)*

Breed	Length at Less Than One Week of Age
Terrier Breeds Continued	
Norwich Terrier	Leave 1/4–1/3
Sealyham Terrier	Leave 1/3–1/2
Soft-Coated Wheaten Terrier	Leave 1/2–3/4
Welsh Terrier	Leave 2/3§
Toy Breeds	
Affenpinscher	Close to body (leave 1/3 in.)
Brussels Griffon	Leave 1/4–1/3
English Toy Spaniel	Leave 1/3
Miniature Pinscher	Leave 1/2 in. (two vertebrae)
Silky Terrier	Leave about 1/3 (about 1/2 in.)
Toy Poodle	Leave 1/2–2/3 (about 1 in.)
Yorkshire Terrier	Leave about 1/3 (about 1/2 in.)
Nonsporting Breeds	
Miniature Poodle	Leave 1/2–2/3 (about 1 1/8 in.)
Schipperke	Close to body‡
Standard Poodle	Leave 1/2–2/3 (about 1 1/2 in.)
Miscellaneous Breeds (not registered by American Kennel Club)	
Cavalier King Charles Spaniel	Optional. Leave at least 2/3. Always leave white tip in broken-colored dogs.
Spinoni Italiani	Leave 3/5

*This list gives *approximate* guides for docking when done before the puppy is 1 week old. If definite information was not given in the official breed standard, *opinions* were obtained from judges, breeders, veterinarians, and professional handlers. Breeds not listed are those not usually docked. Docking disqualifies the Boston terrier, Cardigan Welsh corgi, and West Highland White terrier for showing. An improperly docked tail may ruin a puppy for show purposes. If one is in doubt, consultation with an established breeder is suggested. There may be variations among puppies, and a knowledge of breed characteristics is important in determining the correct length to dock. M. Josephine Deublner, V.M.D., compiled most of these data.

† Taken from official breed standard.

‡May be naturally tail-less.

§The tip of the docked tail should be approximately level with the top of the skull with the puppy in show position.

DEWCLAW REMOVAL

Because dewclaws may become torn during field exercise, they are often removed from all four feet of many hunting and working breeds. Removing dewclaws makes the legs of a dog appear smooth and clean.

Breeds from which dewclaws should be removed include the following: Chesapeake Bay retriever, Vizsla, Weimaraner, Norwegian elkhound, Alaskan malamute, Belgian malinois, Belgian sheepdog, Belgian tervuren, Bernese mountain dog, boxer, Komondor, St. Bernard, Shetland sheepdog, Siberian husky, Cardigan Welsh corgi, Dandie Dinmont terrier, Kerry blue terrier, Lakeland terrier, Papillon, Silky terrier, and Dalmatian. Dewclaws may be removed from the basset hound and Puli. Do not remove dewclaws from the Briard and Great Pyrenees; these breeds must have double dewclaws on the hind leg.

FEEDING DOGS AND CATS

Feeding Methods

Self-feeding is economical, keeps animals quiet, prevents shy animals from being pushed away from food, and discourages coprophagy. About 10 per cent of all dogs will overeat and become obese. Cats rarely have this problem. Only dry-type rations can be self-fed. Rations of less than 1400 cal per lb may be too bulky for growing or lactating dogs. Overeating can cause too rapid growth, which produces skeletal problems in young animals; therefore, an animal should be 80 per cent grown before being self-fed.

Feeding by hand requires regularity and knowledge of exact amounts and feeding times. A good method is to feed a dog the amount of food that it will consume in 20 minutes. Adult dogs and cats can be fed once daily; puppies, toy breeds, pregnant, and lactating animals should be fed at least twice daily. Between-meal snacks may cause obesity unless a measured amount is allotted for each day and calculated in the daily caloric requirement. Table scraps usually are inadequate and may produce an unbalanced diet; however, an amount of wholesome scraps up to 15 per cent of a diet by weight can be added to a top quality balanced diet without unhealthy effects.

Amounts for hand feeding should be obtained from charts of requirements appropriate to an individual animal's weight and matched to ingredient analysis of the specific food to be used. Tables 153 through 155 provide a general guide for hand feeding, but the actual feeding must be further adjusted to the animal's response. The best guideline is to follow a feeding plan that results in maintenance of an ideal constant weight in addition to a good coat and vigor.

Types of Foods

Commercial pet foods come in different forms, which are largely characterized by moisture content (Tables 156 to 158). Most *dry foods* contain 10 to 12 per cent moisture and 1400 to 1700 kcal per lb. They are the most economical but may be low in palatability, quality of protein, caloric density, and quantity of fatty acids. Some premium brands contain as much as 2000 kcal per lb. Value of a diet depends on the ingredients used, not on the form of the food.

Text continued on page 852

Table 153. RECOMMENDED NUTRIENT ALLOWANCES FOR DOGS
(PER LB OR KG OF BODY WEIGHT PER DAY)*

Nutrient	Per Lb	Per Kg
Protein (gm)	2.25	5.0
Fat (gm)	0.70	1.5
Linoleic acid (gm)	0.1	0.22
Carbohydrate†	—	—
Minerals		
Calcium (mg)	120	265
Phosphorus (mg)	100	220
Potassium (mg)	65	144
Sodium chloride (mg)	91	200
Magnesium (mg)	6.4	14
Iron (mg)	0.6	1.32
Copper (mg)	0.07	0.16
Manganese (mg)	0.05	0.11
Zinc (mg)	1.0	2.2
Iodine (mg)	0.015	0.033
Selenium (µg)	1.1	2.42
Vitamins		
Vitamin A (IU)	50	110
Vitamin D (IU)	5	11
Vitamin E (µg)	0.55	1.2
Thiamine (µg)	11.0	24
Riboflavin (µg)	22.0	48
Pyridoxine (µg)	11.0	24
Pantothenic acid (µg)	100	220
Niacin (µg)	114	250
Folic acid (µg)	1.8	4
Vitamin B_{12} (µg)	0.5	1.1
Biotin (µg)	1.0	2.2
Choline (mg)	11.8	26

*1977 modification by Cornell Research Laboratory for Diseases of Dogs; data taken from NAS-NRC Publication No. 8, Nutrient Requirements of Dogs, 1974.

†Carbohydrate as such has not been shown to be required. As a common ingredient of most dog foods, it serves as an excellent source of energy and may be required for reproduction.

From Sheffy, B. E.: Nutrition and nutritional disorders. Vet. Clin. North Am., 8:10, 1978.

Table 154. RECOMMENDED CALORIC ALLOWANCES FOR MAINTENANCE AND DAILY FOOD INTAKES OF AVERAGE ADULT DOGS OF VARIOUS BODY WEIGHTS (IN POUNDS)*

Weight (Lb)	Kcal Me Per Lb Body Weight	Daily Rations of Dog Food in Ounces		
		Dry Type	*Semi-moist*	*Canned*
2	60	1.2	1.5	3.4
5	48	2.4	3.0	6.8
10	40	4.0	5.0	11.0
15	37	5.6	6.9	15.5
20	34	6.8	8.5	19.0
30	32	9.7	12.0	27.0
45	28	12.7	15.8	35.5
75	24	18.2	22.5	50.7
110	22	24.5	30.2	68.0

*Needs for growth may be estimated by multiplying adult requirements by appropriate multiples of maintenance as follows:
Weaning to 40 per cent adult size-weight = 2 × maintenance
40 to 80 per cent adult size-weight = 1.5 × maintenance
80 per cent adult size-weight to maturity = 1.2 × maintenance
From Sheffy, B. E.: Nutrition and nutritional disorders. Vet. Clin. North Am., 8:20, 1978.

Table 155. ESTIMATED DAILY FOOD ALLOWANCES OF CATS

Cat	Weight of Cat, Kg	Dry Type*		Semi-moist†		Canned‡	
		Gm/kg Body Wt	*Gm/Cat*	*Gm/kg Body Wt*	*Gm/Cat*	*Gm/kg Body Wt*	*Gm/Cat*
Kittens							
10 weeks	0.4–1.0	70	28–70	80	32–80	200	80–200
20 weeks	1.2–2.0	36	43–72	42	50–84	104	125–208
30 weeks	1.5–2.7	28	42–76	32	48–86	80	120–216
40 weeks	2.2–3.8	22	48–84	26	57–99	64	141–243
Adults§							
Inactive	2.2–4.5	20	44–90	22	48–99	56	123–252
Active	2.2–4.5	24	53–108	27	59–122	68	150–306
Gestation	2.5–4.0	28	70–112	32	80–128	80	200–320
Lactation	2.2–4.0	70	154–280	80	176–320	200	440–800

*Dry matter, 90 per cent; ME, 3.60 kcal/gm
†Dry matter, 70 per cent; ME, 3.15 kcal/gm
‡Dry matter, 25 per cent; ME, 1.25 kcal/gm
§Fifty weeks of age or older
From Nutrient Requirements of Cats, Publication No. 13. Washington, D.C., National Academy of Sciences–National Research Council, 1978, p. 27.

Table 156. APPROXIMATE RECOMMENDED NUTRIENT CONTENTS OF DRY, CANNED, AND SEMI-MOIST DOG FOODS (IN PERCENTAGE OR SPECIFIC AMOUNTS PER KG)

Nutrient	Dry Type (Per cent)	Canned Meat (Per cent)	Semi-moist (Per cent)
Dry matter	90.0	25.00	67.00
Water	10.0	75.00	33.00
Protein	24.0	12.00	19.95
Fat	9.0	6.00	7.60
Linoleic acid	1.0	0.275	0.825
Fiber	3.6	1.00	3.00
Ash	8.0–9.00	3.00–4.00	6.00
Minerals			
Calcium	1.8	0.40	0.825
Phosphorus	1.4	0.30	0.675
Potassium	0.8	0.25	0.675
Sodium chloride	1.0	0.55	1.30
Magnesium	0.2	0.028	0.075
	Mg/Kg of Food	**Mg/Kg of Food**	**Mg/Kg of Food**
Iron	51.48	15.40	42.90
Copper	6.48	2.00	5.45
Manganese	4.32	1.30	3.63
Zinc	108.90	30.80	90.75
Iodine	1.35	0.04	1.17
Selenium	0.10	0.028	0.083
Vitamins			
Vitamin E (alpha tocopherol)	45	13.70	37.50
Thiamine	0.90	0.28	0.75
Riboflavin	1.98	0.60	1.65
Pyridoxine	0.90	0.28	0.75
Pantothenic acid	9.00	2.75	7.50
Niacin	9.90	3.00	8.25
Folic acid	0.16	0.05	0.135
Biotin	0.09	0.027	0.075
Vitamin B_{12}	0.02	0.006	0.020
Choline	1080.00	330.00	900.00
	IU/Kg of Food	**IU/Kg of Food**	**IU/Kg of Food**
Vitamin A	4500	1375	3750
Vitamin D	450	137	375
Metabolizable energy-Kcal*	3500/kg	1270/kg	2870/kg

*ME calculation from product label: ME kcal/oz = [100 + (% fat × 2.5)] − (% fat + % ash + % moisture) C.A. Banta, Allen Products Company, Allentown, Pennsylvania.

From Sheffy, B. E.: Nutrition and nutritional disorders. Vet. Clin. North Am., 8:13, 1978.

Table 157. CHARACTERISTICS OF THE DIFFERENT FORMS OF COMMERCIAL CAT FOODS

Form	Sold In	Energy Content	Needed Daily for Maintenance*	% Water	% Protein in the Dry Matter	% Fat in the Dry Matter	Digestible Energy (kcal/gm) of Dry Matter
Dry	Sacks	200–300 kcal/cup	1 cup (50–100 gm)	9–12	33–36	8–12	3.9–4.3
Soft-Moist	1.5 oz pkg	125 kcal/pkg	2 pkg (60–120 gm)	27–32	34–41	10–15	4.2–4.6
Canned	12–15 oz can	500 kcal/can	½ can (150/300 gm)	72–78	35–41	9–18	3.9–4.3
	6 oz can	165–225 kcal/can	2 cans	72–78	40–65	15–40	6.0–7.5

*Average amount needed daily for the 8-lb active house cat (30 kcal/lb/day). Increased amounts are needed during pregnancy, lactation (3 × more) and growth (3 × more at 5 weeks of age to 1½ × more at 30 weeks of age), and there is much individual variation.

Modified from Nutrient Requirements of Cats, Publication No. 13. Washington, D.C., National Academy of Sciences–National Research Council, 1978, p. 318.

Table 158. COMPOSITION OF FELINE SCIENCE DIETS (HILLS)

(%)	Maintenance		Growth and Reproduction	
	Dry	Canned	Dry	Canned
Moisture	9.0	70.6	9.0	69.7
Protein	31.5	12.2	34.4	15.1
Fat	21.3	7.4	25.2	9.2
Carbohyrates	35.4	7.9	23.5	3.8
Fiber	1.0	0.2	1.6	0.2
Ash	4.8	1.7	6.3	2.0
Calcium	0.8	0.24	1.2	0.34
Phosphorus	0.8	0.22	1.0	0.31
Magnesium	0.08	0.02	0.096	0.028
Magnesium (Mg)/100 kcal	16	15	19.8	16.6
Sodium	0.29	0.16	0.39	0.16
Calories/gm	4.86	1.6	4.86	1.69
Calories/cup or can	470	670	590	720

Courtesy of Hills Packing Co., Topeka, KS.

Semi-moist foods contain 25 to 30 per cent moisture and 1200 to 1400 kcal per lb (500 kcal/6-oz package). Most contain propylene glycol, sorbic acid, and phosphoric or hydrochloric acid to prevent spoilage. They are available in individual packs, patties, or bulk bags. Frequently soft-moist and dry foods are contained in the same package. Semimoist foods are palatable and highly digestible, which may result in obesity.

Canned foods contain 70 to 80 per cent water and 500 to 600 kcal per lb (not per can, because most cans of dog food weigh 14 to 16 oz). Not all canned products are complete, balanced rations; those products that are not should be avoided. Balanced products are expensive, highly palatable, cannot be used for self-feeding, and do not keep the teeth and gums in good condition.

Most commercial diets are compounded to meet requirements for growth and lactation; however, they may cause owners to overfeed mature or sedentary animals. Consequently, rations lower in protein and total energy are marketed as *maintenance diets* (Fit and Trim—Ralston-Purina, St. Louis, Missouri; Cycle 2, 3, and 4—Gaines Co., White Plains, New York; Science Diet Maintenance—Hill's Pet Products, Topeka, Kansas). The philosophy of feeding rations to meet specific physiologic needs such as growth, lactation, and work is appropriate, but some commercial products meet special needs better than others. In Tables 159 to 168, data are presented concerning typical commercial grocery store foods, premium-priced foods marketed by pet shops and veterinarians, and dietary foods for animals with special problems.

Gourmet canned foods often sold in pet stores deserve special mention. They may be all skeletal muscle but are usually a variety of animal by-products and textured vegetable protein, which is textured soy flour colored red or brown to look like meat. The canned gourmet cat foods may be composed of animal tissue such as shrimp, tuna, kidney, liver, or chicken. Cats may become addicted to a single-ingredient food. In addition, these are not complete, balanced rations, and they must not be fed as the sole food for either dogs or cats. The high protein content forces the animal to use protein for energy, a situation that may be undesirable in some animals. However, because of their excellent palatability and high protein and fat content, these foods may be useful in animals with anorexia, extensive wound healing, and protein-losing nephropathy or enteropathy. When the disease process is resolved in these cases, however, the animals *must* be placed on a balanced diet for long-term feeding.

Estimate the metabolizable energy (ME) from the label data by using the following formulas:

kcal ME per ounce "as is" food = $100 + (\% \text{ fat} \times 2.5) - (\% \text{ moisture} + \% \text{ fat} + \% \text{ ash})$. This is a rough approximation for canned rations.

$$\text{kcal ME per gram of "as is" food} = \frac{\text{kcal per ounce "as is" food}}{28}$$

Homemade diets are rarely balanced and adequate; they should not be used routinely for long periods of time unless they have been carefully compounded by a nutritionist. Even then, most owners will not adhere to a feeding protocol that includes "baked potato and cooked egg" or some of the less common items that may be needed.

Formulating a Diet

The following steps should be taken when formulating a diet:
1. Weigh the patient accurately.
2. Check Table 154 for dogs and Table 169 for cats to determine the basic daily caloric requirement (kcal of ME).
3. Modify the energy needs for growth (2 × base energy requirement), pregnancy (20 per cent above base), lactation (3 × base for a large litter and 2 × base for a small litter), and work (1.5 to 4 × base).
4. Choose the type of balanced commercial food to use, depending on the cost, convenience, palatability, and feeding method.
5. Determine the amount of food to use to meet the daily requirements.
6. Weigh and observe the animal weekly and adjust the diet as indicated to maintain constant weight for mature animals or to attain a conservative growth rate for the breed in young animals.

Special Feeding Problems

Pregnancy

Feed a *good quality* balanced diet for normal maintenance during the first 6 weeks of pregnancy. Increase food in proportion to weight gains during the last 3 weeks (increase approximately 15 to 20 per cent). If a high energy diet is fed during lactation, make the aforementioned changes the last 10 days of gestation to avoid a change at whelping. Provide abundant exercise; do not allow the animal to become soft or overweight.

Lactation

Feed a *good quality* diet that has proved to be nutritionally adequate for reproduction (check label) in sufficient quantity to maintain body weight. Increase the diet 1½ times the first week of lactation, 2 times the second week, and approximately 3 times the third week.

During the next 3 weeks, feed twice the maintenance diet plus 25 per cent for each nursing pup. This increases the diet in proportion to the litter size.

At weaning, decrease food for 3 days. Withhold food the day before weaning. Give ¼ of maintenance level for 3 days, then gradually increase the food normal maintenance.

Text continued on page 868

Table 159. APPROXIMATE CHEMICAL COMPOSITION OF COMMERCIAL DOG FOOD PRODUCTS

	Purina Puppy Chow	Purina Chuck Wagon	Purina Dog Chow[2]	Purina Hi-Pro	Purina Fit & Trim	Purina Field'n Farm	Purina Moist'n Chunky	Purina Mainstay	Purina Praise
Moisture % (max)	12	12	12	12	12	12	34	12	14
Dry matter % (min)	88	88	88	88	88	88	66	88	86
Protein % (min)	27	21	21	26	16[1]	21	18	16[1]	21
Fat % (min)	9	8	8	10	5	7	7	6	8
Linoleic acid %	1.70	1.85	1.75	1.70	1.25	1.75	1.30	1.35	1.60
Fiber % (max)	5.0	5.0	4.5	4.0	10.0	4.5	3.5	8.0	4.0
Ash %	8.5	8.0	7.5	8.5	8.5	7.5	8.0	9.0	7.5
Calcium %	1.7	1.4	1.3	1.6	1.0	1.2	1.3	1.2	1.3
Phosphorus %	1.0	0.90	0.90	0.95	0.80	0.90	0.85	0.80	0.90
Dig. protein %	85	85	83	85	73	80	83	75	83
Dig. energy (cal/lb)	1625	1600	1600	1750	1300	1600	1300	1550	1600
Vitamin A (IU/lb)	8000	8000	8000	8000	8000	8000	8000	8000	8000
Vitamin D (IU/lb)	800	800	800	800	800	800	800	800	800
Vitamin E (IU/lb)	5	5	5	5	5	5	20	5	5
Vitamin K, ppm	0.5	0.5	0.5	0.5	0.5	0.5	0.5	0.5	0.5
Choline, ppm	1100	1100	1100	1100	900	1100	2000	1000	1100
Vitamin B_{12}, ppm	0.025	0.025	0.025	0.025	0.025	0.025	0.025	0.025	0.025

Niacin, ppm	52	39	42	47	40	45	75	40	45
Riboflavin, ppm	4.8	4.4	4.3	4.5	3.0	4.0	6.0	3.5	4.5
Thiamin, ppm	7.8	7.0	7.0	7.3	7.0	7.0	10.0	7.0	7.0
Pyridoxine, ppm	8.0	7.8	7.1	7.0	7.0	7.0	6.0	7.0	7.0
Pantothenic acid, ppm	10	8	8	9	10	9	15	8	9
Biotin, ppm	0.13	0.13	0.13	0.13	0.13	0.10	0.10	0.13	0.13
Folic acid, ppm	1.3	1.3	1.3	1.3	1.3	1.3	1.3	1.3	1.3
Sodium %	0.50	0.45	0.45	0.50	0.40	0.45	0.40	0.35	0.45
Potassium %	0.65	0.65	0.65	0.65	0.55	0.65	0.65	0.65	0.55
Chloride %	0.65	0.60	0.60	0.70	0.55	0.65	0.60	0.50	0.60
Magnesium %	0.15	0.15	0.15	0.15	0.15	0.15	0.12	0.15	0.15
Iron, ppm	250	200	200	200	200	200	200	200	200
Zinc, ppm	110	95	95	95	90	90	90	90	80
Manganese, ppm	55	52	51	56	50	50	50	51	55
Cobalt, ppm	0.75	0.75	0.75	0.75	0.75	0.75	0.75	0.75	0.75
Copper, ppm	14	11	12	13	12	12	10	12	13
Iodine, ppm	2.5	2.1	2.1	2.2	2.0	2.1	2.0	2.0	2.1

The levels of these nutrients equal or exceed levels determined to be required from research at the Purina Pet Care Center.

(1) 18% in California

(2) Same figures apply to Purina Butcher's Blend dog food and Purina Beef, Bacon, and Cheese Blend dog food

Courtesy of Ralston Purina Co., St. Louis, Mo.

Table 160. COMPOSITION OF TYPICAL COMMERCIAL
DRY DOG FOODS

Approximate Composition		Gaines Cycle 1			Gaines Cycle 2			Gaines Cycle 3		
		Guar-antee	As is Basis	Dry Basis	Guar-antee	As is Basis	Dry Basis	Guar-antee	As is Basis	Dry Basis
Food solids	%	—	91.1	100.0	—	90.9	100.0	—	90.3	100.0
Moisture (water)	%	12 mx	8.9	—	12 mx	9.1	—	12 mx	9.7	—
Protein	%	27 mn	27.6	30.2	18 mn	20.2	22.2	18 mn	20.6	22.8
Fat	%	8 mn	11.9	13.1	6 mn	10.9	12.0	5 mn	9.8	10.9
Fiber	%	5 mx	3.7	4.1	5 mx	3.4	3.7	10 mx	7.0	7.8
Ash (minerals)	%	—	7.7	8.5	—	6.8	7.5	—	5.7	6.3
Carbohydrate	%	—	40.2	44.1	—	49.6	54.6	—	47.2	52.2
Metabolizable energy–kcal (as is)										
Per pound			1547			1451			1301	
Per 8-fl oz measuring cup			290			272			244	
Dry matter digestibility	%		76			76			66	
Protein digestibility	%		81			77			76	
Calcium (Ca)	%		1.1			1.0			1.0	
Phosphorus (P)	%		0.9			0.8			0.8	
Salt (NaCl)	%		1.4			1.4			1.0	
		For puppies up to 18 months old; balanced nutrition with extra protein and vitamins.			For adult dogs 1–7 yr of age.			For less active or overweight adult dogs.		

Courtesy of Gaines Division, General Foods, White Plains, NY.

Table continued on opposite page

Table 160. COMPOSITION OF TYPICAL COMMERCIAL
DRY DOG FOODS (*Continued*)

Gaines Cycle 4			Gaines Meal			Gaines Gravy Train			Gaines Complete		
Guar-antee	*As is Basis*	*Dry Basis*	*Guar-antee*	*As is Basis*	*Dry Basis*	*Guar-antee*	*As is Basis*	*Dry Basis*	*Guar-antee*	*As is Basis*	*Dry Basis*
—	90.6	100.0	—	91.2	100.0	—	90.5	100.0	—	92.0	100.0
12 mx	9.4	—	12 mx	8.8	—	12 mx	9.5	—	12 mx	8.0	—
18 mn	19.8	21.9	21 mn	22.0	24.1	21 mn	21.8	24.1	21 mn	23.2	25.2
5 mn	9.7	10.7	5 mn	8.3	9.1	6 mn	10.2	11.3	5 mn	7.0	7.6
8 mx	3.4	3.8	6 mx	3.9	4.3	6 mx	3.6	4.0	6 mx	3.3	3.6
—	7.2	8.0	—	6.9	7.6	—	7.1	7.9	—	8.5	9.2
—	50.5	55.6	—	50.1	54.9	—	47.8	52.7	—	50.0	54.4
	1403			1493			1547			1520	
	263			280			290			285	
	76			75			79			78	
	78			78			79			79	
	0.5			1.0			1.0			1.0	
	0.4			0.8			0.8			0.8	
	0.3			1.4			1.4			1.4	

For dogs over 7 yr. Nutritionally complete and balanced diets for puppies throughout the growth stage and for maintenance of active and inactive adults. Ideal for self-feeding.

Table 161. COMPOSITION OF CANNED CYCLE DOG FOOD (GAINES)

Approximate Composition		Cycle 1			Cycle 2			Cycle 3			Cycle 4		
		Guar- antee	As is Basis	Dry Basis	Guar- antee	As is Basis	Dry Basis	Guar- antee	As is Basis	Dry Basis	Guar- antee	As is Basis	Dry Basis
Food solids	%	—	29.4	100.0	—	26.5	100.0	—	25.8	100.0	—	25.4	100.0
Moisture (water)	%	78 mx	70.6	—	78 mx	73.5	—	78 mx	74.2	—	78 mx	74.6	—
Protein	%	10 mn	11.0	37.4	7 mn	8.3	31.3	7 mn	8.0	31.0	5 mn	6.3	24.8
Fat	%	6 mn	6.7	22.8	5 mn	6.3	23.8	2 mn	3.6	14.0	3 mn	4.6	18.1
Fiber	%	2 mx	0.8	2.7	2 mx	0.6	2.3	5 mx	2.0	7.8	5 mx	2.5	9.8
Ash (minerals)	%	—	2.5	8.5	—	2.5	9.4	—	2.4	9.3	—	2.7	10.6
Carbohydrate	%	—	8.4	28.6	—	8.8	33.2	—	9.8	37.9	—	9.3	36.7
Metabolizable energy-kcal (as is)													
Per pound			568			521			425			442	
Per 3-oz pattie			—			—			—			—	
Per 6-oz packet			—			—			—			—	
Per 14-oz can			497			456			372			387	
Dry matter digestibility	%		81			85			72			71	
Protein digestibility	%		83			84			79			78	
Calcium (Ca)	%		0.35			0.35			0.29			0.29	
Phosphorus (P)	%		0.29			0.29			0.23			0.23	
Salt (NaCl)	%		0.44			0.39			0.39			0.15	
		For puppies up to 18 months old.			For adult dog 1–7 yr.			For less active or over-weight adult dogs.			For dogs over 7 yr.		

Courtesy of Gaines Division, General Foods, White Plains, NY.

Table 162. COMPOSITION OF TYPICAL COMMERCIAL SOFT–MOIST DOG FOODS (GAINES)

Approximate Composition		Puppy Choice			Top Choice			Gaines-Burgers			Prime Variety		
		Guarantee	As is Basis	Dry Basis	Guarantee	As is Basis	Dry Basis	Guarantee	As is Basis	Dry Basis	Guarantee	As is Basis	Dry Basis
Food solids	%	—	75.4	100.0	—	76.2	100.0	—	76.8	100.0	—	76.2	100.0
Moisture (water)	%	36 mx	24.6	—	36 mx	23.8	—	36 mx	23.2	—	36 mx	23.8	—
Protein	%	21 mn	22.5	29.8	18 mn	19.2	25.2	18 mn	19.2	25.0	18 mn	19.2	25.2
Fat	%	7 mn	11.0	14.6	7 mn	11.0	14.4	7 mn	13.2	17.2	7 mn	11.0	14.4
Fiber	%	3 mx	2.3	3.1	3 mx	2.5	3.3	3 mx	2.3	3.0	3 mx	2.5	3.3
Ash (minerals)	%	—	7.2	9.6	—	6.2	8.1	—	6.3	8.2	—	6.2	8.1
Carbohydrate	%	—	32.4	42.9	—	37.3	49.0	—	35.8	46.6	—	37.3	49.0
Metabolizable energy-kcal (as is)													
Per pound			1280			1280			1280			1280	
Per 3-oz pattie			—			—			240			—	
Per 6-oz packet			480			480			—			480	
Per 14-oz can			—			—			—			—	
Dry Matter Digestibility	%		80			80			80			80	
Protein Digestibility	%		80			80			80			80	
Calcium (Ca)	%		0.9			0.84			0.84			0.84	
Phosphorus (P)	%		0.75			0.68			0.68			1.68	
Salt (NaCl)	%		1.14			1.14			1.14			1.14	

Puppy Choice: A nutritionally complete and balanced diet specifically formulated for the growth of puppies. Also ideal for brood bitches in gestation and lactation, working dogs, and dogs under other stress conditions; for presurgical conditioning and postsurgical recovery.

Prime Variety: Nutritionally complete and balanced diets for all stages of life, particularly for maintenance of normally active and inactive adults.

Table 163. APPROXIMATE CHEMICAL COMPOSITION OF TYPICAL CAT FOOD PRODUCTS

	Purina Cat Chow	Purina Special Dinners	Purina Meow Mix	Purina Thrive	Purina Good Mews	Purina Kitten Chow	Purina Tender Vittles	Purina Happy Cat	P100 Land-Based	P100 Poultry-Based	P100 Fish-Based	P100 Comb. Dinners
Moisture, % (max)	12	12	12	12	12	12	34	34	78	78	78	78
Dry matter, % (min)	88	88	88	88	88	88	66	66	22	22	22	22
Protein, % (min)	30	30	30	30	30	35	24	24	12	12	12	13
Dig. protein, %	85	85	85	85	85	85	85	85	85	85	85	85
Dig. energy, (cal/lb)	1700	1650	1725	1725	1650	1750	1300	1300	585	600	560	600
Fat, % (min)	8.0	8.0	8.0	8.0	8.0	8.5	8.5	8.5	2.0	4.0	2.0	4.0
Fiber, % (max)	4.5	4.0	4.0	4.0	4.0	4.0	3.5	3.5	1.0	1.0	1.0	1.0
Linoleic acid, %	1.2	1.2	1.2	1.2	1.2	1.2	1.0	1.0	1.0	1.0	2.0	.75
Ash, %	7.5	7.5	7.75	7.75	7.75	8.5	7.0	7.0	3.5	3.5	3.5	3.5
Ash, % (can diet equiv.)	1.9	1.9	1.9	1.9	1.9	2.1	2.3	2.3	3.5	3.5	3.5	3.5
Calcium, %	1.0	1.2	1.3	1.3	1.2	1.6	1.2	1.2	0.5	0.8	0.4	0.4
Phosphorus, %	0.8	1.0	0.9	0.9	1.0	1.1	1.0	1.0	.45	.40	.35	.35
Vitamin A, (IU/kg)	10,000	10,000	10,000	10,000	10,000	20,000	10,000	10,000	4,400	3,300	2,200	1,650
Vitamin D, (IU/kg)	1,600	1,600	1,600	1,600	1,600	1,600	2,000	2,000	200	220	220	220
Vitamin E, (IU/kg)	10	10	10	10	10	10	10	10	33	33	33	33
Vitamin K, ppm	0.5	0.5	0.5	0.5	0.5	0.5	0.5	0.5	0.25	0.25	0.25	0.25
Choline, ppm	2,200	2,200	3,000	3,000	3,000	3,000	2,500	2,500	800	800	800	800
Vitamin B_{12}, ppm	0.02	0.025	0.025	0.025	0.025	0.025	0.025	0.025	0.05	0.05	0.04	0.05
Niacin, ppm	75	75	80	80	75	90	75	75	50	30	45	45
Riboflavin, ppm	5.0	6.0	6.0	6.0	6.0	7.0	5.0	5.0	5.0	3.0	3.0	2.5
Thiamin, ppm	5	5	5	5	5	7	4	4	4	4	4	4
Pyridoxine, ppm	5.0	5.0	6.0	6.0	5.0	7.0	6.0	6.0	3.0	2.0	3.5	2.5
Pantothenic acid, ppm	20	20	20	20	20	20	14	14	6	6	6	6
Biotin, ppm	0.075	0.075	0.075	0.075	0.075	0.075	0.05	0.05	0.05	0.05	0.03	0.05
Folic acid, ppm	1.0	1.2	1.2	1.2	1.2	1.2	1.5	1.5	1.2	0.3	0.3	0.3
Sodium, %	0.5	0.5	0.5	0.5	0.5	0.5	0.5	0.5	0.25	0.15	0.5	0.2
Chloride, %	0.65	0.65	0.65	0.65	0.65	0.65	0.65	0.65	0.2	0.15	0.5	0.2
Potassium, %	0.65	0.7	0.7	0.7	0.7	0.8	0.6	0.6	0.3	0.25	0.5	0.2
Magnesium, %	0.14	0.14	0.14	0.14	0.14	0.14	0.12	0.12	0.035	0.05	0.05	0.04
Iron, ppm	250	250	300	300	275	350	235	235	160	100	75	120
Zinc, ppm	90	80	90	90	90	110	70	70	40	40	40	40
Manganese, ppm	45	45	45	45	45	45	40	40	15	15	15	15
Copper, ppm	12.0	11.0	14.0	14.0	12.0	15.0	8.0	8.0	2.5	2.5	2.0	2.0
Iodine, ppm	1.5	1.5	1.5	1.5	1.5	1.5	1.5	1.5	0.75	1.0	1.0	0.75

Courtesy of Ralston Purina Co., St. Louis, MO.

Table 164. COMPOSITION OF CANINE SCIENCE DIETS (HILLS)

(%)	Maintenance		Growth		Lactation	Senior		Performance	Maximum Stress
	Dry	Canned	Dry	Canned	Dry	Dry	Canned		
Moisture	9.0	71.7	9.0	69.4	9.0	9.0	72.8	9.0	9.0
Protein	23.0	7.8	27.0	8.9	26.0	17.0	5.3	31.0	28.0
Fat	14.5	5.5	18.5	6.6	18.5	9.8	4.3	24.0	26.5
Carbohydrate	45.9	12.9	34.5	12.2	35.3	57.2	15.7	26.6	26.8
Fiber	3.3	0.4	3.5	0.6	3.7	3.4	0.7	3.2	3.6
Ash	4.3	1.7	7.5	2.3	7.5	3.6	1.2	6.2	6.1
Calcium	0.6	0.24	1.5	0.4	1.5	0.6	0.23	1.3	1.0
Phosphorus	0.6	0.17	1.2	0.31	1.2	0.5	0.13	1.0	0.81
Sodium	0.33	0.13	0.63	0.12	0.61	0.23	0.08	0.45	0.27
Calories/gm	4.3	1.4	4.3	1.5	4.3	4.0	1.3	4.7	4.8
Calories/cup or can	370	620	410	670	400	320	580	600	600

Courtesy of Hills Packing Co., Topeka, KS.

Table 165. COMPOSITION OF CANNED PRESCRIPTION DIETS
(CANINE)

	g/d		k/d		u/d		s/d	
	As Is (%)	Dry Wt (%)	As Is (%)	Dry Wt (%)	As Is (%)	Dry Wt (%)	As Is (%)	Dry Wt (%)
Moisture	7.3	—	73.3	—	72.1	—	71.0	—
Protein	5.0	18.7	4.3	16.1	2.9	10.4	2.2	7.6
Fat	4.7	17.6	7.3	27.3	7.6	27.2	7.6	26.2
NFE	15.4	57.7	14.1	52.8	16.3	58.4	17.2	59.3
Fiber	0.8	3.0	0.2	0.7	0.4	1.4	0.7	2.4
Ash	0.8	3.0	0.8	3.0	0.7	2.5	1.3	4.5
Calcium	0.23	0.86	0.12	0.45	0.11	0.39	0.08	0.27
Phosphorus	0.12	0.45	0.07	0.26	0.04	0.14	0.04	0.13
Potassium	0.1	0.37	0.08	0.3	0.10	0.36	0.13	0.45
Sodium	0.08	0.3	0.06	0.22	0.07	0.24	0.35	1.2
Kcal/can	585	—	660	—	690	—	690	—
% Protein cal.	16.9	—	13.0	—	8.4	—	6.4	—

Courtesy of Hill Packing Co., Topeka, KS.

Table continued on opposite page

Table 165. COMPOSITION OF CANNED PRESCRIPTION DIETS (CANINE) (*Continued*)

h/d		r/d		p/d		d/d		i/d	
As Is (%)	Dry Wt (%)	As Is (%)	Dry Wt (%)	As Is (%)	Dry Wt (%)	As Is (%)	Dry Wt (%)	As Is (%)	Dry Wt (%)
72.6	—	74.2	—	70.7	—	70.8	—	70.1	—
4.8	17.5	7.1	27.5	9.4	32.1	7.7	26.4	7.6	25.4
7.6	27.7	1.7	6.6	7.8	26.6	5.5	18.8	4.4	14.7
13.6	49.6	9.2	35.7	9.6	32.8	13.8	47.3	15.3	51.2
0.2	0.7	5.6	21.7	0.3	1.0	0.1	0.3	0.2	0.7
1.2	4.4	2.2	8.5	2.2	7.5	2.1	7.2	2.4	8.0
0.15	0.55	0.37	1.4	0.38	1.3	0.33	1.1	0.36	1.2
0.12	0.44	0.28	1.1	0.32	1.1	0.27	0.09	0.27	0.9
0.25	0.79	0.28	1.1	0.24	0.82	0.26	0.89	0.33	1.1
0.03	0.09	0.14	0.05	0.17	0.58	0.18	0.62	0.15	0.5
722	—	330	—	690	—	640	—	620	—
16.6	—	36.6	—	26.8	—	23.7	—	24.2	—

Table 166. COMPOSITION OF CANNED PRESCRIPTION DIETS (FELINE)

	k/d As Is (%)	k/d Dry Wt (%)	p/d As Is (%)	p/d Dry Wt (%)	r/d As Is (%)	r/d Dry Wt (%)	h/d As Is (%)	h/d Dry Wt (%)	s/d As Is (%)	s/d Dry Wt (%)	c/d* As Is (%)	c/d* Dry Wt (%)
Moisture	67.5	—	70.6	—	76.6	—	76.7	—	71.0	—	71.5	—
Protein	8.9	27.4	13.0	44.2	8.1	34.6	12.6	43.0	12.0	41.4	12.5	43.8
Fat	10.8	33.2	8.7	29.6	2.0	8.5	7.8	26.6	9.9	34.1	8.5	29.8
NFE	11.2	34.5	5.0	17.0	6.8	29.0	6.7	22.8	5.3	18.3	5.7	20.0
Fiber	0.2	0.6	0.7	2.4	5.2	22.2	0.5	1.7	0.4	1.4	0.4	1.4
Ash	1.4	4.3	2.0	6.8	1.3	5.6	1.7	5.8	1.4	4.8	1.4	4.9
Calcium	0.18	0.55	0.33	1.12	0.22	0.94	0.24	0.82	0.2	0.69	0.2	0.7
Phosphorus	0.16	0.49	0.23	0.78	0.11	0.47	0.23	0.78	0.16	0.55	0.19	0.7
Potassium	0.26	0.80	0.18	0.61	0.13	0.56	0.22	0.75	0.19	0.66	0.17	0.6
Sodium	0.13	0.4	0.17	0.58	0.14	0.6	0.07	0.24	0.23	0.79	0.15	0.42
Magnesium	0.2	0.07	0.023	0.078	0.014	0.06	0.02	0.07	0.014	0.058	0.02	0.07
Kcal/can	800	—	690	—	360	—	675	—	720	—	680	—
% Protein cal.	20.9	—	35.8	—	43.1	—	35.4	—	31.45	—	—	—

*For c/d diet, substitute manganese for sodium.

Table 167. COMPOSITION OF DRY PRESCRIPTION DIETS

	g/d As Is (%)	g/d Dry Wt (%)	k/d As Is (%)	k/d Dry Wt (%)	u/d As Is (%)	u/d Dry Wt (%)	h/d As Is (%)	h/d Dry Wt (%)	r/d As Is (%)	r/d Dry Wt (%)	i/d As Is (%)	i/d Dry Wt (%)	Feline c/d As Is (%)	Feline c/d Dry Wt (%)
Moisture	9.0	—	9.0	—	9.0	—	9.0	—	9.0	—	9.0	—	9.0	—
Protein	16.8	18.5	13.5	14.8	9.5	10.4	16.2	17.8	24.2	26.6	24.8	27.3	31.0	34.0
Fat	9.7	10.7	18.0	19.7	20.0	21.2	19.0	20.9	5.9	6.5	11.7	12.9	23.7	26.0
NFE	57.7	63.4	56.0	61.5	57.0	62.6	50.9	55.9	35.6	39.1	46.5	51.1	30.2	33.2
Fiber	3.1	3.4	0.8	0.9	2.0	2.2	1.0	1.1	19.0	20.9	0.8	0.88	1.6	1.8
Ash	3.7	4.0	2.7	3.0	2.5	2.7	3.9	4.3	6.3	6.9	7.2	7.9	4.5	4.9
Calcium	0.65	0.71	0.36	0.4	0.37	0.4	0.62	0.68	0.9	1.0	1.3	1.4	0.85	0.92
Phosphorus	0.56	0.61	0.28	0.3	0.17	0.18	0.52	0.57	0.6	0.66	1.1	1.2	0.81	0.89
Potassium	0.32	0.35	0.41	0.45	0.4	0.44	0.75	0.82	0.86	0.95	0.86	0.95	0.45	0.49
Sodium	0.26	0.28	0.21	0.23	0.24	0.26	0.05	0.055	0.05	0.55	0.48	0.52	0.42	0.46
Magnesium	0.09	0.1	0.07	0.08	0.04	0.044	—	—	0.12	0.13	—	—	0.07	0.08
Kcal/cup	300	—	380	—	305	—	365	—	186	—	350	—	600	—
% Protein cal.	18.3	—	12.9	—	8.9	—	15.5	—	34.4	—	26.5	—	28.2	—

Courtesy of Hills Packing Co., Topeka, KS.

Table 168. PRESCRIPTION DIET FEEDING GUIDE* (HILLS)

Product	Form	Weight of Dog						
		5 lb	*10 lb*	*20 lb*	*40 lb*	*60 lb*	*80 lb*	*100 lb*
Canine k/d†	Can(s)	1/3	2/3	1	1 3/4	2 1/2	3	3 2/3
	Cup(s) Dry	2/3	1	2	3 1/3	4 1/2	5 1/2	6 2/3
Canine u/d	Can(s)	1/3	2/3	1	1 3/4	2 1/3	3	3 1/2
	Cup(s) Dry	3/4	1 1/3	2 1/3	4	5 1/3	6 3/4	8
Canine s/d	Can(s)	1/3	2/3	1	1 3/4	2 1/3	3	3 1/2
Canine g/d	Can(s)	1/3	2/3	1 1/5	2	2 2/3	3 1/3	4
	Cup(s) Dry	3/4	1 1/3	2 1/3	4	5 1/3	6 2/3	8
Canine h/d	Can(s)	1/3	2/3	1	1 3/4	2 1/2	3	3 2/3
	Cup(s) Dry	2/3	1	2	3 1/3	4 1/3	5 1/2	6 1/2
Canine i/d	Can(s)	1/3	2/3	1	2	2 1/2	3 1/4	3 3/4
	Cup(s) Dry	1/2	1	2	3 1/2	4 1/2	5 3/4	7
Canine r/d	Can(s)	1/3	2/3	1	1 3/4	2 1/3	2 3/4	3 1/3
	Cup(s) Dry	2/3	1	1 3/4	3	4	5	6
Canine d/d	Can(s)	1/3	2/3	1	2	2 1/2	3	3 3/4
	Feed Ad Lib approximate daily intake at age:	Estimated Mature Weight						
		5 lb	*10 lb*	*20 lb*	*40 lb*	*60 lb*	*80 lb*	*100 lb*
Canine p/d	Amount to Feed Daily at Age: 15 3/4 oz can — 6 wk	1/8	1/4	1/2	1 1/8	1 3/4	2 1/2	2 3/4
	8 wk	1/6	1/3	2/3	1 1/3	2	2 2/3	3 1/8
	3 mo	1/4	1/2	3/4	1 2/3	2 3/4	3 1/2	4
	6 mo	1/3	2/3	1	2 1/2	4	5	6

		Weight of Cat			
		5 lb	7–8 lb	10 lb	15 lb
Feline c/d	Can(s), Cup(s) Dry	1/4	1/3	2/5	3/5
Feline k/d	Can(s)	1/5	1/3	2/5	1/2
Feline h/d	Can(s)	1/4	1/3	2/5	3/5
Feline r/d	Can(s)	1/3	1/2	3/5	3/4
Feline s/d	Can(s)	1/4	1/3	2/5	3/5

			Age of Kitten			
		6 wks	2 mos	3 mos	4 mos	5 mos
Feline p/d Can						
Growing Kittens Feed Ad Lib		1/8	1/8	1/5	1/4	1/3

				Age of Kittens				
		1 wk	2 wk	3 wk	4 wk	5 wk	6 wk	7 wk
Lactating	Wt. of Queen:							
Queens	Feed Ad Lib							
	5 lb	1/4	1/4	1/3	2/5	1/2	2/5	1/4
	7–8 lb	1/3	1/3	2/5	1/2	2/3	1/2	1/3
	10 lb	2/5	2/5	1/2	2/3	4/5	2/3	2/5

*These average intakes are useful as starting points only and should be adjusted to maintain optimum body weight. Feeding should be based on *desired weight* rather than *obese weight*. The quantity of food in chart is minimal amount of Feline p/d for a queen with a small litter. Large litters will require more food for the queen. As kittens begin to eat solids, their food is added to these amounts.

†k/d = kidney diet; u/d = urologic diet; h/d = heart diet; i/d = intestinal diet; r/d = reducing diet; d/d = dermatologic diet; g/d = geriatric diet; p/d = protein diet; c/d = cat diet; and s/d = "stone" diet.

From Hill Packing Company, Topeka, KS.

Table 169. RECOMMENDED DAILY METABOLIZABLE ENERGY
ALLOWANCES FOR CATS*

Kittens (wk of age)	Kcal/kg BW†	Adult‡	Kcal/kg BW
10	250	inactive	70
20	130	active	85
30	100	gestation	100
40	80	lactation	250

*Metabolizable energy allowances based on 4 kcal/gm of dietary protein and
carbohydrate (nitrogen-free extract), and 9 kcal/gm of dietary fat. These allowances are
presumed to apply in a thermoneutral environment (approximately 22° C).
†Body weight.
‡Fifty weeks of age and older.
From Nutrient Requirements of Cats. Publication No. 13. Washington, D.C.,
National Academy of Sciences–National Research Council, 1978.

Text continued from page 853

Physical Activity

The objective is to increase the caloric density of the diet, so that a small
volume of highly digestible food provides abundant energy. This is achieved
by adding fat so that caloric density is increased to 2200 to 2500 kcal per lb of
food. Three to 6 tablespoons of fat may be *added* per pound of food, or a
balanced, high fat commercially prepared diet may be fed.

Start feeding the high energy diet 2 to 3 days before activity is begun.
Feed ⅔ of the daily nutrient needs in the morning of activity, and give the
balance in several small feedings during the day.

Feed special foods such as Maximum Stress Diet, Science Diet Performance, ANF, or Eukanuba. See Table 170 for caloric requirements of dogs,
based on physical activity.

Aged Animals

Decreasing metabolic rate with aging means decreased energy requirements. Older animals need highly digestible ingredients, with moderation in
items such as fat, protein, minerals, and salt. There are numerous commercially
prepared diets available that incorporate these dietary modifications. Diet
modification may be needed to accommodate a variety of disease processes in
individual pets.

Growth

Weigh the young weekly, and chart their growth. They should increase in
weight every day from birth. The young should be started on solid food at 3
weeks of age to supplement nursing and to reduce dependence on mother's
milk.

Table 170. CALORIE REQUIREMENTS FOR ADULT DOGS BASED ON
PHYSICAL ACTIVITY AND BREED SIZE*

	Mature Weight Kg.	Lb.	House Dog† Calories	Active Dog‡ Calories	Working Dog§ Calories
	2.3	5	200	250	300
Small	4.5	10	400	500	600
Breeds	6.8	15	600	750	900
	9.1	20	800	1000	1200
	9.1	20	560	700	840
	11.4	25	700	875	1050
	13.6	30	840	1050	1260
	15.9	35	930	1225	1470
	18.2	40	1120	1400	1680
Medium	20.5	45	1260	1575	1890
Breeds	22.7	50	1400	1750	2100
	25.0	55	1540	1925	2310
	27.3	60	1680	2100	2520
	29.5	65	1820	2275	2730
	31.8	70	1980	2450	2940
	34.1	75	2100	2625	3150
	34.1	75	1800	2250	2700
	36.4	80	1980	2400	2880
	38.6	85	2040	2550	3060
	40.9	90	2160	2700	3240
	43.2	95	2280	2850	3420
	45.5	100	2400	3000	3600
	47.7	105	2520	3150	3780
Large	50.0	110	2640	3300	3960
Breeds	52.3	115	2760	3450	4140
	54.5	120	2880	3600	4320
	56.8	125	3000	3750	4500
	59.1	130	3120	3900	4680
	61.4	135	3240	4050	4860
	63.6	140	3360	4200	5040
	65.9	145	3480	4350	5220
	68.2	150	3600	4500	5400

*These are average daily requirements. Animals may vary according to age, breed,
temperature, and degree of activity. Owing to temperament, there is some overlap
between the largest animals of some breeds and the smallest of others.

†Caloric requirements of house dogs = adult dogs maintained in laboratory cages.

‡Active dogs = adult dogs allowed to free run in outside pens, 125 to 480 square
feet in size.

§Working dogs = adult dogs running at 5 mph on a 6 per cent incline for 4 hours
each day.

Data courtesy of Ralston Purina Company, St. Louis, Missouri.

Table 171. RECOMMENDED DAILY CALORIC INTAKE FIRST FOUR
WEEKS OF LIFE

Dog			Cats (Estimated)	
Kcal/oz BW	Kcal/gm BW	Week	Kcal/gm BW	Kcal/oz BW
3.8	0.133	1	0.20	5.7
4.4	0.155	2	0.22	6.3
5.0–5.7	0.175–0.20	3	0.27	7.7
5.7+	0.20+	4	0.29	8.3

After fourth week, see Tables 154 (for dogs) and 169 (for cats).
Amount of formula per day (ml) = weight of young (in gms) times kcal factor (/gm BW)
for age.

Feed only a balanced diet that has proved to be nutritionally adequate for
growth in the amounts indicated in Table 171. Do not overfeed; keep young
animals thin and growing at a conservative normal rate.

Newborn and Orphaned Animals

Feed a milk substitute (as indicated in Table 172) in sufficient amounts to
provide the proper caloric intake (see Table 171). Feed by gavage or baby
bottle (*not* with eye dropper) in 3 or 4 portions during the day.

The following formulas may also be used:

Emergency Formula 1. Refrigerate, but warm and mix well before using.
Use 1 part boiled water, 5 parts evaporated milk, and 1 teaspoon of dicalcium
phosphate per quart of formula (contains 1.0 cal/ml). *Note:* Evaporated milk
must be diluted to give adequate H_2O.

Table 172. COMPOSITION OF MATERNAL MILK AND SUBSTITUTES

	Kcal Per MI	% Solids	Fat	Protein	Carbo-hydrate
Bitch milk	1.5	24.0	44.1	33.2	15.8
Esbilac powder*†	1.0	98.4	44.1	33.2	15.8
Esbilac liquid*	0.9	15.3	44.1	33.2	15.8
Cow milk	0.7	12.0	30.0	25.6	38.5
Evaporated milk‡	1.2	14.0	15.8	13.9	19.5
Cat milk	0.9	18.2	25.0	42.2	26.1
KMR*	0.9	18.2	25.0	42.2	26.1

*Manufactured by Pet-Vet Products, Borden Chemical Company, Borden, Inc.,
Norfolk, Virginia 23501.
†1 volume to 3 volumes water.
‡4 volumes to 1 volume water.

Table 173. TEMPERATURE GUIDE FOR RAISING ORPHANS

Age of Puppy	Environmental Temperature
Birth–5 days	85°F–90°F
6–20 days	80°F
21–28 days	78°F
29–35 days	75°F
After 35 days	70°F

Age of Kitten	Environmental Temperature
Birth–7 days	80°F–92°F
8–14 days	80°F–85°F
15–28 days	80°F
29–35 days	75°F
After 35 days	70°F

Emergency Formula 2. Refrigerate, but warm and mix well before using. Use 8 ounces of homogenized whole milk, 1 teaspoon of salad oil, 1 drop of infant multiple vitamins, and 2 egg yolks (contains 1.2 cal/ml).

Following each feeding, burp the young animal; wash the abdomen and perineum with warm water to stimulate urination and defecation after each feeding. Dry and massage the animal gently.

Keep the young in separate compartments in a thermostatically controlled, heated environment at temperatures listed in Table 173.

Isolate the young, and do not handle them needlessly.

At 3 weeks of age, start the young on semi-solid foods such as gruels made from dry or canned puppy diets. Follow the feeding guides shown in previous tables. Weaning should follow easily at 5 to 7 weeks of age.

SPECIAL PROBLEMS IN FEEDING CATS

Most of the general principles given for feeding dogs also apply to cats. However, the following statements highlight important differences:

1. Never give cats dog food or feed them human-type diets.

   Cats need high-caloric density and high-protein diets.

   Cats cannot convert methionine or cysteine to taurine, and deficiency of the latter causes retinal degeneration.

   Cats need both linoleic and arachidonic acids (the latter is present only in animal fat); dogs need only linoleic acid (present in both animal and vegetable fats).

   Cats cannot convert tryptophan to niacin.

   Cats cannot convert beta carotene to vitamin A.

   Cats must have arginine; dogs do not need it.

2. Feed only balanced and complete cat rations, and *do not supplement* them.

3. Feed a nutritionally adequate (proven by feeding tests) food containing multiple ingredients.

Cats may become addicted to single-ingredient foods (such as liver or tuna) if given exclusively.

Excess amounts of single items may have harmful effects such as (a) liver may produce vitamin A toxicity; (b) fish may produce excess unsaturated fatty acids and a relative vitamin E deficiency; and (c) raw fish contains thiaminase, which destroys thiamine.

4. Dry cat food may be used to self-feed cats. However, if urinary problems develop, foods should be limited to those containing a maximum of 5 per cent ash (0.1 per cent magnesium). It is important to keep the water intake high to help minimize urinary disorders. Always keep fresh water available.

Supportive Alimentation (See p. 582)

Obesity

Frequently seen in older pets, obesity occurs most commonly in animals fed noncommercial diets by older people or highly palatable canned meat–type foods. Protein and fat restriction will reduce caloric intake.

Procedure for Weight Reduction

1. Hospitalize and evaluate the animal for metabolic disorders.
2. Withhold all food, and give the animal only water and vitamin-mineral supplements. This may be a workable but unrealistic method. Instead, it may be better to feed a restricted calorie reducing diet, especially designed for the particular species, in an amount to maintain optimum weight.
3. Provide daily exercise and human companionship.
4. Chart weight at weekly intervals. The animal will lose approximately 4 per cent of its body per week.

After 4 to 8 weeks (or when weight is optimum), start feeding unmoistened, good-quality balanced dry food (not *too* palatable) in the proper amount for ideal weight. Foods such as Fit and Trim, Cycle 3, Dry r/d, and Feline r/d are suitable. Instruct the owner of the animal to chart weight weekly and to continue the diet and exercise regimen, stressing that they give the animal no snacks. The animal may also continue to be fed the reducing diet in larger amounts once the desired weight is achieved. A recipe for a homemade reducing diet is on page 875.

RENAL DISEASE

In the medical management of acute and chronic renal failure, it is desirable to reduce the production of metabolic products that cause the clinical signs and that can cause the renal dysfunction to worsen. The restriction of dietary proteins is indicated to minimize production of waste products from the catabolism of proteins, that is, organic acids and sulfates.

Protein intake must be adjusted depending on the severity of the renal failure. Dogs placed on diets that supply protein below their requirement level will become protein depleted.

The aim of feeding diets that contain reduced protein of high biologic value is to minimize metabolic wastes and to keep the BUN as near normal (20 mg/dl) as possible. Initiate management by feeding Prescription Diet k/d (16.1 per cent protein). If and when the BUN rises to above 50 mg per dl, feed u/d (10.5 per cent protein).

Reducing phosphorus intake to prevent phosphorus retention and hyperparathyroidism is as important as reducing protein intake. Phosphorus has been shown to accelerate the rate of progression of renal failure. Phosphorus must be controlled by feeding a phosphorus-restricted diet. It cannot be completely managed with phosphate binders. The diet should be as low as possible, but in no event should it be above 0.5 per cent phosphorus in the dry matter. See Table 168 for specific feeding guidelines or page 875 for homemade recipes.

Dietary Management of Chronic Polyuric Renal Failure

1. Provide unlimited access to fresh water.
2. Dietary regulation is extremely important. Protein deficiency and excess protein may both have deleterious consequences in the dog with renal disease. Each animal must be evaluated individually, but, for best effect, diet regulation must be started early, when the specific gravity of the urine is decreased. Indications to begin the use of protein restrictive diets are fixed urine specific gravity, development of azotemia, and hyperphosphatemia.
3. Two commercial dietary foods—namely, Prescription Diet k/d (16 per cent protein) and Prescription Diet u/d (10 per cent protein)—are available. Both products contain approximately 250 mg of sodium per 100 gm of dry diet and supply 35 mg of sodium per kg of body weight if fed at a level of 70 kcal per kg of body weight per day. Selection of the diet to be used is dependent on the individual animal's response to treatment and control of azotemia.

   Do not make sudden changes from normal commercial foods that contain higher protein and sodium levels to Prescription Diets. These changes may alter sodium intake too radically, reducing extracellular fluid volume. A more gradual change to lower sodium Prescription Diet k/d or u/d is advocated.
4. Chronic polyuric renal failure is often associated with systemic metabolic acidosis (see p. 125). Measurements of blood bicarbonate, blood pH, or urine pH are guides to whether oral sodium bicarbonate is indicated. Blood bicarbonate concentration less than 18 mEq per L or urine pH of 5.5 or lower are indications for beginning sodium bicarbonate therapy (5–30 grains TID) to bring the blood bicarbonate level to a more normal, 18 to 26 mEq per L range. Administer sodium bicarbonate in gradually increasing amounts.
5. Hyperphosphatemia associated with chronic renal insufficiency should be managed by dietary regulation. In advanced renal disease, administration of oral phosphate binding agents (Amphojel, Basajel) is also indicated. Serum phosphorus levels should be reduced to 3.0 to 4.5 mg per dl. Oral phosphate binders can be administered, 300 to 500 mg TID.

6. Anabolic steroids may be used in chronic renal failure to aid in controlling nonresponsive anemias and to increase general body condition. Use agents such as nandrolene decanoate, testosterone enanthate, stanozolol, and oxymethalone (see p. 928).

CARDIOVASCULAR DISEASE—LOW-SODIUM DIET

A low-sodium diet is used in animals with congestive heart failure. Moderate restriction is less than 300 mg per 100 gm of dry diet; severe restriction is less than 100 mg per 100 gm of dry diet. A ranking of the available diets is as follows: canned foods, 1000 mg per 100 gm of dry diet; soft-moist, 700 mg per 100 gm of dry diet; dry foods, 450 mg per 100 gm of dry diet; k/d, 250 mg per 100 gm of dry weight; canned h/d, 90 mg per 100 gm of dry diet; dry h/d, 50 mg per 100 gm of dry diet; and homemade diet, 50 mg per 100 gm of dry diet. Use the appropriate diet to provide the degree of sodium restriction needed. Avoid "softened water" (or even tap water if above 150 ppm), using distilled water if necessary. Avoid all snacks, tidbits, and treats. See Table 174 for a homemade recipe.

Text continued on page 877

Table 174. RECIPES FOR HOMEMADE DIETARY FOODS

Recipe 1 *Highly Digestible Diet for Dogs*	Recipe 2 *Restricted Protein/Phosphorus Diet for Dogs*
½ cup farina (Cream of Wheat) cooked to make 2 cups 1½ cups creamed cottage cheese 1 large hard-cooked egg 2 T brewers yeast 3 T sugar 1 T vegetable oil 1 t potassium chloride 2 t dicalcium phosphate Balanced supplement that fulfills the canine MDR for all vitamins and trace minerals Cook farina according to package directions. Cool. Add remaining ingredients to farina and mix well. Yield: 2 lb	¼ lb ground beef (regular)* 1 large hard-cooked egg 2 cups cooked rice 3 slices white bread, crumbled 1 t calcium carbonate Balanced supplement that fulfills the canine MDR for all vitamins and trace minerals *Do not use lean ground round or chuck. Braise the meat, retaining fat. Combine all ingredients and mix well. This mixture is somewhat dry and the palatability can be improved by adding some water (not milk). Yield: 1¼ lb

<table>
<tr><td colspan="2" align="center">Analysis</td><td colspan="2" align="center">Analysis</td></tr>
<tr><td>Moisture %</td><td>7.50</td><td>Moisture %</td><td>66.0</td></tr>
<tr><td>Protein %</td><td>7.3</td><td>Protein %</td><td>6.4</td></tr>
<tr><td>Fat %</td><td>3.7</td><td>Fat %</td><td>5.0</td></tr>
<tr><td>Carbohydrate %</td><td>9.6</td><td>Carbohydrate %</td><td>21.0</td></tr>
<tr><td>Calories</td><td>480 kcal/lb</td><td>Ash %</td><td>1.6</td></tr>
</table>

Phosphorus %.................... 0.1
Sodium %........................ 0.1
Calories†.................. 740 kcal/lb

†This diet supplies 17% protein calories, 30% fat calories, and 53% carbohydrate calories.

Recipe 3
Restricted Purine/Phosphorus Ultra Low–Protein Diet for Dogs

2½ cups cooked rice
1 oz vegetable oil
2 large hard-cooked eggs
¼ t calcium carbonate
Balanced supplement that fulfills the canine MDR for all vitamins and trace minerals

Cook rice as per package instructions. Add other ingredients and mix well. Refrigerate between feedings. Yield: 1¼ lb

Analysis

Moisture %..................... 68.6
Protein %...................... 3.5
Fat %.......................... 6.7
Carbohydrate %................. 19.3
Ash %.......................... 1.9
Calcium %...................... 0.10
Phosphorus %................... 0.05
Sodium %....................... 0.05
Calories*.................. 720 kcal/lb

*This diet supplies 12% protein calories, 38% fat calories, and 50% carbohydrate calories.

Recipe 4
Low-Fat-Reducing Diet for Dogs

¼ lb lean ground beef
½ cup cottage cheese, **uncreamed**
2 cups carrots, canned solids
2 cups green beans, canned solids
1½ t calcium phosphate
Balanced supplement that fulfills the canine MDR for all vitamins and trace minerals

Cook beef, drain fat, and cool. Yield: 1¾ lb

Analysis

Moisture %..................... 85.0
Protein %...................... 7.0
Fat %.......................... 1.7
Carbohydrate %................. 5.0
Calories................... 300 kcal/lb

Recipe 5
Low-Sodium Diet for Dogs

¼ lb lean ground beef
2 cups cooked rice
1 T vegetable oil
2 t dicalcium phosphate
Balanced supplement that fulfills the canine MDR for all vitamins and trace minerals

Braise meat, retaining fat. Add the remaining ingredients and mix. Yield: 1 lb

Analysis

Moisture %..................... 70.0
Protein %...................... 8.0
Fat %.......................... 5.6
Carbohydrate %................. 16.0
Sodium* %...................... 0.01
Calories................... 700 kcal/lb

*50 mg of sodium/100 gm of dry diet

Recipe 6
Hypoallergenic Diet for Dogs or Cats

4 oz cooked lamb
1 cup cooked rice
1 t vegetable oil
1½ t dicalcium phosphate
Balanced supplement that fulfills the canine MDR for all vitamins and trace minerals

Do not season meat during cooking, and discard excess fat. Combine all ingredients and mix well. Yield: ¾ lb

Analysis

Moisture % 65.0
Protein % 10.0
Fat % 8.0
Carbohydrates % 15.3
Calories . . . . 800 kcal/lb

Recipe 7
Liquid Diet for Dogs or Cats

8 oz Prescription Diet i/d canned
2 oz vegetable oil
20 oz water
Blend to liquid consistency in a blender.
Yield: 30 oz

Analysis

Moisture % 84.6
Protein % 2.4
Fat % 7.8
Carbohydrate % 5.2
Calories . . . . 30 kcal/oz

Daily dose (dog or cat): 1 oz/lb body weight. Fulfills all normal fluid and nutrient needs. Excessive fluid losses must be replaced by additional water or parenteral fluids.

Recipe 8
Restricted Mineral and Sodium Diet for Cats

1 lb regular ground beef, cooked
¼ lb liver, cooked
1 cup cooked rice
1 t vegetable oil
1 t calcium carbonate

Balanced supplement that fulfills the feline MDR for all vitamins and trace minerals

Combine all ingredients. Yield: 1¾ lb

Analysis

Moisture % 64.0
Protein % 14.1
Fat % 13.8
Carbohydrate % 6.6
Ash % 1.5
Calcium % 0.24
Phosphorus % 0.15
Magnesium % 0.014
Magnesium, mg/100 kcal 8
Sodium % 0.04
Calories . . . . 975 kcal/lb

Recipe 9
Restricted Protein/Phosphorus Diet for Cats

¼ lb cooked liver
1 large hard-cooked egg
2 cups cooked rice
1 T fat (bacon grease or vegetable oil)
1 t calcium carbonate
Balanced supplement that fulfills the feline MDR for all vitamins and trace minerals

Braise the meat, retaining fat. Dice or grind liver and egg. Combine all ingredients and mix well. This mixture is somewhat dry, and the palatability may be improved by adding some water (not milk). Yield: 1¼ lb

Analysis

Moisture %......................66.8
Protein %...................... 8.7
Fat %............................ 6.2
Carbohydrate %................18.3
Ash %......................... 2.0
Calcium %..................... 0.3
Phosphorus %.................. 0.16
Sodium %...................... 0.03
Calories.................. 780 kcal/lb

Recipe 10
Low-Fat-Reducing Diet for Cats

1¼ lb liver, cooked and ground
1 cup cooked rice
1 t vegetable oil
1 t calcium carbonate
Balanced supplement that fulfills the
    feline MDR for all vitamins and
    trace minerals

Combine all ingredients. Yield: 1¾ lb

Analysis

Moisture %......................71.8
Protein %......................15.3
Fat %.......................... 3.4
Ash %......................... 1.4
Calcium %..................... 0.2
Phosphorus %.................. 0.2
Calories.................. 534 kcal/lb

Recipes supplied by Mark Morris Associates, Topeka, KS. See also Lewis, L. D., and Morris, M. L., Jr.: Small Animal Clinical Nutrition, 2nd ed. Topeka, Kansas, Mark Morris Associates, 1984.

Text continued from page 874

HEPATIC DISEASE—(MEAT-FREE, LOW-PROTEIN DIETS)

Dietary Therapy for Chronic Hepatic Insufficiency

The basic premise of this diet is to decrease food residue in the colon by feeding a diet that is almost 100 per cent digestible. It should be balanced and complete, but meat-free and low in protein.

The following diet is based on the recommendations provided by Strombeck and contains the following ingredients as measured in gm per 100 gm of dry weight: casein, 9.0; animal fat, 20.0; sucrose, 32.35; corn starch, 32.35; vitamin mix, 1.0; mineral mix, 5.0; and choline chloride, 0.3.

DIET 1

	Gm (As Is) Per Batch	Oz (As Is) Per Batch	Measurements* (As Is) Per Batch
Instant non-fat dry milk *fortified* with vitamins A and D	208	7 3/8	3 C
Blackstrap molasses†	133	4 3/4	2/5 C (between 1/3 and 1/2 cup)
Wheat germ, raw ground if possible‡	114	4	1 C and 2 T (1 1/8 C)
Bone meal§	37	1 3/10	1/5 C
Safflower oil	100	3 1/2	1/2 C
Animal fat‖	100	3 1/2	1/2 C
Table salt, *iodized***	10	3/8	1 1/2 t
Cornstarch	403	14 1/5	3 C
Vitamin C (ascorbic acid††)	Provide vitamin C as a supplement at 10 mg/lb BW/day.		
Choline‡‡	A dog weighing 33 lb or less should be given 250 mg of choline per day; 500 mg per day should be given to larger dogs.		

*C = cup, T = tablespoon, t = teaspoon. If possible, ingredients should be weighed rather than measured, because weighing is more accurate.

†Blackstrap molasses is available at most health food stores and in some supermarkets. Blackstrap is the most "crude" form of molasses available and is highest in nutritional quality (i.e., has the highest mineral content).

‡Raw wheat germ is available in bulk in most health food stores. The toasted wheat germ available in supermarkets is not acceptable. Raw wheat germ spoils fairly quickly, so it should be bought fresh regularly. If the equipment is available, the wheat germ should be ground into smaller particles, using a coffee mill, mortar and pestle, or blender.

§Bone meal is available at pet care stores. It should be the kind prepared specifically for consumption by animals, i.e., sterilized.

‖Lard or beef tallow may be used. Because the type of fat used is an important component of a diet's palatability, this choice should be tailored to the individual animal's taste.

**If a lower sodium content is desired, the NaCl level may be reduced. However, if the diet is to be fed over a long period of time, an additional source of iodine, an essential nutrient, must be provided. See discussion following Diet 2.

††See discussion following Diet 2.

‡‡Choline tablets (either choline chloride or choline bitartrate) can be bought at health food stores. Also, see discussion following Diet 2.

From Strombeck, D., et al.: *In* Kirk, R. W. (ed.): Current Veterinary Therapy VIII: Small Animal Practice. Philadelphia, W. B. Saunders Company, 1983, pp. 814–821.

In mixing Diet 1, use a blender to mix wheat germ and cold safflower oil. Salt, bone meal, and corn starch should be mixed separately and added. Add dry instant milk and molasses, and mix.

This diet should be refrigerated, and a portion can be frozen. The diet provides 4.6 kcal per gm of dry weight. As described in Diet 1, a batch of this diet will feed one 33-lb dog for 4 days.

Strombeck has also developed a second diet:

DIET 2

	Measurements Per Batch*
Low-fat cottage cheese	2 lb
Animal fat†	1/2 lb
Safflower oil	1/4 C
Sugar	1 lb plus 3 T
Cornstarch	1 lb plus 5 T
Bone meal‡	1 1/3 oz (a little less than 1/4 C)
Salt substitute (KCl) *iodized*§	3 1/4 t
Table salt (NaCl) *iodized*‖	2 t
Vitamin C (ascorbic acid)**	Provided as supplement at 10 mg/lb BW/day
Choline††	Provided as supplement: 33-lb dog or less, 250-mg tablet per day; large dogs, 500 mg per day
Centrum‡‡	High-potency multivitamin and multimineral formula designed for human use; one tablet daily

*C = cup, T = tablespoon, t = teaspoon. If possible, ingredients should be weighed rather than measured, because weighing is more accurate.

†Lard or beef tallow may be used. Because the type of fat used is an important component of a diet's palatability, this choice should be tailored to the individual animal's taste.

‡Bone meal is available at pet care stores. It should be the kind prepared specifically for consumption by animals, i.e., sterilized.

§Only iodized salt (e.g., that manufactured by Schilling) should be used. This addition is important, because the diet would otherwise be very low in K⁺, and dogs with hepatic insufficiency are often depleted of potassium owing to vomiting, diarrhea, increased renal losses, and reduced food intake. Note that salt substitute (KCl) is not the same as "Lite Salt," which is a combination of NaCl and KCl.

‖If a lower sodium content is desired, the NaCl level may be reduced. However, if the diet is to be fed over a long period of time, an additional source of iodine, an essential nutrient, must be provided. See discussion following Diet 2.

**See discussion following Diet 2.

††Choline tablets (either choline chloride or choline bitartrate) can be bought at health food stores. Also, see discussion following Diet 2.

‡‡Centrum (Lederle) is widely available.

From Strombeck, D., et al.: *In* Kirk, R. W. (ed.): Current Veterinary Therapy VIII: Small Animal Practice. Philadelphia, W. B. Saunders Company, 1983, pp. 817–821.

In formulating this diet, mix the sugar, corn starch, bone meal, and salt together. Blend animal fat (at room temperature) with the sugar mixture. Mix the cottage cheese and safflower oil, and blend this into the other ingredients.

This diet must also be refrigerated. It is more expensive to prepare than Diet 1. It provides 4.7 kcal per gm of dry weight and 3.2 kcal per gm of wet weight.

Dry Prescription k/d approximates the above formulas in that it is meat-free and low in protein. However, it has lower digestibility, more fiber, and poorer quality protein.

Special diets for animals with hepatic disease must be continued indefinitely or until the liver function tests have returned to normal.

GASTROINTESTINAL DISEASE—HIGHLY DIGESTIBLE DIET

The highly digestible diet is indicated when it is necessary to provide nutrients that are digested and absorbed with low residue. The diet should be low in fat, low in fiber, and moderate in protein, with easily digested carbohydrates. (For constipation, a high fiber diet is indicated.) Use a commercially available (i/d) or homemade diet such as the one provided on page 875.

ALLERGIC DISEASE—HYPOALLERGENIC DIET

In suspected cases of food-induced allergy, a hypoallergenic diet containing items not commonly fed to the animal is indicated. Avoid all regular commercial foods (they have many ingredients). Semi-moist foods in particular are to be avoided. Give the homemade hypoallergenic diet (p. 875) and distilled water for 2 weeks. Then expose the animal to individual items (such as tap water, beef, or wheat) to determine which are the offending items. If the diet produces no response, food can be ruled out as a cause. *Feed only the test diet,* and *do not give snacks!*

Hypoallergenic Diet.* Use 4 oz of cooked lamb, 1 cup of cooked rice, 1 tsp of corn oil, 1½ tsp of dicalcium phosphate, and a balanced supplement that fulfills the canine MDR for all vitamins and trace minerals. Do not season the meat during cooking, and discard the excess fat. Combine all ingredients and mix well. *Yield:* ¾ lb. *Analysis:* moisture (%), 65.0; protein (%), 10.0; fat (%), 8.0; carbohydrate (%), 15.3; and calories, 800 kcal per lb. Feed 1 lb to a 20-lb dog, 2 lb to a 60-lb dog, and 3 lb to a 100-lb dog.

UROLITHIASIS—CALCULOLYTIC DIETS

Dogs with struvite uroliths (see p. 864) can be managed with Prescription Diet s/d fed twice daily in an amount to maintain optimum body weight (see

---

*Formula for homemade hypoallergenic diet supplied by Mark Morris Associates, Topeka, Kansas.

Table 168). It takes from 2 to 20 weeks, with an average of 8 weeks for the calculi to dissolve. Only struvite calculi can be dissolved by diet, and the client must not supplement the diet with other foods or vitamin-mineral supplements. Because of its high sodium content, s/d diet should not be fed to dogs with heart failure, edema, or ascites. Important points to remember before using a calculolytic diet include:

1. If urinary tract infection is present, obtain a urine culture and treat with appropriate antibiotics.
2. In adult male dogs, determine the probable type of urolith present (see p. 825).
3. Follow the animal's progress with monthly radiographs to observe changes in calculi while on s/d diet. Feed the calculolytic diet for 1 month after the uroliths are no longer visible.
4. After the uroliths have disappeared, change the diet to regular maintenance food. If the uroliths recur, dissolve them with s/d and prevent further recurrence with Prescription Diet u/d.

In forms of urolithiasis other than struvite calculi, mineral and protein restricted diets (u/d or k/d) may help prevent recurrence. Other forms of therapy, including acidification of the urine or the use of sodium bicarbonate, allopurinol, or D-penicillamine, may be indicated (see p. 928).

DALMATIAN DIET—RESTRICTED PURINE, PHOSPHORUS, AND ULTRA LOW-PROTEIN DIET

Used in Dalmatians or other dogs with hyperuricosuria, urate uroliths, and secondary urinary and skin infections. A meat-free rice and vegetable diet supplemented with vitamin B complex, B_{12}, and fat-soluble vitamins is indicated. Two commonly used recipes are included.

Restricted Purine/Phosphorus Ultra Low–Protein Diet. See page 875 for homemade recipe.

Dalmatian Research Foundation Recipe*

1. Prepare vegetable puree and rice as follows:
   a. *Vegetable puree* (multiple batch). Use three #1 cans of carrots†; three #1 cans of peas†; three #1 cans of green beans†; three #1 cans of tomatoes†; one 10-oz package of broccoli (chopped, frozen); and one #1 can of greens† (kale, dock, spinach, or mustard greens). Boil the broccoli in 2 cups of water until tender. Combine with other vegetables in a large kettle, mix, and puree thoroughly until smooth. Fill 18 1-pint plastic containers and freeze.
   b. *Rice* (make as needed). Use 2½ cups of rice (broken bits, cheapest grade); 5 cups of water; ⅓ cup of corn oil; 1 teaspoon of salt; and ¼ cup of bacon fat. Mix the ingredients, and boil vigorously. Reduce heat, and simmer until water is absorbed. Cook (should weigh 4½ pounds).

---

*Dalmatian Research Foundation recipe from Muller, G. H., and Kirk, R. W.: Small Animal Dermatology. Philadelphia, W. B. Saunders Company, 1976, p. 592.
†Do not drain these cans of vegetables.

2. Thaw 1 pint of vegetable puree, and add to rice, mixing thoroughly.
3. Feed adult Dalmatians 1½ to 2 cups, three times daily. Do not overfeed. Keep weight stable. Do not add meat supplements.
4. Thin or vigorous dogs may receive small amounts of cottage cheese (1–2 oz), additional fat, and toast, if needed.

References and Additional Readings

Lewis, L. D., and Morris, M. L., Jr.: Small Animal Clinical Nutrition. Topeka, Kansas, Mark Morris Associates, 1983.

Nutrient Requirements of Cats. Washington, D.C., National Academy of Sciences–National Research Council Publication No. 13, 1978.

Nutrient Requirements of Dogs. Washington, D.C., National Academy of Sciences–National Research Council Publication No. 8, 1974.

Polzin, D. J., and Osborne, C. A.: Conservative management of canine chronic polyuric renal failure. In Kirk, R. W. (ed.): Current Veterinary Therapy VIII: Small Animal Practice. Philadelphia, W. B. Saunders Company, 1983.

Renegar, W. R., et al.: Parenteral hyperalimentation—Use of lipid as prime caloric source. J.A.A.H.A., *151*:411, 1979.

Sheffy, B. E.: Nutrition and nutritional disorders. In Mosier, J. E. (ed.): Symposium on pediatrics. Vet. Clin. North Am., *8*:7, 1978.

Strombeck, D. R.: Diet and nutrition in the management of gastrointestinal problems. In Kirk, R. W. (ed.): Current Veterinary Therapy VIII. Philadelphia, W. B. Saunders Company, 1980, pp. 919–929.

Strombeck, D. R.: Dietary therapy with chronic hepatic insufficiency. In Kirk, R. W. (ed.): Current Veterinary Therapy VIII: Small Animal Practice. Philadelphia, W. B. Saunders Company, 1983.

NORMAL PHYSIOLOGIC DATA

See Tables 175 to 177.

Canine and Feline Growth Curves

See Figures 104 and 105.

A Roster of Normal Values for Dogs and Cats

See Tables 178–186.*

Age, gender, breed, diurnal periodicity, and emotional stress at the time of sampling can be expected to cause variation in normal values. The methodology will also affect the biologic parameters. For this reason, practitioners are

Text continued on page 909

---

*Material (except for Table 178) provided courtesy of John Bentinck-Smith, D.V.M., Ithaca, New York.

Table 175. 63-DAY PERPETUAL GESTATION

In each month pair the top line is the day of conception (1–31) and the line below is the corresponding due date. The middle column names the month into which the later due dates fall; the overflow column gives those high conception days and their due dates in the following month.

Conception	Due (month)	1	2	3	4	5	6	7	8	9	10	11	12	13	14	15	16	17	18	19	20	21	22	23	24	25	26	27	28	29	30	31	Overflow (conception day → due day, next month)
Jan.	March	5	6	7	8	9	10	11	12	13	14	15	16	17	18	19	20	21	22	23	24	25	26	27	28	29	30	31					April: 28→1, 29→2, 30→3, 31→4
Feb.	April	5	6	7	8	9	10	11	12	13	14	15	16	17	18	19	20	21	22	23	24	25	26	27	28	29	30						May: 27→1, 28→2
Mar.	May	3	4	5	6	7	8	9	10	11	12	13	14	15	16	17	18	19	20	21	22	23	24	25	26	27	28	29	30	31			June: 30→1, 31→2
Apr.	June	3	4	5	6	7	8	9	10	11	12	13	14	15	16	17	18	19	20	21	22	23	24	25	26	27	28	29	30				July: 29→1, 30→2
May	July	3	4	5	6	7	8	9	10	11	12	13	14	15	16	17	18	19	20	21	22	23	24	25	26	27	28	29	30	31			August: 30→1, 31→2
June	August	3	4	5	6	7	8	9	10	11	12	13	14	15	16	17	18	19	20	21	22	23	24	25	26	27	28	29	30	31			Sept.: 30→1
July	September	2	3	4	5	6	7	8	9	10	11	12	13	14	15	16	17	18	19	20	21	22	23	24	25	26	27	28	29	30			Oct.: 30→1, 31→2
Aug.	October	3	4	5	6	7	8	9	10	11	12	13	14	15	16	17	18	19	20	21	22	23	24	25	26	27	28	29	30	31			Nov.: 30→1, 31→2
Sept.	November	3	4	5	6	7	8	9	10	11	12	13	14	15	16	17	18	19	20	21	22	23	24	25	26	27	28	29	30				Dec.: 29→1, 30→2
Oct.	December	3	4	5	6	7	8	9	10	11	12	13	14	15	16	17	18	19	20	21	22	23	24	25	26	27	28	29	30	31			Jan.: 30→1, 31→2
Nov.	January	3	4	5	6	7	8	9	10	11	12	13	14	15	16	17	18	19	20	21	22	23	24	25	26	27	28	29	30	31			Feb.: 30→1
Dec.	February	2	3	4	5	6	7	8	9	10	11	12	13	14	15	16	17	18	19	20	21	22	23	24	25	26	27	28					March: 28→1, 29→2, 30→3, 31→4

Table 176. TIME OF EPIPHYSEAL FUSION OF BONES
AS SHOWN BY RADIOGRAPHS*

Tuber scapulae	4½–6 months
Humeral head and tubercles	10–12 months
Condyles and medial epicondyle of humerus	8 months
Radius	
Proximal epiphysis	9–11 months
Distal epiphysis	10–12 months
Ulna	
Olecranon	8–10 months
Distal epiphysis	10–12 months
Epiphysis of accessory carpal bone	4½ months
Distal epiphysis of the metacarpal bones and	
proximal epiphysis of first and second phalanges	6–7 months
Fusion of the ilium, ischium, pubis, and os acetabuli	5–6 months
Proximal end of femur	9–11 months
Distal epiphysis of femur	9–12 months
Epiphysis of tibial tuberosity	
Fuses with proximal epiphysis	6–9 months
Fuses with shaft of tibia	10–14 months
Proximal articular epiphysis of tibia	10–14 months
Proximal articular epiphysis of fibula	9–11 months
Distal epiphysis of tibia	9–11 months
Distal epiphysis of fibula	8–13 months
Epiphysis of tuber calcanei	
With fibular tarsal bone	6 months

*The data in this table were derived from greyhounds and large mongrels. (Chapman[1] has shown that fusion may occur approximately 2 months earlier for all bones in purebred beagles.)

From Habel, R. E.: Applied Veterinary Anatomy, 2nd ed. Ithaca, New York, published by the author, 1981.

[1]Chapman, W. L.: Appearance of ossification centers and epiphyseal closures as determined by radiographic techniques. J.A.V.M.A., *147*, (2):138–141, 1965.

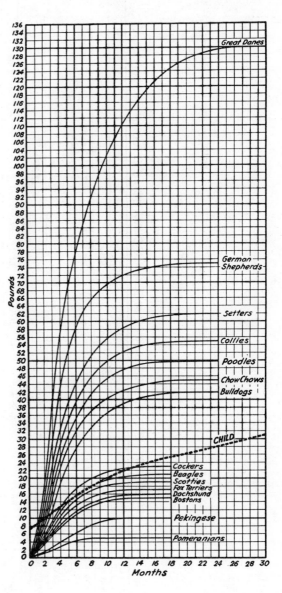

Figure 104. Canine growth chart.

Table 177. USEFUL LABORATORY ANIMAL INFORMATION (SCHUCHMAN)

	Hamster	Rabbit	Mouse	Rat	Gerbil	Guinea Pig
Weight at birth	2 gm	100 gm	1.5 gm	5.5 gm	3 gm	100 gm
Puberty	(F) 28–31 days (M) 45 days (best to breed 70 days)	4–9 months	35 days	50–60 days	(F) 3–5 months (M) 10–12 weeks	(F) 20–30 days (M) 70 days
Duration of estrus cycle*	4 days	15–16 days	4 days	4 days	4 days	16 days
Gestation	16 days	28–36 days	19–21 days	21–23 days	24 days	62–72 days
Separation of adults during parturition and weaning	Yes	Yes	No	No	No (mates for life)	No
Number per litter	4–10	7	10	8–10	1–12	1–4
Eyes open	15 days	10 days	11–14 days	14–17 days	16–20 days	Prior to birth
Wean at	25 days	42–56 days	21 days	21 days	21 days	14–21 days or 160 gm
Postpartum estrus	Within 24 hours	14 days	Within 24–48 hours	Within 24–48 hours	Within 24–72 hours	Within 24 hours

Breeding life	11–18 months	1–3 years (maximum 6 years)	12–18 months	14 months	15–20 months	3–4 years
Adult weight	(F) 120 gm (M) 108 gm	(F) 4 kg (M) 4.3 kg	(F) 30 gm (M) 30 gm	(F) 300 gm (M) 500 gm	(F) 75 gm (M) 85 gm	(F) 850 gm (M) 1000 gm
Life span	2–3 years	5–7 years	3–3½ years	3 years	4 years	4–5 years
Body temperature (°F)	97–101	101–103.2	96.4–100	99.5–100.6	100.8	100.4–102.5
Daily adult water consumption	8–12 ml/day	80 ml/kg body weight	3–3.5 ml/day	20–30 ml/day	4 ml/day	10 ml/100 gm body weight
Daily adult food consumption (varies with age and condition)	7–12 gm/day	150–100 gm/day	2.5–4 gm/day	20–40 gm/day	10–15 gm/day	30–35 gm/day
Diet	Commercial rat, mouse, or hamster chow supplemented with kale,† cabbage,† apples, milk	Commercial rabbit pellets, greens in moderation	Commercial mouse chow	Commercial rat or mouse chow	Commercial mouse or rat chow (lowest fat possible), sunflower seeds	Commercial guinea pig chow, good quality hay, kale, cabbage, fruits (cannot rely on vitamin C levels of commercial ration)
Room temperature (°F)	65–75	62–68	70–80	76–78	65–80	65–75
Humidity (per cent)	50	50	50	50	less than 50	50

*All species listed are seasonal polyestrus.
†Better source of vitamin C than lettuce.

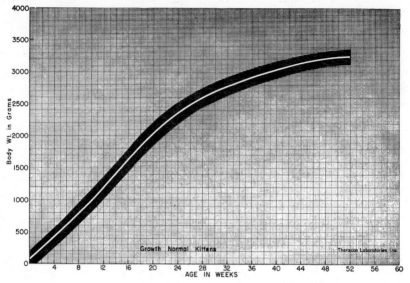

Figure 105. Feline growth chart.

Table 178. SAMPLE REQUIREMENTS FOR LABORATORY TESTS

Test Description	Specimen

These recommendations are only guidelines. Sample requirements may vary depending on each laboratory's protocol. Consult your own laboratory for specific instructions.

Test Description	Specimen
Acid-base balance	3 ml heparinized whole blood (arterial sample preferred)
ACTH (adrenocorticotropic hormone)	12 ml plasma; frozen—separate into two 6-ml vials
A/G ratio (total protein, albumin, A/G)	2 ml serum
ALA (aminolevulinic acid)	20-ml aliquot of 24-hr urine. Add 6N HCl to pH 1–2. Note 24-hr volume.
Albumin	2 ml serum
Alkaline phosphatase	1 ml serum
Alkaline phosphatase isoenzymes	2 ml serum frozen
Ammonia, blood	3 ml heparinized plasma; freeze immediately
Amylase, fluid	1 ml fluid
Amylase serum	1 ml serum
Amylase, urine	10 ml random urine

Table continued on opposite page

Table 178. SAMPLE REQUIREMENTS FOR LABORATORY
TESTS *(Continued)*

Test Description	Specimen
ANA (anti-nuclear antibody)	2 ml serum
Bence Jones protein	30 ml fresh random urine
Bile, urine, qualitative	2 ml random urine
Bilirubin, direct	1 ml serum (do not expose to light)
Bilirubin, total	1 ml serum (do not expose to light)
Bilirubin, urine, qualitative	5 ml random urine
Brucella titer, canine	1 ml serum
BSP (Bromsulphalein)	3 ml EDTA-plasma
Buffy coat preparation	EDTA tube
BUN (blood urea nitrogen)	1 ml serum
Calcium, serum	2 ml serum
Calcium, serum, ionized	3 ml serum
Calcium, urine	25-ml aliquot of 24-hr urine. Add 6N HCl to pH 1–2. Note 24-hr volume.
Carbon dioxide content L (CO_2)	2 ml serum
Carbon monoxide (carboxyhemoglobin)	1 grey top
Chloride, CSF	1 ml CSF
Chloride, fluid	1 ml fluid
Chloride, serum	1 ml serum
Chloride, urine	24-ml aliquot of 24-hr urine. Note 24-hr volume.
Cholesterol by enzymatic method	1 ml serum
Cholinesterase, RBC	2 ml heparinized blood
Cholinesterase, serum	1 ml serum
Coagulation factors	
Activated partial thromboplastin time (APTT)	Plasma, frozen. Two 1-ml aliquots—blue top
Factor VIII	Plasma, frozen. Two 1-ml aliquots—blue top
Factor IX	Plasma, frozen. Two 1-ml aliquots—blue top
Factor XI	Plasma, frozen. Two 1-ml aliquots—blue top
Factor XII	Plasma, frozen. Two 1-ml aliquots—blue top
Factor XIII	Plasma, frozen. Two 1-ml aliquots—blue top
Fibrin split products	Plasma, 2 ml. Collect in special blue-top vial containing thrombin and special enzyme inhibitor.
Fibrin stabilizing factor (factor XIII)	Plasma, frozen. Two 1-ml aliquots—blue top
Fibrinogen titer	Plasma, frozen. Two 1-ml aliquots—blue top
Partial thromboplastin time (see APTT)	Plasma, frozen. Two 1-ml aliquots—blue top

Table continued on following page

Table 178. SAMPLE REQUIREMENTS FOR LABORATORY
TESTS *(Continued)*

Test Description	Specimen
Plasma clot lysis	Plasma, frozen. Two 1-ml aliquots—blue top
Platelet count	EDTA tube
Platelet factor 3	1-ml plasma; need not be frozen. Results not valid if there is any clotting of sample or if corticosteroids are given prior to sample drawing—blue top
Prothrombin consumption time	1 ml serum, frozen. Two 1-ml aliquots
Prothrombin time	Plasma, frozen. Two 1-ml aliquots—blue top
Russell's viper venom time	Plasma, frozen. Two 1-ml aliquots—blue top
Coccidioidomycosis antibody, screening	2 ml serum
Cold agglutinins	2 ml serum
Coombs, direct canine or feline	1 red top
Coombs, indirect canine or feline	1 red top
Copper, serum	2 ml serum
Copper, urine	100-ml aliquot 24-hr urine. Note 24-hr volume.
Cortisol, serum or plasma	3 ml serum or heparinized plasma
Cortisol, urine	10-ml aliquot of 24-hr urine frozen. Note 24-hr volume.
CPK isoenzymes	1 ml serum
Creatine, serum	2 ml serum frozen
Creatine, urine	10-ml aliquot of 24-hr urine frozen. Note 24-hr volume.
Creatine phosphokinase (CPK)	2 ml serum
Creatinine clearance	2 ml serum/10-ml aliquot of specifically timed (12 or 24 hr) urine. Note total volume/time.
Cryoglobulins, qualitative	1 red top
11-Deoxy cortisol (compound S)	3 ml heparinized plasma; separate immediately
11-Deoxy/11-Oxy ratio of 17-ketogenic steroids	100-ml aliquot of 24-hr urine. Note 24-hr volume.
Digitoxin, RIA	2 ml serum
Digoxin, RIA	2 ml serum
Dirofilariasis	EDTA tube
D-Xylose tolerance	100-ml aliquot of 5-hr urine. Note total volume.
Electrolytes (includes sodium, potassium, chloride, carbon dioxide)	2 ml serum
Electrophoresis, CSF	1 ml CSF
Electrophoresis, hemoglobin	EDTA tube

Table continued on opposite page

Table 178. SAMPLE REQUIREMENTS FOR LABORATORY
TESTS *(Continued)*

Test Description	Specimen
Electrophoresis, protein, serum	1 ml serum
Electrophoresis, protein, urine	20-ml aliquot of 24-hr urine. Note 24-hr volume.
Eosinophil count, direct	EDTA tube
Erythropoietin, quantitative	2 ml serum
ESR (erythrocyte sedimentation rate)	EDTA tube
Estradiol, serum, RIA	5 ml heparinized plasma or serum frozen
Fatty acids, free	4 ml serum
Feline leukemia virus	3 thin blood smears
Fibrinogen, quantitative	1 blue top
FIP, Fluid exam	3 ml fluid in EDTA tube, fixed smear of sediment
Gamma globulins, quantitative (immunoglobulins) (includes IgG, IgA, and IgM)	1 ml serum
GGTP (gamma glutamyl transpeptidase)	1 ml serum
Glucose, blood, fasting	1 grey top
Glucose, CSF	1 ml CSF
Glucose, fluid	1 grey top
Glucose, urine, quantitative	25-ml aliquot of 24-hr urine. Add 250 mg NaF to aliquot and mix. Note 24-hr volume.
Glucose tolerance (3 tests)	3 grey tops (indicate time)
Each Additional Glucose	1 grey top (indicate time)
Heavy metal screen (includes antimony, arsenic, mercury, and bismuth)	50 ml random urine
Hemoglobin, free, urine	10 ml random urine
Hemoglobin electrophoresis	1 EDTA tube
Hemogram (includes WBC, RBC, Hgb, Hct, MCV, MCH, and MCHC)	EDTA tube
Histoplasmosis, serological screen only	1 red top
Immunoelectrophoresis	1 ml serum. Avoid hemolysis.
Immunoglobulins, quantitative (includes IgG, IgA, and IgM in most species)	1 ml serum
Insulin, plasma	2 ml serum or plasma frozen
Iron, total, and iron-binding capacity	4 ml serum
Lactic acid	Mix 4 ml blood from grey top with 4 ml 7% perchloric acid. (Remove tourniquet before blood withdrawal.)
LDH (Lactic acid dehydrogenase), serum	1 ml serum (Do not freeze.)
LDH isoenzyme pattern	1 ml serum (Do not freeze.)
LE prep	1 red top (Do not mail.)
Lead, blood	1 green top
Lead, urine	100-ml aliquot of 24-hr urine. Note 24-hr volume.

Table continued on following page

Table 178. SAMPLE REQUIREMENTS FOR LABORATORY
TESTS *(Continued)*

Test Description	Specimen
Leptospira agglutinins	2 ml serum
Lipase	2 ml serum
Lipase, total, serum	2 ml serum
Magnesium, serum	1 ml serum
Methemalbumin (Schumm test)	2 ml serum
Methemoglobin	1 grey top; deliver immediately
Microfilaria	EDTA tube
Mucopolysaccharides, qualitative	30 ml random urine
Ornithine carbamyl transferase (OCT)	3 ml serum
Osmolality, serum	2 ml serum
Osmolality, urine	2 ml urine
Oxalate	50-ml aliquot of 24-hr urine. Note 24-hr volume.
Parathyroid hormone (PTH)	8 ml serum frozen
Phosphatase, alkaline	1 ml serum
Phospholipids	2 ml serum
Phosphorus, serum	1 ml serum
Phosphorus, urine	25-ml aliquot of 24-hr urine. Note 24-hr volume.
Plasma clot lysis	Plasma, frozen. Two 1-ml aliquots.
Platelet factor 3	1 lavender or blue. Sample must be free of any clot formation.
Potassium, fluid	1 ml fluid
Potassium, serum	1 ml serum
Potassium, urine	10-ml aliquot of 24-hr urine. Note 24-hr volume.
Protein, total, CSF	2 ml CSF
Protein, total, urine	100-ml aliquot of 24-hr urine. Note 24-hr volume.
Protein, total, serum	1 ml serum
Protein electrophoresis, serum	1 ml serum
Protein electrophoresis, urine	20 ml random urine

Table continued on opposite page

Table 178. SAMPLE REQUIREMENTS FOR LABORATORY
TESTS *(Continued)*

Test Description	Specimen
Reticulocyte count	EDTA tube
Rheumatoid factor, canine	1 ml serum
Salicylates	1 ml serum
Sedimentation rate (ESR)	EDTA tube
SGOT (transaminase-SGO)	1 ml serum
SGPT (transaminase-SGP)	1 ml serum
Sodium, fluid	1 ml fluid
Sodium, serum	1 ml serum
Sodium, urine	10-ml aliquot of 24-hr urine. Note 24-hr volume.
Specific gravity, fluid	1 ml fluid
T_3 uptake (resin)	1 ml serum
T_4 by RIA	2 ml serum
Free T_4 by equilibrium dialysis	3 ml serum
Testosterone, serum (RIA)	2 ml serum
Testosterone, urine (RIA)	25-ml aliquot of 24-hr urine. Refrigerate sample. Note 24-hr volume.
Thrombin time	Plasma, frozen. Two 1-ml aliquots
Total protein, serum	1 ml serum
Toxoplasma, fluorescent antibody	1 ml serum
Transaminase-SGO	1 ml serum
Transaminase-SGP	1 ml serum
Triglycerides	3 ml serum
Urea nitrogen, blood (BUN)	1 ml serum
Urea nitrogen, urine	10-ml aliquot of 24-hr urine. Note 24-hr volume.
Uric acid, serum	1 ml serum
Uric acid, urine	25-ml aliquot of 24-hr urine. Note 24-hr volume.
Viscosity, serum	6 ml serum
Xylose tolerance	100-ml aliquot of 5-hr urine. Plus 250 mg NaF. Note 5-hr volume.
Zinc, serum	5 ml serum

Table 179. NORMAL BLOOD VALUES[31]

Erythrocytes	Adult Dog	Average	Adult Cat	Average
Erythrocytes (millions/µl)	5.5–8.5	6.8	5.5–10.0	7.5
Hemoglobin (gm/dl)	12.0–18.0	14.9	8.0–14.0	12.0
Packed cell volume (vol %)	37.0–55.0	45.5	24.0–45.0	37.0
Mean corpuscular volume (femtoliters)	66.0–77.0	69.8	40.0–55.0	45.0
Mean corpuscular hemoglobin (picograms)	19.9–24.5	22.8	13.0–17.0	15.0
Mean corpuscular hemoglobin concentration (gm/dl)				
Wintrobe	31.0–34.0	33.0	31.0–35.0	33.0
Microhematocrit	32.0–36.0	34.0	30.0–36.0	33.2
Reticulocytes (%) (excludes punctate retics.)	0.0–1.5	0.8	0.2–1.6	0.6
Resistance to hypotonic saline (% saline solution producing initial and complete hemolysis)				
Minimum	0.40–0.50	0.46	0.66–0.72	0.69
Maximum	0.32–0.42	0.33	0.46–0.54	0.50
Erythrocyte sedimentation rate (mm at 60 min)	PCV 37	13	PCV 35–40	7–27
RBC life span (days)	PCV 50 100–120	0	—	—
RBC diameter (µ)	6.7–7.2	7.0	66–78 5.5–6.3	5.8
Leukocytes (no/µl)	6,000–17,000	11,500	5,500–19,500	12,500
Neutrophils—bands (%)	0–3	0.8	0–3	0.5
Neutrophils—mature (%)	60–77	70.0	35–75	59.0

Table 179. NORMAL BLOOD VALUES[31] (Continued)

Erythrocytes	Adult Dog	Average	Adult Cat	Average
Lymphocyte (%)	12–30	20.0	20–55	32.0
Monocyte (%)	3–10	5.2	1–4	3.0
Eosinophil (%)	2–10	4.0	2–12	5.5
Basophil (%)	Rare	0	Rare	0
Neutrophils—bands (no/µl)	0–300	70	0–300	100
Neutrophils—mature (no/µl)	3,000–11,500	7,000	2,500–12,500	7,500
Lymphocytes (no/µl)	1,000–4,800	2,800	1,500–7,000	4,000
Monocytes (no/µl)	150–1,350	750	0–850	350
Eosinophils (no/µl)	100–1,250	550	0–1,500	650
Basophils	Rare	0	Rare	0

From Bentinck-Smith, J.: A roster of normal values. *In* Kirk, R. W. (ed.): Current Veterinary Therapy VII. Philadelphia, W. B. Saunders Company, 1980, p. 1321.

Table 180. CANINE BLOOD PARAMETERS AT DIFFERENT AGES—AVERAGE VALUES[1]

Age	Millions/µL RBC	Retic. %*	Nucl. RBC/ 100 WBC*	Gm/ dl Hb	Vol % PCV	/dl WBC	/dl Neut.	/dl Bands	/dl Lymph.	/dl Eos.
Birth	5.75	7.1	1.8	16.70	50	16,500	1,300	400	2,500	600
2 weeks	3.92	7.1	1.8	9.76	32	11,000	6,500	100	3,000	300
4 weeks	4.20	7.1	1.8	9.60	33	13,000	8,600	0	4,000	40
6 weeks	4.91	3.6	1.8	9.59	34	15,000	10,000	0	4,500	100
8 weeks	5.13	3.9	0.3	11.00	37	18,000	11,000	234	6,000	270
12 weeks	5.27	3.9	rare	11.60	36	15,300	9,400	115	4,600	322

*See reference 13.

From Bentinck-Smith, J.: A roster of normal values. *In* Kirk, R. W. (ed.): Current Veterinary Therapy VII. Philadelphia, W. B. Saunders Company, 1980, p. 1322.

Table 181. CANINE BLOOD PARAMETERS AT DIFFERENT AGES[26]

	Canine	Birth to 12 mo	Average	1–5 yr	Average	More than 6 yr	Average
Erythrocytes (million/µl)	Male	2.99–8.52	5.09	5.26–6.57	5.92	3.33–7.76	5.28
	Female	2.76–8.42	5.06	5.13–8.6	6.47	3.34–9.19	5.17
Hemoglobin (gm/dl)	Male	6.9–16.5	10.7	12.7–16.3	15.5	14.7–21.2	17.9
	Female	6.4–18.9	11.2	11.5–17.9	14.7	11.0–22.5	16.1
Packed Cell Volume (vol %)	Male	22.0–45.0	33.9	35.2–52.8	44.0	44.2–62.8	52.3
	Female	25.8–55.2	36.0	34.8–52.4	43.6	35.8–67.0	49.8
Leukocytes (thousands/µl)	Male	9.9–27.7	17.1	8.3–19.5	11.9	7.9–35.3	15.5
	Female	8.8–26.8	15.9	7.5–17.5	11.5	5.2–34.0	13.4
Neutrophil Mature %	Male	63–73	68	65–73	69	55–80	66
	Female	64–74	69	58–76	67	40–80	64
Lymphocyte %	Male	18–30	24	9–26	18	15–40	29
	Female	13–28	21	11–29	20	13–45	29
Monocyte %	Male	1–10	6	2–10	6	0–4	1
	Female	1–10	7	0–10	5	0–4	1
Eosinophil %	Male	2–11	3	1–8	4	1–11	4
	Female	1–9	5	1–10	6	0–19	6

From Bentinck-Smith, J.: A roster of normal values. *In* Kirk, R. W. (ed.): Current Veterinary Therapy VII. Philadelphia, W. B. Saunders Company, 1980, p. 1322.

Table 182. FELINE BLOOD PARAMETERS AT DIFFERENT
AGES—AVERAGE VALUES[31]

Age	Millions/μl RBC	Gm/dl Hb	Vol % PCV	/dl WBC	/dl Neut.	/dl Lymph.
Birth	4.95	12.2	44.7	7,500		
2 weeks	4.76	9.7	31.1	8,080		
5 weeks	5.84	8.4	29.9	8,550		
Average*	4.80	7.5	26.2	11,770	4,600	6,970
Range*	3.90–5.70	6.6–8.4	21.0–33.5	7,500–14,500		4,500–9,400
6 weeks	6.75	9.0	35.4	8,420		
8 weeks	7.10	9.4	35.6	8,420		
Average*	5.90	7.5	26.2	12,400	7,500	4,900
Range*	3.30–7.30	7.6–15.0	22–38	6,900–23,100		1,925–10,100

*See reference 2.
From Bentinck-Smith, J.: A roster of normal values. *In* Kirk, R. W. (ed.): Current
Veterinary Therapy VII. Philadelphia, W. B. Saunders Company, 1980, p. 1322.

Table 183. FELINE BLOOD PARAMETERS AT DIFFERENT AGES[25]

	Feline	Birth to 12 mo	Average	1–5 yr	Average	More than 6 yr	Average
Erythrocytes (millions/µl)	Male	5.43–10.22	6.96	4.48–10.27	7.34	5.26–8.89	6.79
	Female	4.46–11.34	6.90	4.45–9.42	6.17	4.10–7.38	5.84
Hemoglobin (gm/dl)	Male	6.0–12.9	9.9	8.9–17.0	12.9	9.0–14.5	11.8
	Female	6.0–15.0	9.9	7.9–15.5	10.3	7.5–13.7	10.3
Packed cell volume (vol %)	Male	24.0–37.5	31	26.9–48.2	37.6	28.0–43.8	34.6
	Female	23.0–46.8	31.5	25.3–37.5	31.4	22.5–40.5	30.8
Leukocytes (thousands/µl)	Male	7.8–25.0	15.8	9.1–28.2	15.1	6.4–30.4	17.6
	Female	11.0–26.9	17.7	13.7–23.7	19.9	5.2–30.1	14.8
Neutrophils— Mature %	Male	16–75	60	37–92	65	33–75	61
	Female	51–83	69	42–93	69	25–89	71
Lymphocyte %	Male	10–81	30	7–48	23	16–54	30
	Female	8–37	23	12–58	30	9–63	22
Monocyte %	Male	1–5	2	1–5	2	0–2	1
	Female	0–7	2	0–5	2	0–4	1
Eosinophil %	Male	2–21	8	1–22	7	1–15	8
	Female	0–15	6	0–13	5	0–15	6

From Bentinck-Smith, J.: A roster of normal values. *In* Kirk, R. W. (ed.): Current Veterinary Therapy VII. Philadelphia, W. B. Saunders Company, 1980, p. 1323.

Table 184. NORMAL BONE MARROW (PERCENTAGE)

Erythrocytic Cells	Dog[31]	Cat[23]
Rubriblasts	0.2 ⎫	1.71
Prorubricytes	3.9 ⎬	12.50
Rubricytes	27.0 ⎭	
Metarubricytes	15.3	11.68
Total erythrocytic cells	46.4	25.89
Granulocytic Cells		
Myeloblasts	0.0	1.74
Progranulocytes	1.3	0.88
Neutrophilic myelocytes	9.0	9.76
Eosinophilic myelocytes	0.0	1.47
Neutrophilic metamyelocytes	7.5	7.32
Eosinophilic metamyelocytes	2.4	1.52
Band neutrophils	13.6	25.80
Band eosinophils	0.9	—
Neutrophils	18.4	9.24
Eosinophils	0.3	0.81
Basophils	0.0	0.002
Total granulocytic cells	53.4	58.542
M:E Ratio—average	1.15:1.0	2.47:1.0
M:E Ratio—range (Schalm)	0.75–2.50:1.0	0.60–3.90:1.0
Other Cells		
Lymphocytes	0.2	7.63
Plasma cells	0	1.61
Reticulum cells	0	0.13
Mitotic cells	0	0.61
Unclassified	0	1.62
Disintegrated cells	0	4.60

From Bentinck-Smith, J.: A roster of normal values. *In* Kirk, R. W. (ed.): Current Veterinary Therapy VII. Philadelphia, W. B. Saunders Company, 1980, p. 1324.

Table 185. BLOOD, PLASMA, OR SERUM CHEMICAL CONSTITUENTS

(B) = Blood, (P) = Plasma, (S) = Serum

Chemical constituents are liable to show markedly different values depending on the methodology used.

Constituent	Adult Dog		Adult Cat	
	Coulter Chemistry[34]	Technicon SMA[36]	Coulter Chemistry[34]	Technicon SMA[36]
Urea N (S) (mg/dl)	8–23	10–22	18–32	5–30
Glucose (S) (mg/dl)	71–115	50–120	66–95	70–150
Total bilirubin (S) (mg/dl)	0.1–0.6	0–0.6	0.15–0.3	0–0.8
Total protein (S) (mg/dl)	5.2–7.0	5.4–7.8	5.9–7.3	5.5–7.5
Albumin (S) (mg/dl)	2.7–3.8	2.2–3.4	2.2–3.0	2.2–3.5
Alkaline phosphatase (S) (IU/L)	10–82	20–120	7–30	10–80
Calcium (S) (mg/dl)	9.8–11.4	9–11.6	8.9–10.6	7.6–11.0
Inorganic phosphorus (S) (mg/dl)	2.8–5.1	3.9–6.3	4.3–6.6	3.2–6.3
LDH (S) (IU/L)	8–89	40–200	33–99	10–200
AST or SGOT (S)	13–93*	5–80†	32–58*	10–60†
ALT or SGPT (S) (IU/L)	15–70	5–25	10–50	10–60
Total CO (S) (mEq/L)	18–25	17–25‡	18–25	16–25‡
Creatinine[2] (S) (mg/dl)	0.5–1.2	0.4–1.5‡	0.5–1.7	1.3–2.1‡
Uric acid (S) (mg/dl)		0.2–0.8‡		0.1–0.7‡
Total cholesterol (S) (mg/dl)	82–282	156–294‡	41–225	116–126‡
Triglycerides (S) (mg/dl)		10–42‡		6–58‡
CPK (S) (IU/L)	12–84	27–93‡	6–130	62–262‡

Chemical Parameters Affected by Age	Dog < 6 mo — SMA[36]	Cat < 6 mo — SMA[36]
Inorganic phosphorus (S) (mg/dl)	3.9–9.0	3.9–8.1
Calcium (S) (mg/dl)	7.0–11.6	7.0–11.0
Alkaline phosphatase (S) (IU/L)	20–200	10–120
LDH (S) (IU/L)	40–400	10–300

Total Protein (S and P) (gm/dl)	Birth to 12 mo	Average	1–5 yr	Average	More than 6 yr	Average
Dogs (S)[26]						
Male	3.90–5.90	5.15	4.90–9.60	6.33	5.5–7.3	6.4
Female	4.00–6.40	5.58	5.50–7.80	6.34	4.7–7.5	6.2
Cats (S)[25]						
Male	4.3–10.0	6.4	6.8–10.0	8.1	6.2–8.5	7.2
Female	4.8–9.1	6.4	6.6–8.9	7.4	6.0–9.0	7.3

Plasma protein	Basenji Dogs[13]	Cats[31]
6–8 wk	5.33 ± 0.29	Lower values for younger animals
9–12 wk	5.87 ± 0.46	Adults, 6–8
4–6 mo	6.60 ± 0.25	
1–2 yr	7.03 ± 0.33	

*Trans Act Units/L (General Diagnostics). 1 Trans Act Unit of GOT activity is the amount of enzyme in one L of sample that will form 1 mM of oxalic acid in 1 minute under specified conditions.
†IU/L.
‡See reference 7.

Table continued on following page

Table 185. BLOOD, PLASMA, OR SERUM CHEMICAL CONSTITUENTS
(B) = Blood, (P) = Plasma, (S) = Serum (*Continued*)

Chemical constituents are liable to show markedly different values depending on the methodology used.

Electrophoresis	Dogs	Cats
Albumin (S) (gm/dl)	2.3–3.4	2.3–3.5
Globulin (S) (gm/dl)	3.0–4.7	2.6–5.0
Alpha 1 (S) (gm/dl)	0.3–0.8	0.3–0.5
Alpha 2 (S) (gm/dl)	0.5–1.3	0.4–1.0
Beta (S) (gm/dl)	0.7–1.8	0.6–1.9
Gamma (S) (gm/dl)	0.4–1.0	0.5–1.5
Albumin/globulin ratio, A/G (S)	0.7–1.1	0.5–1.0

Other Constituents	Adult Dog	Adult Cat
Lipase (S) Sigma Tietz units/ml	0–1	0–1
Roe Byler units (5)	0.8–12	0–5
IU (5)	13–200	0–83
Amylase (S) Harleco units/dl	0–800	0–800
Harding units/dl	1600–2400	0–2700 (5)
Dy Amyl General Diagnostics, Inc.	under 3200 (5)	0–2600 (5)
Caraway units/dl[24]	330–1530	170–1170
Lactic acid (S) (mg/dl)	3–15	
Pyruvate (B) (mEq/L)	0.1–0.2	

	Dogs Coulter[24]	Dogs Technicon[7]	Cats Coulter[34]	Cats Technicon[7]
Cholesterol esters (S) (mg/dl)		84–168		45–120
Free cholesterol (S) (mg/dl)		28–84		15–60
Total lipid (P) (mg/dl)		47–725		145–607
Free glycerol (S) 24-hr fast (mg/dl)[28]		14.2–23.2		
Bromsulphalein retention test (P)		<5%		
Iron (S) (µg/dl)		94–122		68–215
Total iron binding capacity (S) (µg/dl)		280–340		170–400
Lead (B) (µg/dl)		0–35		0–35

Electrolytes	Dogs Coulter[24]	Dogs Technicon[7]	Cats Coulter[34]	Cats Technicon[7]
Sodium (S) (mEq/L)	143–151	144–154	150–162	147–161
Potassium (S) (mEq/L)	4.1–5.7	3.8–5.8	3.7–5.5	3.7–4.9
Magnesium (S) (mEq/L)	1.4–2.4	1.07–1.73	2.2	1.92–2.28
Chloride (S) (mEq/L)	103–115	93–121	114–124	80–158
Sulfate (S) (mEq/L)	2.0			
Osmolality (S) (mOsm/kg)	280–310		280–310	
pH (Corning)	7.31–7.42		7.24–7.40	

Blood Gases	Adult Dog	Adult Cat
PO$_2$ (B) mm Hg (arterial)*	85–95	—
(B) mm Hg (venous)*	40–60	—
PCO$_2$ (B) mm Hg (arterial)*	29–36	—
(B) mm Hg (venous)*	29–42	
Base excess (B) (mEq/L)	± 2.5	± 2.5
Bicarbonate (P) (mEq/L)	17–24	17–24

*Standard temperature and pressure.

Table continued on following page

Table 185. BLOOD, PLASMA, OR SERUM CHEMICAL CONSTITUENTS
(B) = Blood, (P) = Plasma, (S) = Serum (Continued)

Chemical constituents are liable to show markedly different values depending on the methodology used.

Endocrine Secretions	Adult Dog		Adult Cat	
	Resting Level	Post-ACTH*	Resting Level	Post-ACTH*
Cortisol (S) (RIA) (µg/dl)[27]	1.8–4	3–4 × pretreatment	1–3	3–4 × pretreatment[32]
Cortisol (S) (CPB) (µg/dl)[35]	2–6	3–4 × pretreatment[32]	2–5	3–4 × pretreatment[32]
Cortisol (S) (fluorometric) (µg/dl)[32]	5–10	10–20		
	Resting Level	Post-TSH†	Resting Level	Post-TSH
T$_4$ (P) (RIA) (µg/dl)[4]	1.52–3.60	At least 3–4 fold	1.2–3.8	
T$_3$ (P) (RIA) (ng/dl)[4]	48–154	More than 10 ng increase		
Protein-bound iodine[3] (µg/dl)	1.6–3.0	Increase of 3 µg/dl (mean)		

T$_4$ Changes With Age	Dog	Cat
T$_4$ (S) (RIA)	Decrease of 0.07 µg/dl per year[4] of age	No values for cat
T$_4$ (S) (CPB) µg/dl		
10–12 wk[15, 16]	3.24 ± 0.51	2.82 ± 0.73
1 yr[15, 16]	2.25 ± 0.33	2.43 ± 0.55

	Adult Dog		Adult Cat
Thyroid uptake of radioiodine (^{131}I %)[15, 16]	17–30		
Insulin (S) (RIA) μU/ml[37]	0–30		0–50

Hemostatic Parameters (No test should be interpreted without an accompanying normal control.)

	Adult Dog		Adult Cat
Bleeding time			
Dorsum of nose (min)	2–4		1–5[33]
Lip (sec)	85–110		
Ear (min)	2.5–3		
Abdomen (min)	1–2		
Whole blood coagulation time			
Glass (Lee and White) (min)	6–7.5		8 min[33]
Silicone (Lee and White) (min)	12–15		
Capillary tube (min)[11]	3–4		5.2 ± 0.2[21]
Activated coagulation time of whole blood			
Room temp. (sec)	60–125[10]	83–129[19]	A limited number of cats have
37° C (sec)		64–95[19]	shown a range similar to the dog.
Prothrombin time (sec)[11]	6–10		8.6 ± 0.5[21]
Puppies 1–4 hr old (sec)[5]	42.2		
6–12 hr old (sec)	49.1		
16–48 hr old (sec)	36.8		
48 hr old (sec)	24.5		
Russell's viper venom time (sec)[29]	11		9
Partial thromboplastin time (sec)	15–25		
Prothrombin consumption (sec)[28]	20.5		20
Fibrin degradation products (μg/ml)	<10		

*Sample 2 hr after injection, 2 μ ACTH gel IM.
†Sample 4–6 hr after injection, 5 μ TSH IV.

Table continued on following page

Table 185. BLOOD, PLASMA, OR SERUM CHEMICAL CONSTITUENTS
(B) = Blood, (P) = Plasma, (S) = Serum (*Continued*)
Chemical constituents are liable to show markedly different values depending on the methodology used.

Normal Renal Function and Urine Parameters

Urine[22]	Adult Dog	Adult Cat
Specific gravity		
Minimum	1.001	1.001
Maximum	1.060	1.080
Usual limits (normal water and food intake)	1.018–1.050	1.018–1.050
Volume (ml/kg body weight/day)	24–41	22–30
Osmolality urine (mOsm/kg)		
Usual range	500–1200	
Maximal limits	2000–2400	
Osmolality plasma	300	

Urine Constituents[37] (Values markedly affected by degree of concentration)	Adult Dog	Adult Cat
Creatinine (mg/dl)	100–300	110–280
Urea (gm/dl)	1.0–2.5	1.0–3.0
Protein (mg/dl)	0–30	0–20
Amylase (Somogyi units)	50–150	30–120
Sodium (mEq/L)	20–165	
Potassium (mEq/L)	10–120	
Calcium (mEq/L)	2–10	
Inorganic phosphorus (mEq/L)	50–180	

Urinalysis—Semiquantitative Values	Adult Dog	Adult Cat
Protein	0–trace	0–trace
Glucose	0	0
Ketones	0	0
Bilirubin	0	
10–20% dogs—high specific gravity	1+	1+
5% cats—high specific gravity		0–1
Urobilinogen (Ehrlich unit)	0–1	<1:32
(Wallace and Diamond)	<1:32	

Renal Function—Dog[22]

Effective renal plasma flow	266 ± 66 ml/min/m² of body surface	
	13.5 ± 3.3 ml/min/kg of body weight	
Glomerular filtration rate	84.4 ± 19 ml/min/m² of body surface	
	4 ml/min/kg of body weight	

Renal Function Tests—Dog

Phenolsulfonphthalein		
Excretion in urine at 20 min, 6-mg dose[11]	21–66%	
Clearance (P) 1 mg/kg at 60 min	<80 μ/ml	
T½ clearance 5 mg/kg[9]	19.6 min	
Creatinine, endogenous clearance[22]	60 ± 22 ml/min/m² of body surface	
Glomerular Filtration Rate (GFR)	2.98 ± 0.96 ml/min/kg of body weight	

Table continued on following page

Table 185. BLOOD, PLASMA, OR SERUM CHEMICAL CONSTITUENTS

(B) = Blood, (P) = Plasma, (S) = Serum (*Continued*)

Chemical constituents are liable to show markedly different values depending on the methodology used.

Cerebrospinal Fluid[12]	Adult Dog	Adult Cat
Color	Clear, colorless	Clear, colorless
Pressure (mm H_2O)	<170	<100
Cells/μl	<5 lymphocytes	<5 lymphocytes
Protein (ml/dl)	<25	<20
Glucose (mg/dl)	61–116	85

Normal Synovial Fluid—Carpal, Elbow, Shoulder, Hip, Stifle, and Hock Joints[30]	Adult Dog	
	Range	*Mean*
Amount ml	0.01–1.00	0.24
pH	7–7.8	7.33
Leukocytes × 10^3/μl		0.43
Erythrocytes × 10^3/μl	0–2.9	12.15
Neutrophils/μl	0–320	3.63
Neutrophils (%)[30]	0–32	
Monocytes/μl	10	230.77
Lymphocytes/μl	0–838	245.6
Clasmatocytes/μl	0–2436	14.69
Mononuclears (%)[30]	0–166	
Mucin clot	90	
	Tight ropy clump	
	Clear supernate	

From Bentinck-Smith, J.: A roster of normal values. *In* Kirk, R. W. (ed.): Current Veterinary Therapy VII. Philadelphia, W. B. Saunders Company, 1980, pp. 1325–1328.

Table 186. CANINE SEMEN[14]

Regular collection by hand manipulation with a teaser (125 ejaculates from small dogs, mostly beagles)[8]

	Mean	Standard Deviation	Range
Volume (ml)	5	4.3	0.5–20.4
% Motile sperm	75	7.5	30–90
% Normal sperm	86	14.7	34–97
pH	6.72	0.19	6.49–7.10
Concentration/cu mm (10^3)	148	84.6	27.2–388.8
Total sperm per ejaculate (10^6)	528	321.0	94–1428

Fractionated Ejaculates (Based on 65 Ejaculates)			
	Mean	Range	pH
1st Fraction	0.8 ml	0.25–2.00	6.37
2nd Fraction	0.6 ml	0.40–2.00	6.10
3rd Fraction	0.4 ml	1.0–16.3	7.20

Purebred Labrador Retrievers, 18 to 48 Mo[23]		
	Mean	Range
Volume (ml)	2.2*	0.5–6.5
% Motile sperm	93	75–99
% Unstained sperm (eosin nigrosin)	84	61–99
Concentration/cu mm (10^3)	564	103–708

*Only the first two fractions were collected, resulting in smaller volume and higher concentration of sperm/cu mm than would result if all the prostatic fluid (3rd fraction) were obtained.

From Bentinck-Smith, J.: A roster of normal values. *In* Kirk, R. W. (ed.): Current Veterinary Therapy VII. Philadelphia, W. B. Saunders Company, 1980, p. 1329.

Text continued from page 882

well advised to use the normal values supplied by the laboratory that they patronize. However, this laboratory must have determined its normal ranges and means by using a sufficient number of normal samples to provide statistical validity. The laboratory should run control serum samples and provide other means of quality control (see Table 178).

Because biochemical results are most frequently determined on the Technicon SMA, equipment values for this methodology are provided through the courtesy of Dr. A. I. Hurvitz and Dr. Robert J. Wilkins, The Animal Medical Center. Other data are derived from the New York State College of Veterinary Medicine, the Ralston Purina Corporation, Biozyme Veterinary Laboratory—a division of Biozyme Medical Laboratories, Inc.—standard texts, and current literature. References are cited as footnotes within the tables and are listed alphabetically at the end of this discussion.

Inappropriate collection and preparation, length of storage, hemolysis, lipemia, and hyperbilirubinemia may invalidate the laboratory results.

References and Additional Readings

1. Anderson, A. C., and Gee, W.: Normal values in the beagle. Vet. Med., 53:135 and 156, 1958.
2. Anderson, L., Wilson, R., and Hay, D.: Haematological values in normal cats from four weeks to one year of age. Res. Vet. Sci., 12:579, 1971.
3. Baker, H. J.: Laboratory evaluation of thyroid function. *In* Kirk, R. W. (ed.): Current Veterinary Therapy IV. Philadelphia, W. B. Saunders Company, 1971.
4. Belshaw, B. E., and Rijnberk, A.: Radioimmunoassay of Plasma T_4 and T_3 in the Diagnosis of Primary Hypothyroidism in Dogs. J.A.A.H.A., 15:17, 1979.
5. Benjamin, M.: An Outline of Veterinary Clinical Pathology, 3rd ed. Ames, Iowa, Iowa State Press, 1978.
6. Berman, E.: Hemogram of the cat during pregnancy and lactation and after lactation. Am. J. Vet. Res., 35:457, 1974.
7. Biozyme Veterinary Laboratory, a division of Biozyme Medical Laboratories, Inc.: Normal Ranges Chemistry. Olean, New York.
8. Boucher, J. H.: Evaluation of semen quality in the dog and the effects of frequency of ejaculation upon semen quality, libido, and restoration of sperm reserves. M.S. Thesis, Cornell University, Ithaca, New York, 1957.
9. Brobst, D. F., Carter, J. M., and Horron, M.: Plasma phenolsulfonphthalein determination as a measure of renal function in the dog. 17th Gaines Veterinary Symposium, University of Minnesota, 1967, p. 15.
10. Byars, T. D., Ling, G. V., Ferris, N. A., and Keeton, K. S.: Activated coagulation time (ACT) of whole blood in normal dogs. Am. J. Vet. Res., 37:1359, 1976.
11. Coles, E. H.: Veterinary Clinical Pathology, 3rd ed. Philadelphia, W. B. Saunders Company, 1980.
12. deLahunta, A.: New York State College of Veterinary Medicine, Cornell University, Ithaca, New York. Personal communication.
13. Ewing, G. O., Schalm, O. W., and Smith, R. S.: Hematologic values of normal Basenji dogs. J.A.V.M.A., 161:1661, 1972.
14. Revisions and corrections courtesy of Dr. R. H. Foote, Professor of Animal Physiology, Department of Animal Science, New York State College of Life Sciences, Cornell University, Ithaca, New York.
15. Kallfelz, F. A.: Associate Professor of Clinical Nutrition, Department of Large Animal Medicine, Obstetrics and Surgery, New York State College of Veterinary Medicine, Ithaca, New York. Personal communication.
16. Kallfelz, F. A., and Erali, R. P.: Thyroid function tests on domesticated animals. Am. J. Vet. Res., 34:1449, 1973.
17. Kaufman, C. F., and Kirk, R. W.: The sixty-minute plasma phenolsulfonphthalein concentration as a test of renal function in the dog. J.A.A.H.A., 9:66, 1973.
18. Kraft, W.: Schielddrusenfunktionsstörungen beim hund (Thyroid function disturbances in the dog). Thesis, Justus Liebig University, Giessen, West Germany, 1964. Cited by Belshaw.
19. Middleton, D. J., and Watson, A. D. J.: Activated coagulation times of whole blood in normal dogs and dogs with coagulopathies. J. Small Anim. Pract., 19:417, 1978.
20. Miller, J. B., Perman, V., Osborne, C. A., Hammer, R. F., and Gambardella, P. C.: Synovial fluid analysis in canine arthritis. J.A.A.H.A., 10:392, 1974.
21. Osbaldiston, G. W., Stowe, E. C., and Griffith, P. R.: Blood coagulation: comparative studies in dogs, cats, horses, and cattle. Br. Vet. J., 126:512, 1970.
22. Osborne, C. A., Low, D. G., and Finco, D. R.: Canine and Feline Urology. Philadelphia, W. B. Saunders Company, 1972.

23. Penny, R. H. C., Carlisle, C. H., and Davidson, H. A.: The blood and marrow picture of the cat. Br. Vet. J., *126*:459, 1970.
24. Pitman-Moore, Inc., Chemassay Amylase, Washington Crossing, New Jersey.
25. Ralston Purina Company: 1975 Normal Blood Values for Cats. Checkerboard Square, St. Louis, Missouri, Ralston Purina Co., Professional Marketing Services.
26. Ralston Purina Company: 1975 Normal Blood Values for Dogs. Checkerboard Square, St. Louis, Missouri, Ralston Purina Co., Professional Marketing Services.
27. Reimers, T. J.: Assistant Professor and Director of the Endocrinology Laboratory, New York State College of Veterinary Medicine, Cornell University, Ithaca, New York. Personal communication.
28. Rogers, U. A., Donovan, E. F., and Kociba, G. J.: Lipids and lipoproteins in normal dogs and dogs with secondary hyperlipoproteinemia. J.A.V.M.A., *166*:1092, 1975.
29. Rowsell, H. C.: Blood coagulation and hemorrhagic disorders. *In* Medway, W., Prier, J. E., and Wilkinson, J. S. (eds.): Textbook of Veterinary Clinical Pathology. Baltimore, Williams & Wilkins, 1969, p. 247.
30. Sawyer, D. C.: Synovial fluid analysis of canine joints. J.A.V.M.A., *143*:609, 1963.
31. Schalm, O. W., Jain, N. C., and Carroll, E. J.: Veterinary Hematology, 3rd ed. Philadelphia, Lea & Febiger, 1975.
32. Scott, D. W.: Assistant Professor of Medicine, Dept. of Clinical Sciences, New York State College of Veterinary Medicine, Cornell University, Ithaca, New York. Personal communication.
33. Seager, S. W. J., and Fletcher, W. S.: Collection, storage, and insemination of canine semen. Lab. Anim. Sci., *22*:177, 1972.
34. Tasker, J. B.: Reference values for clinical chemistry using the Coulter chemistry system. Cor. Vet., *68*:460, 1978.
35. Wallace, R.: Research Support Specialist, New York State College of Veterinary Medicine, Cornell University, Ithaca, New York. Personal communication.
36. Wilkins, R. J., and Hurvitz, A. I.: Profiling in Veterinary Clinical Pathology. Tarrytown, New York, Technicon Instruments Corp., 1978, pp. 17 and 19.
37. Wilkins, R. J.: Animal Medical Center, 510 East 62nd St., New York, New York. Personal communication.

IMMUNIZATION PROCEDURES

Cats and Dogs

See Tables 187 and 188.

Immunization of Wild Animal "Pets" Against Common Diseases

As with domestic animals, there is no unanimous opinion as to the proper method(s) that should be used in immunizing wild animals. The following information represents current approaches to the problem.

Family Canidae. Coyote, fox, jackal, wolf, dingo, cape hunting dog, and so on.

Table 187. CANINE VACCINE RECOMMENDATIONS

Disease	Type of Vaccine	Route of Administration	Age at First Vaccination (wk)	Age at Second Vaccination (wk)	Age at Third Vaccination (wk)	Revaccination
Distemper	MLV	SC or IM	6–8	10–12	14–16	Annual
Infectious	MLV	SC or IM	6–8	10–12	14–16	Annual
canine hepatitis CAV-1 or CAV-2	Inactivated	SC or IM	6–8	10–12	14–16	Annual
Parvovirus infection	MLV	SC or IM	6–8	10–12	14–16	Annual
	Inactivated	SC or IM	6–8	10–12	14–16	Annual
Bordetellosis	Inactivated	SC or IM	6–8	10–12	14–16	Annual
	Live attenuated	IN	>2	—	—	Biannual
Parainfluenza	MLV	SC, IM, or IN	6–8	10–12	14–16	Annual
Leptospirosis	Inactivated	SC or IM	10–12	14–16	—	Annual
Rabies*	MLV	IM	12–16	—	—	Annual/triennial
	Inactivated	IM	12–16	—	—	Annual/triennial

*To comply with state laws.

From Kirk, R. W.: Current Veterinary Therapy 8: Small Animal Practice. Philadelphia, W. B. Saunders Company, 1983, p. 1141.

Table 188. FELINE VACCINE RECOMMENDATIONS

Disease	Type of Vaccine	Age at First Vaccination (Wk)	Age at Second Vaccination (Wk)	Revaccination	Route of Administration
Panleukopenia (FP)	Inactivated	8–10	12–14	Annual	SC or IM
	MLV	8–10	12–14	Annual	SC or IM
	MLV IN	8–10	12–14	Annual	IN
Viral rhinotracheitis (FVR)	MLV	8–10 (or earlier)	12–14	Annual	SC or IM
	MLV IN	8–10	—	Annual	IN
	Inactivated	8–10 (or earlier)	12–14	Annual	SC or IM
Caliciviral disease (FCV)	MLV	8–10 (or earlier)	12–14	Annual	SC or IM
	MLV IN	8–10	—	Annual	IN
	Inactivated	8–10 (or earlier)	12–14	Annual	SC or IM
Pneumonitis	MLV	8	—	Annual	SC or IM
Rabies	Inactivated	12	—	Annual	IM
	MLV*	12	—	Annual	IM
Feline leukemia (FeLV)	Inactivated	9 (or later)	2–3 later	2–4 months later; then annual	IM

*Approved for use in cats (only one vaccine as of January 1983). Use of nonapproved MLV vaccines in cats can result in vaccine-induced rabies.

Modified from Kirk, R. W.: Current Veterinary Therapy 8: Small Animal Practice. Philadelphia, W. B. Saunders Company, 1983, p. 1128.

Canine distemper—infectious canine hepatitis (ICH). Administer modified live virus (MLV) vaccine as for domestic dogs. Revaccinate annually and prior to anticipated possible exposure if 6 months have elapsed since last vaccination.

Parvovirus. Canine parvovirus vaccines are being used on wild canids, but there are no data to support statements on efficacy or safety.

Rabies. Administer inactivated virus tissue culture vaccine (murine origin). Use according to manufacturer's recommendations. Begin vaccination at 3 to 6 months of age; revaccinate annually.

Family Felidae. Tiger, leopard, lion, cheetah, jaguar, lynx, ocelot, margay, bobcat, mountain lion, jungle cat, golden cat, and so on.

Feline panleukopenia. Wild *Felidae* appear to be exquisitely susceptible to the feline panleukopenia virus. Proper and adequate vaccination is a *must!*

Vaccinate with MLV vaccine containing rhinotracheitis and calicivirus vaccines. Begin vaccination when the animal is 6 to 8 weeks of age, and repeat two or three times at 4-week intervals. Revaccinate adults at 12-month intervals. Use manufacturers' recommendations.

Pneumonitis. The use of MLV pneumonitis vaccine is definitely an *elective procedure* and cannot be recommended as a routine procedure for the individual cat. Pneumonitis vaccine might best be administered to wild *Felidae* with anticipated exposure to other domestic or wild *Felidae* (such as cat shows, etc.). In this situation, the vaccine should be administered 10 to 14 days prior to anticipated exposure.

Rabies. Administer inactivated virus tissue culture vaccine (murine origin). Vaccinate kittens at 3 to 6 months of age; repeat annually in adults. Follow manufacturers' recommendations.

Family Procyonidae. Lesser panda, raccoon, coatimundi, and kinkajou.

Canine distemper. MLV vaccine may be administered according to the manufacturers' recommendations. Adults should be revaccinated annually.

Infectious canine hepatitis. Limited data available; inapparent infection may occur in raccoons. No recommendations.

Feline panleukopenia. Although proven cases have been reported only in the raccoon and the coatimundi, the current trend is to vaccinate all captive members of the family *Procyonidae.* MLV vaccine may be used according to the manufacturers' recommendations. Adults should be revaccinated every 12 months.

Pneumonitis. Elective procedure as per family *Felidae.*

Rabies. Administer inactivated MLV vaccine (murine origin). Initial vaccine may be given at 3 to 6 months of age. Adults should be revaccinated yearly.

Family Viverridae. Binturong, foussa, linsang, mongoose, and civit.

Canine distemper. Cases of proven canine distemper have been reported in the binturong and civit. It is suggested that all captive *Viverridae* be vaccinated for canine distemper as per the family *Canidae.*

Infectious canine hepatitis. No data available.

Feline panleukopenia. Cases are poorly documented, but it has been recommended that at least the binturong if not all captive *Viverridae* be vaccinated for feline panleukopenia as per the family *Felidae.*

Rabies. Vaccinate as per the families *Canidae* and *Felidae*.

Family Ursidae. Bears.

Canine distemper. Although several species of bears are reported to be susceptible to canine distemper, bears are not routinely vaccinated at zoos. Nevertheless, it might be advisable to vaccinate individual pet bears where the risk of exposure is high. MLV vaccine as per family *Canidae*.

Infectious canine hepatitis. Infection of bears with ICH has been described but not confirmed. No recommendations.

Feline panleukopenia. Cases of panleukopenia (not verified by virus isolation) have been reported in young bear cubs. No recommendations can be given at this time as to the advisability of vaccinating bears for feline panleukopenia.

Rabies. No data available.

Family Hyaenidae. Hyenas.

Canine distemper. All species of hyena are susceptible and should be vaccinated for canine distemper as per family *Canidae*.

Infectious canine hepatitis. No data available.

Rabies. As per family *Canidae*.

Family Mustelidae. Ferret, mink, otter, skunk, wolverine, badger, martin, sable, gnison, and fisher.

Canine distemper. The mink, ferret, and skunk are susceptible, and probably all captive *Mustelidae* should be vaccinated for canine distemper using an MLV vaccine as per family *Canidae*.

Infectious canine hepatitis. Limited data available. No recommendations.

Viral enteritis (may be variant of feline panleukopenia). Mink only. Administer autogenous or commercial mink enteritis formalized vaccine or killed feline panleukopenia virus vaccine. Kits, 6 to 8 weeks of age; adults should be revaccinated annually. Follow manufacturers' recommendations.

Feline panleukopenia. It has been suggested that all *Mustelidae* except the ferret are susceptible to feline panleukopenia and should receive vaccine as per the family *Felidae*. Mink should receive either killed panleukopenia vaccine or formalized mink enteritis vaccine. They need not receive both.

Botulism (mink and ferret). *Clostridium botulinum* type C toxoid. Kits can be vaccinated at 10 to 12 weeks of age; adults should be revaccinated yearly.

Rabies. Vaccinate as per family *Felidae*.

Order Marsupialia, Family Didelphidae. Opossum.

The opossum is highly resistant to infection by canine distemper and rabies and probably does not need to be vaccinated for these diseases.

Order primates. Subhuman.

Poliomyelitis (apes only—gorilla, orangutan, chimpanzee, and gibbon). Live oral polio virus vaccine. Adults, one 12-month booster with trivalent vaccine. Initial dose, a child's dose of trivalent vaccine administered twice at 6- to 8-week intervals.

Rabies. Depends on likelihood of exposure. Tissue culture vaccines duck embryo, or preferably diploid cell vaccine. MLV rabies vaccine should be avoided. Revaccinate per manufacturers' recommendations.

Tuberculosis (immunization *not* recommended). Susceptible nonhuman primates should be subjected to periodic tuberculin tests and either eliminated or vigorously treated with appropriate medication if found to be positive. Test procedure (WHO recommendations): Koch's Old Tuberculin (full strength) 0.1 cc. *intradermally* in the upper eyelid. Read test at 24, 48, and 72 hours postinjection; positive test is characterized by swelling and erythema with closure of the eye. Should have three successive negative tests at 2-week intervals.

Measles, smallpox, and so on. Vaccination of primates (especially apes) against the common childhood diseases is an elective procedure and depends on the degree of exposure to which the primate may be subjected. Consult with a pediatrician on the choice of immunizing agent(s).

Hepatitis. Where the possibility of disease exists or where there is known exposure to a hepatitis patient, gamma globulin IM may be administered prophylactically.

Order Rodentia. Mouse, rat, hamster, gerbil, guinea pig, and squirrel.

Rabies. Vaccination is not recommended for these animals if they remain caged.

Ectromelia (mice and rats). Routine vaccination is not recommended, because this viral disease does not appear to be a problem in the United States.

Order Lagamorpha. Rabbit and hare.

See Order *Rodentia.*

References and Additional Readings

Fowler, M. E.: Immunoprophylaxis in nondomestic carnivores. *In* Kirk, R. W. (ed.): Current Veterinary Therapy 8: Small Animal Practice. Philadelphia, W. B. Saunders Company, 1983.

Shipping Regulations for Small Animals*

Interstate Regulations

For the exact requirements regarding the entry of dogs and cats into the various states of the United States and Puerto Rico, inquiry should be made to the State Veterinarian in the state of destination.

Under most circumstances, no animal that is affected with or has recently been exposed to any infectious, contagious, or communicable disease or that originates from a rabies-quarantined area shall be shipped or, in any manner, transported or moved into any state until written permission for such entry is first obtained from the State Veterinarian or chief animal health official of the state to which the animal is to be transported.

Common carriers will usually not accept dogs or cats for interstate movement without health certificates; thus, it would seem advisable, even if

---

*From Kirk, R. W. (ed.): Current Veterinary Therapy VII. Philadelphia, W. B. Saunders Company, 1980, p. 1317.

not specifically required, that such certificates be issued by the accredited practicing veterinarian in the state of origin.

International Regulations

Travelers from the United States to foreign countries on vacations and duty assignments frequently desire to take their pets with them. Similarly, persons returning from abroad need to make arrangements for the reentry of their pets and for animals acquired in other countries. For both importations and exportations, there are usually health requirements with which one must comply.

MOVEMENT INTO FOREIGN COUNTRIES

There are no United States Regulations governing the movement of dogs and cats to any foreign country. The regulations that must be complied with are those of the receiving country. These regulations are many, varied, and subject to change. If pets are to be moved to any foreign country except Canada, the owner should obtain from the nearest consulate of the country of destination that country's regulations and procedural instructions governing the import of pets, such as the number of copies of the health certificate to be furnished, an indication of whether it must be validated by the consulate, and whether certified copies of the pedigree or photograph of the pet must accompany the health certificate.

Dogs from the United States may be imported into Canada through any Canadian customs port of entry when accompanied by a certificate signed by a veterinarian licensed in Canada or the United States. The certificate must show that the dog has been vaccinated against rabies during the preceding 12 months.

IMPORTATION OR REENTRY OF DOGS INTO THE UNITED STATES

The entry of dogs into the United States from all foreign countries is under the jurisdiction of the Public Health Service of the United States Department of Health, Education, and Welfare. An excerpt from the United States Public Health Service regulations regarding importation of dogs is quoted:

Vaccination for rabies shall be accomplished with nerve tissue vaccine more than one month but not more than 12 months before the dog's arrival, or with chicken embryo vaccine more than one month but not more than 36 months before arrival.

DRUG THERAPY
Prescription Writing

A prescription is a written order given by a veterinarian to a pharmacist. Drugs may be prescribed by their official names, which are listed in the *United States Pharmacopeia (USP)* or *National Formulary* (NF); by their nonofficial generic names or *United States Adopted Name (USAN)*; or by manufacturer's trade name. Prescribing drugs by their generic name allows a pharmacist to dispense a more economical product than a trademarked preparation. Some states have "generic drug laws" specifying that a pharmacist must dispense only a generic drug.

A prescription by tradition is written in a certain order and consists of four basic parts.

1. *Superscription*—This is R_x, coming from the Latin abbreviation for recipe, meaning "take thou."
2. *Inscription*—Represents the ingredients and their amounts.
3. *Subscription*—Contains the directions for dispensing.
4. *Signature*—Abbreviated as *sig;* contains the directions on how the drug is to be administered (such as 1 teaspoonful three times a day). The signature should indicate whether the medicine is intended for external, internal, or other special form of application and whether any toxic effects may be produced.

Additionally, the basic parts of the prescription should include the name of the client; the animal's name and some descriptive notation or number; whether the medication is refillable, and if so, how often; and a BNDD number, if indicated. They must be signed by the veterinarian.

Prescriptions are written in English, but Latin abbreviations may be time-saving; the common abbreviations are included in Table 189. (See also Fig. 106.)

Antimicrobial and Antibacterial Therapy

See Tables 190 and 191.

Digitalization Therapy

See Table 192.
1. There is no specific dosage for digitalization.
2. Every cardiac glycoside dose must be adjusted to the individual animal at that particular time.
3. Accumulation of digitalis in the body is dependent on maintenance dose. Rapid loading dose of digitalis should be used only in acute cardiac failure.
4. *Do not* give digitalizing dose to the point of toxicity.
5. Give digoxin on the basis of lean body weight, which is total body weight minus 15 per cent.

Text continues on page 924

NEW YORK STATE VETERINARY TEACHING HOSPITAL
CORNELL UNIVERSITY
ITHACA, NEW YORK 14853

Owner's Name .... Address ....

R
 Animal's Name .... AGE .... WT. .... SEX .... BREED ....

M.D.D.: ....

DATE ....

DEA # ....

REFILL: 0 1 2 3 4 5 .... Times

THIS PRESCRIPTION WILL BE FILLED GENERICALLY UNLESS SIGNED "DISPENSE AS WRITTEN."

_____ DVM   _____ DVM

A DISPENSE AS WRITTEN   SUBSTITUTION PERMISSIBLE

NEW YORK STATE VETERINARY TEACHING HOSPITAL
CORNELL UNIVERSITY
ITHACA, NEW YORK 14853

Owner's Name *Jane Doe* .... Address *5 Pine St, Any City*

R
 Animal's Name *Fido* AGE *5 Y* WT. *30 lb* SEX *M* BREED *Spaniel*

Phenobarbital 30 mg

Tabs No. 60

Sig 1 Tab q 12 h

M.D.D.: *2 Tabs*

DATE *10/10/70*

DEA # *0123456*

REFILL: 0 1 2 ③ 4 5 .... Times

THIS PRESCRIPTION WILL BE FILLED GENERICALLY UNLESS SIGNED "DISPENSE AS WRITTEN."

_____ DVM   *James Smith* DVM

B DISPENSE AS WRITTEN   SUBSTITUTION PERMISSIBLE

Figure 106. A and B, Prescription forms.

Table 189. COMMONLY USED PRESCRIPTION
ABBREVIATIONS

Abbreviation	Meaning
ad lib.	freely; as much as is wanted
aa	of each
a.c.	before meals
aqua	water
aqua dist.	distilled water
b.i.d.	twice daily
caps	capsules
chart.	powder
$\bar{c}$	with
d.t.d.	give such doses
gtt.	a drop, drops
h.	hour
h.s.	hour of sleep; at bedtime
Tr.	tincture
Ung.	ointment
at diet.	as directed
M	mix
non. rep.	do not repeat
No.	number
s.i.d.	once daily
o.h.	every hour
o.d.	right eye
o.s.	left eye
os.	mouth
pil.	pill
$\bar{p}$	after
p.c.	after meals
p.r.n.	according to circumstances; occasionally
q.s.	a sufficient amount
q.i.d.	four times a day
$\bar{ss}$	one-half
sig.	write on label
$\bar{s}$	without
stat	immediately
tab.	tablet
t.i.d.	three times a day

Table 190. USE OF ANTIMICROBIAL AGENTS FOR TREATMENT OF INFECTIONS

Organism	Disease	Drugs of Choice	Alternative Drugs
Actinomyces	Actinomycosis	Penicillin G*	Tetracyclines
Anaerobic organisms *Peptococcus, Peptostreptococcus, Lactobacillus*	Soft tissue infections, granulomas, wound infections after GI surgery	Chloramphenicol, ampicillin, clindamycin/lincomycin	Penicillin, cephaloridine, erythromycin
Bacillus anthracis	Anthrax	Penicillin G	Erythromycin, cephalosporin, tetracyclines
Bacteroides	Wound infections	Chloramphenicol, clindamycin	Tetracycline, cephalosporin
Blastomyces, Candida, Coccidioides, Cryptococcus, Mucor, Aspergillus	Pneumonia, skin and soft-tissue lesions, bone lesions, disseminated disease	Amphotericin B	2 hydroxystilbamide† (*Blastomyces*), flucytosine† (*Candida, Cryptococcus*)
Bordetella bronchiseptica	Respiratory infections	Tetracyclines	Chloramphenicol
Brucella canis	Abortions	Tetracyclines with streptomycin	Chloramphenicol with streptomycin
Chlamydia psittaci	Respiratory infections, conjunctivitis	Tetracyclines	Chloramphenicol
Clostridium tetani	Tetanus	Penicillin G*	Erythromycin
Clostridia (other)	Gas gangrene	Penicillin G*	Tetracyclines
Coccidia	Coccidiosis	Sulfonamides	Nitrofurazone

Table continued on following page

Table 190. USE OF ANTIMICROBIAL AGENTS FOR TREATMENT OF INFECTIONS (Continued)

Organism	Disease	Drugs of Choice	Alternative Drugs
Escherichia coli	Urinary tract infections	Gentamicin, ampicillin	Cephalosporins, nitrofurantoin, chloramphenicol, tetracyclines, sulfonamides, Tribrissen
	Other infections	Ampicillin, chloramphenicol, tetracyclines	Aminoglycosides, polymyxins
Fusobacterium	Ulcerative stomatitis	Penicillin G	Tetracyclines, metronidazole
Giardia	Enteritis	Penicillin G	Quinacrine, glycobiarsol
Haemobartonella	Infectious anemia	Tetracyclines‡	Chloramphenicol‡
Klebsiella, Enterobacter	Respiratory, urinary tract infections	Kanamycin, gentamicin	Cephalosporins, chloramphenicol
Leptospira	Leptospirosis	Penicillin G with streptomycin	Tetracyclines
Microsporum, Trichophyton, Epidermophyton	Skin, hair, and nail bed infections	Griseofulvin	—
Mycobacterium	Tuberculosis	Isoniazid with streptomycin or p-aminosalicylic acid	—
Mycoplasma	Respiratory infection (?), conjunctivitis	Erythromycin	Chloramphenicol, tetracycline
Neorickettsia	Salmon disease	Tetracyclines	Chloramphenicol
Nocardia	Nocardiosis	Sulfonamides with ampicillin or Tribrissen	Ampicillin with erythromycin
Pasteurella multocida	Abscesses, respiratory infections	Penicillin G*	Tetracyclines, ampicillin

Organism	Infection	Drug of Choice	Alternative Drugs
Pentatrichomonas	Trichomonal enteritis	Metronidazole	Glycobiarsol
Pityrosporum	Skin and ear infections	2% "tame" iodine or 25% glyceryl triacetate topically	—
Proteus mirabilis	Urinary tract and soft-tissue infections	Ampicillin, cephalosporin, nitrofurantoin§	Chloramphenicol, aminoglycosides
Pseudomonas	Urinary tract and soft-tissue infections, burns	Gentamicin, tobramycin	Carbenicillin with amikacin
Salmonella	Gastroenteritis	Chloramphenicol	Ampicillin, nitrofurans
Staphylococcus aureus	Pyoderma, endocarditis, osteomyelitis, soft-tissue infections	Penicillin G Sensitive: penicillin G Penicillin G resistant: chloxacillin, erythromycin	Ampicillin, macrolides, lincomycin Cephalosporins, chloramphenicol, lincomycin
Streptococcus	Urinary tract infections, otitis, soft-tissue infections, upper respiratory infections	Penicillin G	Ampicillin, cephalosporins, erythromycin
Toxoplasma	Toxoplasmosis	Pyrimethamine with sulfonamide	—

*Large dosage.
†Used to treat these infections in man; efficacy in dogs and cats uncertain.
‡Efficacy questionable.
§Urinary tract infections only.

Modified from Aronson, A. L., and Kirk, R. W.: Antimicrobial drugs. *In* Ettinger, S. J.: Textbook of Veterinary Internal Medicine. Philadelphia, W. B. Saunders Company, 1975. Also see Watson, A. D. J.: Antimicrobial therapy. *In* Kirk, R. W. (ed.): Current Veterinary Therapy VI. Philadelphia, W. B. Saunders Company, 1977, pp. 18–19.

Table 191. MOST EFFECTIVE pH FOR OPTIMAL ANTIBACTERIAL ACTIVITY

Antimicrobial Drug	pH 5.5	6.0	6.5	7.0	7.5	8.0
ˣAmpicillin	+	+	+			
Cephalothin*		+	+	+	+	+
ˣChloramphenicol*					+	+
ˣColistin					+	+
Erythromycin†						+
Gentamicin					+	+
ˣKanamycin					+	+
Lincomycin					+	
ˣMethenamine mandelate	+	+				
ˣNeomycin†					+	+
ˣNitrofurantoin†		+				
Novobiocin	+	+				
Oxacillin		+				
ˣPenicillin G		+	+			
ˣPolymyxin*						+ (best)
Streptomycin†					+	+
ˣSulfonamides*		+	+	+	+	+
(pH not important except as it affects solubility)						
Tetracycline*		+	+	+		
ˣOxytetracycline*	+	+	+			
Chlortetracycline†		+				

*The pH is not important. Effectiveness of the drug is not highly dependent on pH but (+) indicates optimal range.

†The pH is very important. Effectiveness of the drug is highly dependent on pH; (+) indicates optimal range.

ˣEspecially useful in urinary infections.

Text continued from page 918

6. Larger animals require a smaller dose of digoxin per pound of body weight.
7. Daily maintenance dose of digoxin for older animals should be reduced by 25 to 50 per cent.
8. Digoxin dosage should be reduced 50 per cent for each 50 mg per cent increase in BUN.
9. In cases of renal failure, administer the maintenance dose more frequently—every 4 to 8 hours instead of every 12 hours.
10. When using digoxin elixir, the lean body weight dosage should be reduced an additional 10 per cent.

THERAPEUTIC BLOOD LEVELS OF DIGOXIN IN THE DOG

Determinations of digoxin serum concentrations by radioimmunoassay can be obtained after constant maintenance dosages have been given for at least

Table 192. DIGITALIZATION AND MAINTENANCE GUIDE FOR
VETERINARY DIGOXIN ELIXIR
(LANOXIN—0.05 MG PER CC)

Digitalization (Guide* to 48-Hour Loading Dose Method. Digoxin Given Every 12 Hours for 48 Hours.†)			Maintenance (Guide‡ to Maintenance Dosage. Digoxin Given Every 12 Hours.§)		
Weight in lb	*Dosage in cc*	*Dosage in mg*	*Weight in lb*	*Dosage in cc*	*Dosage in mg*
5	1.2–2.4 cc	0.06–0.12 mg	5	0.45 cc	0.022 mg ± 0.15 cc
10	2.4–4.8 cc	0.12–0.24 mg	10	0.90 cc	0.045 mg ± 0.24 cc
15	3.6–7.2 cc	0.18–0.36 mg	15	1.50 cc	0.075 mg ± 0.36 cc
20	4.8–9.6 cc	0.24–0.48 mg	20	1.80 cc	0.090 mg ± 0.45 cc
30	7.8–9.9 cc	0.40–0.50 mg	30	3.00 cc	0.15 mg ± 0.75 cc
40	9.9–15.0 cc	0.50–0.75 mg	40	3.60 cc	0.18 mg ± 0.90 cc
50	15.0 cc	0.75 mg	50	4.50 cc	0.225 mg ± 1.20 cc
over 50	19.8 cc	1.0 mg	over 50	6.00 cc	0.30 mg ± 1.50 cc
over 100	30.0 cc	1.5 mg	over 100	9.00 cc	0.45 mg ± 3.00 cc

*Guideline means the approximate amount of the glycoside usually required by dogs in each weight group. Individual variations will occur and must be considered.

†Dosage to be given for four full doses unless intoxication develops first. Signs of digitalis intoxication indicate that full digitalization has been reached, regardless of the dose administered.

‡Guideline refers to the approximate amount of the glycoside usually required by dogs in each weight category for daily maintenance therapy. Individual variations require individual titration of the actual dosage.

§Requires twice-daily administration, preferably at 12-hour intervals.

Courtesy of Burroughs Wellcome Company.

3.5 half-lives (10 days) of the drug. Dogs with digoxin levels greater than 3.5 ng per ml are toxic. Dogs with a digoxin level between 1 and 3.0 ng per ml are adequately digitalized. Dogs with digoxin levels less than 1 ng per ml are not adequately digitalized.

THERAPEUTIC BLOOD LEVELS OF DIGOXIN IN THE CAT

The toxic range of digoxin in the cat is 2.4 to 2.9 ng per ml. The mean therapeutic concentration is 1.4 ng per ml and biological half-life is 33 ± 9.5 hours.

Drugs Used to Treat Solid Tumors in Dogs and Cats

See Table 193.

Table 193. DRUGS USED TO TREAT SOLID TUMORS IN DOGS AND CATS

Drug	Suggested Dosages
Plant Alkaloids	
Vincristine (Oncovin, Eli Lilly), 1- and 5-mg vials	0.5 mg/m² weekly or biweekly, IV
	0.0125–0.025 mg/kg weekly, IV
Vinblastine (Velban, Eli Lilly), 10-mg vials	2 mg/m² weekly or biweekly, IV
	0.05–0.1 mg/kg every 7–10 days, IV
Antimetabolites	
Methotrexate (Lederle Labs), 2.5-mg tablets, 5- and 10-mg vials	0.06 mg/kg daily, per os (may vomit)
	2.5 mg/m² daily, per os (may vomit)
	5–10 mg/m² once per day × 4 days weekly, per os or IV
	0.3–0.8 mg/kg weekly, IV
	15 mg/m² for dogs ≤15 kg or 20 mg/m² for dogs ≥16 kg IV every 3 weeks in combination therapy
	DO NOT USE IN CATS
5-Fluorouracil (Roche Labs), 500-mg vials	100–200 mg/m² weekly, IV
	2–5 mg/kg weekly, IV
Alkylating Agents	
Cyclophosphamide (Cytoxan, Mead Johnson), 25- and 50-mg tablets; 100-, 200- and 500-mg vials	50 mg/m² once per day × 3 to 4 days, weekly, IV or per os
	10 mg/kg every 7–10 days, IV
	200 mg/m² or 10 mg/kg, every 3 weeks, IV, in combination therapy
n, n′, n″ Triethylenethiophosphoramide (thio-TEPA, Lederle Labs), 15-mg vials	9 mg/m² as single dose or as 2–4 divided doses on successive days, IV or intracavitary
	0.2–0.5 mg/m² as single dose repeated weekly, IV or intracavitary
	0.2–0.5 mg/kg daily × 5 or 10 days, repeat every 3 weeks

Antibiotics

Actinomycin D (Cosmegan, Merck, Sharp, and Dohme), 500-μg vials

0.015 mg/kg every 3–5 days, IV, wait 3 weeks for marrow recovery

1.5 mg/m² once weekly

Doxorubicin hydrochloride (Adriamycin, Adria Labs), 10- and 50-mg vials

30 mg/m² every 21 days, IV, maximum cumulative dose 300 mg/m², dose every 5 weeks in cats

10 mg/m² once per day × 3–4 days, IV or SQ, repeat weekly, maximum cumulative dosage 200 mg/m²

Bleomycin (Blenoxane, Bristol Labs), 15 units/vial

0.3–0.5 units/kg weekly, IM

Hormones

Adrenal corticosteroids (prednisone)

0.5–1.0 mg/lb divided b.i.d., per os

10–40 mg/m² daily, per os, gradually change to 10–20 mg/m² every 2 days

30 mg/m² once per day, per os, decreasing weekly

Miscellaneous

Dacarbazine (DTIC, Dome Labs), 100- and 200-mg vials

100 mg/m² IV, days 1–5 every 3 weeks in combination therapy

200 mg/m² × 5 days every 3 weeks, IV

300 mg/m² IV, every 3 weeks

From Brown, N.: Management of solid tumors. *In* Kirk, R. W. (ed.): Current Veterinary Therapy 8: Small Animal Practice Philadelphia, W. B. Saunders Company, 1983, p. 416.

TABLE OF COMMON DRUGS: APPROXIMATE DOSES

Drug Name	Dog	Cat
Acetazolamide	10 mg/kg q6h PO	Same
Acetylcysteine (Mucomyst)	*Eye:* Dilute to 2% of soln with artificial tears and apply topically q2h to eye for maximum of 48 hr *Respiratory:* 50 ml/hr for 30–60 min q12h by nebulization	Same
Acetylpromazine (acepromazine)	0.055–0.11 mg/kg IV, IM, SC 0.55–2.2 mg/kg PO	0.055–0.11 mg/kg IM, SC 1.1–2.2 mg/kg PO
Acetylsalicylic acid (aspirin)	*Analgesia:* 10 mg/kg PO q12h *Antirheumatic:* 40 mg/kg PO q18h or 25 mg/kg q8h	*Analgesia:* 10 mg/kg PO q52h *Antirheumatic:* 40 mg/kg q72h
ACTH	2 units/kg/day IM (therapeutic) or 20 units/dog IM (response test; take post sample in 2 hr)	10 units/cat IM (response test)
Actinomycin D (Cosmegan)	0.015 mg/kg/once daily for 5 days	None
Aldactone (spironolactone)	1–2 mg/kg q12h	Same
Allopurinol (Zyloprim)	10 mg/kg PO q8h, then reduce to 10 mg/kg PO daily	None
Amatraz (Mitaban)	10.6 ml in 2 gallons water, dip q2wk for 3 treatments, let dry on	None
Amforol	2–6 tablets/9 kg initially *Maintenance:* 1–3 tabs/9 kg q8h	None
Amikacin	5 mg/kg q8h IM, IV	None
Aminophylline	10 mg/kg q8h PO, IM, IV	6.6 mg/kg q12h PO
Ammonium chloride	100 mg/kg q12h PO	¼ tsp powder/feeding
Amoxicillin	22 mg/kg q12h PO	Same
Amphetamine	4.4 mg/kg IV, IM	Same
Amphotericin B	0.15–1.0 mg/kg dissolved in 5–20 ml 5% dextrose and water given rapidly IV 3× weekly for 2–4 mo. Do not exceed 2.0 mg/kg. Pretreat with antiemetics if needed. Monitor BUN.	Same
Ampicillin (Polyflex, Princillin)	10–20 mg/kg q6h PO; 5–10 mg/kg q6h IV, IM, SC	Same
Amprolium	100–200 mg/kg/day in food or water for 7–10 days	None
Anterior pituitary gonadotropin	*Bitches:* 100–500 units once daily to effect	None
Apomorphine	0.02 mg/kg IV or 0.04 mg/kg SC; ¼–½ tablet in conjunctival sac, flush once emesis begins	None

Ascorbic acid (vitamin C)	100–500 mg/day (maintenance) or 100–500 mg q8h (urine acidifier)	100 mg/day (maintenance) or 100 mg q8h (urine acidifier)
L-Asparginase	10,000–20,000 IU/m² weekly IP or 400 IU/kg weekly	Same
Atropine	0.05 mg/kg q6h IV, SC, IM or 1% soln in eye	Same
	Organophosphate poisoning:	
	0.2–2.0 mg/kg IV, SC, IM. Give ¼ dose IV and remainder IM or SC prn	
Aurothioglucose (Solganol)	First wk 5 mg IM; second wk 10 mg IM; then 1 mg/kg once/wk IM, decreasing to once/mo	First wk, 1 mg IM; second wk, 2 mg IM; then 1 mg/kg once/wk IM, decreasing to once/mo
Azathioprine	2 mg/kg q24h PO	None
BAL	4 mg/kg q4h IM until recovered	None
Betamethasone (Betasone)	0.028–0.055 ml/kg IM. Give only once.	None
Bethanechol (Urecholine)	5–25 mg q8h PO	2.5–5.0 mg q8h PO
Bismuth, milk of	10–30 ml q4h PO	Same
Bismuth (subnitrate, subgallate, or subcarbonate)	0.3–3.0 gm q4h PO	Same
Bleomycin (Blenoxane)	10 mg/m² daily IV or SC for 4 days, then 10 mg/m² weekly to a maximum total dose of 200 mg/m²	None
Blood	20 ml/kg IV or IP or to effect	Same
Brewer's yeast	0.2 gm/kg once daily PO	Same
Bromsulphalein (BSP) (5% solution)	*Test only:* 5 mg/kg IV; post sample in 30 min	None
Bunamidine (Scolaban)	25–50 mg/kg PO. Fast 3 hr before and after administration.	Same
Busulfan (Myleran)	4.0 mg/m² daily PO; 0.1 mg/kg daily	None
Butorphanol	0.055–0.11 mg/kg q6–12h SC up to 7 days; 0.55 mg/kg q6–12h PO	None
Caffeine	0.1–0.5 gm IM	None
Calcium carbonate	1–4 gm/day PO	Same
Calcium chloride (10% solution)	1–2 ml IV, IC	0.05–0.1 ml/kg IV, IC
Calcium EDTA	100 mg/kg diluted to 10 mg/ml in 5% dextrose and given SC in 4 divided doses; continue for 5 days	Same
Calcium gluconate (10% solution)	10–30 ml IV (slowly)	5–15 ml IV (slowly)
Calcium lactate	0.5–2.0 gm PO	0.2–0.5 gm PO

Table continued on following page

TABLE OF COMMON DRUGS: APPROXIMATE DOSES (Continued)

Drug Name	Dog	Cat
Canine DA₂P vaccine	1 vial SC at 8, 12, and 16 wk of age; annual booster	None
Canine parvovirus vaccine (MLV)	1 ml SC 8, 12, 16, and 20 wk; annual revaccination	None
Carbenicillin	15 mg/kg q8h IV	Same
Castor oil	8–30 ml PO	4–10 ml PO
Cephalexin (Keflex)	30 mg/kg q12h PO	Same
Cephalothin sodium	35 mg/kg q8h IM, IV	Same
Cephapirin	10–20 mg/kg q6h IM, IV	Same
Charcoal, activated (Requa)	0.3–5 gm q8–12h PO	Half the canine dose
	Poisoning: 1–2 tsp/10–15 kg in 200 ml tap water. Administer by stomach tube.	
Cheracol	5 ml q4h PO	3 ml q4h PO
Chlorambucil (Leukeran)	0.2 mg/kg PO once daily	Same
	1.5 mg/m² PO as single dose; decrease for repeated dosage	
Chloramphenicol	50 mg/kg q8h PO, IV, IM, SC	Same, except q12h
Chlordane	0.5% solution on dog or premises	None
Chlorethamine	0.2–1.0 gm q8h PO	100 mg q8h PO
Chlorpheniramine	4–8 mg q12h PO	2 mg q12h PO
Chlorpromazine (Thorazine)	3.3 mg/kg PO sid to qid;	Same
	1.1–6.6 mg/kg IM sid to qid;	
	0.55–4.4 mg/kg IV sid to qid	
Chlortetracycline	20 mg/kg q8h PO	Same
Chlorthiazide (Diuril)	20–40 mg/kg q12h PO	Same
Cimetidine (Tagamet)	5–10 mg/kg q6–12h	None
Cloxacillin	10 mg/kg q6h PO, IV, IM	Same
Cod liver oil	1 tsp/10 kg once daily PO	Same
Codeine	*Pain:* 2 mg/kg q6h SC	None
	Cough: 5 mg/dose q6h PO	
Colistimethate (Coly-Mycin)	1.1 mg/kg q6h IM	Same
Cyclophosphamide (Cytoxan)	6.6 mg/kg PO for 3 days, then 2.2 mg/kg PO once daily;	Same

Drug		
Cyclothiazide		None
Cytarabine (Cytosar)	10 mg/kg q7–10 days IV; 50 mg/m² PO, IV once daily for 3–4 days/wk; repeat prn	Same
Dapsone	0.5–1.0 mg/PO once daily	None
Darbazine	5–10 mg/kg once daily for 2 wk, or 30–50 mg/kg IV, IM, SC once/wk; 100 mg/m² once daily IV, IM for 4 days, then 150 mg/m²; 1.1 mg/kg q8h PO; 0.14–0.22 ml/kg q12h SC;	0.14–0.22 ml/kg q12h SC
Delta Albaplex	2–7 kg: 1 #1 capsule q12h PO; 7–14 kg: 1–2 #1 capsules q12h PO; Over 14 kg: 1 #3 capsule q12h PO 3–7 kg: 1–2 tablets/day PO; 7–14 kg: 2–4 tablets/day PO; 14–27 kg: 4–6 tablets/day PO; Over 27 kg: 6–8 tablets/day PO	1 tablet q12h PO
Depo-penicillin	15,000–30,000 units/kg q48h IM, SC	Same
Desoxycorticosterone acetate (Doca)	1–5 mg q24h IM	0.5–1.0 mg q24h IM
Desoxycorticosterone pivalate	Each 25 mg releases 1 mg Doca/day for 1 mo IM dose: 5–10 mg once/mo to effect	Same
Dexamethasone (Azium)	0.25–1.0 mg IV, IM once daily; 0.25–1.25 mg PO once daily; *Shock*: 5 mg/kg IV	0.125–0.5 mg once daily PO, IV, IM *Shock*: same
Dextran	20 ml/kg IV to effect	Same
Dextrose solutions (5% in water, saline, or Ringer's)	40–50 ml/kg q24h IV, SC, IP	Same
Diazepam (Valium)	2.5–20 mg IV, PO; 10-mg bolus IV (slowly) if in status epilepticus; repeat if no effect	2.5–5.0 mg IV, PO
Diazoxide	10–40 mg/kg/day divided PO	None
Dichlorphenamide	2–4 mg/kg q8h PO	10–25 mg q8h PO
Dichlorvos (Task)	26.4–33 mg/kg PO; in risk animals divide dose, give remaining half 8–24 hr later	None
Dicloxacillin (Dicloxin)	11–55 mg/kg q8h PO	Same

Table continued on following page

TABLE OF COMMON DRUGS: APPROXIMATE DOSES (Continued)

Drug Name	Dog	Cat
Diethylcarbamazine (Caricide, Cypip, Filaribits)	*Treatment of ascarids:* 55–110 mg/kg PO *Prevention of ascarids:* (Cypip) 3.3 mg/kg PO once daily *Prevention of heartworms:* (Caricide, Filaribits) 6.6 mg/kg PO once daily	*Treatment of ascarids:* 55–110 mg/kg PO
Diethylstilbestrol (DES)	0.1–1.0 mg/day PO	0.05–0.10 mg/day PO (caution)
Di-Gel (liquid)	30–60 ml PO	Half the canine dose
Digitoxin (Foxalin-Vet)	0.033–0.11 mg/kg PO, divided bid	None
Digoxin (Lanoxin, Cardoxin)	*Digitalization:* 0.028–0.055 mg/kg q12h PO for 2 days *Maintenance:* 0.0055–0.011 mg/kg q12h PO; 0.01 mg/kg IM q6–12h to digitalize (maximum dose 0.04–0.06 mg/kg), then switch to ¼ total amount given q24h for maintenance; 0.044 mg/kg IV to digitalize, then switch to oral maintenance; or 0.01 mg/kg IV q1h to digitalize (maximum dose 0.04–0.06 mg/kg), then switch to ¼ total amount given q24h for maintenance	0.0055 mg/kg q12h (tablet only)
Dihydrocodeinone	5 mg q6h PO	None
Dihydrostreptomycin	10 mg/kg q8h IM, SC	Same
Dihydrotachysterol	0.01 mg/kg/day	1–2 drops q12–24h PO
Dimenhydrinate (Dramamine)	25–50 mg q8h PO	12.5 mg q8h PO
Dioctyl sulfosuccinate (Surfak, Permeatrate)	10–15 ml of 5% soln with 100 ml water q12h PO, per rectum prm; 1 or 2 50-mg capsules q12–24h PO	2 ml of 5% soln with 50 ml water q12h PO, per rectum prm; 1 50-mg capsule q12–24h PO
Diphenhydramine (Benadryl)	2–4 mg/kg q8h PO; 5–50 mg q12h IV	Same
Diphenylhydantoin (Dilantin) See *Phenytoin*		
Diphenylthiocarbazone	60 mg/kg q8h PO for 5 days beyond recovery	None
Dipyrone	25 mg/kg SC, IM, IV, may repeat q8h	Same
Disophenol (DNP)	10 mg/kg SC; may be repeated in 2–3 weeks	None

Disopyramide (Dizan)	6–15 mg/kg q8h PO	None
Dithiazanine (Dizan)	6.6–11 mg/kg PO once daily for 7–10 days	None
Dobutamine HCl (Dobutrex)	250 mg in 1,000 ml 5% dextrose, IV at a rate of 2.5 mcg/kg/min	None
Domeboro's solution	1–2 tablets/pint water; apply topically q8h; store soln no longer than 7 days	Same
Dopamine HCl (Intropin)	40 mg in 500 ml lactated Ringer's, IV at a rate of 2–8 mcg/kg/min	Same
Doxapram (Dopram)	5–10 mg/kg IV	5–10 mg/kg IV
	Neonate: 1–5 mg SC, sublingual or umbilical vein	*Neonate*: 1–2 mg SC, sublingual vein
Doxorubicin (Adriamycin)	30 mg/m² IV q 3 wk	None
Doxylamine succinate	1–2 mg/kg q8h IM	Same
Edrophonium	0.11–0.22 mg/kg IV	None
Emetrol	4–12 ml q15min PO until emesis ceases	Same
Enflurane (Ethrane)	*Induction*: 2–3%	Same
	Maintenance: 1.5–3%	
Ephedrine	5–15 mg PO	2–5 mg PO
Epinephrine (1:1000 soln)	0.1–0.5 ml SC, IM, IV, or intracardiac	0.1–0.2 ml SC, IM, IV, or intracardiac
Erythromycin	10 mg/kg q8h PO	Same
Estradiol cyclopentyl propionate (ECP)	0.25–2.0 mg IM *once*	0.25–0.5 mg IM *once*
Ether	0.5–4.0 ml (*Induction*: 8%; *Maintenance*: 4%; inhalant to effect)	Same
Ethoxzolamide (Cardrase)	4 mg/kg q12h PO	Same
Feline panleukopenia vaccine	Used, but not FDA-approved	1 vial SC at 8, 12, and 16 wk of age; annual booster
Fenbendazole	50 mg/kg/day for 3 days	None
Fentanyl (Sublimaze)	0.02–0.04 mg/kg (preanesthetic) IM, IV, SC	Same, but use with tranquilizer to prevent excitation
Ferrous sulfate	100–300 mg q24h PO	50–100 mg q24h PO
Festal	1–2 tablets PO with or immediately after feeding	1 tablet PO with or immediately after feeding
Flucytosine (Ancobon)	100 mg/kg q12h PO	Same

Table continued on following page

TABLE OF COMMON DRUGS: APPROXIMATE DOSES (Continued)

Drug Name	Dog	Cat
Fludrocortisone (Florinef)	0.2–0.8 mg once daily PO	0.1–0.2 mg once daily PO
Flumethasone (Flucort)	0.06–0.25 mg once daily PO, IV, IM, SC	0.03–0.125 mg once daily PO, IV, IM, SC
Flunixin	0.3 mg/kg IM	None
5-Fluorouracil	5 mg/kg IV q 5–7 days;	None
	200 mg/m^2 IV once daily for 3 days, followed by 100 mg/m^2 IV on alternate days until signs of toxicity appear; then 200–400 mg/m^2 IV weekly	
Folic acid	5 mg/day PO	2.5 mg/day PO
Furosemide (Lasix)	2.5–5.0 mg/kg once or twice daily at 6–8-hr intervals PO, IM, IV	2.5 mg/kg once or twice daily at 6–8-hr intervals PO, IM, IV
Gentamicin	2 mg/kg q8h IM, SC	Same
Glucagon	*Tolerance test:* 0.03 mg/kg IV	None
Glycerin	0.6 ml/kg q8h PO	Same
Glycopyrrolate	0.01 mg/kg IM or SC	None
Griseofulvin	50 mg/kg PO once daily with fat for 6 wk	Same
Halothane (Fluothane)	*Induction:* 3%	Same
	Maintenance: 0.5–1.5%	
Heparin	Initial IV dose: 200 units/kg; continue by SC administration q8h	Same
Hetacillin (Hetacin)	10–20 mg/kg q8h PO	Same
Hydralazine	1 mg/kg q8h PO	None
Hydrochlorothiazide (Hydrodiuril)	2–4 mg/kg q12h PO	Same
Hydrocortisone (Solu-Cortef)	4.4 mg/kg q12h PO	Same
	Shock: 50 mg/kg IV	
Hydrogen peroxide (3%)	5–10 ml q 15 min PO until emesis occurs	Same
Hydroxyurea (Hydrea)	80 mg/kg q 3 days PO; 40–50 mg/kg divided twice daily PO;	Same
Imidazole (DTIC)	20–30 mg/kg PO as a single daily dose	None
	200 mg/m^2 for 5 days IV; repeat 5-day cycle q 3 wk	

Innovar-Vet	0.1–0.14 ml/kg IM; 0.04–0.09 ml/kg IV; Administer with atropine to minimize bradycardia and salivation	CNS excitation—do not use.
Insulin (regular)	2 units/kg q2–6h IV (ketoacidosis), modified to effect *Hyperkalemia:* 0.5–1.0 units/kg with 2 gm dextrose per unit of insulin	3–5 units SC q6h, modified to effect
Insulin (intermediate)	0.5–1.0 units/kg q24h SC, modified as needed	3–5 units q24h SC, modified as needed
Isoproterenol (Isuprel)	0.1–0.2 mg q6h IM, SC; 15–30 mg q4h PO 1 mg in 250 ml 5% dextrose, IV at a rate of 0.01 mcg/kg/min	Same 0.5 mg in 250 ml 5% dextrose, IV to effect
Isuprel	Elixir: 0.44 ml/kg q8h PO	Same
Jenotone	2 mg/kg q12h IM, SC	Same
Kanamycin (Kantrim)	10 mg/kg q6h PO; 7 mg/kg q6h IM, SC	Same
Kaopectate	1–2 ml/kg q2–6h	*Restraint:* 11 mg/kg IM
Ketamine (Vetalar)	None	*Anesthesia:* 22–33 mg/kg IM; 2.2–4.4 mg/kg IV
Ketoconazole	10 mg/kg/day PO	Same
Lactated Ringer's solution	40–50 ml/kg/day IV, SC, IP	Same
Lactulose	1 ml/4.5 kg q8h PO to start, then adjust	*Laxative:* 1–2 ml PO 2–3 days/wk
Laxatone	*Laxative:* 2–4 ml PO 2–3 days/wk	*Hairballs:* 2–4 ml/day PO for 2–3 days; then 1–2 ml 2–3 days/wk
Leucovorin	3 mg/m² within 3h of methotrexate administration	None
Levallorphan (Lorfan)	0.02–0.2 mg/kg IV prn	1 mg/kg IV prn
Levamisole (L-tetramisole)	*Microfilariae:* 10 mg/kg once daily PO for 6–10 days	*Lungworms:* 20–40 mg/kg PO every other day for 5–6 treatments
	Immunostimulant: 0.5–2 mg/kg 3 times weekly PO	None
Levarterenol (norepinephrine)	1–2 ml in 250 ml of drip, IV to effect	None
Levo-Thyroxin	22 mcg/kg q12h PO	0.05–0.1 mg PO once daily

Table continued on following page

TABLE OF COMMON DRUGS: APPROXIMATE DOSES (Continued)

Drug Name	Dog	Cat
Lidocaine (without epinephrine) (Xylocaine)	1–2 mg/kg IV bolus, followed by IV drip, 0.1% soln at 30–50 µg/kg/min	Do *not* use as antiarrhythmic.
Lime sulfur Vlem-Dome (1:16–1:40 dilution of concentrate)	2–5 mg/kg q2h as needed IM 3% solution, dip once a week for 4–6 wk, let dry on	Same
Lincomycin	15 mg/kg q8h PO; 10 mg/kg q12h IV, IM	Same
Lindane	0.025–0.1% aqueous soln topically	None
Liothyronine.	4 mcg/kg q8h PO	None
Lomotil	2.5 mg q8h PO	None
Magnesium hydroxide (milk of magnesia)	*Antacid:* 5–30 ml PO *Cathartic:* 3–5 times the antacid dose	*Antacid:* 5–15 ml PO
Magnesium sulfate (Epsom salts)	8–25 gm PO	2–4 gm PO
Mannitol (20% soln)	1.0–2.0 gm/kg q6h IV	Same
Measles vaccine	1 vial SC to dogs between 6 and 8 wk of age	None
Mebendazole (Telmintic)	22 mg/kg with food q24h for 3 days	None
Meclizine (Bonine)	25 mg once daily PO	12.5 mg once daily PO
Megestrol acetate (Ovaban)	*Skin:* 1 mg/kg/day PO	*Skin:* 5 mg/day PO for 1 wk, then twice weekly
	Behavior: 2–4 mg/kg once daily; reduce to half dose at 8 days for maintenance	*Behavior:* 2–4 mg/kg once daily; reduce to half dose at 8 days for maintenance
	To postpone estrus: In proestrus: 2 mg/kg PO daily for 8 days In anestrus: 0.5 mg/kg PO daily for 32 days False pregnancy: 2.0 mg/kg PO daily for 8 days	
Melatonin	1–2 mg once daily SC for 3 days; repeat monthly as needed	None
Melphàlan (Alkeran)	0.05–0.1 mg/kg PO once daily; 1.5 mg/m² PO once daily for 7–10 days, then no therapy for 2–3 wk	Same

Meperidine (Demerol)	10 mg/kg IM prn	3 mg/kg IM prn
6-Mercaptopurine (6-MP)	50 mg/m² daily PO or 2 mg/kg daily	None
Metamucil	2–10 gm q12–24h in wetted or liquid food	2–4 gm q12–24h in wetted or liquid food
Metaraminol (Aramine)	2–10 mg SC, IM; 10–50 mg/500 ml saline infused IV to effect	None
Methenamine mandelate (Mandelamine)	10 mg/kg q6h PO to effect	None
Methicillin	20 mg/kg q6h IV, IM	Same
DL-Methionine	0.2–1.0 gm q8h PO	0.2 gm q8h PO
Methischol	1 capsule/15 kg q8h PO	1 capsule q12h PO
Methocarbamol	44.4–222.2 mg/kg IV 44.4 mg/kg q8h PO first day, then 22.2–44.4 mg/kg q8h	Same
Methohexital (Brevital)	11 mg/kg IV (2.5% soln)	Same
Methotrexate	0.06 mg/kg once daily PO; 0.3–0.8 mg/kg IV weekly; 2.5 mg/m² once daily PO, IV, IM	Same
Methoxyflurane (Metofane)	Induction: 3% Maintenance: 0.5–1.5%	Same
Methylprednisolone (Medrol, Depomedrol)	See prednisolone 1.0 mg/kg IM every 2 wk	Same 20 mg/cat IM once
Methyltestosterone	0.5 mg/kg q24h PO	Same
Metoclopramide	0.2–0.4 mg/kg q6–8h PO, SC 1.0–2.0 mg/kg/24hr in IV continuous infusion	Same
Metronidazole	60 mg/kg q24h PO for 5 days	Same
Metropine	0.5–1.0 mg q8h PO	None
Mibolerone	30 mcg/0.45–11.3 kg, 60 mcg/11.8–22.7 kg, 120 mcg/23–45.3 kg, 180 mcg/45.8 kg and over daily PO German shepherd and German shepherd mix: 180 mcg all weights daily PO	None
Milk of magnesia. See *Magnesium hydroxide*		
Mineral oil	2–60 ml PO	2–10 ml PO

Table continued on following page

TABLE OF COMMON DRUGS: APPROXIMATE DOSES (*Continued*)

Drug Name	Dog	Cat
Mithramycin	2 μg/kg IV once daily for 2 days	Same
Morphine	1 mg/kg SC, IM prn	0.1 mg/kg SC, IM prn
Nafcillin	10 mg/kg q6h PO, IM	Same
Nalorphine	1.0 mg/kg IV, IM, SC	None
Naloxone (Narcan)	0.04 mg/kg IV, IM, SC	None
Nandrolone decanoate	1.0–1.5 mg/kg/wk IM	
Neo-Darbazine	1 #1 capsule q12h PO (4.5–9 kg)	None
	2 #1 capsules q12h PO (9–13.6 kg)	
	3 #1 capsules or 1 #3 capsule q12h PO (13.6–27.3 kg)	
	1 or 2 #3 capsules q12h PO (over 27.3 kg)	
Neomycin (Biosol)	20 mg/kg q6h PO;	Same
	3.5 mg/kg q8h IV, IM, SC	
Neostigmine (Stiglyn)	1–2 mg IM prn;	None
	5–15 mg PO prn	
Niclosamide (Yomesan)	157 mg/kg PO. Overnight fast. Repeat in 2–3 wk.	Same
Nikethimide (Coramine)	7.8–31.2 mg/kg IV, IM, SC	Same
Nitrofurantoin	4 mg/kg q8h PO;	Same
	3 mg/kg q12h IM	
Novobiocin	10 mg/kg q8h PO	Same
Nystatin	100,000 units q6h PO	Same
Octin	0.5–1.0 ml IM;	0.25–0.5 ml IM;
	1 tablet q8–12h PO	½–1 tablet q12h PO
o,p-DDD(Lysodren)	50 mg/kg once daily PO to effect (approx. 5–10 days), then once every 2 wk	None
Orgotein	5 mg once weekly SC	None
Ouabain	0.02–0.04 mg/kg total dose IV, ¼–½ dose initially, then ¼ dose q30min. Maintenance dose: ¼ of total dose q3h	None

Oxacillin	11–22 mg/kg q8h PO	Same
Oxymetholone	1 mg/kg q8–24h PO	
Oxymorphone (Numorphan)	0.1–0.2 mg/kg SC, IM, IV prn	Same
Oxytetracycline	20 mg/kg q8h PO;	Same
	7 mg/kg q12h IV, IM	
Oxytocin	5–10 units IM, IV; repeat q 15–30 min	0.5–3.0 units IM, IV
2-PAM	40 mg/kg IV over 2-min period, q12h as needed (may be given IM or SC)	None
Pancreatin	2–10 tablets with food	1–2 tablets with food
Pancuronium	0.1 mg/kg IV	None
Papavatrol-10	None	¼–½ tablet q8–12h PO
Paregoric	3–5 ml q6h PO	None
D-Penicillamine (Cuprimine)	10–15 mg/kg q12h	None
Penicillin G, benzathine	40,000 units/kg q 5 days IM	Same
Penicillin G (Na or K)	40,000 units/kg q6h PO (not with food);	Same
	20,000 units/kg q4h IV, IM, SC	
Penicillin G, procaine	20,000 units/kg q12–24h IM, SC	Same
Penicillin V	10 mg/kg q8h PO	Same
Pentazocine (Talwin)	0.5–1.0 mg/kg IM maximum. **Never IV.**	None
Pentobarbital	*Sedation:* 2–4 mg/kg IV	Same
	Anesthesia: 30 mg/kg IV to effect	
Pepto-Bismol	2.2 ml/kg PO	None
Phenethicillin	10 mg/kg q8h	Same
Phenobarbital	*Status epilepticus:*	Same
	6 mg/kg q6–12h IM, IV prn	
	Less severe conditions:	
	2 mg/kg PO bid	
Phenoxybenzamine	0.25–0.5 mg/kg q6–8h PO	Same
Phenylbutazone (Butazolidin)	22 mg/kg q8h IV; total dose not to exceed 0.8 gm/day	None
Phenylephrine (Neo-Synephrine)	0.15 mg/kg IV;	Same
	10% soln topically in eye	
	Antiepileptic: 50–80 mg/kg q8h PO	*Antiepileptic:* 2–3 mg/kg/day;
Phenytoin (Dilantin)	*Antiarrhythmic:* 50–100 mg IV over 5-min period, maximum total dose 24 mg/kg 8–15 mg/kg q8h PO	20 mg/kg/wk
		Antiarrhythmic: None

Table continued on following page

TABLE OF COMMON DRUGS: APPROXIMATE DOSES (Continued)

Drug Name	Dog	Cat
Phthalofyne (Whipcide)	180 mg/kg PO after 24-hr fast; repeat in 3 mo	None
Phthalylsulfathiazole (Sulfathaladine)	50 mg/kg q6h PO; 100 mg/kg q12h PO	Same
Phytonadione (vitamin K₁)	5–20 mg q12h IV, IM, SC	1–5 mg q12h IV, IM, SC
Piperacetazine (Psymod)	Following IV therapy, 5 mg q12h PO for 7 days	
	Tranquilization: 0.11 mg/kg PO bid to qid; 0.11 mg/kg IV, IM, SC	Same
	Sedation: 0.44 mg/kg IV, IM, SC	
Piperazine	110 mg/kg PO, repeat in 21 days	Same
Pitressin (ADH)	10 units IV, IM (aqueous) or 0.5–1.0 ml IM every other day (oil)	Same
Polymyxin B	2 mg q12h IM; Aerosol: Nebulize 300,000 units in 2.5 ml saline q8–12h	Same
Potassium chloride	1–3 gm/day PO IV: maximum 10 mEq/hr and 40 mEq/day/dog	0.2 gm/day PO
Praziquantel (Droncit)	½ tablet/2.3 kg and under	½ tablet/1.8 kg and under
	1 tablet/2.7–4.5 kg	1 tablet/2.3–5.0 kg
	1½ tablets/5–6.8 kg	1½ tablets/5 kg and over
	2 tablets/7.3–13.6 kg	
	3 tablets/14–20.5 kg	
	4 tablets/20.9–27.3 kg	
	5 tablets maximum over 27.3 kg	
Prazosin	1–2 mg q8–12h PO	None
Prednisolone (Solu-Delta-Cortel)	*Allergy:* 0.5 mg/kg bid PO or IM	1.0 mg/kg bid PO or IM
	Immune suppression: 2.0 mg/kg bid PO or IM	3.0 mg/kg bid PO or IM
	Prolonged use: 0.5–2.0 mg/kg every other morning	2.0–4.0 mg/kg every other evening PO
	Shock: 5.5–11.0 mg/kg IV, then q 1, 3, 6, or 10 h prn	Same
Primidone	55 mg/kg PO sid	None

Drug		
Procainamide (Pronestyl)	10–12 mg/kg PO sustained-release (SR)	None
	10–12 mg/kg q8h PO	
	11–22 mg/kg IM q3–6h; 100-mg bolus IV, followed by IV drip at 10–40 µg/kg/min	
Promazine (Sparine)	2.2–4.4 mg/kg IV, IM	Same
Promethazine (Phenergan)	0.2–1.0 mg/kg q8–12h PO, SC	None
Propantheline (Pro-Banthine)	Small: 7.5 mg q8h PO	7.5 mg q8h PO
	Medium: 15 mg q8h PO	
	Large: 30 mg q8h PO	
Propiopromazine (Tranvet)	1.1–4.4 mg/kg PO sid to bid	None
Propranolol (Inderal)	0.2–1.0 mg/kg q8h PO	Same
	.04–.06 mg/kg IV slowly	0.25 mg diluted in 1 ml saline, 0.2-ml IV boluses to effect
Propylthiouracil	11 mg/kg q12h PO	Same
Prussian blue	0.1 gm/kg/day PO q8h	None
Pyrantel pamoate	5 mg/kg PO, repeat in 3 wk	10 mg/kg PO, repeat in 3 wk
Pyrimethamine	1 mg/kg q24h PO for 3 days, then 0.5 mg/kg q24h PO	Same
Quadrinal	¼ to ½ tablet q4–6h PO	¼ tablet q4–6h PO
Quibron	1–3 capsules q8h PO	½ capsule q8h PO
	Elixir: 5 ml/15 kg q8h PO	Elixir: 2 ml q8h PO
Quinacrine (Atabrine)	50–100 mg q12h PO for 3 days, repeat in 3 days	None
Quinidine gluconate (Quinaglute)	8–20 mg/kg q8–12h PO	None
	8–20 mg/kg IM or slow IV q8h	
Quinidine polygalacturonate (Cardioquin)	8–20 mg/kg q8–12h PO	None
Quinidine sulfate	8–20 mg/kg q6–8h PO	None
Rabies vaccine (CEO)	1 vial IM (as per state regulations)	Same
Rabies vaccine (TCO)	1 vial IM (as per state regulations)	Same
Riboflavin	10–20 mg/day PO	5–10 mg/day PO
Ringer's solution	40–50 ml/kg/day IV, IP, SC	Same
Rompun. See *Xylazine*		
Septra	30 mg (combined)/kg q24h PO or 15 mg/kg q12h	None
Sodium bicarbonate	50 mg/kg q8–12h PO (1 tsp powder equals 2 gm)	Same
	1 mEq/kg IV immediately, add 3 mEq/kg to drip	Same

Table continued on following page

TABLE OF COMMON DRUGS: APPROXIMATE DOSES (Continued)

Drug Name	Dog	Cat
Sodium chloride (0.9% soln)	40–50 ml/kg/day IV, IP, SC	Same
Sodium dioctyl sulfosuccinate	100–300 mg q12h PO	100 mg q12–24h PO
Sodium iodine (20% soln)	1 ml/5 kg q8–12h PO, IV	Same
Sodium sulfate (Glauber's salt)	Purgative: 10–25 gm PO	Purgative: 2–4 gm PO
	Laxative: ⅓ the purgative dose	
Spectinomycin	5.5–11 mg/kg q12h IM	None
Stanozolol (Winstrol-V)	½–2 tablets q12h PO	½ tablet q12h PO
	25–50 mg IM weekly	25 mg IM weekly
Styrid-Caricide	1 ml/10 kg once daily PO for heartworm prevention	None
Sulfonamides:		
Phthalylsulfathiazole	100 mg/kg q12h PO (not absorbed)	Same
Sulfadiazine	220 mg/kg initial dose, then 110 mg/kg q12h	Same
Sulfadimethoxine	25 mg/kg q24h PO, IV, IM	Same
Sulfamethazine, sulfamerazine, sulfadiazine (Triple sulfa)	50 mg/kg q12h PO, IV	Same
Sulfasalazine (Azulfidine)	10–15 mg/kg q6h PO	None
Sulfathalidine	100 mg/kg q12h PO (not absorbed)	Same
Sulfisoxazole, sulfamethizole	50 mg/kg q8h PO	Same
Tannic acid (Tannalbin)	1 tablet/5 kg q12h PO; decrease dose for several days after diarrhea is under control	Same
Tan-Sal (5% tannic acid, 5% salicylic acid, and 70% ethyl alcohol)	Topical, q8h; no more than 2 treatments	Same
Temaril-P	1 capsule PO q24h (up to 5 kg)	Same
	2 capsules PO q24h (5–10 kg)	
	4 capsules PO q24h (10–20 kg)	
	6 capsules PO q24h (over 20 kg)	
Testosterone	2 mg/kg once daily q 2–3 days PO up to 30 mg total; 2 mg/kg (up to 30 mg total) IM (repositol) q 10 days	Same
Tetanus antitoxin	100–500 units/kg, maximum 20,000 units (initial test of 0.1–0.2 ml SC 15–30 min prior to IV dose)	Same

Tetracycline	20 mg/kg q8h PO; 7 mg/kg q12h IV, IM	Same
Thenium Closylate	500 mg PO for dogs heavier than 4.55 kg; 250 mg bid for those 2.27–4.55 kg; repeat in 2–3 wk	None
Thiabendazole	50 mg/kg once daily PO for 3 days; repeat in 1 mo	None
Thiacetamide (Caparsolate)	2.2 mg/kg IV bid for 2 days	None
Thiamine	10–100 mg/day PO	5–30 mg/day PO
Thiamylal (Surital, Bio-Tal)	17.5 mg/kg IV (4% soln)	Same, but use 2% soln
6-Thioguanine (6-TG)	1 mg/kg/day PO	Same
ThioTEPA	0.5 mg/kg once daily for 10 days IV or intralesionally; 9 mg/m² as single dose or in 2–4 divided doses on successive days IV or intracavitary	Same
Thyroid (desiccated)	10 mg/kg/day PO	Same
Timolol	1 drop in the eye q12–24h	
Toluene (methylbenzene)	200 mg/kg PO	Same
Tresaderm	Topically, q12h; maximum duration of treatment 7 days	Same
Triamcinolone (Vetalog)	0.25–2 mg once daily PO for 7 days; 0.11–0.22 mg/kg IM, SC	0.25–0.5 mg once daily PO for 7 days 0.11–0.22 mg/kg IM, SC
Trichlorfon (Neguvon)	3% solution to whole body q 3 days	None
Triflumeprazine (Nortran)	0.55–2.2 mg/kg PO, q12–24h	Same
Trimethobenzamide (Tigan)	3 mg/kg q8h IM	None
Trimethoprim plus sulfadiazine (Tribrissen)	15 mg (combined)/kg q12h, or 30 mg (combined)/kg q24h PO, SC	None
Tripelennamine	1.0 mg/kg q12h PO; 1 ml/20 kg IM	Same
Trisulfapyrimidine	50 mg/kg q12h PO	None
TSH (thyroid-stimulating hormone)	1 unit IV (response test); post sample in 4 h	1 unit IM or SC
Tylosin	10 mg/kg q8h PO; 5 mg/kg q12h IV, IM	Same
Verapamil	0.1–0.3 mg/kg IV slowly, not to exceed 5 mg total dose	None
	1–3 mg/kg q6–8h PO	

Table continued on following page

TABLE OF COMMON DRUGS: APPROXIMATE DOSES (Continued)

Drug Name	Dog	Cat
Vermiplex	*Single-dose method:*	Same
	1 #000 capsule/0.23 kg	
	1 #00 capsule/0.57 kg	
	1 #0 capsule/1.14 kg	
	1 #1 capsule/2.27 kg	
	1 #2 capsule/4.55 kg	
	1 #3 capsule/9.1 kg	
	1 #4 capsule/18.2 kg	
	Can be repeated in 2–4 wk	
	Divided-dose method:	
	Divide body weight by 5, and administer appropriate size capsule once daily for 5 days. Can be repeated in 2–4 wk.	Same
Vinblastine (Velban)	3.0 mg/m² weekly IV, or 0.1–0.5 mg/kg weekly	Same
Vincristine (Oncovin)	0.025–0.05 mg/kg q7–10 days; 0.5 mg/m² IV weekly or biweekly	Same
Viokase	Mix into food 20 min prior to feeding; 1–3 tsp/lb of food	Same
Vi-Sorbin	1–3 tsp/day PO	½ tsp/day PO
Vitamin A	400 units/kg/day PO for 10 days	Same
Vitamin B complex	0.5–2.0 ml q24h IV, IM, SC	0.5–1.0 ml q24h IV, IM, SC
Vitamin B₁₂	100–200 µg/day	50–100 µg/day
Vitamin D	30 units/kg/day PO for 10 days	Same
Vitamin E	500 mg/day PO	100 mg/day PO
Xylazine (Rompun)	1.1 mg/kg IV; 1.1–2.2 mg/kg IM, SC	Same

Compiled by Richard Johnson, Reg. Ph.

INDEX

Note: Page numbers in *italics* refer to illustrations; page numbers followed by (t) refer to tables.